Environmental Health

From Global to Local

SECOND EDITION

HOWARD FRUMKIN

EDITOR

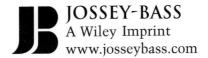

JOSSEY-BASS
A Wiley Imprint
www.josseybass.com

A Wiley Imprint
989 Market Street, San Francisco, CA 94103-1741—www.josseybass.com

Jossey-Bass books and products are available through most bookstores. To contact Jossey-Bass directly call our Customer Care Department within the U.S. at 800-956-7739, outside the U.S. at 317-572-3986, or fax 317-572-4002.

Jossey-Bass also publishes its books in a variety of electronic formats. Some content that appears in print may not be available in electronic books.

Library of Congress Cataloging-in-Publication Data

Environmental health : from global to local / Howard Frumkin, editor. —2nd ed.
    p.;   cm.
    Includes bibliographical references and indexes.
    ISBN 978-0-470-40487-4 (cloth)
       1. Environmental health.   2. Health risk assessment.   I. Frumkin, Howard.
[DNLM: 1. Environmental Health.   2. Environmental Exposure—prevention & control.
3. Environmental Medicine—methods. WA 30.5 E6063 2010]
    RA565.E482 2010
    616.9'8—dc22

                                                          2009044623

Printed in the United States of America
SECOND EDITION

HB Printing   10 9 8 7 6 5 4 3

CONTENTS

PART ONE: METHODS AND PARADIGMS

PART TWO: ENVIRONMENTAL HEALTH ON THE GLOBAL SCALE

PART THREE: ENVIRONMENTAL HEALTH ON THE REGIONAL SCALE

PART FIVE: THE PRACTICE OF ENVIRONMENTAL HEALTH

TABLES, FIGURES, AND EXHIBITS

TABLES

FIGURES

EXHIBITS

I dedicate this book to my children, Gabe and Amara—dedicated environmentalists, great lovers of the outdoors, hard-headed idealists, and two of the most wonderful people I know. They will make giant contributions to a safer, healthier, and more sustainable world.

THE EDITOR

Howard Frumkin is director of the National Center for Environmental Health and Agency for Toxic Substances and Disease Registry (NCEH/ATSDR) at the U.S. Centers for Disease Control and Prevention. NCEH/ATSDR works to maintain and improve the health of the American people by promoting a healthy environment and by preventing premature death and avoidable illness and disability caused by toxic substances and other environmental hazards.

An internist, environmental and occupational medicine specialist, and epidemiologist, Frumkin previously served as professor and chair of the Department of Environmental and Occupational Health at Emory University's Rollins School of Public Health and professor of medicine at Emory Medical School. He also founded and directed Emory's Environmental and Occupational Medicine Consultation Clinic and the Southeast Pediatric Environmental Health Specialty Unit. He has served on the board of directors of Physicians for Social Responsibility, as president of the Association of Occupational and Environmental Clinics, as chair of the Science Board of the American Public Health Association, and on the National Toxicology Program Board of Scientific Counselors, and has participated in workgroups and committees for a number of federal and state agencies. He currently serves on the Institute of Medicine Roundtable on Environmental Health Sciences, Research, and Medicine. He is the author or coauthor of five books and over 160 scientific journal articles and chapters. He received his MD degree from the University of Pennsylvania, his MPH and DrPH degrees from Harvard, his internal medicine training at the Hospital of the University of Pennsylvania and Cambridge Hospital, and his occupational medicine training at Harvard.

THE CONTRIBUTORS

John M. Balbus, MD, MPH
Senior Research Scientist
Department of Global Health
School of Public Health and Health
  Services
George Washington University
Washington, D.C.

Scott M. Bartell, PhD
Assistant Professor
Program in Public Health
University of California, Irvine
Irvine, California

Michelle L. Bell, PhD
Associate Professor, Environmental Health
Yale University
New Haven, Connecticut

H. C. "Chip" Clitheroe, Jr., PhD
Lecturer
School of Social Ecology
University of California, Irvine
Irvine, California

Vincent T. Covello, PhD
Director

Center for Risk Communication
New York, New York

**Andrew L. Dannenberg,
MD, MPH**
Associate Director for Science
Division of Emergency and
Environmental Health Services
National Center for Environmental
  Health
Centers for Disease Control and
  Prevention
Atlanta, Georgia

Henry Falk, MD, MPH
Director
Coordinating Center for Environmental
  Health and Injury Prevention
Centers for Disease Control and
  Prevention
Atlanta, Georgia

Timothy E. Ford, PhD
Vice President for Research and Dean of
  Graduate Studies
University of New England
Biddeford, Maine

Joel Forman, MD
Associate Professor, Pediatrics and
  Community and Preventive Medicine
Mount Sinai School of Medicine
New York, New York

Maida P. Galvez, MD, MPH
Assistant Professor
Department of Community and
  Preventive Medicine
Mount Sinai School of Medicine
New York, New York

Lynn R. Goldman, MD, MPH
Professor, Environmental Health
  Sciences
Johns Hopkins Bloomberg School of
  Public Health
Baltimore, Maryland

George C. Hamilton, PhD
Department Chairman and Extension
  Specialist in Pest Management
Department of Entomology
Rutgers University
New Brunswick, New Jersey

Sarah K. Heaton, MPH
Presidential Management Fellow
National Center for Environmental
  Health
Centers for Disease Control and
  Prevention
Atlanta, Georgia

Douglas A. Henderson, PhD, JD
Partner
Troutman Sanders LLP
Atlanta, Georgia
Adjunct Associate Professor

Department of Health Policy
  and Management
University of Georgia College of Public
  Health
Athens, Georgia

Jeremy J. Hess, MD, MPH
Medical Epidemiologist
National Center for Environmental Health
Centers for Disease Control and
  Prevention
Assistant Professor
Emory University School of Medicine
  and Public Health
Atlanta, Georgia

Don Hinrichsen
Consultant on Environment and
  Population
Institute for War and Peace Reporting
New York and London

Howard Hu, MD, MPH, ScD
NSF International Chair and Professor,
  Environmental Health, Epidemiology,
  Internal Medicine
University of Michigan Schools of Public
  Health and Medicine
Ann Arbor, Michigan

Andrew Jameton, PhD
Professor, Health Promotion, Social &
  Behavioral Health
College of Public Health
University of Nebraska Medical Center
Omaha, Nebraska

Holly Jessop
Graduate Student
Department of Zoology

University of Hawai'i at Manoa
Honolulu, Hawai'i

Markey Johnson, PhD
Epidemiology and Exposure Assessment
  Research Scientist
National Health and Environmental
  Effects Research Laboratory
National Exposure Research Laboratory
U. S. Environmental Protection Agency
Research Triangle Park, North Carolina

James W. Keck, MD, MPH
General Preventive Medicine Resident
Johns Hopkins Bloomberg School of
  Public Health
Baltimore, Maryland

Mark E. Keim, MD
Senior Science Advisor, Preparedness &
  Emergency Response
National Center for Environmental Health
Centers for Disease Control and
  Prevention
Atlanta, Georgia

**Sarah B. Kotchian, PhD,
MPH, EdM**
Sarah Kotchian Consulting
Former Associate Director for Planning
Institute for Public Health
University of New Mexico School of
  Medicine
Albuquerque, New Mexico

Philip J. Landrigan, MD, MSc
Ethel H. Wise Professor and Chairman
Department of Community and
  Preventive Medicine
Professor of Pediatrics

Mount Sinai School of Medicine
New York, New York

Robert J. Laumbach, MD, MPH, CIH
Assistant Professor, Environmental and
  Occupational Medicine
Robert Wood Johnson Medical School
University of Medicine and Dentistry
  of New Jersey
Piscataway, New Jersey

Charles Lee
Director
Office of Environmental Justice
U. S. Environmental Protection Agency
Washington, D.C.

**David McSwane, HSD, REHS,
CP-FS**
Professor, Public and Environmental
  Affairs
School of Public and Environmental
  Affairs
Indiana University
Indianapolis, Indiana

A. Stanley Meiburg, PhD
Deputy Regional Administrator
U. S. Environmental Protection Agency,
  Region 4
Atlanta, Georgia

Jaymie R. Meliker, PhD
Assistant Professor, Preventive Medicine
Graduate Program in Public Health
Faculty Member in Consortium for
  Inter-Disciplinary Environmental
  Research (CIDER)
Stony Brook University
Stony Brook, New York

Gary W. Miller, PhD
Professor, Environmental and
  Occupational Health
Rollins School of Public Health
  of Emory University
Atlanta, Georgia

Christine L. Moe, PhD
Eugene J. Gangarosa Professor of Safe
  Water and Sanitation
Hubert Department of Global
  Health
Emory University
Atlanta, Georgia

Jerome Nriagu, PhD, DSc
Professor, Environmental
  Health Sciences
University of Michigan School
  of Public Health
Ann Arbor, Michigan

Kenneth G. Orloff, PhD
Senior Toxicologist
Agency for Toxic Substances and
  Disease Registry
Centers for Disease Control
  and Prevention
Atlanta, Georgia

Jonathan A. Patz, MD, MPH
Professor, Population Health Sciences
Gaylord Nelson Institute
  for Environmental Studies
University of Wisconsin
Madison, Wisconsin

Melissa J. Perry, ScD, MHS
Associate Professor, Occupational
  Epidemiology

Harvard School of Public Health
Boston, Massachusetts

Junaid Abdul Razzak, MD, PhD
Associate Professor and Chair
Department of Emergency Medicine
Aga Khan University
Karachi, Pakistan

Jason R. Richardson, MS, PhD
Assistant Professor, Environmental
  and Occupational Health
Robert Wood Johnson Medical School
University of Medicine and Dentistry
  of New Jersey
Piscataway, New Jersey

**Mark Gregory Robson, PhD,
MPH, ATS**
Professor and Dean of Agricultural
  and Urban Programs
Rutgers University School of
  Environmental and Biological Sciences
New Brunswick, New Jersey

Sven E. Rodenbeck, ScD, PE, BCEE
Captain, U.S. Public Health Service
Agency for Toxic Substances and
  Disease Registry
Centers for Disease Control and
  Prevention
Atlanta, Georgia

P. Barry Ryan, PhD
Professor, Exposure Science and
  Environmental Chemistry
Department of Environmental and
  Occupational Health
Rollins School of Public Health of
  Emory University

Professor
Department of Chemistry
Emory University
Atlanta, Georgia

Jonathan M. Samet, MD, MS
Professor and Flora L. Thornton Chair
  of Preventive Medicine
Keck School of Medicine
Director
Institute for Global Health
University of Southern California
Los Angeles, California

Wattasit Siriwong, PhD
Academic Lecturer and Assistant Dean
College of Public Health Sciences
Chulalongkorn University
Bangkok, Thailand

Kyle Steenland, PhD
Professor, Environmental and
  Occupational Health
Rollins School of Public Health
  of Emory University
Atlanta, Georgia

Daniel Stokols, PhD
Chancellor's Professor
School of Social Ecology and College
  of Health Sciences
University of California, Irvine
Irvine, California

William A. Suk, PhD, MPH
Director
Center for Risk and Integrated Sciences
Director

Superfund Research Program
National Institute of Environmental
  Health Sciences
National Institutes of Health
Research Triangle Park, NC

Arthur C. Upton, MD
Clinical Professor, Environmental
  and Community Medicine
University of Medicine and Dentistry
  of New Jersey
Robert Wood Johnson Medical School
Piscataway, New Jersey

Lance A. Waller, PhD
Rollins Professor and Chair, Biostatistics
  and Bioinformatics
Rollins School of Public Health of
  Emory University
Atlanta, Georgia

Bruce A. Wilcox, PhD
Professor, Ecology and Health
Department of Public Health Sciences
John A. Burns School of Medicine
University of Hawai'i
Honolulu, Hawai'i

Samuel H. Wilson, MD
Chief, DNA Repair and Nucleic
  Acid Enzymology Section
Environmental Biology Program
Laboratory of Structural Biology
National Institute of Environmental
  Health Sciences
National Institutes of Health
Research Triangle Park, North Carolina

ACKNOWLEDGMENTS

In many religions and cultures teachers are revered. I honor that tradition, as well I should: I have been blessed with more superb teachers than I had any right to expect when I first marched off to school. They didn't know it, but they were all preparing me to envision this book and pull it together. One of the sweetest privileges of an editor—and there have been many—is the chance to thank them.

I express my deep and lasting gratitude to my high school teacher Barbara Leventer, who taught me that writing a research paper means specifying a hypothesis, organizing an outline, finding good sources, and writing clearly (and all of that before the Internet!); my college teachers Ed Beiser, who taught me that there is no excuse for muddled thinking and unclear expression, and Steve Lyons and Hunter Dupree, who taught me the majesty and endless relevance of history; my medical school teachers Paul Stolley, who taught me the power of epidemiological data and who set a standard for principled advocacy, and the late John Eisenberg, who modeled a formidable combination of clinical excellence, astute policy analysis, and great kindness; my residency teacher Bob Lawrence, who taught me that primary care extends from the bedside to the global commons; and my graduate school teachers Richard Monson, John Peters, and David Wegman, who taught me the interface of public health and the environment.

I thank my colleagues and students at Emory University's Rollins School of Public Health, where I had the great good fortune to serve as a faculty member from 1990 to 2005, and where I edited the first edition of this textbook. I also thank my colleagues at the U.S. Centers for Disease Control and Prevention, National Center for Environmental Health and the Agency for Toxic Substances and Disease Registry, where I have served as director since 2005. Although a university and a governmental agency are very different places, both have been wonderful places to work, marked by intellectual stimulation, hard-working, dedicated colleagues, and dear friends. I also thank my colleagues at other agencies, such as the Environmental Protection Agency and the National Institute for Environmental Health Sciences, and at organizations ranging from environmental and community groups to law firms to manufacturing companies, who have taught me more than I can say about the many facets of environmental health. Over the years, I have especially appreciated my friends and colleagues at Physicians for Social Responsibility; the Institute of Medicine Roundtable on Environmental Health, Research, and Medicine; the Clean Air Campaign; the EPA Children's Health Protection Advisory Committee; the Association of Occupational and Environmental Clinics; the American Public Health Association; Sustainable Atlanta; the Children and Nature Forum; and Atlanta's Green Reading Group.

I thank the chapter authors of this book, all of them highly expert and exceedingly busy people. They willingly shared their expertise and time (and gracefully tolerated my prodding and editing) to help compile the kind of book that we would all want to use in our own teaching.

I thank my editors at Jossey-Bass, Andy Pasternack and Seth Schwartz, who believed in this project, generously tolerated delays, and kept me on track. If there is a special place for editors in heaven, Andy and Seth will certainly end up there (although they would probably prefer to stay in San Francisco). I thank my friend Jim Grode, who lent his formidable skills as a writer, editor, analytical thinker, and environmentalist to processing each chapter as it arrived, ranging from image permissions to truth-testing the prose. And I thank copyeditor Elspeth MacHattie, a consummate professional, a pleasure to work with, and an enormous asset to both editions of this book.

I thank the staff at Emory who supported the preparation of the first edition of this book, including Hope Jackson, Robin Thompson, Adrienne Tison, Erica Weaver, Rachel Wilson, and Suzanne Mason. A very special thanks goes to Cheryl Everhart at NCEH/ATSDR. Cheryl has an extraordinary combination of organizational skills, work ethic, faith, kindness, and optimism. She managed the logistics of the second edition of this book impeccably, and that was only one of a thousand balls she juggled.

INTRODUCTION

HOWARD FRUMKIN

Please stop reading.

That's right. Close this book, just for a moment. Lift your eyes and look around. Where are you? What do you see?

Perhaps you're in the campus library, surrounded by shelves of books, with carpeting underfoot and the heating or air-conditioning humming quietly in the background. Perhaps you're home—a dormitory room, a bedroom in a house, a suite in a garden apartment, maybe your kitchen. Perhaps you're outside, lying beneath a tree in the middle of campus, or perhaps you're on a subway or a bus or even an airplane. What is it like? How does it feel to be where you are?

Is the light adequate for reading? Is the temperature comfortable? Is there fresh air to breathe? Are there contaminants in the air—say, solvents off-gassing from newly laid carpet or a recently painted wall? Does the chair fit your body comfortably?

If you're inside, look outside. What do you see through the window? Are there trees? Buildings? Is the neighborhood noisy or tranquil? Are there other people? Are there busy streets, with passing trucks and busses snorting occasional clouds of diesel exhaust?

Now imagine that you can see even farther, to a restaurant down the block, to the nearby river, to the highway network around your city or town, to the factories and assembly plants in industrial parks, to the power plant in the distance supplying electricity to the room you're in, to the agricultural lands some miles away. What would you see in the restaurant? Is the kitchen clean? Is the food stored safely? Are there cockroaches or rats in the back room? What about the river? Is your municipal sewage system dumping raw wastes into the river, or is there a sewage plant discharging treated, clean effluent? Are there chemicals in the river

Howard Frumkin declares no competing financial interests.

water? What about fish? Could you eat the fish? Could you swim in the river? Do you drink the water from the river?

As for the highways, factories, and power plant . . . are they polluting the air? Are the highways clogged with traffic? Are people routinely injured and killed on the roads? Are workers in the factories being exposed to hazardous chemicals or to noise or to machines that may injure them or to stress? Are trains pulling up to the power plant regularly, off-loading vast piles of coal? And what about the farms? Are they applying pesticides, or are they controlling insects in other ways? Are you confident that you're safe eating the vegetables that grow there? Drinking the milk? Are the farmlands shrinking as residential development from the city sprawls outward?

Finally, imagine that you have an even broader view. Floating miles above the earth, you look down. Do you notice the hundreds of millions of people living in wildly differing circumstances? Do you see vast megacities with millions and millions of people, and do you see isolated rural villages three days' walk from the nearest road? Do you see forests being cleared in some places, rivers and lakes drying up in others? Do you notice that the earth's surface temperature is slightly warmer than it was a century ago? Do you see cyclones forming in tropical regions, glaciers and icecaps melting near the poles?

OK, back to the book.

Everything you've just viewed, from the room you're in to the globe you're on, is part of your environment. And many, many aspects of that environment, from the air you breathe to the water you drink, from the roads you travel to the wastes you produce, may affect how you feel. They may determine your risk of being injured before today ends, your risk of coming down with diarrhea or shortness of breath or a sore back, your risk of developing a chronic disease in the next few decades, even the risk that your children or your grandchildren will suffer from developmental disabilities or asthma or cancer.

WHAT IS ENVIRONMENTAL HEALTH?

Merriam-Webster's Collegiate Dictionary first defines *environment* straightforwardly as "the circumstances, objects, or conditions by which one is surrounded." The second definition it offers is more intriguing: "the complex of physical, chemical, and biotic factors (as climate, soil, and living things) that act upon an organism or an ecological community and ultimately determine its form and survival." If our focus is on human health, we can consider the environment to be all the external (or nongenetic) factors—physical, nutritional, social, behavioral, and others—that act on humans.

A widely accepted definition of *health* comes from the 1948 constitution of the World Health Organization (2005): "A state of complete physical, mental, and social well-being and not merely the absence of disease or infirmity." This broad definition goes well beyond the rather mechanistic view that prevails in some medical settings to include many dimensions of comfort and well-being.

Environmental health has been defined in many ways (see Exhibit I.1). Some definitions make reference to the relationship between people and the environment, evoking an ecosystem concept, and others focus more narrowly on addressing particular environmental conditions. Some focus on abating hazards, and others focus on promoting health-enhancing environments. Some focus on physical and chemical hazards, and others extend more broadly to aspects of the social and built environments. In the aggregate the definitions in Exhibit I.1 make it clear that environmental health is many things: an interdisciplinary academic field, an area of research, and an arena of applied public health practice.

EXHIBIT I.1
Definitions of Environmental Health

"[Environmental health] [c]omprises those aspects of human health, including quality of life, that are determined by physical, chemical, biological, social and psychosocial factors in the environment. It also refers to the theory and practice of assessing, correcting, controlling, and preventing those factors in the environment that can potentially affect adversely the health of present and future generations" (World Health Organization [WHO], 2004).

"Environmental health is the branch of public health that protects against the effects of environmental hazards that can adversely affect health or the ecological balances essential to human health and environmental quality" (Agency for Toxic Substances and Disease Registry, cited in U.S. Department of Health and Human Services [DHHS], 1998).

"Environmental health comprises those aspects of human health and disease that are determined by factors in the environment. It also refers to the theory and practice of assessing and controlling factors in the environment that can potentially affect health. It includes both the direct pathological effects of chemicals, radiation and some biological agents, and the effects (often indirect) on health and well-being of the broad physical, psychological, social and aesthetic environment, which includes housing, urban developmental land use and transport" (European Charter on Environment and Health; see WHO, Regional Office for Europe, 1990).

"Environmental health is the discipline that focuses on the interrelationships between people and their environment, promotes human health and well-being, and fosters a safe and healthful environment" (National Center for Environmental Health, cited in DHHS, 1998).

THE EVOLUTION OF ENVIRONMENTAL HEALTH

Human concern for environmental health dates from ancient times, and it has evolved and expanded over the centuries.

Ancient Origins

The notion that the environment could have an impact on comfort and well-being—the core idea of environmental health—must have been evident in the early days of human existence. The elements can be harsh, and we know that our ancestors sought shelter in caves or under trees or in crude shelters they built. The elements can still be harsh, both on a daily basis and during extraordinary events; think of the Indian Ocean earthquake and tsunami of 2004, Hurricanes Katrina and Rita in 2005, the Sichuan earthquake of 2008, and the ongoing drought in Australia.

Our ancestors confronted other challenges that we would now identify with environmental health. One was food safety; there must have been procedures for preserving food, and people must have fallen ill and died from eating spoiled food. Dietary restrictions in ancient Jewish and Islamic law, such as bans on eating pork, presumably evolved from the recognition that certain foods could cause disease. Another challenge was clean water; we can assume that early peoples learned not to defecate near or otherwise soil their water sources. In the ruins of ancient civilizations from India to Rome, from Greece to Egypt to South America, archeologists have found the remains of water pipes, toilets, and sewage lines, some dating back more than 4,000 years (Rosen, [1958] 1993). Still another environmental hazard was polluted air; there is evidence in the sinus cavities of ancient cave dwellers of high levels of smoke in their caves (Brimblecombe, 1988), foreshadowing modern indoor air concerns in homes that burn biomass fuels or coal.

An intriguing passage in the biblical book of Leviticus (14:33–45) may refer to an environmental health problem well recognized today: mold in buildings. When a house has a "leprous disease" (as the Revised Standard Version translates this passage),

> . . . then he who owns the house shall come and tell the priest, "There seems to me to be some sort of disease in my house." Then the priest shall command that they empty the house before the priest goes to examine the disease, lest all that is in the house be declared unclean; and afterward the priest shall go in to see the house. And he shall examine the disease; and if the disease is in the walls of the house with greenish or reddish spots, and if it appears to be deeper than the surface, then the priest shall go out of the house to the door of

the house, and shut up the house seven days. And the priest shall come again on the seventh day, and look; and if the disease has spread in the walls of the house, then the priest shall command that they take out the stones in which is the disease and throw them into an unclean place outside the city; and he shall cause the inside of the house to be scraped round about, and the plaster that they scrape off they shall pour into an unclean place outside the city; then they shall take other stones and put them in the place of those stones, and he shall take other plaster and plaster the house. If the disease breaks out again in the house, after he has taken out the stones and scraped the house and plastered it, then the priest shall go and look; and if the disease has spread in the house, it is a malignant leprosy in the house; it is unclean. And he shall break down the house, its stones and timber and all the plaster of the house; and he shall carry them forth out of the city to an unclean place.

As interesting as it is to speculate about whether ancient dwellings suffered mold overgrowth, it is also interesting to consider the "unclean place outside the city"—an early hazardous waste site. Who hauled the wastes there, and what did that work do to their health?

Still another ancient environmental health challenge, especially in cities, was rodents. European history was changed forever when infestations of rats in fourteenth-century cities led to the Black Death (Zinsser, 1935; Herlihy and Cohn, 1997; Cantor, 2001; Kelly, 2005). Modern cities continue to struggle periodically with infestations of rats and other pests (Sullivan, 2004), whose control depends in large part on environmental modifications.

Industrial Awakenings

Modern environmental health further took form during the age of industrialization. With the rapid growth of cities in the seventeenth and eighteenth centuries, *sanitarian* issues rose in importance. "The urban environment," wrote one historian, "fostered the spread of diseases with crowded, dark, unventilated housing; unpaved streets mired in horse manure and littered with refuse; inadequate or nonexisting water supplies; privy vaults unemptied from one year to the next; stagnant pools of water; ill-functioning open sewers; stench beyond the twentieth-century imagination; and noises from clacking horse hooves, wooden wagon wheels, street railways, and unmuffled industrial machinery" (Leavitt, 1982, p. 22).

The provision of clean water became an ever more pressing need, as greater concentrations of people increased both the probability of water contamination and the impact of disease outbreaks. Regular outbreaks of cholera and yellow fever in the eighteenth and nineteenth centuries (Rosenberg, 1962) highlighted the need for water systems, including clean source water, treatment including filtration, and distribution through pipes. Similarly, sewage management became a pressing need, especially after the provision of piped water and the use of toilets created large volumes of contaminated liquid waste (Duffy, 1990; Melosi, 2000).

The industrial workplace—a place of danger and even horror—gave additional impetus to early environmental health. Technology advanced rapidly during the late eighteenth and nineteenth centuries, new and often dangerous machines were deployed in industry after industry, and mass production became common. Although the air, water, and soil near industrial sites could become badly contaminated, in ways that would be familiar to modern environmental professionals (Hurley, 1994; Tarr, 1996, 2002), the most abominable conditions were usually found within the mines, mills, and factories.

Charles Turner Thackrah (1795–1833), a Yorkshire physician, became interested in the diseases he observed among the poor in the city of Leeds. In 1831, he described many work-related hazards in a short book with a long title: *The Effects of the Principal Arts, Trades and Professions, and of Civic States and Habits of Living, on Health and Longevity, with Suggestions for the Removal of Many of the Agents which Produce Disease and Shorten the Duration of Life.* In it he proposed guidelines for the prevention of certain diseases, such as the elimination of lead as a glaze in the pottery industry and the use of ventilation and respiratory protection to protect knife grinders. Public outcry and the efforts of early Victorian reformers such as Thackrah led to passage of the Factory Act in 1833 and the Mines Act in 1842. Occupational health did not blossom in the United States until the early twentieth century, pioneered by the remarkable Alice Hamilton (1869–1970). A keen firsthand observer of industrial conditions, she documented links between toxic exposures and illness among miners, tradesmen, and factory workers, first in Illinois (where she directed that state's Occupational Disease Commission from 1910 to 1919) and later from an academic position at Harvard. Her books, including *Industrial Poisons in the United States* and *Industrial Toxicology*, published in 1925 and 1934, respectively, helped establish that workplaces could be dangerous environments for workers.

A key development in the seventeenth through nineteenth centuries was the quantitative observation of population health—the beginnings of epidemiology. With the tools of epidemiology, observers could systematically attribute certain diseases to certain environmental exposures. John Graunt (1620–1674), an English merchant and haberdasher, analyzed London's weekly death records—the "bills of mortality"—and published his findings in 1662 as *Natural and Political Observations Upon the Bills of Mortality.* Graunt's work was one of the first formal analyses of this data source and a pioneering example of demography. Almost two centuries later, when the British Parliament created the Registrar-General's Office (now the Office of Population Censuses and Surveys) and William Farr

(1807–1883) became its compiler of abstracts, the link between vital statistics and environmental health was forged. Farr made observations about fertility and mortality patterns, identifying rural-urban differences, variations between acute and chronic illnesses, and seasonal trends, and implicating certain environmental conditions in illness and death. Farr's 1843 analysis of mortality in Liverpool led Parliament to pass the Liverpool Sanitary Act of 1846, which created a sanitary code for Liverpool and a public health infrastructure to enforce it.

If Farr was a pioneer in applying demography to public health, his contemporary Edwin Chadwick (1800–1890) was a pioneer in combining social epidemiology with environmental health. At the age of thirty-two, Chadwick was appointed to the newly formed Royal Commission of Enquiry on the Poor Laws, and helped reform Britain's Poor Laws. Five years later, following epidemics of typhoid fever and influenza, he was asked by the British government to investigate sanitation. His classic report, *Sanitary Conditions of the Labouring Population* (1842), drew a clear link between living conditions—in particular overcrowded, filthy homes, open cesspools and privies, impure water, and miasmas—and health, and made a strong case for public health reform. The resulting Public Health Act of 1848 created the Central Board of Health, with power to empanel local boards that would oversee street cleaning, trash collection, and water and sewer systems. As sanitation commissioner, Chadwick advocated such innovations as urban water systems, toilets in every house, and transfer of sewage to outlying farms where it could be used as fertilizer (Hamlin, 1998). Chadwick's work helped establish the role of public works—essentially applications of sanitary engineering—to protecting public health. As eloquently pointed out by Thomas McKeown (1979) more than a century later, these interventions were to do far more than medical care to improve public health and well-being during the industrial era.

The physician John Snow (1813–1858) was, like William Farr, a founding member of the London Epidemiological Society. Snow gained immortality in the history of public health for what was essentially an environmental epidemiology study. During an 1854 outbreak of cholera in London, he observed a far higher incidence of disease among people who lived near or drank from the Broad Street pump than among people with other sources of water. He persuaded local authorities to remove the pump handle, and the epidemic in that part of the city soon abated. (There is some evidence that it may have been ending anyway, but this does not diminish the soundness of Snow's approach.) Environmental epidemiology was to blossom during the twentieth century (see Chapter Three) and provide some of the most important evidence needed to support effective preventive measures.

Finally, the industrial era led to a powerful reaction in the worlds of literature, art, and design. In the first half of the nineteenth century, Romantic painters, poets, and philosophers celebrated the divine and inspiring forms of nature. In Germany painters such as Caspar David Friedrich (1774–1840) created meticulous images of the trees, hills, misty valleys, and mercurial light of northern Germany, based on a close observation of nature, and in England Samuel Palmer (1805–1881) painted landscapes that combined straightforward representation of nature with religious vision. His countryman John Constable (1776–1837) worked in the open air, painting deeply evocative English landscapes. In the United States, Hudson River School painters, such as Thomas Cole (1801–1848), took their inspiration from the soaring peaks and crags, stately waterfalls, and primeval forests of the northeast. At the same time, the New England transcendentalists celebrated the wonders of nature. "Nature never wears a mean appearance," wrote Ralph Waldo Emerson (1803–1882) in his 1836 paean, *Nature.* "Neither does the wisest man extort her secret, and lose his curiosity by finding out all her perfection. Nature never became a toy to a wise spirit. The flowers, the animals, the mountains, reflected the wisdom of his best hour, as much as they had delighted the simplicity of his childhood." Henry David Thoreau (1817–1862), like Emerson a native of Concord, Massachusetts, rambled from Maine to Cape Cod and famously lived in a small cabin at Walden Pond for two years, experiences that cemented his belief in the "tonic of wildness." And America's greatest landscape architect, Frederick Law Olmsted (1822–1903), championed bringing nature into cities. He designed parks that offered pastoral vistas and graceful tree-lined streets and paths, intending to offer tranquility to harried people and to promote feelings of community. These and other strands of cultural life reflected yet another sense of *environmental health*, forged in response to industrialization: the idea that pristine environments were wholesome, healthful, and restorative to the human spirit.

The Modern Era

The modern field of environmental health dates from the mid-twentieth century, and no landmark better marks its launch than the 1962 publication of Rachel Carson's *Silent Spring. Silent Spring* focused on DDT, an organochlorine pesticide that had seen increasingly wide use since the Second World War. Carson had become alarmed at the ecosystem effects of DDT; she described how it entered the food chain and accumulated in the fatty tissues of animals, how it indiscriminately killed both target species and other creatures, and how its effects persisted for long periods after it was applied. She also made the link to human health, describing how DDT might increase the risk of cancer and birth defects. One of Carson's lasting contributions was to place human health in the context of larger environmental processes. "Man's attitude toward nature," she declared in

1963, "is today critically important simply because we have now acquired a fateful power to alter and destroy nature. But man is a part of nature, and his war against nature is inevitably a war against himself. . . . [We are] challenged as mankind has never been challenged before to prove our maturity and our mastery, not of nature, but of ourselves" (*New York Times*, 1964).

The recognition of chemical hazards was perhaps the most direct legacy of *Silent Spring*. Beginning in the 1960s, Irving Selikoff (1915–1992) and his colleagues at the Mount Sinai School of Medicine intensively studied insulators and other worker populations and showed that asbestos could cause a fibrosing lung disease, lung cancer, mesothelioma, and other cancers. Outbreaks of cancer in industrial workplaces—lung cancer in a chemical plant near Philadelphia due to bis-chloromethyl ether (Figueroa, Raszkowski, and Weiss, 1973; Randall, 1977), hemangiosarcoma of the liver in a vinyl chloride polymerization plant in Louisville (Creech and Johnson, 1974), and others—underlined the risk of carcinogenic chemicals. With the enormous expansion of cancer research, and with effective advocacy by such groups as the American Cancer Society (Patterson, 1987), environmental and occupational carcinogens became a focus of public, scientific, and regulatory attention (Epstein, 1982).

But cancer was not the only health effect linked to chemical exposures. Herbert Needleman (1927–), studying children in Boston, Philadelphia, and Pittsburgh, showed that lead was toxic to the developing nervous system, causing cognitive and behavioral deficits at levels far lower than had been appreciated. When this recognition finally helped achieve the removal of lead from gasoline, population blood lead levels plummeted, an enduring public health victory. Research also suggested that chemical exposures could threaten reproductive function. Wildlife observations such as abnormal genitalia in alligators in Lake Apopka, Florida, following a pesticide spill (Guillette and others, 1994) and human observations such as an apparent decrease in sperm counts (Carlsen, Giwercman, Keiding, and Skakkebaek, 1992; Swan, Elkin, and Fenster, 1997) suggested that certain persistent, bioaccumulative chemicals (persistent organic pollutants, or POPs) could affect reproduction, perhaps by interfering with hormonal function. Emerging evidence showed that chemicals could damage the kidneys, liver, and cardiovascular system and immune function and organ development.

Some knowledge of chemical toxicity arose from toxicological research (see Chapter Two) and other insights resulted from epidemiological research (see Chapter Three). But catastrophes—reported first in newspaper headlines and only later in scientific journals—also galvanized public and scientific attention. The discovery of accumulations of hazardous wastes in communities across the nation—Love Canal in Niagara Falls, New York (Gibbs, 1998; Mazur, 1998); Times Beach, Missouri, famous for its unprecedented dioxin levels; Toms River,

New Jersey, and Woburn, Massachusetts, where municipal drinking water was contaminated with organic chemicals; "Mount Dioxin," a defunct wood treatment plant in Pensacola, Florida; and others—raised concerns about many health problems, from nonspecific symptoms to immune dysfunction to cancer to birth defects. And acute disasters, such as the isocyanate release that killed hundreds and sickened thousands in Bhopal, India, in 1984, made it clear that industrialization posed real threats of chemical toxicity (Kurzman, 1987; Dhara and Dhara, 2002; Lapierre and Moro, 2002).

In tandem with the growing awareness of chemical hazards, environmental health during the second half of the twentieth century was developing along another promising line: *environmental psychology*. As described in Chapter Five, this field arose as a subspecialty of psychology, building on advances in perceptual and cognitive psychology. Scholars such as Stephen Kaplan and Rachel Kaplan at the University of Michigan carried out careful studies of human perceptions and of reactions to various environments. An important contribution to environmental psychology was the theory of biophilia, first advanced by Harvard biologist E. O. Wilson in 1984. Wilson defined *biophilia* as "the innately emotional affiliation of human beings to other living organisms." He pointed out that for most of human existence, people have lived in natural settings, interacting daily with plants, trees, and other animals. As a result, Wilson maintained, affiliation with these organisms has become an innate part of human nature (Wilson, 1984). Other scholars extended Wilson's concept beyond living organisms, postulating a connection with other features of the natural environment—rivers, lakes, and ocean shores; waterfalls; panoramic landscapes and mountain vistas (Kellert and Wilson, 1993; Kellert, 1997; see Chapter Twenty-Four). Environmental psychologists studied not only natural features of human environments but also such factors as light, noise, and way-finding cues to assess the impact of these factors. They increasingly recognized that people responded to various environments, both natural and built, in predictable ways. Some environments were alienating, disorientating, or even sickening, whereas others were attractive, restorative, and even salubrious.

A third development in modern environmental health was the continued integration of ecology with human health, giving rise to a field called *ecohealth*. Ancient wisdom in many cultures had recognized the relationships between the natural world and human health and well-being. But with the emergence of formal complex systems analysis and modern ecological science, the understanding of ecosystem function advanced greatly (see Chapter One). As part of this advance the role of humans in the context of ecosystems was better and better delineated. On a global scale, for example, the concept of *carrying capacity* (Wackernagel and Rees, 1995) helped clarify the impact of human activity on ecosystems and permitted evaluation of the ways ecosystem changes, in turn, affected human health and well-being (Rappaport and others, 1999; McMichael, 2001; Aron and Patz, 2001; Martens and McMichael, 2002; Alcamo and others, 2003; Waltner-Toews, 2004; Brown, Grootjans, Ritchie, and Townsend, 2005). Ecological analysis was also applied to specific areas relevant to human health. For example, there were advances in medical botany (Lewis and Elvin-Lewis, 2003; van Wyk and Wink, 2004), in the understanding of biodiversity and its value to human health (Grifo and Rosenthal, 1997; Chivian and Bernstein, 2008) and in the application of ecology to clinical medicine (Aguirre and others, 2002; Ausubel with Harpignies, 2004). These developments, together, reflected a progressive synthesis of ecological and human health science, yielding a better understanding of the foundations of environmental health.

A fourth feature of modern environmental health was the expansion of health care services related to environmental exposures. Occupational medicine and nursing had been specialties in their respective professions since the early twentieth century, with a traditional focus on returning injured and ill workers to work and, to some extent, on preventing hazardous workplace exposures. In the last few decades of the twentieth century, these professional specialties incorporated a public health paradigm, drawing on toxicological and epidemiological data, using industrial hygiene and other primary prevention approaches, and engaging in worker education (see Chapter Twenty-Seven). In addition, the occupational health clinical paradigm was broadened to include general environmental exposures. Clinicians began focusing on such community exposures as air pollutants, radon, asbestos, and hazardous wastes, emphasizing the importance of taking an environmental history, identifying at-risk groups, and providing both treatment and preventive advice to patients. Professional ethics expanded to recognize the interests of patients (both workers and community members) as well as those of employers, and in some cases even the interests of unborn generations and of other species (see Chapter Seven). Finally, a wide range of alternative and complementary approaches—some well outside the mainstream—arose in occupational and environmental health care. For example, an approach known as *clinical ecology* postulated that overloads of environmental exposures could impair immune function, and offered treatments including "detoxification," antifungal medications, and dietary changes purported to prevent or ameliorate the effects of environmental exposures (Randolph, 1976, 1987; Rea, 1992–1998).

Environmental health policy also emerged rapidly. With the promulgation of environmental laws beginning in the 1960s, federal and state officials created agencies and assigned them new regulatory responsibilities (see Chapter Thirty). These agencies issued rules that aimed to reduce emissions from smokestacks, drainpipes, and tailpipes; control hazardous wastes; and achieve clean air and water. Although many of these laws were oriented to environmental preservation, the protection of human health was often an explicit rationale as well. Ironically, the new environmental regulations created a schism in the environmental health field. Responsibility for environmental health regulation had traditionally rested with health departments, but this was now transferred to newly formed environmental departments. At the federal level, the U.S. Environmental Protection Agency (EPA) assumed some of the traditional responsibilities of the Department of Health, Education, and Welfare (now Health and Human Services), and corresponding changes occurred at the state level. Environmental regulation and health protection became somewhat uncoupled from each other.

Environmental regulatory agencies increasingly attempted to ground their rules in evidence, using quantitative risk assessment techniques (see Chapter Twenty-Nine). This signaled a sea change in regulatory policy. The traditional approach had been simpler; dangerous exposures were simply banned. For example, the 1958 Delaney clause, an amendment to the 1938 federal Food, Drug, and Cosmetic Act, banned carcinogens in food. In contrast, emerging regulations tended to set permissible exposure levels that took into account anticipated health burdens, compliance costs, and technological feasibility. Moreover, regulations tended to assign the burden of proof of toxicity to government regulators. As the scientific and practical difficulties of this approach became clear in the late twentieth century, an alternative approach emerged: assigning manufacturers the burden of proving the safety of a chemical. Based philosophically in the *precautionary principle* (see Chapter Twenty-Six), this approach was legislated in Europe as part of the European Union's REACH (Registration, Evaluation, Authorisation and Restriction of Chemical substances) initiative, which entered into force in 2007 (European Commission, 2009).

At the dawn of the twenty-first century, then, while traditional sanitarian functions remained essential, the environmental health field had moved well beyond its origins. Awareness of chemical toxicity had advanced rapidly, fueled by discoveries in toxicology and epidemiology. At the same time, the complex relationships inherent in environmental health—the effects of environmental conditions on human psychology, and the links between human health and ecosystem function—were better and better recognized. In practical terms, clinical services in environmental health had developed, and regulation had advanced through a combination of political action and scientific evidence.

Emerging Issues

Environmental health is a dynamic, evolving field. Looking ahead, we can identify at least five trends that will further shape environmental health: environmental justice, a focus on susceptible groups, scientific advances, global change, and moves toward sustainability.

Beginning around 1980, African American communities identified exposures to hazardous waste and industrial emissions as matters of racial and economic justice. Researchers documented that these exposures disproportionately affected poor and minority communities, a problem that was aggravated by disparities in the enforcement of environmental regulations. The modern *environmental justice* movement was born, a fusion of environmentalism, public health, and the civil rights movement (Bullard, 1994; Cole and Foster, 2000; see also Chapter Eight). Historians have observed that environmental justice represents a profound shift in the history of environmentalism (Shabecoff, 1993; Gottlieb, 1993; Dowie, 1995). This history is commonly divided into waves. The first wave was the conservation movement of the early twentieth century, the second wave was the militant activism that blossomed in 1970 on the first Earth Day, and the third wave was the emergence of large, "inside-the-beltway" environmental organizations such as the Environmental Defense Fund, the League of Conservation Voters, and the Natural Resources Defense Council, which had gained considerable policy influence by the 1980s. Environmental justice, then, represents a fourth wave, one that is distinguished by its decentralized, grassroots leadership, its demographic diversity, and its emphasis on human rights and distributive justice. The vision of environmental justice—eliminating disparities in economic opportunity, healthy environments, and health—is one that resonates with public health priorities. It emphasizes that environmental health extends well beyond technical solutions to hazardous exposures to include human rights and equity as well. It is likely that this vision will be an increasingly central part of environmental health in coming decades.

Environmental justice is one example of a broader trend in environmental health—a *focus on susceptible groups*. For many reasons, specific groups may be especially vulnerable to the adverse health effects of environmental exposures. In the case of poor and minority populations, these reasons include disproportionate exposures, limited access to legal protection, limited access to health care, and in some cases compromised baseline health status (see Chapter Eight). Children make up another susceptible population, for several reasons (see Chapter Twenty-Five). They eat more food, drink more water, and breathe more air per unit of body weight than adults do and are therefore heavily exposed to any contaminants in these media. Children's behavior—crawling on floors, placing their hands in their mouths, and so on—further increases their risk of exposure. With developing organ systems and immature biological defenses, children are less able than adults to withstand some exposures. And with more years of life ahead of them, children have more time to manifest delayed toxic reactions (National Research Council, Committee on Pesticides in the Diets of Infants and Children, 1993). These facts have formed the basis for research and public health action on children's environmental health.

Women bear some specific environmental exposure risks, both in the workplace and in the general environment, due both to disproportionate exposures (for example, in health care jobs) and to unique susceptibilities (for example, to reproductive hazards). Elderly people also bear some specific risks, and as the population ages, this group will attract further environmental health attention. For example, urban environments will need to take into account the limited mobility of some elderly people and provide ample sidewalks, safe street crossings, and accessible gathering places to serve this population. People with disabilities, too, require specific environmental health attention to minimize the risks they face. In coming decades environmental health will increasingly take account of susceptible groups as the risks they face and their needs for safe, healthy environments become better recognized.

A third set of emerging issues in environmental health grows out of *scientific advances*. In toxicology better detection techniques have already enabled us to recognize and quantify low levels of chemical exposure and have supported major advances in the understanding of chemical effects (see Chapter Two). Innovative toxicological approaches, including physiologically based pharmacokinetic modeling (PBPK) (Kim and Nylander-French, 2009) and high-throughput computational techniques (Schoonen, Westerink, and Horbach, 2009; Nigsch, Macaluso, Mitchell, and Zmuidinavicius, 2009), offer rapid insights into chemical toxicity. Advances in data analysis techniques have supported innovative epidemiological analyses and the use of large databases. In particular the use of geographic information systems (GISs) has yielded new insights on the spatial distribution of environmental exposures and diseases (see Chapter Twenty-Eight). Perhaps the most promising scientific advances are occurring at the molecular level, in the linked fields of genomics, toxicogenomics, epigenetics, and proteomics (Schmidt, 2003; Pognan, 2004; Waters and Fostel, 2004; Li, Aubrecht, and Fornace, 2007; Reamon-Buettner, Mutschler, and Borlak, 2008; see also Chapter Six). New genomic tools such as microarrays (or gene chips) have enabled scientists to characterize the effects of chemical exposures on the expression of thousands of genes. Databases of genetic responses, and the resulting protein and metabolic pathways, will yield much information on the effects of chemicals and on the variability in responses among different people. Scientific advances related to environmental health will have profound effects on the field in coming decades.

Moving from the molecular scale to the global scale, a fourth set of emerging environmental health issues relates to *global change*. This broad term encompasses many trends, including population growth, climate change, urbanization, changing patterns of energy use, and the increasing integration of the world economy (Friedman, 2008). These trends will shape environmental health in many ways.

The world population is now approximately 6.5 billion and is expected to plateau at roughly 9 billion during the twenty-first century (see Chapter Nine). Most of this population growth will occur in developing nations, and much of it will be in cities. Not only this population growth but also the increasing per capita demand for resources such as food, energy, and materials will strain the global environment (Brown, 2008), in turn affecting health in many ways. For example, environmental stress and resource scarcity may increasingly trigger armed conflict, an ominous example of the links between environment and health (Homer-Dixon, 1999; Klare, 2001; Friedman, 2008). Global climate change, which results in large part from increasing energy use (see Chapter Thirteen), will threaten health in many ways, from infectious disease risks to heat waves to severe weather events (see Chapter Ten). As more of the world's population is concentrated in dense urban areas, features of the urban environment—noise, crowding, vehicular and industrial pollution—will come to be important determinants of health (United Nations Centre on Human Settlements, 2001; see also Chapter Fourteen). And with integration of the global economy—through the complex changes known as globalization—hazards will cross national boundaries (Ives, 1985; see also Chapter Eleven), trade agreements and market forces will challenge and possibly undermine national environmental health policies (Low, 1992; Runge, 1994; Brack, 1998; Nordstrom and Vaughan, 1999), and global solutions to environmental health challenges will increasingly be needed (Huynen, Martens, and Hilderink, 2005).

Sustainability has been a part of the environmental health vernacular since the 1980s. In 1983, the United Nations formed the World Commission on Environment and Development to propose strategies for sustainable development. The commission, chaired by then Norwegian prime minister Gro Harlem Brundtland, issued its landmark report, *Our Common Future,* in 1987. The report included what has become a standard definition of sustainable development: "development that meets the needs of the present without compromising the ability of future generations to meet their own needs." In 1992, several years after the publication of *Our Common Future,* the United Nations Conference on Environment and Development (UNCED), commonly known as the Earth Summit, convened in Rio de Janeiro. This historic conference produced, among other documents, the Rio Declaration on Environment and Development, a blueprint for sustainable development. The first principle of the Rio declaration placed environmental health at the core of sustainable development: "Human beings are at the centre of concerns for sustainable development. They are entitled to a healthy and productive life in harmony with nature" (United Nations, 1992).

Like environmental justice the concept of sustainable development blends environmental protection with notions of fairness and equity. As explained on the Web site of the Johannesburg Summit, held ten years after the Earth Summit:

> The Earth Summit thus made history by bringing global attention to the understanding, new at the time, that the planet's environmental problems were intimately linked to economic conditions and problems of social justice. It showed that social, environmental and economic needs must be met in balance with each other for sustainable outcomes in the long term. It showed that if people are poor, and national economies are weak, the environment suffers; if the environment is abused and resources are over consumed, people suffer and economies decline. The conference also pointed out that the smallest local actions or decisions, good or bad, have potential worldwide repercussions [United Nations Department of Economic and Social Affairs, 2006].

The concept of sustainability has emerged as a central theme, and challenge, not only for environmentalism but for environmental health as well. In the short term, sustainable development will permit improvement in the living conditions and therefore the health of people across the world, especially in the poor nations. In the long term, sustainable development will protect the health and well-being of future generations. Some of the most compelling thinking in environmental health in recent years offers social and technical paths to sustainable development (Hawken, Lovins, and Lovins, 1999; Brown, 2001, 2008; McDonough and Braungart, 2002; Ehrlich and Ehrlich, 2004; Brown and others, 2005; Anastas and Beach, 2007). These approaches build on the fundamental links among health, environment, technological change, and social justice. Ultimately, they will provide the foundation for lasting environmental health.

SPATIAL SCALES, FROM GLOBAL TO LOCAL

The concept of spatial scale is central to many disciplines, from geography to ecology to urban planning. Some phenomena unfold on a highly local scale— ants making a nest, people digging a septic tank. Some phenomena spread across regions—the pollution of a watershed from an upstream factory, the sprawl of a city over a 100-mile diameter. And some phenomena, such as climate change, are truly global in scale. Al Gore, in describing environmental destruction in his 1992 book, *Earth in the Balance*, borrowed military categories to make this point, distinguishing among "local skirmishes," "regional battles," and "strategic conflicts."

Spatial scale is important not only in military and environmental analysis but also in environmental health. Some environmental factors that affect health operate locally, and the environmental health professionals who address these factors work on a local level; think of the restaurant and septic tank inspectors who work for the local health department or the health and safety officer at a manufacturing facility. Other environmental factors affect health at a regional level, and the professionals who address these problems work on a larger spatial scale; think of the state officials responsible for enforcement of air pollution or water pollution regulations. At the global level such problems as climate change require responses on the national and international scales. These responses are crafted by professionals in organizations such as the World Health Organization and the Intergovernmental Panel on Climate Change. So useful is the concept of spatial scales in environmental health that it provides the framework for this book. After introducing the methods and paradigms of environmental health in the first eight chapters, we address specific issues, beginning with global scale problems in Chapters Nine to Eleven, moving to regional scale problems in Chapters Twelve to Fifteen, and ending with local problems in Chapters Sixteen to Twenty-Five. The final seven chapters (Chapters Twenty-Six to Thirty-Two) describe the practice of environmental health, ranging from the use of tools such as geographic information systems to activities such as risk communication and health care services.

It is clear that environmental health professionals work on different spatial scales, but it is not always so clear who is an environmental health professional. Certainly, the environmental health director at a local health department; the director of environment, health, and safety at a manufacturing firm; an environmental epidemiology researcher at a university; or a physician working for an environmental advocacy group would self-identify and be recognized by others as an environmental health professional. But many other people work in fields that have an impact on the environment and human health. The engineer who designs power plants helps to protect the respiratory health of asthmatic children living downwind if she includes sophisticated emissions controls. The transportation planner who enables people to walk instead of drive also protects public health by helping to clean up the air. The park superintendent who maintains urban green spaces may contribute greatly to the well-being of people in his city. In fact much of environmental health is determined by "upstream" forces that seem at first glance to have little to do with environment or health.

THE FORCES THAT DRIVE ENVIRONMENTAL HEALTH

Public health professionals tell the emblematic story of a small village perched alongside a fast-flowing river. The people of the village had always lived near the river, they knew and respected its currents, and they were skilled at swimming, boating, and water rescue. One day they heard desperate cries from the river and noticed a stranger being swept downstream past their village. They sprang into action, grabbed their ropes and gear, and pulled the victim from the water. A few minutes later, as they rested, a second victim appeared, thrashing in the strong current and gasping for breath. The villagers once again performed a rescue. Just as they were remarking on the coincidence of two near drownings in one day, a third victim appeared, and they also rescued him. This went on for hours. Every available villager joined in the effort, and by mid-afternoon all were exhausted. Finally, the flow of victims stopped, and the villagers collapsed, huffing and puffing, in the town square.

Just at that moment another villager strode whistling into the town square, relaxed and dry. He had not been seen since the first victims were rescued and had not helped with any of the rescues. "Where were you?" his neighbors demanded of him. "We've been pulling people out of the river all day! Why didn't you help us?"

"Ah," he replied. "When I noticed all the people in the river, I thought there must be a problem with that old footbridge upstream. I walked up to it, and sure enough, some boards had broken and there was a big hole in the walkway. So I patched the hole, and people stopped falling through."

PERSPECTIVE
A Prevention Poem: A Fence or an Ambulance

Like the story of the villagers who saved drowning victims, this poem emphasizes that prevention may lie with root causes. These root causes are often environmental—like the hole in the village's bridge or, in this case, an unguarded cliff edge.

'Twas a dangerous cliff, as they freely confessed,

Though to walk near its crest was so pleasant;

But over its terrible edge there had slipped

A duke, and full many a peasant;

Upstream thinking has helped identify the root causes of many public health problems, and this is nowhere more true than in environmental health. Environmental hazards sometimes originate far from the point of exposure. Imagine that you inhale a hazardous air pollutant. It may come from motor vehicle tailpipes, from power plants, from factories, or from any combination of these. As for the motor vehicle emissions, the amount of driving people do in your city or town reflects urban growth patterns and available transportation alternatives, and the pollutants generated by people's cars and trucks vary with available technology and prevailing regulations. As for the power plants, the amount of energy they produce reflects the demand for energy by households and businesses in the area they serve, and the pollution they emit is a function of how they produce energy (are they coal, nuclear, or wind powered?), the technology they use, and the regulations that govern their operations. Hence a full understanding of the air pollutants you breathe must take into account urban growth, transportation, energy, and regulatory policy, among other upstream determinants. This book contains chapters on many of the upstream forces that affect environmental health, including population growth, transportation, and energy.

These ideas are at the core of a useful model created by the World Health Organization, Regional Office for Europe (2004) (see Figure I.1). The DPSEEA (driving forces-pressures-state-exposure-effects-actions) model was developed as a tool both for analyzing environmental health hazards and for designing indicators useful in decision making. The driving forces are the factors that motivate environmental health processes. In our air pollution example, these factors might

So the people said something would have to be done,

But their projects did not at all tally.

Some said: "Put a fence round the edge of the cliff;"

Some, "An ambulance down in the valley."

But the cry for the ambulance carried the day,

For it spread through the neighboring city.

A fence may be useful or not, it is true,

But each heart became brimful of pity

PERSPECTIVE (Continued)

For those who slipped over that dangerous cliff;

And dwellers in highway and alley,

Gave pounds or gave pence, not to put up a fence,

But an ambulance down in the valley.

(For the cliff is all right if you're careful," they said,

"And if folks even slip and are dropping,

It isn't the slipping that hurts them so much

As the shock down below when they're stopping."

So day after day as those mishaps occurred,

Quick forth would those rescuers sally,

To pick up the victims who fell off the cliff

With the ambulance down in the valley.

Then an old sage remarked, "It's a marvel to me

That people gave far more attention

To repairing results than to stopping the cause,

When they'd much better aim at prevention.

Let us stop at its source all this mischief," cried he;

"Come, neighbors and friends, let us rally;

If the cliff we will fence, we might also dispense

With the ambulance down in the valley."

"Oh he's a fanatic," the others rejoined;

"Dispense with the ambulance? Never!

He'd dispense with all charities too if he could.

    No, no! We'll support them forever!

Aren't we picking up folks just as fast as they fall?

    And shall this man dictate to us? Shall he?

Why should people of sense stop to put up a fence

    While their ambulance works in the valley?"

But a sensible few who are practical too,

    Will not bear with such nonsense much longer.

They believe that prevention is better than cure;

    And their party will soon be the stronger.

Encourage them, then, with your purse, voice, and pen,

    And (while other philanthropists dally)

They will scorn all pretense and put a stout fence

    On the cliff that hangs over the valley.

Better guide well the young than reclaim them when old,

    For the voice of true wisdom is calling;

To rescue the fallen is good, but it's best

    To prevent other people from falling;

Better close up the source of temptation and crime

    Than deliver from dungeon or galley;

Better put a strong fence 'round the top of the cliff,

    Than an ambulance down in the valley.

—Joseph Malins (1895)

FIGURE I.1   The DPSEEA Model

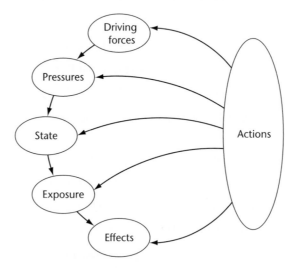

Source: WHO, Regional Office for Europe, 2004.

include population growth; consumer preferences for energy-consuming homes, appliances, and vehicles; and sprawl that requires traveling over long distances. The driving forces result in pressures on the environment, such as the emission of oxides of nitrogen, hydrocarbons, particulate matter, and other air pollutants. These emissions, in turn, modify the state of the environment, accumulating in the air and combining to form additional pollutants such as ozone. However, this deterioration in the state of the environment does not invariably threaten health; human *exposure* must occur. In the case of air pollutants, exposure occurs when people are breathing when and where the air quality is low. (Some people, of course, sustain higher exposures than others; an outdoor worker, an exercising athlete, or a child at play receives relatively higher doses of air pollutants than a person in an air-conditioned office.) The hazardous exposure may lead to a variety of health effects, acute or chronic. In the case of air pollutants, these effects may include coughing and wheezing, asthma attacks, heart attacks, and even early death. The DPSEEA model is further discussed in Chapter Twenty-Six, where it is linked with concepts of prevention.

Finally, to eliminate or control environmental hazards and protect human health, society may undertake a wide range of actions, targeted at any of the upstream steps. For example, protecting the public from the effects of air pollution might include encouraging energy conservation to reduce energy demand and designing live-work-play communities to reduce travel demand (addressing driving forces), providing mass transit or bicycle lanes to reduce automobile use, requiring emissions controls on power plants or investing in wind turbines to reduce emissions from coal-fired power plants (addressing pressures), requiring low-sulfur fuel (addressing the state of the environment), warning people to stay inside when ozone levels are high (addressing exposures), and providing maintenance asthma medications (addressing health effects). The most effective long-term actions, however, are those that are preventive, aimed at eliminating or reducing the forces that drive the system (see Chapter Twenty-Six). This theme is universal in public health, applying both to environmental hazards and to other health hazards.

CONFLICTS OF INTEREST

In recent years, increasing attention has been focused on integrity in scientific publishing. A principal stimulus to this concern has been the pharmaceutical industry. Editors of such prominent medical journals as the *Lancet*, the *New England Journal of Medicine*, and the *British Medical Journal* have lamented the relationship between the pharmaceutical industry and medical journals (Smith, 2005), and empirical research has demonstrated an association between funding source and pharmaceutical research findings (Lexchin, Bero, Djulbegovic, and Clark, 2003). Certainly, environmental health experiences many of the same pressures as the pharmaceutical sector, and conflicts of interest must be recognized as a real concern in this field too.

Conflicts of interest have been defined as "conditions in which professional judgment concerning a primary interest (such as a patient's welfare or the validity of research) tends to be unduly influenced by a secondary interest (such as financial gain)" (Thompson, 1993). Conflicts of interest, real or perceived, can derail the quest for truth, have a corrosive effect on scientific data (Bekelman, Li, and Gross, 2003), and undermine public faith in science (Friedman, 2002; Kennedy, 2004).

Those who publish or report on science have increasingly tackled the challenge of conflicts of interest (Maurissen and others, 2005). Transparency is a leading solution, recalling Justice Brandeis's adage that "Sunshine is the best disinfectant." Most medical journals now require disclosures of potential conflicts of interest when publishing papers (Krimsky and Rothenberg, 2001; Ancker and Flanagin, 2007). (Examples of such conflicts are discussed in Campbell, 2001; Davidoff and others, 2001; DeAngelis and others, 2001.) Such disclosures serve a purpose; they inform readers' views of what they read (Chaudhry, Shroter, Smith, and Morris, 2002). Many (but not enough) reports of scientific results in the popular media now mention funding sources (Cook, Boyd, Grossman, and Bero, 2007). Many universities require faculty to disclose potential conflicts of interest (Boyd and Bero, 2000). But it is rare for textbooks to adopt such procedures. This omission is curious given the wide readership of textbooks, the tendency of textbook chapters to draw broad conclusions, and the fact that student readers may be rather impressionable.

The second edition of *Environmental Health: From Global to Local* has addressed this concern by asking each chapter author to report real or perceived conflicts of interest. Following excellent guidelines from a Natural Resources Defense Council workshop (Sass, 2009) and major journals, each author of each chapter was asked to disclose relationships occurring during the last three years, currently active, or reasonably anticipated to occur in the foreseeable future "with companies that make or sell products or services discussed in the chapter, companies that make or sell related products or services, and other pertinent entities with an interest in the topic, specifying the type of relationship." These relationships were defined as including (but not limited to)

Grant support
Employment (past, present, or firm offer of future)
Stock ownership or options
Payment for serving as an expert witness or giving testimony
Personal financial interests on the part of the author, immediate family members, or institutional affiliations that might gain or lose financially through publication of the chapter
Other forms of compensation, including travel funding, consultancies, honoraria, board positions, and patent or royalty arrangements
Employment by a for-profit, nonprofit, foundation, or advocacy group

Each author's declaration appears at the bottom of the first text page of his or her chapter. I am not aware of another major textbook that has implemented such a policy. I hope this helps to ensure the integrity of every chapter in this book and becomes more common in scientific textbooks in coming years.

REFERENCES

Aguirre, A. A., and others (eds.). *Conservation Medicine: Ecological Health in Practice.* New York: Oxford University Press, 2002.

Alcamo, J., and others. *Ecosystems and Human Well-Being: A Framework for Assessment.* Millennium Ecosystem Assessment. Washington, D.C.: Island Press, 2003.

Anastas, P. T., and Beach, E. S. "Green Chemistry: The Emergence of a Transformative Framework." *Green Chemistry Letters and Reviews*, 2007, *1*, 9–24.

Ancker, J. S., and Flanagin, A. "A Comparison of Conflict of Interest Policies at Peer-Reviewed Journals in Different Scientific Disciplines." *Science and Engineering Ethics*, 2007, *13*, 147–157.

Aron, J. L., and Patz, J. A. (eds.). *Ecosystem Change and Public Health: A Global Perspective.* Baltimore, Md.: Johns Hopkins University Press, 2001.

Ausubel, K., with Harpignies, J. P. (eds.). *Ecological Medicine: Healing the Earth, Healing Ourselves.* San Francisco: Sierra Club Books, 2004.

Bekelman, J. E., Li, Y., and Gross, C. P. "Scope and Impact of Financial Conflicts of Interest in Biomedical Research. A Systematic Review." *JAMA*, 2003, *289*, 454–465.

Boyd, E., and Bero, L. "Assessing Faculty Financial Relationships with Industry. *JAMA*, 2000, *284*, 2209–2214.

Brack, D. (ed.). *Trade and Environment: Conflict or Compatibility?* London: Earthscan, 1998.

Brimblecombe, P. *The Big Smoke: A History of Air Pollution in London Since Medieval Times.* London: Routledge, 1988.

Brown, L. R. *Eco-Economy: Building an Economy for the Earth.* New York: Norton, 2001.

Brown, L. R. *Plan B 3.0: Mobilizing to Save Civilization.* New York: Norton, 2008.

Brown, V. A., Grootjans, J., Ritchie, J., and Townsend, M. *Sustainability and Health: Supporting Global Ecological Integrity in Public Health.* London: Earthscan, 2005.

Bullard, R. D. *Dumping in Dixie: Race, Class, and Environmental Quality.* (2nd ed.) Boulder, Colo.: Westview Press, 1994.

Campbell, P. "Declaration of Financial Interests." *Nature*, 2001, *412*, 751.

Cantor, N. *In the Wake of the Plague: The Black Death and the World It Made.* New York: Free Press, 2001.

Carlsen, E., Giwercman, A., Keiding, N., and Skakkebaek, N. "Evidence for Decreasing Quality of Semen During Past 50 Years." *British Medical Journal*, 1992, *305*, 609–613.

Chaudhry, S., Shroter, S, Smith, R., and Morris, J. "Does Declaration of Competing Interests Affect Readers' Perceptions? A Randomized Trial." *British Medical Journal*, 2002, *325*, 1391–1392.

Chivian, E., and Bernstein, A. *Sustaining Life: How Human Health Depends on Biodiversity.* New York: Oxford University Press, 2008.

Cole, L. W., and Foster, S. R. *From the Ground Up: Environmental Racism and the Rise of the Environmental Justice Movement.* New York: New York University Press, 2000.

Cook, D. M., Boyd, E. A., Grossman, C., and Bero, L. A. "Reporting Science and Conflicts of Interest in the Lay Press." *PLoS ONE*, 2007, *2*(12): e1266, doi:10.1371/journal.pone.0001266.

Creech, J. L., and Johnson, M. N. "Angiosarcoma of the Liver in the Manufacture of PVC." *Journal of Occupational Medicine*, 1974, *16*, 150–151.

Davidoff, F., and others. "Sponsorship, Authorship, and Accountability." *JAMA*, 2001, *286*, 1232–1234.

DeAngelis, C. D., Fontanarosa, P. B., and Flanagin, A. "Reporting Financial Conflicts of Interest and Relationships Between Investigators and Research Sponsors." *JAMA*, 2001, *286*, 89–91.

Dhara, V. R., and Dhara, R. "The Union Carbide Disaster in Bhopal: A Review of Health Effects." *Archives of Environmental Health*, 2002, *57*, 391–404.

Dowie, M. *Losing Ground: American Environmentalism at the Close of the Twentieth Century.* Cambridge, Mass.: MIT Press, 1995.

Duffy, J. *The Sanitarians: A History of American Public Health.* Urbana: University of Illinois Press, 1990.

Ehrlich, P., and Ehrlich, A. *One with Nineveh: Politics, Consumption, and the Human Future.* Washington, D.C.: Island Press, 2004.

Epstein, S. *The Politics of Cancer.* New York: Random House, 1982.

European Commission. "What Is REACH?" http://ec.europa.eu/environment/chemicals/reach/reach_intro.htm, 2009.

Figueroa, W. G., Raszkowski, R., and Weiss, W. "Lung Cancer in Chloromethyl Methyl Ether Workers." *New England Journal of Medicine*, 1973, 288, 1096–1097.

Friedman, P. "The Impact of Conflict of Interest on Trust in Science." *Science and Engineering Ethics*, 2002, 8, 413–420.

Friedman, T. *Hot, Flat, and Crowded: Why We Need a Green Revolution and How It Can Renew America.* New York: Farrar, Straus & Giroux, 2008.

Gibbs, L. M. *Love Canal: The Story Continues.* Gabriola Island, B.C.: New Society, 1998.

Gore, A. *Earth in the Balance.* Boston: Houghton Mifflin, 1992.

Gottlieb, R. *Forcing the Spring: The Transformation of the American Environmental Movement.* Washington, D.C.: Island Press, 1993.

Grifo, F., and Rosenthal, J. (eds.). *Biodiversity and Human Health.* Washington, D.C.: Island Press, 1997.

Guillette, L. J., Jr., and others. "Developmental Abnormalities of the Gonad and Abnormal Sex Hormone Concentrations in Juvenile Alligators from Contaminated and Control Lakes in Florida." *Environmental Health Perspectives*, 1994, *102*, 680–688.

Hamlin, C. *Public Health and Social Justice in the Age of Chadwick: Britain, 1800–1854.* New York: Cambridge University Press, 1998.

Hawken, P., Lovins, A., and Lovins, L. H. *Natural Capitalism: Creating the Next Industrial Revolution.* Boston: Little, Brown, 1999.

Herlihy, D., and Cohn, S. K. *The Black Death and the Transformation of the West.* Cambridge, Mass.: Harvard University Press, 1997.

Homer-Dixon, T. F. *Environment, Scarcity and Violence.* Princeton, N.J.: Princeton University Press, 1999.

Hurley, A. "Creating Ecological Wastelands: Oil Pollution in New York City, 1870–1900." *Journal of Urban History*, 1994, *20*, 340–364.

Huynen, M. M., Martens, P., and Hilderink, H. B. "The Health Impacts of Globalisation: A Conceptual Framework." *Globalization and Health*, 2005, *1*, 1–14.

Ives, J. H. (ed.). *The Export of Hazard: Transnational Corporations and Environmental Control Issues.* New York: Routledge, 1985.

Kellert, S. R. *Kinship to Mastery: Biophilia in Human Evolution and Development.* Washington, D.C.: Island Press, 1997.

Kellert, S. R., and Wilson, E. O. (eds.). *The Biophilia Hypothesis.* Washington, D.C.: Island Press, 1993.

Kelly, J. *The Great Mortality: An Intimate History of the Black Death, the Most Devastating Plague of All Time.* New York: HarperCollins, 2005.

Kennedy, D. "Disclosure and Disinterest." *Science,* 2004, *303,* 15.

Kim, D., and Nylander-French, L. A. "Physiologically Based Toxicokinetic Models and Their Application in Human Exposure and Internal Dose Assessment." *EXS,* 2009, *99,* 37–55.

Klare, M. T. *Resource Wars: The New Landscape of Global Conflict.* New York: Henry Holt, 2001.

Krimsky S, Rothenberg L. Conflict of Interest Policies in Science and Medical Journals: Editorial Practices and Author Disclosures. *Science and Engineering Ethics,* 2001, 7, 205-218.

Kurzman, D. *A Killing Wind: Inside Union Carbide and the Bhopal Catastrophe.* New York: McGraw-Hill, 1987.

Lapierre, D. , and Moro, J. *Five Past Midnight in Bhopal: The Epic Story of the World's Deadliest Industrial Disaster.* New York: Warner Books, 2002.

Leavitt, J. W. *The Healthiest City: Milwaukee and the Politics of Health Reform.* Princeton, N.J.: Princeton University Press, 1982.

Lewis, W. H., and Elvin-Lewis, M.P.F. *Medical Botany: Plants Affecting Human Health.* (2nd ed.) New York: Wiley, 2003.

Lexchin, J., Bero, L. A., Djulbegovic, B., and Clark, O. "Pharmaceutical Industry Sponsorship and Research Outcome and Quality." *British Medical Journal,* 2003, *326,* 1167–1170.

Li, H. H., Aubrecht, J., and Fornace, A. J., Jr. "Toxicogenomics: Overview and Potential Applications for the Study of Non-Covalent DNA Interacting Chemicals." *Mutation Research,* 2007, *623* (1–2), 98–108.

Low, P. (ed.). *International Trade and the Environment.* World Bank Discussion Papers 159. Washington, D.C.: World Bank, 1992.

Martens, P., and McMichael, A. J. (eds.). *Environmental Change, Climate and Health: Issues and Research Methods.* New York: Cambridge University Press, 2002.

Maurissen, J. P., and others. "Workshop Proceedings: Managing Conflict of Interest in Science. A Little Consensus and a Lot of Controversy." *Toxicological Sciences,* 2005, *87,* 11–14.

Mazur, A. *A Hazardous Inquiry: The Rashomon Effect at Love Canal.* Cambridge, Mass.: Harvard University Press, 1998.

McDonough, W., and Braungart, M. *Cradle to Cradle: Remaking the Way We Make Things.* New York: North Point Press, 2002.

McKeown, T. *The Role of Medicine: Dream, Mirage, or Nemesis?* Princeton, N.J.: Princeton University Press, 1979.

McMichael, T. *Human Frontiers, Environments and Disease.* New York: Cambridge University Press, 2001.

Melosi, M. V. *The Sanitary City: Urban Infrastructure in America from Colonial Times to the Present.* Baltimore, Md.: Johns Hopkins University Press, 2000.

National Research Council, Committee on Pesticides in the Diets of Infants and Children. *Pesticides in the Diets of Infants and Children.* Washington, D.C.: National Academies Press, 1993.

New York Times. "Rachel Carson Dies of Cancer; 'Silent Spring' Author Was 56." http://www.nytimes.com/learning/general/onthisday/bday/0527.html, Apr. 15, 1964. (Statements quoted originally aired on *CBS Reports,* Apr. 3, 1963.)

Nigsch, F., Macaluso, N. J., Mitchell, J. B., and Zmuidinavicius, D. "Computational Toxicology: An Overview of the Sources of Data and of Modelling Methods." *Expert Opinion on Drug Metabolism & Toxicology,* 2009, 5, 1–14.

Nordstrom, H., and Vaughan, S. *Trade and Environment*. Special Studies 4. Geneva: World Trade Organization, 1999.

Patterson, J. T. *The Dread Disease: Cancer and Modern American Culture*. Cambridge, Mass.: Harvard University Press, 1987.

Pognan, F. "Genomics, Proteomics and Metabonomics in Toxicology: Hopefully Not 'Fashionomics.'" *Pharmacogenomics*, 2004, *5*, 879–893.

Randall, W. *Building 6: The Tragedy at Bridesburg*. Boston: Little, Brown, 1977.

Randolph, T. G. *Human Ecology and Susceptibility to the Chemical Environment*. Springfield, Ill.: Thomas, 1976.

Randolph, T. G. *Environmental Medicine: Beginnings and Bibliographies of Clinical Ecology*. Fort Collins, Colo.: Clinical Ecology, 1987.

Rappaport, D. J., and others. "Ecosystem Health: The Concept, the ISEH, and the Important Tasks Ahead." *Ecosystem Health*, 1999, *5*, 82–90.

Rea, W. J. *Chemical Sensitivity*. 4 vols. Boca Raton, Fla.: Lewis, 1992–1998.

Reamon-Buettner, S. M., Mutschler, V., and Borlak, J. "The Next Innovation Cycle in Toxicogenomics: Environmental Epigenetics." *Mutation Research*, 2008, *659*(1–2), 158–165.

Rosen, G. *A History of Public Health*. (Expanded ed.) Baltimore, Md.: Johns Hopkins University Press, 1993. (Originally published 1958.)

Rosenberg, C. *The Cholera Years: The United States in 1832, 1849, and 1866*. Chicago: University of Chicago Press, 1962.

Runge, C. F. *Freer Trade, Protected Environment: Balancing Trade Liberalization and Environmental Interests*. New York: Council on Foreign Relations Press, 1994.

Sass, J. *Effective and Practical Disclosure Policies: NRDC Paper on Workshop to Identify Key Elements of Disclosure Policies for Health Science Journals*. Natural Resources Defense Council. http://www.nrdc.org/health/disclosure, 2009.

Schmidt, C. W. "Toxicogenomics: An Emerging Discipline." *Environmental Health Perspectives*, 2003, *110*, A750–A755.

Schoonen, W. G., Westerink, W. M., and Horbach, G. J. "High-Throughput Screening for Analysis of in Vitro Toxicity." *EXS*, 2009, *99*, 401–452.

Shabecoff, P. *A Fierce Green Fire: The American Environmental Movement*. New York: Hill & Wang, 1993.

Smith, R. "Medical Journals Are an Extension of the Marketing Arm of Pharmaceutical Companies." *PLoS Medicine*, 2005, *2*, e138, doi:10.1371/journal.pmed.0020138.

Sullivan, R. *Rats: Observations on the History and Habitat of the City's Most Unwanted Inhabitants*. New York: Bloomsbury, 2004.

Swan, S. H., Elkin, E. P., and Fenster, L. "Have Sperm Densities Declined? A Reanalysis of Global Trend Data." *Environmental Health Perspectives*, 1997, *105*, 1228–1232.

Tarr, J. A. *The Search for the Ultimate Sink: Urban Pollution in Historical Perspective*. Akron, Ohio: University of Akron Press, 1996.

Tarr, J. A. "Industrial Waste Disposal in the United States as a Historical Problem." *Ambix*, 2002, *49*, 4–20.

Thompson, D. F. "Understanding Financial Conflicts of Interest." *New England Journal of Medicine*, 1993, *329*, 573–576.

United Nations. Report of the United Nations Conference on Environment and Development: Annex I: *Rio Declaration on Environment and Development*. http://www.un.org/documents/ga/ conf151/ aconf15126-1annex1.htm, 1992.

United Nations Centre for Human Settlements (UN-Habitat). *Cities in a Globalizing World: Global Report on Human Settlements 2001*. London: Earthscan, 2001.

United Nations Department of Economic and Social Affairs. *Johannesburg Summit 2002*. http://www .un.org/jsummit/html/basic_info/unced.html, 2006.

U.S. Department of Health and Human Services. *An Ensemble of Definitions of Environmental Health*. http://web.health.gov/environment/DefinitionsofEnvHealth/ehdef2.htm, Nov. 1998.

van Wyk, B.-E., and Wink, M. *Medicinal Plants of the World: An Illustrated Scientific Guide to Important Medicinal Plants and Their Uses*. Portland, Ore.: Timber Press, 2004.

Wackernagel, M., and Rees, W. *Our Ecological Footprint: Reducing Human Impact on the Earth*. Gabriola Island, B.C.: New Society, 1995.

Waltner-Toews, D. *Ecosystem Sustainability and Health: A Practical Approach*. New York: Cambridge University Press, 2004.

Waters, M. D., and Fostel, J. M. "Toxicogenomics and Systems Toxicology: Aims and Prospects." *Nature Reviews: Genetics*, 2004, *5*, 936–948.

Wilson, E. O. *Biophilia: The Human Bond with Other Species*. Cambridge, Mass.: Harvard University Press, 1984.

World Commission on Environment and Development. *Our Common Future*. New York: Oxford University Press, 1987.

World Health Organization. *Protection of the Human Environment*. http://www.who.int/phe/en, 2004.

World Health Organization. *Governance: Constitution of the World Health Organization*. http://www .who.int/governance/en, 2005.

World Health Organization, Regional Office for Europe. *Environment and Health: The European Charter and Commentary*. WHO Regional Publications European Series No. 35. Copenhagen: World Health Organization, Regional Office for Europe, 1990.

World Health Organization, Regional Office for Europe. *Environment and Health Information System: The DPSEEA Model of Health-Environment Interlinks*. http://www.euro.who.int/EHindicators/ Indicators/20030527_2, 2004.

Zinsser, H. *Rats, Lice and History: Being a Study in Biography, Which, After Twelve Preliminary Chapters Indispensable for the Preparation of the Lay Reader, Deals with the Life History of Typhus Fever*. Boston: Little, Brown, 1935.

PART ONE

METHODS
AND
PARADIGMS

CHAPTER ONE

ECOLOGY AND ENVIRONMENTAL HEALTH

BRUCE WILCOX

HOLLY JESSOP

KEY CONCEPTS

- Ecology is a rigorous scientific discipline in which the interactions between biological organisms and their biotic and abiotic environments can be quantified and described; from this information predictions can be made and hypotheses tested.

- Humans exist within, and are not separate from, ecosystems and ecological interactions.

- Ecosystem functioning is driven by material and energy cycles, as biological and physical components interact both hierarchically and in circular feedback loops. As human activities alter these flows, the pace of global climate change increases, with concomitant public health impacts.

- Ecosystem functioning affects whether toxins and pathogens in the environment are broken down or concentrated and whether they may lead to environmental health risks.

- Biodiversity strongly influences ecosystem functioning, such as system capacity to regulate weather, break down hazardous agents, provide physical buffers against environmental disasters, and be resilient under both human and natural stresses.

- Populations have minimum size limits, set primarily by availability of resources and intrinsic characteristics. Below these limits they are easily extinguished by chance events. Populations also have maximum size limits, set primarily by extrinsic environmental factors.

- Abnormally rapid rates of environmental change, driven primarily by human population growth and unplanned development and overexploitation of natural resources, are altering ecological systems on an unprecedented scale. Among the environmental health consequences are emerging and reemerging infectious diseases.

THIS chapter introduces the science of ecology, its general principles, and the relevance of these principles to environmental health. **Ecology** is defined as the study of the interactions between organisms and their environments, including both the living (biotic) and nonliving (abiotic) components.

Ecology involves subject matter that is often readily observable and evident all around us. From the moment of birth, each of us interacts with the environment. We begin our life's journey by developing relationships both with other humans and with nonhuman organisms and by engaging in interactions with our physical surroundings.

Most ecologists study wildlife, wetlands, forests, fisheries, or parts of these and other natural systems. The concepts and principles that make up the ecological sciences deal with how nature works. Nearly everybody at one time or another actively observes and even ponders nature, making almost everybody an ecologist of sorts. This is true even for someone who has lived entirely in an urban environment. Ecology is also a broad scientific discipline. In fact the development of ecological thought has involved subsuming numerous ideas from such other sciences as geology, physics, sociology, and economics.

In spite of our intimate connections with the environment and awareness of nature, our processes of determining the scientific concepts of ecology are not always intuitive—and this is just as true when we are working in physics and economics. Every organism interacts with a multitude of other organisms, contributes to the flow of energy and materials (the currency of ecological systems), and responds to the physical environment in myriad subtle ways. We humans, the most conscious species, are unconscious of most of the ways in which we influence and are influenced by our environment; they are in effect invisible to us. For example, most people know little of the organisms and processes that underlie the ecological systems responsible for the oxygen we breathe, the water we use, the food we eat, and the infectious illnesses we contract.

It would take a book at least as big as this one to describe thoroughly the ecological basis of human health and well-being. This chapter focuses on the ecological concepts and principles most relevant to human health and the ways in which they can help us understand specific environmental health problems. Before proceeding, let us briefly consider the purpose, approaches, and perspectives encompassed by the field of ecology.

Bruce A. Wilcox and Holly Jessop declare no competing financial interests.

THE FIELD OF ECOLOGY

Ecology aims to understand how natural systems such as plant and animal communities are organized and function. This includes investigating the subsystems and other parts of natural systems, the relationships among them, and the processes at and above the level of the individual organism that allow biological systems to persist and evolve as dynamic entities. Modern ecology emerged from the study of **natural history**, which focused primarily on compiling descriptions and catalogues of plants and animals and which generally considered biological systems (including species) to be static entities. After Charles Darwin's *On the Origin of Species* was published in 1859, the fact that living organisms undergo change through the process of **natural selection** began to be incorporated into ecological study of the dynamics of natural systems. Thus ecology and **evolutionary biology** are closely allied and are considered one field by many biologists.

In fact Ernst Haeckel, the German zoologist (and Darwin's contemporary) who coined the term *ecology* in 1866, was an interpreter of Darwin's work. Haeckel created the new term to draw attention to the study of organisms in their environments, in contrast to their study only in the laboratory: the *eco* in ecology (from the Greek word *oikos*) means "home" or "place of dwelling" (Keller and Golley, 2000).

Although ecology developed during the nineteenth and twentieth centuries as a natural science, many of its concepts and principles have been applied to other fields, ranging from human social development (Bronfenbrenner, 1979) to social and cultural systems (Park, 1952; Bennett, 1993) and to epidemiology (Last, 1998). Also the traditional focus on the study of natural systems such as forests, grasslands, wetlands, rivers, lakes, and oceans has increasingly been extended beyond purely natural systems. For example, the application of ecological thinking began expanding by the mid-twentieth century to encompass human-built and "hybrid" human-natural systems such as cities and cultivated landscapes (Nevah and Lieberman, 1994). Recently, a **social-ecological systems perspective** (Berkes, Colding, and Folke, 2003) and **resilience theory** (Gunderson and Holling, 2002) have developed within the field of ecology to deal explicitly with humans and nature as a single, integrated, and complex system. This integrative approach to understanding living systems has been found necessary to meaningfully address issues such as **sustainability**, a concept that implies the dependence of human health and well-being on healthy ecosystems. In this way ecology has become as much a worldview as a scientific discipline (Keller and Golley, 2000).

Ecology is built on three different but complementary perspectives often considered its major subdisciplines: **ecosystem ecology, community ecology,** and **population ecology** (Begon, Harper, and Townsend, 2008). In addition, landscape ecology helps link these concepts across different scales, especially in applied contexts. The fundamentals of the three main subdisciplines of ecology are summarized in the following section. These and other lines of ecological research are then further discussed in the context of specific environmental health challenges.

Ecosystems, Communities, and Populations

Ecosystem ecology stresses energy flows and material cycles, including the ways in which energy and materials are modified by human activities. It aims to understand how energy and materials (such as water, carbon, nitrogen, phosphorus, and other elements) essential to growth and metabolism—from the organism level to the entire ecosystem—flow in, out, and through and are compartmentalized and transformed.

The **ecosystem** is in many ways the most important concept and functional entity in ecology, much as the cell is in physiology. An ecosystem is formed by the interactions of living organisms with their physical environment. Much as particular kinds of cells make up tissues and organ systems, various kinds of ecosystems make up Earth's living environmental systems. Collectively, these ecosystems constitute the **biosphere**, a central concept in ecology. The biosphere is the largest known ecosystem, in which all other ecosystems are embedded; it consists of all the Earth's living organisms interacting with the physical environment.

Understanding the idea of the biosphere and its development is fundamental to understanding life on Earth and the dependence of our health and well-being on natural systems. For example, it is critically important to understanding environmental health issues such as global climate change. Remarkably, its original conception a century ago included many insights relevant to environmental health today, such as recognition of the risks as well as benefits of an economy based on fossil fuels (such as coal, petroleum, and natural gas) and associated synthetic compounds (such as plastics, pharmaceuticals, and pesticides). The biosphere concept also highlighted the ubiquitous character of life in the form of microorganisms, occurring everywhere and within every living thing. Indeed, microorganisms constitute most of the free-living biomass on Earth, driving or regulating the biogeochemical cycles that make the biosphere possible, and forming an integral part of the ecology of every living organism. For example, every human supports hundreds of species of known microorganisms (mainly bacteria and viruses), ranging from the beneficial bacterial flora of our gastrointestinal tracts (without which we could not live) to the harmful influenza viruses that can cause disease.

PERSPECTIVE
The Biosphere

The term biosphere was coined in 1885 by the pioneering nineteenth-century earth scientist Eduard Suess. The idea was expanded and elaborated by Vladimir Vernadsky in 1925 in an extraordinary two-volume essay, *Biosphera*. As well described by Vaclav Smil (2002), Vernadsky presented a number of the key ideas that make up modern ecology as well as the earth sciences, such as the idea that balanced carbon exchange between the Earth's surface and atmosphere contributes to our planet's habitability. His idea led to the discovery that this balance is changing, due primarily to anthropogenic burning of fossil fuels and deforestation, which in turn is contributing to changes in the Earth's climate system. (The myriad direct and indirect effects of global climate change on health are discussed in Chapter Ten.)

What is the biosphere and how does it relate to ecological understanding? The biosphere is the layer of living matter—microbes, plants, and animals—that has been described as a "film" on the surface of the planet. It is sandwiched between the relatively thick lithosphere (the outer rocky layer of Earth) and the troposphere (the lowermost portion of the Earth's atmosphere). Life penetrates rocks and also the ocean depths and the highest mountain peaks where only tiny microorganisms adapted to extreme environmental conditions can exist. However, it is only within a relatively narrow zone of the biosphere that the transformation of solar energy through photosynthesis is possible.

Organisms have not only developed and adapted to conditions within the Earth's biosphere. They have also created the biological and physical conditions of the biosphere. For example, the original environment on the Earth's surface would have been completely uninhabitable and fatal to most organisms living on the Earth today. However, the evolution of photosynthesizing organisms, which generate oxygen, ultimately led to today's atmosphere. Such modifications to the biosphere have allowed subsequent life forms to evolve, survive, and even flourish. Indeed, many contemporary life forms, including humans, now depend on the oxygen generated by photosynthesis. And without today's protective tropospheric shield, very few kinds of organisms could survive the intense ultraviolet radiation and temperature extremes that would otherwise exist on the Earth's surface.

As a central paradigm in ecology, the biosphere provides us with a way of thinking about life framed in a large view, along with an understanding of the processes that make it possible for life to have evolved and to survive on Earth. Today we call this a *systems view*, with the Earth seen as a single unit of interacting living and nonliving parts and related processes. The idea of the biosphere provides the framework that allows us to begin to make sense of the complexity of human-nature interactions. The idea of the biosphere also links directly to the idea of the ecosystem, which is central to understanding the ecological basis of environmental health.

TABLE 1.1   The Major Subdisciplines of Ecology

Subdiscipline	Focus
Ecosystem ecology	Whole systems view; ecosystem as unit of study; emphasis on energy and material cycles.
Community ecology	Interactions of species; emphasis on species' composition and diversity.
Population ecology	Population-level processes; emphasis on population dynamics and regulation, and on interspecies interactions.

The other two major branches of ecology view nature from the perspective of component parts above the level of species that make up ecosystems. Community ecology deals with *ecological communities*, which are defined as assemblages of interacting plants, animals, and microbes coexisting in a particular location. Its aim is to understand the factors and mechanisms that determine the composition and diversity of species found in a particular place. Community and ecosystem ecologies overlap. However, community ecology focuses less on energy and material transfers and more on processes and factors that determine species' composition and diversity.

Population ecology attempts to explain the dynamics of species populations and interactions among species as well as relationships between species and their physical environment. The overlap of community ecology and population ecology becomes apparent when we consider that interspecies interactions—competition, predation, and parasitism—are some of the key determinants by which species coexist in a particular place (that is, make up a community).

In sum, ecosystem ecologists are mainly interested in how ecosystems are organized and function, community ecologists in why communities have the number and assortment of species that they do, and population ecologists in what determines the abundance and distribution of a species. The perspectives and research foci of the major subdisciplines of ecology are summarized in Table 1.1.

Core Questions of Ecology

The subdisciplines of ecology are complementary. All address an overarching question that has motivated natural historians and ecologists from the beginning: what determines why and how ecological systems form, species assemblages develop, and populations survive in the environments that they do? Scientists began focusing on this question in earnest beginning with Alfred Russell Wallace, Darwin's contemporary and a codiscoverer of the principle of evolution by natural selection. Wallace was the first (in a work published in 1876) to map the world's "zoogeographic realms," comprehensive distributions of known animal species. This in turn led generations of ecologists to investigate what determines the geographic distribution of major types of ecosystems and communities. In addition, countless ecologists have studied individual species' interactions with each other and with the physical environment.

Certain critical features determine the character of ecosystems. Prime among them are the amount of precipitation, the temperature, and the availability of soil nutrients. These features in turn predict the kind of vegetation that grows, defining the major ecological zones, or **biomes** (Figures 1.1 and 1.2). Basically, biomes are the world's major geographic regions defined by characteristic ecosystem type. Major biome types include tundra, boreal forest, temperate forest, tropical forest, scrubland, grassland and savannah, and desert (Table 1.2); these are divided into subtypes such as coniferous or deciduous forest, semiarid or tropical scrubland, and so on. The traits of the organisms that make up a biome or ecosystem type and the physical structure of the vegetation, including its height and density, are responses to evolutionary and ecological constraints and to opportunities posed largely by climate.

Local circumstances such as geology and landscape (topography) can also have a strong influence on the ecosystem type that develops in an area. But even these **abiotic** factors are ultimately shaped or determined in part by biological, or **biotic**, factors. For example, the reshaping of rocks and landforms, or **geomorphology**, is partly a consequence of the interaction of vegetation cover and rainfall. Vegetation influences not only rainfall but also the rates of erosion in uplands and sedimentation in lowlands, including deposition of sediments and soil downstream in river systems.

Understanding the internal workings of ecosystems related to these observed biogeographic patterns has provided critical insights into the mechanisms underlying a number of important environmental health problems. For example, not the least of these is how changing human land use and industrial activity have altered the natural cycling, storage, and release of carbon in its different forms (solid and gaseous). The net decrease in carbon stored in ecosystems such as tropical forests and the increase in carbon dioxide in the Earth's atmosphere are key contributors to global warming and its associated health impacts (discussed further in Chapter Ten). Observing how different biomes and ecosystems vary in their organization, functioning, and component organisms has also helped to reveal mechanisms underlying other environmental health challenges. For example, studies of how energy and matter are transferred from lower to higher levels in the food chains of

FIGURE 1.1   Map of Western Hemisphere Biomes

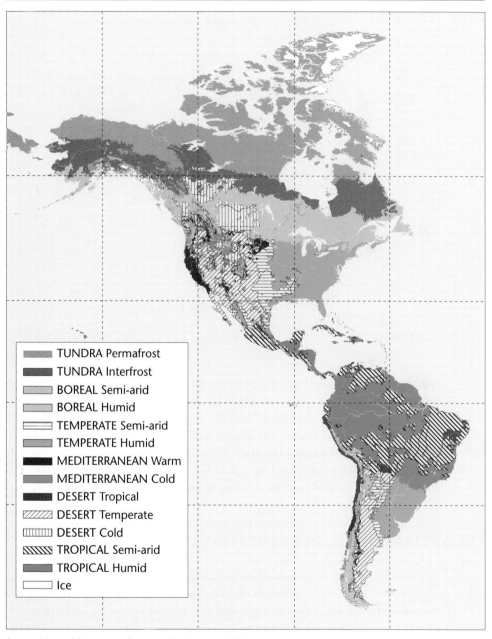

Legend:
- TUNDRA Permafrost
- TUNDRA Interfrost
- BOREAL Semi-arid
- BOREAL Humid
- TEMPERATE Semi-arid
- TEMPERATE Humid
- MEDITERRANEAN Warm
- MEDITERRANEAN Cold
- DESERT Tropical
- DESERT Temperate
- DESERT Cold
- TROPICAL Semi-arid
- TROPICAL Humid
- Ice

Source: Natural Resources Conservation Service, 2003.

Major biomes include desert, grassland, tropical rainforest, and taiga.

FIGURE 1.2   "Cloud" Diagram of the Six Major Terrestrial
Biomes Plotted by Mean Annual Temperature (in Degrees F)
and Precipitation (in Inches)

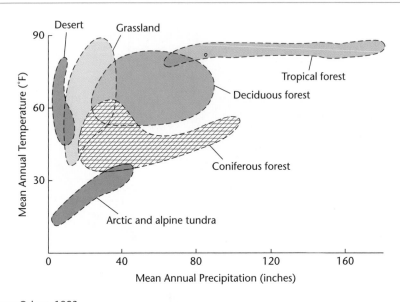

Source: Odum, 1993.

aquatic ecosystems explains such phenomena as biomagnification. As described later, biomagnification can result in unsafe levels of toxins in seafood. Similarly, studies of ecosystem "physiology" and discovery of factors that control biomass production in aquatic ecosystems have helped to explain how nutrient pollution can cause **harmful algal blooms**. Other research on the regulatory functions of forest ecosystems has helped to explain how deforestation releases vectors and pathogens from natural controls, leading to **emerging infectious diseases**.

ECOSYSTEM PROCESSES AND FUNCTIONING

Naturally mediated and regulated ecological processes, such as the breakdown of organic waste and the recycling of chemical elements, are part of what is called ecosystem functioning. For example, key processes in the back-and-forth movement of materials between living and nonliving biosphere components are the **hydrologic cycle** (Figure 1.3) and the biogeochemical cycles, which include the **carbon cycle** and **nitrogen cycle** (Figures 1.4 and 1.5).

TABLE 1.2   Major Ecosystem Types and Biomes

Ecosystem Type	Biomes
Marine ecosystems	Open ocean (pelagic)
	Continental shelf water (inshore water)
	Upwelling regions (fertile areas with productive fisheries)
	Deep sea (hydrothermal vents)
	Estuaries (coastal bays, sounds, river mouths, salt marshes)
Freshwater ecosystems	Lentic (standing water): lakes and ponds
	Lotic (running water): rivers and streams
	Wetlands: marshes and swamp forests
Terrestrial biomes	Tundra: arctic and alpine
	Boreal coniferous forests
	Temperate deciduous forests
	Temperate grassland
	Tropical grassland and savanna
	Chaparral: winter rain–summer drought regions
	Desert: herbaceous and shrub
	Semi-evergreen tropical forest: pronounced wet and dry seasons
	Evergreen tropical rain forest
Domesticated ecosystems	Rural techno-ecosystems (transportation corridors, small towns, industries)
	Agro-ecosystems
	Urban-industrial techno-ecosystems (metropolitan districts)

Source: Adapted from Odum, 1993.

Such cycling of water and elements is central to the functioning of ecosystems and the biosphere. Indeed, these processes are the basis of Earth's life support system, and thus are essential to human health. For example, they make possible the wetlands, marshes, and mangrove forests that provide key **ecosystem services** such as natural waste recycling, water filtration, barriers against storm surges and saltwater intrusion, and nurseries for fish and shellfish. The degradation of ecosystems and the alteration of their functioning can have severe health consequences. This relationship of ecological functioning to human health is a recurrent theme in this chapter and is discussed further in the context of other processes and properties of ecosystems, communities, and populations.

PERSPECTIVE
Ecosystem Services

As described in a synthesis report from the Millennium Ecosystem Assessment (2005), the benefits provided by ecosystems are indispensable to the well-being of people throughout the world. These benefits include food, natural fibers, a steady supply of clean water, regulation of some pests and diseases, medicinal substances, recreation, and protection from natural hazards such as storms and floods. Yet because of the complexity of ecosystems, the innumerable ways in which human well-being is linked to ecosystem productivity, and the limitations of economic methods and data, it is not yet possible to accurately measure the economic value of goods and services provided by ecosystems (Daily and others, 2003). The report divides ecosystem services into four categories: provisioning services, regulating services, supporting services, and cultural services. The functions particularly relevant to environmental health are the regulating services: provision and purification of water, recycling of wastes, and regulation of climate and of infectious diseases. Here are summaries of the report's findings in these areas.

Provision of clean water. Ecosystems, especially forests, act both as reservoirs, holding water much like giant sponges, and as pumps. Through the process of evapotranspiration, forest vegetation draws water from the ground and releases it into the atmosphere. These functions, which contribute much to the hydrologic cycle, effectively recycle used as well as unused surface water, remove impurities, and deliver fresh water to places from which it can be harvested. Fresh water is a key resource for human health, vital for growing food, drinking, washing, cooking, and diluting and recycling wastes. Unfortunately, as a result of ecosystem degradation, population growth, and inadequate water treatment and distribution infrastructure, over a billion people in the world do not have access to clean water. Overall, the annual burden of disease resulting from inadequate water, sanitation, and hygiene totals 1.7 million deaths and the loss of more than 54 million healthy life years.

Waste recycling (nutrients, pathogens, and breakdown of toxins). As suggested earlier, ecosystem processes resulting in the breakdown of organic wastes and the filtering of suspended material, including pathogens, are effective mechanisms for cleansing the environment of wastes. Natural ecosystems can be so effective at purifying and detoxifying wastewater that some municipalities have restored wetlands in order to use them for tertiary sewage treatment. The filtering and microbial degradation properties of wetlands, such as marshes, swamps, and streamside, or riparian, zones consisting of soil perennially saturated with water, are capable of physically removing or breaking down even the most toxic chemicals and heavy metals as well as human pathogens. Despite their value, wetlands are among the world's most endangered ecosystems, as coastal wetlands and their upstream tributary rivers and streams are often filled and paved over for urban development or are otherwise functionally destroyed by misdirected flood management programs. The loss of this waste-recycling capacity has now led to local and sometimes global waste accumulation, as the ecosystems that remain are unable to absorb and remove the onslaught of contaminants. For example, the loss of this recycling capacity, along with fertilizer-laden runoff in the Mississippi River Basin, is responsible for the eutrophic dead zone in the Gulf of Mexico.

Regulation of infectious disease. An ecosystem's characteristics, particularly its landscape ecology, strongly influence the incidence of zoonotic and vector-borne diseases in local human populations and the potential for the emergence of new, epidemiologically significant diseases. Intact ecosystems, with their innumerable interspecies relationships and heterogeneous landscape structures, offer a series of checks and balances that tend to moderate population dynamics and prevent any particular species (including host, vector, or pathogen species) from dispersing widely or becoming superabundant, or both. This moderating function tends to break down with the clearing or fragmenting of natural ecosystems, such as the logging of forests or the expansion of cropland and pasture. Artificial changes in the distribution and availability of surface waters, such as occur through dam construction, irrigation, and stream diversion, have a similar effect. Intensification of animal husbandry and livestock production practices resulting in increased concentration, movement, and novel mixing of animal species and of animal products and waste facilitates the cultivation and maintenance of new pathogens strains, as evidenced in the development of avian influenza (H5N1).

Regulation of climate. Natural ecosystems regulate the global climate system by acting as sinks for greenhouse gasses. In particular, the clearing and burning of tropical forests around the world has been a major contributor to the accelerated increase in carbon dioxide in the Earth's atmosphere and thus to global warming in recent decades. At the regional and local levels, natural and managed ecosystems strongly influence climate due to physical properties that affect the flows of energy and rainfall. For example, the conversion of vegetated land cover to hardened surfaces associated with urbanization produces the *urban heat island* effect, elevating the temperature of a city and the surrounding region. In this way ecosystems may moderate or intensify extreme weather events such as heat waves, freezing weather, storms, and associated floods and coastal storm surges—events thought to be increasing due to anthropogenic global climate change. Intact ecosystems limit the degree and extent of adverse weather impacts on public health, directly through reducing deaths and injuries and indirectly through limiting economic disruption, infrastructure damage, and population displacement. Ecosystems and the ways they are managed can also have a strong negative or positive impact on air quality and its associated health risks.

FIGURE 1.3   Hydrologic Cycle

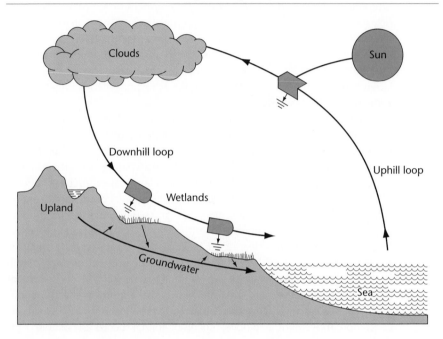

Source: Odum, 1993.

Water continually moves through various states. The uphill loop is driven by solar energy, and the downhill loop provides goods and services such as rainfall. (In Odum's notation, the pointed icon on the uphill loop represents the interaction of energy flows to produce higher quality energy, and the bullet-shaped icons on the downhill loop represent conversion and concentration of solar energy.)

Ecosystem Organization

As alluded to earlier, the term *ecosystem* may refer to a theoretical idea or paradigm on the one hand or to a particular entity on the other—a lake, a forest patch, or a coral reef, for example. Realizing this distinction, the great ecologist Eugene Odum pointed to organizational integrity as the defining criterion for an ecosystem. He defined an ecosystem as "any unit that includes all of the organisms (*i.e.* the 'community') in a given area interacting with the physical environment so that a flow of energy leads to clearly defined trophic structure, biotic diversity, and material cycles (*i.e.* exchange of materials between living and nonliving parts) within the system" (Odum, 1971, p. 8).

FIGURE 1.4 Carbon Cycle

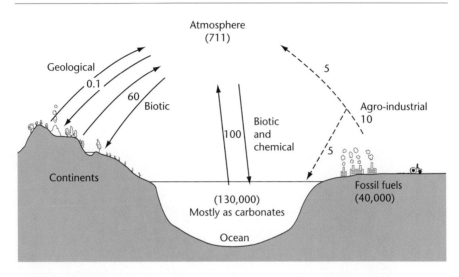

Source: Odum, 1993.

Estimates of the amounts of carbon dioxide (in 10^9 tons) are shown in four major compartments: the atmosphere, oceans, terrestrial biomass, and soils and fossil fuels. Flux rates between compartments are shown by arrows. Note that the atmospheric pool of carbon is relatively small, especially in comparison to the fossil fuel reservoir, but it is active and changing. Most flows are balanced, as shown by pairs of solid lines, but there is a net transfer from fossil fuels to the atmosphere and oceans (shown by dotted lines) dating from the early industrial age.

   The two most significant organizational aspects of any ecosystem, aspects to which ecosystem functioning is tied, are trophic structure and the associated material cycles of nutrients (such as carbon, nitrogen, phosphorus, and potassium), trace essential minerals (such as iron, sulfur, zinc, and selenium), and water. **Trophic structure** refers to the organization of ecosystems by feeding levels, often conveniently conceptualized as a pyramid. A **trophic level** is the position that an organism occupies on this pyramid or to put it another way, in a food chain—what it eats, and what eats it ("trophic" derives from *trophe*, the Greek word for feeding). As shown in Figure 1.6, organisms such as plants and algae that use photosynthesis to convert solar energy into stored chemical energy (in the form of carbohydrates) can be represented as **primary producers**, or **autotrophs**, because they make their own energy. These kinds of organisms constitute the base of the trophic pyramid and, at the same time, the bottom of the food chain.

FIGURE 1.5   Nitrogen Cycle

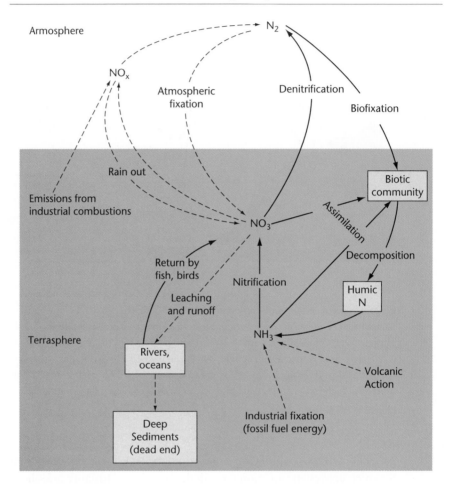

Source: Odum, 1993.

Note: NO_x = nitrogen oxides; NO_2 = nitrogen dioxide; NO_3 = nitrate; NH_3 = ammonia.

Vital to all life on Earth, nitrogen is a key component of DNA and amino acids. Although nitrogen is bountiful in the atmosphere, usable forms are produced only by a few specialized microbes (*diazotrophs*) that are able to *fix* nitrogen (and by lightning, combustion, and industrial processes). Nitrogen is returned to the atmosphere via denitrification by both biotic and abiotic processes. Solid lines indicate natural biotic flows of nitrogen, and dashed lines indicate flows influenced by humans or other physical processes. Oxides of nitrogen in the atmosphere contribute to air pollution (as discussed in Chapter Twelve).

FIGURE 1.6   Solar Energy Flow Through a Biological Food Chain (in kcal/m²/year)

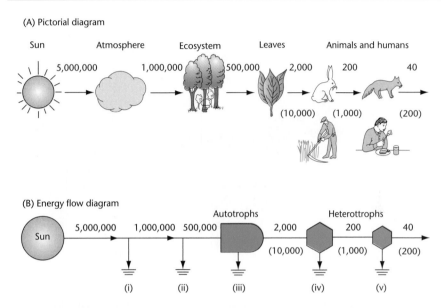

Source: Odum, 1993.

Energy is lost as solar energy passes through the biosphere performing work (and being dissipated as heat) at each step. For example, only about 1 percent (up to 5 percent under optimal conditions) of the energy that reaches a green layer is converted to organic matter through photosynthesis. It is the flow of energy that drives the flow of materials. (In Odum's notation, the bullet-shaped icon represents a producer that converts and concentrates solar energy, and the hexagon represents a consumer that uses converted energy.) Figures in parentheses are energy levels "subsidized" by other sources such as fuel.

Producers are fed upon by **primary consumers** (herbivore species) that in turn are fed upon by secondary consumers, and so on. **Secondary consumers** are also called **heterotrophs**, because they get their energy from feeding on other organisms (both plants and animals). The amount of biomass found at a trophic level (that is, the cumulative mass of all the individual organisms of all the species at a particular trophic level) decreases by roughly an order of magnitude with each step up the pyramid. This occurs because, as energy is transferred from one trophic level to the next (producers→herbivores→carnivores), a portion of the energy is lost as heat (a consequence of the second law of thermodynamics).

FIGURE 1.7   Nutrient Cycling and One-Way Energy Flow
Through an Ecosystem

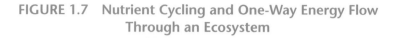

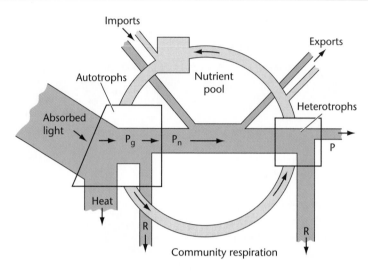

Source: Odum, 1993.

The biogeochemical cycle is superimposed on a simplified energy flow diagram, showing that the energy flow drives the biogeochemical cycle. P_g = gross primary production, P_n = net primary production, P = secondary production, and R = respiration.

In fact the amount of energy gathered from solar radiation and stored in plant biomass is relatively small compared to the total solar energy reaching Earth. Thus we can easily understand why top predators such as sharks or tigers tend to have relatively small population sizes even under the best of circumstances. These naturally small population sizes are the reason why these top predators can so easily become endangered through overharvesting or habitat loss.

The relationships among trophic structure, **nutrient cycles**, and energy flow displayed in Figure 1.7 illustrate how the one-way flow of energy, entering the ecosystem as sunlight, drives the cycling of nutrients such as nitrogen. The compartments in Figure 1.7 represent pools of nutrients and the biomass of organisms (autotrophs and heterotrophs). In a healthy ecosystem the energy flow, nutrient cycles, and biomass are relatively stable. These compartments represent the *stocks* of energy and materials, and the pathways are their *flows*. As we will see later in this chapter, human activities can dramatically alter these quantities and

TABLE 1.3   Levels of Organizational Hierarchies

Sociopolitical	Ecological
World	Biosphere
Nation (or region)	Biome (or biogeographic province)
State or province	Landscape
County or district	Ecosystem
Municipality	Biotic community
Household	Population (species)
Individual	Organism

Source: Adapted from Odum, 1993.

processes, resulting in serious imbalances that can lead to severe environmental health consequences.

One important consequence of trophic structure is that some pollutants can become concentrated in organisms at the higher trophic levels (higher on the food chain)—in predator species, for example. Examples of this phenomenon are discussed in the Perspective titled "Toxins and Biomagnification."

Hierarchy and Scale

Ecosystems, and biological systems in general, have been found to exhibit properties consistent with all so-called complex systems. The most obvious of these properties is hierarchical organization. As illustrated in Table 1.3, ecological systems, like sociopolitical systems, self-organize in a nested pattern, in which larger entities (or subsystems) that exist on one scale contain subsystems that exist on a smaller scale (and that operate on shorter time or smaller spatial scales).

This hierarchical property of complex systems—the scaled, nested arrangement of parts—has functional implications. The function of the whole system—the biosphere in the case of ecological systems—both constrains the behavior of the parts (or subsystems) and is a consequence of them. For example, carbon dioxide uptake and oxygen release by the autotrophic organisms within communities and ecosystems help to determine the atmospheric concentrations of these gasses, which in turn drive weather patterns globally. As illustrated in Figure 1.2, the average precipitation and temperature of different weather patterns themselves influence ecological processes to the extent of determining biomes and the types of primary producers present in a regional ecosystem.

PERSPECTIVE
Toxins and Biomagnification: Mercury and POPs.

Unlike energy, a significant portion of which is lost as it is transferred from one trophic level to the next in an ecosystem, some substances increase in concentration as they are transferred up a food chain. This phenomenon is called **biomagnification**. Biomagnification is based on **bioaccumulation**, which occurs when organisms (including humans) take up contaminants more rapidly than their bodies can eliminate them. Over time, of course, an organism consumes a vastly greater amount of biomass than that represented by its own body, effectively amassing the exposures of many organisms in its food chain. An organism can thus potentially assimilate and concentrate a toxic substance at much greater levels than occur in its environment. Persistent chemicals are especially likely to bioaccumulate. Moreover, the higher an organism's trophic level, the greater is the concentration of a bioaccumulated substance.

These processes are responsible for the potentially harmful levels of toxic substances found in some species of fish. Similarly, terrestrial predators feeding at the tops of food pyramids may accumulate environmental toxins that have become increasingly concentrated in prey organisms. Such chemical hazards arise from natural as well as "unnatural" human disturbances and inputs into fresh water, marine, and terrestrial environments.

Mercury provides a key example of biomagnification of a toxic substance. Mercury is well known as an environmental pollutant with serious human health consequences. Fish and other wildlife in various ecosystems commonly have concentrations

Complex systems are replete with these kinds of circular feedback mechanisms, leading to nonlinear responses to natural and human ecosystem perturbations. Because the outcomes of these perturbations are extremely difficult to predict accurately, they can also be easy to ignore or deny. This is often the case with climate change. The massive conversion of the world's natural ecosystems to urban ecosystems over the past three centuries, along with fossil fuel burning, is causing a dramatic change in the atmospheric concentration of greenhouse gasses—and this is just one of many ecological consequences of the transformation of the biosphere through human activities (Smil, 2002; also see Chapter Ten). Because this change has been gradual and because science cannot predict its outcomes precisely, policymakers and the public have frequently been surprised by these outcomes. However, experts knowledgeable about ecological systems are often anything but surprised.

of mercury of toxicological concern when eaten by humans. Mercury enters ecosystems as a result of both natural processes and human activities (especially coal combustion, because coal may be contaminated with mercury) and is converted to various forms, including the highly toxic organic form methylmercury, which can bioaccumulate. Many of the details of how mercury compounds form and circulate in an ecosystem remain unknown. However, what is known is that mercury has the potential to be a serious health hazard and that human-derived emissions are increasing.

Persistent organic pollutants (POPs) provide another example of toxic chemical substances that can dangerously biomagnify. With slow or no degradation, such substances persist in the environment and can be transported by wind or water. Like mercury, POPs can threaten both wildlife and human health. For example, many widely used pesticides (such as DDT), chemicals such as polychlorinated biphenyls (PCBs), and combustion by-products such as dioxins, are POPs that can be toxic even at very low levels of exposure. As with mercury, the mechanism driving biomagnification of POPs is bioaccumulation within the trophic pyramid of ecosystems: autotrophs and primary consumers accumulate POPs in their tissues, resulting in concentrations greater than those found in the surrounding environment. When these organisms are themselves consumed by heterotrophs, POPs become even more concentrated. Thus low-level POPs in the environment can quickly become dangerously concentrated in organisms that feed at higher trophic levels. Unfortunately, POPs are becoming ubiquitous in the biosphere, an outcome deriving almost solely from human-generated effluents entering the Earth's hydrologic cycle.

Crawford (Buzz) Holling and his colleagues have shown how this pattern of denial and surprise applies to many environmental crises and failures of environmental management in areas ranging from attempts to establish sustainable forests and fisheries to efforts to control pest- and vector-borne disease. Building on earlier research on ecosystem organization, behavior, and management, Holling and colleagues have developed a useful framework based on complexity theory and case studies (Holling, 1978, 1986; Gunderson, Holling, and Light, 1995; Gunderson and Holling, 2002; Berkes and others, 2003). A central feature of this framework is the **adaptive renewal cycle** (Figure 1.8), a model that describes the repeated cycles of change exhibited by ecological, economic, and institutional systems—as coupled human-natural systems—through four distinct phases: exploitation, conservation, release, and reorganization.

FIGURE 1.8   Adaptive Renewal Cycle

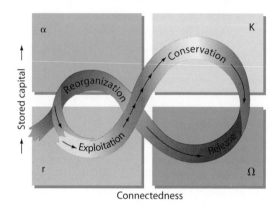

As indicated on the diagram, the r phase represents growth and exploitation, the K phase represents conservation, the Ω phase represents release, and the α phase represents reorganization.

Unlike traditional ecosystem models that treat humans as external components, the adaptive renewal cycle model acknowledges the reality of what has been called the total human ecosystem (Nevah and Lieberman, 1994)—the idea that humans and their environment form a single entity to be studied in its totality. This model incorporates feedback relationships within and between the human and natural system components. This includes relationships that link the institutional and natural parts of the system and that involve "signals" that provide feedback (information) about the status of the stocks and flows of energy and materials.

A classic example of such feedback is the information gathered by fishery biologists on the status of the target fish population(s) being harvested. This information typically is gathered and provided to decision makers who then decide how to adjust harvesting rates, through such approaches as limiting the number of permits issued, constraints on fishing gear, and other measures. Ideally, the feedback mechanism thus triggers institutional behavior that results in a sustainable harvesting regime, with functionally intact fish populations, healthy ecosystems, and economically productive fishing industries.

This system of cyclical monitoring and adjusting was named **adaptive management** (Holling, 1978; Walters, 1986). It is the central idea of **ecosystem**

management and involves monitoring key indicators of the health of the ecosystem, such as measures of nutrient flow and animal stocks, and adjusting human actions accordingly. The idea of adaptive management has more recently been extended to environmental health risk management (Carpenter, 1997).

Chesapeake Bay offers one of the best cases of adaptive management. This ecosystem has long been one of eastern North America's most important environmental resources, owing to its fisheries, recreational uses, and other valued characteristics. Accordingly, pollutant discharges into the bay and its upstream drainages had long been a concern. In the 1970s, when major federal and state environmental protection laws were promulgated in the United States, governmental agencies began monitoring the state of this aquatic ecosystem, using increasingly sophisticated ecological indicators and indicators of environmental health risk. They looked, for example, at concentrations of toxic metals and organic compounds in waters, sediments, fish, and shellfish.

An adaptive management system has evolved since the 1970s through a dynamic relationship between science and governance (Hennessey, 1994). This ultimately led to a comprehensive set of measures indicating the state of health of the bay ecosystem and its resources, and the risks to human health. These risks include exposure to toxic chemicals, infection by pathogens, and frequency and intensity of production of biotoxins by harmful algae (Boesch, 2000). The Chesapeake Bay Program has become a model for large-scale environmental restoration and management that involves stakeholders' participation at all levels of government and an extensive research community. The evolving suite of ecosystem health indicators has at times included more than eighty-two separate metrics adapted to different management needs: condition indicators, evaluation indicators, diagnostic indicators, communication indicators, and futures indicators (Hershner, Havens, Bilkovic, and Wardrop, 2007).

Biological Diversity and Ecosystem Functioning

The concept of biological diversity is closely intertwined with the organizational hierarchy of biological systems and complex ecosystem functioning, including some ecological processes that affect human health. Biological diversity, or **biodiversity** as it often called, refers both to organismic variety at the various levels of the organizational hierarchy and to genetic diversity among individual organisms (Grifo and Rosenthal, 1997; Chivian and Bernstein, 2008). Ecosystems with greater numbers of species or with species populations harboring greater differences in their genetic makeup are said to have greater biodiversity.

Ecosystems that retain higher levels of biological diversity often retain superior air, water, and soil quality and regulate pathogens more effectively. Moreover, greater biological diversity makes ecosystems more resilient and better able to assimilate environmental stressors, such as physical restructuring, invasive species, extreme weather events, overharvesting, or pollution (Folke and others, 2004). Overall, greater biodiversity offers numerous benefits for human health.

Unfortunately, biodiversity is eroding at unprecedented and alarming rates, largely through the degradation of ecosystems (especially tropical forests), species extinctions, and the reduction of genetic diversity within species. Among higher organisms such as birds, mammals, reptiles, and amphibians, whose status can be relatively well monitored (in contrast to the status of millions upon millions of invertebrate species), species are now being extinguished due to human activities at least a thousand times faster than new species are being created.

COMMUNITIES AND SPECIES

Community ecology focuses on the determinants of the number and composition of species in an ecological community. These determinants include resources, space, species-specific characteristics, and interspecies interactions.

Assembling Communities

The amount of space in a habitat plays a key role in determining the number of species present. As habitat area increases, so do two important environmental variables: the amount of resources and the variety of resources, termed **habitat diversity**. A large and geographically dispersed population ensures against any number of natural and human threats to species survival, and such a population is likely to have demographic and genetic assets that can lead to long-term persistence. Greater extent and diversity of habitat translates into a larger number of species supported.

This fact is a reflection of one of the most fundamental principles in ecology, known as the **species-area relationship** (Figures 1.9 and 1.10). Ecologists surveying study plots of different sizes that are nested or arrayed separately across landscape or that are completely ecologically isolated, areas such as mountain ranges separated by valleys or the islands of an archipelago, invariably find the same pattern. Regardless of the taxonomic group or ecosystem—species of ants, butterflies, passerine birds, rodents, orchids, or palm trees—the number of different species plotted against the size of the area sampled approximates the power function form (Rosenzweig, 1995). This is shown in Figure 1.9.

The species-area relationship is normally presented as a log-log plot that produces a straight line, as shown in Figure 1.10, which is based on real data on the

FIGURE 1.9   Species-Area Curve

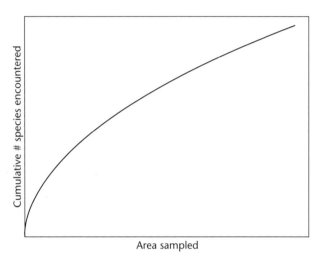

Larger areas are associated with a higher number of species, that is, with more biodiversity.

FIGURE 1.10   Log-Log Species Area Plot

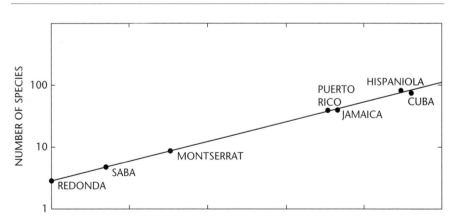

Source: MacArthur and Wilson (1967), adapted from Darlington, (1957).

The number of species of amphibians and reptiles found on seven West Indies islands varies with island size.

FIGURE 1.11   MacArthur's Warblers

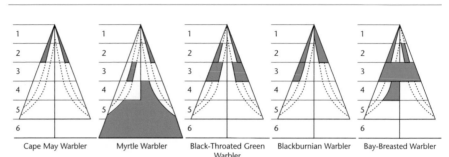

| Cape May Warbler | Myrtle Warbler | Black-Throated Green Warbler | Blackburnian Warbler | Bay-Breasted Warbler |

Source: Adapted from MacArthur, 1958.

MacArthur found that different warbler species tended to allocate their time to different parts of a tree—one toward the outside of the top, another mostly around the middle interior, and so on. In this diagram, the zones that accounted for 50 percent of each species feeding activity are blackened.

number of reptile and amphibian species for islands of varying size in the West Indies. This particular finding for these West Indies fauna led zoogeographer P. J. Darlington (1957) to point out that "division of area by ten divides the fauna by two," a formula that has become known as **Darlington's Rule**. The species-area relationship helps to explain why shrinking habitat by converting native forests and other natural habitats to domestic land uses decreases the number of species. More than this though, reducing habitat alters species composition and reduces biodiversity. With less biodiversity, an ecosystem has less resilience and less functional capacity.

The particular needs of a species (the unique set of conditions to which it is adapted) and its role in its community are collectively known as its **niche**. A niche is like the occupation of a species, whereas its habitat is like its address. The niche concept is central in ecology. It links community ecology and population ecology and is also critical to evolutionary biology. A species' niche is molded through natural selection over evolutionary time and dynamically adjusted through physiological and behavioral adaptations. The driving forces for evolutionary change include both abiotic factors and biotic factors such as competition, predation, parasitism, and disease. The biotic circumstance of a species is a particularly important aspect of niche theory, in which the **competitive exclusion principle** comes into play. This principle states that no two species can occupy the same niche. A classic example is ecologist Robert MacArthur's finding that five species of wood warblers—insect-eating birds that live in coniferous forests—occupied distinct niches within the same trees (Figure 1.11). Ecologists have found that in nature, as well as in the laboratory, when populations of two species are forced to exploit the same resource, one species eventually eliminates the other through direct interference, more efficient resource use, or both.

Predators, parasites, and disease all play important roles in determining the presence or absence of a species in a community. *Competition* is an especially powerful factor in determining the composition of communities when the extent of available habitat is limited. This helps explain why large islands can support more species than small islands (Figure 1.10); with more options for dividing up the available space and resources (such as food, shelter, and breeding sites), more species can be supported. Structural diversity is also generally a good surrogate for habitat diversity. Thus tropical forests and coral reefs, with their intricate architectures, tend to have high numbers of species.

Besides the *area effect* just described, the species numbers on islands also often exhibit a *distance effect*, in which more remote islands tend to have fewer species. The distance effect is especially important when distances are great (as in the case of oceanic islands) or when the members of the species of interest are poor dispersers. Although most forest birds can easily fly across moderate expanses of open water, some species are behaviorally resistant to crossing even small expanses of uninhabitable land or water. Yet given the vastness of time and the numerous accidents and contingencies that occur, even the most remote islands assemble communities surprisingly rich in species, including relatively poorly dispersing species. A classic case is Krakatau, an Indian Ocean island completely sterilized by a volcanic explosion in 1883. In less than a century it had been recolonized by hundreds of plant, invertebrate, and vertebrate species. In addition to "volunteer" immigrants, the new arrivals included birds that had been blown off course by storms and invertebrate species, small mammals, reptiles, and amphibians that floated in on "rafts" of vegetative debris. As the island filled up, untold competitive, predator-prey, and parasite-host relationships unfolded as species sorted out their roles. Such a sorting out may include some populations being cut from the team, so to speak.

The presence in a habitat of the resources for a particular species' niche is no guarantee that the species will survive. The habitat area must also be large enough to ensure survival given the vicissitudes of abiotic and biotic circumstances over time. Usually, effective insurance against devastating chance events (such as storms or disease) requires that multiple populations exist, as a bet-hedging "strategy." Even long-established island or continental communities experience regular extinctions, especially in smaller islands or areas where bet-hedging opportunities are few. However, in stable ecosystems populations can be kept topped up over the long term with the ongoing arrival of new immigrants.

FIGURE 1.12   Population Equilibrium in Island Biogeography

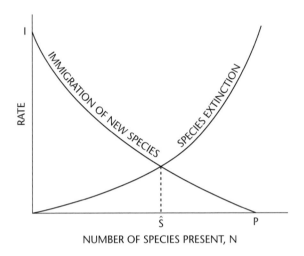

Source: MacArthur and Wilson, 1963.

This simplified chart of the immigration rate for new species and the extinction rate for established species illustrates that as the number of species present increases, immigration rates decline but extinction rates increase. The intersection defines the equilibrium species number.

Piecing these facts together led to one of most important ideas of modern ecological science, the **equilibrium theory** of island biogeography. This theory, developed by Robert MacArthur and E. O. Wilson (1967), points out that the number of species in an isolated place can be described in terms of the rates of immigration and extinction, as shown in Figure 1.12.

Moreover, this theory does not apply only to true islands; it applies to ecosystems in general, whether true islands or *habitat islands*, patches of a particular habitat within a larger landscape. For example, forest patches within grassland, cropland, or city are ecosystems that operate in accord with the island biogeography theory. So are patches of habitat that are cut off from other patches by highways or other human-made barriers. As land is fragmented, increasingly small and isolated fragments can become functional islands.

Disassembling Communities

An equilibrium number of species is maintained in a community only if the habitat remains intact and a pool of potential immigrants exists within dispersal distance. MacArthur and Wilson anticipated that neither of these conditions would exist for long, especially in a world where the loss of natural habitat has been accelerating. Later this line of research coalesced into the field of conservation biology (Soulé and Wilcox, 1980) and research into the wholesale collapse of communities due to habitat loss (through tropical deforestation, for example). The implications for genetic as well as species diversity and for the sustainability of ecosystems and ultimately the biosphere have focused scientists' attention on the idea of biological diversity and its relationship to health and well-being.

A key area of conservation biology research today remains investigating patterns and processes involved in the disassembly of communities. The breakdown of community relationships due to habitat loss or other stresses is not fully understood. However, some effects are clear (Laurance and Bierregaard, 1997). The species most vulnerable to habitat loss and degradation are those at high trophic levels, especially predators. Examples include mammals in the cat, dog, weasel, and mongoose families and birds that are raptors, such as hawks and eagles. As these species decline, the principal effect is reduced population control of prey species. As a result, prey species such as deer, antelope, pigs, and rodents often become more abundant. This loss of top-down control and often a corresponding hyperabundance of animal populations at lower trophic levels results in a number of consequences for ecosystem functioning, with particular implications for human health. With predation reduced, primary consumers overgraze available vegetation and create imbalances within ecosystems that undermine the normal regulation of pathogens and disease. For example, when herbivore species overgraze or otherwise disturb vegetation cover, they may cause soil erosion and disrupt the normal capture and filtration of materials contained in runoff. These materials enter streams and rivers and, ultimately, lakes, reservoirs, and coastal waterways. This can result in chronic as well as acute episodes of non-point-source releases of toxins and pathogens into drinking water and recreational waters. Thus pollution of the environment by toxins, pathogens, and excess nutrients can result from loss of the filtering, recycling, and digestion ecosystem services provided by vegetation and healthy community relationships.

A second consequence of disturbances to ecosystem community equilibrium is enhanced pathogen transmission. Species are more prone to become pathogen reservoirs when they exceed critical threshold population densities and may be more likely to have contact with humans and spread disease when they are hyperabundant. Lyme disease is a prime example (as described in the accompanying Perspective).

PERSPECTIVE
Landscape Change and Lyme Disease

Lyme disease in North America is a classic case of ecological changes playing a primary role in the emergence of an infectious disease and of habitat alteration affecting a pathogen's transmission cycle (Ostfeld, Keesing, Schauber, and Schmidt, 2002). Lyme disease is caused by pathogenic bacteria (of the genus *Borrelia*), which are transmitted to humans and other mammals by a tick vector. Causing fever, rashes, and fatigue, as well as more serious joint, heart, and nervous system damage when left untreated, Lyme disease is especially prevalent in the Northeastern region of the United States. In many parts of the Northeast, deforestation and suburban sprawl have produced a fragmented landscape, which in turn has caused incomplete assemblages of species at upper trophic levels and reduced predation. Combined with reduced habitat availability, this has led to abnormally high densities of prey species such as deer and rodents. At such high densities, deer and rodent populations function as more efficient reservoirs for Lyme disease bacteria. The white-footed mouse (*Peromyscus leucopus*) and white-tailed deer (*Odocoileus virginianus*) have become especially hyperabundant in the Northeast. In addition, as shown by ecologists Richard Ostfeld and Felicia Keesing, these species are highly competent pathogen hosts (meaning that they are especially capable of transmitting the infecting bacteria from themselves to a tick vector such as the common black-legged tick, *Ixodes scapularis*). Thus tick populations flourish with plentiful hosts upon which to feed, and Lyme disease bacteria flourish with plentiful host reservoirs and easy transmission from host to host via ticks. The result has been increased incidence of Lyme disease in humans, due ultimately to ecosystem community disassembly as a result of altered landscapes, along with an increase in human populations living near *edge habitats* (such as where forest and grassland meet).

THE ECOLOGY OF POPULATIONS

Population ecology is in many ways at the core of all ecological science. The ecological definition of a population is "a group of interbreeding individuals in a particular locality." The processes and mechanisms operating at the population level determine the abundance and distribution of species, which in turn define communities and ecosystems.

Ecological science has long been interested in precisely how population size changes, including the mathematical details of such life history parameters as

FIGURE 1.13 Human Population Growth Since Prehistoric Times

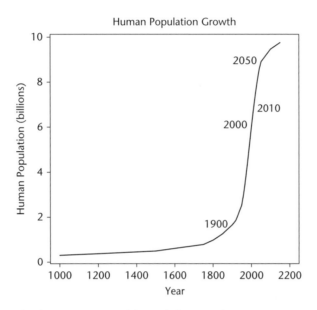

This is an example of a steep, exponential population growth curve.

birthrate, death rate, reproductive age, and longevity. In many cases it is not clear why the numbers of a particular organism are what they are at any given time. Yet this understanding is important not only for forest, wildlife, and fishery management but also for the control of organisms responsible for human disease as well as other pathogens and so-called pests injurious to livestock, crops, and food stocks.

The elemental population processes are births, deaths, immigration, and emigration. Thus the population ecologists' formally phrased question, What determines the abundance and distribution of a species? can be more simply stated as, How does the environment affect the elemental processes of birth, death, immigration, and emigration? Ultimately, the answer will explain why a species occurs in some places and not in others. This knowledge can be of critical public health importance when managing the abundance and distribution of both beneficial and harmful species. The latter include host and vector populations responsible for many reemerging and newly emerging infectious diseases.

The potential for a species to increase in numbers at an extremely rapid rate is perhaps best demonstrated by the Earth's swelling human population (Figure 1.13). This can be juxtaposed with examples of species undergoing catastrophic population declines, which have become near-daily news items. Historically, the American passenger pigeon (*Ectopistes migratorius*) and American bison (*Bison bison*) provide useful examples of species declines. Both numbered in the millions before being extinguished in the wild by habitat loss and hunting in the nineteenth century. Even in captivity the passenger pigeon never recovered, and the last individual died in a zoo. The remaining American bison live only as managed populations on national parks and some private lands. In the cases of humans, pigeons, and bison, the causes of their population changes are fairly evident. However, the population dynamics of most species, including the underlying mechanisms responsible for abundance or scarcity, are usually more subtle and complex. The basic properties of population growth and regulation described in the Perspective "Population Growth and Minimum Viable Populations" are a sampling of the most fundamental aspects of population ecology.

There is an important distinction between the role of other species and the role of the physical environment in a species' population regulation. These biotic and abiotic factors are associated with two different modes of population regulation: **density-independent regulation** and **density-dependent regulation**. Abiotic factors such as temperature, humidity, and rainfall operate independently of population size, whereas biotic factors such as competition, predation, and parasitism tend to have greater impact with greater population density.

Mosquitoes that act as disease vectors provide a useful example of these population ecology concepts in practice. In tropical and subtropical regions of the Americas, the geographic distributions of diseases such as dengue fever, yellow fever, and malaria largely follow the distributions of *Aedes* and *Anopheles* mosquitoes. Species of these genera are typically most abundant in wet tropical areas where there is plentiful rainfall, numerous natural or artificial water containers, and ideal temperature and humidity for these species. Such abiotic factors provide optimal conditions for mosquito growth and survival. In contrast, mosquito populations diminish, and sometimes disappear altogether, at higher altitudes and latitudes, where breeding, egg laying, and larval growth are limited by low temperatures, low humidity, and scant rainfall. However, even in places where the abiotic conditions are optimal, biotic factors can control mosquito population sizes. For example, both adult and larval mosquitoes are subject to competition, predation, and parasitism. Indeed, these biotic factors can play an important role in regulating mosquito numbers. Spraying of nonspecific pesticides intended for mosquito control can actually result in greater mosquito abundance by eliminating the natural predators, competitors, and parasites that keep a population in check. That is, pesticides can negatively disrupt the biotic factors that normally regulate the density of mosquito populations (Ellis and Wilcox, 2009).

Most species consist of many, more or less discrete local populations occupying areas of suitable habitat across a limited geographic range. The exceptions are large-bodied animals, especially land predators such as lions and bears and ocean predators such as sharks and swordfish, that are habitat generalists and whose individual home ranges encompass relatively large areas.

We often use the term population loosely to describe all the individuals of a species in a certain area. However, when the area of interest is large relative to the typical dispersal distance of an individual of the species in question, population is technically a misnomer. Ecologists often find that such "regional populations" actually consist of multiple local populations separated by gaps of habitat less suitable to their needs. The term **metapopulation** is better used to describe such a population structure.

Moreover, habitat patches tend to vary in terms of resource quality and quantity. The bigger and better a habitat patch in terms of resources, the more robust the population residing there. The more robust populations tend to "export" their excess individuals, and the less robust populations occupying the smaller and less productive patches tend to be the recipients of these dispersing individuals. The flow of immigrants from *source* patches may be the only reason a patch of marginal habitat even has a population, that is, the marginal habitat behaves as a *sink*. Source-sink dynamics are thought to be fundamental to understanding why particular species (including pest species) persist in some landscapes and not others (Hanski, 1991).

LANDSCAPES AND LAND USE CHANGE

A convenient way to grasp systemic changes that operate and link processes across scales—from ecosystem to populations—is through the perspective of landscape ecology. Studies in this area focus on the structure of the landscape, particularly on spatial patterns uncovered through remote sensing and geographic information systems. These patterns can be studied analytically, using quantitative methods to assess findings that are biologically meaningful (Turner and others, 1993).

The composition and arrangement of landscape features (such as natural and anthropogenic vegetation cover) and of human land use (such as urban, agricultural, watershed, and conservation uses) have a large and often unappreciated effect on human health and well-being. Examples range from altered landscapes that contribute to environmental disasters such as Hurricane Katrina to landscape features that influence the environmental mobility and fate of toxins and pathogens. In fact the resurgence of existing infectious diseases and the emergence of new ones can largely be attributed to the transformation of landscapes on a global scale (Patz and others, 2004).

PERSPECTIVE
Population Growth and Minimum Viable Populations

The study of population ecology began in earnest in the early nineteenth century, after Thomas Malthus published *An Essay on the Principle of Population* (1798), in which he focused attention on the problem of population regulation and the limits to population growth imposed by the environment. Malthus became famous for pointing out the "geometric tendency" of an accelerating human population increase and contrasting it to the more slowly growing and limited food supply. His ideas inspired several generations of scientists, whose work ultimately became the foundation of modern population ecology, and also encouraged scholars and popular authors to write about environmental carrying capacity. **Carrying capacity** is the population size that can be supported in a given area within the limits of available food, habitat, water, and other needed resources.

Later, the physicist Alfred Lotka (1925) used calculus to formalize the fundamental principles of population growth and regulation. In general, the size of a population can be expressed as

$$dN/dt = f(N)$$

which simply states that the rate of change in the number of individuals (N) over time (t) depends in some way on the number of individuals present. For an ideal population, this becomes

$$N = e^{rt}$$

which is the **exponential equation for population growth**, where r represents the unrestricted rate of increase per individual (birth rate minus death rate) and e is constant (2.72). Figures 1.13 and 1.14(a) show growth curves for populations increasing in size exponentially.

However, in the real world of resource limitations, population growth is eventually limited. For example, Malthus reasoned that food production could not increase exponentially and this meant eventual deprivation and even starvation for human populations that had increased exponentially. Population growth of organisms, including humans, is also potentially limited by many factors other than food. Lotka's exponential expression was therefore expanded to acknowledge these limiting factors by adding a second term:

$$dN/dt = rN[(K - N)/K]$$

or

$$N = K/(1 + e^{-rt.})$$

This is the logistic equation for population growth, where K represents carrying capacity. As shown in Figure 1.14(b), population size increases rapidly at first, but then

FIGURE 1.14   Exponential and Logistic Curves Describing
Population Growth

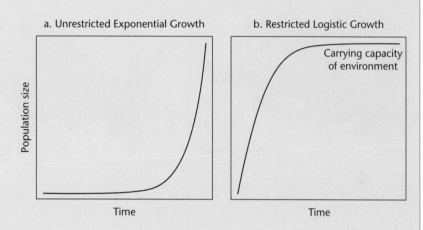

slows as it approaches the value of K, producing a sigmoid-shaped curve. This is
the simplest possible model of density-dependent population regulation.

However, real populations rarely increase in size smoothly and then stay at
a particular level. Rather, because environmental conditions such as the abundance of food and other resources are never constant, population sizes fluctu-
ate around their environment's carrying capacity. These fluctuations result from
factors whose effects are independent of population size, such as weather and
catastrophic events.

A viable population is one that has the demographic and genetic profile necessary for that population to persist over time and in the face of chance events
and environmental change (Morris and Doak, 2002). The lower limits of a viable
population can be viewed as a threshold line, something like the K of the logistic
curve, except that it operates in the opposite way: instead of being elastically
pulled below a threshold K where it regains a positive rate of change, a population
that dips below its viability threshold continues in a downward spiral. For example,
a population might be initially reduced by overharvesting or habitat destruction.
Once this population falls below its threshold, factors such as chance events in the
lives of individuals and loss of genetic variability, and thus of capacity to adapt to
environmental changes, abruptly reduce the probability that the population will
persist for many generations. This threshold is highly species and situation specific.
However, for most vertebrate species it is believed to be on the order of several
hundred to over a thousand individuals. Population sizes of large-bodied wildlife
species in national parks and other protected areas are often smaller than this,
which does not bode well for their future.

FIGURE 1.15   Forest Fragmentation in the Upper Paraná
Region, 1900–2000

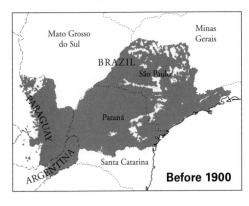

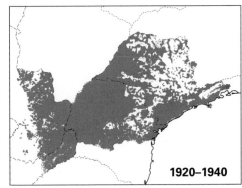

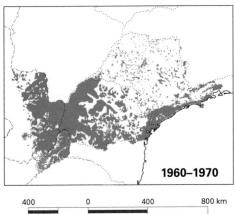

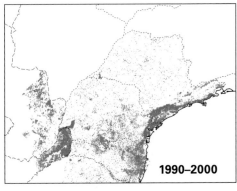

Forest cover data: Fundação S.O.S. Mata Atlântica (Brazil), Fundación Moisés Bertoni
(Paraguay), Dirección de Ordenamiento Territorial (Ministerio de Agricultura de Paraguay),
Carrera de Ingeniería Forestal de la Universidad Nacional de Asunción, Fundación Vida
Silvestre Argentina, and Bozzano & Weik 1992.

Source: Galindo-Leal and Camara, 2003.

Dark areas represent intact forest.

A concept associated with landscape ecology and having special relevance to
human health is **landscape heterogeneity.** In this context, *heterogeneity* refers
to irregular spatial patterning, including variability in the distribution of habitat
types. For example, natural landscapes tend to have greater heterogeneity than
agricultural landscapes, which often consist of relatively large areas with only

FIGURE 1.16 Factors That Interact and Culminate in the Emergence of Infectious Diseases

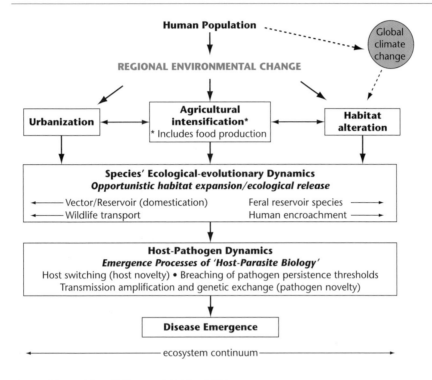

Source: Adapted from Wilcox and Gubler, 2005.

The initiating driver for disease emergence is human population, which has direct implications for regional environmental change. Regional change can be characterized according to a continuum of landscape types, from urban areas and agricultural land to more natural ecosystems that are nonetheless undergoing myriad habitat alterations. The level of regional environmental change then affects the ecological and evolutionary dynamics among species in varying ways and degrees. For example, biological vectors that are reservoirs for pathogens may become domesticated, or opportunistic wildlife (such as rodents or blood-feeding insects) may invade domestic areas. Conversely, feral reservoir species, such as cats, mice, or pigs, may invade natural habitats, disrupting ecosystem equilibrium and services. In either case, human encroachment facilitates contact with pathogens and their vector reservoirs and drives additional environmental change and disruption of ecological dynamics. As ecological dynamics are modified, so too are host-pathogen dynamics, promoting disease emergence. For example, pathogens have more frequent opportunities to switch hosts (for example, from pigs to humans), are transmitted more frequently between vectors and hosts, and benefit from greater densities via increased genetic diversity and capacity to evolve more virulent strains.

one kind of land cover (one particular crop). In general, heterogeneity tends to constrain ecological processes involving energy and material flows, including population growth and organism dispersal. For example, pest outbreaks that would be spatially limited in a heterogeneous landscape, can readily spread and may even become catastrophic in a homogeneous landscape of agricultural monoculture.

How the landscape patterns of natural vegetation, especially forests, change with the expansion of human land uses across a region has become an important area of applied ecological research that meshes with community ecology. As discussed earlier, the landscape perspective is especially valuable in understanding how land use patterns, including human-created fragmented forests, affect infectious disease epidemiology. With urbanization, suburban sprawl, and

PERSPECTIVE
Ecology and Emerging Infectious Diseases

The resurgence (or reemergence) of "old" infectious diseases and the emergence of new ones, together referred to as **emerging infectious diseases** (EIDs), represents one of the most significant environmental health challenges today. In 2002, an estimated 26 percent of deaths worldwide were attributable to infectious and parasitic diseases (Fauci, 2005), and 249 percent of the global burden of disease was caused by infectious diseases (World Health Organization, 2008).

Ecological science is increasingly being recognized as having a critically important role in EID research, intervention, and control. As Wilcox and Colwell (2005) point out, the vast majority of EIDs recognized by the World Health Organization and the U.S. Centers for Disease Control and Prevention are **zoonotic** (that is, transmitted from animals to humans). It follows that environmental factors play a key role in disease emergence. Host life cycles, pathogen transmission dynamics, and therefore disease incidence are all largely a function of ecological factors.

What is responsible for the current surge in EIDs? During the twentieth century we made great progress in the control and eradication of infectious diseases that had afflicted people throughout human history. New drugs, vaccines, insecticides, treatments, and control strategies reinforced public health programs already in place and provided the tools necessary to control many of the worst diseases, including smallpox, typhus, yellow fever, malaria, dengue fever, and others. By the late 1960s, the "war on infectious diseases" was declared expansion of cropland, the clearing of natural habitat, especially wetlands and forests, has been pervasive and dramatic in recent decades. The current scale and intensity of landscape change in the world's tropics, driven by a demand for land and resources fueled by human population growth and globalization, is historically unprecedented (Figure 1.15). The associated forest fragmentation is not only sharply reducing the total habitat area available to species but is also isolating the remnant habitat patches from one another. Such landscape patchiness can have profound negative consequences for biodiversity and human health (Laurance and Bierregaard, 1997). The ways in which urbanization, agricultural intensification, and habitat alteration interact to bring about ecological changes at genetic, population, and landscape levels, resulting in pathogen emergence, are illustrated in Figure 1.16 and discussed further in the accompanying Perspective.

won both by leading experts in the field and by the Surgeon General of the United States.

However, two sets of factors have contributed to a startling reversal of this situation, which began to appear just as the premature claims of victory were being made. These factors were a shift in attention and resources away from infectious disease prevention, and explosive human population growth. The human population explosion has resulted in environmental change in the form of uncontrolled and unplanned urbanization, intensification of agricultural production, deforestation, and biodiversity loss. Thus these two factors, along with the accelerated local, regional, and global movement of people, goods, and thus pathogens have been major and interrelated drivers of the reemergence of epidemic infectious diseases (Gubler, 1998; Wilcox and Gubler, 2005).

Old diseases that were once effectively controlled have reappeared or are now beginning to reappear in epidemic as well as endemic forms. These EIDs include dengue fever, Japanese encephalitis, West Nile virus, yellow fever, measles, plague, cholera, tuberculosis, leishmaniasis, and malaria. In addition, we are beginning to experience epidemics of numerous newly recognized diseases, such as HIV/AIDS, hemorrhagic fevers, diseases caused by hantaviruses and arenaviruses, avian influenza, Hendra and Nipah encephalitis, severe acute respiratory syndrome (SARS), Lyme disease, Chikungunya fever, and ehrlichiosis. In addition to the ecological factors mentioned previously, evolutionarily derived resistance of pathogens to antibiotics and of mosquitoes to insecticide is also playing a role in the emergence and reemergence of infectious diseases as a global public health problem (Gubler, 1998, 2001; Smolinski, Hamburg, and Lederberg, 2003).

In the larger environmental scheme, the ecological phenomena associated with habitat losses are only part of the environmental transformation that occurs as agricultural activity and urbanization expand and intensify. The hydrologic cycle and biochemical cycles are modified as well. Also, with intensified agriculture, industry, and other human activities come increasing waste streams containing gaseous pollutants and air pollution, solid waste, and toxic and hazardous wastes.

SUMMARY

Ecology is the study of interactions between organisms and their environment, including both the living (biotic) and nonliving (abiotic) components. Ecologists emphasize various interacting aspects of the environment, including ecosystems, communities, populations, and landscapes. Ecological changes of concern range from habitat destruction to disruptions of food supplies. These changes may in turn affect human health in many direct and indirect ways.

KEY TERMS

abiotic

adaptive management

adaptive renewal cycle

autotroph

bioaccumulation

biodiversity

biogeochemical cycle

biomagnification

biome

biosphere

biotic

carbon cycle

carrying capacity

community ecology

competitive exclusion
    principle

Darlington's rule

density-dependent
    regulation

density-independent
    regulation

ecology

ecosystem

ecosystem ecology

ecosystem functioning

ecosystem management

ecosystem services

emerging infectious
    diseases

energy flow

equilibrium theory

evolutionary biology

exponential equation for
    population growth

genetic diversity

geomorphology

habitat diversity

heterotroph

hydrologic cycle

landscape heterogeneity

logistic equation for population growth

material cycle

metapopulation

minimum viable
population

natural history

natural selection

niche

nitrogen cycle

nutrient cycle

persistent organic
pollutant

population

population ecology

primary consumer

primary producer

resilience theory

secondary consumer

social-ecological
systems perspective

species-area relationship

sustainability

total human ecosystem

trophic level

trophic structure

zoonotic

DISCUSSION QUESTIONS

1. Identify an ecosystem near where you live. What are its major features?

2. Identify an example of ecosystem management. What is the relevance of this effort to human health?

3. Thomas Malthus predicted that human population would grow exponentially, outstripping the ability of the world to feed itself and resulting in major famines. Was Malthus right or wrong? Why? What do you think the Earth's carrying capacity is for Homo sapiens, and why?

4. What are the ways in which large-scale agriculture might affect ecological factors and human health?

5. List at least three ecosystem services from which you have benefitted today. Do you think it is currently technically possible for humans to build infrastructure that can substitute for these services? Would the monetary cost be likely to be reasonable or prohibitive?

6. What are three infectious diseases with the potential for high incidence where you live? Are any of the infectious diseases in your area influenced by globalization? By landscape changes? By climate change?

7. The Gaia hypothesis proposes that, with all the world's myriad life forms closely integrated with each other and with the Earth's physical features, the Earth should be viewed as a single living organism. Please offer some arguments and examples both for and against this idea.

REFERENCES

Begon, M., Harper, J. L., and Townsend, C. R. (eds). *Ecology: Individuals, Populations, and Communities.* (4th ed.). Oxford, U.K.: Blackwell Science, 2008.

Bennett, J. W. *Human Ecology as Human Behavior.* New Brunswick, N.J.: Transaction, 1993.

Berkes. F., Colding. J., and Folke, C. (eds.). *Navigating Social-Ecological Systems: Building Resilience for Complexity and Change.* Cambridge, U.K. New York: Cambridge University Press, 2003.

Boesch, D. F. "Measuring the Health of the Chesapeake Bay: Toward Integration and Prediction." *Environmental Research, Section A,* 2000, *82,* 134–142.

Bronfenbrenner, U. *The Ecology of Human Development: Experiments by Nature and Design.* Cambridge, Mass.: Harvard University Press, 1979.

Carpenter, R. A. "*The Case for Continuous Monitoring and Adaptive Management Under NEPA.*" In R. Clark and L. W. Canter (eds.), *Environmental Policy and NEPA: Past, Present, and Future* (pp. 163–174). Boca Raton, Fla.: St. Lucie Press, 1997.

Chivian, E., and Bernstein, A. (eds.). *Sustaining Life: How Human Health Depends on Biodiversity.* New York: Oxford University Press, 2008.

Daily, G. C., and others. "The Value of Nature and the Nature of Value." *Science,* 2003, *289*(5478), 395–396.

Darlington, P. J. *Zoogeography: the Geographical Distribution of Animals.* New York: John Wiley, 1957.

Di Bitetti, M. S., Placci, G. Y., and Dietz, L. A. *A Biodiversity Vision for the Upper Paraná Atlantic Forest Ecoregion: Designing a Biodiversity Conservation Landscape and Setting Priorities for Conservation Action.* Washington, D.C.: World Wildlife Fund, 2003.

Ellis, B., and Wilcox, B. A. "The Ecological Dimensions of Vector-Borne Disease Research and Control." *Cadernos de Saúde Pública/Reports in Public Health,* 2009, *25*(suppl. 1), S155–S167.

Fauci, A. S. "Emerging and Reemerging Infectious Diseases: The Perpetual Challenge." *Academic Medicine,* 2005, *80*(12), 1079–1085.

Folke, C. S., and others. "Regime Shifts, Resilience, and Biodiversity in Ecosystem Management." *Annual Review of Ecology, Evolution, and Systematics,* Dec. 2004, *35,* 557–581.

Galindo-Leal, C., and Camara, I. de G, Eds. *The Atlantic Forest of South America: Biodiversity Status, Threats, and Outlook. Conservation International.* Washington D.C.: Island Press, 2003.

Grifo, F., and Rosenthal, J. (eds.). *Biodiversity and Human Health.* Washington, D.C.: Island Press, 1997.

Gubler, D.J. "Resurgent Vector-Borne Diseases as a Global Health Problem." *Emerging Infectious Diseases,* 1998, *4*(3), 442–450.

Gubler, D. J. "Prevention and Control of Tropical Diseases in the 21st Century: Back to the Field." *American Journal of Tropical Medicine and Hygiene,* 2001, *65*(1), v–xi.

Gunderson, L. H., & Holling, C. S. (eds.). *Panarchy: Understanding Transformations in Human and Natural Systems.* Washington, D.C.: Island Press, 2002.

Gunderson, L. H., Holling, C. S., and Light, S. S. (eds.). *Barriers and Bridges to the Renewal of Ecosystems and Institutions.* New York: Columbia University Press, 1995.

Hanski, I. "Single-Species Metapopulation Dynamics: Concepts, Models and Observations." *Biological Journal of the Linnean Society,* 1991, *42,* 17–38.

Hennessey, T. M. "Governance and Adaptive Management for Estuarine Ecosystems: The Case of Chesapeake Bay." *Coastal Management,* 1994, *22,* 119–145.

Hershner, C., Havens, K., Bilkovic, D.M., and Wardrop. D.H. "Assessment of Chesapeake Bay Program Selection and Use of Indicators." *EcoHealth* 2007, *4*, 187–193.

Holling, C. S. (ed.). *Adaptive Environmental Assessment and Management.* Hoboken, N.J.: Wiley, 1978.

Holling, C. S. "*The Resilience of Terrestrial Ecosystems: Local Surprise and Global Change.*" In W. C. Clark and R. E. Munn (eds.), *Sustainable Development of the Biosphere* (pp. 292–397). New York: Cambridge University Press, 1986.

Keller, D. R., and Golley, F. B. (eds.). *The Philosophy of Ecology: From Science to Synthesis.* Athens:, GA: University of Georgia Press, 2000.

Last, J. M. *Public Health and Human Ecology.* Stamford, Conn.: Appleton & Lange, 1998.

Laurance, W. F., and Bierregaard, R. O. (eds.). *Tropical Forest Remnants: Ecology, Management, and Conservation of Fragmented Communities.* Chicago: University of Chicago Press, 1997.

Lotka, A. J. *Elements of Physical Biology.* Philadelphia: Lippincott Williams & Wilkins, 1925.

MacArthur, R.H. Population Ecology of Some Warblers of Northeastern Coniferous Forests." *Ecology*, 1958, *39*(4), 599–619.

MacArthur, R. H., and Wilson, E. O. "An Equilibrium Theory of Insular Zoogeography." *Evolution*, 1963, *17*(4), 373–387.

MacArthur, R. H., and Wilson, E. O. *The Theory of Island Biogeography.* Princeton, N.J.: Princeton University Press, 1967.

Millennium Ecosystem Assessment. *Ecosystems and Human Well-Being: Synthesis Report.* Washington, D.C.: Island Press, 2005.

Morris, W. F., and Doak, D. F. *Quantitative Conservation Biology: Theory and Practice of Population Viability Analysis.* Sunderland, Mass.: Sinauer Associates, 2002.

Natural Resources Conservation Service. "Major Biomes Map." http://soils.usda.gov/use/worldsoils/mapindex/biomes.html, Sept. 2003.

Nevah, Z., and Lieberman, S. *Landscape Ecology: Theory and Application.* New York: Springer-Verlag, 1994.

Odum, E. P. *Fundamentals of Ecology.* Philadelphia: Saunders, 1971.

Odum, E. P. *Ecology and Our Endangered Life-Support Systems.* Sunderland, Mass.: Sinauer Associates, 1993.

Ostfeld, R. S., Keesing, F., Schauber, E.M., and Schmidt. K.A."*The Ecological Context of Infectious Disease: Diversity, Habitat Fragmentation, and Lyme Disease Risk in North America.*" In: A. Aguirre, R. S. Ostfeld, C. A. House, G. Tabor, and M. Pearl, eds. *Conservation Medicine: Ecological Health in Practice.* New York: Oxford University Press, 2002.

Park, R. E. *Human Communities: The City and Human Ecology.* New York: Free Press, 1952.

Patz, J. A., and others. "Unhealthy Landscapes: Policy Recommendations on Land Use Change and Infectious Disease Emergence." *Environmental Health Perspectives*, 2004, *112*(10), 1092–1098.

Rosenzweig, M. L. *Species Diversity in Space and Time.* New York: Cambridge University Press, 1995.

Smil, V. *The Earth's Biosphere: Evolution, Dynamics, and Change.* Cambridge, Mass.: MIT Press, 2002.

Smolinski, M. S., Hamburg, M. A., and Lederberg, J. (eds.). *Microbial Threats to Health: Emergence, Detection, and Response.* Washington, D.C.: National Academies Press, 2003.

Soulé, M. E. and Wilcox, B. A. *Conservation Biology: An Evolutionary-Ecological Perspective.* Sunderland, MA: Sinauer, 1980.

Turner, B. L., and others (eds.). *The Earth as Transformed by Human Action: Global and Regional Changes in the Biosphere over the Past 300 Years.* New York: Cambridge University Press, 1993.

Walters, C. J. *Adaptive Management of Renewable Resources.* New York: Macmillan, 1986.

Wilcox, B. A., and Colwell, R. R. "Emerging and Reemerging Infectious Diseases: Biocomplexity as an Interdisciplinary Paradigm." *EcoHealth*, 2005, *2*(4), 244–257.

Wilcox, B. A., and Gubler, D. J. "Disease Ecology and the Global Emergence of Zoonotic Pathogens." *Environmental Health and Preventive Medicine*, 2005, *10*(5), 263–272.

World Health Organization. *The Global Burden of Disease: 2004 Update. Geneva: WHO, 2008. http://www. who.int/healthinfo/global_burden_disease/2004_report_update/en/index.html.*

FOR FURTHER INFORMATION

Books

Several major textbooks provide excellent introductions to ecology. They vary in the extent to which they address human health issues.

Begon, M., Townsend, C. A., and Harper, J. L. *Ecology: From Individuals to Ecosystems.* (4th ed.) Malden: Mass.: Wiley-Blackwell, 2006.

Krebs, C. J. *Ecology: The Experimental Analysis of Distribution and Abundance.* (6th ed.) San Francisco: Pearson Benjamin Cummings, 2008.

Odum, E., Brewer, R., and Barrett, G. W. *Fundamentals of Ecology.* (5th ed.) Philadelphia: Saunders, 2004.

Also useful and interesting are books that focus on philosophical and policy issues related to ecology.

Collinge, S. K., and Ray, C. (eds.). *Disease Ecology: Community Structure and Pathogen Dynamics*. New York: Oxford University Press, 2006.

Keller, D. R., and Golley, F. B. (eds.). *The Philosophy of Ecology: From Science to Synthesis*. Athens: University of Georgia Press. 2000.

Levin, S. A. *Fragile Dominion: Complexity and the Commons*. New York: Basic Books, 2000. Several texts books address the links between ecology and human health.

Mayer, K. H., and Pizer, H. F. (eds.). *Social Ecology of Infectious Diseases*. San Diego, Calif.: Academic Press, 2007.

McMichael, T. *Human Frontiers, Environments and Disease*. New York: Cambridge University Press, 2001.

Reports and Programs

Millennium Ecosystem Assessment, http://www.millenniumassessment.org. This important effort, which was called for by United Nations Secretary-General Kofi Annan in 2000, is assessing the consequences of ecosystem change for human well-being and the scientific basis for action needed to enhance the conservation and sustainable use of specific ecosystems and their contribution to human well-being. The findings to date, downloadable from the organization's Web site, consist of five technical volumes and six synthesis reports, providing a scientific appraisal of conditions and trends in the world's ecosystems and the services they provide (such as clean water, food, forest products, flood control, and natural resources) and the options to restore, conserve, or enhance the sustainable use of ecosystems.

Toxic Substances Hydrology Program, http://toxics.usgs.gov/index.html. Toxic Substances Hydrology Program A U.S. Geological Survey program that provides scientific information on chemical contamination of ecosystems. Publications and other information can be downloaded from the program Web site.

Organizations

Ecological Society of America, http://www.esa.org. The major professional organization of ecologists in the United States.

International Association for Ecology and Health, http://www.ecohealth.net. A smaller professional organization that focuses directly on links between ecology and health.

CHAPTER TWO

TOXICOLOGY

Jason R. Richardson

Gary W. Miller

KEY CONCEPTS

- Toxicology is an interdisciplinary field that studies the adverse effects of chemicals on biological systems.

- All substances have the potential to be toxic, so it is important to determine which compounds pose the most likely human exposures, are most potent, and are most likely to harm human health.

- Route of exposure is an important determinant of toxic outcomes.

- The structure of a chemical can provide clues as to its relative level of toxicity and selectivity.

- Through the process of metabolism, chemicals can be modified to forms that are either more or less toxic than the parent chemical.

- Basic toxicology testing is critical to proper risk assessment.

TOXICOLOGY (from the Greek *toxinos*, meaning "poison") is the study of the adverse effects of chemicals on biological systems. These adverse effects can range from mild skin irritation to liver damage, birth defects, and even death. Both natural and man-made chemicals are studied. The breadth of topics in toxicology requires the field to take an interdisciplinary approach, borrowing techniques and methods from numerous scientific fields (Figure 2.1). The term *biological system* can be broadly defined, and so a toxicologist might study the effects of pesticides on insect physiology, of herbicides on plant development, of antibiotics on bacterial growth, or of pollution on an entire ecosystem (the latter has evolved into a separate discipline termed **ecotoxicology**; see Walker, Hopkin, and Sibly, 2006). However, most work in the field of toxicology is focused on the adverse effects of chemicals on human health. This chapter examines these adverse effects with an emphasis on the impact of environmental agents on human health, such as the deleterious effects of reactive gases on pulmonary function, environmental estrogens on reproductive function, and pesticides on neuronal function.

Typically, a toxicologist has earned a PhD degree in toxicology or a related field (such as biochemistry, pharmacology, or environmental health) and has received additional training in laboratory science during postdoctoral fellowships. Toxicologists are employed in academia, industry, and government positions. Academic toxicologists perform basic research on the adverse effects of chemicals, train the next generation of toxicologists, and teach toxicology to public health, medical, pharmacy, and veterinary students. Toxicologists in pharmaceutical companies seek to identify adverse effects of new drugs before these drugs move into clinical trials, and they may suggest ways these drugs can be modified to minimize toxicity. A toxicologist at an agricultural company may work to develop safer and more effective pesticides. On the government side, toxicologists at the Food and Drug Administration, the Environmental Protection Agency, and the Centers for Disease Control and Prevention ensure that companies are following federal regulations, determine the relative safety of drugs or chemicals, provide resources to the general public regarding toxic exposures, and advise the government on policy decisions regarding industrial products. Indeed, the subdiscipline of regulatory toxicology has been developed to address specific issues involved in decision making by governmental agencies, but it is grounded in the basic foundations of the discipline of toxicology described in the following pages.

Jason R. Richardson declares no competing financial interests. Gary W. Miller declares receiving grants from the National Institutes of Health, Omeros, Inc., and Neuronova, Inc. In addition, he has served as a consultant and expert witness for several legal cases involving toxicology issues.

FIGURE 2.1   Interdisciplinary Nature of Toxicology

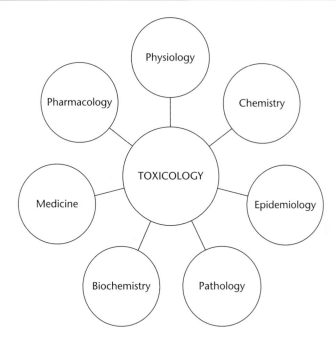

Toxicology borrows from several disciplines to characterize the adverse effects of chemicals.

A basic tenet of toxicology is that all substances have the potential to be toxic. Paracelsus, the father of toxicology, was the first to articulate this concept. Although poisons such as strychnine, cyanide, or nerve gas come readily to mind, every compound can cause toxicity. Of course all compounds are not equally toxic; some have effects at minuscule doses and others require very high doses. For example, table salt (sodium chloride) used in moderation is fine in the human diet, but consuming half a cup of salt a day would eventually cause significant electrolyte and kidney problems and possibly death (Exhibit 2.1). Conversely, ingestion of even a small amount of potassium cyanide (one gram) can kill a human. It is the job of the toxicologist to determine the relative toxicity of various compounds. This information, when combined with information about the potential benefits of a compound, aids regulatory bodies in deciding whether a

PERSPECTIVE
"The Dose Makes the Poison"—Paracelsus

Philippus Aureolus Theophrastus Bombastus von Hohenheim (1493–1541; his friends called him Paracelsus) was a respected physician of his day. He stated, *Alle Ding sind Gift und nichts ohn Gift; alein die Dosis macht daß ein Ding kein Gift ist* ("All things are poison and nothing is without poison; only the dose makes a thing not a poison"). This may be paraphrased as, all substances are toxic; the dose differentiates a remedy from a poison—or even more simply, the dose makes the poison.

EXHIBIT 2.1
LD$_{50}$ for Various Compounds

The **LD$_{50}$**, or lethal dose for 50 percent, is the dose of a chemical that kills 50 percent of those exposed to it in a defined time frame. A low LD$_{50}$ for a chemical indicates that compared to other compounds less of this chemical is needed to cause toxicity—that it is more potent, or in common terms, that it is more poisonous. Here, for example, are the LD$_{50}$s and the structures for several chemicals; LD$_{50}$s are expressed in terms of dose per kilogram of body weight.

Glyphosate (Roundup): 5,600 mg/kg

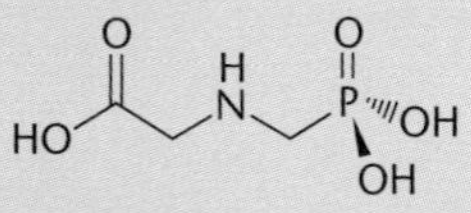

Table salt (sodium chloride): 2,400 mg/kg

NaCl

Pseudoephedrine: 660 mg/kg

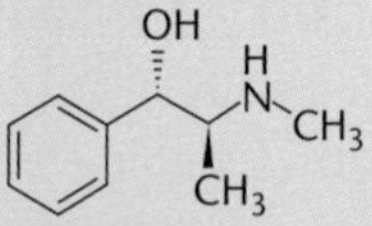

Acetaminophen (Tylenol): 500 mg/kg

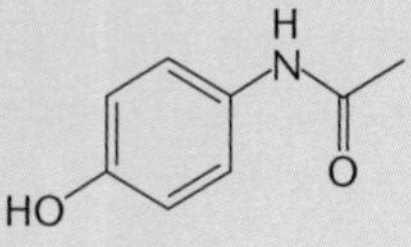

compound is acceptable for a particular use and what doses (for a medication) or exposures (for other chemicals) are permissible. For example, the general public (and regulatory agencies) would not tolerate a cold remedy that caused mild liver or kidney damage in 10 percent of users or a food additive that caused cancer in 1 in 1,000 consumers. However, if a new chemotherapeutic agent cured cancer in 80 percent of the cases, some mild liver or kidney damage might be found to be acceptable. Toxicology helps researchers to characterize the adverse effects that form part of the risk-benefit balance for a given chemical, and defining the **dose-response relationship** is perhaps the most critical aspect of this process.

Chlorpyrifos (Dursban): 118 mg/kg

Sodium cyanide:10 mg/kg

NaCN

VX nerve gas:1 mg/kg

Saxitoxin (shellfish toxin): 0.003 mg/kg

The dose-response relationship quantitatively describes the association between exposure to a compound and the toxic effects produced by that exposure. In order for a chemical to exert a toxic effect, the chemical or its active metabolite must reach the site in the body where it can exert its adverse actions, it must do so at a concentration sufficient to cause an effect, and it must persist at this site long enough to exert the effect. In order to assess the toxicity of a given chemical, we need to know not only about the toxic effects it produces but also how an individual might be exposed to the compound and how frequently that exposure occurs (exposure is examined further in Chapter Four). **Dermal exposure, ingestion**, and **inhalation** are the major routes by which humans can be exposed to chemicals, and the route of administration can have a significant effect on the toxicity of certain chemicals. For example, the pesticide **chlorpyrifos** is ten times more toxic via oral administration than dermal application.

Several issues must be considered when evaluating a dose-response relationship. First and foremost, it must be known that the response observed is due to the exposure to the compound. Second, the magnitude of the response should be a function of the dose administered. Finally, there should be a quantitative method for measuring the response (Eaton and Gilbert, 2007).

Decades ago many compounds could be detected only at relatively high concentrations, for example, in parts per million. Today's detection systems, such as gas and liquid chromatography, mass spectrometry, and atomic absorption spectrometry, are up to a million times more sensitive. As a result, dangerous chemicals are now often detected in environmental samples; however, they may be present at extremely low levels. It is essential to remember that the dose, and not the mere presence of a toxicant in a sample, makes the poison. If it takes a concentration of 10 parts per billion of a particular compound to cause any toxicity and if that compound is detected at 1 part per trillion, it is very unlikely to cause an effect. Thus one of the most important questions to ask is, How much of the compound is in the environment? As described in Chapter Four, this is the domain of an exposure assessment professional, often working in conjunction with a toxicologist or chemist.

TOXICOLOGY AND ENVIRONMENTAL PUBLIC HEALTH

Toxicology is an essential part of environmental health and of public health more generally. Public health professionals manage resources necessary to maintain health, prevent disease, and treat illnesses. A chemical or other environmental contaminant that harms humans at levels found in the environment raises obvious public health concern.

The field of toxicology helps determine the conditions under which a given compound may cause adverse effects, so it is important for public health professionals to understand key concepts that toxicologists use to make these determinations. Once exposure has occurred, through what routes does the compound enter the body? How much of the compound enters? Where in the body does it go? What does it do once it reaches a particular organ? What physiological effects follow, and if appropriate, what forms of treatment exist? How does the body handle the compound? Is it stored in particular organs, and is it metabolized and cleared? Armed with the scientific principles of toxicology, the public health professional can find answers to these questions and make prudent decisions on how to manage a particular exposure.

Toxicology is integrated into public health practice in several ways. For example, in providing safe drinking water to a community, it is important to understand both the adverse effects of organisms found in the water and the adverse effects of chemicals used to kill the organisms. As discussed in Chapter Fifteen, chlorination is an effective means of reducing microbiological contamination in water, but it can result in the presence of chlorinated organic compounds known as *disinfection by-products*. Toxicology can help in identifying these compounds, assessing the risk they pose, and balancing that risk against the risk of microbiological contaminants. Once again, the collaboration between professionals in related disciplines, risk assessment in this case, becomes critical in protecting the public.

Another reason that a student in any discipline, especially environmental health, should develop an appreciation for toxicology is that it is highly relevant to his or her own health. We are exposed to a myriad of chemicals every day. We ingest chemical residues in the food we eat, and we inhale particles in the air we breathe. Many people voluntarily ingest pharmaceutical and recreational drugs with little or no knowledge of the potential adverse effects. An understanding of toxicology can clarify some of these issues and help us make healthy choices. For example, a student who has a basic understanding of toxicology will realize that a claim that a product—whether a vitamin, an herbal supplement, an agricultural chemical, a medication, or an illegal drug—has no side effects is erroneous and misleading. Virtually no agent is completely free of adverse effects, given sufficient doses and circumstances. Similarly, a student who thinks in terms of toxicological action will realize that *natural* is not the same as *safe*. Nature produces some highly toxic compounds, such as arsenic, many snake venoms, and the carcinogenic toxins produced by some molds. Many psychogenic compounds are completely natural but can have dramatic and long-term adverse effects on brain chemistry. Natural is not necessarily safe.

TOXICANT CLASSIFICATIONS

Toxic compounds are categorized in three major ways: by chemical class, by source of exposure, and by effects on human health, or more specifically, on specific organ systems (Table 2.1). A knowledge of each category helps in understanding toxicology.

TABLE 2.1   Examples of Toxicants Classified in Three Ways

Chemical class	Alcohols
	Solvents
	Heavy metals
	Oxidants
	Acids
Source of exposure	Industrial wastes
	Agricultural chemicals
	Waterborne toxicants
	Air pollutants
	Food additives
Organ system affected	Kidney (nephrotoxins)
	Liver (hepatotoxins)
	Heart (cardiotoxins)
	Nervous system (neurotoxins)
	DNA (mutagens, carcinogens)

PERSPECTIVE
A Train Crash That Released Chlorine Gas

On January 6, 2005, a train hauling forty-two cars, three of which were tankers filled with chlorine gas, collided with a locomotive with two cars parked on a side track near a mill in Graniteville, South Carolina. The crash derailed sixteen cars, including the three chlorine tankers. Fortunately, only one of the chlorine tankers was damaged, but it sustained a four-inch hole in its side. A cloud of chlorine gas spread throughout the area, exposing hundreds of people in the following hours.

Chlorine is a yellow-greenish gas with intermediate water solubility. It can combine with water to form hydrochloric acid and hypochlorous acid:

$$Cl_2 + H_2O = HCl + HOCl$$

Thus, when chlorine gas is inhaled, it can react with the moisture in a person's eyes, mouth, and airways to form corrosive acids. The initial symptoms include irritation and pain of the conjunctivas (linings of the eyelids) and the mucosal linings of the nose, pharynx, larynx, trachea, and bronchi. The irritation of the airway mucosa leads to local edema (swelling). When the reaction is severe, pulmonary edema can occur, with the lungs filling with fluid, impairing breathing. This is precisely what was seen in the people exposed in Graniteville. Those exposed to low levels of the gas complained of eye and throat irritation, and those closer to the accident scene had significant breathing difficulties.

Fortunately, local and federal response teams had information on how to deal with a chlorine release. Much of our knowledge of the toxicological consequences of

Chemical Class

Examples of chemical classes are heavy metals, alcohols, and solvents. In essence the rules of chemistry create the classes, based on such features as functional groups, the presence of metallic elements, and physical properties, such as vapor pressure. Chemical classification may also address physical state, that is, whether a toxicant exists as a liquid, solid, gas, vapor, dust, or fume.

Source of Exposure

The second system of categorization is functional and is based on the source of exposure. Examples are industrial pollutants, waterborne toxicants, air pollutants, and pesticides. These categories are useful in identifying the source of a problem and are commonly used by environmental health professionals. However, chemicals used in similar ways may vary greatly in their mechanism of toxicity. Because this categorization system groups together chemicals with little chemistry in common, it can obscure connections based on molecular structure. To the toxicologist this system ignores the biological mechanisms that underlie toxicity.

chlorine gas has, sadly, come from dramatic human suffering. During World War I, at Ypres, the German army used chlorine gas (and a related chemical, phosgene) as a chemical weapon, killing over 40,000 soldiers. Chlorine gas is heavier than air, so it settled into the trenches. The soldiers trapped there died of massive pulmonary edema. Since then, there have been several industrial incidents in which storage tanks or railway tank cars have released significant quantities of chlorine gas.

The response in Graniteville had several components. A hazardous materials (or **HAZMAT**) team, wearing suitable protective equipment, was able to patch the leak before all the chlorine escaped. The exposed area was cleared, and chlorine levels were monitored until the gas had dissipated. Affected individuals were taken to medical facilities where they were clinically evaluated with physical examinations, chest X-rays, and pulmonary function testing, and were treated when necessary with such interventions as supplemental oxygen and bronchodilators. Clinical follow-up monitored them for the presence of persistent respiratory problems, including a condition called *reactive airways dysfunction syndrome*, which can follow acute irritant inhalation exposures.

From a historical perspective the incident at Graniteville stands out as one of the worst chlorine gas releases in the United States. Over 5,000 people were evacuated, 250 people were injured, and 9 people died. Those who were injured may continue to have breathing difficulties for years. The community of Graniteville was devastated by this incident, which resulted in the closing of the mill and the loss of many jobs in addition to the immediate injuries and deaths. This incident illustrates the acute toxicity of irritating inhaled materials and how this exposure may occur both in the workplace and in the general environment. It also illustrates the trade-offs inherent in environmental health; although chlorine gas is highly toxic, chlorine has an important, and arguably essential, public health role in water purification.

Organ System Affected

The third system of categorization looks at the organ system in which toxic effects are most pronounced (the **target organ**). For example, toxins that damage the liver are referred to as **hepatotoxins** and those that target the kidney are called **nephrotoxins**. Compounds that damage the nervous system, whether peripheral or central, are **neurotoxins**. Chemicals that disrupt DNA structure or function

PERSPECTIVE
Endocrine Disruptors

Over the past several years, toxicologists have been observing that chemicals in the environment may act in a manner analogous to that of endogenous hormones in wildlife and humans. Such chemicals are termed **endocrine disruptors** and can be defined as exogenous substances or mixtures that alter the function of the endocrine system and cause adverse health effects. Although this concept has received heightened attention in recent years, it is not new. Rachel Carson's book *Silent Spring*, published in 1962, is widely considered to have foreshadowed the current interest in endocrine disruption. Carson suggested that widespread and heavy use of the insecticide DDT was causing problems in bird reproduction, and that if not stopped DDT use would devastate bird populations and lead to a "silent spring." More recently, in *Our Stolen Future*, Colburn, Dumanoski, and Myers (1996) directly addressed the issue of endocrine disruption and asserted that environmental endocrine disruptors may threaten future generations.

The endocrine disrupters that have gained the most attention mimic endogenous estrogen; they are often termed *environmental estrogens* or *xenoestrogens* (Dickerson and Gore, 2007). Estrogen is the predominant female reproductive hormone. It exerts its physiological actions by binding to nuclear receptors and activating gene transcription in target tissues such as the breast, uterus, and brain. Environmental estrogens may disrupt normal estrogen function by binding to these same receptors and eliciting a similar, although usually smaller, response as the endogenous hormone or by blocking normal estrogen binding to these receptors. Chemicals that may act this way include the pesticide **DDT** and **polychlorinated biphenyls** (PCBs). Evidence of this phenomenon in the environment includes observations of feminized male fish downstream from pulp mills, associated with high concentrations of chlorophenolic compounds produced during the pulp bleaching process, and male feminization and reproductive failure among alligators in Lake Apopka, Florida, associated with elevated levels of DDT and its metabolite **DDE** following a pesticide spill. There is some evidence linking human trends such as menarche at younger ages and declining sperm counts with environmental estrogens, although this finding remains controversial.

In addition to man-made chemicals that may act as estrogen mimics, there are also naturally occurring estrogen mimics, such as the isoflavones that are synthesized by plants as a defense against pathogens and herbivores. Indeed, high levels of isoflavones in clover have been linked to the infertility in sheep termed clover disease. High levels are classed as **genetic toxicants, mutagens**, or **carcinogens**, depending on their specific effects. Other organ systems that can be the targets of toxicity include the respiratory system, cardiovascular system, skin, reproductive system, endocrine system, immune system, and blood. Fetal development is more a process than an organ system, but it too is often viewed as a target of toxic exposures.

of isoflavones have also been found in soy milk. Excretion of natural hormones, the use of estrogen-containing pharmaceuticals, and the use of veterinary medication may also contribute to the levels of estrogens in the environment.

Estrogens are not the only hormones whose action may be disrupted by environmental chemicals. The androgenic pathway has also been suggested to be a target for a variety of environmental toxicants, including phthalates, vinclozolin, and DDE. These chemicals may interfere with androgen-mediated events such as formation of the male genitalia during embryogenesis. Indeed, recent animal studies have demonstrated that in utero exposure to vinclozolin results in transgenerational toxicity to the testes (Anway, Cupp, Uzumcu, and Skinner, 2005).

The thyroid system is another major endocrine target of environmental toxicants. Various chemicals have been demonstrated to interfere with thyroid function, primarily in laboratory tests. For example, PCBs, polybrominated diphenyl ethers, and perchlorate have all been demonstrated to affect thyroid function. Because thyroid hormones are critical in neurodevelopment and metabolic control, there is increasing concern over the effects such chemicals might have on the human population and whether such exposures might contribute to cognitive dysfunction, decreased IQ, obesity, or diabetes (Tan and Zoeller, 2007). Here are the structures of six suspected endocrine-disrupting chemicals.

Isoflavone

Vinclozolin

Estradiol

DDE

PCB

PBDE

Organ system classification of toxicants is favored by most toxicologists. When working to protect human health, one needs to consider how a chemical will affect a particular physiological function, whether it be blood pressure, respiration, memory, or urine production. Because each of these functions is controlled by a particular organ system (or systems), organ system classification provides a logical framework for toxicologists; indeed toxicologists often specialize in the actions of compounds on a specific organ system. Also, even though compounds that affect a specific system may differ in their chemical composition, they often share the features that lead them to target that system. A public health professional should not be satisfied with knowing that a particular substance is toxic, but should ask, What does it do to the body? What system is it disrupting? What are the expected effects? The organ system approach is especially helpful in answering such questions.

To evaluate the toxic effects of a chemical on a particular organ system, one needs a general understanding of how that system works. For example, the main function of the kidneys is to maintain fluid and electrolyte homeostasis in the body. This is accomplished by the reabsorption of material filtered from the blood, including water, ions, and nutrients, and by the excretion of waste material. The kidneys receive a disproportionate amount of the body's blood flow, approximately 20 percent of cardiac output, considering that they represent less than 1 percent of the total body weight. This high blood flow, in combination with the numerous transport mechanisms within the kidney, renders the kidneys exquisitely sensitive to damage by blood-borne toxicants. Of all the cell types in the kidney, one of the most common targets of toxicant-induced injury is the proximal tubule. The renal proximal tubule is divided into three morphologically distinct segments, designated S1, S2, and S3. S1 is characterized by a thick brush border and high rates of metabolism and transport. S2 contains fewer mitochondria than S1 and has a less developed brush border. S3 contains sparse amounts of mitochondria and in most species the brush border is shorter than that of S2. The proximal tubule reabsorbs 99 percent of the glomerular filtrate. The numerous transport mechanisms in the proximal tubule allow reabsorption of amino acids, sugars, proteins, bicarbonate, sodium, potassium, chloride, phosphate, and other solutes. Damage to the proximal tubules by toxicant exposure can lead to deterioration of renal function and ultimately renal failure. Exposure to **mercury**, for example, is known to damage S3 segments of the proximal tubule. Enzymes involved in S3 brush border functions may slough off into the urine, providing a biomarker for this type of injury. A toxicologist interested in identifying how mercury alters renal function might isolate proximal tubules in the laboratory and perform toxicity tests on these isolated cellular sections. Another approach would be to study animals, evaluating renal function from urine clearance studies and post mortem examination.

TOXICANTS IN THE BODY

After a person is exposed to a **xenobiotic** (a chemical foreign to the body), a sequence of steps determines the response to the chemical: **absorption** into the body, **distribution** throughout the body, **metabolism**, and **excretion**. Along the way, toxic effects may occur. Understanding the risks of a chemical exposure and how to reduce these risks requires understanding **toxicokinetics**, that is, the processes in this toxicological sequence.

Absorption

Once a person has come in contact with a toxic compound, that compound may gain access to the body. It is not enough for this compound to contact the skin, be inhaled into the lungs, or enter the intestinal track; it must actually traverse the biological barrier. Each of these pathways exhibits characteristics that affect absorption.

The gastrointestinal system is designed for nutrient absorption, and it has a large surface area with numerous transport mechanisms. Many toxicants can take advantage of this system to enter the body. Toxicants can also be absorbed through the pulmonary alveoli. The alveoli are the functional units of the lung and the sites of gas exchange between the air and the blood supply. Alveoli allow diffusion of most water-soluble compounds. In addition, water-soluble compounds dissolve in the mucous lining of the airways and may be absorbed from there. Lipid-soluble (fat-soluble) gases can also cross into the bloodstream via the alveoli. Large particles and aerosol droplets of a toxicant may be deposited in the upper part of the lungs, where cilia attempt to excrete them. Smaller particles and aerosols penetrate more deeply, reaching the alveoli, where absorption is very efficient. The skin represents a third key route of toxicant exposure. Many occupational exposures occur via this route. Although intact skin offers an effective barrier against water-soluble toxicants, fat-soluble toxicants can readily penetrate the skin and enter the bloodstream.

Distribution

Once in the bloodstream a toxicant can be distributed throughout the body. If the toxicant is lipid soluble, it is often carried through the aqueous environment of the bloodstream in association with blood proteins, such as albumin. Toxicants generally follow the laws of diffusion, moving from areas of high concentration to areas of low concentration. Chemicals absorbed in the intestine are shunted to the liver through the portal vein, in a *first-pass* process, and may undergo metabolism promptly. A limited number of chemicals may be excreted unchanged into bile or by the kidneys into urine.

Metabolism

Once in the body most toxicants undergo metabolic conversion, or **biotransformation**, a process mediated by enzymes. The majority of biotransformation reactions occur in the liver, which is rich in metabolic enzymes. However, nearly all cells in the body have some capacity for metabolizing xenobiotics. In general, metabolic transformations lead to products that are more polar and less fat soluble. The metabolic product is therefore more soluble in urine, which facilitates its excretion. For example, benzene is oxidized to phenol, and glutathione combines with halogenated aromatics to form nontoxic and more polar mercapturic acid metabolites. However, metabolic transformations sometimes yield increasingly

PERSPECTIVE
Chemical Carcinogenesis

That cancer can result from chemical exposure has been known for over two centuries. Cancer is pathologically defined as uncontrolled cell growth, growth that reflects alterations in the cell's genome or gene expression (or both). Chemically induced carcinogenesis is thought to proceed in stages. The first stage, **initiation**, is associated with an irreversible change in cell genotype or phenotype. At this time the cell either moves to the next stage in the process or is destroyed, typically through programmed cell death (apoptosis). In the initiation stage the chemical carcinogen may act through a genotoxic mechanism and directly damage DNA. Alternatively, the carcinogen may alter signal transduction pathways, resulting in altered phenotype. Chemicals that act in this latter manner are termed **epigenetic**. The second stage, **promotion**, involves factors that facilitate cell growth and replication, such as dietary and hormonal factors. Promotion is not required for all chemical carcinogens, and unlike initiation, it is reversible. An example of a promoting agent is the hormone estrogen, which activates gene expression pathways in target organs such as the breast and thereby promotes tumor growth. Another example of a promoter is any chemical that inhibits the programmed cell death that would normally terminate an initiated cell. The third stage, **progression**, is irreversible and involves morphological alterations in the genomic structure and growth of altered cells. In the final stage, **metastasis**, the affected cell population spreads from its immediate microenvironment to invade other tissues.

Many of the known environmental chemical carcinogens must be bioactivated in order to exert their damaging effects. An example is **benzo[a]pyrene**, which must be toxic products. One example is the oxidation of methanol (a relatively nontoxic compound in its native form) to formaldehyde and formic acid (a compound that is quite toxic to the optic nerve and causes blindness).

The idea that metabolism may increase the toxicity of a compound is well established in the field of **carcinogenesis. Vinyl chloride**, known to cause liver and other tumors, is oxidized to a reactive epoxide intermediate, which is actually the proximate carcinogen. Similar transformations probably occur with **trichloroethylene**, vinylidene chloride, vinyl benzene, and chlorobutadiene. In fact a major mechanism of carcinogenicity in aromatic compounds is conversion to reactive epoxides, which in turn combine with cellular nucleophiles, like DNA and RNA.

converted to its epoxide metabolite in order to damage DNA, as displayed in the following graphic. Other chemical carcinogens include metals (such as **arsenic, chromium**, and **nickel**), minerals (such as **asbestos**), aliphatic compounds (such as **formaldehyde** and **vinyl chloride**), and aromatic compounds (such as coke oven emissions and naphthylamines).

Benzo(a)pyrene — CYP → Benzo(a)pyrene 7,8 epoxide — EH → Benzo(a)pyrene 7,8 diol — CYP → Benzo(a)pyrene 7,8 diol-9,10 epoxide

Although many chemicals have the potential to induce cancer, a number of defense mechanisms can mitigate cell damage. Many enzyme systems can detoxify reactive toxicants before they can interact with their target molecules. DNA repair mechanisms can often repair damage caused by toxicants. If DNA is not repaired, the cell may undergo programmed cell death before the altered DNA can be replicated. Finally, the immune system can seek out and destroy transformed cells that have escaped the other mechanisms of defense.

Traditionally, metabolic transformations are divided into four categories: **oxidation, reduction, hydrolysis**, and **conjugation**. Transformations in the first three of these reaction categories, known as **phase I reactions**, generally increase the polarity of substrates and can either increase or decrease toxicity by revealing functional sites. Many compounds undergo **bioactivation** at this stage. In conjugation, the only **phase II reaction**, polar groups are added to the products of phase I reactions. Most chemicals pass sequentially through these two phases, although some are directly conjugated. The spectrum of reactions of each type can be found in any toxicology text, and only a few examples, of environmental health interest, are presented here.

Oxidation is the most common biotransformation reaction. There are two general kinds of oxidation reactions: direct addition of oxygen to the carbon, nitrogen, sulfur, or other bond, and dehydrogenation. Most of these reactions are mediated by microsomal enzymes, although there are mitochondrial and cytoplasmic oxidases as well. Reduction is a much less common biotransformation than oxidation, but it does occur with substances whose redox (oxidation-reduction) potentials exceed that of the body. Conjugation involves combining a toxin with a normal body constituent. The result is generally a less toxic and more polar molecule, which can be more readily excreted. However, conjugation can be harmful if it occurs in excess and depletes the body of an essential constituent. Hydrolysis is a common reaction in a variety of biochemical pathways. Esters are hydrolyzed to acids and alcohols, and amides are hydrolyzed to acids and amines.

As mentioned earlier, various combinations of these reactions may be assembled in response to the same toxicant. Metabolic strategies for a particular toxin may vary widely among species, so an animal study, to be applicable to humans, should use a species with pathways similar to those of humans. The most prominent enzyme system for performing phase I reactions is the cytochrome 450 system, also known as the mixed-function oxygenase system. These enzymes are found in the endoplasmic reticulum of hepatocytes and other cells. In recent years advances in molecular biology have greatly expanded our understanding of **cytochrome P450**. Dozens of distinct P450 genes have been identified and sequenced. They have been grouped into eight distinct families, and for many, specific functions have been identified. For example, the enzyme CYP1A1 metabolically activates **polycyclic aromatic hydrocarbons (PAHs)**; the enzyme CYP2D6 is responsible for metabolizing such medications as beta-blockers, tricyclic antidepressants, and **debrisoquin**, an antihypertensive; and the enzyme CYP2E1 bioactivates **vinyl chloride, methylene chloride**, and **urethane**.

These insights in turn have helped explain why people may vary widely in their metabolic activity following similar exposures. Polymorphism in the genes that code for various P450 proteins has been shown to result in different metabolic phenotypes (see Chapter Six). For example, people whose CYP2D6 phenotype makes them poor metabolizers of debrisoquin are at risk of various adverse drug reactions, whereas extensive metabolizers are at increased risk of lung cancer, probably because of carcinogenic metabolites they produce.

Any enzyme system has a finite capacity. When a preferred pathway experiences **saturation**, the remaining substrate may be handled by alternative pathways (most substrates can be metabolized by more than one enzyme system). However, in some instances when a preferred metabolic pathway is saturated, the substrate may persist in the body and exert toxic effects. One form of enzyme saturation is **competitive inhibition**. This may be a mechanism of toxicity, as when organophosphate pesticides compete with acetylcholine for the binding sites on cholinesterase molecules, or when metals such as beryllium compete with magnesium and manganese for enzyme ligand binding. However, competitive inhibition is also important in metabolizing toxins. For example, methyl alcohol is oxidized by the enzyme alcohol dehydrogenase to the optic nerve toxin formaldehyde. This process can be blocked by large doses of ethanol, which competes for the binding sites of the enzyme and slows the formation of the toxic metabolite. The drug fomepizole acts in the same way, by selectively inhibiting **alcohol dehydrogenase**. This drug has been used to treat ethylene glycol poisoning, preventing the formation of the toxic metabolites glycolic acid and oxalic acid.

The enzyme systems that metabolize xenobiotics are not static. When the demand is high, their synthesis can be enhanced in a process called **enzyme induction**. The resulting increase in enzyme activity helps the organism respond to subsequent exposures not only to the original xenobiotic but to similar substances as well. DDT and methylcholanthrene are examples of substances known to induce metabolic enzymes. People vary in their capacity for biotransformation in several ways. Two areas of variation have already been mentioned: genetic factors and enzyme induction. Other factors that account for interindividual differences in metabolism are general health, nutritional status, and concurrent medications.

Excretion

Biotransformation tends to make compounds more polar and less fat soluble; the beneficial outcome of this process is that toxins can be more readily excreted from the body. The major route of excretion of toxins and their metabolites is through the kidneys. The kidneys handle toxins in the same way that they handle any serum solutes: passive glomerular filtration, passive tubular diffusion, and active tubular secretion. Smaller molecules can reach the tubules through passive glomerular filtration, because the glomerular capillary pores will allow molecules of up to about 70,000 daltons to pass through. However, this excludes substances bound to large serum proteins; these substances must undergo active tubular secretion to be excreted. The tubular secretory apparatus apparently has separate processes for organic anions and organic cations, and, as with any active transport system, these processes can be saturated and competitively blocked. Finally, passive tubular diffusion out of the serum probably occurs to some extent, especially for certain organic bases. Passive diffusion also occurs in the opposite direction, from the tubules to the serum. As in any of the membrane crossings discussed previously, lipid-soluble molecules are reabsorbed from the tubular lumen much more readily than are polar molecules and ions, which explains the practice of alkalinizing the urine to hasten the excretion of acids. The daily volume of filtrate produced is about 200 liters—five times the total body water—in a remarkably efficient and thorough filtration process.

A second major organ of excretion is the liver. The liver occupies a strategic position because the portal circulation promptly delivers compounds to it following gastrointestinal absorption. Furthermore, the generous perfusion of the liver and the discontinuous capillary structure within it facilitate its filtration of the blood. Thus excretion into the bile is potentially a rapid and efficient process. Biliary excretion is somewhat analogous to renal tubular secretion. There are specific transport systems for organic acids, organic bases, neutral compounds, and possibly metals. These are active transport systems with the ability to handle protein-bound molecules. Finally, reuptake of lipid-soluble substances can occur after secretion, in this case through the intestinal walls. Toxicants that are secreted with the bile enter the gastrointestinal tract and, unless reabsorbed, are secreted with the feces. Materials ingested orally and not absorbed and materials carried up the respiratory tree and swallowed are also passed with the feces. All of this may be supplemented by some passive diffusion through the walls of the gastrointestinal tract, although that is not a major mechanism of excretion.

Volatile gases and vapors are excreted primarily by the lungs. The process is one of passive diffusion, governed by the difference between plasma and alveolar vapor pressure. Volatiles that are highly fat soluble tend to persist in body reservoirs and take some time to migrate from adipose tissue to plasma to alveolar air. Less fat-soluble volatiles are exhaled fairly promptly, until the plasma level has decreased to that of ambient air. Interestingly, the alveoli and bronchi can sustain damage when a vapor such as gasoline is exhaled, even if the initial exposure occurred percutaneously or through ingestion.

Other routes of excretion, although of minor significance quantitatively, are important for a variety of reasons. Excretion into mother's milk obviously introduces a risk to the infant, and because milk is more acidic (pH 6.5) than serum, basic compounds are concentrated in milk. Moreover, owing to the high fat content of breast milk (3 to 5 percent), fat-soluble substances such as DDT can also be passed to the infant. Some toxins, especially metals, are excreted in sweat or laid down in growing hair, which may be of use in diagnosis. Finally, some materials are secreted in the saliva and may then pose a subsequent gastrointestinal exposure hazard.

Toxicokinetics

It is a useful exercise to track a potentially toxic compound from the environment (water, air, soil, food) into and then through the body all the way to its molecular site of action. This process is referred to as toxicokinetics. Suppose that a given compound is generated as a by-product of a particular industrial process. Whereas an exposure assessor measures the concentrations of the compound in the air and an epidemiologist studies the incidence of certain diseases in the surrounding community, the toxicologist is concerned with how the compound gets into the body and what it does once it is there. For example, the compound may be inhaled into the lungs. Once there, it rapidly crosses the alveolar membrane and enters the pulmonary circulation. It travels through the pulmonary vein to the left side of the heart and then circulates throughout the entire body. A large proportion of the compound goes to the liver, where it is activated into a reactive epoxide. This metabolite then finds its way to the kidney, where it is reabsorbed along with salts and other polar compounds and transported across the cellular membrane of the proximal tubule. There it accumulates and damages cellular macromolecules.

If the toxicologist can show that this compound damages the kidney and if the epidemiologist identifies an exposure-related increase in the incidence of renal failure in a population, regulatory steps may be taken to eliminate or limit the use of this compound. Toxicology can also be very useful in monitoring the development of new compounds. If a toxicologist shows that a new compound has an effect in rats or mice similar to the effect of a known toxicant, the new compound is likely to show the same toxicity in humans, so a manufacturer would be wise to discontinue development of that compound. Thus the understanding of mechanisms can lead to the development of safer chemicals and drugs. In fact, toxicology can inform developments in **Green Chemistry**, the design of chemical products and processes that reduce or eliminate the use or generation of hazardous substances.

TOXICOLOGICAL SPECIFICITY

Chemicals can exhibit an amazing level of **toxicological specificity**. A chemical that can be extremely toxic to one cell type or organ can be harmless to another. The most dramatic differences in specificity are found between species. **Glyphosate** (Roundup) is used to kill unwanted or nuisance vegetation (for example, grass in sidewalk cracks). This compound was specifically designed to inhibit 5-enolpyruvylshikimate-3-phosphate synthase, an enzyme involved in a biochemical pathway (the shikimate pathway) in the chloroplasts of higher plants, that produces aromatic amino acids. This pathway is essential for plant function, and when it is blocked, the plant dies. Animals, in contrast, rely on their diet for aromatic amino acids; they therefore do not have the molecular target of glyphosate and do not exhibit toxicity until extremely high exposures occur.

A different example is the piscicide **rotenone**, which is used to kill unwanted fish. Rotenone disrupts mitochondrial function by disabling complex I of the mitochondrial electron transfer chain (ETC). It exerts this action in humans just as it does in fish. Thus, unlike glyphosate, rotenone is not species specific. Species specificity therefore relates closely to the mechanism of toxic action.

Another kind of specificity is target organ specificity. Toxicants, whether endogenous or exogenous, are distributed to many cells and tissues but often cause toxicity in only a specific type of cell or organ. This may be due in part to greater accumulation of the toxicant in a particular cell type or organ. Some cells may be specifically affected owing to their genetic or biological makeup or the level of activity at which they function. For example, the heart and lung may be particularly vulnerable because they receive the largest blood volumes of all the organ systems. Conversely, the brain and testes may be protected from a number of toxicants because of the presence of the blood-brain and blood-testes barriers. However, the brain is extremely sensitive to toxicants that affect energy metabolism, due to its high requirement for ATP (adenosine triphosphate), the primary cellular energy source.

Some toxicants interact with targets that are shared by a number of cells, tissues, or organs. Good examples of this type of toxicant are compounds such as **carbon monoxide** and **cyanide**, which affect the cellular utilization of oxygen or the supply of high-energy compounds such as ATP. Because every cell and tissue requires oxygen and energy, these compounds have the ability to damage many cell and tissue types. However, the organ systems that require the most oxygen and energy are the most vulnerable to these toxicants. Thus the heart and brain are considered uniquely sensitive to the toxic effects of cyanide and carbon monoxide.

In contrast, some toxicants are more selective and are especially toxic for particular cell types or organ systems. For example, the herbicide **paraquat** specifically targets the lung via selective uptake by the diamine/polyamine transporter. Once in the lung, paraquat readily undergoes oxidation-reduction reactions, generating free radicals. This can result in lung fibrosis and ultimately in death because of reduced respiratory capacity. Exposure of humans to less than three grams of paraquat has been demonstrated to be lethal. Another example of this is the different toxicities observed with different forms of mercury. Organic mercury, typically **methylmercury**, readily crosses the blood-brain barrier and targets the central nervous system. However, inorganic mercury concentrates in the kidney and cause renal toxicity. This organ-specific toxicity is based on the physicochemical properties of the two forms of mercury. The organic mercury is **hydrophobic**, allowing it readily to cross into the lipid-rich brain, whereas inorganic mercury is **hydrophilic** and is filtered into the kidney, where it can concentrate and cause damage. Other toxicants are specifically designed to target a particular organ system, as is the case with insecticides. Most insecticides are designed to kill insects through hyperexcitation of the nervous system. For example, the oxon metabolites of **organophosphate** insecticides inhibit the enzyme acetylcholinesterase, with predictable physiological effects. Unfortunately, humans have the same acetylcholinesterase enzyme as insects, giving rise to the possibility of harm to humans.

All the previous examples have focused on acute toxicity, often at high doses. However, humans are more commonly exposed to low levels of toxicants for long periods of time, raising the possibility of chronic toxicity as opposed to acute toxicity. An example of chronic toxicity is the development of emphysema or lung cancer following years of cigarette smoking. In this situation the compounds contained in cigarette smoke do not cause an immediate acute toxic outcome. However, years of exposure to the compounds in cigarette smoke may overwhelm the protective defenses of the body and result in damage to the lung. Another example is the possible outcome of long-term exposure to the chemical **acrylamide**, which is often used as a waterproofing agent and to remove solids from water, as in sewage treatment plants. Acrylamide is a neurotoxicant that attacks the sensory and motor nerves, primarily in the extremities. It may cause damage following a single high exposure; however, it has been demonstrated in laboratory animals and in some occupationally exposed individuals that longer-term, lower-level exposures can result in similar damage. In 2002, considerable concern followed media reports of acrylamide in french fries. Some public health advocates have called for more stringent regulation of acrylamide levels in food (Becalski, Lau, Lewis, and Seaman, 2003). The Food and Drug Administration (FDA) is currently evaluating historical and ongoing studies to determine where there should be more stringent regulation.

PERSPECTIVE
Organophosphate Insecticides

Organophosphorus insecticides, commonly referred to as organophosphates, were first synthesized by Gerhardt Schrader, in Germany, prior to World War II. Although Schrader's interests were in the development of effective pesticides, the high toxicity and volatility of some of the early compounds led to their development by the German army as chemical warfare agents. After the war the interest in organophosphates as insecticides was renewed, and following the banning of organochlorine pesticides in the 1970s, organophosphates became the primary class of pesticides, with numerous uses in agricultural and household settings (see Chapter Seventeen). Recently, for example, the organophosphate insecticide **malathion** was used in New York City to combat mosquitoes thought to carry the West Nile virus.

Organophosphate insecticides exert their toxicity by inhibiting the enzyme acetylcholinesterase, which elevates levels of the neurotransmitter acetylcholine. This results in hyperstimulation of cholinergic receptors in the central and peripheral nervous system, leading to the characteristic signs of cholinergic poisoning: hypersecretion (including diarrhea and excess production of saliva, tears, and urine), constricted pupils, and spasm of the airways. With severe acute intoxication, organophosphates cause death through depression of the respiratory center of the brain and paralysis of the diaphragm.

In the body most organophosphates are converted to their oxon metabolites, the active compound. This conversion occurs primarily in the liver and is catalyzed by the cytochrome P450 family of enzymes. An example of this conversion, starting with the pesticide chlorpyrifos, is shown in Figure 2.2. Chlorpyrifos may be converted to the active oxon (chlorpyrifos-oxon), in a reaction termed desulfuration, a phase I reaction. Alternatively, a detoxication reaction called dearylation may occur giving rise to 3,5,6-trichloropyridinol and either diethyl phosphate or diethyl phosphorothioate. This is also a phase I reaction and demonstrates the molecular complexity of biotransformation in the body as it relates to exposure to toxic compounds.

The organophosphates provide a good example of trade-offs in environmental health. Many of them are highly toxic and have had their uses restricted. However, this

TESTING COMPOUNDS FOR TOXICITY

How does a toxicologist determine that one compound is more toxic than another? Several decades ago toxicologists used a rather crude method for determining the relative toxicity of compounds. By exposing laboratory animals to compounds and determining the dose that killed half the animals, they calculated the "lethal

FIGURE 2.2 Biotransformation Pathways of Chlorpyrifos

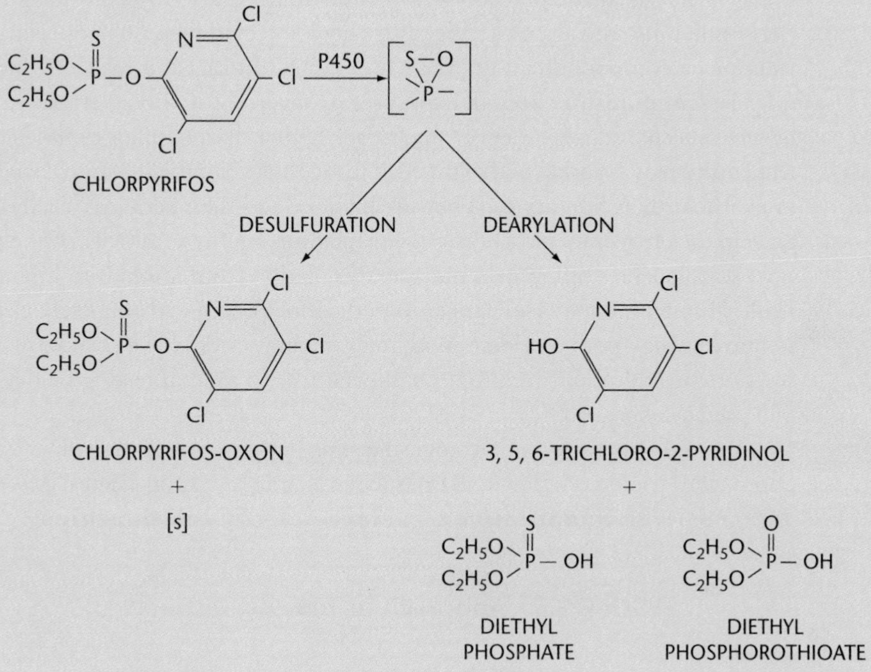

CHLORPYRIFOS

DESULFURATION

DEARYLATION

CHLORPYRIFOS-OXON

+

[s]

3, 5, 6-TRICHLORO-2-PYRIDINOL

+

DIETHYL PHOSPHATE

DIETHYL PHOSPHOROTHIOATE

class of pesticides has reduced insect-borne disease and insect-related crop losses over the past fifty years. Maximizing crop yield and safety and minimizing disease require a combination of toxicological knowledge and systems thinking, as described in Chapter Twenty-Six.

dose for 50 percent," or LD_{50}, an index that allowed comparisons among several unrelated compounds. Although crude, the LD_{50} has some important scientific strengths. The exposure is well defined (unlike the exposure in most human situations), the outcome is unambiguous, the measure can be applied across different compounds, and it can lead to a useful practical conclusion: if a compound is lethal at very low doses then human exposures should be prevented or strictly controlled.

Animal testing is also used to study chronic toxicities, such as cancers. In a typical study, animals are exposed to a suspected carcinogen at several dose levels. There is also a placebo group. The animals are observed for a defined period of time and then sacrificed to check for evidence of neoplasm. If, for example, a compound causes excess liver cancer in rats at a relatively low dose, it is prudent to restrict human exposures. Conversely, if rodent studies show no adverse effects at doses orders of magnitude higher than humans experience, then a chemical may be approved to proceed through development. Animal studies are not without their limitations. They use higher doses than people typically experience in the environment, a necessity for maximizing the sensitivity of the testing. Species-to-species differences make extrapolation from animals to humans difficult. Human life spans are longer than those of rodents, so long-term outcomes in humans may not be evident in animals. Finally, critics have pointed to animal welfare considerations, urging that alternatives to animal testing be developed and used (Meyer, 2003).

A tiered approach to toxicological testing has now emerged, with at least two approaches used alongside (and often before) animal testing (Figure 2.3). *Desktop analysis* relies on **quantitative structure-activity relationships** (QSARs);

FIGURE 2.3   Approach to Toxicity Testing

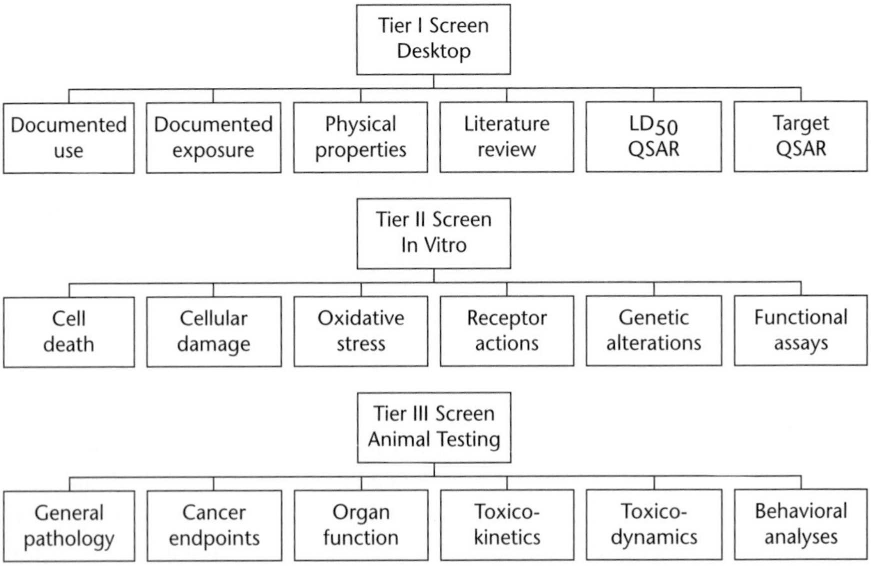

if the toxicologist notes that a particular chemical structure has a particular toxicity, then other chemicals with related structures are assessed for the potential to cause similar effects. **In vitro testing** involves exposure of cell systems, such as bacteria or cultured human cells, to a potential toxin. Cellular responses such as mutation are observed and help to predict human responses. Desktop and in vitro studies are less expensive and more rapid than animal testing, but the need to extrapolate to human responses, with all the assumptions required in that exercise, make them less definitive methods than animal testing and epidemiological studies. However, they are extensively used by pharmaceutical companies in screening libraries of compounds for potential therapeutic use. QSARs have also been used extensively in toxicology to ascertain molecular mechanisms of action and identify compounds most likely to cause potential health effects in living organisms. Another exciting development is the use of so called -omic technologies in toxicity testing. The advent of genomic, proteomic, and metabolomic tests provide an opportunity to examine genes, proteins, and metabolites on a global scale (see Chapter Six).

REGULATORY TOXICOLOGY

Toxicology can generate vast amounts of data on how chemicals affect human health, but in order to improve public health this information must be integrated into public policy. These issues fall into the domain of **regulatory toxicology**, which is closely aligned with the field of risk assessment (see Chapter Twenty-Nine for more information on how toxicological information is used in assessing risk). However, the basic principles of the dose-response relationship described earlier in the chapter are a critical part of the process. The shape of the dose-response curve has many important implications for the assessment of toxicity. One of the most important determinations that can be made from the shape of the dose-response curve is whether or not a **threshold** exists for the expression of toxicity. The threshold concept is built on the observation that for many chemicals there is a dose below which no toxicity is observed. Although the presence of a threshold is well established for a number of compounds, genotoxic carcinogens (those that directly damage DNA) are considered to exhibit a no-threshold phenomenon. Thus there is assumed to be no dose without risk.

Through evaluation of dose-response curves generated during animal testing, as described previously, several values can be determined that can be a basis for regulatory decisions. One of the most important values determined in such studies is the **no-observed adverse effect level**, or NOAEL. This is the highest dose administered for which no harmful effects are observed. The NOAEL is used by the Environmental Protection Agency in establishing the **reference dose (RfD)**, which is an estimate of the daily oral dose of a chemical that is likely to be without appreciable risk for an individual when taken over a lifetime. Several factors must be taken into account in calculating such a value; when used quantitatively these are termed **uncertainty factors**. The first uncertainty factor (Uf) reflects possible human-animal differences, and introduces a margin of safety to account for such interspecies differences. Second, there may be intraspecies differences in the response. Finally, other uncertainty factors may need to be incorporated. A good example is the recognition that sensitive subpopulations exist. Although this factor was thought to be addressed by the intraspecies uncertainty factor, recent data demonstrating the unique susceptibility of children have led to the inclusion of an additional safety factor for chemicals that may more disproportionately children. Thus an RfD would be derived as follows:

$$RfD \ (mg/kg/day) = \frac{NOAEL \ (mg/kg/day)}{Uf_{inter} \times Uf_{intra} \times Uf_{other}}$$

For the inter- and intraspecies difference, the Ufs are typically set at 10. So in general the NOAEL derived from animal studies would be divided by 100 to establish the RfD, if no other Ufs were deemed to be required.

More recently, toxicologists, risk assessors, and regulators have noted that the monotonic dose-response curve typically considered in risk assessment may not be correct for all chemicals. For example, essential nutrients such as vitamins exhibit a U-shaped dose-response curve. At very low levels of consumption, vitamin D deficiency causes toxic effects such as rickets. Once intake rises above the deficiency level, a region of homeostasis is achieved. However, vitamin D in excess of that level can result in kidney damage. Although this U-shaped curve was initially described for radiation effects and nutrients, there is emerging evidence that environmental toxicants may also exhibit similar dose-response relationships. This concept is termed **hormesis,** and is often attributed to a pattern of low-dose stimulation and high-dose inhibition, which produces the characteristic U- or J-shaped dose-response curve (Calabrese, 2005). An emerging literature on **bisphenol A**, an endocrine disruptor, suggests an inverted U-shaped dose-response curve, with effects at very low doses and fewer effects at high doses—implying that traditional risk assessment approaches may need to be reconsidered ((Weltje, vom Saal, and Oehlmann, 2005; vom Saal and Hughes, 2005). Although it is well established that toxicants can have very different effects depending on the dose, there is still significant debate over the interpretation that low doses may actually be beneficial. However, the biological mechanisms behind hormetic effects are not currently well established, which brings the concept of applying hormesis to the risk assessment process into question. This is currently an area of intense investigation by toxicologists and risk assessors (Holsapple and Wallace, 2008).

SUMMARY

Toxicology is the study of the adverse effects of chemicals on biological systems. Environmental and occupational toxicology is the study of how chemical exposures in the workplace, air, water, food, and other environmental media may threaten human health. Toxicologists think in terms of an exposure sequence, from exposure to absorption to distribution to metabolism to excretion, and analyze the end-effects on organs that may occur during this process. They are interested in identifying mechanisms of toxicity and levels of exposure that are safe or unsafe. This information is directly informative to regulators and others who work to identify the safest chemicals for our use and to set acceptable levels of exposure for chemicals that may be dangerous.

KEY TERMS

absorption
acetaminophen
acrylamide
alcohol dehydrogenase
animal testing
arsenic
asbestos
benzo[a]pyrene
bioactivation
biotransformation
bisphenol A
carbon monoxide
carcinogenesis
carcinogens

chlorine
chlorpyrifos
chromium
competitive inhibition
conjugation
cyanide
cytochrome P450
DDE
DDT
debrisoquin
dermal exposure
distribution
dose-response relationship
ecotoxicology

endocrine disruptors
enzyme induction
epigenetic
excretion
formaldehyde
genetic toxicants
glyphosate
Green Chemistry
HAZMAT
hepatotoxins
hormesis
hydrolysis
hydrophilic (polar, or
    water-soluble)

hydrophobic (nonpolar, or fat-soluble)

in vitro testing

ingestion

inhalation

initiation

LD_{50}

malathion

mercury

methylcholanthrene

methylene chloride

methylmercury

metabolism

metastasis

mutagens

nephrotoxins

neurotoxins

nickel

no-observed adverse effect level (NOAEL)

organophosphates

oxidation

paraquat

phase I reactions

phase II reactions

polychlorinated biphenyls

polycyclic aromatic hydrocarbons (PAH)

progression

promotion

pseudoephedrine

quantitative structure-activity relationships

reduction

reference dose (RfD)

regulatory toxicology

rotenone

saturation (of a metabolic pathway)

saxitoxin

target organ

threshold

toxicant

toxicokinetics

toxicological specificity

toxicology

trichloroethylene

uncertainty factors

urethane

vinyl chloride

VX

xenobiotic

DISCUSSION QUESTIONS

1. Toxicologists study both acute and chronic toxic effects. Acute effects are easier to study, and regulations have traditionally been based on acute toxicity, although in recent years more emphasis has been given to chronic outcomes. Why do you think the initial emphasis was on acute effects?

2. Why might you and your classmates have different responses to the same exposure to a chemical?

3. Pick a toxic effect that interests you, such as reproductive toxicity, endocrine disruption, or another effect. Look up the methods toxicologists use to test for this outcome, and describe these methods.

4. Compare and contrast the information that can be gleaned from a study of a particular chemical in animals and in isolated cells. Why do you think scientists continue to rely on animal studies when evaluating the adverse effects of a chemical?

5. People may be exposed to mercury in a number of forms. Two of the primary forms of concern—methylmercury and inorganic mercury—exert their toxicity on different organ systems (the nervous system and the kidneys, respectively). What factors do you think might contribute to this difference in target organ toxicity?

6. Aspects of human physiology as well as particle composition and size need to be considered when investigating the potential toxicological effects of airborne particulate matter. How do you think particulate matter size and composition could affect the amount of human exposure?

REFERENCES

Anway, M. D., Cupp, A. S., Uzumcu, M., and Skinner, M. K. "Epigenetic Transgenerational Actions of Endocrine Disruptors and Male Infertility." *Science*, 2005, *308*, 1466–1469.

Becalski, A., Lau, B. P., Lewis, D., and Seaman, S. W. "Acrylamide in Foods: Occurrence, Sources, and Modeling." *Journal of Agricultural and Food Chemistry*, 2003, *51*(3), 802–808.

Calabrese, E. J. "Toxicological Awakenings: The Rebirth of Hormesis as a Central Pillar of Toxicology." *Toxicology and Applied Pharmacology*, 2005, *204*, 1–8.

Carson, R. *Silent Spring*. Boston: Houghton Mifflin, 1962.

Colburn, T., Dumanoski, D., and Myers, J. P. *Our Stolen Future: Are We Threatening Our Fertility, Intelligence, and Survival?* New York: Dutton, 1996.

Dickerson, S. M., and Gore, A. C. "Estrogenic Environmental Endocrine-Disrupting Chemical Effects on Reproductive Neuroendocrine Function and Dysfunction Across the Life Cycle." *Reviews in Endocrine & Metabolic Disorders*, 2007, *8*(2), 143–159.

Eaton, D. L., and Gilbert, S. G. "*Principles of Toxicology*." In C. D. Klaasen (ed.), *Casarett and Doull's Toxicology: The Basic Science of Poisons*. New York: McGraw-Hill, 2007.

Holsapple, M. P., and Wallace, K. B. "Dose Response Considerations in Risk Assessment: A Recent Overview of ILSI Activities." *Toxicology Letters*, 2008, *180*, 85–92.

Meyer, O. "Testing and Assessment Strategies, Including Alternative and New Approaches." *Toxicology Letters*, 2003, *140–141*, 21–30.

Tan, S. W., and Zoeller, R. T. "Integrating Basic Research on Thyroid Hormone Action into Screening and Testing Programs for Endocrine Disruptors." *Critical Reviews in Toxicology*, 2007, *37*, 5–10.

vom Saal, F. S., and Hughes, C. "An Extensive New Literature Concerning Low-Dose Effects of Bisphenol A Shows the Need for a New Risk Assessment." *Environ. Health Perspect.*, 2005, *113*, 926-933.

Walker, C. H., Hopkin, S. P., and Sibly, R. M. *Principles of Ecotoxicology*. (3rd ed.) Boca Raton, Fla.: CRC Press, 2006.

Weltje, L., vom Saal, F. S., and Oehlmann, J. "Reproductive Stimulation by Low Doses of Xenoestrogens Contrasts with the View of Hormesis as an Adaptive Response." *Human and Experimental Toxicology*, 2005, *24*, 1–7.

FOR FURTHER INFORMATION

Books

Goldstein, B. D. "Toxicology and Risk Assessment in the Analysis and Management of Environmental
    Risk." In R. Detels, R. Beaglehole, M. A. Lansang, and M. Gulliford (eds.), *Oxford Textbook of
    Public Health.* (5th ed.) New York: Oxford University Press, 2008.
Klaasen, C. D. (ed.). *Casarett and Doull's Toxicology: The Basic Science of Poisons.* New York: McGraw-Hill,
    2007.

Organizations

Agency for Toxic Substances and Disease Registry (ATSDR), http://www.atsdr.cdc.gov. ATSDR
    maintains data on hazardous chemicals at http://www.atsdr.cdc.gov/toxfaq.html and http://
    www.atsdr.cdc.gov/toxpro2.html.
Center for Alternatives to Animal Testing (CAAT) at Johns Hopkins University, http://caat.jhsph.edu.

CHAPTER THREE

ENVIRONMENTAL AND OCCUPATIONAL EPIDEMIOLOGY

KYLE STEENLAND

CHRISTINE MOE

KEY CONCEPTS

- Epidemiology is the study of the distribution and determinants of health and disease in human populations.

- Environmental epidemiology and occupational epidemiology study the role of exposures in the general environment and in the workplace, respectively. The two employ many similar methods.

- In environmental and occupational health, epidemiological data complement other kinds of data, such as toxicological data.

- There are many kinds of epidemiological study designs. The optimal study design depends on features of the population being studied, the exposure of interest, the disease of interest, and other factors.

- The strongest epidemiological conclusions come from studies that use large populations, and accurate and precise measurements of exposure and disease.

- Epidemiologists work to achieve results that are free of bias (confounding, selection bias, and information bias).

- Epidemiological data are invaluable in risk assessment, standard-setting and other policymaking, and dispute resolution, in environmental and occupational health.

A PRIMER ON EPIDEMIOLOGY

Epidemiology is the study of the distribution and determinants of health and disease in human populations. Epidemiologists study exposures in relation to disease, to answer a simple but important question: whether a given exposure, or set of exposures, causes a certain disease. Obviously, if we can show that an exposure causes disease, we have a chance to intervene and prevent disease occurrence, which is our ultimate goal.

Epidemiology can give us the tools, the techniques of study design and analysis, to determine whether a given exposure is associated with a given disease. How do we judge that an association is causal (a process sometimes called **causal inference**)?

A general philosophical framework for judging causality, accepted by most epidemiologists, stems from the writings of the philosopher **Karl Popper** (for a good discussion, see Rothman and Greenland, 1998, pp. 16–28). This framework posits that observations (especially repeated observations) that one event (A) is followed by another (B) enable the epidemiologist to form a hypothesis, that is, a proposition that A causes B. The key to Popperian philosophy is that all hypotheses (or theories of causation) are tentative and may be disproved by further testing. Hypotheses that are tested many times and hold up tend to become accepted as scientific facts (for example, we accept that cigarettes cause lung cancer), but over the course of time many accepted hypotheses are overthrown by new scientific insights (we now know that miasma or foul air does not cause cholera).

On a practical level, a famous set of criteria set out by Austin Bradford Hill (1965) is commonly used by epidemiologists to judge whether a particular causal hypothesis is plausible, whether the observed association between A and B makes it likely that in fact A causes B. Hill set out nine criteria. Only one—the proper **temporal relationship**—is absolutely required: the exposure must precede the disease. Although it seems this should always be easy to know, sometimes it is not clear. Other commonly used Hill criteria that favor causality are **consistency** (the association is repeated in many studies), a large **effect size** (the exposed have much more disease than the nonexposed), a positive **dose-response** relationship (more exposure causes more disease), and **biological plausibility** (some biological explanation makes it reasonable that A causes B).

Regulators and risk assessors must conclude from the weight of the epidemiological evidence, applying criteria such as these, whether an association

Kyle Steenland and Christine L. Moe declare no competing financial interests.

is likely to be causal. A number of agencies, such as the International Agency for Research on Cancer (IARC), the National Toxicology Program (NTP), the Institute of Medicine (IOM, a part of the National Academy of Sciences), and the Environmental Protection Agency (EPA), regularly review epidemiological evidence and publish summaries in which they evaluate whether associations are likely to be causal. Epidemiology has provided evidence judged as causal that many environmental and occupational exposures are associated with diseases, including evidence associating lead with cognitive impairment in children, trihalomethanes (in water) with bladder cancer, particulate air pollution with cardiorespiratory disease, radon gas with cancer, and ergonomic stress with low back pain, to name just a few.

Kinds of Epidemiological Studies

Epidemiological studies can be divided into categories that reflect their design.

Descriptive Studies   At the simplest level there are descriptive studies, which characterize a disease by factors such as age, sex, time, and geographical region. These studies do not formally test a hypothesis that a specific exposure (or risk factor) is associated with a disease but rather describe patterns in disease occurrence in terms of broad demographic and other variables. These studies are often first steps and may provide clues about factors that cause disease. For example, the fact that malaria occurs mainly in tropical areas provides a clue that warm climate may play a role in its transmission. The fact that heart disease occurs at a later age in women than men may provide a clue that endogenous estrogen plays a protective role.

Correlational, or Ecological, Studies   Descriptive studies are a close cousin to **correlational studies**, or **ecological studies**, which study the correlation between disease rates and some specific exposure, but at the level of groups rather than individuals. For example, one can correlate breast cancer rates in countries around the world with degree of socioeconomic development; breast cancer incidence is higher in richer, more urbanized countries. Like descriptive studies, ecological studies often provide clues about possible risk factors for disease, factors that can then be examined further in studies of individuals. Generally, ecological studies are viewed as weaker than studies of individuals, because across a population, individuals with the risk factors are not necessarily the same individuals who contract the disease. As a result ecological studies are often called *hypothesis-generating studies*. However, in some instances an ecological design is the design of choice. One example is time series studies of air pollution, in which pollution levels are correlated with disease rates on a day-to-day basis. Such studies have the advantage of looking at a population that is presumably stable over time (eliminating most confounding). The only variables changing on a daily basis are the exposure variable of interest (air pollution levels) and the outcome of interest (daily disease rates), although seasonal variation in temperature also needs to be taken into account.

Etiologic, or Analytical, Studies   **Etiologic studies**, or **analytical studies,** are generally studies of individuals in which the investigators seek to test a specific hypothesis about exposure and disease, for example, whether pesticide exposure is associated with Parkinson's disease. These studies are often undertaken after descriptive and correlational studies have indicated that they are worth doing, that is, after a plausible hypothesis has emerged that needs to be tested.

Analytical studies can in turn be divided into two types, clinical trials and observational studies.

Clinical Trials. Clinical trials, usually called **randomized clinical trials**, are in a sense the model for rigorous epidemiological studies. They are often done to compare one medication or treatment to another. They are controlled experiments, because they assign treatment (or exposure) randomly to one group and not another. The treated and untreated groups are therefore likely to be comparable with regard to other variables (such age, weight, sex, and education) that might affect the disease outcome; therefore any difference in subsequent disease rates can be assumed to be due to exposure. Both treated and untreated groups are followed prospectively over time.

Randomized clinical trials are generally impractical for studying environmental and workplace exposures, because one cannot ethically administer a suspected toxin to a human population. Clinical trials are restricted to comparing a treatment suspected to be beneficial to a conventional treatment or to no treatment. Therefore, the epidemiologist interested in studying suspected occupational and environmental toxins needs to conduct observational studies. There is an important exception: for environmental toxins already known to cause disease, randomized intervention trials to measure the effect of lowering exposures can be conducted (Rogan and others, 2001).

Observational Studies. Observational studies are uncontrolled studies, or **natural experiments**, of which the epidemiologist takes advantage. For example, the epidemiologist wants to study the effect of lead on cancer, so he or she observes a cohort of lead-exposed workers over time and compares their cancer rates to those of the general population. However, the workers and the general population may differ in some important respects, such as smoking habits or diet, that may in turn affect cancer rates (such variables are called **confounders**). The epidemiologist may be able to adjust or control for the effects of such confounders, but if he or she cannot, these effects may distort the findings about the effect of exposure on disease. For this reason observational studies are viewed as less definitive than clinical trials. A famous recent example of different findings for clinical trials and for observational studies can be seen in the case of postmenopausal estrogen replacement therapy and the risk of heart disease (Whittemore and McGuire, 2003).

The three principal designs for observational studies are cohort, case-control, and cross-sectional. **Cohort studies** start with an exposed group and a nonexposed group, both disease free, and follow them forward in time to observe disease incidence or mortality rates. Disease rates in the exposed and nonexposed can be then compared using a **rate ratio** or a rate difference. The observation period in cohort studies may start in the past and move forward to the present (**retrospective studies**), or start in the present and move into the future (**prospective studies**). The former is quicker and usually cheaper: for example, to study lung cancer among welders and nonwelders one can identify a cohort as of 1950 and trace its members' lung cancer mortality until the present. The disadvantage of the retrospective approach is having to depend on historical information about exposure levels and about potential confounders (for example, smoking habits). Although prospective studies take a long time and are often expensive, they are more appropriate when one wants to measure exposure levels and confounding variables at baseline, or when biological samples such as blood tests are required. Prospective studies may also be needed to study diseases that are difficult to ascertain in retrospect, such as spontaneous abortions (whose occurrence and date of occurrence may be difficult to remember accurately). Cohort studies can consider disease events per person (**cumulative incidence**, or **risk**) or disease events per person-time (**rates**, such as **incidence** or **mortality**). The former are appropriate for short follow-up periods and *fixed* cohorts, in which everyone can be followed for the whole follow-up period. The latter are appropriate for long follow-up periods and *dynamic* cohorts, in which individuals may enter follow-up at different times and be lost to follow-up at any time and are therefore followed for different periods of time. Cohort studies are good for rare exposures and common diseases, because one begins with assembling an exposed group and hence can readily assemble an adequate number of exposed subjects (for example, welders); conversely, when the disease is rare, a very large number of subjects may need to be assembled to yield an appreciable number of cases.

Case-control studies use an opposite approach to that of cohort studies. Here, the epidemiologist begins with diseased and nondiseased groups and looks backward in time. For example, bladder cancer patients (*cases*) and people free of bladder cancer (*controls*) can be asked about their past consumption of water treated with chlorine, which results in trihalomethane formation (trihalomethanes are suspected bladder carcinogens). The investigator determines the odds of exposure in each group, and compares them—if a is the number exposed, and b is the number nonexposed, then $a/(a + b)$ is the proportion exposed, and a/b is the odds of exposure. If the odds of exposure are higher among the cases than among the controls, then one judges that the exposure is associated with the disease. The usual measure of effect is the **odds ratio**. Case-control studies are more subject to bias than cohort studies because it is sometimes difficult to choose cases and controls who are representative of the overall diseased and nondiseased populations (this is particularly true for the controls) and because it is often difficult to measure past exposure accurately. **Recall bias**, for example, can occur if cases tend to remember more about past exposures than controls. However, if cases and controls are chosen properly, a case-control study should give the same answer as would a cohort study about the exposure-disease relationship.

Case-control studies are useful for rare diseases and common exposures, the opposite of cohort studies. Case-control studies can be carried out in the general population or in hospitals or can be nested within cohorts.

Cross-sectional studies, or prevalence studies, tend to measure exposure and disease at the same time. For example, lead exposure in relation to performance on tests of intelligence in children may be studied by measuring lead in blood at the time of the neurological testing, or cadmium levels in the urine of smelter workers can be measured at the same time as small protein in the urine (a measure of kidney damage). Cross-sectional studies are often done when the outcome of interest is subclinical or asymptomatic disease. In the workplace, cross-sectional studies will miss symptomatic cases if workers with the disease have left work.

A typical problem of cross-sectional studies is determining whether exposure in fact preceded the health outcome. For example, in the case of the smelter workers, if those with higher levels of cadmium in the urine were also excreting more small protein, it would not be known whether the protein excretion preceded or followed the presence of cadmium in the urine. The same would be true for neurological tests in relation to lead levels in children. Interpretation of positive findings in the latter study would be made even more difficult by the fact that socioeconomic status (SES) is an important confounder that is difficult to control; children of low SES have higher lead exposure and perform worse on neuropsychological tests. Cross-sectional studies tend to be seen as a somewhat weaker design than cohort and case-control studies, although they are often the only possible design and can provide valid results, which can then be confirmed in cohort or case-control studies.

Bias

Bias refers to the distortion of the true relationship between exposure and disease. The most important sources of bias are selection bias, confounding, and information bias.

Selection bias occurs when the relationship between exposure and disease in the study population is not representative of the true relation between exposure and disease in the general population because the investigator has selected the study population in a nonrepresentative way. For example, in a study of ethylene oxide (a sterilant gas) and breast cancer, suppose only 20 percent of the individuals in the target population answer a questionnaire about breast cancer occurrence. These self-selected study participants may differ from the rest of the target population: for example, perhaps they have more breast cancer (motivating them to participate) and higher exposures (making them concerned that exposure may have caused their disease and again motivating participation). This would result in demonstrating an association between exposure and disease might not have been found if the entire target population had participated. This kind of bias cannot be corrected in the analysis. In fact one cannot even be sure of the direction of such a bias based on the 20 percent of the population studied, because the rate of occurrence of breast cancer in the remaining 80 percent of subjects cannot be known. The study conclusions will thus be suspect. The **healthy worker effect** is another kind of selection bias, occurring when workers are compared to the general population. Workers are healthier than the general population, so study results will be biased against finding adverse health effects among the workers. This is another example of a selection bias that cannot be readily fixed at the analysis stage.

Confounding refers to the distortion of the exposure-disease relationship by a third variable that is associated both with exposure and with disease. For example in the study of welders in relation to lung cancer, if the welders smoke more than nonwelders do, then smoking (strongly associated with lung cancer) would act as a confounder. Adjustment for the effect of smoking can be made during analysis by stratifying the groups into smokers and nonsmokers, determining the exposure-disease relationship in each group, and then forming a weighted average of the exposure-disease relationship across both groups. Adjustment can also be accomplished using one of several statistical approaches that involve **multivariate analysis**. However, this can be done only when adequate data on smoking have been collected in both exposed and nonexposed groups.

The welding-lung cancer relationship might also differ between smokers and nonsmokers: one could imagine, for example, that only smokers show a welding effect, because smoking injures the lung epithelium permitting a carcinogenic effect from the metal fumes. This situation is called **effect modification** because the third variable (smoking) modifies the effect of the exposure variable of interest (welding). Effect modification is different from confounding. In this circumstance the investigator cannot calculate the weighted average of exposure-disease associations across both strata of the third variable and instead must report results for each stratum separately. No adjustment for confounding is possible, as no weighted average of exposure effect across levels of the confounder should be conducted.

Finally, once the study population has been selected, **information bias** can occur when information obtained about either exposure or disease is incorrect. One of the main sources of information bias in epidemiological studies is **mismeasurement** or **misclassification** of exposure. When exposure is measured incorrectly (for a continuous exposure variable) or misclassified (for a categorical exposure variable), one can expect the exposure-disease association to be distorted. When exposure is measured or classified equally poorly for both diseased and non-diseased groups (called **nondifferential error** or **misclassification**), then the effect is usually to bias the finding toward the **null hypothesi**s (toward finding no exposure-disease association). Conversely, if the mismeasurement or misclassification is greater for either the diseased or the nondiseased, bias away from the null can occur. This problem is typical of retrospective exposure assessment in case-control studies, when cases may recall past exposures more often than controls do (recall bias), biasing the study toward finding an association (away from the null).

Data Analysis

Methods of analysis in epidemiology typically depend on whether the exposure variable and the disease variable are **continuous variables** or **categorical variables**. Most of the approaches described previously consider disease to be a categorical (yes/no) variable (often called a **dichotomous variable**). This is typically true of a specific disease: you either get the disease or you don't. However, many studies consider a continuous disease variable, such as blood pressure or the concentration of a small protein in the urine. In some instances these variables can be transformed into categorical variables (for example, high blood pressure might be defined as a systolic pressure greater than 140), especially when there are medical guidelines for such cutpoints. Exposure variables may also be continuous (for example, cadmium in the urine) or categorical (welder or nonwelder).

When both exposure and disease variables are dichotomous, then one usually calculates the measures referred to previously, such as a rate ratio or an odds ratio. These categorical analyses may be stratified to control for confounding, as indicated earlier. However, when both the disease and the exposure are **continuous variables**, typically a **regression analysis** is conducted (for example, linear regression), in which the outcome is disease and the predictors include exposure and any other confounder variables about which the investigator has data. One seeks to know if the exposure is a significant predictor of disease, as reflected by a regression coefficient for the exposure variable that differs significantly from the null value of zero.

In addition, mixtures of these situations can arise. A **linear regression** analysis for a continuous outcome may also be calculated with the exposure variable categorized in the regression. Furthermore, even when the disease variable is dichotomous, one can employ a type of regression called **logistic regression** in which the measure of interest remains the odds ratio and either categorical or continuous variables may be included among the predictors.

One important feature of any data analysis is the **precision** of the estimate of effect (for example, the rate ratio, the odds ratio, or the regression coefficient for the exposure variable). Large **sample sizes** confer greater **statistical power** to detect associations, and lead to high precision. Precision is often presented by a **confidence interval**, which represents a range of plausible values for the measure of effect. For example, an odds ratio in a case-control study of bladder cancer and water supply (public water versus private wells) might be 2.00, indicating that those who use public water (more trihalomethanes) versus private wells (fewer trihalomethanes) have a doubling of bladder cancer risk. If the study is based on 20 cases and 20 controls, it will have low precision and the 95 percent confidence interval for the odds ratio of 2.00 might be 0.50 to 8.00, indicating a wide range for plausible values. If the study were based on 2,000 cases and 2,000 controls, the 95 percent confidence interval might be 1.90 to 2.30, indicating a narrow range of plausible values. The precision of the estimate is a reflection of what is called *random error*, the error likely to result from choosing a sample of the total population of interest (in this case, all users of water).

Precision is related to **statistical significance**. Statistically significant usually means that the estimate of effect is different from the null value and that the difference is unlikely to have occurred by chance. Typically, a finding is judged to be statistically significant when the difference from the null value has less than a 1 in 20 likelihood of having occurred by chance (usually stated as a **p value** of less than 0.05). A 95 percent confidence interval that excludes the null value (for example, the null value of 1.00 for an odds ratio, which indicates no difference in risk of disease between exposed and nonexposed), corresponds to a p value of less than 0.05. Epidemiologists now prefer to express the precision of study results with confidence intervals rather than with p values and tests of statistical significance, partly because a range of plausible values is more informative than a single test of statistical significance.

ENVIRONMENTAL AND OCCUPATIONAL EPIDEMIOLOGY

Environmental and occupational epidemiology uses few truly unique epidemiological techniques but is simply an area of epidemiology defined by the exposures it studies.

Environmental epidemiology concerns environmental agents to which large numbers of people are exposed involuntarily. This area of concern usually excludes voluntary exposures such as alcohol, cigarettes, and medications. However, it usually includes environmental ("secondhand") tobacco smoke and infectious agents in water supplies. Although this definition is sometimes a bit arbitrary, and although environmental epidemiology thus defined can sometimes overlap with other areas of epidemiology, nonetheless it is useful. Some examples of environmental agents (and their associated outcomes) are radon in homes in relation to lung cancer, environmental tobacco smoke in relation to lung cancer, arsenic in water in relation to low birthweight, chlorination by-products in water supplies in relation to bladder cancer, pesticide residues in food in relation to cancer, particulate matter in the air in relation to cardiovascular disease, and lead in soil in relation to neurological deficits. These exposures are often low level and relatively homogenous across large numbers of people, making them particularly difficult to study. The differences in risk between those with more exposure and those with less exposure are usually small and therefore hard to detect reliably, often requiring large sample sizes.

Environmental exposures can be thought of as contributing either to **epidemics** or to **endemic diseases** Epidemics are unusual outbreaks of disease clearly above a normal level and often caused by known agents, although sometimes the agent is initially unknown. For example, the cholera outbreaks in Peru a few years ago had a known cause. However, other causes of recent disease outbreaks have not been initially known, including the cause of the 1981 outbreak of neuropathy in Madrid (eventually found to be due to an oil contaminant), of the 1993 gastrointestinal illness outbreak in Milwaukee (due to cryptosporidium), and of the 1976 pneumonia outbreak in Philadelphia (due to Legionnaire's disease). In contrast, endemic diseases exist at constant, low (or *background*) levels and may or may not have an environmental cause. Examples are the possible contribution of radon in homes to lung cancer, the contribution of dioxin in the diet to cancer rates, the contribution of low-level air pollution to cardiovascular disease, and the contribution of lead in the environment to neurological deficits in children. Possible associations between environmental agents and background levels of disease are more and more often the subject of environmental epidemiology, especially in developed countries, and these associations are difficult to detect.

Occupational epidemiology is the epidemiological study of illness or injury associated with workplace exposures. Examples include the association of stressful repetitive motion and carpal tunnel syndrome, welding and lung cancer, silica exposure and kidney disease, and poor office ventilation and respiratory illness. Occupational epidemiology often involves relatively high exposures in relatively small numbers of people, often geographically isolated at a worksite.

This context makes for easier studies from a scientific standpoint (the workplace exposure is a natural experiment). However, workplace studies also involve vested economic interests and are sometimes politically controversial. It may be difficult to gain access to the workers or their worksite, for example.

Historically, occupational studies were carried out in the context of very high exposures. Early studies revealed silicosis and asbestosis resulting from silica and asbestos exposure respectively. Historical occupational studies are also responsible for the discovery of many carcinogens, including asbestos, aniline dyes, silica, nickel, cadmium, arsenic, dioxin, beryllium, acid mists, radon gas, and diesel fumes (Steenland, Loomis, Shy, and Simonsen, 1996; Rom and Markowitz, 2006). Most of these agents occur in the general environment as well, where people are exposed at much lower levels. Whether associations seen in the workplace also occur in the general environment is an empirical question. For example, it is unclear whether dioxin or diesel fumes in the general environment cause cancer. However, radon in homes and arsenic in water are believed to be environmental carcinogens.

Today, workplace exposures to suspected toxins are much lower than in the past, at least in industrialized countries, and they are less often the focus of occupational epidemiology. For example, occupational cancer is less commonly studied today, as many of the most obvious suspected carcinogens in the workplace have already been studied and controlled. More commonly today, occupational studies involve issues more difficult to study, such as possible relationships between job stress and heart disease or lifting and back strain.

Understanding Clusters

One aspect of both environmental and occupational epidemiology that deserves special mention is the occurrence of clusters. A **cluster** is an apparently elevated number of cases of disease in a limited area over a limited period of time, suggesting some common cause (Rothman, 1990); typically the number of cases in the cluster is small, on the order of ten or twenty rather than hundreds. Clusters typically come to the attention of public health authorities, who must first determine whether a cluster in fact represents an unusually high occurrence of disease. This is more difficult than it might seem, particularly for environmental clusters whose geographical and temporal boundaries are not clear. For example, three cases of childhood leukemia on the same street might be unusual if the denominator at risk is taken to be all the children on that street but might not appear excessive if the boundary is the local neighborhood composed of a dozen streets. Assuming that investigators can determine that a cluster does in fact represent a high rate of disease, the next step is to determine whether there is a common cause. (Some clusters will occur simply as random events.) A common cause is more likely when the cases of disease are restricted to a specific diagnosis, such as childhood leukemia, rather than a general category, such as childhood cancer; cancer includes many diseases with many different causes. But even when the cases represent a narrow and specific diagnosis, they will often have many possible causes, and an epidemiological study will often not be able to pinpoint a specific cause. One reason for this is that such a study is typically restricted to a small number of cases (often using a case-control design), and the power to detect an association is low, even if that association is quite strong.

Most investigations of environmental clusters do not find a common cause for the cluster. Caldwell (1990) summarized 108 cancer clusters investigated by the Centers for Disease Control and Prevention and concluded that no clear, single cause was found for any of them. Similarly, Schulte, Ehrenberg, and Singal, (1987) summarized 61 occupational clusters and found that only 16 were confirmed, and in none was a specific cause discovered.

Nonetheless, despite the long odds, cluster investigations have from time to time provided important clues that have later been confirmed in larger studies. Among the famous clusters that have led to discovery of new associations are the 1976 cluster of Legionnaire's disease in a hotel in Philadelphia (environmental), the clusters of asthma cases in Barcelona in the early 1980s that were eventually tied to soybean dust (environmental), the 1973 cluster of angiosarcoma cases among workers in a single vinyl chloride plant (occupational), and the 1977 cluster of infertility in a plant making a pesticide called dibromochloropropane (DBCP) (occupational). Studies of clusters have more chance of leading to the discovery of a specific cause when the disease in question is extremely rare. Occupational clusters have somewhat more of a chance than environmental clusters of representing a common cause because they have a natural boundary (the worksite) and therefore avoid the boundary problem inherent in environmental clusters.

Measuring Exposure

Measuring exposure with as much accuracy as possible is key to valid epidemiological studies (for a fuller discussion see Chapter Four). Accurate exposure assessment is essential to detecting and quantifying a dose-response relationship, for example, which is one of the key elements supporting a **causal relationship**. Mismeasured exposure (as a continuous variable) usually leads to flattening, or *attenuating*, a true dose-response. Misclassification of dichotomous exposure status (exposed versus nonexposed) can severely bias results toward the null.

In cross-sectional or prospective studies current exposure can be measured more or less easily, depending on the agent of interest. However, it is often difficult to assess exposure accurately when exposure must be estimated in the past, as in case-control studies, in retrospective cohort studies, and in cross-sectional studies of the impact of past exposures on current outcomes. Therefore we focus here on the problem of retrospective exposure assessment. In case-control studies of bladder cancer and drinking water, for example, subjects may be trying to remember their pattern of drinking-water consumption over the past fifty years. In cross-sectional studies of lead and neurologic deficits in children, one may wish not only to measure current lead levels via the blood but also to assess prior exposure to lead via its measurement in bone. In retrospective cohort studies, investigators may be estimating past silica exposure for workers in a specific plant. As can be seen in these examples, in some instances investigators attempt to measure external exposure (water drinking patterns, silica in workers' breathing zone) and in others they seek a biomarker of internal exposures (blood and bone lead). Below we discuss both these scenarios.

First, let us consider more thoroughly the example of assessment of past exposure to silica among workers in a retrospective cohort study. Suppose there are some existing silica exposure measurements made during the past twenty years for some workers in some jobs. Such a relatively short record is typically the case, as exposure measurements were not often made until somewhat recently. However, the cohort may have been employed over the past forty or fifty years, and because investigators seek to conduct an exposure-response analysis, they require an estimate of past exposure for all workers across all jobs at all points in time. This may not be possible at all in many retrospective cohort studies. However, in some instances it may be possible to construct a **job-exposure matrix** (JEM), which is simply a cross classification of jobs and exposure levels across time. This can be done if industrial hygienists can extrapolate beyond more recent exposure data to make a good guess about exposure further back in time, based on process changes at the plant. Typically, plants were dirtier further back in time. The industrial hygienist will also need to divide jobs in the cohort into categories on the basis of their presumably sharing the same exposure level and of their having at least some past measurements. Then all workers in all jobs in this category, at any given point in time, can be assigned the same exposure level. If all this is possible, a JEM can be constructed (Figure 3.1), and all workers in a given job at a given point in time can be assigned a level of exposure by the JEM. This will in turn enable an estimate of cumulative exposure to silica for each worker. Cumulative exposure is often the measure of interest for chronic disease outcomes such as silicosis, lung cancer, or kidney disease.

An alternative to estimating external exposure is to use a **biomarker of exposure**. Examples of such biomarkers are dioxin in blood, cotinine (a metabolite

FIGURE 3.1   Construction of a JEM for a Retrospective
Cohort Study

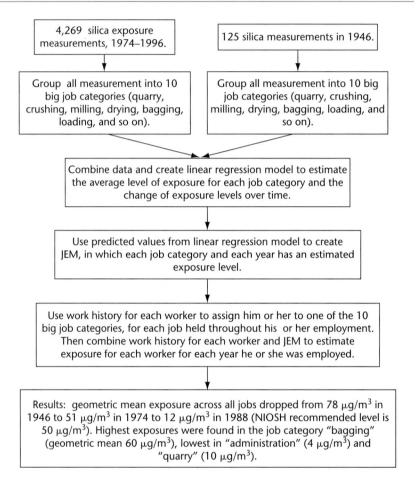

Source: Adapted from Steenland, Sanderson, and Calvert, 2001; Sanderson, Steenland, and
Deddens, 2000.

of nicotine) in blood, and lead in bone. Such biomarkers can be useful because
they measure internal dose rather than external exposure. They may therefore
take into account variation in absorption and metabolism of the external dose,
possibly providing a more accurate estimate of the biologically relevant dose that
can cause disease. However, there are many problems that may make a measure

of the internal dose less desirable than a measure of the external exposure, including wide individual variation, difficulty in obtaining accurate laboratory measurements of the biomarker, and possibly choosing the wrong biomarker in a metabolic pathway that features several candidate toxins. Perhaps more important in the case of retrospective exposure assessment, few biomarkers of exposure persist long enough to be useful for such a study.

For example, in a case-control study of Parkinson's disease in which serum from the cases is available, it would be ideal to be able to measure past exposure to pesticides (organophosphates and organochlorines), as well as other organochlorines such as polychlorinated biphenyls (PCBs). However, organophosphate pesticides, thought to play a role in chronic neurological disease partly because of their acute effects on the nervous system, are rapidly metabolized. Therefore blood levels of these compounds cannot be used to measure exposure beyond a few days in the past. Organochlorine pesticides and PCBs are also of interest because they have been shown to decrease dopamine levels in the brain in animal studies, and dopamine loss is the hallmark of Parkinson's disease. Organochlorines have half-lives that are measured in years. Some may be measured in the serum long after exposure has ceased, and therefore may be more useful in detecting exposures above background levels. DDE, for example, the principal metabolite of the pesticide DDT, can be measured today in the serum of most of the U.S. population even though use of DDT in this country was phased out in the 1970s. On the other hand, many other organochlorine pesticides phased out at the same time, such as dieldrin and aldrin, have shorter half-lives and are nondetectable in most of the U.S. population. PCBs were also phased out in the 1970s. The heavier PCBs (more highly chlorinated) can be measured in older Americans, but the lighter ones are usually not detectable.

Another important example is lead, often measured in the blood, where it reflects exposure over the previous two or three months. However, lead also accumulates in the bone where it provides a good indicator of cumulative exposure over time, even long after exposure ceases. This has been important in measuring the association between lead and neurological deficits in children. This association has been controversial for several reasons. Most studies are cross-sectional, and current blood lead levels may not reflect past exposure. Lead and SES are closely related, and SES in turn is closely related to performance on cognitive tests. Lead in teeth shed by children has been useful in establishing prior lead exposure and can act as a measure of the level of exposure in groups that are identical in SES. Similarly, bone lead measured by radiographic techniques has been important in studies of past lead exposure in adults in relation to blood pressure and other long-term effects of lead.

PERSPECTIVE
An Occupational Epidemiology Example

This perspective continues the example of the retrospective cohort study of silica-exposed workers that was introduced earlier in discussing silica exposure estimation over time. It has long been known that silica cause silicosis, a nonmalignant respiratory disease. In this cohort, there were two additional outcomes of interest, lung cancer and kidney disease (Steenland, Sanderson, and Calvert, 2001, Steenland and Sanderson, 2001). There was considerable debate about whether silica could cause these diseases.

There were 4,626 workers in the cohort, exposed to silica while producing industrial sand from the 1940s to the 1980s. The average length of exposure was nine years. Complete work history was obtained from company personnel records, which also provided information on social security number, birth date, race, and sex. The cohort was 99 percent male. Follow-up began at the time of first exposure and continued through 1996. Cause of death, needed to determine who died of lung cancer, was obtained from death certificate information using the **National Death Index**, a national registry of deaths. In addition to lung cancer mortality, the incidence of nonmalignant kidney disease was studied by matching the cohort with a national registry of patients with end-stage kidney disease. These are patients whose kidneys have failed; in the United States the government pays for the expensive treatment, either dialysis or transplant, for these patients. As a result there is a national registry of end-stage kidney patients, virtually the only national disease registry in the United States. Other countries have many such national registries, facilitating epidemiology.

This was a dynamic cohort, which means that workers could enter and exit the cohort at any time. Exit occurred at death or the end of the study in 1996. Workers were followed and were at risk of lung cancer and kidney disease after they left work. (For acute outcomes such as work-related injuries, the follow-up period might end when employment ends.) Because workers were followed for different amounts of time, the investigators studied lung cancer *rates* (rather than *risks*) in the exposed cohort, so that the denominator was person-time rather than people.

The comparison population was the U.S. population, with **stratification** used to control possible confounding by age, race, sex, and calendar time. Lung cancer death rates for the United States are available from vital statistics. U.S. kidney disease incidence rates are available from the same U.S. registry of end-stage kidney disease used to determine who in the cohort had had kidney disease.

There were 109 deaths from lung cancer, with 68 expected, resulting in a rate ratio of 1.60 (95 percent CI 1.23 to 1.93). The workers had a 60 percent higher lung cancer death rate than the U.S. population of a similar age, race, and sex did. Given that workers smoke more than the general population and that smoking is by far the most important known risk factor for lung cancer, one might question whether the excess lung cancer rate was due to smoking or to silica. Limited smoking data on 346 men in the cohort were available for the years 1978 to 1989. Such limited data are typical for retrospective studies based on company personnel records. These data indicated that among cohort members aged twenty-four to sixty-four, 24 percent were never smokers, 41 percent were current smokers, and 35 percent were former smokers. The corresponding data for the U.S. male population aged twenty-five to sixty-four in the 1980s were 37 percent, 35 percent, and 28 percent, respectively. These smoking differences would be expected to lead to an approximately 10 percent higher lung cancer rate among the silica-exposed workers compared to the U.S. population, suggesting that silica exposure rather than cigarette smoking was responsible for most of the observed 60 percent higher lung cancer rate among the workers.

Twenty-three cases of end-stage kidney disease occurred in the cohort versus the 11.7 cases expected for the U.S. population of similar age, race, and sex (rate ratio 1.97, 95 percent CI 1.25 to 2.06).

The availability of exposure estimates enabled the investigators to conduct detailed exposure-response analyses in this study, which were important in assessing causality as well as in conducting quantitative risk assessment (discussed later in this chapter and in Chapter Twenty-Nine). Exposure-response data for lung cancer, silicosis, and kidney disease in relation to estimated cumulative exposure to silica are shown in Table 3.1. Cumulative exposure was divided into quartiles for analysis, and workers in the lowest quartile served as the comparison population (rate ratio of 1.0). For lung cancer, cumulative exposure was estimated using a fifteen-year lag, under the assumption that exposures in the last fifteen years before the end of follow-up could not yet be causing lung cancer (that is, allowing for a fifteen-year **latency period**). All three outcomes showed a positive trend with increased cumulative exposure, strengthening the case for causality. Silicosis deaths were included as a kind of validity check on the exposure estimates, since they would be expected to show a positive trend (the numbers of silicosis deaths are small, but many more workers had silicosis than died from it). The probabilities that the observed positive linear trends in lung cancer, end-stage kidney disease, and silicosis occurred by chance (trend tests) were 0.07, 0.0004, and 0.00001.

TABLE 3.1   Cohort Rate Ratios for Lung Cancer and Silicosis Mortality and for End-Stage Kidney Disease Incidence

	Exposure levels			
Outcomes	**Lowest Quartile**	**Quartile 2**	**Quartile 3**	**Highest Quartile**
Lung cancer (15-year lag)	1.00 (17 deaths)	0.78 (21 deaths)	1.51 (20 deaths)	1.57 (16 deaths)
End-stage kidney disease	1.00 (2 cases)	3.09 (5 cases)	5.22 (6 cases)	7.79 (5 cases)
Silicosis	1.00 (1 death)	1.22 (2 deaths)	2.91 (4 deaths)	7.39 (7 deaths)

Source: Data from Steenland, Sanderson, and Calvert, 2001; Steenland and Sanderson, 2001.

PERSPECTIVE
An Environmental Epidemiology Example

Studies of recreational water quality provide an interesting example of many of the principles and challenges of environmental epidemiology. The number of gastroenteritis outbreaks associated with recreational water exposure increased three- to fourfold from 1978, when the surveillance for these outbreaks started, to 2004 (Dziuban and others, 2006) and prompted closer examination of the risk factors leading to both endemic and epidemic waterborne disease associated with exposure to recreational waters (see Chapter Fifteen). Many epidemiological studies of recreational water quality and gastrointestinal illness have been conducted (see reviews by Pruss, 1998; Wade, Pai, Eisenberg, and Colford, 2003). The basic research approach is typically a cohort study. Swimmers and nonswimmers are recruited into the study at a recreational water site and interviewed about their swimming exposure on that day. Water samples may be collected. Participants are later interviewed regarding disease incidence following their visit to the water site, and swimmers are compared to nonswimmers.

Gastroenteritis is the most common health outcome of water contamination and has been the most frequently studied. Most studies have collected data on self-reported symptoms, using a standardized questionnaire or interview. The exposure of interest is water with fecal contamination, because of the fecal-oral transmission route of enteric pathogens.

Misclassification or mismeasurement of exposure is likely to be the most common problem in these studies and may be due to error in assessing water quality (from the use of poor microbial indicators or poor water sample storage and analyses) or in classifying the degree of individual water contact. This bias is likely to be random and nondifferential, biasing results toward the null.

Selection bias may occur in several ways. Recruitment of the study population at a beach may result in a study population that is not representative of the general population. For example, tourist populations at the beach may have higher attack rates than local populations, affecting **generalizability** of results (**external validity**). Regarding **internal validity**, selection of a nonexposed group that systematically differs from the exposed group for some unmeasured confounder may cause bias that cannot be corrected by controlling for measured confounders in the analysis. There is a debate whether the nonexposed group should be nonswimmers or swimmers in cleaner water.

Confounding may occur, for example, due to exposures to enteric pathogens through alternative routes (food and drink) or due to socioeconomic factors that may be related both to exposure and to disease. Seasonality and water temperature may also act as confounders if the study takes place over different seasons or over different days with different water temperatures.

An epidemiological study by Haile and others (1999) illustrates the concepts just discussed. The purpose of this study was to examine the risks of gastrointestinal illness associated with swimming in marine waters that received untreated runoff from storm drains in Santa Monica Bay, near Los Angles. The specific study questions were these:

1. Are there different risks of adverse health outcomes among subjects swimming at different distances from the storm drains?
2. Are risks of specific health outcomes associated with the concentration of specific bacterial indicators of water quality or with the presence of enteric viruses?

The study team interviewed subjects at three beaches in Santa Monica Bay that had a wide range of microbial indicator concentrations in the water and high swimmer density. A total of 22,085 subjects were interviewed between June 25 and September 14, 1995, and 17,253 of these were eligible and able to participate. Subjects were eligible if they had a telephone, spoke English or Spanish, and had not been swimming at the study beaches or in heavily polluted areas in the seven days before the beach interview. A total of 15,492 subjects (90 percent of the eligible subjects) agreed to participate in the study and were asked to provide information about their age, residence, and swimming experience (location, immersion of head into water) on that day.

The locations of the storm drains were identified, and the interviewer categorized the swimmer's location by distance from the storm drain (categories were 0, 1–50, 51–100, and 400 yards from the drain) and noted the gender and race of each subject. Follow-up interviews, conducted by telephone nine to fourteen days after the beach interview, included questions about the occurrence of fever, chills, eye discharge, earache, ear discharge, skin rash, infected cuts, nausea, vomiting, diarrhea, diarrhea with blood, stomach pain, coughing, nasal congestion, and sore throat. *Highly credible gastrointestinal illness* (HCGI) was defined as one or more of the following: (1) vomiting, (2) diarrhea and fever, or (3) stomach pain and fever. The investigators were able to contact 13,278 subjects (86 percent) for follow-up interviews. During these interviews, 1,485 subjects were excluded because they had swum at a study beach or in heavily polluted waters between the day of the beach interview and the telephone follow-up and it would not be possible to determine whether any symptoms they reported at the interview were due to their exposure on the day of the beach interview (when the water quality was measured) or to subsequent exposures. An additional 107 subjects were excluded because they did not immerse their faces in ocean water during swimming.

Water samples were collected on the same days that subjects were recruited at the beaches. Samples were collected from each exposure category location (distance from drains) and were analyzed for commonly used microbial indicators of water quality: total coliforms, fecal coliforms, enterococci, and *E. coli* using standard membrane filtration techniques. Additional water samples were collected on weekends from three storm drain sites and analyzed for culturable enteric viruses.

Because the study population was restricted to swimmers, the analyses compared symptom rates and HCGI rates among groups of swimmers. One approach compared swimmers more than 400 yards from a storm drain with swimmers closer to a storm drain. A second approach compared swimmers in waters with different prespecified levels of microbial indicators. For example, enterococci exposure categories were set to ≤35 colony-forming units (cfu) per 100 ml (the U.S. EPA (1986) guideline for marine recreational water), 35–104 cfu/100 ml, and >104 cfu/100 ml. All analyses were adjusted for the following potential confounders: age (categorical), sex, beach, race, California resident versus out-of-state resident, and concern about potential health hazards at the beach (categorical).

The study found that the rates of several symptoms and of HCGI (331 cases) were higher among people who swam near the drains than among those who swam at least 400 yards away from the drains. The adjusted relative risks ranged from about 1.2 for eye discharge, sore throat, and HCGI to 2.3 for earache. Positive associations were also observed between various symptoms and higher levels of specific microbial indicators. Swimmers within 50 yards of the storm drains on days when enteric viruses were detected in the water samples (386 swimmers) reported elevated rates of HCGI and several other symptoms compared to those who swam near the storm drains on days when enteric viruses were not detected ($n = 3,168$). Adjusted relative risks ranged from about 1.2 for cough, diarrhea, and chills to 1.9 to 2.3 for eye discharge, vomiting, and HCGI. However, there were no clear dose-response patterns across increasing levels of microbial indicators, and none of the elevated relative risks were statistically significant. The investigators concluded that the strength and consistency of the associations they observed across several measures of exposure suggest that there is an increased risk of adverse health effects associated with swimming in marine waters that receive untreated urban runoff, despite the lack of dose-response patterns (possibly due to misclassification of exposure) and the lack of statistical significance.

Although this study had the advantage of a large sample size, it seems likely that there were problems with misclassification of exposure. No data were provided on the results of the microbiological analyses of the beach water. What was the range of water quality to which study subjects were exposed? How much variation was there between water samples taken at different locations from a single beach on a single day, and how well do these samples reflect the water quality to which a swimmer is actually exposed at the location and time he or she is swimming? There can be substantial temporal and spatial variation in water quality, especially in open bodies of water with currents. How frequently were high levels of microbial contamination measured, and how closely did those levels reflect the presence of fecal contamination and microbial pathogens?

Individuals in the low-exposure reference group, those who swam at the greatest distance from the drains, may have been exposed to high levels of pathogens either because they swam near the drains without observing that they did so or because water currents moved slugs of contaminants to the area where they were swimming. It is also possible that classification of exposure on the basis of bacterial indicator organisms, especially total and fecal coliforms, is a poor surrogate for exposure to the pathogens that actually caused the infections suffered by the swimmers in the contaminated water. There is considerable debate in the scientific community about which microbial indicators are sufficiently similar to microbial pathogens in terms of their movement and persistence in the aquatic environment (National Research Council, 2004). Several previous studies have reported no significant relationships between symptom rates and fecal indicator bacteria, and Pruss (1998) asserts that the use of microbial indicators is one of the major sources of bias in epidemiological studies of recreational water quality and health. In this study the investigators attempted to measure enteric viruses in water but did not show any data on how frequently they detected these viruses in the water samples and the efficacy of their virus detection methods. Detection and quantification of enteric viruses in environmental water samples is difficult.

A recent meta-analysis of twenty-seven studies of recreational water quality and gastrointestinal illness (Wade and others, 2003) concluded that despite significant heterogeneity among the studies, the results generally supported the EPA's guideline levels for *E. coli* in freshwater and enterococci in marine waters. The authors noted that the studies that reported elevated relative risks tended to be those that used a nonswimming control group, focused on children, or used study populations found at athletic or other recreational events instead of populations recruited at a beach. This observation shows how study design features can affect the observed association between water quality and gastrointestinal illness, presumably by introducing selection biases affecting either external or internal validity. Wade and others (2003) argue that if measuring the risks associated with swimming is the goal of the study, then nonswimmers are the appropriate control group and that using a control group of swimmers may underestimate the risk of recreational water contact and result in insufficiently protective regulatory guidelines. Nonswimming controls used by other studies have been family members or others at the beach who did not swim, bystanders, organizers of athletic or organized recreational water events, or participants in a related recreational event that did not include swimming (Wade and others, 2003). However, Haile and others (1999) defended their use of a swimming control group (those who swam >400 yards away from the storm drains, or those in the lowest bacterial indicator exposure category) on the grounds that restricting the study to swimmers reduced the potential for confounding (that is, subjects who swim are different from subjects who choose not to swim). Future studies could attempt to collect more information on swimmers and nonswimmers in order to ensure that these groups have similar age distributions and risk factors.

EPIDEMIOLOGY AND RISK ASSESSMENT

The results of occupational and environmental epidemiological studies can affect public health by alerting policymakers to new hazards and possibly by triggering regulations about permissible levels of exposure. Sometimes a single large and definitive study is deemed sufficient to change public policy, but in other instances regulators want to see a study's results replicated (recall Hill's criterion of consistency). When a number of studies point in the same direction, public authorities are more likely to act.

In the past, qualitative literature reviews were used to summarize the evidence across many studies. Today one is more likely to see a **quantitative meta-analysis** that provides a weighted average of quantitative results across studies. Meta-analyses were originally used for clinical trials but have been used extensively for observational studies in the last decade. They can combine results from different study designs, such as rate ratios from cohort studies and odds ratios from case-control studies. For example, a meta-analysis may give a weighted average of lung cancer rate ratios or odds ratios across many studies of silica and lung cancer (actually the logarithms of the ratio measures are used, and then results are converted back to the original scale at the end). The weights are typically the inverse of the variance of each study's result; this means that the largest studies with the narrowest confidence intervals, those that are estimated more precisely, will have the lowest variance and be accorded the most weight.

Meta-analyses do not require access to the original study data; they can use results from the published literature. A variant method to summarize data across studies is a **pooled analysis**, in which the raw data for each study are obtained and the combined data then reanalyzed. Pooled analyses are much more time consuming but have the advantage of providing more flexibility in the analysis. Meta-analyses are most often done to determine a common ratio measure of disease rates (for example, a rate ratio) in the exposed versus the nonexposed. However, they may also be done to determine a common exposure-response coefficient across a number of exposure-response analyses.

Exposure-response analyses are of particular interest to public health authorities who seek to determine a permissible exposure level for the public or for workers. The determination of a permissible exposure level is based on **risk assessment** (and is discussed in detail in Chapter Twenty-Nine). Risk assessment may be based on animal data or human data. The former requires extrapolation from animals to humans and hence involves a considerable amount of uncertainty. For this reason, human (epidemiological) data are preferred, but they may not exist for the agent in question. When epidemiological data do exist, results giving the increased rate of disease per unit of exposure (exposure-response data) for an exposed population must typically be converted to the excess risk of disease over a lifetime for an individual who received a specific exposure. The exposure associated with a specific level of excess lifetime risk, typically somewhere in the range of 1 in 100,000 to 1 in 1,000, is then determined to be permissible. For workers, the U.S. Occupational Safety and Health Administration (OSHA) typically seeks to limit risk to 1 in 1,000,000, a higher risk than is usually accepted by the EPA, under the assumption that workers voluntarily accept a somewhat higher risk. Rates can be converted to risk using simple formulas.

Two issues of concern arise for risk assessors working with epidemiological exposure-response models. The first is the shape of the exposure-response curve. When data are sparse, and sometimes even when they are not, it may be difficult to choose among competing models for setting permissible limits, models that can have very different consequences.. Typical questions involving model selection might be whether the exposure-response shows a linear increase in disease rates per unit of exposure, whether there is a threshold below which there is no risk followed by an increase, or conversely, whether there is a cutpoint above which disease risk begins to flatten out or even decrease. A second question typical of risk assessment is the nature of the exposure-response relationship in the low-dose region, where there may be few data. This question often arises when occupational epidemiological studies (high exposure) are used for risk assessment for general environmental exposures such as diesel fumes, dioxin, or asbestos.

An example in which both these issues occurred is a risk assessment for cancer subsequent to dioxin exposure, based on a study of 3,538 workers (Steenland, Deddens, and Piacitelli, 2001). Most workers were exposed to dioxin several orders of magnitude above typical environmental levels, raising the issue of whether results could be extrapolated to low-dose levels. However, there were some data in the low-dose range, yielding more confidence in such extrapolation. The model using the logarithm of cumulative exposure produced estimated risks from low-dose exposure that were ten times higher than the risks predicted by the linear model. A doubling of background levels in the serum (10 ppt versus 5 ppt), such as might occur due to high fish consumption (dioxin intake in the general public comes primarily from diet), resulted in an increase in lifetime risk of cancer mortality of about 0.9 percent according to a model with the logarithm of cumulative exposure, and of about 0.05 percent according to a two-piece linear model. The background risk of cancer death by age seventy-five is 12 percent for males and 11 percent for females. In this case the two-piece linear model was the better model to use in the low-dose region, given that the logarithmic model by definition invariably results in an extremely high slope in this region.

FUTURE DIRECTIONS

Occupational epidemiology is becoming less and less concerned with exposures to toxins, which are becoming less and less prevalent in the workplace. Instead, interest is now focusing more on other types of exposures that affect a large number of workers. One such exposure is job stress, which is difficult to measure but which may have large consequences via increasing blood pressure or cardiovascular disease, or both. Results to date for a link between job stress and blood pressure are tantalizing but far from conclusive; potential confounding by socioeconomic status is a major issue in studies of job stress. Shift work and a noisy workplace are related exposures that may result in stress and increased blood pressure. Another related exposure is loss of employment, which may in turn increase stress and predict poor health in other ways.

Yet another area of large concern is ergonomics. Musculoskeletal injuries such as low back pain and carpal tunnel syndrome are extremely common in the workplace and result in a large economic burden of disability. Epidemiological studies relating specific work practices to these musculoskeletal outcomes are difficult to design and conduct. Nonetheless the evidence to date clearly implicates forceful repetitive motion in the development of carpal tunnel syndrome. The epidemiological evidence for low back pain is somewhat less conclusive but also points to awkward lifting postures as contributors.

When toxins do continue to be of concern in the workplace, epidemiologists are increasingly concerned with risks of subclinical outcomes among the exposed workers, outcomes that may or may not have long-term consequences. Examples of these outcomes are cytogenetic changes such as sister-chromatid exchange and chromosomal aberrations (future cancer risk?), excess small protein in the kidney (future kidney disease?), and the presence of autoantibodies in the serum (future autoimmune disease?).

Another trend is the assessment of gene-environment interactions. For example, subjects with high levels of PCBs in their serum may be at risk for Parkinson's disease only if they have a certain genetic polymorphism. (This possibility and its implications for public health are discussed in Chapter Six.)

The trends discussed here are occurring primarily in developed industrialized countries (where the practice of epidemiology is more common). In less developed countries, large numbers of people still sustain very high levels of exposure to the classic occupational toxins. In many of these cases, however, what is needed is hazard surveillance and control rather than new epidemiological studies.

One problem that affects occupational epidemiology in the United States, and to some extent all countries, is the increasing difficulty of conducting workplace studies at all. In many instances, permission from the employer is required, and the spread of market economies, coupled with weakness of organized labor, has meant less emphasis on workplace health and safety and more barriers to conducting occupational studies.

As for environmental epidemiology, low-level exposure to common toxins continues to be of interest in determining whether such exposure contributes to background endemic disease rates. Arsenic in the water, PCBs in the diet, mercury in the air, and small particulates in the air are just a few of the agents of interest. A new class of toxins of concern is fluorocarbons such as perfluorooctanoic acid (PFOA). This industrial chemical does not exist in nature, but it is now present in the serum of virtually all inhabitants of industrialized countries. The route of exposure is still not clear. Although use of PFOA is now being phased out, it has been employed in common products such as Teflon and Scotchgard. It persists indefinitely in the environment and has been found by the EPA to be a probable human carcinogen. The difficulty of conducting conclusive epidemiological studies on such agents, combined with their large potential public health consequences, continues to lead to more sophisticated study methods.

In addition to these classic problems, newer issues are demanding attention. Global climate change is now largely accepted as a real trend by the scientific community (see Chapter Ten). However, the health effects of climate change are challenging to study and have yet to be fully documented. Indeed, the endpoints for such studies are not always clear, and the appropriate study designs may not be apparent. Lack of a protective ozone layer in certain parts of the world is another example of a recent and challenging issue. Other issues are even newer, such as how to measure the health effects of urban environment features such as parks, pedestrian infrasturcture, and pavement (see Chapter Fourteen).

SUMMARY

Epidemiology is the study of the distribution and determinants of health and disease in human populations, and epidemiologists are dedicated to studying whether a given exposure or set of exposures causes a certain disease. Environmental epidemiology and occupational epidemiology study the role of exposures in the general environment and in the workplace, respectively. Investigators in these two fields use many similar methods.

There are many kinds of epidemiological study designs. Examples include ecological studies, cohort studies, and case-control studies. In each case, epidemiologists work to define and measure exposures, to define and measure the health outcomes of interest, and to define and measure other factors that may bear on the association of interest. They also work to eliminate or control sources of bias that may skew their findings, including confounding, selection bias, and information bias.

Epidemiological data are invaluable in risk assessment, in standard setting and other policymaking, and in dispute resolution in environmental and occupational health.

KEY TERMS

analytical studies

biological plausibility (Hill criterion)

biomarker of exposure

case-control studies

categorical variable

causal inference

causal relationship

clinical trials

cluster

cohort studies

confidence interval

confounding

consistency (Hill criterion)

continuous variable

correlational studies

cross-sectional studies

cumulative incidence

descriptive studies

dichotomous variable

dose-response (Hill criterion)

ecological studies

effect modification

effect size (Hill criterion)

endemic disease

environmental epidemiology

epidemic

epidemiology

etiologic studies

external validity

generalizability

healthy worker effect

Hill's criteria

incidence

information bias

internal validity

job-exposure matrix

Karl Popper

latency period

linear regression

logistic regression

meta-analysis

misclassification

mismeasurement

multivariate analysis

National Death Index

natural experiment

nondifferential error

null hypothesis

observational studies

occupational epidemiology

odds ratio

p value

pooled analysis

precision

prevalence

prospective studies

quantitative meta-analysis

randomized clinical trials

rate

rate ratio

recall bias

regression analysis

retrospective studies

risk

risk assessment

sample size

selection bias

statistical power

statistical significance

stratification

temporal relationship (Hill criterion)

DISCUSSION QUESTIONS

1. Perfluorooctanoic acid (PFOA) is present at background levels of about 5 ng/ml in the blood of the general U.S. population. Operations at a Teflon plant in Parkersburg, West Virginia, resulted in contaminated drinking water in nearby parts of West Virginia and Ohio. Approximately 70,000 residents living in six water districts near the plant had their blood levels measured in 2005 and 2006 as part of the settlement of a class action lawsuit; blood levels averaged 80 ng/ml (with a very wide range). In addition, approximately 1,000 workers at the chemical plant had been measured in 2004 and had blood levels on the order of 500 ng/ml at that time. Data on emissions of PFOA over time are available. PFOA is an animal carcinogen (liver, testicular, pancreatic, and perhaps breast cancer) and causes fetal loss in mice. Data on cancer in people in possible relation to PFOA are sparse and inconsistent. There is some evidence of a modest correlation between mothers' PFOA blood levels and lower birthweight in infants, and also between increased cholesterol and PFOA. What kinds of studies would you conduct in the populations just described, assuming you had access to data from both the general population and the workers and could count on their cooperation? What measure of exposure would you use? How would you estimate past exposure?

2. Suppose you want to study whether environmental tobacco smoke (ETS) causes heart disease. ETS exposure occurs among both smokers and non-smokers who are around tobacco smoke. However, smokers take in much higher levels of chemicals from cigarettes than the levels encountered by nonsmokers exposed to ETS. In what population would you choose to study ETS? Who would be the exposed and who would be the nonexposed? How would you measure exposure? What would be your heart disease outcome, and how would you measure it? What study design would you use?

3. We rely on both human evidence (from epidemiology) and animal evidence (from toxicology) to clarify the health effects of toxic exposures. Each provides valuable information, and each has both advantages and disadvantages. Please compare and contrast the two kinds of evidence and explain their relative merits.

REFERENCES

Caldwell, G. "Twenty-Two Years of Cancer Cluster Investigations at the Centers for Disease Control." *American Journal of Epidemiology*, 1990, *132*(suppl. 1), S43–S62.

Dziuban, E. J., and others. (2006). "Surveillance for Waterborne Disease and Outbreaks Associated with Recreational Water—United States, 2003–2004." *Morbidity and Mortality Weekly Report*, 2006, *55*(SS-12), 31–58.

Haile, R.W., and others. "The Health Effects of Swimming in Ocean Water Contaminated by Storm Drain Runoff." *Epidemiology*, 1999, *10*, 355–363.

Hill, A. B. "The Environment and Disease: Association or Causation?" *Proceedings of the Royal Society of Medicine*, 1965, *58*, 295–300.

National Research Council. *Indicators for Waterborne Pathogens*. Washington, D.C.: National Academies Press, 2004.

Pruss, A. "Review of Epidemiological Studies on Health Effects from Exposure to Recreational Water." *International Journal of Epidemiology*, 1998, *27*, 1–9.

Rogan, W., and others. "Treatment of Lead-Exposed Children Trial Group: The Effect of Chelation Therapy with Succimer on Neuropsychological Development in Children Exposed to Lead." *New England Journal of Medicine*, 2001, *344*, 1421–1426.

Rom, W., and Markowitz, S. (eds.). *Environmental and Occupational Medicine*. (4th ed.). Philadelphia: Lippincott Williams & Wilkins, 2006.

Rothman, K. "A Sobering Start for the Cluster Busters' Conference." *American Journal of Epidemiology*, 1990, *132*(suppl. 1), S6–S13.

Rothman, K., and Greenland, S. *"Causation and Causal Inference."* In K. Rothman and S. Greenland, *Modern Epidemiology* (2nd ed., pp 7–28). Philadelphia: Lippincott-Raven, 1998.

Sanderson, W., Steenland, K., and Deddens, J. "Historical Respirable Quartz Exposures of Industrial Sand Workers: 1946–1996." *American Journal of Industrial Medicine*, 2000, *38*, 389–398.

Schulte, P., Ehrenberg, R., and Singal, M. "Investigation of Occupational Cancer Clusters: Theory and Practice." *American Journal of Public Health*, 1987, *77*, 52–56.

Steenland, K., Deddens, J., and Piacitelli, L. "Risk Assessment for 2,3,7,8-*p*-dioxin (TCDD) Based on an Epidemiologic Study." *American Journal of Epidemiology*, 2001, *154*, 451–458.

Steenland, K., Loomis, D., Shy, C., and Simonsen, N. "A Review of Occupational Lung Carcinogens." *American Journal of Industrial Medicine*, 1996, *29*, 474–490.

Steenland, K., and Sanderson, W. "Lung Cancer Among Industrial Sand Workers Exposed to Crystalline Silica." *American Journal of Epidemiology*, 2001, *153*, 695–703.

Steenland, K., Sanderson, W., and Calvert, G. "Kidney Disease and Arthritis Among Workers Exposed to Silica." *Epidemiology*, 2001, *12*, 405–412.

U.S. Environmental Protection Agency. *Bacteriological Water Quality Criteria for Marine and Fresh Recreational Waters*. EPA-440/5-84-002. Cincinnati, Ohio: U.S. Environmental Protection Agency, Office of Water Regulations and Standards, 1986.

Wade, T. J., Pai, N., Eisenberg, J. N., and Colford, J. M. "Do US Environmental Protection Agency Water Quality Guidelines for Recreational Waters Prevent Gastrointestinal Illness? A Systematic Review and Meta-Analysis." *Environmental Health Perspectives*, 2003, *111*, 1102–1109.

Whittemore, A., and McGuire, V. "Observational Studies and Randomized Trials of Hormone Replacement Therapy: What Can We Learn from Them?" *Epidemiology*, 2003, *14*, 8–110.

FOR FURTHER INFORMATION

Textbooks

Many excellent epidemiology textbooks are available, some providing a general overview of the field and others focusing on environmental and occupational epidemiology. Here are some examples.

General Epidemiology

Aschengrau, A., and Seage, G. R. *Essentials of Epidemiology in Public Health*. (2nd ed.) Sudbury, Mass.: Jones & Bartlett. 2007.

Gordis, L. *Epidemiology*. (4th ed.) Philadelphia: Saunders, 2008.

Koepsell, T. D., and Weiss, N. S. *Epidemiologic Methods: Studying the Occurrence of Illness*. New York: Oxford University Press, 2003.

Rothman, K. J. *Epidemiology: An Introduction*. New York: Oxford University Press, 2002.

Rothman, K. J., Greenland, S., and Lash, T. L. *Modern Epidemiology*. (3rd ed.) Philadelphia: Lippincott Williams & Wilkins, 2008.

Szklo, M., and Nieto, F. K. *Epidemiology: Beyond the Basics*. (2nd ed.) Sudbury, Mass.: Jones & Bartlett, 2006.

Environmental and Occupational Epidemiology

Baker, D., and Nieuwenhuijsen, M. J. (eds.). *Environmental Epidemiology: Study Methods and Application*. New York: Oxford University Press, 2008.

Checkoway, H., Pearce, N., and Kriebel, D. *Research Methods in Occupational Epidemiology*. (2nd ed.) New York: Oxford University Press, 2004.

Friis, R., and Sellers, T. *Epidemiology for Public Health Practice*. (4th ed.) Sudbury, Mass.: Jones & Bartlett, 2008.

Merrill, R. M. *Environmental Epidemiology: Principles and Methods*. Sudbury, Mass.: Jones & Bartlett, 2007.

Steenland, K. *Case Studies in Occupational Epidemiology*. New York: Oxford University Press, 1992.

Steenland, K., and Savitz, D. (eds.). *Topics in Environmental Epidemiology*. New York: Oxford University Press, 1997.

Journals

Many journals publish epidemiological research. These include general medical and public health journals and also specialty journals such as the following:

American Journal of Epidemiology
Annals of Epidemiology
Epidemiologic Reviews
Epidemiology
International Journal of Epidemiology
Journal of Epidemiology and Community Health

Organizations

American College of Epidemiology, http://www.acepidemiology.org. A professional organization dedicated to continuing education and advocacy for epidemiologists in support of their efforts to promote public health.

Conference of State and Territorial Epidemiologists, http://www.cste.org. A professional association of public health epidemiologists working in states, local health agencies, and territories.

International Society for Environmental Epidemiology, http://www.iseepi.org. A group with members from over fifty countries that provides a professional forum for discussing problems unique to the study of health and the environment.

Society for Epidemiologic Research, http://www.epiresearch.org. A forum in which professionals can share epidemiological research.

CHAPTER FOUR

EXPOSURE ASSESSMENT, INDUSTRIAL HYGIENE, AND ENVIRONMENTAL MANAGEMENT

P. BARRY RYAN

KEY CONCEPTS

■ Assessing environmental exposures is key to identifying hazards, understanding the effects of hazards on health, controlling hazards, and monitoring the success of control efforts.

■ Industrial hygiene is a discipline that involves the anticipation, recognition, evaluation, and control of workplace hazards.

■ Industrial hygiene uses many measurement techniques, such as air sampling and biomonitoring.

■ Industrial hygiene uses a hierarchy of control strategies, such as substitution, ventilation, and personal protective equipment.

■ Exposure science is an emerging field that applies many of the tools of industrial hygiene to the general environment.

THIS chapter introduces a set of concepts and activities that are at the core of environmental health: recognizing, measuring, and ultimately controlling hazardous **exposures**. Our account begins with **industrial hygiene**, a technical field that evolved in industrial workplaces. It then moves beyond industrial hygiene, to describe a modern field active both in the workplace and the general environment: **exposure assessment**.

Industrial hygiene and exposure assessment share a common task: quantifying hazardous exposures. This task is relevant both to public health practice and to research. In public health practice, quantifying exposures helps assess potential problems, direct preventive efforts and monitor their success, and check compliance with regulations. Quantifying exposures is also essential in research, because it allows investigators to quantify the association between the exposures and health outcomes. Knowing, for example, that carbon monoxide is an asphyxiant is only so useful. Knowing *how much* carbon monoxide exposure can be tolerated and how much is dangerous, and knowing how to measure the exposures where and when they occur, enables us to understand the biological effects more completely, identify acceptable levels and set standards accordingly, and monitor environments to be sure they are safe.

But even though they share a common task, industrial hygiene and exposure assessment differ in an important way. Industrial hygiene has traditionally moved beyond measuring exposures to controlling them. An industrial hygienist in a factory typically monitors air levels of, say, hazardous solvents, and if they are excessive in a particular part of the factory, she or he implements controls, such as substituting a safer solvent, upgrading the ventilation system, or providing personal protective equipment for affected workers. An exposure assessor, in contrast, specializes only in measuring and quantifying exposures (often in a research setting), whereas responsibility for controlling excessive exposures rests with other professionals.

ANTICIPATION, RECOGNITION, EVALUATION, AND CONTROL

Industrial hygiene has been defined as the "science and art devoted to the anticipation, recognition, evaluation, and control of those environmental factors or stresses arising in or from the workplace that may cause sickness, impaired health and well-being, or significant discomfort among workers or among citizens of the community" (American Industrial Hygiene Association, quoted in Plog, Niland, and Quinlan, 1996). Industrial hygienists are the professionals who manage workplace risks, together with allied professionals such as occupational physicians and nurses.

P. Barry Ryan declares no competing financial interests.

Industrial hygiene has been practiced in the United States for almost one hundred years. Historically, the profession's paradigm was summarized as "recognition, evaluation, and control," but in recent years it has been expanded to "anticipation, recognition, evaluation, and control." Under this paradigm, the industrial hygienist aims to predict and then recognize hazards in the workplace, measure the magnitude of exposure, and implement appropriate control strategies. Koren and Besesi (1996) have developed concise definitions of each part of this paradigm. They define **anticipation** of hazards as "proactive estimation of health and safety concerns that are commonly, or at least potentially, associated with a given occupational or environmental setting." **Recognition** of occupational hazards is the "identification of potential and actual hazards in a workplace through direct inspection," a definition that emphasizes that empirical observation is at the heart of industrial hygiene. **Evaluation** includes measuring exposures through "visual or instrumental monitoring of a site." Finally, **control** is the "reduction of risk to health and safety through administrative or engineering measures." Industrial hygiene is by its nature a field discipline, and industrial hygienists spend much of their time in workplaces, observing, measuring, and problem solving. As they do so, each element of the paradigm is part of their approach.

Anticipation

Anticipation may be viewed as the "pre-preliminary" assessment before going into the field. Prior to visiting a workplace the industrial hygienist typically receives some information about it, such as the history of the site, the manufacturing processes in place, job titles, and chemicals in use. Based on this information and on general knowledge of the industry, the hygienist can develop a preliminary list of potential health and safety hazards, including those confined to the workplace—*occupational hazards*—and those that may migrate over the fence line to nearby rivers, woodlands, or communities, becoming environmental hazards.

Industrial hygienists divide occupational hazards into two focus areas: safety and health. Examples of **safety hazards** include insufficient emergency egress, slippery surfaces and other risks of trips and falls, and chemical storage posing fire or explosion risk. Moving machinery, unguarded catwalks, and moving vehicles such as forklifts also come under this general heading. Although these concerns are the domain of a related profession, **safety engineering**, many industrial hygienists handle safety concerns as part of their job, especially at smaller facilities where they need to be jacks-of-all-trades.

Health hazards in the workplace are highly varied. They may include **physical hazards** such as high noise levels, elevated temperatures and humidity, and radiation. Physical hazards may also include repetitive motion such as typing or hand tool use, which can increase the risk of work-related musculoskeletal injuries such as shoulder pain or carpal tunnel syndrome. **Chemical hazards** can also result from many workplace processes and may be acute or chronic. Acute high-level exposures to certain highly toxic chemicals, such as chlorine gas, may result in both acute and chronic health effects, disability, and even death. Such events must be clearly anticipated and controlled. More common are long-term exposures leading to chronic effects. Some effects, such as neurological damage from solvent exposure, have been well established through occupational epidemiological investigations. For example, long-term exposure to benzene increases the risk of bone marrow dysfunction and aplastic anemia, a blood disease characterized by reduced amounts of several lines of blood cells. Other examples include increased risk of asbestosis in asbestos workers, silicosis in foundry workers, and lung cancer in uranium miners.

In modern industrial hygiene, the industrial hygienist is often called upon to anticipate **environmental hazards** as well as hazards in the workplace. Environmental hazards may endanger safety (as when a chlorine tank ruptures and neighbors are exposed to toxic gas), health (as when a plume of organic wastes from improper disposal at a factory contaminates groundwater and enters people's wells), and welfare (as when smokestack emissions damage nearby trees or homes). Environmental effects may also include ecological damage (such as damaging the oxygen-carrying ability of a local water supply) and economic damage (such as contaminating nearby land with heavy metals, industrial solvents, or pesticides to the point that the land can no longer be used for residential or recreational purposes). The industrial hygienist should anticipate such possibilities, and design a preliminary investigation to address such concerns. This may include reviewing many aspects of a factory's operations. For example, if records or employee interviews suggest that hazardous materials were stored inappropriately in years past, then these materials might have seeped into the ground and migrated off site, contaminating groundwater. The hygienist who suspects such widespread contamination may consult an environmental specialist with expertise in environmental exposure assessment.

The two accompanying Perspectives present examples of evaluations that might be performed by an industrial hygienist, emphasizing the opportunities to anticipate hazards. The examples show that even with minimal information, the industrial hygienist can anticipate hazards and devise a reasonable plan of attack prior to visiting a facility. This strategy depends on examining all available information before visiting the site: the industrial process description, the job titles of workers in the facility, the chemicals in use at the facility (this information is often available on material safety data sheets), and the history of the site. Using this information the industrial hygienist develops a list of potential health and safety hazards, perhaps in checklist form to permit recording of observations during the walk-through visit. During the plant visit, unanticipated hazards may of course become apparent as well.

PERSPECTIVE
Assessing an Electronics Manufacturing Facility: The Role of Anticipation

An industrial hygienist is asked to evaluate an electronic manufacturing facility and to focus on occupational hazards. She is told of several operations with potential health impacts that are performed at this workplace. Solvent degreasing (to clean metal pieces) and acid etching may expose workers to chemicals, various machines and cutting tools are in use, and some workers perform repetitive operations with their hands and arms.

Solvents such as trichloroethylene, acetone, and Stoddard solvent, are used extensively for degreasing in industry. Most facilities have a single room in which these materials are used. The prudent industrial hygienist anticipates the potential in this room for spillage, respiratory exposure (perhaps due to inadequate ventilation), and skin contact (perhaps due to improper handling or inadequate personal protective equipment). Further, on-site storage areas for solvents may result in occupational exposure and, over time, contamination of the surrounding environment. The industrial hygienist plans for close inspection of solvent use and storage areas in this facility. Anticipated concerns with acid-etching activities are similar, although occupational and environmental outcomes are likely to be different. The industrial hygienist is concerned with the specific activities associated with acid etching, the storage of used materials and acids on site, and the potential for environmental contamination and effects.

At least some workers perform repetitive operations as part of their jobs, and the industrial hygienist anticipates problems associated with such activities. She arranges to observe the repetitive activities to assess the potential for associated musculoskeletal damage. This is an essential part of her *walk-through* visit to the facility. Similarly, she plans to inspect machine operations for electrical safety, the presence of unguarded cutting edges, risks of crush injury, and so on.

The industrial hygienist will also review administrative procedures that may bear on risk. Are workers trained in safety procedures? Do records of injuries on the job suggest an excess? Are chemical inventories carefully tracked and accounted for?

Finally, the industrial hygienist will anticipate hazards that may not have been mentioned in the initial request, hazards of which the company may be unaware or that personnel may take for granted. Examples include safety hazards such as fire exits, fire potential, and potential for trips and falls. The walk-through visit should include attention to all such hazards.

This facility may be viewed as a prototype of an industrial manufacturing setting. In such a case the industrial hygienist may visit the facility with a checklist of potential or expected hazards. Some of these potential hazards may be present in a specific situation, others may be absent, and still others may be controlled. Only direct inspection (or evaluation, as discussed later in this chapter) can lead to a direct conclusion about control strategies.

PERSPECTIVE
Assessing Leaking Underground Storage Tanks: The Role of Anticipation

An industrial hygienist is asked to evaluate an abandoned gas station in a residential setting where, he is told, gasoline and oil leakage has been noted. Further, he is told that there is housing nearby and associated with this housing is a drinking-water well field that supplies drinking water for some part of the local area. How does he anticipate potential hazards in such a situation?

Although this is not a classical industrial hygiene problem, it is one that more and more industrial hygienists are seeing in their daily work. This facility is no longer in operation and therefore does not have any occupational hazards associated with it; it is now in the realm of *environmental hygiene*. Because of this, the industrial hygienist may wish to contact an environmental consultant for added insight. However, the industrial hygienist can identify numerous anticipated hazards.

From the information given, the most important consideration is the leakage of gasoline and oil from the facility. It is critical, then, to evaluate the magnitude of the leakage and the time over which it has occurred. Underground storage tanks may leak undetected for months or even years. Because there is nearby housing and a superficial well field close to the location, such leakage has the potential for serious environmental consequences. These outcomes may include property damage, well contamination, and even closure of the wells. The industrial hygienist therefore plans to evaluate the extent of the contamination when he reaches the site. Has the contaminant plume migrated off site? If so, how far? Are homes in danger? Is there sufficient hazard to merit evacuation and immediate cleanup? Has the well field been affected? If so, are all wells contaminated? Time is of the essence in addressing these concerns.

Recognition

Once the industrial hygienist has anticipated the potential hazards associated with a facility, the next step is recognition of the actual hazards. The initial recognition phase is usually accomplished during a site visit or **walk-through**, a visual inspection of the facility. The purpose of the walk-through is to gather both qualitative and quantitative information about occupational and environmental hazards. The industrial hygienist reviews the various processes and procedures at the facility, the job categories, the number of workers in each job category and their job descriptions, and any health and safety programs in place at the plant.

She or he identifies hazardous physical, chemical, and biological exposures and also ergonomic, mechanical, and psychological factors affecting the workplace. Visual inspection might reveal such hazards as exposed machinery, pinch points, sharp edges or blades, unsecured tip-over hazards, high noise levels, and the presence of chemicals. A similar review of environmental hazards may be undertaken with an emphasis on off-site emissions.

Another important aspect of the walk-through is recognition of the subpopulations in the facility. For example, certain workers may be exposed to ergonomic hazards because they perform lifting activities or repetitive movements as part of their jobs. A second group may experience few of these hazards but may work in a high-temperature area and be subject to heat stress. A third group may confront neither of these exposures but may work with industrial machinery and thereby be exposed to safety hazards. During a walk-through the industrial hygienist notes these subpopulations and might choose to evaluate hazards differently for different groups.

At the end of the recognition phase the industrial hygienist should have a detailed picture of the manufacturing processes, a listing of the associated hazards, and a plan for evaluating these hazards. This plan is written down and a detailed protocol developed for the next phase, the evaluation of the hazards.

Evaluation

At this point the industrial hygienist has a list of potential hazards in the facility but no quantitative information about the degree of worker exposure. Even if a metalworking facility uses toxic degreasing solvents, for example, the risk of exposure may be minimal with proper storage and handling and appropriate ventilation. The evaluation phase actually begins during the walk-through, and there is a smooth transition from the recognition of hazards to their evaluation.

The evaluation component focuses on quantifying the degree of exposure. As described later in the section on exposure assessment, the hygienist may choose to measure exposures in a part of the workplace (**area sampling**), in the immediate vicinity of individual workers (**personal sampling**), or even in the bodies of individual workers (**biological sampling**).

Population Sampling for Exposure Evaluation   Initially, the hygienist needs to determine which workers' exposures to study. The focus may be on certain workers with specific job titles. For example, degreasers may be monitored for solvent exposure whereas forklift drivers or package handlers may be monitored for ergonomic exposures. In some industries, especially those with widespread or serious hazards, evaluation may involve all employees at a facility or even all workers in a specific industry. Examples include workers in asbestos-related industries or in industries using radiation, such as nuclear power generation. In industrial settings monitoring is sometimes performed at the request of a local union. In this case the union may have specific concerns and may ask for monitoring of all its members. Although the industrial hygienist may offer guidance and suggest monitoring only specific subpopulations, she or he may have to defer to the requirements of the union.

Once the population has been selected, the next choice is the type of population sample to be taken. In small facilities or in facilities where regulation requires it, a *census* sample should be taken. In such a sample all potentially exposed individuals are monitored. However, in larger facilities this can be very expensive, and a statistically representative subsample can characterize the exposure of a larger group. Each individual monitored thus represents a known number of individuals in the same class. For example, if a given airline has 10,000 flight attendants, it may be impractical to monitor each of them for exposure to ozone during flights. The industrial hygienist may choose to monitor a subset of, say, 500 individuals, selected to be statistically representative of the full 10,000. This type of measurement is subject to sampling error because not all the exposed people are monitored. However, techniques are available to estimate the magnitude of this error. The industrial hygienist, working with statistical colleagues, can determine the adequacy of any sample size for characterizing exposures for the entire population.

A third type of population often used is the so-called convenience sample. Often such a sample consists of volunteers or of individuals with a particular complaint. Convenience sampling is subject to bias; there is no reason to believe that volunteers or those with complaints typify all members of the group. This sampling strategy should be avoided. However, a related sampling strategy may have a role. The hygienist may select *worst-case* sampling—sampling those workers at highest risk of exposure or sampling at times when exposures are most likely, or doing both, on the assumption that if these workers' exposures are shown to be well controlled, then the remaining workers are also unlikely to be overexposed.

Exposure Evaluation Instruments   Two general types of instruments are available for measuring environmental exposures: direct reading instruments and sample collection instruments. Direct reading instruments provide real-time measurements of the parameter of interest, and sample collection instruments, as the name implies, collect samples for later analysis.

Direct reading instruments are useful for measuring many physical hazards, such as temperature, noise, and radiation. These instruments typically have a digital readout, and some have the ability to store data collected over a period of time for later downloading. Common examples are digital thermometers to measure temperature, hygrometers to measure relative humidity, noise monitors, and direct reading radiation monitors based on the Geiger counter principle. Such instruments are portable, often weighing less than a kilogram, and are usually enclosed in a rugged carrying case, allowing easy transport to field sites.

Direct reading instruments are also available for measuring levels of many airborne pollutants, including gases, vapors, and particles. For example, organic vapors are measured with photoionization detectors or portable gas chromatographs (*GC-on-a-chip*), and particulate matter with light-scattering devices. Other types of monitors are also available for specific compounds. A limitation in using these instruments is that the character of the airborne pollutant must be known before monitoring can be carried out. In industrial hygiene applications, this often poses little difficulty as, typically, one specific compound is of concern or a particle of a specific size is produced by the process under investigation.

Sample collection instruments are used instead of direct reading instruments when multiple airborne pollutants are present or further analysis on samples is desirable. In this case the instrument collects a sample of air—with whatever contaminants are in it—on an absorbing medium. The absorbing medium is then taken to the laboratory and the amounts of the compounds of interest are determined.

These air delivery/absorber systems are generally one of two types, active or passive. In the *active sampling devices*, air is drawn through the absorbing medium by an electric pump. The amount of air drawn through is controlled by the pump and can be varied. The total volume of air sampled can be calculated by multiplying the air flow rate by the duration of sampling, and when the mass of contaminant on the sampling medium is later quantified, its concentration in air, in units of mass per volume, can be readily calculated. The sampling time period can be shortened by increasing the pump flow rate, thereby delivering the same amount of air in less time—a useful maneuver if exposure durations occur over short periods of time or are highly variable.

There are distinct disadvantages to **active sampling**. Chief among these is the presence of the pump, which requires electricity to run and is often bulky. These drawbacks make such devices unsuited to many kinds of personal sampling. Often, active sampling is limited to area sampling, which is by its very nature not what the individual worker experiences as contaminant exposure. Two active sampling devices are shown in Figure 4.1. The sampling devices themselves (for ozone and particulate matter) and the pump are located inside the box at the bottom of the apparatus. The vertical pipe with the metal cone on top is a device designed to collect particles that are inhalable deeply into the lung. The

**FIGURE 4.1   Air Pollution Sampling Apparatus for Ozone
and Particulate Matter**

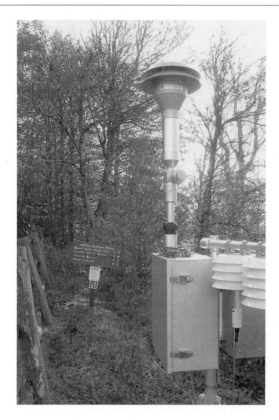

device includes a size-selection sampling head designed to allow particles smaller than a certain diameter to pass through to the particulate sampler. Ozone is sampled off the same air stream.

Passive sampling devices require an absorbing medium that removes the compound of interest from the air by reaction or absorption. This process takes advantage of the concentration gradient between the air to be sampled and the surface of the absorbing medium. Because of this concentration gradient, the compound of interest diffuses from the air to the surface of the absorbing medium, from which it is then removed. Analysis of the concentration is accomplished in a manner similar to active sampling analysis; the amount found in the absorbing medium is determined in the laboratory and the amount of air delivered to the surface is computed using Fick's Law of Diffusion. The concentration in the air during the sampling period is then calculated by dividing the amount of material on the absorbing medium, determined in the laboratory, by the volume of air passed through the system to the absorber. Many industrial hygiene applications make use of this type of system.

Passive devices have the advantage of not requiring a pump but the disadvantage of low sampling rates, often 1,000-fold slower than active samplers. Thus the amount of material sampled in a given time is also substantially lower. However, in occupational settings concentrations are often sufficiently high to allow use of passive devices and still achieve excellent results. Further, improved laboratory analytical procedures have substantially reduced the amount of material that must be collected to yield accurate quantification of many compounds of interest. When available and of sufficient precision and accuracy, passive sampling devices can be the method of choice. The industrial hygienist developing a monitoring system should be cautious, however. Passive devices do not exist for every contaminant of interest. In particular, passive devices for particulate matter are not yet of sufficient precision and accuracy to merit their use in typical occupational settings, although this too is changing with improved technology.

Biological monitoring, discussed later in this chapter, is of interest to the industrial hygienist as well. In such monitoring programs, biological samples, such as hair, saliva, blood, or urine, are collected from potentially exposed individuals and analyzed for either the compound of interest or a metabolite of that compound. In circumstances where such techniques exist, they often offer the best solution for a monitoring program.

Control

The final component of the industrial hygiene paradigm is control of the hazards. In public health terms this corresponds to *primary prevention*, a central goal. Industrial hygienists use several approaches to modify the workplace environment: substitution, isolation, and ventilation. **Substitution** involves replacing a hazardous material or process with a less hazardous one. For example, benzene (a bone marrow toxin) might be replaced by toluene. **Isolation** involves containing or limiting access to the hazardous process. For example, a metal cage may be placed around moving parts to reduce the likelihood of clothes catching on the parts and subsequent injuries to a worker. For certain hazards, most notably chemical and heat-related hazards, **ventilation** offers a viable control strategy. For example, the introduction of fresh air, local exhaust ventilation, or cool air may significantly alter the risk associated with exposure to these hazards.

Protective devices are often used to control safety hazards. For example, a worker operating a cutting machine may need to push two buttons, one

FIGURE 4.2   Personal Protective Equipment for
                        Solvent Exposure

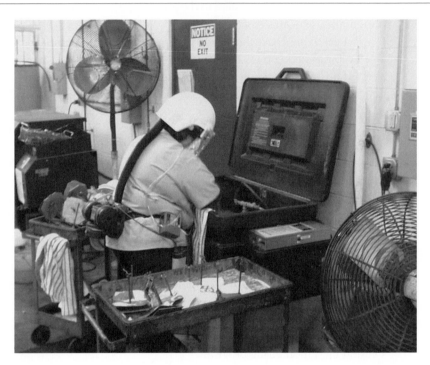

Source: Courtesy of Phillip L. Williams, Dean and Professor, University of Georgia College of
Public Health.

with each hand, to initiate a cut; this guarantees that his or her hand cannot be
in the cutting zone when the machine functions. Similarly, a power cutoff may
be installed, automatically cutting the electrical supply to a machine when it is
entered for maintenance. This prevents unintentional startup of the machine,
which would endanger maintenance workers. The so-called lockout/tagout procedures are an example of this strategy; a worker places a lock on the machinery
in such a fashion that it cannot be started until he or she removes that lock,
and the lock is located so as to keep the worker safely away from the hazardous
part of the machine. **Personal protective equipment**, such as respirators,
gloves, safety glasses, hardhats, safety harnesses, and steel-toed boots may also be
recommended, although this approach is less preferable than the environmental
changes described previously. Figure 4.2 shows an example of personal protective
equipment in use. Working at a solvent degreasing tank, the worker is subjected

to elevated levels of vapor exposures if not protected. The worker wears personal protective equipment consisting of a face shield to protect the face from splashed solvent and a fresh air supply (delivered by a pump, on the worker's back) and a plastic hose) to dilute the solvent vapors being breathed. The exposure is monitored using the pump and the collection device mounted on the worker's hip.

Administrative strategies, such as rotating workers through dangerous jobs to limit any individual's aggregate exposures (an approach used, for example, with radiation workers) sometimes have a role as well. (These strategies, and the philosophy that guides choosing among them, are discussed in further detail in Chapter Twenty-Six.)

EXPOSURE SCIENCE

Industrial hygiene focuses on workplace exposures. Although such exposures are often quite high and therefore of great scientific and public health interest, they affect only a subset of the population. Environmental health scientists are also concerned about the community as a whole. The study of exposures in nonoccupational settings grew out the industrial hygiene experience. As early as the 1950s, environmental health scientists began turning their attention from high-level workplace exposures to lower-level community exposures to the same chemicals. These efforts gave rise to the field of exposure science.

Exposure science focuses on quantifying the contaminant exposures people experience as they go about their daily activities, evaluating factors that influence these exposures, and exploring new and innovative measurement methods designed to quantify exposure and effect. **Exposure assessment**, one aspect of exposure science, is concerned with the quantification of exposures in both occupational and environmental settings. In performing this quantification, assessors attend to such key concepts as concentration, exposure, and dose (as discussed in the related Perspective).

Magnitude, Frequency, and Duration of Exposure

An important aspect of exposure is its time course, sometimes referred to as the *exposure profile*. Intuitively, one might suppose that a brief but high-level exposure to a contaminant would have a health impact different than the health impact of exposure to a modest concentration over an entire work shift, even assuming equivalent total exposures. For example, one worker may be welding for 15 minutes in an enclosed space and be subjected to a concentration of metal fumes of 40 mg/m^3, receiving an exposure of $(40 \text{ mg/m}^3)(0.25 \text{ h}) = 10 \text{ mg/m}^3 \cdot \text{h}$. After

PERSPECTIVE
Understanding Concentration, Exposure, and Dose

A starting point for exposure assessment is to ask how much of a contaminant is found in environmental media—what, for example, is the level of lead in workplace air or the level of pesticides in food? These parameters are usually measured as **concentration**, expressed in units of mass per mass or mass per volume. Air contaminants such as particulate matter, for example, may be quantified in units of micrograms (μg) of contaminant per cubic meter of air (m^3), that is, $\mu g/m^3$. In measuring air concentrations of gases, the units often express a mixing ratio—the fraction of total air that is made up of the contaminant gas, usually expressed as parts per million (ppm) or parts per billion (ppb.) For example, suppose a carbon monoxide (CO) level is measured at 1 ppm. This means that in a given volume of air divided into 1 million portions of equal volume, 1 part would be CO and the remaining 999,999 parts something else. In 1 cubic meter (m^3) of air, 1 cubic centimeter (cm^3, or cc) would be CO (and nitrogen and oxygen would represent about 780,000 cc and 210,000 cc, respectively). Of course, all of these parts are mixed together; the CO is not all contained in a single cc, instead it is dispersed throughout the entire m^3. Although 1 ppm sounds like a very low concentration, for many air contaminants it is sufficient to threaten health.

Concentrations are measured similarly in other environmental media, including water, soil, and food. Contaminant concentrations in water are expressed in terms of either micrograms of contaminant per cubic meter of water or micrograms of contaminant per gram of water. The first is similar to air concentrations, and the second is analogous to the mixing ratio in air (because 1 μg of contaminant per gram of water is a ratio of masses, corresponding to 1 ppm). Similarly, soil or food, both being solids, can be described using either unit.

But concentration is different from exposure; the mere presence of a contaminant at some concentration does not necessarily imply that people will be exposed. **Exposure** is defined as contact between the environmental contaminant and a boundary of the subject of interest. Even though ecological exposure assessment is an important area, this discussion focuses on human exposures. Thus the boundaries of interest are tissues such as skin, alveolar surfaces, and the gastrointestinal tract lining, which separate the "inside" of a human receptor from the "outside," the rest of the environment. Exposure requires the simultaneous presence of a contaminant in the environment and a human receptor in the same environment.

If a person is indeed exposed, the exposure is a function of the concentration and of time. Therefore exposures are expressed in units of concentration multiplied by time, such as micrograms per cubic meter multiplied by hours: $(\mu g/m^3)$(hours). When a contaminant is ingested, the temporal component appears in the computation as the number of meals or the total mass taken into the body during, say, a twenty-four-hour period.

Just as concentration is different from exposure, exposure is different from dose. The **dose** is the amount of contaminant that crosses the epithelial barrier and gets inside the body. Suppose a person is exposed to an air contaminant concentration of 100 $\mu g/m^3$ for a period of 10 hours, and suppose that inhalation is the only significant exposure route; ingestion and dermal contact do not contribute. At this concentration (100 $\mu g/m^3$), the exposure is (100 $\mu g/m^3$)(10 hours) = 1,000 ($\mu g/m^3$)(hours) of exposure. What is the dose? Here additional information is needed. The dose is delivered to the lungs through breathing. A typical breathing rate (depending on the person's size, level of activity, and other factors) might be 1,100 cc/breath and 15 breaths per minute, or approximately 1 m^3 of air per hour. During a 10-hour period, this person would breathe in 10 m^3 of air. The dose is the product of the concentration, the **duration of exposure**, and the rate at which the material reaches the appropriate boundary:

$$Dose = 100 \; \frac{\mu g \; (contaminant)}{m^3(air)} \times 10 \; (hours \; of \; exposure) \times \frac{1 \; m^3(air \; breathed)}{Hour \; of \; exposure}$$

$$Dose = 1,000 \; \mu g \; (contaminant \; breathed)$$

In this case, 1,000 μg of contaminant has reached the body boundary. This is the potential dose. Assuming all the material crosses the boundary, this is the actual dose. Note that the units correspond to the amount of mass delivered across the boundary. There is no explicit time dimension.

From an exposure assessment point of view, evaluators often stop at the potential dose, that is, the amount of material that reaches the body boundary over a fixed period of time. However, absorption is typically incomplete, and the **biologically relevant dose** or **target organ dose** may be lower than the entire potential dose. Toxicologists, physicians, and other health scientists may focus specifically on the actual dose absorbed as they study the relationship between exposure and health effects (see Chapter Two).

Suppose a worker is required to enter a tank that was formerly filled with a volatile solvent. The enclosed space is saturated with the solvent vapor. What is the concentration in the tank, the worker's exposure, and her dose?

The concentration in the tank is relatively simple to understand; it is the saturation vapor pressure of the organic solvent. This can be readily measured using appropriate instrumentation.

What is the worker's exposure? This is a more difficult question. In an occupational setting such as the one described, the worker would doubtless be fitted with a respirator that supplied air from outside the tank, as it would be much too dangerous to send an individual into such an enclosed space without such a

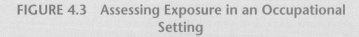

FIGURE 4.3   Assessing Exposure in an Occupational
Setting

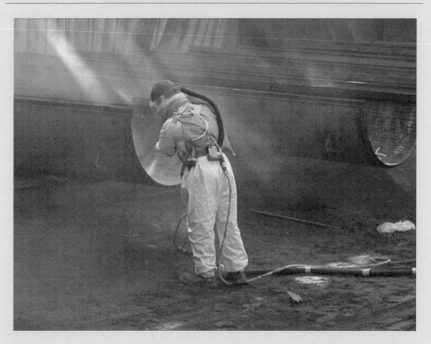

Source: Courtesy of Phillip L. Williams, Dean and Professor, University of Georgia College of Public Health.

welding, he goes on to different activities in a different part of the facility in which he experiences no further exposure to welding fumes. His coworker, working in the welding area but not exposed directly to the fumes, remains for the entire 8-hour shift. Measurement of metal fume concentrations over the course of the day in the coworker's location shows a concentration of 1.25 mg/m^3. The worker in this location receives an identical total exposure $[(1.25 \text{ mg/m}^3)(8 \text{ h}) = 10 \text{ mg/m}^3 \cdot \text{h}]$, but the exposure profile is different.

This issue is important because some contaminants are relatively readily metabolized or cleared at low levels of exposure but toxic at higher levels of exposure. In other words, the **dose rate** may affect the health outcome. To account for such differences, exposure assessors focus on the **magnitude**, **frequency**, and **duration of exposure**, asking such questions as these: What is the **peak** device. Under these conditions (assuming a functioning respirator), her **inhalation exposure** would be zero since no solvent vapor would reach her lung epithelium. However, she might receive an exposure to her skin, and dermal exposure may be an important route for the substance of concern. It is important to consider all routes and attempt to identify all pathways to exposure.

And what is her dose? The definition of dose requires an understanding of how much material actually crosses the boundary and gets inside the body. If the worker did not wear a respirator, one could infer the inhaled dose by knowing the concentration and breathing rate. To estimate dose, one would need information regarding the efficiency of transfer across the alveolar membranes in the lungs. Similarly, calculating the dermal dose would combine information about the concentration in the air, the skin area exposed, and the efficiency of skin absorption. To combine these routes, a biomarker of exposure—say, blood levels of the solvent or urinary levels of its metabolite—would provide an integrated estimate of dose.

Figure 4.3 shows an example of exposure measurement. Here a worker is using a sandblaster to remove silica-containing material from a pipe. Because inhalation of silica can cause severe respiratory problems, the worker is using an airline respirator that supplies fresh air through the pipe going off to the right; the worker sustains no exposure to silica dust. However, the worker is still exposed to potentially hazardous noise from the sandblaster. To test for this hazard, the worker wears a noise monitor (the small rectangular box attached near the small of the worker's back).

concentration experienced during the monitoring period? Does it differ significantly from the mean concentration? How frequently are high concentration peaks found? Are the concentrations relatively stable, or is there variability from minute to minute or hour to hour? Do the peaks recur regularly or episodically? What is the duration of the exposure? Is it short followed by no exposure, or does it occur at moderate levels for a long period? Such information can prove invaluable in addressing potential effects and control strategies.

Exposure scientists distinguish acute exposures from chronic exposures. **Acute exposures** are brief, and when they occur at high levels, poisoning or other acute responses may follow. **Chronic exposures** occur over months, years, or even decades. Chronic exposures at low levels may manifest nonacute health outcomes such as carcinogenesis, long-term lung damage, or similar effects. Intermediate between these two are **subchronic exposures**, which may occur over intermediate time scales, often weeks or months, and also may be episodic and recurring.

Routes and Pathways of Exposure

As explained in Chapter Two, environmental contaminants enter the body through one of three principal routes of exposure: **inhalation**, **ingestion**, and **dermal**. (Other routes, such as injection or ocular absorption, may be important in some circumstances, and transplacental transfer is important with regard to fetal exposures.) It is important to distinguish between these routes of exposure and the **exposure pathway**, or the path by which the contaminant moves from a source to a human receptor. For example, sulfur dioxide exposure may result from distinct pathways. It may be generated through the combustion of sulfur-containing coal, followed by the concomitant release of this gas from the combustion facility and by advection and dispersion in the air. Alternatively, an industrial process might use sulfurous acid, with the concomitant release of sulfur dioxide at an individual workstation, exposing the worker directly. These two pathways differ substantially and require entirely different control strategies to reduce exposure.

Exposure Assessment Methods

Just as there is a continuum of a kind from concentration to exposure to dose (see the previous Perspective), there is a corresponding continuum of exposure assessment methods. The ideal method would quantify the amount of contaminant reaching the target organ of interest in each individual of interest, but this is of course not feasible in most cases. Four broad categories of exposure assessment methods can be identified: imputing or modeling exposures, measuring environmental exposures, measuring personal exposures, and measuring biomarkers. In general these methods become increasingly expensive, and increasingly accurate, as one moves along the continuum. In addition we look at aggregate and cumulative exposure assessment in this section.

Imputing or Modeling Exposures   To impute exposures, scientists use **indirect exposure assessment** methods that either forgo direct measurements of the exposures of interest or employ partial data. For example, in a study of air pollution exposure, researchers might identify various microenvironments thought to have relatively homogeneous concentrations and measure those concentrations. Research subjects could record the amount of time spent in each of the microenvironments (or the researchers could estimate this). The scientists would them multiply the concentrations by the amount of time spent in each microenvironment and sum the results for an estimate of each subject's overall exposure. For other routes of exposure, a similar approach can be used. For example, for ingestion, concentrations of selected contaminants can be measured in each of many foods. A research subject would then record types and amounts of foods eaten, using a food diary. Summing over all the foods eaten gives the dietary exposure.

An alternative strategy, called **exposure scenarios**, does without direct measurement. In this strategy, an activity pattern for an individual is assumed, perhaps based on observational data about population activity patterns. Available monitoring data for each activity and location can then be combined with activity data to model estimates of individual exposures. This approach is less expensive to implement because no individuals actually have their exposures measured and no specific activities are recorded. Exposure scenarios are used extensively in risk assessment.

A special case of indirect exposure assessment is the **job-exposure matrix**, as described in Chapter Three. Suppose an occupational epidemiologist wants to study the health effects of silica exposure in a working population, using a retrospective cohort approach. Consulting old employment records, the epidemiologist might identify ten job categories, each with characteristic tasks, and fifteen workplace zones, each with its own silica concentration. (Historical industrial hygiene monitoring results may be of use in reconstructing this information and in estimating concentrations in each zone of the workplace.) The epidemiologist then constructs a job-exposure matrix, with an exposure level assigned retrospectively to each worker, based on job assignment and location in the workplace. If the workplace has changed over time, as is typical, then the epidemiologist creates a job-time-exposure matrix, classifying each worker's exposure according to job title, location in the plant, and calendar year. In this fashion the epidemiologist can impute an exposure profile to each member of the cohort. This method is often the only available way to assess exposures in retrospective epidemiological studies. However, it is painstaking and time consuming, and records are not always accurate or complete enough to support accurate exposure assessment.

Although less satisfying than direct exposure assessment, these indirect approaches are often substantially easier to implement, and large populations can be studied more effectively in this manner. Further, for retrospective studies—studies for which it is impossible to take measurements—indirect approaches are the only methods available.

Measuring Environmental Exposures   Direct exposure assessment methods may occur at an area level or an individual level, as described earlier in the context of industrial hygiene. An example of environmental measurement is air pollution monitoring, which is carried out in most major cities. Not only does ongoing measurement of air pollutants (ozone, NOx [nitrogen oxides], SOx [sulfur oxides], and particulate matter) help monitor compliance with regulations, it also provides exposure information that can be used to warn the public of dangerous exceedances, to monitor the success of interventions, and to support health research.

Measuring Personal Exposures   Personal exposure assessment involves outfitting an individual with a monitor that measures exposures during daily activities, exactly as is done in the workplace. This is most easily visualized for airborne contaminants. In this case an air monitor collects a sample of the air breathed by the individual over a period of time and that air sample is analyzed for the contaminant of interest, either on a real-time or time-integrated basis. Similar monitors may be envisioned for exposures occurring via the ingestion or dermal pathways as well, using, for example, duplicate diet sampling or absorbent patches worn on the skin, respectively. With such direct methods, actual exposures experienced by an individual can be observed. This is a major strength in accessing exposure and is generally desirable. However, portable monitors may not exist for the particular contaminant under investigation, or using the monitor may unduly influence the activity patterns of the individual, with the result that the activities monitored are not her or his typical ones.

Aggregate and Cumulative Exposure Assessment   The forgoing discussion has implicitly focused on the simplest of exposure scenarios, namely, the investigation of a single contaminant, nominally found in a single environmental medium. The Food Quality Protection Act of 1996 has expanded this one-at-a-time approach to exposure assessment by introducing the new concepts of aggregate exposure and cumulative exposure (also see Chapters Eight and Twenty-Nine). In **aggregate exposure** scientists consider *simultaneously* all routes and pathways that may have been involved in an exposure to a single compound. Consider the case of an agricultural worker. This worker may receive exposure to a certain pesticide through both inhalation and dermal exposure at his workplace. This may be compounded by additional exposure he receives through ingestion of food containing the same pesticide as a residue from agricultural processes. Further, there may be residual contamination of clothing that he wore during his work and that he has brought back to his home. Consideration of only one route and pathway, such as inhalation during agricultural spraying, underestimates his total exposure, perhaps even substantially. Consideration of all routes and pathways simultaneously—aggregate exposure assessment—is necessary in order to quantify the hazard properly. Most modern environmental assessments look at aggregate exposure because each of the multiple routes and pathways may contribute significantly to the total exposure. This may be less true in occupational settings where exposure through a single route and pathway is assumed to dominate. However, this assumption can only be verified through aggregate exposure assessment.

Even more complexity can be envisioned. This is encompassed in the definition of **cumulative exposure** as aggregate exposure to a series of compounds (or nonchemical exposures) that affect health through similar mechanisms. The standard example of cumulative exposure focuses on exposure to organophosphorus pesticides such as chlorpyrifos, malathion, and diazinon, which have a common mechanism of toxicity, namely acetylcholinesterase inhibition. Acetylcholine is a messenger molecule that aids in the transmission of nerve signals. In a healthy nerve system, acetylcholine passes across the nerve synapse, thereby transmitting a nerve impulse, and is then inactivated by an enzyme called acetylcholinesterase. Organophosphorus pesticides (OPs) interfere with this process by inhibiting the action of acetylcholinesterase, resulting in continued firing of the neuron. All OPs operate by this mechanism and thus are all to some degree toxic. In order to understand the impact of exposure to this type of toxic compound, one must consider exposure not just to a single OP, for example, chlorpyrifos, but rather to all pesticides operating through acetylcholinesterase inhibition. This is a new way of thinking about exposure and requires measurement of either all of the compounds simultaneously, or measurement of some effect, such as acetylcholinesterase inhibition, that integrates over all exposures. As can be easily envisioned, this is a complex process. It can be even more complex when nonchemical exposures, such as stress or malnutrition, operate, perhaps compounding the effects of chemical exposures.

This leads us to the next stage of exposure assessment. How can exposure scientists measure the exposure to a number of compounds, possibly related, at the same time? Is it best to do this by measuring multiple environmental media for multiple chemical compounds, or is there a more parsimonious and useful approach?

Measuring Biomarkers Exposure to environmental contaminants requires the simultaneous presence of a contaminant concentration and a human subject to receive the exposure. The methods described so far assume that exposure occurs if these two conditions exist. However, the only way to verify this assumption is to measure contaminant levels in humans themselves. This is what exposure assessors do when they use **biological markers** (sometimes referred to as **biomarkers**) of exposure. They sample biological material, such as exhaled breath, urine, blood, feces, or hair, for contaminants of interest. These samples may be analyzed for the contaminant itself, called the *parent compound*, a metabolite, or a biological response known to reflect exposure. For example, blood lead levels are measured to quantify lead exposure, levels of urinary cotinine (a metabolite of nicotine) are measured to quantify exposure to environmental tobacco smoke, and blood carboxyhemoglobin levels are measured to quantify exposure to carbon monoxide. Pesticide exposure offers another example. Blood samples can be analyzed for organochlorine pesticide parent compounds to ascertain exposure to this class of compound. For organophosphorus pesticides, the direct parent compound can be determined in serum or, alternatively, metabolites produced through hydrolysis, such as dialkyl phosphates, can be used to infer the magnitude and timing of exposures.

PERSPECTIVE
Assessing Exposure to Carbon Monoxide

Carbon monoxide (CO) is a colorless, odorless gas that competes with oxygen for binding sites on hemoglobin. CO binds avidly with hemoglobin, effectively disabling the hemoglobin's oxygen-carrying capacity. If enough CO is inhaled, death can ensue due to asphyxiation.

Although some CO is produced endogenously, environmental exposure to CO occurs through a single route, inhalation. The pathways are numerous but all involve incomplete combustion; CO is produced when too little oxygen is present to permit complete conversion of hydrocarbons and oxygen to carbon dioxide and water. Specific pathways often associated with the production of CO leading to CO poisoning are improperly vented combustion appliances (such as gas heaters), improperly vented gasoline engines (such as automobiles running in closed spaces), and cigarette smoke.

Exposure to CO is easily measured in two ways. Relatively simple air samplers are available that sample for CO either actively or passively. In active mode, real-time analyzers can give second-by-second readings of CO concentration. Exposure is determined by noting the amount of time spent in the location being measured. An alternative strategy is to use a biological marker of exposure, the blood concentration of carboxyhemoglobin, the CO adduct to hemoglobin. Unexposed people typically have about 1 percent carboxyhemoglobin in their blood due to endogenous production of CO. Smokers carry a higher percentage, as high as 4 percent, due to inhalation of CO in cigarette smoke. Symptoms such as headaches are observed in most people with levels above about 10 percent, and levels above 40 percent are life threatening.

Exposure as defined previously does not tell the full story with respect to carbon monoxide's effects. People in industrial societies are exposed to modest levels

Biomarkers of exposure have important advantages. Detection of a biomarker of exposure proves that absorption of the compound measured (or its parent in the case of metabolites) has occurred—a conclusion that environmental measurements cannot confirm. Further, biomarkers account for bioavailability. A compound may enter the body through, for example, ingestion, but if transfer across the gut epithelium is inefficient, the biological significance of exposure is unclear. Biomarkers overcome this difficulty; in order for the compound to be measured in the biological medium, it must have crossed the boundary, signaling that the exposure was "effective" in delivering a dose to the body. Biomarkers integrate over all routes of exposure. For these reasons, Sexton, Needham, and Pirkle (2004) have referred to **biomonitoring** as the "gold standard" for exposure assessment.

of CO. Regulations are in place to ensure that these levels are kept low enough to maintain carboxyhemoglobin levels below a threshold at which health could be affected. However, many scenarios could give rise to the same cumulative exposure. Exposure to 1 ppm of CO for 10,000 hours would give the same exposure as 10,000 ppm of CO for one hour. However, these two scenarios would yield completely different effects. The long-term, low-level would cause no problems at all, while the brief, intense exposure would surely result in death. In addition, the previous discussion does not address other more subtle characteristics of exposure and its effects. For example, the establishment of equilibrium between carboxy-hemoglobin and ambient CO is not instantaneous, nor are the effects. There is a kinetic component associated with the gas being taken up through inhalation, crossing the lung epithelial barrier, and then binding with hemoglobin. Moreover, once ambient concentrations are reduced, there is a similar kinetic component associated with decarboxylation of hemoglobin, and elimination of CO through exhalation. Thus although effects may be delayed while concentrations are increasing, the adverse impact of CO may persist for some time after the exposure ends.

This example illustrates the importance of considering the magnitude and duration of the exposure in estimating effects. Further, it emphasizes the importance of understanding the toxicology of the effect under investigation. CO binds reversibly to hemoglobin, albeit with a very long half-life. If only a little CO is around, a person will still have plenty of hemoglobin left to bind oxygen and carry it to the cells. However, if there is a lot of CO around and it displaces oxygen from hemoglobin, then a person may not have enough oxygen being delivered to the cells and asphyxiation can result. The effect of noninstantaneous uptake and release of CO from hemoglobin complicates the challenge of proper exposure assessment further.

The Centers for Disease Control and Prevention have taken a leadership role in developing and implementing biomarker monitoring in the exposure assessment and exposure science field (www.cdc.gov/biomonitoring).

The use of biomarkers of exposure is not above criticism, however. The primary strength of biomarkers as an exposure assessment tool, namely their ability to integrate over all routes and pathways, is also a major shortcoming. For example, once a molecule, say a pesticide, is in the body and is metabolized, its source is no longer identifiable. One cannot determine if the exposure came from inhalation of airborne pesticide, dermal contact with sprays, or through ingestion of small amounts found in the food supply. As described in Chapter Thirty, regulatory responsibility in the United States is partitioned among different agencies—the Food and Drug Administration, the Department of Agriculture, the Consumer Product Safety Commission, the Environmental Protection Agency, and others—that tend to focus on one or another route or pathway. Because biomarkers integrate over multiple sources, regulators are hard-pressed to use them to control exposure.

There are other problems associated with biomarker use in exposure assessment. Often the biomarker of exposure is a metabolite of the parent compound; this is true of OPs for example. This can result in two problems. First, multiple compounds can yield the same biomarker. For OPs, dialkyl phosphates of varying structures can result from exposures to many different OP parent compounds that have the same chemical moiety that is being measured. This result precludes distinguishing among exposures to different OPs that give rise to the same metabolite.

An additional and somewhat related problem occurs when individuals display different abilities to metabolize a toxic substance, due to, for example, a genetic polymorphism. Consider two individuals exposed to identical concentrations of a parent pesticide. Further, suppose that the parent pesticide is more toxic than the metabolite used as the biomarker of exposure. And suppose that one person is an average metabolizer of the pesticide and the other person is a slow metabolizer of the pesticide. Biomarker levels in these two people would likely be quite different, despite identical exposures, resulting in misclassification of exposure in at least one of the people. Further, because we are assuming that the parent molecule is more toxic than the biomarker, the second person, despite having a lower level of the biomarker in the urine, likely would experience a greater effect—a misclassification of risk to the individual as well.

Despite these cautions, biomonitoring and the use of biomarkers of exposure are likely to increase in the future. The information provided by biomonitoring is invaluable. Further, development of new biomarkers of exposure is advancing rapidly, with new, more accurate measures appearing in the literature every month. Current research suggests that panels of biomarkers, measuring multiple markers at once, may be able to overcome many of the shortcomings listed here while giving new and powerful insight into mechanisms of toxicity and control strategies for exposure (Ryan and others, 2007).

Ingestion and Skin Absorption: Challenges for Exposure Assessment

Much of exposure assessment developed around inhalation exposures. However, the two remaining principal routes of entry, ingestion and skin absorption, are important in many circumstances and also pose special challenges for exposure assessment.

One approach to assessing **ingestion exposure** is to collect duplicate portions of food as eaten and then analyze the food for contaminant levels— an approach known as a **duplicate diet study**. Typically, a researcher would homogenize all of the food eaten, creating a single sample; weigh the sample to determine total mass; and analyze an aliquot for contaminant content and concentration. Multiplication of the concentration in the food by the amount eaten yields the total amount of material ingested during the time period—the exposure. (This is not yet a dose because it only measures what was ingested, not what was absorbed across the epithelial layer, the gut lining.) This straightforward method is an example of the direct method of exposure assessment described earlier.

In a second approach to ingestion exposure assessment, people are asked to keep dietary diaries. Simultaneously, the researcher purchases various foods at local grocery stores and brings them back to the laboratory for analysis. A data set is then compiled listing each type of food and its contaminant concentration. The food diary data set can then be combined with the concentration data set to determine the amount of contaminant ingested by each study participant. Because the food actually eaten by the person is never measured, this method is an example of indirect exposure assessment. This technique is quite useful in that food diaries are much easier to administer than duplicate diet studies and thus can be implemented on a large scale. Further, fewer food samples have to be analyzed as once all individual food items have been assessed, no further analysis is needed. The principal disadvantage of this method is that the individual food items consumed by the participants are not analyzed. If the concentrations in those items differ from those purchased at the grocery store, this causes error in the exposure estimate proportional to the variability in pollutant concentrations in various food items.

Dermal exposures are quite difficult to study. In one method, people are asked to wear a skin patch that absorbs the material of interest, such as pesticides, and to carry out activities while exposed to air containing the pesticides. This may occur for research purposes in a laboratory setting, with known concentrations of pesticide in the air, or it may occur in actual exposure situations. Either way, the patches are removed from the person's skin following exposure and analyzed for pesticide concentration. Knowing the size of the patch relative to the total exposed skin surface, one can estimate overall skin exposure. A second method uses cadaver skin. Pesticide is placed on one side of the cadaver skin and the penetration of the material through the skin surface is measured.

Each of these techniques has limitations. Experimental use of the patch method is contrived and offers little insight about real-world exposures. Use of the patch in the real world, however, suffers in that many exposures are below the detection limit of the analytical process yet still will incur the large costs associated with analysis. Although of interest, the cadaver skin method measures dose and provides little information on exposure. Further, cadaver skin may not act the same way living skin does with a given exposure level, calling into question the dose determination.

SUMMARY

Industrial hygiene, the anticipation, recognition, evaluation, and control of workplace hazards, presents a paradigm for the study of the more general discipline of environmental exposure assessment. Many of the tools of industrial hygiene are easily transferable to environmental exposure science, but this science requires some new tools as well. The four-step paradigm must be integrated into the community setting. Sampling strategies, compliance with monitoring protocols, and field implementation are often more difficult in community exposure assessment studies than in workplace studies, and they call for statistical sampling techniques more commonly found in epidemiological studies. Exposure science is a rapidly growing area, ripe for contributions from professionals in many areas of environmental health. Research and professional practice will continue to grow for the foreseeable future.

KEY TERMS

active sampling

acute exposure

administrative strategies

aggregate exposure

anticipation

area sampling

biological markers

biomarkers

biological monitoring

biomonitoring

biological sampling

biologically relevant dose

chemical hazard

chronic exposure

concentration

control

cumulative exposure

dermal exposure

direct reading instruments

dose

dose rate

duplicate diet study

duration of exposure

environmental hazard

evaluation

exposures

exposure assessment

exposure pathway

exposure scenarios

exposure science

frequency of exposure

health hazard

indirect exposure
   assessment

industrial hygiene

ingestion exposure

inhalation exposure

isolation

job-exposure matrix

magnitude of exposure

modeling of exposures

passive sampling

peak concentration

personal protective
   equipment

personal sampling

physical hazard

protective devices

recognition

safety engineering

safety hazard

sample collection
   instruments

subchronic exposure

substitution

target organ dose

ventilation

walk-through

DISCUSSION QUESTIONS

1. The challenges exposure assessment faces in the community setting are different from those found in the workplace setting. What are these differences?
2. Exposure assessment is essential to environmental epidemiology. Do you agree or disagree with this statement? Explain your answer.
3. Biomarkers of exposure offer many advantages over environmental sampling. What are these advantages?
4. Biomarkers of exposure may function very differently in the age of genomics. Do a literature search on the role of genetic polymorphisms in interpreting biomarker data, and summarize your findings.

REFERENCES

Koren, H., and Bisesi, M. *Handbook of Environmental Health and Safety: Principles and Practices*. 2 vols. (3rd ed.) Boca Raton, Fla.: CRC Press, 1996.

Plog, B. A., Niland, J., and Quinlan, P. J. *Fundamentals of Industrial Hygiene*. (4th ed.) Itasca, Ill.: National Safety Council, 1996.

Ryan, P. B., and others. "Using Biomarkers to Inform Cumulative Risk Assessment." *Environmental Health Perspectives*, 2007, *115*(5), 833–840.

Sexton, K., Needham, L. L., and Pirkle, J. L. "Human Biomonitoring of Environmental Chemicals: Measuring Chemicals in Human Tissues Is the 'Gold Standard' for Assessing People's Exposure to Pollution." *American Scientist*, 2004, *94*(1), 38–45.

FOR FURTHER INFORMATION

Books and Articles

Standard References in Industrial Hygiene

In addition to Koren and Bisesi (1996) and Plog, Niland, and Quinlan (1996), see

Harris, R. L. (ed.). *Patty's Industrial Hygiene*. 4 vols. (5th ed.) Hoboken, N.J.: Wiley, 2001.

Overviews of Exposure Assessment

Lioy, P. "Assessing Total Human Exposure to Contaminants." *Environmental Science & Technology, 1990,* 24, 938–945.

Zartarian, V. G., Ott, W. R., and Duan, N. "A Quantitative Definition of Exposure and Related Concepts." *Journal of Exposure Analysis and Environmental Epidemiology,* 1997, *7*(4), 411–437.

Reviews of Exposure Biomarkers

Godschalk, R. W., Van Schooten, F. J., and Bartsch, H. "A Critical Evaluation of DNA Adducts as Biological Markers for Human Exposure to Polycyclic Aromatic Compounds." *Journal of Biochemistry and Molecular Biology,* 2003, *36*(1), 1–11.

Metcalf, S. W., and Orloff, K. G. "Biomarkers of Exposure in Community Settings." *Journal of Toxicology and Environmental Health, Part A,* 2004, *67*(8–10), 715–726.

Wessels, D., Barr D. B., and Mendola, P. "Use of Biomarkers to Indicate Exposure of Children to Organophosphate Pesticides: Implications for a Longitudinal Study of Children's Environmental Health." *Environmental Health Perspectives,* 2003, *111*(16), 1939–1946.

Wilson, S. H., and Suk, W.A. (eds.). *Biomarkers of Environmentally Associated Disease: Technologies, Concepts, and Perspectives.* Boca Raton, Fla.: Lewis, 2002.

In addition the Centers for Disease Control and Prevention maintains a Web site with useful information on biomonitoring, at http://www.cdc.gov/biomonitoring.

Reviews of Job-Exposure Matrices

Coughlin, S. S., and Chiazze, L., Jr. "Job-Exposure Matrices in Epidemiologic Research and Medical Surveillance." *Occupational Medicine,* 1990, *5*(3), 633–646.

Plato, N., and Steineck, G. "Methodology and Utility of a Job-Exposure Matrix." *American Journal of Industrial Medicine,* 1993, *23*(3), 491–502.

Organizations

Information on Industrial Hygiene

American Conference of Governmental Industrial Hygienists (ACGIH), http://www.acgih.org.

American Industrial Hygiene Association (AIHA), http://www.aiha.org.

Information on Exposure Assessment

International Society of Exposure Science (ISES), http://www.iseaweb.org.

U.S. Environmental Protection Agency (U.S. EPA), *Exposure Assessment Tools and Models.* http://epa.gov/opptintr/exposure, 2009.

CHAPTER FIVE

ENVIRONMENTAL PSYCHOLOGY

DANIEL STOKOLS

CHIP CLITHEROE

KEY CONCEPTS

- Environmental psychology expands the scope of environmental health by considering health and behavior in their sociophysical context.

- Environmental psychology emphasizes both environmental hazards and environmental conditions that can promote good health.

- Environmental psychology considers both objectively measurable environmental conditions and subjective perceptions of the environment.

- Environmental psychology considers both immediate and remote environmental conditions, the cumulative effect and interaction of different environments over time, and the interaction of objective and subjective factors.

E NVIRONMENTAL psychology focuses on behavior in its sociophysical context. The field of environmental psychology assumes that a dynamic and reciprocal relationship exists between individuals and groups and the environments in which they live, work, play, learn, recreate, and travel (as displayed in the Perspective "A Trio of Tripping Pedestrians"). To an environmental psychologist, environmental health and well-being are the result of an appropriate and supportive fit between an individual or group and the places and people with whom they interact as they go about their lives.

PERSPECTIVE
A Trio of Tripping Pedestrians

Pat tripped first. She had stepped off this curb hundreds of times, and if you'd asked her, she would have told you that it was a little higher than the normal curb. But today she'd been seriously distracted—she was deeply involved in a conversation with her boyfriend who had asked her to marry him the night before.

Joe stumbled next. He was new to the big city. He had been gawking at the fast-moving traffic, tall buildings, and rushing throngs on their way to work. In the quiet suburbs where he lived, there weren't many pedestrians, and the curbs were all exactly the same height.

Mark was the last to stumble. He considered himself an excellent athlete but had twisted his ankle last night sliding into second base, trying to stretch a single into a double in the recreational softball league, and was using one of his father's canes this morning. He didn't misgauge the height of the curb—he planted the cane awkwardly in the street and almost lost his balance.

The street maintenance workers watching these behaviors concluded that the curb was unsafe and needed modification because it was a public health hazard.

Environmental psychologists study the myriad ways in which sociophysical **contexts** affect the behavior and health of individuals and groups. The contextual factors involved may include the kind of dwelling in which an individual resides, social and physical aspects of his or her neighborhood, and features of his or her commute between home and work. But environmental psychology is about more than objective descriptions of these factors. An individual's perceptions or feelings about each of these factors are likely to have an important bearing on his

Daniel Stokols and Chip Clitheroe declare no competing financial interests.

or her emotional and physical well-being, and these perceptions and feelings are also within the province of environmental psychology.

Environmental psychologists approach contexts as holistic, complex, naturally occurring, time-dependent entities. Moreover, they view the social and the physical dimensions of settings as highly interdependent (hence the term **sociophysical environment**) and as jointly influencing an individual's psychological and physical well-being. In contrast to traditional to public health, environmental psychology focuses on all those factors that might influence an individual's health, including aspects of the physical and ambient environments, social relationships, and anything else that might result in environmental stress. A more encompassing term, **environment and behavior studies** (EBS), is sometimes used to refer to this field (Stokols, 1995).

This chapter explores key concepts, methods, and findings in the field of environmental psychology and their relevance to environmental health. The following approaches are typical of the field of environmental psychology:

- Research in the field of environmental psychology is centrally concerned with the behavioral, emotional, and health outcomes of people's transactions with their everyday environments (or *settings*). These environments may include residential, occupational, educational, recreational, public, and virtual places (Barker, 1968; Bechtel, 1997; Gifford, 1997; Proshansky, Ittelson, and Rivlin, 1976; Stokols and Montero, 2002).
- Research in this field favors naturalistic field studies over controlled laboratory experiments.
- Environmental psychology emphasizes a multidisciplinary perspective, incorporating ideas from all the branches of psychology, environmental design (architecture, landscape architecture, interior design, and urban planning), geography, sociology, human ecology, natural resources management, government, and public health.
- Environmental psychologists study behavioral and health outcomes in relation to both the objective features and the subjective meanings of built and natural environments.
- Environmental psychology focuses on users. A user is anyone who comes in contact with, is affected by, or interacts with a context.
- Environmental psychologists examine behavior within relevant time intervals. These *events* have naturally occurring beginnings and endings, and the relationship between contextual factors and health conditions and outcomes can change during the course of an event (Altman and Rogoff, 1987; Clitheroe, Stokols, and Zmuidzinas, 1998).
- Environmental psychologists emphasize a holistic and longitudinal approach to understanding the environment's impact on individuals; that is, they

consider the effects of multiple settings and contextual factors over time and these factors' cumulative or joint influences on health.

• The field of environmental psychology has always been committed to understanding and responding to important societal issues, including public health.

The field of environmental psychology thus offers a valuable reservoir of conceptual insights, methodological tools, and empirical findings for broadening the scope of environmental health practice and assisting it in becoming even more relevant to the present and future concerns of the field of public health.

PERSPECTIVE
The Trio of Tripping Pedestrians Revisited

Pat's, Joe's, and Mark's well-being was apparently threatened by a curb. But was this an accurate conclusion? Pat had stepped off that curb successfully hundreds of times; her well-being was in fact threatened this morning by a lack of attention that had nothing to do with the physical setting. Joe's well-being was threatened by his being a first-time visitor to the big city—in environmental psychological terms, by his lack of an adequate cognitive schema describing a dense urban setting and his status as a first-time way finder. Mark's health had already been affected by his recreational escapades of the night before. His stumbling had nothing to do with the curb but rather with his temporary disabled status and inability to plant the cane tip firmly in the street. The environmental psychologists who had also been observing this behavior had chosen to observe the interaction between the setting and its users from a distance, so that they wouldn't affect the natural interaction occurring in the context. They concluded that the curb at this location was not really the problem but that modifying it and adding wheelchair-accessible, curb-cut ramps would facilitate safer interactions between the curb and all its users.

EXPANDING THE PERSPECTIVE OF ENVIRONMENTAL HEALTH

The field of environmental health has focused largely on the deleterious effects of people's exposure to toxins, pathogens, radiation, and other hazardous conditions of the physical environment (Detels, McEwen, Beaglehole, and Tanaka, 2002; Koren and Bisesi, 2002; Yassi, Kjellström, de Kok, and Guidotti, 2001). Environmental psychology is more broadly concerned with conceptualizing, measuring, and evaluating complex environmental settings such as buildings, neighborhoods, and public places and the ways these settings influence behavior, health, and well-being. Environmental psychologists consider health to be more than the absence of illness or injury and to include both physical and psychological well-being, or wellness.

The field of environmental health began to expand beyond its long-standing concern with the negative health effects of physical hazards, toxins, and pathogens at the same time the field of environmental psychology began to emerge as a viable discipline—in the turbulent social change and expanding ecological awareness of the 1960s. During this period, for example, Cassel (1964, 1976) urged public health researchers to give greater attention to the crucial role of social relationships in moderating individuals' resistance to hazardous environments. Cassel's research signaled a shift from germ theory accounts of health and illness (focusing on the adverse effects of specific pathogens once they invaded a human host) toward a social epidemiological model of public health and disease prevention, one that studies social determinants of health as well as physical and biological determinants.

During the 1980s, Lindheim and Syme (1983) reiterated Cassel's call for greater emphasis on social factors in health and highlighted the joint influence of multiple environmental dimensions (that is, the natural, social, symbolic, and built environments) on emotional and physical well-being. More recently, Frumkin (2001; see also Chapter Twenty-Four) described the "greening of environmental health" and underscored the importance of documenting the positive health outcomes associated with people's exposure to natural landscapes and wilderness settings. He has also identified several facets of healthy places and cited evidence suggesting that individuals' sense of place substantially affects their mental and physical well-being (Frumkin, 2003).

These and other efforts among researchers to broaden the scope of the field of environmental health reflect a convergence with some of the basic principles and themes of environmental psychology—especially an emphasis on salutogenic as well as pathogenic processes (Antonovsky, 1987) as they occur in relation to natural as well as built, social as well as physical, and subjective as well as objective dimensions of human environments (Bechtel and Churchman, 2002; Stokols and Altman, 1987).

The Sociophysical Context of Health

Environmental psychology assumes that the health effects of our surroundings result from the confluence of a variety of contextual factors. The negative health effects of routine exposure to residential density and noise, for example, are more severe in poor households than in affluent ones due to the cumulative effects of multiple environmental stressors faced by low-income families (Evans, 2004). Field experiments, similarly, have shown that persons exposed to cold viruses are much more likely to develop cold symptoms when they are experiencing high levels of stress in one or more areas of their lives (for example, in their relationships with family members, friends, or coworkers) than when they are reporting low levels of chronic stress (see, for example, Cohen and others, 1997a, 1998).

Clearly, a large number of life circumstances can affect the ways in which people respond to particular environmental demands. Yet identifying the many contextual factors that influence a person's health is a dauntingly complex task due to the large number of settings in which individuals participate on a day-to-day basis and the diverse physical and social factors they encounter in each setting. Moreover, each of these environmental factors can be considered in relation to diverse health criteria, ranging from the absence of physical injury and illness to states of complete wellness reflected in exceptionally high levels of emotional, physical, spiritual, and social well-being (O'Donnell, 1989; World Health Organization, 1986, 1997).

In establishing a basis for mapping sociophysical contexts of health, it is useful to begin by identifying a relatively small number of analytical categories, each of which subsumes a much larger set of environmental variables (Clitheroe and others, 1998; Magnusson, 1981). The basic units of environmental analysis are arrayed on different levels, or scales, ranging from specific stimuli that are part of the situations immediately experienced by persons in a particular setting or place (for example, being stuck in rush hour traffic, with horns honking and tempers flaring) to more complex life domains (for example, residential, employment, and educational environments) that are themselves clusters of multiple situations and settings (Table 5.1).

Stimuli are defined as observable features of objects or discrete conditions in an environment, such as the color of a table, the temperature level in a room, a sudden flash of light, or the occurrence of a loud noise (Pervin, 1978). **Situations** are sequences of individual or group activities and events that occur at a particular time and place (Forgas, 1979). **Settings** are socially structured and geographically bounded locations where certain kinds of activities and events recur on a regular basis—for example, the college classroom to which one reports for a particular course at the same time each week or the favorite coffee shop one visits several times each month for a mocha Frappuccino (Barker, 1968; Schoggen, 1989; Stokols and Shumaker, 1981). **Life domains** are larger, more encompassing spheres of a person's life, such as all those activities, relationships, and settings that involve family, education, religion, recreation, or employment (Campbell, 1981). An even broader unit of contextual analysis can be defined,

TABLE 5.1   Levels of Environmental Analysis

Elemental	Water, air, earth, food, germs, physical substances, solids, gases, liquids.
Individual	An individual's (1) body and physical, perceptual, and cognitive abilities, and (2) intellectual abilities, personal beliefs, values, attitudes, emotions, memories, and experiences.
Stimuli	Discernible (by any sense) features of an environment that cause a personal perception or physical or psychological reaction, or both.
Situation	Sequences of individual or group activities and events that occur at a particular time and place—these may be unique or may occur at regular intervals.
Setting	Socially structured and geographically bounded locations where certain kinds of activities and events recur on a regular basis.
Life domain	Spheres of a person's life that encompass multiple situations and settings, for example, home, work, or school.
Societal	Overarching systems of beliefs and values, social and cultural norms, and social, political, and economic institutions that integrate life domains for large groups of people.

usually referred to as a person's overall life situation, that encompasses all the major life domains in which the individual is involved during a particular period of his or her life (Chapin, 1974; Magnusson, 1981; Michelson, 1985).

Altman and Rogoff (1987), in a seminal book chapter, describe four different "world views" in psychology: trait, interactional, organismic, and transactional. A **trait worldview** tries to understand and predict the enduring, consistent features of physical settings and people as individual factors. Most scientific disciplines start with this worldview by describing the basic units that will constitute their scope of interest. An **interactional worldview** posits stable relationships among traits and proposes basic "laws" that describe these relationships. In this worldview, once basic units are defined, scientific inquiry begins to look for simple and then increasingly complex relationships between these basic factors. An **organismic worldview** tries to understand larger, more complete, more complex aggregates of factors (for example, a community or a geographic region), acknowledging that these factors may change or evolve over time. In this worldview, after enough relationships among basic units are identified and explored, scientific inquiry begins to assemble holistic, complete models of the phenomena being considered. A **transactional worldview** proposes that the factors that affect behavioral phenomena are part of a constant, dynamic, reciprocal milieu. In this approach it becomes necessary to define a relevant period of time that includes the phenomena of interest. Altman and Rogoff propose that a transactional worldview attempts to understand the world around us as a series of "events": a confluence of social and environmental factors with a natural beginning and a natural ending point in time. A good example of a smaller, more contained event is a localized epidemic. A good example of a very complex, large-scale event is the preparation for and response to a natural disaster, such as Hurricane Katrina.

Implied in a transactional approach to understanding natural disasters is that no two disasters are alike; they will differ in location, duration, warning, force, extent of damage, response, and impact. Thus it is important to learn from each event by understanding it as completely as possible and applying what is learned to potential contexts for future similar disasters. (An in-depth examination of

PERSPECTIVE
Hurricane Katrina: A Transactional Event

Assessments of the impact of Hurricane Katrina are uniformly bleak. As one commentator put it, "Katrina did not merely lay waste to a geographic region [Figure 5.1]; it also exposed every public policy failure essential to community and population health" (Rosenbaum, 2006). Why was the failure so endemic? Environmental psychologists would propose that the planning and preparation for natural disasters in the New Orleans area had been conducted at an interactional or possibly organismic level, whereas a hurricane is best conceptualized as a transactional event. The event that was Hurricane Katrina had three parts: (1) awareness and preparation, (2) immediate response, and (3) aftermath.

Environmental psychology can contribute a more comprehensive approach to understanding each phase of this event. Concepts that could be usefully applied to the entire event include **sense of place** (the unique characteristics of a place and the feelings or perceptions a place evokes in people) (Relph, 1976), **place attachment** (emotional bonding between people and their life spaces) (Stokols & Shumaker, 1981), and **contextual transformation** (sudden and dramatic context changes, resulting in fundamental behavior modification) (Clitheroe and others, 1998). The awareness and preparation phase focuses on risk perception and communication (Vaughan, 1993) and attitude change (Fishbein and Ajzen, 1975). The response phase focuses on the use of common setting features as **"affordances"** (possibilities for action that are latent in an environment) (Gibson, 1977) and that could prove useful during the immediate response. The aftermath phase focuses on environmental and psychological stress (Evans and Kantrowitz, 2002); individual, the event that was, and continues to be, Hurricane Katrina is beyond the scope of this chapter. Among those beginning to explore this tragic event in detail are Rosenbaum, 2006, and Brunsma, Overfelt, and Picou, 2007.)

Three Principles of Contextual Analysis

Three basic principles of **contextual analysis** are common to environmental psychology.

　　1. *The relationship between environment and health is influenced by interdependencies among immediate situations, immediate settings, and more remote environmental conditions.*

FIGURE 5.1　Destruction Following Hurricane Katrina

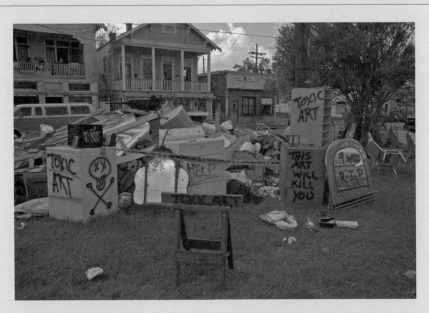

Source: FEMA/Marvin Nauman.

family, and community adaptation; and helping behavior norms and exceptions (Baum and Fleming, 1993). The aftermath phase of the 2005 Hurricane Katrina event is, unfortunately, ongoing.

Stimuli and situations are nested within larger units such as organized settings and places that are themselves subsumed by individuals' life domains, community activity systems, and societal conditions and trends (in, for example, economic, political, or cultural arenas). As environmental analyses shift their focus from smaller and simpler to larger and more complex levels, the potential range of contextual influences on mental and physical health expands dramatically due to the hierarchically nested structure of human environments.

For instance, when unemployment rates in a community are high, psychological and organizational stress associated with job insecurity is more prevalent and disruptive among coworkers at companies in that region (Dooley, 2003; Dooley, Fielding, and Levi, 1996). At the same time, workplace health and safety at the local level are directly influenced by state and national regulations aimed at protecting environmental quality and employee health (Stokols, McMahan, Clitheroe, and Wells, 2001). A more dramatic and tragic example of the interdependencies between local and remote environments is the syndrome of chronic emotional stress and health impairment triggered by the terrorist attacks of September 11, 2001, not only among Americans residing in or near New York City, Washington, D.C., and Shanksville, Pennsylvania, but also among those living hundreds or thousands of miles away from the attack sites (Silver and others, 2002). These examples suggest a second principle of contextual analysis.

2. *The different environments in which an individual participates exert a cumulative, synergistic effect on his or her health.*

Bronfenbrenner (1979) emphasized the ways in which functional linkages between two or more settings (such as an individual's family and occupational environments) and connections with other more distant settings in which an individual does not directly participate (for example, the workplaces of a child's parents) can affect development and well-being. Such multilevel, integrative analyses can identify subtle relationships affecting health (for example, stressful experiences at work that impair the quality of parents' interactions with their children at home). Particularly important in a world of expanding communication and entertainment media is Bronfenbrenner's concept that the overarching societal system of beliefs, social and cultural norms, and political and economic institutions and events surrounding individuals and groups also influences the health and well-being of those individuals and groups. (This relates to the concept of cumulative risk assessment, as discussed in Chapter Eight.)

The combined influence of multiple settings and life domains on individuals' health has been observed in several studies and is recognized in the third general principle of contextual analysis.

3. *Health is the result of an interaction among the objective features of the environments in which individuals participate, individuals' perceptions of those features, and individuals' personal attributes.*

That is, the impact of particular stimuli, situations, settings, and life domains on a person's health depends not only on the objective features of an environment but also on the person's individual attributes (for example, genetic heritage, psychological dispositions, and coping resources) and on his or her subjective interpretation of the environments in which he or she participates. For instance, when children are exposed to environmental stressors such as crowding and noise in both their home and school environments, these exposures cause additive effects on their health (for example, elevated systolic and diastolic blood pressure) and academic performance (Cohen, Evans, Stokols, and Krantz, 1986). In other studies, employees' perception that they lacked the flexibility to schedule children's doctor visits during working hours led to their underutilization of employer-provided family health benefits (Fielding, Cumberland, and Pettitt, 1994), with long-term negative health consequences for the family. Studies have also documented both the negative health consequences of work-family conflict and the positive effects of spousal support in buffering work-related stressors (O'Neil and Greenberger, 1994).

More precise hypotheses about the links between environmental factors and their effects on health can be derived by developing and testing more specific theories of the relationship between persons and their environment that identify (1) those situations and settings in a person's life that have the greatest impact on his or her health and (2) the ways in which personal attributes or individual differences (involving, for example, personality, cognition, gender, age, education, or income) mediate the effects of environmental conditions on emotional and physical well-being. These are examples of applying an interactional worldview.

Understanding these multiple settings and environments and their interaction constitutes a daunting research challenge. It requires data on individuals nested within areas or neighborhoods (Diez Roux, 2001). Analytical methods able to assess these complex relationships are emerging from the fields of environmental health (multilevel analysis), urban planning (geographic information systems, or GISs), and the behavioral sciences (hierarchical linear analysis).

HEALTH EFFECTS OF THE CHANGING NEIGHBORHOOD

The **neighborhood** is an especially appropriate context in which to consider the links between environment, behavior, and health, for at least three reasons. First, the neighborhood is a sufficiently broad contextual unit to encompass a variety of stimuli, situations, settings, and life domains relevant to health. Second, the concept of neighborhood is not peripheral to people's day-to-day activities and concerns but plays a central and meaningful role in determining individuals' physical and psychological well-being and quality of life. And third, although the neighborhood has been long regarded as a geographically, psychologically, and socially meaningful unit of analysis in the fields of sociology, public health, planning, and community and environmental psychology, the concept of neighborhood is currently undergoing fundamental rethinking and change among scholars in several fields due to the advent of digital and mobile communications.

A person's neighborhood is no longer viewed simply as a contiguous, geographically delimited, relatively stable arena of his or her daily activities. People now participate concurrently in multiple, separate, and sometimes isolated geographically defined places and in a number of independent socially defined networks. Some of these places and networks are real (involving a physical space or place), and others are less real (involving a virtual space) and more mobile. Thus consideration of contemporary changes in the structure and functions of the neighborhood offers an opportunity to explore exciting new lines of research concerning the impact of digital communications and virtual communities on people's psychological attachment to places and their overall well-being (see, for example, Blanchard and Horan, 1998; Meyrowitz, 1985; Stokols, 1999; Wellman and Haythornthwaite, 2002).

Traditional definitions of neighborhood emphasize geographic location, unique physical features (such as architectural styles and public parks), the social attributes of residents, and residents' objective participation in and subjective identification with the area (Altman and Wandersman, 1987). For instance, Rivlin (1987) states:

> When we speak of contemporary neighborhoods, we are talking about a very heterogeneous unit based on the nature of the geography, the numbers and kinds of people there, the socioeconomic status of these people, their ages, cultural background, and housing form. . . . The criterion of a neighborhood is the acknowledgment by residents, merchants, and regular users of an area that a locality exists. It presumes some agreement on boundaries and a name and the recognition of distinguishing characteristics of the setting. . . . The recognition by people of a bounded territory as having an integrity and personal meaning is, in my view, the necessary requirement of a neighborhood [pp. 2–3].

Researchers are, however, beginning to recognize that neighborhood contexts may be related to public health in ways independent of place-based attributes (Diez Roux, 2001). According to this emerging view, people's communications and relationships with others are no longer constrained by geography but occur instead within highly personalized digital communication networks unbounded by space and time (Negroponte, 1995; Rheingold, 1993). For instance, Wellman (2001) observes that the "importance of a communication site as a meaningful place will diminish even more. The person—not the place, household, or workgroup—will become even more of an autonomous communication node" (p. 233).

In this discussion, rather than adopting either the traditional view that local neighborhoods are the most important context of people's day-to-day transactions with their surroundings or the revisionist view that place-based neighborhoods are no longer important sources of community and well-being, we offer an integrative conceptualization of neighborhood. It recognizes the complementarity of geographically bounded and virtually dispersed neighborhood functions.

Specifically, we define the new neighborhood as consisting of those people, places, and technologies that enable the sociophysical interactions that define everyday life. This definition assumes that people's psychological ties with local, place-based environments are an important source of their identity and well-being (Proshansky, Fabian, and Kaminoff, 1983; Unger and Wandersman, 1985), but it also recognizes that the number and scope of individuals' psychologically meaningful neighborhoods (such as those based at home, at school, at work, or in public community settings) have expanded and that in addition to being linked by physical proximity individuals can now be closely linked with each other through the Internet and mobile digital communications (Brill and Weidemann, 2001; Wellman and Haythornthwaite, 2002). This emerging view of neighborhoods incorporates both the real and the virtual aspects of an individual's or a family's experience of neighborhood, both of which respond to the same basic human needs (Table 5.2).

TABLE 5.2 Functions of Both Real and Virtual Neighborhoods

Affiliation	Facilitate communication and interaction between individuals and groups.
Identity	Provide a definable group character (name, style, real or virtual landmarks) for assimilation by individuals and an opportunity to contribute to the development of that character and to the individual's own self-concept.
Social support	Offer psychologically reinforcing interactions between individuals or within groups.
Community	Offer a connection to the opportunities provided and demands made by larger social units.
Information	Provide awareness of and access to information the individual finds essential to successful daily life and the accomplishment of personal goals.
Daily life	Assist with the basics: acquisition and maintenance of food, shelter, safety, convenience, and comfort.
Recreation	Supply opportunities to physically or mentally refresh, to play, to explore, to challenge oneself, to learn and grow.

Features of Neighborhoods

A person's neighborhood includes all those physical and virtual settings he or she uses regularly. Some of these settings are located inside buildings, some are located outdoors, and some are virtually located in cyberspace. Virtual neighborhoods arise when people routinely communicate and congregate electronically, with no need for a physical, geographically defined place in which to come together. The following discussion of neighborhood settings presents several examples of environmental psychology's concepts and research that describe contextual factors related to public health. We start with physical settings and conclude with virtual ones.

Indoor Neighborhood Settings   Indoor neighborhood settings include dwellings, classrooms, workspaces, indoor recreation facilities, places for socialization, places for worship, and local commercial settings such as markets, shops, and restaurants. Physical characteristics include building design and furnishings, entrances, exits, and windows. Ambient conditions include lighting, air quality, temperature, humidity, sound, and color. Social conditions include the solitary individuals or groups who use or in some way interact with a place.

Environmental **stress** is any demand made on an individual by an environment (physical or social). Thus environmental stressors may be considered stimuli, requiring a physical or psychological response. Pioneering work by Selye (1956) defined the physiological response to injury, illness, or other environmental stressors: elevated blood pressure, enlarged adrenal glands, both increases and decreases in gastrointestinal secretions and motility, and impaired immune function. Psychological stress can occur when perceived environmental demands exceed the individual's perceived ability to cope with them. Such stress may be caused by experiences of isolation, irritability, or interpersonal conflict. The individual's subjective interpretation of an environment (for example, whether or not its demands seem overwhelming or manageable) plays a major role in determining the severity and persistence of psychological stress reactions.

Research on environmental stress has shown, for example, that chronic exposure to high levels of noise leads to a variety of health impairments. For instance, when children living in noisy dwellings near congested roadways or attending schools under the flight path of a busy airport (Figure 5.2) were compared to children occupying quieter environments, chronic noise exposure was found to be associated with impaired hearing and reading skills, lower levels of academic achievement, and elevated blood pressure (Bronzaft, 2002; Cohen and others, 1986; Cohen, Glass, and Singer, 1973; Evans and others, 2001; Hygge, Evans, and Bullinger, 2002). Similarly, prolonged experiences of crowding in dormitories, apartments, and homes have been linked to dysfunctional social behavior, feelings of isolation, and emotional distress (Baum and Epstein, 1978; Baum and Valins, 1977; Evans and Lepore, 1993).

FIGURE 5.2   Airplane Coming In for Landing over
an Elementary School in Los Angeles

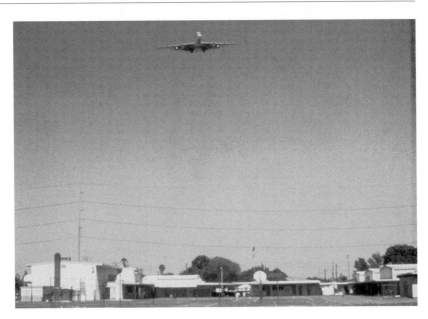

One of the reasons why noisy or crowded interior spaces provoke psychological stress among their occupants is that they typically lead to prolonged feelings
of stimulation overload, distraction, frustration, and fatigue (Baum and Epstein,
1978; Evans and Johnson, 2000; Milgram, 1970). In settings with large numbers
of people (spatially dense settings), an additional source of psychological stress is
the difficulty occupants encounter in their efforts to regulate interpersonal privacy
and personal space (Altman, 1975; Sommer, 1969). Coresidents and coworkers
who are able to establish and maintain effective guidelines for the use of shared
spaces (for example, through personalization and decoration of spaces in a shared
residence or workspace) are better able to remain individually and collectively
productive and to avoid interpersonal conflict and distress (Brill and Weidemann,
2001; Sundstrom and Sundstrom, 1986; Taylor, 1988).

To the extent that individuals can gain some measure of real or perceived
control over environmental stressors such as noise, crowding, and infringements
on privacy, they are able to avoid both the immediate and delayed effects of these
stressors on their performance and well-being (Cohen, 1980; Evans, 2001; Glass
and Singer, 1972). Perceptions of environmental controllability and predictability

enable individuals to maintain high levels of emotional and physical well-being, even in the context of highly demanding settings. For instance, elderly persons living in institutionalized residential care facilities who were encouraged by staff members to take personal responsibility for the maintenance and beautification of their own living spaces (for example, by caring for plants placed in their bedrooms) exhibited higher levels of emotional and physical well-being than those who were not encouraged to assume those responsibilities (Langer and Rodin, 1976; Rodin and Langer, 1977; also see Schulz and Hanusa, 1978).

Outdoor Neighborhood Settings   Just as physical conditions such as noise and high spatial density influence the quality of social interactions indoors, an interdependence between physical and social conditions is evident in outdoor spaces (Alexander and others, 1977; Altman, 1975). For instance, loud noise (at or above 85 decibels) from a lawnmower operating near the sidewalk in a suburban neighborhood significantly reduced pedestrians' attentiveness to the needs of others (specifically, to the needs of a person wearing an arm cast who had dropped a stack of books near his car) and their willingness to stop and render assistance (Mathews and Canon, 1975).

In another study the linear distance between the front doors of apartments in a Massachusetts Institute of Technology student housing complex (a physical dimension) reliably predicted which residents happened to meet each other and eventually became friends (Festinger, Schachter, and Back, 1950). Moreover, neighbors whose apartments were further apart but who met regularly at group mailboxes, a basketball court, or in the parking lot (social dimensions) were more likely to form friendships than those who lived far apart and did not "run into" each other regularly.

The influence of sociophysical environmental factors on friendship formation has important health implications. Most immediately, the presence of friends who live close by and can render assistance when called upon improves the sociability, or social climate, of the neighborhood (Moos, 1979). A positive social climate is in turn seen as a form of social capital and can contribute to residents' perceptions of security and neighborhood safety (Putnam, 2000). Other research suggests that socially isolated individuals are more susceptible to illnesses of various kinds—even premature death—than are those who are actively involved in mutually supportive friendship, family, religious, and professional networks (Berkman and Syme, 1979; Cohen and others, 1997b, 2003).

The sociability of neighborhoods can be undermined by the presence of physical and social incivilities. **Physical incivilities** include the presence of litter, graffiti, protective bars on windows, evidence of street disrepair (for example, broken curbs and potholes), poor building and exterior maintenance (for example, peeling paint, unkempt yards, and overgrown landscaping), and damage to buildings (for example, broken windows) (Nasar and Fisher, 1993; Perkins, Wandersman, Rich, and Taylor, 1993). **Social incivilities** include displays of public drunkenness, the presence of gangs or prostitutes, excessive numbers of liquor stores, stores offering pornography, and a generally unfriendly or threatening atmosphere in the neighborhood (Holman and Stokols, 1994).

One consequence of environmental incivilities is the stigmatization of a neighborhood, accompanied by reduced social and economic investment in the area, greater fear of crime, and higher rates of victimization and injury among residents and visitors. Neighborhoods, such as South Central Los Angeles, that have experienced widely publicized civil violence are particularly prone to this downward spiral of stigmatization, disinvestment, and crime. Concerted efforts to remove physical cues such as disrepair and to encourage the development of prosocial events, including street and cultural fairs, drama or music festivals, and community gardening programs, can reverse this negative trend (Garland and Stokols, 2002; Lewis, 1979).

Other architectural and site-planning strategies can be applied to create outdoor spaces that enhance the social climate and security of residential and commercial areas. **Defensible space** (Newman, 1973) refers to those features of an environment that "combine to bring it under the control of its residents" (p. 3). For instance, apartment buildings can be sited on blocks so as to create natural buffer zones easily surveyed by residents, and apartment windows can be positioned to facilitate surveillance of semipublic areas adjacent to the building. Changes in elevation, landscaping, and signage also can be used to mark transitions between public and private areas (Alexander and others, 1977). In a study of Salt Lake City neighborhoods, Brown (1985) found that homes characterized by defensible space design (for example, the presence of actual or symbolic barriers such as fences or hedges surrounding the property and physical traces of residents' presence (such as lights on in the home) were less likely to have been burglarized than were residences lacking those features. This body of environmental psychology research has become institutionalized in the form of guidelines promoted by police departments and adopted by cities and counties throughout the United States (Newman, 1966).

Neighborhoods as Wholes A neighborhood can be described not only in terms of buildings, sidewalks, open areas, parks, shops, and streets but also in terms of larger factors that contribute to its distinctive identity or overall atmosphere (Ittelson, 1973). For instance, Lynch (1960) defines **imageability** as an environment's memorability, its capacity to evoke strong visual memories of its physical features among residents and visitors. According to Lynch, the likelihood that an environment will evoke a vivid image in an observer depends on its visual clarity, or "legibility—the ease with which its parts can be recognized and organized into a coherent pattern" (p. 3). The imageability and **legibility** of a place derive not only from its physical features but also from social meanings. In a study of Parisians' cognitive maps, Milgram and Jodelet (1976) found that certain areas of the city were remembered more for their social and historical meanings than their distinctive physical or visual attributes.

Both the social and the physical imageability of a neighborhood can affect the well-being of residents and visitors in at least two ways. First, visually legible environments are less confusing and easier to navigate than others, enabling pedestrians and drivers to feel more secure, to arrive at their destinations more efficiently, to enjoy their experience of the neighborhood, and to avoid potentially unsafe areas; these are all experiences that decrease environmental stress. Second, the presence of widely recognized and shared cultural or symbolic meanings can contribute positively to the sociability and supportive climate of a place, thereby increasing social capital and promoting norms of cooperativeness, trust, and engagement with others (see, for example, Putnam, 2000) while also reducing crime rates and fear of crime in the area. All of these factors contribute to the health of the neighborhood and of the people who live, work, and play there.

An important neighborhood quality that contributes to its social climate is the number and diversity of its behavioral settings, including recreational, commercial, cultural, educational, and civic places (Barker and Schoggen, 1973; Jacobs, 1961). The presence of multiple settings geared to the interests and activities of diverse groups of residents and visitors (children, adolescents, young adults, elderly persons, and various cultural and ethnic groups) promotes active interchange among these groups and contributes to the overall vitality of the neighborhood and the quality of life for its residents and visitors. Conversely, an overabundance of certain settings, such as fast-food restaurants, may have a negative influence on residents' well-being. In a recent study of the "economics of obesity," Rashad and Grossman (2004) found that a major factor in the rise of obesity in the United States between 1980 and the present is the dramatic growth in the per capita number of fast-food and full-service restaurants during those years. According to this research, as much as two-thirds of the increase in adult obesity since 1980 can be explained by the rapid expansion of the restaurant industry and the increasing tendency of U.S. adults and children to eat their meals at fast-food and full-service restaurants (Figure 5.3). Thus a prevalence of fast-food settings (which generally serve high-fat, high-calorie meals) and abundant opportunities for families to dine out in a neighborhood may have a deleterious effect on residents' health.

Among the most important neighborhood settings are what Oldenburg (1999) refers to as **third places**—"the variety of public places that host the regular,

FIGURE 5.3   Cars Waiting in Line for Fast-Food Service

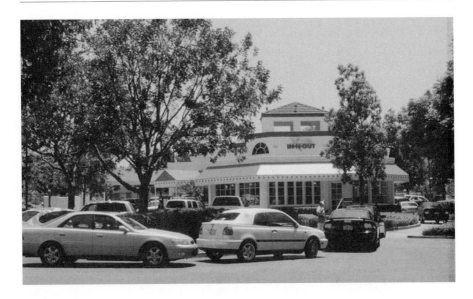

voluntary, informal, and happily anticipated gatherings of individuals beyond the realms of home and work" (p. 16). (Home and work are, respectively, individuals' first places and second places.) Third places such as local bookstores, coffee shops, parks, and other popular hangouts (such as Ghirardelli Square in San Francisco, shown in Figure 5.4) serve as "core settings of informal life." Oldenburg contends that third places offer people escape and relief from the psychological stress of work and family responsibilities and strengthen their sense of belonging to the community and thus their overall well-being. Interestingly, Florida's (2002) research on the **creative class** suggests that regional economic growth and job opportunities in the United States are fueled by where creative people, who represent 30 percent of the workforce, choose to live. One of the attributes creative people seek when deciding whether to move to a particular area is a diverse mix of third places—neighborhood settings that offer recreational resources such as a vibrant nightlife and opportunities for social and cultural exchange.

In some localities schools may become third places. A recent positive example of neighborhood change involved the conceptualization of neighborhood public schools as places that can "improve overall health in densely populated communities" when they are designed as "mixed-use, neighborhood-centered" facilities that provide "much needed, neighborhood-based health and human services . . . [and] safe, convenient spaces for children and their families to walk, run, participate in sports and otherwise enjoy being outdoors" (Abel and Fielding, 2004, p. M2).

FIGURE 5.4   Ghirardelli Square in San Francisco

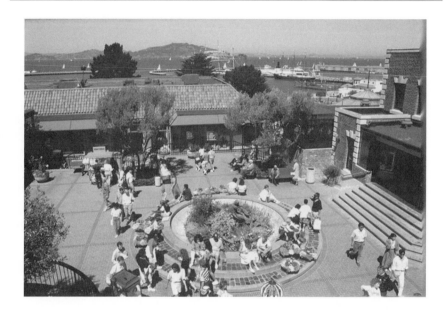

In addition to third places, the aesthetic quality of neighborhood environments, the presence of nature (for example, lakes or forested parks) at all environmental levels (see Table 5.3 and Figure 5.5), and the provision of resources for
physical activity (for example, bike trails and public parks) all contribute positively
to residents' mental and physical health and to the neighborhood's sense of place.
Natural areas in a neighborhood offer residents a respite from their daily work
routines as well as opportunities for emotional restoration and recovery from
mental fatigue (Kaplan and Kaplan, 1989). Similarly, urban design features can
either encourage or discourage residents' engagement in physical activity, activity that could be an antidote to the obesity pandemic currently rampant in the
U.S. population (Frank, Engelke, and Schmid, 2003). (The links between access
to nature and well-being and between urban design and physical activity patterns
are discussed more fully in Chapters Fourteen and Twenty-Four.)

Virtual Neighborhoods   We now consider the ways in which the Internet and digital communications have given rise to fundamentally new type of neighborhood—
virtual communities located in cyberspace, that complement (and sometimes
complicate) people's transactions with their place-based environments.

The computing revolution and the rapid expansion of the Internet during
the 1980s and 1990s (Kiesler, 1997; Kling and Iacono, 1991) have dramatically

TABLE 5.3 The Presence of Nature

Elemental	Natural scents (incense)
	Natural objects (driftwood, shells, stones, plants)
Individual	Clothing choices
	Eating choices
Stimuli	Natural sounds (birdsong, rain, wind in trees)
	Natural surfaces (wood, rock, grass, sand, water)
	Natural colors and textures (earth tones, burlap)
	Views of nature through windows
	Natural images (pictures of natural places)
Situation	Outdoor meetings, meals, and entertainment
	Gardening
Setting	Outdoor recreation
	Outdoor relaxation or meditation
Life domain	Outdoor occupations
	Location of residence and workplace
	Mode of transportation and routes
Societal	Nature preserves and wilderness areas
	Protected seashores, rivers, and lakes
	Regional, national, and international ecological conventions and agreements

FIGURE 5.5 Neighborhood Green Space in Irvine, California

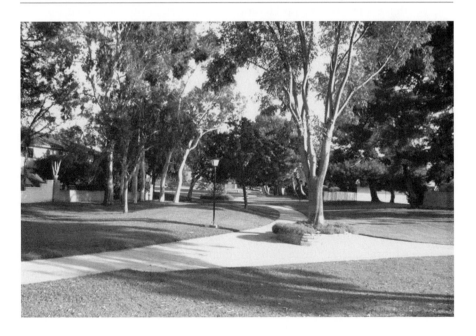

altered people's transactions with their environments in at least three ways. First, the emergence of the Internet and digital communications has made it much easier for individuals to be in contact even when they are geographically or temporally remote from each other. Second, the Internet has facilitated the development of virtual behavioral settings and virtual neighborhoods such as chat rooms, listservs, bulletin boards, information pooling sites such as Wikipedia, social networking sites such as Facebook and Twitter, and electronic commerce sites such as eBay and Amazon.com, each located at a particular "address" (URL) in cyberspace. Like real places, these virtual settings are frequented by users or members on a regular basis, and these individuals develop widely shared norms concerning appropriate social behavior and etiquette (Blanchard, 1997; Blanchard and Horan, 1998). Moreover, the members of virtual communities (such as the Palace and the Well) tend to identify strongly with these sites and fellow members (Rheingold, 1993). Third, because individuals are present in or at a specific physical place at the same time that they are participating in a virtual setting via computer contact or cell phone conversation, they must simultaneously pay attention to information from both their immediate sociophysical environment and their virtual environment.

This concurrent processing of information generated by place-based and virtual settings raises the possibility that certain conflicts between these two realms of experience will occur and that negative health impacts (such as traffic crashes caused by the use of cell phones while driving) may be a consequence of those conflicts. The proliferation of real-virtual situations incorporating at least one real setting (place-based) and one virtual setting (accessed from a desktop computer, laptop, hand-held device, or cell phone), raises novel questions about the relationships between environment, behavior, and health (see, for example, Stokols, 1999). For example, real-virtual conflicts arise when parents engage in chat room activities on a home computer and become less responsive to the needs of their children, or when employees inappropriately "surf the Internet" while at their workplaces, arousing the resentment of coworkers and supervisors who are more focused on job-related tasks. These examples illustrate the kinds of interpersonal, family, and organizational strains that may result from a conflict between real and virtual settings.

Social strains and interpersonal conflicts are not the only health problems prompted by the overlap of real and virtual settings. Another major threat to an individual's well-being is the **stimulation overload** (see, for example, Milgram, 1970) that results from chronic multitasking, such as simultaneously communicating with a person in a real setting and a person in a virtual setting in an attempt to accomplish diverse tasks in a short period of time. The digital electronic revolution has subjected large segments of the population to an onslaught of communications transmitted via desktop and laptop computers, hand-held devices, cell phones, and fax machines. The rapid rise in e-mail communications—both more users and more e-mail messaging per user—has been recorded in a number of recent studies (for example, International Technology and Trade Associates, 2000; Lyman and Varian, 2000; Nie and Erbring, 2000; Wellman and Haythornthwaite, 2002; Messagingonline, 2000). This communications explosion has resulted in individuals' becoming more susceptible to distraction, information overload, and mental fatigue (Mark, Gudith, and Klocke, 2005; Mark, Gonzalez, and Harris, 2005). When these conditions persist, individuals can experience **attentional fatigue**, which has been closely linked to greater irritability, reduced sensitivity to the needs of others, and errors in occupational settings—for example, situations involving physicians, nurses, air traffic controllers, and automobile drivers that threaten health and life (Cohen, 1980; Kaplan and Kaplan, 1989; Kohn, Corrigan, and Donaldson, 2000).

Although conflicts between uses of real and virtual settings are common, place-based neighborhoods can also benefit from residents' participation in virtual communities. Blanchard and Horan (1998), for instance, distinguish two types of virtual communities: place-based and geographically dispersed. Place-based communities of interest are exemplified by the Blacksburg Electronic Community (www.bev.net), an Internet site developed by the residents of Blacksburg, Virginia, for the purposes of facilitating social and commercial exchanges among individuals and groups in the city and enhancing the sense of community and sense of place in Blacksburg. Geographically dispersed communities of interest are those in which most participants do not communicate face to face or even by telephone. Examples include health support groups on the Internet as well as Web sites featuring hobbies or shared intellectual, political, artistic, literary, or recreational interests. Even though these virtual communities do not directly reinforce a sense of place, they do enrich the quality of life in place-based neighborhoods by delivering valuable information, services, and support to neighborhood residents.

Not all members of place-based neighborhoods, however, have access to virtual settings, due to limited financial resources or educational backgrounds. The rift between information-rich and information-poor segments of the population is referred to as the **digital divide** (Garces, 2000; National Telecommunications and Information Administration, 2000; Servon, 2002; Mossberger, Tolbert, and Stansbury, 2003). People who find themselves on the wrong side of this divide are frequently caught in a downward spiral of increasing poverty because they have little access to job opportunities that require training in information technology. If this problem is not redressed, the resulting social divisions and inequity may provoke the same sort of social conflict, community destabilization, and health impairments (including lack of access to health care) that led to widespread social upheaval in the 1960s. Thus, narrowing the digital divide remains an important priority for future environmental and health research and public health policy.

Summing Up the Example of Neighborhoods

A focus on neighborhoods highlights the unique contributions of environmental psychology to public health.

- Neighborhoods are large enough to reveal the complex relationships between the physical environment and people that constitute "real life," and yet small enough that most social and physical factors influencing a target behavior (for example, childhood obesity) can be effectively considered and synthesized.
- Although varying widely across cultures and locales, neighborhoods contain many common elements that allow useful comparisons: climate; geography; natural ecological status; residential types, styles, and amenities; transportation modalities and routes; commercial enterprises; public utilities; economic relationships; educational facilities; religious and other social organizations; public governance; and cultural heritage.
- The effects of these and other neighborhood factors on individual and group physical and psychological health and well-being can be effectively modeled and analyzed, and the results generalized to a broader societal context.
- A neighborhood focus allows researchers in environmental psychology to employ useful perspectives from many disciplines—such as sociology, environmental design, political science, urban planning, anthropology, social psychology, and of course public health—and to use other fields' tools as well, such as GISs.
- The concept of neighborhoods is proving useful to understanding the impact of modern telecommunication and computing technology on social and sociophysical relationships—that is, to understanding the differences between real environments and virtual environments—and to exploring the emerging perspective on neighborhood that integrates both real and virtual environments.

LOCAL TO GLOBAL LEVELS OF ANALYSIS

Environmental psychology encompasses multiple levels of analysis. From the smallest microlevel context to the largest holistic context, environmental psychology brings the same focus to bear: environmental influences on the cognition, behavior, and well-being of human participants in that context.

Global climate change offers an excellent example of the range of levels of analysis encompassed by environmental psychology. Global climate change is best approached from an organismic perspective, that is, as a very large, complex, and slowly evolving set of environmental conditions with a wide range of ecological and human impacts. The recent worldwide focus on this global challenge is likely only to become more intense, especially as the connections between different levels of analysis and the potentially catastrophic results of the changes become better defined (Gore, 2006; see also Chapter Ten). Moreover, the "public health response to [climate change] requires a holistic understanding of disease and the various external factors influencing public health. It is within this larger context where the greatest challenges and opportunities for protecting and promoting public health occur" (Gerberding, 2007, p. 1).

TABLE 5.4   Behavioral Impacts of Displacement Due to Climate Change: From Global to Local

Level of Analysis	Climate Change	Behavioral Impact
Global (continental)	Global temperature rise leads to rise in sea level and magnifies impact of natural disasters	Massive population dislocation
National (subcontinental)	Heat, prolonged drought	Changes to and disruption in food production and distribution
Regional (state)	Greater ozone and particulate air pollution	Increased cardiovascular and respiratory disease
Community	Long-term infrastructure damage, especially for public utilities and transportation	Functional disruption leading to scarcity of necessary resources (potable water, electricity, gas, sanitation), damage to and inaccessibility of health care facilities
Neighborhood	Disproportionate social and economic impacts	Inability of neighborhood to recover, neighborhood decay, disruption of social networks, permanent displacement of population
Residential (family)	Loss of shelter, of social and public support, and of contact with extended family	Family separation, conflict, deprivation, long-term negative economic impact, educational disruption, exacerbation of medical conditions
Individual	Disruption of life domains due to all of the factors listed here	Dramatic increase in environmental (psychological) stress, malnutrition, loss of income, poverty, inadequate medical care

Global climate change can have, in fact is already beginning to have, a number of serious public health impacts (in environmental psychology terms, *behavioral outcomes*), including death and illness from heat waves; death and injuries from severe weather events such as hurricanes, tornadoes, and floods; increased levels of air pollutants and allergens, aggravating respiratory and cardiovascular diseases; reduced water quality and quantity; and increased risk of vector-, food- and waterborne diseases (see Chapter Ten).

Although many of these impacts are experienced by the affected population in situ, other impacts, especially catastrophic events, result in the **displacement** of large numbers of people under very difficult circumstances. The study of displacement is not new (Pastalan, 1983). Fullilove (2004) thoroughly explores the communal, family, and personal impacts of large-scale displacement due to U.S. urban renewal programs in the 1960s and 1970s. Displacement due to catastrophic events presents an effective, if unfortunate, opportunity to describe the full range of behavioral impacts on affected populations.

SUMMARY

This chapter has presented the field of environmental psychology as a useful vantage point for understanding a wide variety of relationships between environment and health. Several important topics that expand the conceptualization of environmental health have been introduced:

- Theory and research in environmental psychology are providing a broader conceptualization of the sociophysical context of health than has been typical of the traditional focus of the field of environmental health on the adverse effects of exposure to specific toxins, pathogens, and hazardous conditions of the physical environment.
- Similarly, environmental psychology is adopting a broader stance toward

health itself, considering *good health* to be both the absence of injury or illness and the presence of well-being for individuals and groups.

- Environmental psychology adopts a concept of the environment that includes both objective and subjective perspectives and physiological and psychological health outcomes.
- A revised understanding of neighborhood has been developed in this chapter and used to introduce a wide range of concepts, research, and findings related to individual and social behavioral outcomes as they, in turn, influence personal and population health outcomes.
- The discussion of real and virtual settings and communities has revealed

several potentially adverse as well as beneficial impacts on individuals and groups that have direct consequences for the safety and health of neighborhood residents.

The incorporation of environmental psychology concepts and research results can enlarge the scope and effectiveness of public health programs and policies. Studies of environment and health should give greater attention to health-enhancing as well as pathogenic processes as they occur in relation to the natural and built environments, and to the cumulative influence of conditions experienced by individuals across multiple settings and life domains. This more fully contextual perspective, incorporating the joint influence of multiple environmental settings and factors on health, is exemplified by recent studies of the adaptive burdens faced by individuals, especially members of low-income and ethnic minority groups—burdens resulting from their chronic exposure to multiple social, physical, and economic environmental stressors (Bullard, 1990; Evans, 2004; McEwen and Stellar, 1993; Taylor, Repetti, and Seeman, 1997; see also Chapter Eight). Finally, the rapidly expanding prevalence of telecommunications and virtual communities (incorporated here into an expanded definition of neighborhood) and the multifaceted role of the Internet as both a resource for health promotion and a source of health problems have emerged as important topics for future environmental health research.

KEY TERMS

affordance

attentional fatigue

context

contextual analysis

contextual transformation

creative class

defensible space

digital divide

displacement

environment and behavior studies

imageability

interactional worldview

legibility

life domains

neighborhood

organismic worldview

physical incivilities

place attachment

sense of place

settings

situations

social incivilities

sociophysical environment

stimulation overload

stimuli

stress

third places

trait worldview

transactional worldview

virtual communities

DISCUSSION QUESTIONS

1. Make a list of the ways that you communicate with your friends and acquire information about the world. Then make lists of the ways your parents and grandparents communicated and acquired information when they were your age. Then add to your lists the places that facilitate or enable (in your case) and facilitated or enabled (in your grandparents' case) these communication and information activities. What are the potential health consequences of the changes you note in these lists? (Hint: consider the factors listed in Table 5.2.)

2. What physical and social factors that differ between low-income and high-income neighborhoods have implications for the health of residents? (Hint: Think about the quantity, variety, and quality of the first, second, and third places available to residents of each type of neighborhood.)

3. Draw a large circle on a piece of paper. Around the *left* side of the circle, write words or phrases that describe important physical aspects of your current home or residential environment (for example, "private bedroom," "outside garden/ yard," "comfortable," "spacious" or "cramped," "relaxing"). Around the *right* side of the circle, write words or phrases that describe important *social* aspects of your current home or residential environment (for example, "no privacy," "safe," "quiet," "great for parties," "good for quiet dinners," and so forth). Then draw lines (always going through at least part of the circle) to connect items strongly related to each other (such as "garden" and "relaxing"). A line may connect a physical and a social aspect, two physical aspects, or two social aspects. How complex are the relationships between these sociophysical factors in your residential setting? Which seem most important: that is, which exhibit the most connections to other factors? (To extend this discussion, consider these questions: Which factors might be related to the health of the residents of your home environment? Which of these factors is the most important?)

4. Consider the route you take most often to get to and from school. Do you consider it stressful or relaxing? Why? What do you listen to, that is, what kind of information do you absorb along the way? What options are available to you on this route (fast-food restaurants, natural views, dense urban scenes, light traffic, and so forth)? How does each of these contextual factors affect your mood, your expectations about the day ahead, your readiness to learn, and your overall health?

5. Select one of the following significant issues with important public health impacts: AIDS in Africa, war in the Middle East, destruction of rainforests, global financial recession, international terrorism, dependence on carbon fuels (oil), or poverty in major metropolitan areas. Using Table 5.4 as a template, identify specific impacts and related behavioral or health outcomes for each level of analysis, from global to local.

REFERENCES

Abel, D., and Fielding, J. "If You Want to Build a Better Community, It Takes a School." *Los Angeles Times,* Jan. 25, 2004, p. M2.

Alexander, C., and others. *A Pattern Language.* New York: Oxford University Press, 1977.

Altman, I. *The Environment and Social Behavior.* Pacific Grove, Calif.: Brooks/Cole, 1975.

Altman, I., and Rogoff, B. "World Views in Psychology: Trait, Interactional, Organismic, and Transactional Perspectives." In D. Stokols and I. Altman (eds.), *Handbook of Environmental Psychology* (pp. 7–40). Hoboken, N.J.: Wiley, 1987.

Altman, I., and Wandersman, A. (eds.). *Human Behavior and Environment,* Vol. *9: Neighborhood and Community Environments.* New York: Plenum, 1987.

Antonovsky, A. *Unraveling the Mystery of Health: How People Manage Stress and Stay Well.* San Francisco: Jossey-Bass, 1987.

Barker, R. G. *Ecological Psychology: Concepts and Methods for Studying the Environment of Human Behavior.* Palo Alto, Calif.: Stanford University Press, 1968.

Barker, R. G., and Schoggen, P. *Qualities of Community Life.* San Francisco: Jossey-Bass, 1973.

Baum, A., and Epstein, Y. M. *Human Response to Crowding.* Mahwah, N.J.: Erlbaum, 1978.

Baum, A., and Fleming, I. "Implications of Psychological Research on Stress and Technological Accidents." *American Psychologist,* 1993, *48*(6), 665–672.

Baum, A., and Valins, S. *Architecture and Social Behavior: Psychological Studies of Social Density.* Mahwah, N.J.: Erlbaum, 1977.

Bechtel, R. B. *Environment & Behavior: An Introduction.* Thousand Oaks, Calif.: Sage, 1997.

Bechtel, R. B., and Churchman, A. (eds.). *Handbook of Environmental Psychology.* Hoboken, N.J.: Wiley, 2002.

Berkman, L. F., and Syme, S. L. "Social Networks, Host Resistance, and Mortality: A Nine-Year Follow-Up Study of Alameda County Residents." *American Journal of Epidemiology,* 1979, *109*, 186–204.

Blanchard, A. "Virtual Behavior Settings: An Application of Behavior Setting Theories to Virtual Communities." Unpublished manuscript, Center for Organizational and Behavioral Sciences, Claremont Graduate University, 1997.

Blanchard, A., and Horan, T. "Virtual Communities and Social Capital." *Social Science Computer Review,* 1998, *16*, 293–307.

Brill, M., and Weidemann, S. *Disproving Widespread Myths About Workspace Design.* Buffalo, N.Y.: BOSTI Associates, 2001.

Bronfenbrenner, U. *The Ecology of Human Development: Experiments by Nature and Design.* Cambridge, Mass.: Harvard University Press, 1979.

Brunsma, D. L., Overfelt, D., and Picou, J. (eds.). *The Sociology of Katrina: Perspectives on a Modern Catastrophe.* Lanham, Md.: Rowman & Littlefield, 2007.

Bronzaft, A. L. "Noise Pollution: A Hazard to Physical and Mental Well-Being." In R. B. Bechtel and A. Churchman (eds.), *Handbook of Environmental Psychology.* Hoboken, N.J.: Wiley, 2002.

Brown, B. "Residential Burglaries: Cues to Burglary Vulnerability." *Journal of Architectural Planning and Research,* 1985, *2*, 231–243.

Bullard, R. D. *Dumping in Dixie: Race, Class, and Environmental Quality.* Boulder, Colo.: Westview Press, 1990.

Campbell, A. *The Sense of Well-Being in America.* New York: McGraw-Hill, 1981.

Cassel, J. "Social Science Theory as a Source of Hypotheses in Epidemiological Research." *American Journal of Public Health,* 1964, *54*, 1482–1488.

Cassel, J. "The Contribution of the Social Environment to Host Resistance." *American Journal of Public Health*, 1976, *104*, 107–123.

Chapin, F. S. *Human Activity Patterns in the City: Things People Do in Time and in Space*. Hoboken, N.J.: Wiley, 1974.

Clitheroe, C., Stokols, D., and Zmuidzinas, M. "Conceptualizing the Context of Environment and Behavior." *Journal of Environmental Psychology*, 1998, *18*, 103–112.

Cohen, C., Evans, G. W., Stokols, D., and Krantz, D. S. *Behavior, Health, and Environmental Stress*. New York: Plenum, 1986.

Cohen, S. "Aftereffects of Stress on Human Performance and Social Behavior: A Review of Research and Theory." *Psychological Bulletin*, 1980, *88*, 82–108.

Cohen, S., Glass, D. C., and Singer, J. E. "Apartment Noise, Auditory Discrimination, and Reading Ability in Children." *Journal of Experimental Social Psychology*, 1973, *9*, 407–422.

Cohen, S., and others. "Chronic Social Stress, Social Status, and Susceptibility to Upper Respiratory Infections in Nonhuman Primates." *Psychosomatic Medicine*, 1997a, *59*(3), 213–221.

Cohen, S., and others. "Social Ties and Susceptibility to the Common Cold." *JAMA*, 1997b, *277*, 1940–1944.

Cohen, S., and others. "Types of Stressors That Increase Susceptibility to the Common Cold in Healthy Adults." *Health Psychology*, 1998, *17*(3), 214–223.

Cohen, S., and others. "Sociability and Susceptibility to the Common Cold." *Psychological Science*, 2003, *14*(5), 389–395.

Detels, R., McEwen, J., Beaglehole, R., and Tanaka, H. (eds.). *Oxford Textbook of Public Health*. (4th ed.) New York: Oxford University Press, 2002.

Diez Roux, A. V. "Investigating Neighborhood and Area Effects on Health." *American Journal of Public Health*, 2001, *91*, 1783–1789.

Dooley, D. "Unemployment, Underemployment, and Mental Health: Conceptualizing Employment Status as a Continuum." *American Journal of Community Psychology*, 2003, *32*(1–2), 9–20.

Dooley, D., Fielding, J., and Levi, L. "Health and Unemployment." *Annual Review of Public Health*, 1996, *17*, 449–465.

Evans, G. W. "Environmental Stress and Health." In A. Baum, T. Revenson, and J. E. Singer (eds.), *Handbook of Health Psychology*. Mahwah, N.J.: Erlbaum, 2001.

Evans, G. W. "The Environment of Childhood Poverty." *American Psychologist*, 2004, *59*(2), 77–92.

Evans, G. W., and Johnson, D. "Stress and Open-Office Noise." *Journal of Applied Psychology*, 2000, *85*(5), 779–783.

Evans, G. W., and Kantrowitz, E. "Socioeconomic Status and Health: The Potential Role of Environmental Risk Exposure." *Annual Review of Public Health*, 2002, *23*, 303–331.

Evans, G. W., and Lepore, S. J. "Household Crowding and Social Support: A Quasi-Experimental Analysis." *Journal of Personality and Social Psychology*, 1993, *65*, 308–316.

Evans, G. W., and others. "Community Noise Exposure and Stress in Children." *Journal of the Acoustical Society of America*, 2001, *109*(3), 1023–1027.

Festinger, L., Schachter, S., and Back, K. *Social Pressures in Informal Groups*. New York: HarperCollins, 1950.

Fielding, J. E., Cumberland, W. G., and Pettitt, L. "Immunization Status of Children of Employees in a Large Corporation." *JAMA*, 1994, *271*, 525–530.

Fishbein, M., and Ajzen, I. *Belief, Attitudes, Intention, and Behavior: An Introduction to Theory and Research.* Upper Saddle River, N.J.: Addison-Wesley/Pearson Education, 1975.

Florida, R. *The Rise of the Creative Class.* New York: Basic Books, 2002.

Forgas, J. P. *Social Episodes: The Study of Interaction Routines.* San Diego: Academic Press, 1979.

Frank, L. D., Engelke, P. O., and Schmid, T. L. *Health and Community Design: The Impact of the Built Environment on Physical Activity.* Washington, D.C.: Island Press, 2003.

Frumkin, H. "Beyond Toxicity: Human Health and the Natural Environment." *American Journal of Preventive Medicine,* 2001, *20*(3), 234–240.

Frumkin, H. "Healthy Places: Exploring the Evidence." *American Journal of Public Health,* 2003, *93,* 1451–1456.

Fullilove, M. D. *Root Shock: How Tearing Up City Neighborhoods Hurts America, and What We Can Do About It.* New York: Ballantine, 2004.

Garces, R. F. Experts Propose Policies to Bridge California's Digital Divide, Improve Health. California Center for Health Improvement. http://www.cchi.org/pdf/WrkHlth2.pdf, 2000.

Garland, C. A., and Stokols, D. "The Effect of Neighborhood Reputation on Fear of Crime and Inner City Investment." In J. I. Arragones, G. Francescato, and T. Garling (eds.), *Residential Environments: Choice, Satisfaction, and Behavior.* Westport, Conn.: Greenwood, 2002.

Gerberding, J. L. "Climate Change and Public Health." Testimony before the Committee on Environment and Public Works, United States Senate, Oct. 23, 2007.

Gibson, J., 1977. "The Theory of Affordances." In R. Shaw and J. Bransford (eds.), *Perceiving, Acting, and Knowing: Toward an Ecological Psychology* (pp. 76–82). Mahwah, N.J.: Erlbaum.

Gifford, R. *Environmental Psychology: Principles and Practice.* (2nd ed.) Boston: Allyn & Bacon, 1997.

Glass, D. C., and Singer, J. E. *Urban Stress.* San Diego: Academic Press, 1972.

Gore, A. *An Inconvenient Truth: The Planetary Emergency of Global Warming and What We Can Do About It.* Emmasus, Penn.: Rodale Books, 2006.

Holman, E. A., and Stokols, D. "The Environmental Psychology of Child Sexual Abuse." *Journal of Environmental Psychology,* 1994, *14,* 237–252.

Hygge, S., Evans, G. W., and Bullinger, M. "A Prospective Study of Some Effects of Aircraft Noise on Cognitive Performance in Schoolchildren." *Psychological Science,* 2002, *13*(5), 469–474.

International Technology and Trade Associates. *State of the Internet 2000.* http://www.itta.com/internet2000.htm, 2000.

Ittelson, W. H. *Environment and Cognition.* New York: Seminar Press, 1973.

Jacobs, J. *The Death and Life of Great American Cities.* New York: Random House, 1961.

Kaplan, R., and Kaplan, S. *The Experience of Nature: A Psychological Perspective.* New York: Cambridge University Press, 1989.

Kiesler, S. (ed.). *Culture of the Internet.* Mahwah, N.J.: Erlbaum, 1997.

Kling, R., and Iacono, S. "Making a Computer Revolution." In C. Dunlop and R. Kling (eds.), *Computerization and Controversy: Value Conflicts and Social Choices.* San Diego: Academic Press, 1991.

Kohn, L. T., Corrigan, J., and Donaldson, M. S. *To Err Is Human: Building a Safer Health System.* Washington, D.C.: National Academies Press, 2000.

Koren, H., and Bisesi, M. *Handbook of Environmental Health. 2* vols. (4th ed.) Boca Raton, Fla.: CRC Press, 2002.

Langer, E. J., and Rodin, J. "The Effects of Choice and Enhanced Personal Responsibility for the Aged: A Field Experiment in an Institutional Setting." *Journal of Personality and Social Psychology*, 1976, *34*, 191–198.

Lewis, C. A. "Comment: Healing in the Urban Environment: A Person/Plant Viewpoint." *Journal of the American Planning Association*, 1979, *45*, 330–338.

Lindheim, R., and Syme, S. L. "Environments, People, and Health." *Annual Review of Public Health*, 1983, *4*, 335–359.

Lyman, P., and Varian, H. R. How Much Information? Berkeley School of Information Management and Systems, University of California. http://www.sims.berkeley.edu/how-much-info, Oct. 20, 2000.

Lynch, K. *The Image of the City*. Cambridge, Mass.: MIT Press, 1960.

Magnusson, D. "Wanted: A Psychology of Situations." In D. Magnusson (ed.), *Toward a Psychology of Situations: An Interactional Perspective*. Mahwah, N.J.: Erlbaum, 1981.

Mark, G., Gonzalez, V., and Harris, J. "No Task Left Behind? Examining the Nature of Fragmented Work." Proceedings of the Association on Copmuting Machinery Special Interest Group on Computer-Human Interaction (SIGCHI) Conference on Human Factors in Computing Systems, Portland, Oregon, April 2-7, 2005. http://portal.acm.org/citation.cfm?id51055017.

Mark, G., Gudith, D., and Klocke, U. "The Cost of Interrupted Work: More Speed and Stress." Proceedings of the Association on Copmuting Machinery Special Interest Group on Computer-Human Interaction (SIGCHI) Conference on Human Factors in Computing Systems, Portland, Oregon, April 2-7, 2005. http://portal.acm.org/citation. cfm?id51357054.1357072.

Mathews, K.E.J., and Canon, L. K. "Environmental Noise Level as a Determinant of Helping Behavior." *Journal of Personality and Social Psychology*, 1975, *32*, 571–577.

McEwen, B. S., and Stellar, E. "Stress and the Individual: Mechanisms Leading to Disease." *Archives of Internal Medicine*, 1993, *153*, 2093–2101.

Messagingonline. "AOL Per-User Email Figures Climb 60 Percent in 1999." http://www.messagingon-line.net/mt/html/feature020400.html, Oct. 29, 2000.

Meyrowitz, J. *No Sense of Place: The Impact of Electronic Media on Social Behavior*. New York: Oxford University Press, 1985.

Michelson, W. H. *From Sun to Sun: Daily Obligations and Community Structure in the Lives of Employed Women and Their Families*. Lanham, Md.: Rowman & Littlefield, 1985.

Milgram, S. "The Experience of Living in Cities." *Science*, 1970, *167*, 1461–1468.

Milgram, S., and Jodelet, D. "Psychological Maps of Paris." In H. M. Proshansky, W. H. Ittelson, and L. G. Rivlin (eds.), *Environmental Psychology*. (2nd ed.) Austin, Tex.: Holt, Rinehart and Winston, 1976.

Moos, R. H. "Social Ecological Perspectives on Health." In G. C. Stone, F. Cohen, and N. E. Adler (eds.), *Health Psychology: A Handbook*. San Francisco: Jossey Bass, 1979.

Mossberger, K., Tolbert, C.J., and Stansbury, M. *Virtual Inequality: Beyond the Digital Divide*. Washington: Georgetown University Press, 2003.

Nasar, J. L., and Fisher, B. "Hot Spots of Fear and Crime: A Multimethod Investigation." *Journal of Environmental Psychology*, 1993, *13*, 187–206.

National Telecommunications and Information Administration. "Americans in the Information Age Falling Through the Net." http://www.ntia.doc.gov/ntiahome/digitaldivide, 2000.

Negroponte, N. P. *Being Digital*. New York: Vintage Books, 1995.

Newman, O. *Creating Defensible Space*. Rockville, Md.: U.S. Department of Housing and Urban Development, 1966.

Newman, O. *Defensible Space*. New York: Macmillan, 1973.

Nie, N. H., and Erbring, L. Internet and Society: A Preliminary Report. Stanford Institute for the Quantitative Study of Society. http://www.stanford.edu/group/siqss/Press_Release/Preliminary_Report.pdf, 2000.

O'Donnell, M. P. "Definition of Health Promotion, Part III: Expanding the Definition." *American Journal of Health Promotion*, 1989, *3*, 5.

Oldenburg, R. *The Great Good Place: Cafés, Coffee Shops, Bookstores, Bars, Hair Salons, and Other Hangouts at the Heart of a Community*. (2nd ed.) New York: Marlowe, 1999.

O'Neil, R., and Greenberger, E. "Patterns of Commitment to Work and Parenting: Implications for Role Strain." *Journal of Marriage and the Family*, 1994, *56*, 101–112.

Pastalan, L. A. "Environmental Displacement: A Literature Reflecting Old Person-Environment Transactions." In G. D. Rowles and R. J. Ohta (eds.), *Aging and Milieu: Environmental Perspectives on Growing Old*. San Diego: Academic Press, 1983.

Perkins, D., Wandersman, A., Rich, R., and Taylor, R. "The Physical Environment of Street Crime: Defensible Space, Territoriality, and Incivilities" *Journal of Environmental Psychology*, 1993, *13*, 29–49.

Pervin, L. A. "Definitions, Measurements, and Classifications of Stimuli, Situations, and Environments." *Human Ecology*, 1978, *6*, 71–105.

Proshansky, H. M., Fabian, A. K., and Kaminoff, R. "Place Identity: Physical World Socialization of the Self." *Journal of Environmental Psychology*, 1983, *3*, 57–83.

Proshansky, H. M., Ittelson, W. H., and Rivlin, L. G. (eds.). *Environmental Psychology*. (2nd ed.) Austin, Tex.: Holt, Rinehart and Winston, 1976.

Putnam, R. D. *Bowling Alone: The Collapse and Revival of American Community*. New York: Simon & Schuster, 2000.

Rashad, I., and Grossman, M. "The Economics of Obesity." http://www.thepublicinterest.com/archives/2004summer/article3.html, 2004.

Relph, E. C. (1976). *Place and Placelessness*. London: Pion.

Rheingold, H. *The Virtual Community: Homesteading on the Electronic Frontier*. Upper Saddle River, N.J.: Addison-Wesley/Pearson Education, 1993.

Rivlin, L. G. "The Neighborhood, Personal Identity, and Group Affiliations." In I. Altman and A. Wandersman (eds.), *Human Behavior and Environment*, Vol. *9*: *Neighborhood and Community Environments*. New York: Plenum, 1987.

Rodin, J., and Langer, E. J. "Long-Term Effects of a Control-Relevant Intervention with the Institutionalized Aged." *Journal of Personality and Social Psychology*, 1977, *35*, 897–902.

Rosenbaum, S. "US Health Policy in the Aftermath of Hurricane Katrina." *JAMA*, 2006, *295*, 437–440.

Schoggen, P. *Behavior Settings: A Revision and Extension of Roger G. Barker's Ecological Psychology*. Palo Alto, Calif.: Stanford University Press, 1989.

Schulz, R., and Hanusa, B. H. "Long-Term Effects of Control and Predictability-Enhancing Interventions: Findings and Ethical Issues." *Journal of Personality and Social Psychology*, 1978, *36*, 1194–1201.

Selye, H. *The Stress of Life*. New York: McGraw-Hill, 1956.

Servon, L.J. *Bridging the Digital Divide: Technology, Community, and Public Policy*. Malden, MA: Blackwell, 2002.

Silver, R. C., and others. "Nationwide Longitudinal Study of Psychological Responses to September 11." *JAMA*, 2002, *288*, 1235–1244.

Sommer, R. *Personal Space: The Behavioral Basis of Design*. Upper Saddle River, N.J.: Prentice Hall, 1969.

Stokols, D. "The Paradox of Environmental Psychology." *American Psychologist*, 1995, *50*, 821–837.

Stokols, D. "Human Development in the Age of the Internet: Conceptual and Methodological Horizons." In S. L. Friedman and T. D. Wachs (eds.), *Measuring Environment Across the Lifespan: Emerging Methods and Concepts*. Washington, D.C.: American Psychological Association, 1999.

Stokols, D., and Altman, I. (eds.). *Handbook of Environmental Psychology*. 2 vols. Hoboken, N.J.: Wiley, 1987.

Stokols, D., McMahan, S., Clitheroe, H.C.J., and Wells, M. "Enhancing Corporate Compliance with Worksite Safety and Health Legislation." *Journal of Safety Research*, 2001, *32*, 441–463.

Stokols, D., and Montero, M. "Toward an Environmental Psychology of the Internet." In R. B. Bechtel and A. Churchman (eds.), *Handbook of Environmental Psychology* (pp. 661–675). Hoboken, N.J.: Wiley, 2002.

Stokols, D., and Shumaker, S. "People in Places: A Transactional View of Settings." In J. Harvey (ed.), *Cognition, Social Behavior, and the Environment*. Mahwah, N.J.: Erlbaum, 1981.

Sundstrom, E., and Sundstrom, M. G. *Work Places: The Psychology of the Physical Environment in Offices and Factories*. New York: Cambridge University Press, 1986.

Taylor, R. B. *Human Territorial Functioning*. New York: Cambridge University Press, 1988.

Taylor, S. E., Repetti, R. L., and Seeman, T. "Health Psychology: What Is an Unhealthy Environment and How Does It Get Under the Skin?" *Annual Review of Psychology*, 1997, *48*, 411–447.

Unger, D. G., and Wandersman, A. "The Importance of Neighbors: The Social, Cognitive, and Affective Components of Neighboring." *American Journal of Community Psychology*, 1985, *13*(2), 139–160.

Vaughan, E. "Individual and Cultural Differences in Adaptation to Environmental Risks." *American Psychologist*, 1993, *48*(6), 673–680.

Wellman, B. "Physical Place and Cyberplace: The Rise of Personalized Networking." *International Journal of Urban and Regional Research*, 2001, *25*(2), 227–252.

Wellman, B., and Haythornthwaite, C. A. (eds.). *The Internet in Everyday Life*. Malden, Mass.: Blackwell, 2002.

World Health Organization. Ottawa Charter for Health Promotion. Declaration from the 1st International Conference on Health Promotion. http://www.who.int/hpr/NPH/docs/ottawa_charter_hp.pdf, 1986.

World Health Organization. Jakarta Declaration on Leading Health Promotion into the 21st Century. Declaration from the 4th International Conference on Health Promotion. http://www.who.int/hpr/NPH/docs/jakarta_declaration_en.pdf, 1997.

Yassi, A., Kjellström, T., de Kok, T., and Guidotti, T. *Basic Environmental Health*. New York: Oxford University Press. 2001.

FOR FURTHER INFORMATION

Journals

Environment and Behavior, http://eab.sagepub.com.
Journal of Environmental Psychology, http://www.elsevier.com/wps/find/journaldescription.
cws_home/622872/description#description.
Journal of Architectural and Planning Research, http://www.lockescience.com.

Academic Programs

City University of New York, Department of Psychology. Research-based interdisciplinary PhD pro-
gram in environmental psychology (a subprogram of CUNY's PhD program in psychology).
http://web.gc.cuny.edu/dept/psych/environmental/index.htm.
Georgia Institute of Technology, College of Architecture. Ph.D. program in Architecture, Culture and
Behavior. http://www.publicarchitecture.gatech.edu/acb/
University of California-Irvine, School of Social Ecology. PhD program in social ecology. http://www
.seweb.uci.edu.
University of Sydney, Faculty of Architecture, Design & Planning. Environment, Behaviour, & Society
(EBS) research. http://www.arch.usyd.edu.au/research/env_behaviour.shtml.

Professional Organizations

American Psychological Association, Division 34, Population and Environmental Psychology, http://
apa34.cos.ucf.edu.
American Sociological Association, Environment and Technology Section, http://www.asanet.org/
sections/environ.html; Community and Urban Sociology Section, http://www.asanet.org/
sections/commun.html.
Canadian Psychological Association, Environmental Section, http://www.cpa.ca/environmental.
Environment-Behaviour Research Association of China, http://www.ebra2004.com/home.htm.
Environmental Design Research Association (EDRA), http://www.edra.org.
International Association for Applied Psychology (IAAP), Environmental Psychology Division, http://
www.psy.gu.se/iaap/envpsych.htm.
International Association for People-Environment Studies (IAPS), http://www.iaps-association.org.

CHAPTER SIX

GENETICS AND ENVIRONMENTAL HEALTH

SAMUEL H. WILSON

WILLIAM A.SUK

KEY CONCEPTS

- The risk of disease is a function of both genetic and environmental factors. Gene-environment interactions are central to a full understanding of disease.

- Multifaceted approaches are now available to measure environmental exposures and to study how genetic factors affect the impact of those exposures.

- The variation in genetic risk raises a host of ethical, legal, and social issues that must be addressed.

THE same amount of exposure to organophosphate pesticide can make one child sick but pose little harm to another. Why? Studies have shown that susceptibility to organophosphate pesticide poisoning, as well as to vascular disease, can be traced to variations in a **gene** involved in toxicant metabolism (Davies and others, 1996; Jarvik and others, 2003; Li and others, 2000). Our growing knowledge that the interaction between our environment and our genes is often at the root of disease and our individual susceptibility to it is making possible major advances in environmental health and **personalized medicine**. But it is also making scientific questions, issues, and investigations infinitely more complex.

The concept of **gene-environment interaction** has gained wide acceptance in the scientific community and is central to the future of both **genetics** and environmental health (Collins, 2004; Potter, 2004). These two fields, once separate and distinct, are now inextricable. Genetics, the study of individual genes, has expanded to include **genomics**, which is the study of all the genes that make up an organism; a complete genome is present in every cell and governs an individual's unique characteristics and responses. Similarly, the definition of what constitutes the environment has evolved. Currently, and particularly as it relates to gene-environment interactions, the environment is considered to be anything outside the body that can affect an individual's health. This includes air, water, soil, and climate, of course, but also takes into account elements such as the food, drink, and medicine we ingest; our behavioral choices, such as consuming tobacco and alcohol; our exposure to infectious agents; our socioeconomic status; our age or developmental status; the stress we experience; and even the structures and infrastructure around us (the so-called built environment) (Hanna and Coussens, 2001; also see Chapter Fourteen).

EXPLORING SUSCEPTIBILITY, RISK, AND EXPOSURE

The questions of what causes disease and what can we do to prevent it, cure it, or minimize its impact on quality of life have been central to medicine from time immemorial. Today these questions propel the mission of biomedical science to understand and characterize gene-environment interactions. The vast majority of human disease arises when something is wrong in the relationship between

The authors wish to thank science writer Angela Spivey for her instrumental role in the preparation of this chapter. In addition, Samuel H. Wilson and William A. Suk declare no competing financial interests.

a person's body and the environment. Such miscues can occur in the blink of an eye, as in the case of acute exposures to toxic agents, or can take decades to develop, as in illnesses such as cancer or Alzheimer's disease.

Although certain inherited disorders, such as Huntington's disease, cystic fibrosis, and Tay-Sachs disease, arise from mutation in a single gene, such disorders are relatively rare, accounting for no more than 5 percent of human disease. Thus the risk of such a disease for a person with a disease-specific gene variant (referred to as an **allele**) is relatively high, but the incidence of such *monogenic* diseases in the general population is low. Instead, many common human diseases appear to be *polygenic*, resulting from complex interactions of several genes. A variant of one gene might not be detrimental, but it might become detrimental in combination with specific alleles of other genes. Such susceptibility-conferring genes increase disease risk only a few-fold, but because these genes occur so frequently in the human population, they can have a large effect on the incidence of a disease. However, **susceptibility genes** alone are not sufficient to cause disease; they modify risk in combination with other genes and with exposure to environmental agents (Figure 6.1).

Because every organism is continually exposed to hazardous agents in its environment, organisms have evolved sophisticated pathways that can minimize the biological consequences of such exposures. These pathways constitute the **environmental response machinery**. All human genes, including those that

FIGURE 6.1   Gene-Environment Interaction and
Disease Burden

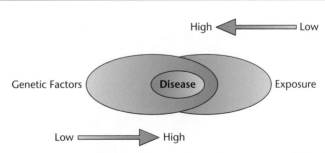

This image represents the hypothesis that combinations of genetic susceptibility factors and environmental exposures (and not genetic or exposure factors alone) account for the majority of the U.S. disease burden. Understanding the multitude of gene-environment combinations that are associated with common diseases is considered an important research approach for the future.

encode components of the environmental response machinery, are subject to genetic variability, which may be associated with altered efficiency of the gene product (usually an enzyme or protein) and ultimately with a biological pathway. So a person's risk for developing an illness as a result of an environmental exposure might depend on the efficiency of his or her own unique set of environmental response genes. These genes might, for example, determine how an individual responds to and metabolizes drugs or carcinogenic compounds after exposure.

Determining how genetic susceptibility contributes to disease risk from environmental exposures is a main focus of today's environmental health research. In the quest to characterize gene-environment interactions, however, the picture is immensely complicated. Not only are combinations of genes typically involved but there are also issues of combinations of exposures, the time periods over which exposures have occurred (relative to physiological development and age), and the detection and identification of chronic low-level exposures (Figure 6.2). The large array of variables affecting gene-environment interactions is daunting. But advances in research technologies and methods and in computational abilities have given environmental health scientists new tools that should spawn major improvements in public health. One important recent achievement was the mapping of the human genome.

FIGURE 6.2   Environmental Exposure and Genetic Variation
as a Consequence of Aging

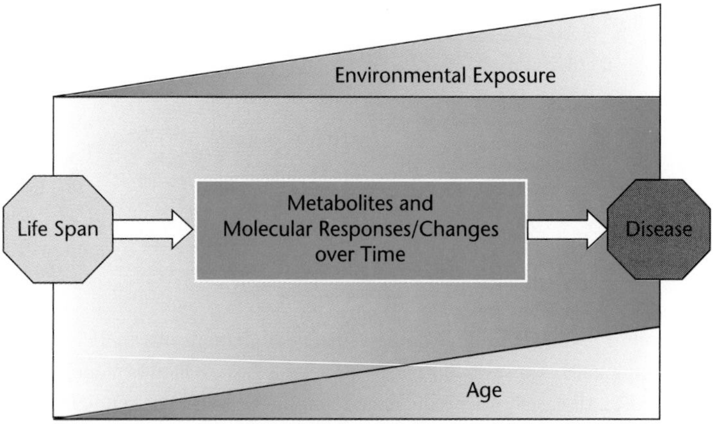

As age and environmental exposure increase over time, so do the progressive molecular responses and changes that are linked to pathogenesis.

PERSPECTIVE
ELSIs

Most people today are at least nominally familiar with the **ethical, legal, and social implications** (ELSIs) of genetics such as the potential for genetic discrimination by employers or insurers and confidentiality issues.

As science and technology rapidly progress and the fields of genomics and environmental health converge, many thorny issues will need to be dealt with forthrightly in the public debate.

Our advancing knowledge of risk and susceptibility, which will eventually enable routine determination of an individual's susceptibility to a wide variety of environmentally induced diseases, will require real-world answers to ethical, legal, and social questions that today are still largely anticipatory and theoretical. For example, if you are found through genotyping to have an increased susceptibility to a specific disease, a risk that is increased by exposure to a specific material, do you have the right to be employed in a workplace likely to expose you to that material? Does the employer have the right to deny you employment based on your genotype, or is the employer obligated to provide a workplace, potentially at great expense, in which you will be protected from occupational exposure to the agent? This is just one among many lines that will soon need to be drawn to ensure that all stakeholders are adequately, responsibly, and ethically informed and protected.

From its inception in 1990, the Human Genome Project recognized the need to address these issues and allocated a significant proportion of its overall budget to research and outreach activities to address ELSIs. The ELSIs program was a successful instance of the scientific community taking its responsibility to the public seriously. It stands today as a model for future initiatives (including a proposed independent and nonprofit genomic policy organization) designed to ensure that as we learn more and more about gene-environment interactions and as that learning influences public and private policies, the rights of every person to privacy, personal freedom, and fair treatment will not be compromised (for review, see Sharp, Yudell, and Wilson, 2004).

THE HUMAN GENOME PROJECT

In 2001, just fifty years after Watson and Crick reported the structure of the DNA double helix (Watson and Crick, 1953), scientists in the **Human Genome Program** (HGP) completed the sequencing of the human genome, providing a complete roadmap to the locations of the approximately 30,000 human genes (Collins, 2001). This will probably stand as one of the most significant achievements in the history of science, but it is clear that the genomic information has not, in and of itself, resulted in answers to the many questions about the genetic basis of disease. The genome sequence information will be used as a reference in the process of learning about individual human **genetic variation**; the sequence can be viewed as a dictionary that gives researchers the framework needed to flesh out "the grammar and syntax of the language of disease." Large questions, such as what is the actual extent of the genetic variation, or **polymorphism**, between human beings, and how much genetic variation is acquired as we age, must still be answered.

GENETIC VARIATION

In our efforts to understand disease, it is characterizing the genetic variations among individuals or groups that will provide the most useful information. Variations in genes or groups of related genes result in **phenotypes**. Phenotypes can describe physical traits such as hair color, behavioral features such as anxiety, and specific physiological susceptibilities or responses to gene-environment interactions. Our collective individual phenotypes make us who we are as individuals—determining whether we are at greater risk than the general population of contracting a disease or whether a particular drug will work, prove ineffective, or even be toxic for us.

Genetic variation among individuals is typically due to insertions and deletions of DNA known as **indels**, and **single nucleotide polymorphisms (SNPs)**, which are normal variations of one letter of the genetic code. Identifying these DNA sequence variations, and characterizing how they determine or influence phenotypes, is the focus of an enormous amount of current research and is the starting point for arriving at a useful understanding of gene-environment interactions and their myriad effects on human health.

It has been estimated that there are roughly 11 million SNPs in the human population (Kruglyak and Nickerson, 2001), of which several million have been identified and catalogued by various research efforts. To be recognized as a SNP, a single-letter variation in DNA sequence must occur in at least 1 percent of the population. SNPs with a frequency of 10 percent or more are thought of as common. SNPs tend to occur in patterns, or blocks, of associated, inherited alleles called **haplotypes**. The identification of haplotypes can in some cases obviate the need to document individual SNPs, as the haplotype is considered to be the inherited functional unit that ultimately influences physiology. A public-private research consortium called the International HapMap Project (2005) aims to map all the haplotypes in the human genome. The HapMap, the second phase of which was completed in 2007, is a powerful new tool for researchers to use in identifying genetic variations that affect disease susceptibility, drug

PERSPECTIVE
Genetic Variability and Susceptibility to Lead Toxicity

Lead has long been recognized to be highly toxic to humans. Although environmental levels of the metal have been greatly reduced over the past few decades, due in large measure to its elimination from gasoline and paint, lead toxicity is still a major public health problem, especially in children who live in housing retaining lead-based paint residues or who reside in lead-contaminated localities, such as areas close to smelters or battery factories. The problem is exacerbated by the fact that lead accumulates in the body and that lead acquired early in life can be released into the bloodstream to wreak physiological havoc much later in life, such as during menopause.

Environmental health scientists have determined that polymorphisms in certain genes can make some individuals far more susceptible to the damaging effects of lead poisoning by affecting the absorption, accumulation, and transport of the toxin. Variants of the gene coding for δ-**aminolevulinic acid dehydratase** (ALAD), an enzyme involved in heme biosynthesis, for example, appear to adversely affect bone and blood levels of lead. Polymorphisms of the vitamin D receptor (VDR) gene have been implicated in increased accumulation of lead in bone. Also variants of the hemochromatosis gene coding for the HFE protein, which is involved in iron transport in the body, may influence lead absorption and transport (Onalaja and Claudio, 2000). Discovery and characterization of these and other genetic markers of increased susceptibility to lead toxicity are key scientific milestones in the effort to reduce, treat, or prevent gene-environment interactions that cause disease and dysfunction associated with lead poisoning.

response, infectious disease resistance, and longevity. Although initiatives designed to establish comprehensive databases of SNPs, indels, and haplotypes take the genome sequence data compiled by the HGP a step further, they still do not yield knowledge that will translate directly into beneficial new treatment, prevention, or therapeutic paradigms. That step will require more information about the nature of the association between human genetic variation and phenotypes.

THE NEW GENERATION IN ENVIRONMENTAL HEALTH RESEARCH

Polymorphisms in an individual's environmental response genes can modify the risk of environmentally induced disease. To achieve an understanding of that relationship and its implications in gene-environment interactions, the National Institutes of Health launched an initiative in 1997 called the **Environmental Genome Project** (EGP) (2005). The EGP uses the candidate gene approach to identify and characterize human genetic variability in selected genes thought to be involved in susceptibility to toxicant-induced disease (Olden and Wilson, 2000; Wilson and Olden, 2004). By resequencing the selected candidate genes in a set of DNA samples representative of the U.S. population, the project aims to discover SNPs and other variants that are relevant to environmental responses, and eventually to yield knowledge that will have implications for medical and environmental policymaking and regulation.

The environmentally responsive genes selected for study by the EGP tend to fall into eight categories: **cell cycle**, **DNA repair**, **cell division**, **cell signaling**, **cell structure**, **gene expression**, **apoptosis**, and **metabolism**. Cell cycle and cell division genes regulate the ability of a cell to proliferate, grow, and differentiate. Changes in the progression of a cell through the cell cycle can increase the cell's ability to survive stress, for example, by allowing cellular damage to be repaired prior to cell division. Cell signaling and gene expression pathways have effects on all cellular functions, including cell proliferation and differentiation. Metabolic pathways are crucial determinants of the outcome of exposure. An innocuous compound may be metabolically converted into a reactive species that causes cellular damage; alternatively, some metabolic pathways destroy toxic compounds by changing the compounds' chemical structure. DNA repair genes can influence the outcome of exposure to environmental agents that cause DNA damage. Individuals with higher or lower capacity for DNA repair have decreased or increased risk, respectively, of certain types of environmentally induced disease. Heavily damaged cells often die by the process known as apoptosis, or programmed cell death. Apoptosis protects the organism by removing damaged or aberrant cells, and failure to execute this process is associated with adverse health effects, such as cancer.

To date about 1,000 candidate genes, mostly metabolism, DNA repair, and cell cycle genes, have been resequenced by the EGP. Another accomplishment was the compilation of the publicly accessible GeneSNPs database, which lists the thousands of new SNPs now made available for research use (GeneSNPs, 2005; EGP, 2005). The EGP has also turned researchers' attention to the functional significance of polymorphisms, in an effort to establish whether or not each polymorphism is an active component in exposure-associated disease. One method of tying SNPs and indels to function is to develop and examine mouse models of human gene variants, and the EGP is currently doing this in a project known as the Comparative Mouse Genomics Centers Consortium. The mouse

PERSPECTIVE
EGP Cases in Point

Using the candidate gene approach, the Environmental Genome Project has already yielded significant information about genes implicated in gene-environment interactions at the root of human disease. EGP investigators Clement Furlong and colleagues have conducted detailed studies of polymorphisms (as briefly alluded to earlier) in the paraoxanase gene PON1 (Davies and others, 1996; Jarvik and others, 2003; Li and others, 2000). The gene regulates production of the enzyme paraoxanase (PON1), which metabolizes toxic organophosphates and some pharmaceutical agents, such as the cholesterol-lowering statin drugs. Furlong's group discovered that certain SNPs influence PON1 activity, altering production of the enzyme. Their study clearly demonstrated that an individual's PON1 status has implications for susceptibility to environmentally associated diseases, including organophosphate toxicity and cardiovascular disease. PON1 status also is suspected to be involved in susceptibility to Gulf War syndrome (as well as Parkinson's disease), although studies of that association have shown conflicting results (Kelada and others, 2003; Kondo and Yamamoto, 1998; Taylor, Le Couteur, Mellick, and Board, 2000; Akhmedova, Anisimov, Yakimovsky, and Schwartz, 1999; Akhmedova, Yakimovsky, and Schwartz, 2001; Wang and Liu, 2000).

EGP researcher Martyn Smith of the University of California at Berkeley examined gene-environment interactions in blood-related cancers, including leukemia, lymphoma, and myeloma. Many leukemia cases are thought to be induced by environmental factors, including exposure to benzene, radiation, and chemotherapeutic agents. Genetic factors are also thought to play a significant role, especially in pathways controlling DNA repair and oxidative DNA damage. Smith and his collaborators identified one candidate gene that appears to be involved in the etiology of leukemia, namely, the gene encoding NAD(P)H:quinone acceptor oxireductase 1 (NOQ1). This enzyme plays a role in preventing oxidative damage caused by exogenous and endogenous quinines, which are biologically active compounds found in natural substances such as vitamins, aloe, and henna and in chemicals such as photographic fixatives and dyes. The C609T polymorphism of that gene, which occurs in 5 to 20 percent of the population, results in complete loss of enzyme activity in homozygotes (people with two copies of the variant gene). Case-control studies indicate a 1.5- to 2.5-fold increased odds ratio for several types of leukemia in association with the 609T variant (Smith and others, 2001, 2002; Krajinovic and others, 2002). Although this effect is relatively small, adverse environmental exposure may interact with this genetic variant and lead to significantly increased risk of disease.

models produced in this project will be subject to phenotypic analysis in tests of susceptibility to environmental exposures.

The significance of individual polymorphisms can be elucidated by population-based research, in which large numbers of people are screened for variants and the data are analyzed to determine associations between polymorphisms, disease susceptibility, and exposures (Altshuler, Kruglyak, and Lander, 1998). The effects of solitary gene polymorphisms are believed to be relatively weak, and the environmentally induced diseases under study are believed to be polygenic, involving interactions of multiple genetic variants and exposures. Due to these factors the population studies will need to be very large to identify subgroups at increased risk of disease because of their particular genotypes. This will undoubtedly be a challenging aspect of the EGP, but it is this type of knowledge that will yield the largest public health benefits.

LINKING GENES AND ENVIRONMENTAL EXPOSURES

Given that most human disease is now understood to involve complex interactions among genetic predispositions (due to genetic variants), environmental exposures (both acute and chronic—that is, both short- and long-term), and aging or physiological development, characterizing the relationships among these elements in a useful way (although an extraordinarily complicated undertaking) is the pathway that will eventually lead to a new age of medicine and disease prevention. An era of personalized medicine is possible, but the road toward achieving it is still very long and most realistically measured in decades. The assurance of progress requires that multiple research approaches be used for linking exposures with clinical disease (Figure 6.3).

The traditional approach to environmental exposure assessment (see Chapters Two and Four), working from the release of a toxicant into the general environment to human exposure to internal dose to biological effect and eventually to disease, has proven to be an extremely effective framework for environmental health research (Suk and Wilson, 2002). Its component methodologies have matured, and innovative measurement and assessment techniques continue to be developed. In the hazard assessment approach to exposure, advanced techniques are employed to characterize the relationship between the dose of an agent and the adverse response of a model organism. Obviously, the starting point for this type of investigation is the agent itself, along with a variety of questions: Is the agent toxic? At what levels of exposure is it toxic? What are the biological effects of such an exposure? How do genotypes modulate the impacts of those effects? And the ultimate question of course is, How can this information be interpreted

FIGURE 6.3   Research Approaches to Link Environmental Exposures with Disease

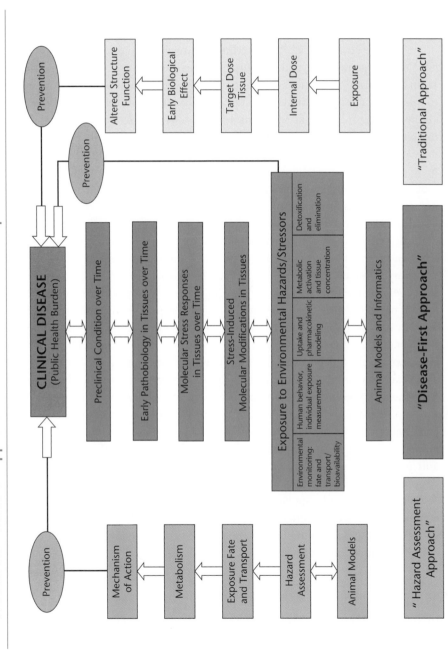

This diagram contrasts the traditional and hazards assessment approaches to environmental health research with the "disease-first" approach, which begins with clinical disease and the public health burden it represents, and then drives inquiry toward the molecular characterization of disease and the underlying exposure responses. Adapted from Wilson and Sule, 2005.

to accurately predict human health outcomes following exposure to environmentally relevant doses? These can be extremely complicated questions, but methodologies are emerging to characterize dose-response curves at the molecular level (such as gene expression, **protein expression**, metabolism, and so forth). High-throughput analytical tools along with the computational tools necessary to interpret massive amounts of data have allowed the development of the scientific paradigm known as **systems biology**. In systems biology the goal is to understand the functioning and responses of the entire organism by integrating information about its elements (such as genes and proteins) with knowledge about these elements' interrelationships. Many laboratories are using high-throughput tools to gain an understanding of how the system operates, while refining information about dose-response relationships.

To understand linkages between disease and environmental exposures, several distinct categories of information must be pursued simultaneously, such as the measurement of general atmospheric pollutants and toxicants, the fate and transport of hazardous agents in the ecosystem, the burden and metabolism of such agents in the human body, and the biomarkers of exposure. Yet all this information needs to be clearly related to the disease burden. This creates the need for another exposure-disease approach that can provide accurate, consistent health status endpoints that can be measured precisely over many years. The disease-oriented approach, which is currently emerging as a new construct in the field, takes a clinical disease and the public health burden it represents as its starting point, or surrogate of exposure, and then directs inquiry toward the molecular characterization of disease and the underlying exposure responses. This approach is presently being used to investigate gene-environment interactions in major diseases influenced by environmental exposures, such as breast cancer, Parkinson's disease, and autism. The disease-oriented approach relies on both exposure research and large-scale studies of the health status of the general population over long periods of time, to identify subpopulations at risk and groups of unaffected individuals for comparison. Research initiatives using this approach will initially be large scale and lengthy, but will eventually become more efficient and cost effective and have a positive impact on health care costs.

The Genes, Environment, and Health Initiative

In 2007, the U.S. Congress funded a major effort to develop genetic data and exposure assessment tools to be used to discover how genetic susceptibility and environmental factors combine to produce disease. This effort, the **Genes, Environment and Health Initiative** (GEI), has two parts: the Genetics Program, which analyzes genetic variation in groups of patients with specific illnesses, and the Exposure Biology Program, which produces and validates new methods for monitoring environmental exposures that may interact with a genetic variation to result in human disease. The Genetics Program, led by the National Human Genome Research Institute, will focus analysis efforts on SNPs. As noted earlier, some of these small variations alter the function of a gene, and many such alterations in the right combination may increase the risk of certain diseases. To identify the sets of SNPs that contribute to disease risk, researchers are conducting genomewide association studies, using high-throughput genotyping of patient samples to find SNPs that occur more frequently in people with certain diseases. Data are made available in a central, controlled-access database established by the National Center for Biotechnology Information (NCBI) for free and broad research use.

Under the Exposure Biology Program, led by the National Institute of Environmental Health Sciences (NIEHS), scientists are developing innovative sensors for measurement of chemical exposure, improved measures of dietary intake and physical activity, tools for measuring exposures to psychosocial stressors and addictive substances, and indicators of biological responses to exposures. For all these aspects of the environment, the goal is to develop methods that provide more accurate, targeted measures than a simple measure of ambient levels of chemicals in the air or water, for example, can provide. For many of these measures, the effort focuses on development of automated and miniaturized personal devices that will enable more accurate information collection and be comparatively easy for study participants to use. For instance, to measure individual chemical exposures, development of small, personal sensors to measure near real-time exposures to several pollutants is under way. Rather than tracking diet with cumbersome questionnaires, new methods may enable study participants to use cell phones to record their daily food intake via photos and voice notes. Physical activity could be measured by devices that include integrated motion sensors. Development of these more sophisticated methods of environmental monitoring is an important step toward more accurately characterizing gene-environment interactions (Schwartz and Collins, 2007).

Challenges of Investigating Gene-Environment Interactions

Use of the tools and knowledge generated by such initiatives as the GEI in large population-based or clinical studies holds promise for discovering how the complex interplay between gene and environment results in disease. But such research is confined in many cases to investigations of a targeted hypothesis involving a particular exposure and a particular gene or gene pathway. This highly targeted approach is necessary, but it limits discovery by assuming that our current understanding of what causes diseases such as asthma or diabetes is correct. For example, a feasible gene-environment study of diabetes might begin by investigating a hypothesis that a genetic variation thought to decrease insulin production interacts over time with consumption of foods that spike blood sugar (such as soft drinks) to increase predisposition to diabetes. A more agnostic approach, such as genotyping a population of people with diabetes for all possible genetic differences and measuring their exposure to all possible environmental factors, might be preferable, and in a perfect world it would be doable. But it would require such a large sample size and large amount of genotyping and exposure assessment that in the real world the cost would be prohibitive.

The -omics Technologies

Many significant advances seen in environmental health sciences over the past several years have been facilitated by the availability of an improved scientific toolbox: improved cellular and animal models; new, more precise experimental methods, materials, and computational tools; and perhaps most of all, new scientific specialties known collectively as the -**omics technologies**. Just as genetics has embraced genomics, many of the traditional fields in biology have now embraced an -omics component, a capability of studying biological phenomena on the genome scale. For example, **pharmacogenetics**, which examines the response of individual genes to medicines, now includes **pharmacogenomics**, which looks at drug response over the entire genome and is in widespread use to identify drug targets, screen compounds for medicinal activity, and characterize response phenotypes. Pharmacogenomics is part of the push toward personalized medicine. Although such an application of pharmacogenomics is still over the horizon for most people, the field is already having some impact on certain individuals' medical care. The breast cancer drug trastuzumab (trade name Herceptin) is marketed in tandem with a diagnostic test that determines whether it will work in individual patients; if a patient's tumor is found to be of a type that will respond to the drug, therapy is commenced; if not, other treatments are employed. Individualized response (or lack of response or hyperresponse) to medication is certainly one very important manifestation of gene-environment interaction. But given the broad definition of environment, there are many more. The investigation of relationships between environmental exposures and genotypes has engendered the relatively new field called **toxicogenomics**. Toxicogenomics has its roots in traditional toxicology, but again, the current ability to examine (or interrogate) all of the genes in a genome simultaneously allows researchers to take a systems biology approach to an organism's response to an environmental insult. Genomewide screenings, which document which genes are expressed in response to a particular exposure, can shed light on the pathways and **signaling networks** that are relevant to outcomes. Now that a number of animal genomes have been sequenced (including mouse, rat, yeast, zebra fish, and nematode genomes), researchers are also pursuing inquiries in a field known as comparative toxicogenomics. They compare genomic responses to identical exposures among animal species and humans as a fruitful method of discovering and describing cellular mechanisms in the environmental response machinery (Mattingly and others, 2004).

Each step along the pathway of cellular response has its own specialized field of study within the -omics universe (for a complete glossary of the -omics, see Cambridge Healthtech Institute, 2005). For the purposes of this chapter's broad overview of genomics and environmental health, two more of these -omics areas should be described: proteomics and metabolomics. **Proteomics** is the study of the proteome, the global expression of proteins in a cell. Unlike the genome, which is more or less static, finite, and can be completely mapped, the proteome is constantly changing in response to the cellular environment, and proteins are constantly interacting with one another in a highly complex fashion. So a cellular proteome is unlikely ever to be fully mapped; it is too dynamic and almost infinitely variable. But a point of proteomics is to gain information about which proteins are expressed by which genes, when and where in the cell this occurs, and at what level, and in response to what stimuli it occurs. Vast amounts of useful information are expected to emerge from this field as these questions are addressed, protein-protein interactions are characterized, and signature patterns of response are derived. Proteomics also aims to classify differences in protein expression between known samples, such as diseased and nondiseased or exposed and unexposed. Unique proteomic patterns of disease can be identified, without necessarily identifying the specific proteins involved. This approach appears promising in the area of clinical diagnostics, as encouraging results have already been seen in the early detection of some forms of cancer (Petricoin and others, 2002) and the ability to predict the metastatic fate of lung tumors (Yanagisawa and others, 2004).

Functional proteomics seeks to uncover the functions of proteins and subsets of proteins by describing their interactions and functional importance in signaling networks, disease mechanisms, and various other biological processes. *Structural proteomics* involves mapping of the three-dimensional structures of proteins as they exist within the architecture of the cell. Such information can elucidate disease states and cellular functions and also point to strategies for the design of therapeutic agents. And finally, **toxicoproteomics** is a field in its own right, with researchers using the methodologies of proteomics to uncover cellular and subcellular mechanisms behind responses to environmental toxicants and other stressors at the protein level. Each proteomics specialty uses extremely sophisticated bioinformatics to accomplish its tasks.

Metabolomics (also referred to as *metabonomics* and as *metabolic profiling*) is another step in the pathway from disease to exposure, or vice versa. Enzymes govern the production of metabolites, which are often the biochemical endpoints in the response process. Metabolomics involves the identification of metabolites, or suites of metabolites, in body fluids as they relate to particular responses. This information can provide fingerprints that serve as biomarkers of response; in this process the identity of the compounds themselves is a secondary consideration.

All of these -omics pursuits play an important role in the grand design of achieving a grasp of systems biology and systems toxicology. As the experimental technologies continue to advance, along with the bioinformatics tools required to glean useful knowledge from the enormous data sets generated, the overarching field of environmental health sciences should move closer to an understanding of the entire range of gene-environment interactions, on both sides of the gene-environment equation (Figure 6.4).

FIGURE 6.4   Advanced Tools for Understanding Gene-Environment Responses Leading to Disease

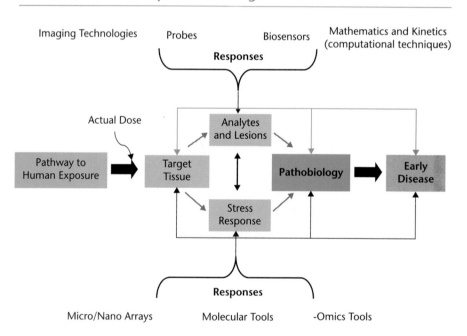

The precise measurements of -omics responses play important roles in conceptualizing and implementing a systems biology and systems toxicology approach to pathobiology and disease.

Beyond the DNA Sequence: Epigenetics

Scientists have begun to realize the importance of yet another route by which environmental exposures can lead to disease—via changes that happen not to the core DNA sequence but to mechanisms such as messenger RNA that carry out the instructions written in the genetic code. These changes can happen as a result of individuals' normal development, exposure to environmental chemicals, ingestion of pharmaceuticals, or diet. The study of these types of modifications to single genes or sets of genes is known as **epigenetics**. Analysis of these changes across the entire genome is referred to as **epigenomics**. Diseases suspected to be associated with epigenetic changes include cancer, autoimmune disease, mental disorders, and diabetes.

Normally, DNA is transcribed to RNA, which is then assembled into messenger RNA, which helps in the manufacture of proteins (the workhorses of the cell). Epigenetic changes can modify any of the steps along this path. These changes include DNA methylation (addition of a methyl group), modifications to the protein-DNA complexes known as chromatin, methylation or other modifications to the proteins that make up chromatin (histones), and control of messenger RNA expression by noncoding RNAs. These changes can activate or repress vital mechanisms such as gene pathways, messenger RNA, or protein expression. For example, DNA repair pathways, which play a major role in protecting against the cytotoxic and mutagenic effects of endogenous, environmental, and clinical DNA-damaging agents, can be inactivated by a particular type of methylation. DNA repair capacity has also been shown to decrease with age, perhaps increasing the likelihood of age-related disease, although the mechanism by which this occurs remains unknown. Researchers have hypothesized that central epigenetic changes that lead to dysregulation of DNA repair gene expression will be associated with disease development, particularly cancer, and aging.

Fetal development is particularly vulnerable to epigenetic changes; an exposure during this period that influences gene expression can result in enduring changes that affect DNA transcription throughout an individual's life. Epigenetic changes can also be passed on across generations, when cells or individuals reproduce. For example, researchers have found that feeding rats extra amounts of choline during gestation results in particular methylations in offspring, who when treated with a chemical that causes breast cancer develop slower growing tumors than rats whose mothers consumed no choline (Kovacheva and others, 2008).

Scientists are beginning to investigate ways that knowledge about epigenetic changes can be used as predictors of disease outcome and treatment response. For instance, a small study found that former smokers who had developed lung cancer showed significant differences in DNA methylation compared to former smokers who had not developed the disease (Vucic and others, 2008).

The NIH Roadmap for Medical Research includes an Epigenomics Program (http://nihroadmap.nih.gov/epigenomics/), led by the National Institute on Drug Abuse and the National Institute of Environmental Health Sciences. Through this program researchers are working to identify specific ways in which gene expression is altered under a variety of environmental conditions, and how the altered expression influences disease risk. Ongoing research investigates such topics as age-related epigenetic effects, transcriptional responses to environmental exposures, how endocrine disruptors cause epigenetic effects in fetal germ cells, how particles and metals cause epigenetic effects that influence cardiac health, and how DNA methylation differs between identical twins with different environmental exposures.

SUMMARY

There will be many new opportunities in environmental health services, research, policy, and outreach in coming years as the recognition of the critical role of the environment in global health emerges at an all-time high. Addressing the opportunities afforded by this enhanced recognition will involve integration of novel information and advances in genetic measurements and environmental factor measurements. This chapter introduces many of the considerations in these areas that environmental health scientists and professionals should master as the field moves forward.

KEY TERMS

allele

apoptosis

cell cycle

cell division

cell signaling

cell structure

δ-aminolevulinic acid dehydratase

DNA repair

Environmental Genome Project

environmental response machinery

epigenetics

epigenomics

ethical, legal and social implications

gene

gene-environment interaction

gene expression

Genes, Environment and Health Initiative

genetic variation

genetics

genomics

haplotype

Human Genome Project

indel

metabolism

metabolomics

omics technologies

personalized medicine

pharmacogenetics

pharmacogenomics

phenotype

polymorphism

protein expression

proteomics

signaling networks

single nucleotide
polymorphism (SNP)

susceptibility gene

systems biology

toxicogenomics

toxicoproteomics

DISCUSSION QUESTIONS

Information on a gene (allele) linked to human disease susceptibility is likely to be developed and quantified in terms of a *risk factor* established through epidemiology studies. Consider the following questions:

1. How could a public health professional communicate the concept of increased or decreased risk factor for disease susceptibility to the lay public?

2. How could a health professional translate information obtained from a large epidemiology cohort to the task of providing advice to an individual patient or client?

3. With what degree of certainty could a public health professional translate risk factor data obtained from a large epidemiology cohort to the issue of causation if he or she were testifying in a courtroom?

REFERENCES

Akhmedova, S., Anisimov, S., Yakimovsky, A., and Schwartz, E. "Gln]Arg 191 Polymorphism of Paraoxonase and Parkinson's Disease." *Human Heredity*, 1999, *49*, 178–180.

Akhmedova, S. N., Yakimovsky, A. K., and Schwartz, E. I. "Paraoxonase 1 Met-Leu 54 Polymorphism Is Associated with Parkinson's Disease." *Journal of the Neurological Sciences*, 2001, *184*, 179–182.

Altshuler, D., Kruglyak, L., and Lander, E. "Genetic Polymorphisms and Disease." *New England Journal of Medicine*, 1998, *338*, 1626.

Cambridge Healthtech Institute. *-Omes and -Omics Glossary & Taxonomy*. http://www.genomicglossaries.com/content/omes.asp, 2005.

Collins, F. S. "Contemplating the End of the Beginning." *Genome Research*, 2001, *11*(5), 641–643.

Collins, F. S. "The Case for a US Prospective Cohort Study of Genes and Environment." *Nature*, 2004, *429*, 475–477.

Davies, H. G., and others. "The Effect of the Human Serum Paraoxonase Polymorphism Is Reversed with Diazoxon, Soman, and Sarin." *Nature Genetics*, 1996, *14*, 334–336.

Environmental Genome Project. [Home page.] http://www.niehs.nih.gov/envgenom/home.htm, 2005.

GeneSNPs. [Home page.] http://www.genome.utah.edu/genesnps, 2005.

Hanna, K., and Coussens, C. *Rebuilding the Unity of Health and the Environment, A New Vision of Environmental Health for the 21st Century: A Workshop Summary for the Institute of Medicine's Roundtable on Environmental Health Sciences, Research, and Medicine*. Washington, D.C.: National Academies Press, 2001.

International HapMap Project. [Home page.] http://www.hapmap.org, 2005.

Jarvik, G. P., and others. "Novel Paraoxonase (PON1) Nonsense and Missense Mutations Predicted by Functional Genome Assay of PON Status." *Pharmacogenetics*, 2003, *13*, 291–295.

Kelada, S. N., and others. "Paraoxonase 1 Promoter and Coding Region Polymorphisms in Parkinson's Disease." *Journal of Neurology, Neurosurgery, and Psychiatry*, 2003, *74*(4), 546–547.

Kondo, I., and Yamamoto, M. "Genetic Polymorphism of Paraoxonase 1 (PON1) and Susceptibility to Parkinson's Disease." *Brain Research*, 1998, *806*, 271–273.

Kovacheva, V. P. and others. "Raising Gestational Choline Intake Alters Gene Expression in DMBA-Evoked Mammary Tumors and Prolongs Survival." *FASEB Journal*, Dec. 1, 2008. (Epub ahead of print.).

Krajinovic, M., and others. "Role of NOQ1, MPO and CYP2E1 Genetic Polymorphisms in the Susceptibility to Childhood Acute Lymphoblastic Leukemia." *International Journal of Cancer*, 2002, *97*, 230–236.

Kruglyak, L., and Nickerson, D. A. "Variation Is the Spice of Life." *Nature Genetics*, 2001, *27*, 234–236.

Li, W. F., and others. "Catalytic Efficiency Determines the in-Vivo Efficacy of PON1 for Detoxifying Organophosphorus Compounds." *Pharmacogenetics*, 2000, *10*, 767–779.

Mattingly, C. J., and others. "Promoting Comparative Molecular Studies in Environmental Health Research: An Overview of the Comparative Toxicogenomics Database (CTD)." *Pharmacogenomics Journal*, 2004, *4*(1), 5–8.

Olden, K., and Wilson, S. "Environmental Health and Genomics: Visions and Implications." *Nature Reviews: Genetics*, 2000, *1*(2), 149–153.

Onalaja, A., and Claudio, L. "Genetic Susceptibility to Lead Poisoning." *Environmental Health Perspectives*, 2000, *108*(suppl. 1), 23–28.

Petricoin, E. F., and others. "Use of Proteomic Patterns in Serum to Identify Ovarian Cancer." *Lancet*, 2002, *359*, 572–577.

Potter, J. D. "Toward the Last Cohort." *Cancer Epidemiology, Biomarkers, and Prevention*, 2004, *13*, 895–897.

Schwartz, D. A., and Collins, F. S. "Environmental Biology and Human Disease." *Science*, 2007, *316*, 695–696.

Sharp, R. R., Yudell, M. A., and Wilson, S. H. "Shaping Science Policy in the Age of Genomics." *Nature Reviews: Genetics*, 2004, *5*, 311–316.

Smith, M. T., and others. "Low NAD(P)H:Quinone Oxidoreductase 1 Activity Is Associated with Increased Risk of Acute Leukemia in Adults." *Blood*, 2001, *97*, 1422–1426.

Smith, M. T., and others. "Low NAD(P)H:Quinone Oxidoreductase Activity Is Associated with Increased Risk of Leukemia with MLL Translocations in Infants and Children." *Blood*, 2002, *100*, 4590–4593.

Suk, W. A., and Wilson, S. H. "*Overview and Future of Molecular Biomarkers of Exposure and Early Disease in Environmental Health.*" In S. H. Wilson and W. A. Suk (eds.), *Biomarkers of Environmentally Associated Disease, Technologies, Concepts, and Perspectives*. Boca Raton, Fla.: Lewis, 2002.

Taylor, M. C., Le Couteur, D. G., Mellick, G. D., and Board, P. G. "Paraoxonase Polymorphisms, Pesticide Exposure and Parkinson's Disease in a Caucasian Population." *Journal of Neural Transmission*, 2000, *107*, 979–983.

Vucic, E. A., and others. "*Contribution of DNA Methylation in Development of Lung Cancer in Former Smokers.*" Abstract A27. In *Seventh Annual AACR International Conference on Frontiers in Cancer Prevention Research* (p. 77). Washington, D.C.: AACR, 2008.

Wang, J., and Liu, Z. "No Association Between Paraoxonase 1 (PON1) Gene Polymorphisms and Susceptibility to Parkinson's Disease in a Chinese Population." *Movement Disorders*, 2000, *15*, 1265–1267.

Watson, J. D., and Crick, F.H.C. "The Structure for Deoxyribose Nucleic Acid." *Nature*, 1953, *171*, 737–738.

Wilson, S. H., and Olden, K. "The Environmental Genome Project: Phase 1 and Beyond." *Molecular Interventions*, 2004, *4*(3), 147–156.

Wilson, S. H., and Sule, W. A. "Framework for Environmental Exposure Research: The Disease-Finder Approach." *Molecular Interventions*, 2005, *5*, 262–267.

Yanagisawa, K., and others. "Proteomic Patterns of Tumour Subsets in Non-Small-Cell Lung Cancer." *Lancet*, 2004, *362*, 433–439.

FOR FURTHER INFORMATION

Articles

These articles provide further background on genomics in general and on gene-environment interactions.

Hunter, D. J. "Gene-Environment Interactions in Human Disease." *Nature Reviews: Genetics*, 2005, *6*(4), 287–298.

Thayer, A. M. "The Genomics Evolution." *Chemical and Engineering News*, Dec. 8, 2003.

Project

Environmental Genome Project (EGP), http://www.niehs.nih.gov/envgenom/home.htm. A project initiated by the National Institute of Environmental Health Sciences (NIEHS) in 1998 to improve the understanding of human genetic susceptibility to environmental exposures. The EGP Web site provides a good overview of current research in this field.

CHAPTER SEVEN

ENVIRONMENTAL HEALTH ETHICS

ANDREW JAMETON

KEY CONCEPTS

- Principles of ethics and morals extend beyond empirical concerns; they also establish important values and expectations of professional conduct.

- Most professions, including those engaged in environmental health, have an established code of ethics that outlines the main ethical ideals and standards of the profession.

- Environmental health professionals play an increasingly important role in mediating between the current health needs of humans and the long-term needs of humans and of the natural world.

- When working with clients, environmental health professionals have an important responsibility to advocate the sustainability of human and environmental health in all activities.

W**E** most often discuss ethics when a controversy or dilemma arises. However, ethical concerns are unobtrusively and globally present in the everyday fabric of life: Everyday actions taken by environmental health professionals typically depend on a commitment to such ethical values as service, improved human health, and concern for the environment.

DEFINING ETHICS AND MORALS

Ethics can be defined most conveniently in contrast with morals. The term **morals**, or **morality**, means the set of core beliefs or commitments of a person or society that identifies what is most important, valuable, or right with regard to conduct and character. The term **ethics** refers to a more formal version of morality. Ethics can mean

- A reasoned or systematic approach to figuring out what is the right or wrong action or position
- Professional morality, as expressed in widely accepted codes and statements, in contrast to personal morality
- The scholarly study of morality by philosophers

When ethical challenges arise in professional life, individuals may need to make use of any of these formal concepts of morality. Because ethics is mostly discussed when making decisions, ethics is not simply about describing the morality of a person, association, or culture. Instead, it is a normative process of deciding what we should do or ought to do.

Ethics is intrinsically social, and not individual. Beginning students of ethics often think of moral beliefs as essentially private and consider it inappropriate to make moral judgments about the conduct of others, but they soon learn that friends and professional colleagues often have genuinely useful and justifiable ideas as to what is right for themselves and others. People are social creatures who live in social contexts, and most environmental health decisions involve and affect many people and the environment. Accordingly, what is "right" in environmental health can never be simply the opinion of a single individual. Written statements

The author thanks Susanna von Essen, professor, Internal Medicine, Section of Pulmonary and Critical Care, University of Nebraska Medical Center, and Kenneth W. Goodman, director, Bioethics Program, codirector, Ethics Programs, University of Miami, for their help. In addition, Andrew L. Jameton declares no competing financial interests.

of ethics in environmental health practice represent the consensus of professional groups and committees authorized to compose principles of practice.

When we make decisions we always go beyond the bare facts and use language and ideas that cannot be resolved entirely by scientific or objective methods. Nevertheless we can think objectively to some degree in ethics. Thinking objectively in ethics is usually characterized by

- Being reasonable and not doctrinaire
- Listening actively to others
- Letting the best reasons determine judgments
- Staying close to the practical issues at hand on which consensus is possible, while avoiding larger philosophical issues on which disagreement is likely
- Remaining calm and optimistic in the face of controversy
- Being realistic about the situations and choices that we face
- Considering the approaches of other cultures involved in the situation

Ethics can be challenging in that its statements and discussions are less precise than the language of scientific discussion and open to persistent controversies. Nevertheless we all need to have a sense of integrity and meaning in our daily lives, and there is no way to achieve this without considering our actions in a broad moral context.

HISTORY OF ETHICS IN ENVIRONMENTAL HEALTH

The environmental health professions are diverse and still in the process of acquiring a common sense of identity. So formal statements of environmental health ethics are in formation and draw on diverse sources. This section sketches the history of environmental health ethics and identifies some of its sources.

Reflection on the connections among health, the environment, and ethics has an ancient history. In classical times, scholars reflected on the relationship of humans to the Earth and debated the extent to which the Earth was created to provide its bounty for human welfare and the extent to which humans have a responsibility to perfect nature for human use. Medieval reflection considered whether environmental damage to the Earth resulted from human sins, and early modern reflection, as science and industry entered their infancy, considered the prospects for human domination over nature (Glacken, 1973).

Modern environmental health has a varied and complex professional structure, dating from the development of statistics and health surveillance in the seventeenth century; the rise of demography and macroeconomics in the early nineteenth century; the occupational health, sanitarian, and public health movements of the nineteenth century; and the modern medical revolution of the early twentieth century (Porter, 1999; Rosen, 1993). The twentieth century was also marked by rapid growth in the number and specialization of all health professions.

Many environmental health professional organizations formed during the early and middle years of the twentieth century. Most of these were associated with industrial and occupational health. One of the first medical subspecialty associations was the American College of Occupational and Environmental Medicine (ACOEM), founded as the American Association of Industrial Physicians and Surgeons in 1916. The American Association of Occupational Health Nurses (AAOHN) was established in 1942 as the American Association of Industrial Nurses. As the environmental revolution took off in the 1970s, many new environmental agencies were founded (such as the U.S. Environmental Protection Agency). Environmental regulation widened, along with rapidly increasing recognition of environmental problems. These developments spurred the creation of new environmental health professions.

Professional Codes of Ethics

The development of ethics in environmental health is closely associated with the growth of ethics in the health professions generally. Although each profession has its own approach to codes, oaths, and ethics statements, all tend to share a set of common concerns and principles (Exhibit 7.1).

EXHIBIT 7.1
Typical Elements of Professional Codes of Ethics

1. Dedication to service to the client
2. Respect for other professionals
3. Assurance of high levels of competence
4. Protection of confidentiality
5. Performance with honesty and integrity
6. Avoidance of conflicts of interest
7. Informed consent and cooperation with clients
8. Service to the community
9. Promotion of the profession itself

Professions adopt ethical codes because professionals

- Provide a socially valued service, such as protecting the health of the community.
- Possess a high degree of autonomy at work as a result of their special expertise, and are not easily supervised by others.
- Have a skill or craft that if incompetently conducted would be harmful.
- Depend on the trust and confidence of clients to function effectively.
- Need to cooperate with others toward common goals.

Each profession's ethics code represents a consensus among leading members of the profession. Although the statements in these codes are useful in organizing the profession and public support for it, they remain subject to interpretation and improvement. Codes are not static; they continue to be revised and recrafted to clarify their meaning and to help professionals in making decisions.

Several ethics codes exist for professionals in environmental health. The Code of Ethics for Members of the National Environmental Health Association (NEHA, 2004) states that the goal of the environmental health profession is, "To prolong life, eliminate and/or control disease, and create and maintain an environment that is conducive to humankind's full development." The ACOEM Code of Ethical Conduct (1993) sets a high priority on safety, scientific integrity, and honesty. It emphasizes confidentiality and privacy of the individual worker while balancing these needs with giving appropriate but limited information to employers. (Many professional codes must find similar balances between some-times competing interests.) It accepts a responsibility to let individuals and groups know of work-related health risks and discusses chemical dependency and abuse. The AAOHN Code of Ethics (AAOHN, 2004) reads very much like the Code for Nurses of the American Nurses Association (ANA). It contains a nondiscrim-ination statement, urges collaboration with other professions, protects privacy, champions community service and public health, and urges members to maintain competence and to participate in educational and scientific efforts. Like many nursing professional codes, it promises that the professional will safeguard clients and the public from unethical or illegal conduct. The American Public Health Association adopted an ethics code in 2002. Although the principles of the APHA code do not address the environment, the introduction includes a key clause rel-evant to environmental health, recognizing that "[p]eople and their physical envi-ronment are interdependent" (Public Health Leadership Society, 2002).

Ethical codes are valuable and should be read carefully. Their main purpose is to indicate the general direction of professional purpose and commitment and to express professional idealism while at the same time setting criteria that define minimal standards of conduct. So an idealistic environmental health professional could, for instance, use such a code to support advocating tighter limits on the release of particulate matter into the air (referring to a clause in a typical ethics code regarding high-quality service to the public), whereas a licensing board could use the same code to support criticizing a professional who accepted bribes in order to suppress health data potentially costly to an industry (referring to a clause requiring high levels of integrity or legal conduct).

When professionals must make decisions on hard cases, however, ethics codes are of limited value. Codes represent a broad consensus, and realms of controversy tend to be omitted. Codes have a way of focusing on the nitty-gritty details of daily work and steering clear of the larger ideals of the profession. Because of this limitation, additional fields of ethics have developed that address broad issues of controversy and change. Two of these fields arose during the 1970s. The first, the field of *bioethics*, was named around 1969 by Van Rensselaer Potter (Potter, 1971; Reich, 1995). Potter's thesis was that biology and the humanities need to be brought together to respect and to integrate human health and the environment in order for humans to be able to survive the environmental crisis with dignity. Intense theoretical and case study of the ethics of the health professions and clinical care grew under the rubric of bioethics. Bioethics assumes that codes of professional ethics need to be grounded in larger principles of ethics (see Exhibit 7.2

EXHIBIT 7.2
Selected Ethical Theories

Deontology. The position that individual autonomy is key, but that responsible choice requires obedience to a common moral law (Kant, [1785] 1998).

Utilitarianism. The position that that act is right which maximizes the likely balance of happiness over unhappiness (Mill, [1863] 1998).

Bioethics. A set of principles for health care ethics that emphasizes beneficence (doing good), nonmaleficence (avoiding harm), respect for patient autonomy, and justice (Beauchamp and Childress, 2008).

Feminist ethics. The principle of care, with a priority that process and relationships, not abstract principles, should dominate ethics (Clement, 1996; Tong, 1997).

Religious ethics. Positions founded in traditions of belief and community practices rooted in a personal perspective on the order of the universe, usually in reference to a God or gods.

for selected ethical theories). It has also been influential in specifying details, laws, and procedures that refine the concepts of respect for patients, confidentiality, informed consent, care of the dying, and so on. As a result, codes of professional ethics now tend to address these issues with increasing care.

The second field that addresses broad issues of controversy and change is **environmental ethics**. Stimulated by the increasing rate of environmental change and decline, ethical thinkers began in the mid-twentieth century to articulate new and revolutionary ideas about the human relationship with nature. Three important concepts in this field are

- *Sustainability* and *resilience*, which place limits on human activity in order to respect long-term consequences to the natural world and future generations
- *Global health*, which places local health concerns in an interconnected global context

Because environmental consciousness has grown in the last century and is changing rapidly, the environmental health professions are just beginning to integrate these ideas into professional codes and position statements. In 1990, for example, McCally and Cassel asserted that the medical profession must begin to accept more global environmental responsibilities. The environmental health professions are beginning to take the same position (World Health Organization (WHO), 1989).

A number of groups in civil society actively promote environmental awareness in the health professions and sciences. Among these groups are the Canadian Association of Physicians for the Environment (CAPE), Health Care Without Harm (HCWH), the Science and Environmental Health Network (SEHN), Hospitals for a Healthy Environment (H2E), Physicians for Social Responsibility (PSR), Union of Concerned Scientists (UCS), and many others. Major environmental groups, such as the Environmental Defense Fund, the Natural Resources Defense Council, and the Sierra Club, have human health platforms or programs, or both. Churches and religious groups are becoming increasingly active in addressing environmental health issues and promoting public action. Virtually all of the major religions have active environmental programs, and this work is complemented by ecumenical groups such as the National Religious Partnership for the Environment, the Evangelical Climate Initiative, and Interfaith Power and Light.

The environmental responsibilities of health professions are often expressed in position statements separate from codes of ethics, sometimes by the professions themselves and sometimes by activist groups. Statements by major social groups on environment and health are especially useful, inspiring, and clarifying.

EXHIBIT 7.3
Examples of Consensus Statements

From the Earth Charter

> The resilience of the community of life and the well-being of humanity
> depend upon preserving a healthy biosphere with all its ecological systems,
> a rich variety of plants and animals, fertile soils, pure waters, and clean air.
> The global environment with its finite resources is a common concern of all
> peoples. The protection of Earth's vitality, diversity, and beauty is a sacred
> trust [Earth Charter Initiative, 2000].

From the Rio Declaration on Environment and Development

> Human beings are at the centre of concerns for sustainable development. We
> are entitled to a healthy and productive life in harmony with nature [United
> Nations Conference on Environment and Development (UNCED), 1992].

For example, the Declaration of the Environment Leaders of the Eight on
Children's Environmental Health (Environment Leaders of the Eight, 1997)
states, "We increasingly understand that the health and well-being of our families
depends upon a clean and healthy environment." The Earth Charter provides an
important statement promoting a unified struggle for both human and environmental health, as does the Rio Declaration on Environment and Development
(see Exhibit 7.3). Such statements not only add specificity and idealism to the
environmental health professions but also lend authority to their actions and
recommendations.

Indeed, the world faces a global environmental crisis. The human population (6.7 billion in 2009) continues to grow, even though it is beginning to level
off as decreasing birth rates and increasing death rates approach equilibrium
(see Chapter Nine). Globally, we live (or aspire to live) at a level beyond the
Earth's capacity to sustain itself (Hails, 2008; Wackernagel and others, 2002). A
deteriorating global environment is an inevitable consequence (United Nations
Development Programme, United Nations Environment Programme, World
Bank, and World Resources Institute, 2000), with deeply worrisome implications
for public health, including environmental health (Weisman, 2007; Diamond,
2005). Many environmental concerns operate "upstream" from health problems,
and have multiple and widespread effects. Global climate change is the prime

example of such a problem; it could conceivably wipe out much of the human population and yield a very different Earth in the next one hundred years or so (Lynas, 2008). Given that environmental health professionals often focus on specific, relatively manageable environmental health problems, what should the broader ethical principles of environmental health work look like?

GENERAL PRINCIPLES OF ETHICS

Most environmental health work involves population health and the relationships of populations to the environment. Accordingly, environmental health ethics needs to be somewhat different from traditional individual-centered professional ethics, as illustrated by the seven environmental health ethical principles outlined in the following sections: sustainability, healthfulness, interconnectedness, respect for all life, global equity, respectful participation, and realism.

Sustainability

Conduct environmental health work in such a way that it meets the needs of both the present and future generations.

> "An acceptable system of ethics is contingent on its ability to preserve the ecosystems which sustain it."
> —*Elliott, 1997*

This statement of the principle of **sustainability** derives from language used by the World Commission on Environment and Development (1987), often referred to as the Brundtland Commission, to describe sustainable development: "development that meets the needs of the present generation without compromising the needs of future generations." Both statements indicate that ethical discussion needs to be multigenerational in scope. Why is this principle important to environmental health?

- Many environmental health technologies and projects, such as those dealing with sewage, agriculture, bridge and levee construction, energy production, and nature restoration, are designed to serve multiple generations.
- Human health needs are lifelong and relatively stable, so considering health over the normal life span commits us to planning for most of a century.
- We care about the future welfare of humanity, and people in the future will have similar health needs and concerns.
- Many of the health problems of our own children can only be solved by addressing the blunt end environmental problems affecting the lives of all children.

- Currently, Earth's declining ecosystems are profoundly reducing the ability of the environment to support human health. These declines are taking place in time frames of decades to centuries.

So environmental health professionals must think for the future as well as the present and press their clients to do so as well. A concern for sustainability has three immediate implications for environmental health practice.

First, methods of cost accounting that discount the future should be avoided. Discounting tends to diminish the significance of events a few decades ahead to nothing, when in fact they are significant and may become irremediable unless we take present action. The significance of the long term has also been expressed in more cultural and religious terms, such as the Iroquois injunction to consider the effects of current actions on the seventh generation yet to come (LaDuke, 1999).

Second, the full life cycle cost of environmental health measures must be included. Life cycle costs stretch from costs of extracting and processing the materials through the costs of transporting, packaging, and using materials and products to the costs of disposing of supplies, tools, equipment, and buildings when they are retired. So, for example, if a municipality plans to build a sewage plant, it must consider not only local health benefits but also the carbon cost to the atmosphere of fuel expenditures to process the sewage and the environmental costs of mining and harvesting materials, producing energy, and shipping supplies in order to build the plant in the first place. As another example, many of the proposals to build new alternate energy sources involve using materials that are potentially toxic, such as the silicates and rare earths used in solar energy collectors; environmental health professionals need to anticipate potential health problems and help to reduce their impact. Once the full environmental costs are considered, initially attractive projects may not prove to offer the best long-term approaches to public health.

Third, many have observed a strong correspondence between the wealth of a nation and the average health of its citizens (World Bank, 1993). However, if in maintaining the current welfare of its population, a nation overburdens its environment or the environments of other nations and of the globe, that nation will undermine everyone's health in the long run. Thus immediate health gains must be judged within limits set by long-term sustainability. To achieve sustainability in the long term, it may be important to change current practices significantly; thus some prefer to use the term **resilience**, which emphasizes the dynamic side of sustainability.

Finding the right economic and public policies to address sustainability is a challenge. As Garrett Hardin (1968) pointed out in a classic article, sharing the global commons without rules limiting consumption inevitably results in a decline of the commons. Some have argued that privatization of parcels of the commons will tend to protect resources better, but ownership of property in a market society does not necessarily protect resources because resources must ultimately be sold to pay for investment in the property and owners are not necessarily farsighted.

Healthfulness

The health of humans and the environment needs to be restored, balanced, and harmonized.

We should think not just of improving human health but of improving human health in the setting of a healthy global environment. Careful thinkers have rightly noted that the meaning of the term *health* cannot be as read-ily applied to the natural environment as to humans. It is not immediately clear what a healthy polar landscape should be like, nor is a polar landscape friendly to humans. Yet as noted earlier, ethics concepts are meant to link values into a coherent whole, and healthy ecosystems are necessary to maintain human health in the long run. Thus the use of such toxic substances as cleaners, pesticides, and herbicides poses a dilemma for environmental health practice. Although these substances may protect human health in the short run, they may damage the environment in the long run. So in addition to their indirect toxic effects on humans, their impact on the environment can also harm human health.

> "Ecological medicine is a new field of inquiry and action to reconcile the care and health of ecosystems, populations, communities, and individuals."
> —*SEHN, 2002*

Moreover, we should think in terms of the restoration of human and environmental health. In many parts of the world, human and environmental health are declining in tandem. Africans bear the cost of many of the environmental practices of the developed nations, and some African regions have fallen to radically low levels of life expectancy. Some island nations are experiencing hurricanes, floods, landslides, and chronic salinization of agricultural and forest land due to climate change.

However, health is only one value among a panoply of ethical values. Many individuals have willingly sacrificed their own health to serve larger community purposes. Most societies generally give higher status to other values, such as liberty, justice, and service. Nevertheless, health is one of the most basic human values and is especially important as a measure of the welfare of the population as a whole. Moreover, healthiness is good in itself. It is a feature of the abundance and thriving of life and not just a means to accomplish other social ends. Thus an environmental health professional should speak to the key value of health and the dependency of achieving other values on health, while recognizing that health is not the only value. This means that environmental health work requires collaborating with others to harmonize health values with other cultural and community goals.

Interconnectedness

"Health depends on everything, all the time."
—*Evans and Stoddart, 2003, p. 374*

Environmental health actions have far-reaching consequences.

A strong sense of interconnectedness does not so much constitute a rule of ethical rightness and wrongness as it speaks to the basic concept of moral responsibility. Much of modern ethical philosophy has been dominated by the notion that the moral responsibility of each individual can be separated from the needs and concerns of others (Mill, [1869] 2003; Lane, Rubinstein, Cibula, and Webster, 2000). Indeed, much has been achieved and won on the basis of individualism and individual rights. And the protection of the individual, and his or her capacity to meet his or her needs, from the weight of collective social needs continues to be essential.

However, the doctrine of individualism has overemphasized the satisfaction of personal wants as a basis of happiness, at considerable environmental cost. In actuality most of us are happiest when we work with others in the service of our families, communities, and meaningful social goals. So a substantial element of an individual's life is a sense of responsibility and connectedness. In fact, one can imagine a modern ethics based on the idea of the maternal-child bond or of families, rather than on the image of the isolated single (male) individual (Ruddick, 1989). At the root of individual choice are our responsibilities and our interest in the care of others, not simply our personal satisfaction.

Interconnectedness has long been a central message of many religions, which see all humans as being related through a relationship with God. Temporal interconnectedness has also been emphasized in religions through their appeal to thousand-year traditions, an afterlife, and a cosmos ordered through an eternal deity. It is also expressed in a sense of care for children through multiple generations, care for the vulnerable, and a sense of service to community. Religions also make modest consumption meaningful by redirecting attention from material things to families and communities. Most traditional religions have endorsed modest consumption in one form or another (Durning, 1992, p. 144). At the same time, religious practices may or may not be green. On one hand, large meeting spaces in churches can be costly in energy consumption, cremation puts carbon in the atmosphere, and pilgrimages may require transportation. On the other hand, vegetarianism helps to reduce the methane output of agriculture, anti-iconic traditions reduce the material costs of churches, and so on.

Our sense of interconnectedness has been greatly amplified by our increasing understanding of the Earth as a coherent ecological system (Lovelock, 1979). For many in the environmental movement, this is largely expressed by awareness of the strong biological and physical interconnections among Earth's ecosystems:

- Greenhouse gases released in the Northern Hemisphere spread everywhere, including the Southern Hemisphere, with the result that those least responsible for climate change suffer most from its effects (Patz and others, 2007).
- Fertilized agricultural areas of the Midwest release nitrogen into rivers; this nitrogen then overloads and kills areas of the Gulf of Mexico.
- Toxic chemical pollutants, such as dioxins, can be found in the ice and snow of polar regions.
- Streams and groundwater in the United States show detectable levels of antibiotics, caffeine, fire retardants, estrogens, and other complex medical, agricultural, and industrial chemicals (Kolpin and others, 2002).
- Much of the lead pollution in Europe is attributable to the use of lead in pipes and other technologies in ancient Roman times. Not only is the world spatially interconnected, it is interconnected over long periods of time as well.
- No longer can physicians diagnose fevers, rashes, and diarrhea in the Midwestern United States without considering the possibility of distant sources of disease.

Interconnectedness is not only biological and physical. It is social and economic as well. The combination of travel, immigration, trade, and transportation has led to a high level of exposure in all populations to diseases that may have had their origins anywhere on the globe. Likewise, global environmental problems require international and global political and economic solutions. One of the important achievements in environmental health in recent decades was the 1987 Montreal Protocol on Substances That Deplete the Ozone Layer (United Nations Environment Programme, 2000), which limited the use of chlorofluorocarbons (CFCs) and other chemicals damaging to stratospheric ozone. Although the Earth's protective ozone layer is still vulnerable, it is believed that this international agreement has done much to reverse a dangerous situation. Many other international treaties, agreements, and statements have addressed environmental and health issues. Numerous international nongovernmental organizations (NGOs) are active in environmental health areas and are influencing environmental health globally.

Respect for All Life

Environmental health work should be conducted with respect for both human and nonhuman life.

Respect for human life and proscriptions against taking it are nearly universal in human culture. Similarly, respect for animal life is widespread and ancient. It appears strongly in Hindu and Buddhist doctrines. And respect for all life is experiencing a rebirth in Western ethical traditions, which have tended during the modern period to subordinate the natural world to the needs of humans and to permit its open-ended exploitation (White, 1967).

A debate has raged among environmental philosophers in recent decades over whether the value of nature depends on its value to humans or whether nature has value independent of human welfare. This is a complex and significant debate, with consequences for choices that environmental health professionals must make. On the side of **anthropocentrism** is a perspective that views us humans as focused on meeting our own needs and limited in our ability to care for nature in itself. This perspective holds that it is unreasonable for us to respect ethical rules that consider Earth's welfare apart from our own. Anthropocentric arguments in defense of nature ultimately rest on the impact of the natural world on humans. The nonanthropocentric approach regards humans as one species situated among others in Earth's larger ecosystems. Nonanthropocentric approaches to nature emphasize its complexity, long history, capacity for adaptation and change, beauty and splendor, and potential for growth and change far into the future. Humans, such a theory might claim, are on Earth in part to care for the natural world, much as Plato ([c. 360 BCE], 1992) argued that a guardian class was expected to care for the society it served.

Some nonanthropocentric theories emphasize the sentience of other species (why, if causing unnecessary pain is unethical, shouldn't the pain of a baby octopus also be considered?) and the fact that many animals seem to act with intention or purpose, such as to protect themselves and their young (Singer, 2002). However, nonanthropocentric theories do not necessarily rest on the sentience of individual animals. They may also rest on a sense of the coherence of the natural world as a whole and as a changing, reactive network of many beings, sentient or not. Indeed the vast bulk of living things are (apparently) not conscious. Microorganisms alone outweigh humans by tens of thousands of times. Plant biomes, plankton, fungal structures, worms, barnacles, and the many senseless creatures of nature make up most of the biological world. It would be foolish of humans to underestimate the importance of these organisms, not only to human health but to the health of other sentient earthly beings as well (Darwin, [1881] 1966; Quammen, 1988, pp. 10–16).

Religious positions vary widely on this debate. Although most religious thought maintains a steady focus on humans and human communities (seldom even including much on domestic animals), they do not differ from modernity in this way. Indeed, some nonreligious environmental works have much of the flavor of, and closely parallel, religious discussions of duties to nature (Naess, 1973; Leopold, 1949; Lovelock, 1979; Berry, 1990; Fox, 2006). Religions have the capacity to propel environmental concern by seeing nature as God's creation, and so religious thought has expressed environmental duties through the notion of stewardship (Bernstein, 1998; Hill, 2006; Tucker and Grim, 1994).

Indeed, care for the Earth can be raised to a high religious order, where the Earth itself becomes the main locus of worship, as it is in some versions of paganism.

The anthropocentric versus nonanthropocentric debate is heartfelt and often leads to differing positions on environmental health issues. Differences are to a degree reflected in what one regards as an environmental health problem. Most anthropocentric in perspective are those who deal with the health hazards and toxicities of the built environment, with concentration on social determinants of health and the most controllable and immediate factors in health, and those who regard environmental concern as a distraction or even threat to justice. Others are conscious of the effects of toxics on the natural world and the consequent loss of nature's services to humans. An even larger view would consider the effects of toxics on the wilderness (especially the hazards of loss of pollinators to wilderness projects). A concern for climate change tends to mix all of these concerns, because this change affects both humans and wilderness into the future.

Nonanthropocentrists are likely to favor nature restoration, even where human health risks are involved. Good examples are the debates over major carnivores. Some naturalists would like to see wolf and tiger habitats preserved and restored, even though this involves risks to human beings. If the loss of habitat for polar bears and walruses were the only harmful consequence of climate change, it would be hard to motivate the significant public commitment needed for climate mitigation. Another good example is wetlands restoration. For environmental and health reasons, including protection of the hydrologic cycle, one may want to restore wetlands. But wetland restoration also tends to encourage the breeding of mosquitoes, notorious vectors of disease. The anthropocentrist would likely take fewer risks on behalf of mosquitoes than would the nonanthropocentrist.

These two sides, however, have much in common. Whether for the sake of humans in the long run or for nature itself, both consider maintenance of a healthy natural world as key. Both sides oppose the notion that human health is best protected by eliminating all predators and oppose using any means, however toxic to nature, to promote human development. So the anthropocentrism debate need not be resolved for environmental health activists to speak strongly on behalf of the natural world.

The middle ground in this debate takes various forms. One course, as discussed in Chapter Twenty-Four, is to emphasize the positive effects of exposure to the natural world on human health. This view can be seen as arising in part from humans' love of the living world, what E. O. Wilson (1984) has termed **biophilia**. If it is in our nature to love the natural world, then it is simultaneously in our interest and our duty to care for it. Another middle course is to set priorities (Shrader-Frechette, 1991). In this view, we should seek first to meet the needs of humans, which include basic human health. Then we should meet the needs of nature. Then, if it does not damage the needs of nature, we can also seek less necessary goods for humans. However, there are three important limitations to this approach:

- Human needs must be met in ways that tread as lightly as possible on the needs of nature.
- Basic human health needs must be understood to be founded on a healthy natural environment.
- The shift to economies that focus on basic goods will require an immense social and philosophical struggle.

Global Equity

Everyone is entitled to just and equal access to the basic resources needed for an adequate and healthy life.

Modern ethical theories do not privilege the needs of one person or community over another. Because humans are interconnected on a limited planet and have roughly equal needs and capacities, it is difficult to justify anything but modest and equal access to basic resources, especially those in the global commons, such as the atmosphere, the oceans, our genetic heritage, and the wilderness.

Arguments that justify differential access to resources usually rest on our local power to influence events close to us, our history of ownership and contribution to society, our specific needs and handicaps as individuals, and the role each of us plays in neighborhoods and communities. Most philosophers would justify some level of difference in access to resources in order to reward meritorious contributions to the community and to discourage harming it. How much difference to tolerate and how to reconcile conflicts over activities that allocate environmental benefits and burdens is subject to debate.

Inequality is harmful to public health. Stratified societies excite envy, hinder self-expression, and tend to create conditions so limited for some that they are unable to meet their basic health needs. Thus among wealthy nations the average level of public health corresponds less to the average level of wealth than to the average level of economic equality (Wilkinson, 1996). Overprivileging one group in relationship to another is probably unhealthy for both groups. For the group left in poverty the environmental health risks are obvious. But for the comfortable there are the risks of overconsumption (such as inactivity and obesity) and the less tangible costs of guarding and justifying their positions. Equality, even apart from its ethical strength, is a public health measure. As a result, environmental health professionals need to consider

- How economic schemes to promote health, such as industrial developments, also affect income inequality.
- What the costs are to others of environmental measures that benefit specific populations.

For example, if a hospital is to be kept clean with strong antibacterial agents, it is important that these agents not be caustic or carcinogenic to the workers who handle and apply them (Pierce and Jameton, 2004).

On a larger scale, a recent WHO commission report on global social determinants of health linked health equity with climate change in its major recommendations: "Ensure that economic and social policy responses to climate change and other environmental degradation take into account health equity" (Commission on Social Determinants of Health, 2008, p. 4). The report also noted that because of the environmental decline with which it is connected, economic growth may not be the key to reducing inequalities: "Coupled with the constraints on global growth associated with climate change, and the disproportionately adverse net impact of climate change on the poor, this casts serious doubt on the dominant view that global growth should be the primary means of poverty reduction. Rather than growth, policies and the global economic system should focus directly on achieving social and environmental objectives" (p. 120).

Ethically speaking, considerations of equity cross national borders. People worldwide share both an entitlement to Earth's resources and the obligation to protect them. **Global health** and income inequality are among the greatest problems the world now faces (Farmer, 2003). Although the World Bank in 2008 reported substantial progress in alleviating poverty globally, rapid rises in food prices undermined these achievements (Chen and Ravallion, 2008). Accordingly, when local decisions have global consequences, the equity considerations may also be global. For example, in the American Midwest an environmental health activist not only might fight for filters and scrubbers on a new coal-fired electric power plant but also might oppose building the plant at all. A new coal-fired plant would increase the burden that Midwesterners place on the Earth's atmosphere, a resource that the developed world already exploits disproportionately. Further, greater local public health gains might be achieved by stressing a reduction in the consumption of electricity and restoration of prairie regions to support wildlife.

One activist group has proposed an outline of distributive targets in order to establish an equitable order for mitigating climate change. EcoEquity has proposed the Greenhouse Development Rights plan (Baer, Athanasiou, Kartha, and Kemp-Benedict, 2008). This and similar proposals hold that to achieve equity in mitigation, the lion's share of fossil fuel reductions must take place in the developed world. On an optimistic note, several countries (India, China, Brazil, South Africa, and Mexico) committed themselves to equity goals in their support for climate change mitigation after the G8 meeting in the summer of 2008. These countries stated: "Negotiations . . . , including a long-term global goal for greenhouse gases (GHG) emissions reductions, must be based on an equitable burden sharing paradigm that ensures equal sustainable development potential for all citizens of the world and that takes into account historical responsibility and respective capabilities as a fair and just approach" (Third World Network, 2008).

Respectful Participation

Respect the considered and responsible choices of stakeholders, whether individuals or organizations (adapted from Lambert and others, 2003).

Those with a stake in environmental health need to participate in the decisions of environmental health professionals. We can generalize about common human health needs, but individuals and organizations have widely varying interpretations of their own environmental health needs. This presents difficulties for environmental health professionals asked by their clients to support unwise choices.

Perhaps the problem of disagreement with patients, employers, and stakeholders is best resolved through the concept of leadership. When consulted, a professional with environmental health expertise is expected to lead others to what the profession would recommend as the healthiest course of action. However, leadership must be balanced. One must chart a course between paternalism, that is, coercive leadership, and abandonment, that is, failing to give direction. Working with stakeholders with whom one disagrees calls upon a professional's deepest skills and sensitivities.

One key way to reconciling potential conflicts between individual choices and professional recommendations is to press for the **right to know**. Although the principle of the right to know takes many forms, its main thrust is to urge that people who are affected by environmental hazards and toxins should be made aware of the nature of the risks to which they are exposed. This principle has many advantages. Assuming that we are reasonable, we can make our own decisions about the risks to which we are exposed. Such communication builds trust among all parties. It also affords the opportunity, for those of us who prefer to do so, to operate more independently. The principle of the right to know strengthens when the hazards to which individuals are exposed are great.

This principle has some weaknesses and complexities. Realistic risk assessment is often intellectually and emotionally difficult. Some information is proprietary and confidential, so the right to know must be weighed against the rights of those who own information or who feel exposed to legal or economic risk if information is disseminated. Some information has been distorted by the media, as is the case with climate change, with the result that reasonable people may confidently hold false beliefs. Moreover, some information involves complex and unpredictable risks for a wide community, as in the case of environmental genomics, and so it is difficult to know who should be informed and whether some would prefer not to know or hear about dangers from which we can do little to protect ourselves (Beritic, 1993; Michaels and others, 1992; Sattler, 1992; Jardine and others, 2003; Beierle, 2004). Moreover, what is known or discovered may affect people with whom the environmental health professional lacks a relationship. Although the needs of those who employ or consult the environmental health professional should presumptively be foremost in the professional's consideration, professionals can educate their clientele about the need to weigh seriously the environmental costs to others and the need to make responsible choices. More difficult is knowing what to do when the environmental health professional encounters clients' needs that conflict with the community's. Although some ethicists argue that professional ethics requires the environmental health professional to insulate the client as much as possible from outside concerns, the spirit of environmental health recommends striving to work in an interconnected manner with the larger community.

Realism

Environmental health ethics should be founded on a realistic understanding of the health sciences and the risks and benefits of proposed activities and investments (adapted from Weed and McKeown, 2003).

Our discussion concludes with this principle because the strong emphasis in the earlier sections on the fate of the Earth's environment may make the principles discussed so far seem idealistic and unrealistic. However, they are realistic; the Earth and its human population are facing a wrenching crisis of resource limits, increasing poverty, and health threats. A realistic ethics takes these concerns into account and expresses them explicitly in the ethical commitments of the environmental health professions. And even if these principles are somewhat idealistic, we must remember that ethical principles are supposed to be idealistic, so that we can strive to do better than we would otherwise. Not being perfect or not achieving the maximal good is not a failure; it is ethically adequate to do the best one can.

Critics of health activists often argue that economic and political realities stand in the way of health improvements. A company may argue that it is too expensive to protect workers' health or to make a safer product. However, the history of many environmental and health campaigns shows that economic and political actors can adapt to the needs of the public and the environment. The point of economics and politics is not that humans should serve the economy and society first. The responsibility is the other way: economics and politics need to adapt to serve the health needs and ideals of communities. Resource limits are real; appreciating the Earth's limits is thus part of realism and not simply a defeatist provocation against economic development. Meeting the basic health needs of humans is not necessarily elaborate or expensive. It is ethically more fundamental that these needs be met than that grander visions be realized (Maslow, 1970). It is clear that humans now consume more in a year than the Earth's natural processes can replace during the year. Some societies clearly consume more than others. A rough measure, the **ecological footprint**, estimates each person's use of global resources. Judging by their footprint, North Americans consume on average at least five or six times what the Earth can provide for the entire human population at the same level of resource consumption (Venetoulis and Talberth, 2005). As global population grows, the environment declines, climate change continues apace, and energy resources become more expensive, it will become very difficult to maintain the environmentally costly lifestyle of the average North American.

This will be very challenging for environmental health professionals and activists. Those aware of environmental health issues and the human dependence on nature will need to educate the population in how to continue to maintain health in a less abundant environment. This will require technological innovation, but it will also involve shifting to philosophies of wellness that include both a philosophy of prevention and a more global sense of how to live well on limited resources.

Realistic risk assessments are also needed in environmental health ethics. Many analyses omit modernity's full costs and the difficulty in managing the environmental risks of otherwise beneficial activities. For instance, many people believe more oil and coal are needed to promote public health and welfare, but the resulting climate change from greater oil and coal consumption is likely to defeat progress (Martens and McMichael, 2002; see also Chapter Ten). Some believe that nuclear power will be needed to replace fossil fuels; yet the proliferation of nuclear waste materials is an unsolved health and security risk (Lovins and Sheikh, 2008). Technological optimists should examine whether the risks of new technologies can be managed over the relevant periods of time, particularly the vast time scales of nuclear technologies. Such revision in modern technological progressivism has already resulted in the increasingly widespread adoption of the **precautionary principle** as a mode of realistic risk assessment. The precautionary principle states that "when an activity raises threats of harm to human health or the environment, precautionary measures should be taken even if some cause and effect relationships are not fully established scientifically" (SEHN, 1998; Raffensperger and Tickner, 1999). This principle

- Recommends better study of the risks of industrial innovations before each new practice or new chemical becomes widespread. For example, those opposed to the development of genetically modified organisms (GMOs) are concerned that these may make potentially disastrous nonpoint sources of toxins if not properly managed.
- Shifts the burden of proof so that proponents (such as manufacturers) must demonstrate that a practice is safe and sustainable, rather than requiring critics to prove it is not.
- Assumes that it is more important to avoid harm than to incur benefits.
- Takes a long-term view.
- Presumes a certain amount of historical and sociological knowledge about the management of toxic materials and risks. Although the risks of a technology may be readily managed in a tightly controlled test environment, they often increase when the technology becomes widely used.

CONTROVERSIES IN ENVIRONMENTAL HEALTH ETHICS

Because environmental and health concerns are involved in most human activities, many ethical questions, dilemmas, and controversies arise in environmental health ethics (see Exhibit 7.4 for a brief list).

These controversies share several similarities. Ethical doubts, dilemmas, and struggles tend to arise when the following elements are present:

- *New technologies with uncertain risks.* New technologies notoriously generate unexpected effects (Tenner, 1996). People may reasonably differ over whether the risks are known, whether they can be well managed, and whether those developing or using the technology can be trusted.

EXHIBIT 7.4
Case Problem Areas

Air pollution. How should we balance the health costs and the benefits of air-polluting activities, and deal with the politics of risk estimation, the involvement of multiple jurisdictions, and uncertainties about health risks?

Water pollution. How can the focus on upstream and downstream ownership be turned to a focus on clean water for all? How should we apply what we are learning about the tensions between groundwater and surface water? How do we face the reality that human uses of water are in conflict with natural habitats?

Vegetarianism. This is a healthy diet with the least environmental impact, but how do we cope with the fact that it is culturally unacceptable in many parts of the world?

Cultural conflict. Many cultures prize activities that are in conflict with both health and the environment. How should health be prioritized in relationship to other cultural values? How do we deal with the dilemma that, for example, driving automobiles and watching television at current levels is not good for us or our world?

Fossil fuels and climate change. How should the short-term gains of using fossil fuels be weighed against major long-term losses (not only from climate change but also from the toxicity of fossil fuels)? As the environmental urgency to limit fossil fuel use increasingly challenges our capacity for rapid social change, how shall we maintain active advocacy for change in balance with increasing pessimism?

Genetically modified organisms. Is it acceptable to copyright living material? Are particular modifications appropriate? How will we deal with unexpected health risks and confront the lack of trust among all the parties involved? How can we direct genetic modifications in directions that reduce human conflict with the environment, and how can we prevent their deliberate misuse as new weapons technologies?

Nuclear power. This would be the solution to our energy problems except that we need to ask, What are the risks of nuclear materials being used for war

- *Social relationships with predictable conflicts*. Confidentiality, informed consent, and environmental justice problems all arise from controversies over respectful treatment of others. These problems are by no means confined to environmental health issues.

or terrorism, and can we solve the problem of safely sequestering radioactive wastes for tens of thousands of years?

Pesticides. Surely we need an ample food supply, and we compete with weeds and insects for food, but what are the health and environmental costs of releasing billions of pounds of toxic materials into the environment? For instance, a controversy has arisen about resuming the use of DDT to control mosquitoes that spread malaria (See Chapter 17, pp. 626–627).

Slaughter of animals. To decrease the risk of pandemic flu, millions of domestic animals have been slaughtered in Asia and elsewhere. Is this excessive, since killing animals is wrong? Consider the somewhat different cases of culling deer or wild horses.

Obesity, undernutrition, starvation. The existence of these conditions reveals a problem in environmental justice. Indeed, should we be regarding many of the conflicts of the world as between the fat and the undernourished?

Environmental exposures and the human genome. Should we conduct genetic testing of job applicants and allow only those most resistant to toxic materials to work in certain occupational environments?

Confidentiality, informed consent, and the right to know. How shall we collect needed epidemiological information without invading the privacy of individuals? To what extent should individuals be able to consent to surveillance for environmental health purposes?

War. Is there any way to conduct human conflict without wrecking the public health and environmental conditions in a region for decades thereafter? Ironically and suicidally, while the world needs to abandon intensive use of fossil fuels, violent regional conflicts are increasing over new fossil fuel sources, including the now melting arctic.

Research ethics. When we ask individuals to subject themselves to experiments for long-term human health gains, are we unfairly using them as a means to an end? What is appropriate consent? What is appropriate oversight? Is it fair to use individuals in particular communities for research when those communities may never see the benefits of the research?

- *Risks and benefits that need to be rationally balanced.* Some of the debates in this area involve disagreements over the value of activities (Do we really need another suburban hospital when the proposed building footprint diminishes local food-growing capacity?). Some of the debates are simply over how to weigh risks rationally: How much more important are safety and avoiding harm than finding new ways to benefit people? And mistrust among groups with different interests makes it difficult to rely on common estimates of risks.

- *Competing goods.* Health is one of many goods. All environmental health discussions must take place in the context of commitments to other values, some of which are difficult to harmonize with health.
- *Cultural differences.* Although there are many human universals, from the maternal-child bond to poetry (Brown, 1991), different cultures tend to use slightly different social concepts and to set out problems and arguments in differing styles. Moreover, different geographic locations tend to expose people to different environmental risks.
- *Different views of our place in and relationship to nature.* While we debate our place in nature, the global environment is deteriorating at an increasing pace. Environmental health professionals need to consider how to balance service to humans with protection of the environment.
- *Complexity.* Many long-standing ethical debates persist simply because they are complex and involve many parties, factors, and issues.

There is no magic formula, no final or ultimate ethical theory for resolving moral problems. Because most environmental health issues involve a community of people and the natural world, there will inevitably be ethics controversies. This means that environmental health professionals need to work respectfully and patiently with others to achieve the environmental health ideals for which they stand. Because the natural world is in decline and maintaining global population health is becoming more challenging, environmental health professionals occupy an increasingly important place in the world and need to speak out clearly and actively for their profession's ethical ideals.

The environmental health professions have a potential for tragedy; population growth, consumption, and environmental limits may well make environmental health an impossible ideal. Although we should strive in everyday professional practice to do the best we can over the long run, the codes of ethics and missions statements of the environmental health professions lend only weak support to these larger aspirations. One approach for professionals is to express their more idealistic concerns in advocacy, in concert with any of the thousands of environmentally active groups, a few of which were mentioned earlier. One great contribution environmental health professionals can make is their professional knowledge, which is very valuable to social action. A regrettable gulf in knowledge between activists and professionals needs to be bridged if the environmental crisis is to be resolved.

In engaging in ethical activism, the key political aim is to seek the *moral high ground*—the place from which one can articulate an ideal strongly enough that it has practical political and economic consequences ("Rules for Radicals," n.d.). Sound scientific knowledge is a component of the moral high ground. As the environmental bottleneck narrows during this century, those of us in the environmental professions will be forced, if we wish to occupy the moral high ground, to become more active and to make our codes and principles more responsive to the depth of the environmental crisis. Although this might threaten the potential for organizational consensus, we must remember that as the crisis worsens, a consensus will grow that major changes in practice and philosophy are needed. As the world becomes more interconnected and our temporal perspective broadens, both the need and the tendency to agree on common actions should increase despite large philosophical differences among us. Professionals can draw inspiration from the many leaders who have shown that what at first seems impossible can be achieved through years of organization and dedication (McCally, 2002; Maathai, 2007; King, 2001; Gandhi, [1930] 2005; Debs, [1890] 2006). Increasingly our global circumstances on Earth require faithfulness to the core foundations of ethics.

SUMMARY

Ethical issues are a constant feature of life. *Morals* are the core beliefs that identify what is most important, valuable, or right with regard to conduct and character. *Ethics* refers to a more formal version of morality. In environmental health, important moral values—reflecting the traditions of both bioethics and environmental ethics—include sustainability, healthfulness, interconnectedness, respect for all life, global equity, respectful participation, and realism. Several professional codes of ethics are relevant to environmental health practice.

KEY TERMS

anthropocentrism

bioethics

biophilia

deontology

ecological footprint

environmental ethics

ethics

feminist ethics

global health

morality

morals

precautionary principle

religious ethics

resilience

right to know

sustainability

utilitarianism

DISCUSSION QUESTIONS

1. Why are some ethical principles stated in professional codes of ethics while other principles are not? Look over one of the codes of ethics relevant to environmental health. Would you add anything? Would you leave anything out? Why? Also, should there be sanctions for those professionals who violate their organization's code of ethics?

2. What are some analogies between human health and the health of the environment? What are some ways in which they are not analogous?

3. Hospitals incur public health risks (through power production, incineration, cleaning agents, disposal of drugs and supplies, and so on). How should these risks be balanced against health gains?

4. Select a debated issue in environmental health ethics. What are some of the reasons (on both sides) that explain why the debate persists? Are there any scientific facts that, if the parties knew them for certain, would likely settle the issue for them?

5. Do you have some personal values that harmonize well with the professional ethics of environmental health? Do you have some that conflict with these ethics?

6. How might you go about reducing the ecological footprint of your personal life? How might you relate your efforts to reduce your personal environmental impact to reducing the impact of your professional work and that of your clients?

7. What ideas in our religious traditions help us to make concern for environmental health paramount and meaningful?

8. What are some cases in which it would be ethical to encourage a stakeholder to think beyond his or her immediate needs and to consider broader human and environmental needs? What are some cases in which it would be unethical to do so? What are the broader social responsibilities of environmental health professionals to advocate environmental health in the political, social, and economic spheres?

REFERENCES

Alinsky, S.D. *Rules for Radicals: A Practical Primer for Realistic Radicals.* New York, Random House, 1971.

American Association of Occupational Health Nurses. "Code of Ethics and Interpretive Statements." *AAOHN Journal, 52*(4). http://www.aaohn.org/practice/ethics.cfm, 2004.

American College of Occupational and Environmental Medicine. *Code of Ethical Conduct.* http://www.acoem.org/code/default.asp, Aug. 1993.

Baer, P., Athanasiou, T., Kartha, S., and Kemp-Benedict, F. *The Greenhouse Development Rights Framework: The Right to Development in a Climate Constrained World*. (2nd ed.) Heinrich Böll Foundation, Christian Aid, EcoEquity and the Stockholm Environment Institute. http://www.ecoequity.org/docs/TheGDRsFramework.pdf. 2008.

Beauchamp, T. L., and Childress, J. F. *Principles of Biomedical Ethics*. (6th ed.) New York: Oxford University Press, 2008.

Beierle, T. C. "The Benefits and Costs of Disclosing Information About Risks: What Do We Know About the Right-to-Know?" *Risk Analysis*, 2004, *24*(2), 335–346.

Beritic, T. "Workers at High Risk: The Right to Know." *Lancet*, 1993, *341*, 933–934.

Bernstein, E., Ed. *Ecology and the Jewish Spirit: Where Nature and the Sacred Meet*. Woodstock, Vermont: Jewish Lights Publishing, 1998.

Berry, W. *What Are People For?* London: Rider Books, 1990.

Brown, D. E. *Human Universals*. Philadelphia: Temple University Press, 1991.

Chen, S., and Ravallion, M. *The Developing World Is Poorer Than We Thought, but No Less Successful in the Fight Against Poverty*. Policy Research Working Paper Series 4703. Washington, D.C.: World Bank, 2008.

Clement, G. *Care, Autonomy, and Justice: Feminism and the Ethic of Care*. Boulder, Colo.: Westview Press, 1996.

Commission on Social Determinants of Health. *Closing the Gap in a Generation: Health Equity Through Action on the Social Determinants of Health*. Final Report of the Commission on Social Determinants of Health. Geneva: World Health Organization, 2008.

Darwin, C. *Darwin on Humus and the Earthworm: The Formation of Vegetable Mould, Through the Action of Worms, with Observations on their Habits*. London: Faber and Faber, 1966. (Originally published 1881 as *The Formation of Vegetable Mould, Through the Action of Worms, with Observations on their Habits*.)

Debs, E. V. "Agitation & Agitators." *Locomotive Fireman's Magazine*, 1890. http://www.marxists.org/history/usa/unions/blf/1890/0800-debs-agitation.pdf, 2006.

Diamond, J. *Collapse: How Societies Choose to Fail or Succeed*. New York: Viking, 2005.

Durning, A. *How Much Is Enough? The Consumer Society and the Future of the Earth*. The Worldwatch Environmental Alert Series. New York: Norton, 1992.

Earth Charter Initiative. *The Earth Charter*. http://www.earthcharter.org/files/charter/charter.pdf, Mar. 2000.

Elliott, H. *A General Statement of the Tragedy of the Commons*. http://www.dieoff.com/page121.htm, Feb. 26, 1997.

Environment Leaders of the Eight. *1997 Declaration of the Environment Leaders of the Eight on Children's Environmental Health*. http://www.g8.utoronto.ca/environment/1997miami/children.html, 1997.

Evans, R. G., and Stoddart, G. L. "Models for Population Health: Consuming Research, Producing Policy?" *American Journal of Public Health*, 2003, *93*, 371–379.

Farmer, P. *Pathologies of Power: Health, Human Rights, and the New War on the Poor*. Berkeley: University of California Press, 2003.

Fox, W. A. *Theory of General Ethics: Human Relationships, Nature, and the Built Environment*. Cambridge, Mass.: MIT Press, 2006.

Gandhi, M. [Speech made on March 11, 1930 at Ahmedabad.] In mahatma.com, "Dandi March." http://www.mahatma.com/php/showNews.php?newsid=4&linkid=12, 2005.

Glacken, C. J. *Traces on the Rhodian Shore: Nature and Culture in Western Thought from Ancient Times to the End of the Eighteenth Century*. Berkeley: University of California Press, 1973.

Hails, C., (ed. in chief). *Living Planet Report 2008*. WWF International, Institute of Zoology, and Global Footprint Network. http://www.panda.org/news_facts/publications/living_planet_report/lpr_2008/index.cfm, 2008.

Hardin, G. "The Tragedy of the Commons." *Science*, 1968, *162*, 1243–1248.

Hill, B. Christian Faith and the Environment: Making Vital Connections. Eugene, Oregon: Wipf & Stock, 2006.

Jardine, C., and others. "Risk Management Frameworks for Human Health and Environmental Risks." *Journal of Toxicology and Environmental Health, Part B, Critical Reviews*, 2003, *6*(6), 569–720.

Kant, I. *Groundwork of the Metaphysics of Morals*. New York: Cambridge University Press, 1998. (Originally published 1785.)

King, M. L. *A Call to Conscience: The Landmark Speeches of Dr. Martin Luther King, Jr.* (eds. C. Carson and K. Shepard). New York: IPM (Intellectual Properties Management) in association with Warner Books, 2001.

Kolpin, D. W., and others. "Pharmaceuticals, Hormones, and Other Organic Wastewater Contaminants in U.S. Streams, 1999–2000: A National Reconnaissance." *Environmental Science & Technology*, 2002, *36*, 1202–1211.

LaDuke W. *All Our Relations: Native Struggles for Land and Life*. Cambridge, Mass.: South End Press, 1999.

Lambert, T. W., and others. "Ethical Perspectives for the Public and Environmental Health: Fostering Autonomy and the Right to Know." *Environmental Health Perspectives*, 2003, *111*, 133–137.

Lane, S. D., Rubinstein, R. A., Cibula, D., and Webster, N. "Towards a Public Health Approach to Bioethics." *Annals of the New York Academy of Sciences*, 2000, *925*, 25–36.

Leopold, A. *A Sand County Almanac and Sketches Here and There*. New York: Oxford University Press, 1949.

Lovelock, J. E. *Gaia: A New Look at Life on Earth*. New York: Oxford University Press, 1979.

Lovins, A. B., and Sheikh, I. "The Nuclear Illusion." http://www.rmi.org/images/PDFs/Energy/E08-01_AmbioNuclIllusion.pdf, 2008.

Lynas, M. *Six Degrees: Our Future on a Hotter Planet*. Washington, D.C.: National Geographic, 2008.

Maathai, W. "The Cracked Mirror." *Resurgence*. http://greenbeltmovement.org/a.php?id=28, Nov. 11, 2007.

Martens, P., and McMichael, A. J. (eds.). *Environmental Change, Climate and Health: Issues and Research Methods*. New York: Cambridge University Press, 2002.

Maslow, A. H. *Motivation and Personality*. (2nd ed.) New York: HarperCollins, 1970.

McCally, M. "Medical Activism and Environmental Health." *Annals of the American Academy of Political and Social Science. 584.*http://ann.sagepub.com/cgi/reprint/584/1/145, 2002.

McCally, M., and Cassel, C. K. "Medical Responsibility and Global Environmental Change." *Annals of Internal Medicine*, 1990, *113*, 467–473.

Michaels, D., and others. "Workshops Are Not Enough: Making Right-to-Know Training Lead to Workplace Change." *American Journal of Industrial Medicine*, 1992, *22*(5), 637–649.

Mill, J. S. *Utilitarianism*. New York: Oxford University Press, 1998. (Originally published 1863.)

Mill, J. S. *On Liberty*. New Haven, Conn.: Yale University Press, 2003. (Originally published 1869.)

Naess, A. "The Shallow and the Deep, Long-Range Ecology Movement." *Inquiry*, 1973, *16*, 95–100.

National Environmental Health Association. *Code of Ethics for Members*. http://www.neha.org/member, 2004.

Patz, J. A., and others. "Climate Change and Global Health: Quantifying a Growing Ethical Crisis." *EcoHealth*, 2007, *4*, 397–405.

Pierce, J., and Jameton, A. *The Ethics of Environmentally Responsible Health Care.* New York: Oxford University Press, 2004.

Plato. *Republic.* Indianapolis: Hackett, 1992. (Written c. 360 BCE.)

Porter, D. *Health, Civilization, and the State: A History of Public Health from Ancient to Modern Times.* New York: Routledge, 1999.

Potter, V. R. *Bioethics: Bridge to the Future.* Upper Saddle River, N.J.: Prentice Hall, 1971.

Public Health Leadership Society. *Principles of the Ethical Practice of Public Health.* Version 2.2. http://209.9.235.208/CMSuploads/PHLSethicsbrochure-40103.pdf, 2002.

Quammen, D. *The Flight of the Iguana: A Sidelong View of Science and Nature.* New York: Simon & Schuster, 1988.

Raffensperger, C., and Tickner, J. (eds.). *Protecting Public Health and the Environment: Implementing the Precautionary Principle.* Washington, D.C.: Island Press, 1999.

Reich, W. T. "The Word 'Bioethics': The Struggle over Its Earliest Meanings." *Kennedy Institute of Ethics Journal*, 1995, *5*(1), 19–34.

Rosen, G. A. *History of Public Health.* (Expanded ed.) Baltimore, Md.: Johns Hopkins University Press, 1993.

Ruddick, S. *Maternal Thinking: Toward a Politics of Peace.* Boston: Beacon Press, 1989.

Sattler, B. "Rights and Realities: A Critical Review of the Accessibility of Information on Hazardous Chemicals." *Occupational Medicine*, 1992, *7*(2), 189–196.

Science and Environmental Health Network. *The Wingspread Statement on the Precautionary Principle.* http://www.sehn.org/state.html#w, Jan. 1998.

Science and Environmental Health Network. *Ecological Medicine: A Call for Inquiry and Action.* http://www.sehn.org, Feb. 2002.

Shrader-Frechette, K. "Ethics and the Environment." *World Health Forum*, 1991, *12*, 311–321.

Singer, P. *Animal Liberation.* New York: Ecco, 2002. (Originally published 1975.)

Tenner, E. *Why Things Bite Back: Technology and the Revenge of Unintended Consequences.* New York: Knopf, 1996.

Third World Network. "G8 and G5 Leaders Issue Different Climate Messages." http://www.twnside.org.sg/title2/climate/info.service/climate.change.20080702.htm, July 14, 2008.

Tong, R. *Feminist Approaches to Bioethics: Theoretical Reflections and Practical Applications.* Boulder, Colo.: Westview Press, 1997.

Tucker, M.E. and Grim, J.A., Eds. *Worldviews and Ecology: Religion, Philosophy, and the Environment.* Maryknoll, New York: Orbis, 1994.

United Nations Conference on Environment and Development. *Rio Declaration on Environment and Development.* http://www.un.org/documents/ga/conf151/aconf15126-1annex1.htm, 1992.

United Nations Development Programme, United Nations Environment Programme, World Bank, and World Resources Institute. *World Resources 2000–2001: People and Ecosystems, the Fraying Web of Life.* Amsterdam: Elsevier Science, 2000.

United Nations Environment Programme, Ozone Secretariat. *Montreal Protocol on Substances That Deplete the Ozone Layer: As Either Adjusted and/or Amended in London 1990, Copenhagen 1992, Vienna 1995, Montreal 1997, Beijing 1999.* http://www.unep.org/ozone/pdfs/Montreal-Protocol2000.pdf, 2000.

Venetoulis, J., and Talberth, J. *Ecological Footprint of Nations: 2005 Update.* Redefining Progress. http://www.rprogress.org/publications/2006/Footprint%20of%20Nations%202005.pdf, 2006.

Wackernagel, M., and others. "Tracking the Ecological Overshoot of the Human Economy." *Proceedings of the National Academy of Sciences of the United States of America*, 2002, *99*(14), 9266–9271.

Weed, D. L., and McKeown, R. E. "Science and Social Responsibility in Public Health." *Environmental Health Perspectives*, 2003, *111*, 1804–1808.

Weisman, A. *The World Without Us.* New York: Thomas Dunne Books, 2007.

White, L., Jr. "The Historical Roots of Our Ecological Crisis." *Science*, 1967, *155*, 1203–1207.

Wilkinson, R. *Unhealthy Societies: The Afflictions of Inequality.* New York: Routledge, 1996.

Wilson, E. O. *Biophilia: The Human Bond with Other Species.* Cambridge, Mass.: Harvard University Press, 1984.

World Bank. *World Development Report 1993: Investing in Health.* New York: Oxford University Press, 1993.

World Commission on Environment and Development. *Our Common Future.* New York: Oxford University Press, 1987.

World Health Organization, Regional Office for Europe. *European Charter on Environment and Health.* http://www.euro.who.int, 1989.

FOR FURTHER INFORMATION

Books and Online Publications

Athanasiou, T. *Divided Planet: The Ecology of Rich and Poor.* Boston: Little, Brown, 1996.

Attfield, R. *Environmental Ethics: An Overview for the Twenty-First Century.* Cambridge, U.K.: Polity, 2003.

Barlett, P. F., and Chase, G. W. (eds.). *Sustainability on Campus: Stories and Strategies for Change.* Cambridge, Mass.: MIT Press, 2004.

Beauchamp, D. E., and Steinbock, B. (eds.). *New Ethics for the Public's Health.* New York: Oxford University Press, 1999.

Brown, N. J., and Quiblier, P. (eds.). *Ethics and Agenda 21: Moral Implications of a Global Consensus.* New York: United Nations, 1994.

Callahan, D. *False Hopes: Why America's Quest for Perfect Health Is a Recipe for Failure.* New York: Simon & Shuster, 1998.

Online Ethics Center for Engineering and Science. National Academy of Engineering. Safety and the Environment. http://www.onlineethics.org/CMS/enviro.aspx.

Chesworth, J. (ed.). *The Ecology of Health: Identifying Issues and Alternatives.* Thousand Oaks, Calif.: Sage, 1996.

Costanza, R., Norton, G. B., and Haskell, B. D. (eds.). *Ecosystem Health: New Goals for Environmental Management.* Washington, D.C.: Island Press, 1992.

Crocker, D. A., and Linden, T. (eds.). *Ethics of Consumption: The Good Life, Justice, and Global Stewardship.* Lanham, Md.: Rowman & Littlefield, 1998.

Daily, G. C. (ed.). *Nature's Services: Societal Dependence on Natural Ecosystems.* Washington, D.C.: Island Press, 1997.

Farmer, P. *Infections and Inequalities.* Berkeley: University of California Press, 1999.

Fox, W. (ed.). *Ethics and the Built Environment.* New York: Routledge, 2000.

Gorz, A. *Ecology as Politics*. Boston: South End Press, 1980.

Harvard Medical School, Center for Health and the Global Environment (CHGE). *Human Health and Global Environmental Change*. http://www.med.harvard.edu/chge/textbook/index.htm, 2004.

International Commission on Occupational Health (ICOH). *International Code of Ethics for Occupational Health Professionals*. http://www.icoh.org.sg. 2004.

Jamieson, D. (ed.). *A Companion to Environmental Philosophy*. Malden, Mass.: Blackwell, 2001.

Light, A., and Rolston, H. (eds.). *Environmental Ethics: An Anthology*. Malden, Mass.: Blackwell, 2003.

Lubchenco, J. "Entering the Century of the Environment: A New Social Contract for Science." *Science*, 1998, *279*, 491–497.

McCally, M. (ed.). *Life Support: The Environment and Human Health*. Cambridge, Mass.: MIT Press, 2002.

McKeown, T. *The Role of Medicine: Dream, Mirage, or Nemesis?* Princeton, N.J.: Princeton University Press, 1979.

McKibben, B. *The End of Nature*. New York: Doubleday, 1989.

Meadows, D., Randers, J., and Meadows, D. *Limits to Growth: The Thirty Year Update*. White River Junction, Vt.: Chelsea Green, 2004.

Newton, L. *Ethics and Sustainability: Sustainable Development and the Moral Life*. Upper Saddle River, N.J.: Prentice Hall, 2003.

Partridge, E. (ed.). *Responsibilities to Future Generations: Environmental Ethics*. Buffalo, N.Y.: Prometheus Books, 1981.

Pedersen, D. "Disease Ecology at a Crossroads: Man-Made Environments, Human Rights and Perpetual Development Utopias." *Social Science and Medicine*, 1996, *43*, 745–758.

Pimentel, D., and Lehman, H. (eds.). *The Pesticide Question: Environment, Economics, and Ethics*. New York: Chapman & Hall, 1993.

Ponting, C. *A Green History of the World: The Environment and the Collapse of Great Civilizations*. New York: St. Martin's Press, 1991.

Proctor, R. N. *Cancer Wars: How Politics Shapes What We Know and Don't Know About Cancer*. New York: Basic Books, 1995.

Rachels, J. *The Elements of Moral Philosophy*. (4th ed.) Boston: McGraw-Hill Humanities, 2002.

Shiva, V. *Staying Alive: Women, Ecology and Development*. London: Zed Books, 1989.

Shrader-Frechette, K., and McCoy, E. D. *Method in Ecology: Strategies for Conservation*. New York: Cambridge University Press, 1993.

Singer, P. "Famine, Affluence, and Morality." In W. Aiken and H. LaFollette (eds.), *World Hunger and Morality* (pp. 26–38). (2nd ed.) Upper Saddle River, N.J.: Prentice Hall, 1996.

Wackernagel, M., and Rees, W. E. *Our Ecological Footprint: Reducing Human Impact on the Earth*. Gabriola Island, B.C.: New Society, 1996.

Westra, L. *Living in Integrity: A Global Ethic to Restore a Fragmented Earth*. Lanham, Md.: Rowman & Littlefield, 1998.

Zwaan, B. van der, and Petersen, A. (eds.). *Sharing the Planet: Population, Consumption, Species: Science and Ethics for a Sustainable and Equitable World*. Delft, The Netherlands: Eburon, 2003.

Organizations

American Association of Occupational Health Nurses (AAOHN), http://www.aaohn.org.

American College of Occupational and Environmental Medicine (ACOEM), http://www.acoem.org.

American Nurses Association (ANA), http://www.nursingworld.org.

American Public Health Association (APHA), http://www.apha.org.

American Society for Bioethics and Humanities (ASBH), http://www.asbh.org.

Association for the Advancement of Sustainability in Higher Education (AASHE), http://www.aashe.org.

Canadian Association of Physicians for the Environment (CAPE), http://www.cape.ca.

CleanMed, an annual conference for greening health care, http://www.cleanmed.org.

Climate Action Network (CAN), http://www.climatenetwork.org.

Collaborative on Health and the Environment, http://www.cheforhealth.org.

Doctors for Global Health (DGH), http://www.dghonline.org.

Environmental Health Perspectives (EHP), http://ehp.niehs.nih.gov.

Environmental Working Group (EWG), http://www.ewg.org.

Health Care Without Harm (HCWH), http://www.noharm.org.

Hospitals for a Healthy Environment (H2E), http://www.h2e-online.org.

International Association for Environmental Philosophy (IAEP), http://www.environmentalphilosophy.org.

International Association of Bioethics (IAB), http://www.bioethics-international.org.

International Society for Ecology and Culture (ISEC), http://www.isec.org.uk.

International Society for Environmental Ethics (ISEE), http://www.cep.unt.edu/ISEE.html.

National Environmental Health Association (NEHA), http://www.neha.org.

National Wildlife Federation (NWF), Campus Ecology, http://www.nwf.org/campusecology.

The Natural Step (TNS), http://www.naturalstep.org.

Nightingale Institute for Health and the Environment (NIHE), http://www.nihe.org.

Northwest Environment Watch, http://www.northwestwatch.org.

Partners in Health, http://www.pih.org/index.html.

Physicians for Human Rights (PHR), http://www.phrusa.org.

Physicians for Social Responsibility (PSR), http://www.psr.org.

Rachel's Environment and Health News, http://www.rachel.org/home_eng.htm.

Redefining Progress, http://www.rprogress.org.

Science and Environmental Health Network (SEHN), http://www.sehn.org.

Second Nature, Education for Sustainability, http://www.secondnature.org.

Union of Concerned Scientists (UCS), http://ucsusa.org.

University of Nebraska Medical Center, Green Health Center Project, http://www.unmc.edu/green.

University of Pennsylvania, Center for Bioethics, http://www.bioethics.upenn.edu.

World Resources Institute, http://www.wri.org.

CHAPTER EIGHT

ENVIRONMENTAL JUSTICE

CHARLES LEE

KEY CONCEPTS

- Environmental justice is a movement that represents the convergence of civil rights and environmentalism.

- Environmental justice is based on the concept that hazardous environmental exposures have disproportionate impacts on people of color and poor communities.

- Environmental justice concerns extend beyond hazardous environmental exposures to disparities in social determinants of health and in access to environmental assets such as parks, transportation, and well-designed communities.

- Collaborative and integrated problem solving at the community level is key to addressing environmental justice concerns.

ENVIRONMENTAL **justice** represents the convergence of two of the greatest social movements of the latter half of the twentieth century, the civil rights movement and the environmental movement. (Other roots of the Environmental Justice movement include public health, labor, farmworker, and native land rights initiatives; see Faber and McCarthy, 2001). It is appropriate, therefore, that a comment attributed to the venerable civil rights activist Fannie Lou Hamer has come to embody the feelings of communities in the environmental justice movement: "*I am sick and tired of being sick and tired.*" This poignant plea by environmentally overburdened people of color, low-income, and tribal communities in the United States reflects profound disappointment with the status of their health, frustration with the public health community's failure to assist in improving their health, anger over the attitude of the many businesses complacent about their regulatory obligations and unresponsive to the health problems their neighbors face, and bewilderment at the government's failure to understand and correct these shortcomings. For many communities facing stresses from factors beyond their control and living with a myriad of polluting facilities, the affront is compounded by the impacts of racial and economic discrimination (National Environmental Justice Advisory Council, 2004).

This chapter begins with a short description of the roots of the environmental justice movement. It then explores three core concepts of environmental justice, concepts at the nexus of civil rights and environmentalism.

- *The meaning of disproportionate impacts*, a concept originally centered on disproportionate exposure and since expanded to encompass cumulative environmental hazards, vulnerability, inequities in regulatory enforcement, and disparities in socioeconomic status, power, and health.
- *The legal, public policy, and research challenges* inherent in the concept of environmental justice, particularly those related to integrating civil rights and social justice concepts into an environmental law paradigm.
- *The community-based, collaborative problem-solving strategies and tools* needed to address the interrelated environmental, health, economic, and social concerns of disadvantaged, underserved, and overburdened communities.

These three concepts are key to integrating environmental justice into the mainstream of environmental and public health practice. (In addition, the

The views expressed in this chapter are solely those of the author. No official support or endorsement by the Environmental Protection Agency or any other agency of the federal government is intended or should be inferred. In addition, Charles Lee declares no competing financial interests.

environmental health and public health fields themselves need to unify; see Lee, 2002.) The first concept deals with issues of assessment—of environmental exposures, of community assets and liabilities, and of disparities. It illuminates the underlying complexities that the second and third concepts must address. The second reflects the paradigmatic conflicts between civil rights law and environmental law. If these conflicts are not recognized and addressed, then civil rights and social justice concepts may be marginalized in environmental policy. Finally, the third concept is strategic. As communities address complex environmental justice issues with many stakeholders, collaborative problem-solving strategies and tools are needed. These three concepts have been conundrums in the evolution of environmental justice theory and practice, and they have enormous historical implications for the future viability of environmental justice.

THE ROOTS OF ENVIRONMENTAL JUSTICE

PERSPECTIVE
Roots of Environmental Justice in Warren County, North Carolina

"[E]ven in 1982 we knew that where we lived, where we worked, and where we played was really our environment. When the state of North Carolina decided that it was going to put PCB into a community that was 65 percent African Americans, we said 'No.' We said we will put our lives on the line.

"And we did it by laying our bodies in front of the trucks, but as we lay there we knew that we were neither politically or economically empowered enough to stop the trucks. . . . As we lay our bodies in front of the trucks and were hauled off to jail by the bus load, we didn't know that the media was going to publicize [our plight]. . . . We didn't know that hundreds of people were going to come and demonstrate with us.

"We only knew in our hearts that we were doing the right thing. We knew in our hearts that God required of us to do justice. We hoped and prayed that our going to jail would not be in vain. And we feel that it was not in vain because many good things happened as a result of our going to jail. For the first time, blacks and whites in Warren County united. African Americans determined that henceforth and forever more we will have some say in the government that was controlling our destiny."

Source: Burwell, 1992.

Although the concept of environmental justice is relatively recent, many would argue that environmental injustice has existed in the Western Hemisphere since the first European settlement more than 500 years ago (Mankiller, 1992). For example, the trans-Atlantic slave trade began as a west-to-east passage, with Christopher Columbus bringing 500 Arawak Indians from the island of Puerto Rico to Spain for sale after his second journey to the Western Hemisphere (Konig, 1976). The workplace environment has long confronted workers with disparate hazardous exposures. For example, the disaster at Gauley Creek, West Virginia, during the Great Depression of the 1930s was perhaps the worst occupational health disaster in U.S. history. Some 500 African American workers died and more than 1,500 were disabled due to silicosis while digging a tunnel for the New Kanawha Power Company, a subsidiary of the Union Carbide Corporation. The deceased were buried in unmarked graves, sometimes two and three to a hole (Cherniak, 1987).

The modern environmental justice movement dates from around 1980. In 1979, the African American community of North Hollywood, in Houston, Texas, filed suit, in *Bean* v. *Southwestern Waste Management*, to prevent the siting of a solid waste landfill. In 1982, the predominantly African American community in Warren County, North Carolina, protested the siting of a PCB landfill. This incident brought together the environmental and civil rights communities and attracted national attention. It gave rise to the landmark 1987 United Church of Christ (UCC) study, *Toxic Wastes and Race in the United States*, the first national study of the demographic patterns associated with the location of hazardous waste sites (United Church of Christ Commission for Racial Justice, 1987; Lee, 1993). The Reverend Benjamin F. Chavis Jr., director of the UCC's Commission for Racial Justice, introduced the term **environmental racism** to describe the tendency of toxic waste sites and emitters to be located near communities of color. The UCC study found that race was the most significant variable in differentiating between areas with and without treatment, storage, and disposal facilities (TSDFs).

In late October 1991, the First National People of Color Environmental Leadership Summit coalesced a national movement on environmental justice. Leaders and activists gathered for the first time in a dramatic display of community-based environmental and social justice activism. To the planners of the conference, the juxtaposition of the words "people of color," "environment," and "leadership" provided a synergy that spoke for itself. When District of Columbia congresswoman Eleanor Holmes Norton spoke at the summit of defining great movements, she said, "We have all the names we need in there" (Norton, 1992). Many people, both persons of color and whites, viewed the summit as a historic turning point in the environmental movement in the United States (Lee, 1992). Within less than three years, the U.S. Environmental Protection Agency (EPA) had established an Office of Environmental Equity (later renamed the Office of Environmental Justice) and the president of the United States had signed an executive order titled "Federal Actions to Ensure Environmental Justice in Minority Populations and Low-Income Populations" (Executive Order No. 12898, 1994).

PERSPECTIVE

Would Dr. King Have Become an Environmental Justice Advocate?

I think all of you know the answer to that question. Dr. King dedicated his life to fighting racial discrimination and social inequity in the United States. He fought racial discrimination during the Birmingham bus boycotts. He fought racial discrimination in education, in employment, in housing, in health care, in the courts, and at the ballot box. Dr. King went to jail to secure for African Americans and other people the right to participate in the political process. Given all this, there is absolutely no doubt in my mind that, if he were living today, Dr. King would be a staunch and committed advocate for environmental justice.

In fact, Dr. King gave his life in 1968 around an environmental justice struggle to advance the rights and working conditions of sanitation workers in Memphis, Tennessee. Were he living today, Dr. King not only would have become an outspoken advocate for environmental justice but, as history tells us, he *always was* an environmental justice advocate and his historical legacy *includes* environmental justice. Indeed, Dr. King gave his life *as a champion for environmental justice.*

_____

Source: Based on Lee, 1994.

These events provided impetus for the emerging consciousness about environmental conditions in low-income, people of color, and tribal communities. A groundswell of activity around a vast array of issues began to take place within these communities, including issues such as toxics, lead poisoning, housing, land use, air quality, workplace heath and safety, transportation, and economic development. Examples of specific struggles are shown in Table 8.1.

In a little over a decade a loose alliance of community-based activists, church-based civil rights leaders, and academic researchers grew into a vibrant social movement. It sought to examine systematically the environmental degradation in people of color, poor, and tribal communities and to develop proactive strategies to address these problems. Initially, the focus was on where hazardous waste sites and other polluting facilities were sited, with the emphasis on demonstrating that they were located disproportionately in communities of color. However, as public discourse over issues of race, poverty, and the environment expanded, environmental justice concerns ranged more widely. For example, a landmark article in

TABLE 8.1 Examples of Community-Based Environmental Justice Issues

Community	Location	Organization(s)	Demographics	Issues
Altgeld Gardens	Chicago, Illinois	People for Community Recovery	African American, poor, urban, industrial	Public housing project, with population of 10,000, built on top of landfill in 1940s and now surrounded by polluting industries, landfills, incinerators, smelters, steel mills, chemical companies, paint manufacturing plant, municipal sewage treatment facility; also known as Chicago's "toxic donut." Led to formation of nation's first environmental organization in a public housing project.
Barrio Logan	San Diego, California	Environmental Health Coalition	Latino, urban, border	City zoning decisions of 1950s made neighborhood a repository for incompatible, noxious land uses (metal plating, auto body shops, highways) and air pollution. In 2002, community-led effort resulted in a city council resolution to develop a new land use and zoning plan for area.
West Harlem	New York City	West Harlem Environmental Action (WE ACT)	African American, urban	Northern Manhattan is the site of North River Sewage Treatment Plant, hosts 5 of 6 bus depots in Borough of Manhattan, and has high rates of asthma and respiratory illness. Partnership between WE ACT and Columbia University School of Public Health is a leading example of community-based participatory research.
Norco	Norco, Louisiana	Concerned Citizens of NORCO	African American, industrial	Homes within feet of a mammoth Shell oil refinery and chemical plant were concerned about health and safety. Area subject to major explosions and spills. After community residents traveled to the Netherlands to confront company executives at a conference, Shell agreed to relocate residents in 2002.
Alaska Native villages	Alaska	Alaska Federation of Natives	Alaska Native rural villages	More than 648 military installations, active and abandoned, pollute land, groundwater, wetlands, streams, and air with fuel spills, pesticides, solvents, munitions, and radioactive materials. Unique and intractable cleanup issues confront the Alaska Native population of approximately 100,000.

Triana	Triana, Alabama	[Not applicable]	African American, rural	DDT and PCB contamination of Alabama River affected nearly 1,200 local residents who use the river for subsistence fishing. Some of highest levels of DDT in humans ever recorded. 1982 lawsuit against Olin Corporation resulted in $24 million settlement.
Townships of North Carolina	North Carolina	Concerned Citizens of Tillary	African American, rural	Proliferation of "hog farms" in concentrated animal feeding operations (CAFOs) throughout state led to multiple major health and environmental impacts. Study by Concerned Citizens of Tillary and University of North Carolina found CAFOs more likely to be located in poor and nonwhite areas of North Carolina.
Asian immigrant women workers	San Francisco, California	Asian Immigrant Women Advocates	Asian, urban	Non-English-speaking immigrant workers in garment, hotel, electronics industries suffer assorted health impacts ranging from exposure to toxic substances to poor work conditions, long hours, and accidents. Participatory action research conducted by hotel workers, union, and University of California Labor Occupational Health Program led to demands for workload reductions at contract negotiations.
Barrio Boca	Guanyanilla, Puerto Rico	Centro de Accion Ambiental, Inc.	Puerto Rican, rural	Pesticide drift caused by aerial spraying on mango and banana plantation owned and operated by Tropical Fruit Company. Community actions resulted in court order to restrict spraying to only optimal weather conditions.
Tucson Airport Superfund Site	Tucson, Arizona	Tucsonians for a Clean Environment	Latino, urban	TCE, an industrial solvent, seeped into aquifer and created toxic groundwater plume five miles long and two miles wide and designation by EPA as a Superfund Site. Class action lawsuit resulted in a settlement with Hughes of $84.5 million. Local residents also secured a health clinic.

the *National Law Journal* in 1994 documented inequities in the enforcement of environmental laws. "There is a racial divide," the authors declared, "in the way the U.S. government cleans up toxic waste sites and punishes polluters. White communities see faster action, better results and stiffer penalties than communities where blacks, Hispanics, and other minorities live. The unequal protection occurs whether the community is wealthy or poor" (Lavelle, Coyle, and MacLachlan, 1994). Poor and people of color communities demanded that the issues they confronted—unemployment, poor public services, poor housing, and others—be linked to environmental policy. As the environmental justice paradigm matured, it became more holistic, increasingly viewing individual and community health as a product of physical, social, cultural, and spiritual factors.

Environmental justice represents a vision borne out of a community-driven process. At its core is a transformative public discourse over what constitutes truly healthy, livable, sustainable, and vital communities for all peoples. It has given birth to a broad definition of the environment as "the place where we live, where we work, and where we play" (Gauna, n.d.). It sees the ecosystem that forms the basis for life and well-being as being composed of four interrelated environments: natural, built, social, and cultural/spiritual (Lee, 1996). It has made clear the necessity for public participation and accountability in formulating environmental policy. It has expanded environmental health discourse to include issues of multiple, cumulative, and synergistic risks. It has pressed for a new paradigm for community-driven science and holistic, place-based, systems-wide environmental protection. It is searching for concepts and tools that are at the same time holistic, bottom-up, community-based, multi-issue, cross-cutting, interdependent, integrative, and unifying.

Historians of the environmental movement have referred to environmental justice as the defining feature of the fourth wave of the environmentalism. The first and longest wave grew out of the conservation movement of the late nineteenth and early twentieth centuries. The activist second wave resulted in the protective legislation of the 1970s and '80s. During the third wave, well-funded mainstream environmental groups operated primarily from "inside the Beltway," relying heavily on legal and political strategies. In the fourth wave, environmental justice emerged as the first truly grassroots form of environmentalism, one that links environmental issues to social and economic inequality and has the potential to be socially transformative (Shabecoff, 1993; Dowie, 1995).

THE MEANING OF DISPROPORTIONATE IMPACTS

The concept of environmental justice arose out of evidence that hazardous environmental exposures and their health consequences differed among different populations, based on race, ethnicity, and income. This pattern was first described in racial terms (hence the term **environmental racism**), when early studies suggested that people of color communities were disproportionately exposed to environmental hazards. Later studies focused on poverty as an additional risk factor for disproportionate exposures. The concept of **disproportionate impacts**, however, is far more complicated than exposures alone. There is a complex interplay of factors at work in communities with a history of social and economic disadvantage, inadequate services, and environmental exposures. Thus, disproportionate impacts may refer to inequities in levels of harmful environmental exposures, deficient services or benefits, diminished ability to withstand or mitigate harms, or any combination of these. This section briefly discusses the components of disproportionate impact and their implications for the theory and practice of environmental justice.

Proximity to Pollution Sources

At the simplest level adverse human health and environmental effects can be understood in terms of differential proximity to environmental hazards. During the 1980s, most environmental justice research focused on the proximity of people of color and low-income populations to environmental hazards. These studies examined a wide spectrum of exposure sources, including waste sites, industrial facilities, ambient air pollution, transportation thoroughfares, garbage transfer stations, hog farms, and all types of so-called **locally undesirable land use** (LULU). Over time the studies established a pattern of disproportionate exposure that convinced even skeptical observers. For example, political scientists James Lester, David Allen, and Kelly Hill (2001) wrote, "We must admit that at the outset in 1994 we were skeptical of many of the *strident* claims regarding environmental injustice. However, our analyses (as well as our findings) over the past five years have caused us to reconsider our original positions." (p. xv)

These proximity studies became far more sophisticated over time, deploying location data in geographic information system (GIS) software (Maantay, 2002; Brulle and Pellow, 2006; also see Chapter Twenty-Eight). GISs have proved helpful in multistressor, multimedia, and multi-issue analyses of communities. For example, GIS has been used to examine the distribution of socioeconomic, racial, ethnic, and class variables, exposure to air pollutants, and occurrence of respiratory disease, in places as diverse as the Bronx (Maantay, 2007), Massachusetts (McEntee and Ogneva-Himmelberger, 2008), Durham, North Carolina (Dolinoy and Miranda, 2004), Phoenix (Grinelski, 2007), and West Oakland (Fisher, Kelly, and Romm, 2006). This is becoming a widely available tool. The EPA's publicly available Environmental Justice Geographic Assessment Tool (www.epa.gov/compliance/whereyoulive/ejtool.html) permits users without advanced training to map demographic factors such as population density, income, and percentage below the poverty line, in relation to certain sources of pollution.

However, proximity to a source is an inexact surrogate for actual contact with a toxicant (see Chapter Four) (Institute of Medicine, 1999). For a full and accurate picture of human health and environmental effects, proximity data must be augmented with exposure studies based on modeling, actual monitoring, or other approaches. In its first report on environmental justice, the EPA concluded:

> There are clear and dramatic disparities among ethnic groups for death rates, life expectancy, and disease rates. There is also a surprising lack of data on human exposure to environmental pollutants for Whites as well as for ethnic and racial minorities. One exception is lead exposures in children, and the data are unequivocal. Black children have disproportionately higher blood lead levels than White children even when socioeconomic variables are factored in. For other pollutants, available information suggests that racial minorities may have a greater *potential* for exposure to some pollutants because they tend to live in urban areas, are more likely to live near a waste site, or exhibit a greater tendency to rely on subsistence fishing for dietary protein [U.S. EPA, 1992; emphasis in original].

Unique Exposure Pathways

Some communities sustain unique environmental exposures because of practices linked to socioeconomic status or cultural background. A good example is **subsistence fishing**. On the one hand, for some indigenous peoples and some Asian and Pacific Islander immigrant populations, this is a culturally specific practice based on a worldview that values a human connection to the environment in both physical and spiritual well-being (Arquette and others, 2002). On the other hand, economic deprivation may compel rural or urban poor people to fish in polluted waters to supplement their diets. West found that African Americans in Detroit engaged in higher levels of subsistence fishing from the contaminated Detroit River compared to the general population of Detroit (West, 1992). Another example is pica, the habit among malnourished young children of eating dirt or paint chips because they are hungry. The issues of socioeconomic status and racial discrimination are embedded in unique exposure pathways. In describing the famous 1982 case involving contamination and subsistence fish consumption in Triana, Alabama, a resident called this yet another example of how "pollution follows the path of least resistance" (Taylor, 1982).

Susceptible and Sensitive Populations

From the perspective of environmental justice, it is necessary to look not only at *intrinsic* factors related to susceptibility, such as age, sex, genetics, and race or ethnicity, but also at *acquired* factors, which may include chronic medical conditions, health care access, nutrition, fitness, other pollutant exposures, and drug and

PERSPECTIVE
Social Position and Susceptibility to Air Pollution Exposure

"People in lower socioeconomic circumstances may be more susceptible to air pollution for reasons directly related to their relative disadvantage and psychosocial stress. For example, they may lack access to grocery stories that sell fresh fruits and vegetables or the income to buy them, resulting in reduced intake of anti-oxidant vitamins that can protect against adverse consequences of air pollution exposure. Another possibility is reduced access to medical care, so poor people may not have the appropriate prescription for a respiratory condition such as asthma. Medication can alleviate symptoms aggravated by pollution exposure, and more consistent use of corticosteroids lowers baseline inflammation, potentially lowering responsiveness to proinflammatory pollutants. An additional hypothesis is that psychosocial stress and violence, which can be higher among those of low SEP (socioeconomic position), can increase susceptibility.

"Characteristics of neighborhoods can affect susceptibility. In four U.S. communities, residence in a disadvantaged neighborhood was associated with coronary heart disease (CHD) incidence, even after controlling for established CHD risk factors and personal income, education, and occupation. With current emphasis on cardiac effects of air pollution, this finding is particularly relevant to the study of air pollution and socioeconomic interaction. Because lower-income people are more likely to live near roadways, there is also evidence that increased traffic density has been associated with lack of neighborhood communication and collaboration (thereby reducing available social networks).

"Another potential mechanism of susceptibility directly related to social position is coexposure to other pollutants, include indoor pollutants. A person with a relatively high dose of other pollutants may be 'weakened' and less able to withstand the additional insult of ambient air pollution. People with less wealth are more likely to be employed in dirtier occupations and in developing countries, they may also be more likely to be exposed to pollutants indoors from heating and cooking. Workers in blue-collar occupations may also be more exposed to environmental tobacco smoke than are white-collar workers in cases where regulations limiting indoor smoking in the workplace are not applied consistently. Housing stock in poorer communities with high rates of crowding can have higher levels of certain allergens as well as other risk factors for asthma sensitization and exacerbation."

Source: O'Neill and others, 2003.

alcohol use (Sexton, 1997). The Perspective "Social Position and Susceptibility to Air Pollution Exposure" presents an excerpt from a recent review paper that explains an important social aspect of susceptibility.

Multiple and Cumulative Effects

Disadvantaged and underserved communities are likely to suffer a wide range of environmental burdens, ranging to poor air to poor housing. For example, a study by the Columbia Center for Children's Environmental Health found that African American women in the South Bronx exposed to auto exhaust, cigarette smoke, and incinerators in the third trimester of pregnancy tended to give birth to smaller babies with smaller head circumferences (Perera and others, 2004). The label **toxic hot spots** is often associated with environmental justice. Risk assessment and risk management have traditionally been unable to address these pockets of multiple and cumulative exposures, owing to a history of typically taking an individual, chemical-by-chemical approach and being geared toward controlling sources of pollution through technology-based regulation (see Chapters Twenty-Nine and Thirty). In this context the U.S. Environmental Protection Agency's 2003 *Framework for Cumulative Risk Assessment* represents a milestone for both **cumulative risk** assessment and environmental justice. It is significant for environmental justice because of the following features:

- It takes a broad view of risk, including areas outside the EPA's regulatory authority, and poses questions for which quantitative methods do not yet exist.
- It uses a population-based and place-based analysis, rather than an agent-to-receptor analysis.
- It promotes a comprehensive and integrated assessment of risk.
- It recognizes multiple stressors, including both chemical and non–chemical stressors, as well as social factors that may affect risk.
- It posits an expanded definition of vulnerability, including both biological and social factors.
- It places a premium on community involvement and partnerships.
- It emphasizes the importance of planning, scoping, and problem formulation.
- It links risk assessment to risk management within the context of prevention and intervention strategies to meet community health goals.

Fundamental to the framework's contribution to the discourse on risk assessment and environmental justice is its recognition that there needs to be an iterative process that involves the affected community and all relevant stakeholders, including government and business, as articulated in the National Academy of Sciences report *Understanding Risk* (Stern and Fineberg, 1996) and in the report of the Presidential/Congressional Commission on Risk Assessment and Risk Management (Presidential Commission, 1997).

Social Vulnerability

Underserved and disadvantaged communities have numerous liabilities that may contribute to the way environmental exposures affect health. These factors may affect a community's ability to prevent, withstand, or recover from the effects of environmental insult. Research by Manuel Pastor and his colleagues revealed an intriguing example. They found a strong correlation between periods of greatest community demographic change and the introduction of noxious land uses. These transition periods seem to be low points for community **social capital**, in terms of stable leaders, networks, and institutions. Pastor, Sadd, and Hipp (2001) coined a term to describe this phenomenon, **ethnic churning**. Social factors such as employment status, access to health insurance, language ability, and access to social capital can play a major role in determining the response to environmental insult. Lack of health care can be a major factor. Poverty, poor nutrition, and psychosocial stress may affect the strength of one's coping systems. Isolation, whether economic, racial, linguistic, or otherwise, leads to fewer connections, less access to information or influence, and thus less ability to prevent, withstand, or recover from environmental stressors. Social problems such as these may significantly limit meaningful involvement in the environmental decision-making process. Indexes that measure such isolation, such as disparity and dissimilarity indexes, may be useful in this area.

Environmental justice work in recent years has increasingly recognized the need to consider issues beyond toxic exposures. Researchers and practitioners have focused on such disparities as access to transportation (Bullard, Johnson, and Torres, 2004), neighborhood walkability (Greenberg and Renne, 2005), and access to recreational facilities (Taylor, Floyd, Whitt-Glover, and Brooks, 2007).

Two major points are highlighted by the foregoing discussion. First, disproportionate impacts cannot be characterized solely or primarily in terms of disparities in exposure to environmental hazards. It is necessary to look at both sides of the risk equation—the magnitude and severity of exposures and the nature of the receptor population. Both biological and social aspects of vulnerability must be taken into account. Second, there is a functional relationship between socioeconomic and cultural factors and environmental risk. Disadvantaged, underserved, and environmentally overburdened communities confront both physical and social vulnerability. Environmental justice is predicated on the fact that certain communities come to the table with preexisting deficits of both a physical and social nature that make the effects of environmental pollution more, and in some cases unacceptably, burdensome. This implies a broad view of **vulnerability**, as proposed by Kasperson and others (1995) and adopted in EPA's 2003 *Framework for Cumulative Risk Assessment*. In this view, vulnerability consists of susceptibility, exposure, preparedness, and ability to respond and recover. The concept of vulnerability is central to the meaning of environmental justice (deFur and others, 2007).

New frameworks for understanding the relationships among vulnerability, racial residential segregation, and various indicators of environmental health inequalities have emerged. Figure 8.1 illustrates an ecosocial, or biosocial, framework that connects a spatial form of social inequality (that is, racial segregation) to community-level conditions that disproportionately expose communities of color to environmental hazards and stressors. These stressors potentially amplify individual-level vulnerability to the toxic effects of pollution. The figure illustrates the multifaceted and multilevel dynamic that may partially explain persistent racial and class-based **health disparities** that are environmentally mediated (Morello-Frosch and Lopez, 2006).

Two important conclusions are embedded in the concept of disproportionate impacts. First, it is complex, a fact that researchers and practitioners are only now fully appreciating. A comprehensive, robust, conceptual framework for understanding disproportionate impacts—one that includes disparities in exposure, susceptibility, law enforcement, and health, and accounts for multiple and cumulative impacts—is emerging. This conceptual framework will greatly enhance the development of research and policy agendas needed to redress such impacts. Second, a focus on pollution and its prevention may be too narrow; it is necessary to address concurrently the myriad social, economic, and cultural realities of disadvantaged, underserved, and overburdened communities. A community's well-being depends on success in many different sectors, including economic development, housing, transportation, arts, green space, and recreation. Public health and environmental justice advocates must think holistically, seeking comprehensive, integrative paradigm changes to promote truly healthy and sustainable communities for all peoples.

LEGAL, PUBLIC POLICY, AND RESEARCH CHALLENGES

Once disproportionate impacts are more fully understood, environmental justice researchers and advocates face a second challenge: crafting legal and policy responses. An important barrier to meeting this challenge has been the divergence between the civil rights and environmental law paradigms.

FIGURE 8.1 Ecosocial Framework of Disproportionate Exposure to Environmental Hazards and Stressors

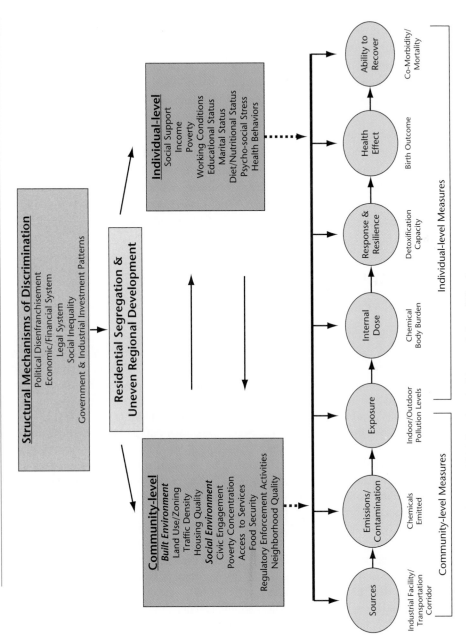

Source: Morello-Frosch and Lopez, 2006. Reprinted with permission of Elsevier.

Just seven years after the 1987 publication of *Toxic Wastes and Race*, on February 11, 1994, President Clinton signed Executive Order No. 12898, "Federal Actions to Address Environmental Justice in Minority Populations and Low-Income Populations." Because Executive Order 12898 was one of the first public policy statements in the arena of environmental justice, it is worth analyzing various interpretations of its key clause, which reads as follows: "To the greatest extent practicable and permitted by law . . . each Federal agency shall make environmental justice part of its mission by identifying and addressing, as appropriate, the disproportionately high and adverse human health and environmental effects of its programs, policies, and activities on minority populations and low-income populations."

Under the prevailing interpretation the executive order has been viewed as a directive to identify minority and low-income populations. These would be defined as "protected groups," on whose behalf protective actions could presumably then be taken. This interpretation is understandable given the legal framework of civil rights,

PERSPECTIVE
Science and Environmental Justice at the EPA

In 1992, a number of environmental justice advocates, including this chapter author, met as members of the Michigan Coalition with then EPA Administrator William Reilly. Administrator Reilly informed us of EPA's plans to establish an Office of Environmental Equity (later renamed Office of Environmental Justice in 1994). I asked Administrator Reilly, "How will EPA ensure that the Office of Environmental Equity not be marginalized like the Office of Civil Rights was?" This encounter presaged the historical significance of the proper interpretation of the language in Executive Order 12898 and the challenges of operationalizing civil rights and social justice concepts within the mission of an environmental agency like the EPA.

It is instructive to recount the testimony of William Ruckelshaus, the first EPA Administrator, before Congress at the time the agency was being established. He was asked how EPA was going to address matters of civil rights and social equity. As I recall, Administrator Ruckelshaus said that as important as these issues were, EPA was primarily a science agency and its first priority was to build its science foundation. Two decades later the United Church of Christ Commission for Racial Justice sent a copy of *Toxic Wastes and Race* to EPA, to which the agency's response was that "EPA addresses issues of technology, not sociology." I wonder where we would be today if Ruckelshaus's answer had been that the EPA would systematically incorporate concerns of civil rights and social equity into its "sound science base" and make such concerns a part of the analytical and operational paradigm within the context of the laws the agency is authorized to administer.

which is premised on the notion of *protected classes*, such as people of color, women, the disabled, and others. However, the intent of Executive Order 12898 extended well beyond identifying target populations; it was action oriented. The order directed agencies to "identify and address disproportionately high and adverse human health and environmental effects." Moreover, it called for actions to be pursued "to the greatest extent practicable and permitted by law." The order created no new rights or obligations, but an often overlooked accompanying presidential memorandum referred to the use of existing statutes to achieve the goals of the order.

Thus it is not surprising that during the decade after this executive order, most community activists, advocates, researchers, industry groups, and governmental agencies operated from the premise of identifying *environmental justice communities*, consisting of disproportionately high-minority and low-income populations. This interpretation fails to recognize that the nation's environmental laws are not premised on the concept of protected classes but on "human health and environmental effects." (Interestingly, the U.S. Department of Justice, whose mission is enforcing the nation's laws, focuses on the concept of "disproportionately high and adverse human health and environmental effects.")

This distinction is important because it bears directly on the use of environmental laws (Gerrard and Foster, 2008). The designation of environmental justice communities, while descriptive, does not trigger specific provisions of applicable laws. Hence, it is often unclear what actions, other than more study or efforts to ensure public participation, an agency should undertake once a determination that an environmental justice community exists is made. *Environmental justice issues* is a far more useful analytical concept, as it incorporates the idea of disproportionate human health and environmental effects (Payne-Sturgess and Gee, 2006). The more clear the nexus between identifying such effects and triggering specific provisions, the more readily legal remedies follow. This emphasizes the importance of fully characterizing the disproportionate human health and environmental effects, as discussed previously.

This discussion recalls the notion of environmental justice as the convergence of the civil rights and environmental movements. Such a convergence does not mean simply transplanting civil rights premises to the environmental arena. Rather it requires an understanding that civil rights law and environmental law bring two very different paradigms to environmental justice issues (Targ, 2002). This distinction has tremendous historical significance, helping explain why the concepts advanced by the civil rights movement have been largely marginalized within the nation's federal and state environmental protection regimes. Although this is an issue that surely will unfold over time, its significance should not be underestimated (as the Perspective "Science and Environmental Justice at the EPA" points out).

These issues bear directly on developing a research agenda that meets the needs of policymakers. It is not surprising that most environmental justice research in the first twenty years of the movement focused on proximity studies, demonstrating that communities of color and low-income communities are disproportionately located near environmental hazards. However, the next generation of research should focus on understanding the functional relationships between socioeconomic factors and environmental exposure and on developing innovative measures of disproportionate health and environmental effects.

PERSPECTIVE
ReGenesis Revitalization Project, Spartanburg, South Carolina

Harold Mitchell grew up in a house near an abandoned hazardous waste site in the impoverished Arkwright section of Spartanburg, South Carolina. Members of his family, like others in the neighborhood, suffered what seemed a disproportionately high number of cancers, respiratory diseases, and miscarriages. Mitchell's leadership helped to transform this concern over environmental insults into a broad vision for community revitalization. Since its inception in 1998, the ReGenesis Revitalization Project has grown to include more than 100 partners. Its vision includes housing, health facilities, recreation facilities and green space, transportation, job creation, and green business development, at the site of a former municipal dump and a shuttered fertilizer factory. Within five years, the project had leveraged more than $5 million in public and private funding. In February 2004, a Swiss bio-technology firm announced plans to locate a plastics alternatives plant in the area. The project is a prime example of Mary Nelson's observation about "turning a corner in the fight for environmental justice." Nelson is Executive Director of Bethel New Life, Inc., a renowned faith-based community development corporation in the West Garfield section of Chicago, Illinois. Nelson believes that communities are understanding that "it is not enough to stand against something. We are now moving to the stage where we can say what we want and formulate a vision for healthy, sustainable communities."

Source: U.S. EPA, Office of Policy, Economics, and Innovation, 2003.

COLLABORATIVE AND INTEGRATED PROBLEM SOLVING

The growing theoretical and practical understanding of disproportionate impacts, as well as related legal, public policy, and research challenges, is helping to identify the strategies and tools best suited to addressing such complex issues. As noted earlier, people of color, indigenous, and low-income communities often suffer adverse and disproportionate exposure to environmental and occupational hazards. Moreover, these populations tend to be more vulnerable by virtue of the social environment, such as housing, land use, transportation, health care, and other factors. Finally, the inability to employ a range of capacities (that is, to make use of human, technical, financial, social, and political capital) within affected communities presents great obstacles to positive change. How can communities and public health professionals work both to improve environmental health and to eliminate disparities related to disproportionate impacts (Freudenberg, 2004)?

The vision of environmental justice is the development of a holistic, community-based, participatory, and integrative paradigm for achieving healthy and sustainable communities for all peoples. This holistic approach aligns with the World Health Organization's view of community health, as a positive concept that includes the totality of environmental, social, and economic resources together with emotional and physical capacities available to people in a particular place (World Health Organization, 1986. Environmental justice also calls for a holistic analysis of the problems that impair the health of people in communities, including social, economic, environmental, political, emotional, and biological determinants, as discussed throughout this chapter.

Roz D. Lasker and Elisa S. Weiss of the New York Academy of Medicine build on this point when introducing the concept of collaboration in community problem solving. They write that the "growing interest in using collaboration stems from the fact that many of these problems are complex; consequently, they go beyond the capacity, resources, or jurisdiction of any single person, program, organization, or sector to change or control. Without sufficiently broad-based collaboration, it has been difficult for communities to understand the underlying nature of these kinds of problems or to develop effective and locally feasible solutions to address them" (Lasker and Weiss, 2003, p 18). Problems that require comprehensive actions have been difficult to solve when essential participants are not involved or when programs, organizations, or policies work at cross-purposes. The tremendous diversity in populations affected by health problems and in the local contexts in which these problems occur limit the effectiveness of top-down, one-size-fits-all solutions.

Both affected communities and public health practitioners must engage in a dialogue about what is needed to apply **collaborative problem solving** to the task of achieving environmental justice and healthy communities (Lee, 2005). Three premises motivate this conclusion:

- Environmental justice advocates and practitioners must develop a conceptual framework that moves the environmental justice discourse from a primary focus on problem identification to a focus that is also solution oriented.

- Environmental justice issues are enormously complex. Environmentally, economically, and socially distressed communities require human, technical, legal, and financial resources to properly address these issues. Environmental justice groups must harness these necessary resources. This speaks to the need for social capital, consensus building, dispute resolution, collaborative problem solving, and civic capacity.
- Environmental justice strategies need to address economic and social factors such as housing, transportation, economic development, job creation, green space, and recreation—factors that make up the larger environment and contribute to overall well-being.

Collaborative and integrative problem solving arose because it is a better way of dealing with complex ecological and organizational systems and with the information needs associated with complex societal problems. There is an emerging literature on collaborative problem solving in arenas such as environmental health, community development, planning, law, and natural resource management. For example, Kathryn Kohm and Jerry Franklin (1997), of the University of Washington, apply this approach to natural resource management. By appreciating the complexity of systems and managing for wholeness rather than for the efficiency of individual components, they place forestry in the context of the broad movement toward systems thinking.

The complex nature of environmentally, economically, and socially distressed communities and tribes requires holistic and integrated problem solving. Julia Wondolleck and Steven Yaffee (2000), writing about collaboration in natural resource management, call for strategies that "focus on the problem in new and different ways." They suggest "rethinking" problems in ways that (1) integrate geographically, (2) integrate functionally, and (3) integrate different elements of the problem.

Applying these lessons to environmental justice will require real community-based experience and authentic partnerships. It will also require an appreciation of the power imbalances and tensions that exist when people are trying to work through complex problems that may require both confrontational and collaborative approaches. A notable example of such collaborative decision making in an environmental justice context is the Los Angeles International Airport (LAX) Expansion Community Benefits Agreement (Los Angeles Alliance for a New Economy, 2004). The legally binding, $500 million agreement, signed in December 2004, was the product of months of discussions involving the City of Los Angeles, Los Angeles World Airports, Inc., and more than twenty community groups, environmental organizations, school districts, and labor unions. Its provisions were designed to address known impacts to surrounding communities through improvements to environmental, labor, noise, and health conditions. The agreement established a national precedent for community improvements around large-scale development projects.

Community benefits agreements are legally enforceable contracts, typically negotiated between a developer and community organizations, that specify benefits that the developer must provide to the community. These benefits include local employment opportunities, affordable housing units, mitigation of environmental impacts, recreational and greenspace development, and other items of importance to the community. Communities began to view community benefits agreements as a viable tool after the Figueroa Corridor Coalition for Economic Justice negotiated a major community benefits agreement with developers of the Los Angeles Sports and Entertainment District in May 2001. Because public dollars were involved and city council approval was required, the neighborhood coalition enjoyed a window of opportunity and some comparative negotiating advantages (Gross, LeRoy, and Janis-Aparicio, 2005).

One goal of such collaborations is to build the strategic thinking, planning, and problem-solving capacity of communities, as well as of other parties. Strategic approaches should build on community visioning and local planning processes. Such collaborative models should employ asset-building and mapping methods, recognizing that no matter how deficit- and problem-ridden a given community may be, it still has many untapped resources to harness. Mary Nelson, the director of Bethel New Life and a leading practitioner of asset building, calls for "turning environmental liabilities into community assets and opportunities." In 2003, Bethel broke ground on a transit-oriented commercial development that will incorporate photovoltaics, a living roof, recycled materials, super insulation, and energy efficiency measures. It was built on a formerly contaminated brownfield site.

When research is needed, environmental justice collaborative models may employ **community-based participatory research** (CBPR), as the two approaches share many principles and methods (see Exhibit 8.1). Moreover, such collaborative models may expand the reach of CBPR by providing the venues and stakeholders that can apply research results to real problems. These models also make use of consensus building and dispute resolution methods, including the "mutual gains approach to negotiations" (Susskind, Levy, and Thomas-Larmer, 2000). Such models build on the concepts in the EPA's cumulative risk framework by promoting proactive, comprehensive, multimedia risk reduction efforts. They have wide applicability for areas including but not limited to community development, transportation, **brownfields** redevelopment, smart growth, and comprehensive community revitalization initiatives.

Social capital—the networks, norms, and trust that facilitate coordination and cooperation for mutual benefit (Putnam, 2000)—is critically important to

EXHIBIT 8.1
Community-Based Participatory Research

- *Builds on and reinforces community capacity.* Dimensions include leadership, participation, skills, resources, social and organizational networks, sense of community and of partnership identity, understanding of community history, community power, shared values, and critical reflection.
- *Promotes active collaboration and participation at every stage of research.* CBPR fosters equal participation from all partners. It provides all participants with an equal sense of ownership over the research and the outcomes.
- *Fosters co-learning.* CBPR provides an environment in which both community residents and researchers contribute their respective expertise and where partners learn from each other. Community members acquire new skills in conducting research, and researchers learn about community networks and concerns—information that can be used to inform hypothesis generation and data collection.
- *Ensures projects are community driven.* Research questions in CBPR are guided by the environmental health issues or concerns of community members. CBPR recognizes that for research and prevention or intervention strategies to be successful, they must address the concerns of community residents.
- *Disseminates results in useful terms.* Upon completion of CBPR projects, results are communicated to all partners in culturally appropriate, respectful, and understandable terms.
- *Ensures research and intervention strategies are culturally appropriate.* With active participation of community residents from the beginning, research and prevention or intervention strategies are likely to be based in the cultural context of the community that they are intended to benefit.
- *Defines community as a unit of identity.* NIEHS *translational research* programs promote collaboration among academic scientists and community partners from underserved communities. In the case of these projects, community is typically characterized by a sense of identification and emotional connection to other members through common interests and a commitment to address shared concerns, such as harmful environmental exposures or environmental injustice.

Source: Compiled from O'Fallon and Dearry, 2002; Minkler and Wallerstein, 2002; National Institute of Environmental Health Sciences (NIEHS) (2002); Minkler, Vasquez, Tajik, and Petersen, 2008.

environmental justice collaborative problem solving. The challenge of linking resources with needs (an apt practical definition of collaboration) is especially salient in disadvantaged and underserved communities, where groups must harness necessary human, technical, legal, institutional, and financial resources to address complex issues. Marshaling the necessary resources requires the efforts of different people from different backgrounds representing all the different sectors of society. It is harder for people not to work toward resolving issues once they have sat at a table together, engaged in dialogue, and come to know each other on a human level. Once social capital is built, it leverages other forms of capital investments—financial, institutional, infrastructural, and environmental. In Robert Putnam's words, "Social connections are also important for the rules of conduct that they sustain. Networks involve (almost by definition) mutual obligations; they are not interesting as mere 'contacts.' Networks of community engagement foster sturdy norms of reciprocity. . . . A society characterized by generalized reciprocity is more efficient than a distrustful society. . . . Trustworthiness lubricates social life. Frequent interaction among a diverse set of people tends to produce a norm of generalized reciprocity. Civic engagement and social capital entail mutual obligation and responsibility for action" (Putnam, 2000, pp. 20–21).

Indeed, the emergence of the idea of using collaborative models to achieve environmental justice and healthy communities reflects a similar movement in many arenas, including community development and community health. In public health, for example, **social determinants of health** are factors in the social environment that influence health, such as income distribution, discrimination, access to education, and housing policies. Public health professionals increasingly recognize that addressing these factors will require innovative research and intervention strategies, collaboration across disciplinary groups, and engagement of community members (Schulz, Galea, and Kreiger, 2002; Wilkinson and Marmot, 2003; Marmot, 2005). The following appraisal of public health practice, from which the ideas of community-based participatory research and social determinants of health emerged, resonates strongly with the vision of environmental justice.

Recognition of the inequities in health status associated with, for example, poverty, inadequate housing, lack of employment opportunities, racism, and powerlessness, has led to calls for a focus on an ecological approach that recognizes that individuals are embedded within social, political, and economic systems that shape behaviors and access to resources necessary to maintain health.

> Researchers and practitioners alike have called for increased attention to the complex issues that compromise the health of people living in marginalized communities; for more integration of research and practice; for greater community involvement and control, for example, through partnerships among academic, health practice, and community organizations; for increased sensitivity to and competence in working with diverse cultures; for expanded use of both qualitative and quantitative research methods; and for more focus on health and quality of life, including the social, economic, and political dimensions of health and well-being [Israel, Schulz, Parker, and Becker, 1998, p. 174].

Indeed, it is enlightening to ponder the vast array of prevention and intervention strategies that can be made available to public health practitioners through a holistic understanding of the natural, built, social, and cultural and spiritual environments—the approach implicit in the concept of environmental justice.

SUMMARY

Nobel laureate Amartya Sen's work has made it clear that vulnerability to environmental change is a major shaper of global risk. Risk is closely tied to vulnerability and can be viewed as a product of environmental stress and human and ecological vulnerability. Authoritative bodies such as the World Commission on Environment and Development have underscored the intertwined nature of poverty and environmental threat. These are the same complex and multidimensional issues, albeit on a global scale, that gave rise to the concept of environmental justice. In a very short period of time both the theory and the practice of environmental justice have evolved to include an impressive array of concepts, players, and types of endeavors. They include new models of community organizing and empowerment, community-based participatory research, environmental impact assessment, utilization of existing laws, and strategies to achieve healthy and sustainable communities domestically and internationally. Issues of environmental justice make up a complex web of public health, environmental, economic, and social concerns that require multiple, holistic, integrative, and unifying strategies. The achievement of a vision of healthy and sustainable communities for all peoples necessitates not only the articulation of new concepts, new strategies, new models, and new partnerships but also a critical appraisal of where progress has been made and what obstacles stand in the way. This will require committed individuals willing and able to provide foresight, analysis, and leadership.

KEY TERMS

brownfields

collaborative problem solving

community-based participatory research

cumulative risk

disproportionate impacts

environmental justice

environmental racism

ethnic churning

health disparities

locally undesirable land use

social capital

social determinants of health

subsistence fishing

toxic hot spot

vulnerability

DISCUSSION QUESTIONS

1. What evidence exists to show that race and poverty contribute to negative environmental health effects?
2. What factors can exacerbate the effects of environmental exposures on populations with low socioeconomic status?
3. Why is involving the affected community important to achieving solutions to environmental justice issues?
4. What are some global implications of environmental justice?
5. What is an example of an environmental justice concern in your own city? Explain that concern.
6. Identify and discuss the ideas that inform this statement: Environmental justice must be concerned not only with disproportionate exposure to hazards but also with disproportionate deprivation of assets such as parks and mass transit.

REFERENCES

Arquette, M., and others. "Holistic Risk-Based Environmental Decision Making: A Native Perspective." *Environmental Health Perspectives*, 2002, *110*(suppl. 2), 259–264.

Brulle, R. J., and Pellow, D. N. "Environmental Justice: Human Health and Environmental Inequalities." *Annual Review of Public Health*, 2006, *27*, 103–124.

Bullard, R. D., Johnson, G. S., and Torres, A. O. (eds.). *Highway Robbery: Transportation Racism and New Routes to Equity*. Cambridge, Mass.: South End Press, 2004.

Burwell, D. "Reminiscences from Warren County, North Carolina." In C. Lee (ed.), *Proceedings of the First National People of Color Environmental Leadership Summit.* New York: United Church of Christ Commission for Racial Justice, 1992.

Cherniak, M. *The Hawk's Nest Incident: America's Worst Industrial Disaster.* New Haven, Conn.: Yale University Press, 1987.

deFur, P. L., and others. "Vulnerability as a Function of Individual and Group Resources in Cumulative Risk Assessment." *Environmental Health Perspectives,* 2007, *115,* 817–824.

Dolinoy D. C., and Miranda, M. L. "GIS Modeling of Air Toxics Releases from TRI-Reporting and Non-TRI-Reporting Facilities: Impacts for Environmental Justice." *Environmental Health Perspectives,* 2004, *112*(17), 1717–1724.

Dowie, M. *Losing Ground: American Environmentalism at the Close of the Twentieth Century.* Cambridge, Mass.: MIT Press, 1995.

Executive Order No. 12898. "Federal Actions to Address Environmental Justice in Minority Populations and Low-Income Populations." *Federal Register, 59,* 7629 (1994).

Faber, D. R., and McCarthy, D. *Green of Another Color: Building Effective Partnerships Between Foundations and the Environmental Justice Movement.* Philanthropy and Environmental Justice Research Project, Northeastern University. Boston: Northeastern Environmental Justice Research Collaborative, Apr. 10, 2001.

Fisher, J. B., Kelly, M., and Romm, J. "Scales of Environmental Justice: Combining GIS and Spatial Analysis for Air Toxics in West Oakland, California." *Health & Place,* 2006, *12*(4), 701–714.

Freudenberg, N. "Community Capacity for Environmental Health Promotion: Determinants and Implications for Practice." *Health Education & Behavior,* 2004, *31,* 472–490.

Gauna, J., Co-director of the SouthWest Organizing Project, quoted in Rodriguez R. "Going Green." Color Lines, March/April 2008. http://www.colorlines.com/article.php?ID=280

Gerrard, M. B., and Foster, S. R. (eds.). *The Law of Environmental Justice: Theories and Procedures to Address Disproportionate Risks.* (2nd ed.) Chicago: American Bar Association, Section of Environment, Energy and Resources, 2008.

Greenberg, M. R., and Renne, J. "Where Does Walkability Matter the Most? An Environmental Justice Interpretation of New Jersey Data." *Journal of Urban Health,* 2005, *82*(1), 90–100.

Grinelski, S. E. "Incorporating Health Outcomes into Environmental Justice Research: The Case of Children's Asthma and Air Pollution in Phoenix, Arizona." *Environmental Hazards,* 2007, *7,* 360–371.

Gross, J., LeRoy, G., and Janis-Aparicio, M. *Community Benefits Agreements: Making Development Projects Accountable.* Washington, D.C.: Goods Jobs First and California Partnership for Working Families. http://www.goodjobsfirst.org/pdf/cba2005final.pdf, 2005.

Institute of Medicine. *Toward Environmental Justice: Research, Education, and Health Policy Needs.* Washington, D.C.: National Academies Press, 1999.

Israel, B. A., Schulz, A. J., Parker, E. A., and Becker, A. B. "Review of Community-Based Research: Assessing Partnership Approaches to Improve Public Health." *Annual Review of Public Health,* 1998, *19,* 173–202.

Kasperson, J. X., Kasperson, R. E., and Turner, B. L. *Regions at Risk: Comparisons of Threatened Environments.* UNU Studies of Critical Environmental Regions. Tokyo: United Nations University Press, 1995.

Kohm, K. A., and Franklin, J. F. *Creating a Forestry for the 21st Century: The Science of Ecosystem Management.* Washington, D.C.: Island Press, 1997.

Konig, H. *Columbus: His Enterprise.* New York: Monthly Review Press, 1976.

Lasker, R. D., and Weiss E. S. "Broadening Participation in Community Problem Solving: A Multidisciplinary Model to Support Collaborative Practice and Research." *Journal of Urban Health,* 2003, *80,* 14–47.

Lavelle, M., Coyle, M., and MacLachlan, C. "Unequal Protection: The Racial Divide in Environmental Law." *National Law Journal,* Sept. 21, 1994, p. S1.

Lee, C. "Introduction." In C. Lee (ed.), *Proceedings of the First National People of Color Environmental Leadership Summit.* New York: United Church of Christ Commission for Racial Justice, 1992.

Lee, C. "Beyond Toxic Wastes and Race." In R. D. Bullard (ed.), *Confronting Environmental Racism: Voices from the Grassroots.* Boston: South End Press, 1993.

Lee, C. "A Dream Deferred: 30 Years After the Passage of the Civil Rights Act of 1964." Speech presented at a U.S. Department of Justice Symposium, Washington, D.C., Nov. 30, 1994.

Lee, C. "Environmental Justice, Urban Revitalization, and Brownfields: The Search for Authentic Signs of Hope." Presentation at the U.S. Environmental Protection Agency National Brownfields Workshop, Washington, D.C., Feb. 13–14, 1996.

Lee, C. "Environmental Justice: Building a Unified Vision of Health and Environment." *Environmental Health Perspectives,* 2002, *110*(suppl. 2), 141–144.

Lee, C. "Collaborative Models to Achieve Environmental Justice and Healthy Communities." In D. Pellow and R. Brulle (eds.), *People, Justice, and the Environment: A Critical Appraisal of the Environmental Justice Movement.* Cambridge, Mass.: MIT Press, 2005.

Lester, J. P., Allen, D. W., and Hill, K. M. *Environmental Injustice in the United States: Myths and Realities.* Boulder, Colo.: Westview Press, 2001.

Los Angeles Alliance for a New Economy. "Council Approves $500 Million Agreement to Help Communities Near LAX." http://www.laane.org/pressroom/releases/lax041214.html, Dec. 14, 2004.

Maantay, J. "Mapping Environmental Injustices: Pitfalls and Potential of Geographic Information Systems in Assessing Environmental Health and Equity." *Environmental Health Perspectives,* 2002, *110*(suppl. 2), 161–171.

Maantay, J. "Asthma and Air Pollution in the Bronx: Methodological and Data Considerations in Using GIS for Environmental Justice and Health Research." *Health & Place,* 2007, *13*(1), 32–56.

Mankiller, W. "Native American Historical and Cultural Perspectives on Environmental Justice." In C. Lee (ed.), *Proceedings of the First National People of Color Environmental Leadership Summit.* New York: United Church of Christ Commission for Racial Justice, 1992.

Marmot, M. "Social Determinants of Health Inequalities." *Lancet,* 2005, *365,* 1099–1104.

McEntee, J. C., and Ogneva-Himmelberger, Y. "Diesel Particulate Matter, Lung Cancer, and Asthma Incidences Along Major Traffic Corridors in MA, USA: A GIS Analysis." *Health & Place,* 2008, *14*(4), 817–828.

Minkler, M., and Wallerstein, N. *Community-Based Participatory Research for Health.* San Francisco: Jossey-Bass, 2002.

Minkler, M., Vasquez, V. B., Tajik, M., and Petersen, D. "Promoting Environmental Justice Through Community-Based Participatory Research: The Role of Community and Partnership Capacity." *Health Education & Behavior,* 2008, *35*(1), 119–137.

Morello-Frosch, R., and Lopez, R. "The Riskscape and the Colorline: Examining the Role of Segregation in Environmental Health Disparities." *Environmental Research*, 2006, *102*(2), 181–196.

National Environmental Justice Advisory Council Cumulative Risks/Impacts Work Group. *Ensuring Risk Reduction for Communities with Multiple Stressors: Environmental Justice and Cumulative Risks/Impacts.* Washington, D.C.: National Environmental Justice Advisory Council, 2004.

National Institute for Environmental Health Sciences. *Health Disparities Research.* http://www.niehs.nih.gov/translat/hd/healthdis.htm, 2002.

Norton, E. H. "Perspectives from the District of Columbia." In C. Lee (ed.), *Proceedings of the First National People of Color Environmental Leadership Summit.* New York: United Church of Christ Commission for Racial Justice, 1992.

O'Fallon, L. R., and Dearry, A. "Community-Based Participatory Research as a Tool to Advance Environmental Health Sciences." *Environmental Health Perspectives*, 2002, *110*(suppl. 2), 155–159.

O'Neill, M. S., and others. "Health, Wealth, and Air Pollution: Advancing Theory and Methods." *Environmental Health Perspectives*, 2003, *111*, 1861–1870.

Pastor, M., Jr., Sadd, J., and Hipp, J. "Which Came First? Toxic Facilities, Minority Move-In, and Environmental Justice." *Journal of Urban Affairs*, 2001, *23*(1), 1–21.

Payne-Sturges, D., and Gee, G. C. "National Environmental Health Measures for Minority and Low-Income Populations: Tracking Social Disparities in Environmental Health." *Environmental Research*, 2006, *102*, 154–171.

Perera, F. P., and others. "Molecular Evidence of an Interaction Between Prenatal Environmental Exposures and Birth Outcomes in a Multiethnic Population." *Environmental Health Perspectives*, 2004, *112*(5), 626–630.

Presidential/Congressional Commission on Risk Assessment and Risk Management. *Framework for Environmental Health Risk Assessment: Final Report.* Vol. *1.* Washington, D.C.: Presidential/Congressional Commission on Risk Assessment and Risk Management, 1997.

Putnam, R. D. *Bowling Alone: The Collapse and Revival of American Community.* New York: Simon & Shuster, 2000.

Schulz, A. J., Galea, S., and Kreiger, J. (eds.). "Community-Based Participatory Research—Addressing Social Determinants of Health: Lessons from the Urban Research Centers." *Health Education and Behavior*, 2002, *20*(3, special issue).

Sexton, K. "Sociodemographic Aspects of Human Susceptibility to Toxic Chemicals: Do Class and Race Matter for Realistic Risk Assessment?" *Environmental Toxicology and Pharmacology*, 1997, *4*, 261–269.

Shabecoff, P. *A Fierce Green Fire: Environmentalism in the 21st Century.* New York: Hill & Wang, 1993.

Stern, P. C., and Fineberg, H. V., (eds.). *Understanding Risk: Informing Decisions in a Democratic Society.* Washington, D.C.: National Academies Press, 1996.

Susskind, L., Levy, P., and Thomas-Larmer, J. *Negotiating Environmental Agreements: How to Avoid Escalating Confrontations, Needless Costs, and Unnecessary Litigation.* Washington, D.C.: Island Press, 2000.

Targ, N. "A Third Policy Avenue to Address Environmental Justice: Civil Rights and Environmental Quality and the Relevance of Social Capital Policy." *Tulane Environmental Law Journal*, 2002, *16*, 167–174.

Taylor, R. "Do Environmentalists Care About the Poor?" *U.S. News and World Report*, Apr. 2, 1982, pp. 51–52.

Taylor, W. C., Floyd, M. F., Whitt-Glover, M. C., and Brooks, J. "Environmental Justice: A Framework for Collaboration Between the Public Health and Parks and Recreation Fields to Study Disparities in Physical Activity." *Journal of Physical Activity and Health*, 2007, *4*(suppl. 1), S50–S63.

United Church of Christ Commission for Racial Justice. *Toxic Wastes and Race in the United States: A National Study on the Racial and Socio-Economic Characteristics of Communities Surrounding Hazardous Waste Sites.* New York: United Church of Christ, 1987.

U.S. Environmental Protection Agency. *Environmental Equity: Reducing Risk for All Communities.* EPA230-R-92-008. Washington, D.C.: U.S. Environmental Protection Agency, June 1992.

U.S. Environmental Protection Agency. *Framework for Cumulative Risk Assessment.* EPA/630/P-02/001F. Washington, D.C.: U.S. Environmental Protection Agency, May 2003.

U.S. Environmental Protection Agency, Office of Policy, Economics, and Innovation. The ReGenesis Partnership: A Case Study. Excerpted from Towards an Environmental Justice Collaborative Model: Case Studies of Six Partnerships Used to Address Environmental Justice Issues in Communities (EPA/100-R-03-002). January, 2003. http://www.epa.gov/evaluate/regenesis.pdf.

West, P. C. "Invitation to Poison? Detroit Minorities and Toxic Fish Consumption from the Detroit River." In B. Bryant and P. Mohai (eds.), *Race and the Incidence of Environmental Hazards: A Time for Discourse.* Boulder, Colo.: Westview Press, 1992, pp. 96–99.

Wilkinson, R., and Marmot, M. (eds.). *Social Determinants of Health: The Solid Facts.* (2nd ed.) Copenhagen: World Health Organization, 2003.

Wondolleck, J. M., and Yaffee, S. L. *Making Collaboration Work: Lessons from Innovation in Natural Resource Management.* Washington, D.C.: Island Press, 2000.

World Health Organization. A discussion document on the concept and principles of health promotion. *Health Promotion.* 1986, *1*, 73–78.

FOR FURTHER INFORMATION

Books

A large library of environmental justice materials has emerged in recent years. Some of the best books are listed here.

Adamson, J., Evans, M. M., and Stein, R. *The Environmental Justice Reader: Politics, Poetics and Pedagogy.* Tucson: University of Arizona Press, 2002.

Bryant, B. *Environmental Justice: Issues, Policies and Solutions.* Washington, D.C.: Island Press, 1995.

Bullard, R. D. (ed.). *The Quest for Environmental Justice: Human Rights and the Politics of Pollution.* San Francisco: Sierra Club Books, 2005.

Camacho, D. (ed.). *Environmental Injustices, Political Struggles: Race, Class, and the Environment.* Durham, N.C.: Duke University Press, 1998.

Cole, L. W., and Foster, S. R. *From the Ground Up: Environmental Racism and the Rise of the Environmental Justice Movement.* New York: NYU Press, 2001.

Corburn, J. *Street Science: Community Knowledge and Environmental Health Justice.* Cambridge, Mass.: MIT Press, 2005.

Pellow, D. N., and Brulle, R. J. (eds.). *Power, Justice, and the Environment: A Critical Appraisal of the Environmental Justice Movement.* Cambridge, Mass.: MIT Press, 2005.

Sandler, R., and Pezzullo, P. C. *Environmental Justice and Environmentalism: The Social Justice Challenge to the Environmental Movement.* Cambridge, Mass.: MIT Press, 2007.

Review Articles

Gee, G. C., and Payne-Sturges, D. C. "Environmental Health Disparities: A Framework Integrating Psychosocial and Environmental Concepts." *Environmental Health Perspectives*, 2004, *112*(17), 1645–1653.

Mohai, P., and Saha, R. "Reassessing Racial and Socioeconomic Disparities in Environmental Justice Research." *Demography*, 2006, *43*(2), 383–399.

Olden, K., and White, S. L. "Health-Related Disparities: Influence of Environmental Factors." *Medical Clinics of North America*, 2005, *89*, 721–738.

Programs, Centers, and Organizations

Academic Centers

Deep South Center for Environmental Justice, Dillard University, New Orleans, http://www.dscej.org.

Environmental Justice Resource Center, Clark Atlanta University, Atlanta, http://www.ejrc.cau.edu.

Environmental Justice Program, University of Michigan, Ann Arbor, http://sitemaker.umich.edu/snre-ej-program/home.Governmental Programs

U.S. EPA Environmental Justice program, http://www.epa.gov/environmentaljustice.

California EPA Environmental Justice program, http://www.calepa.ca.gov/EnvJustice.

Nongovernmental Organizations

National Black Environmental Justice Network, http://www.nbejn.org.

National Hispanic Environmental Council, http://www.nheec.org.

Community-Based Organizations

Southwest Network for Environmental & Economic Justice, Albuquerque, N.M., http://www.sneej.org.

Community Coalition for Environmental Justice, Seattle, Wash., http://www.ccej.org.

Concerned Citizens of South Central Los Angeles., Los Angeles, Calif., http://www.ccscla.org.

Detroiters Working for Environmental Justice, Detroit, Mich., http://www.dwej.org.

West Harlem Environmental Action—WE ACT, Inc., West Harlem, NY, http://www.weact.org.

PART TWO

ENVIRONMENTAL HEALTH ON THE GLOBAL SCALE

CHAPTER NINE

POPULATION PRESSURE

DON HINRICHSEN

KEY CONCEPTS

- Although fertility rates are falling in some regions, global population continues to grow.

- This growth is concentrated in poor countries.

- Global population is also becoming increasingly urban.

- Population growth, together with affluence and technology (both reflecting resource use), exerts major pressures on natural resources and on ecosystem integrity.

- The ecological footprint is an approach to measuring the impact of population and resource use on the ecosystem.

- Carrying capacity refers to the number of people an ecosystem, or the entire Earth, can support.

- Both limiting population growth and reducing per capita resource use play a role in achieving environmental health.

A S the twenty-first century unfolds, population trends underlie much of the troubled relationship between humanity and the environment. The global population is growing, and much of this growth is in the poorest parts of the world. In addition, the world's population is redistributing from rural areas to cities. These changes place enormous pressure on resources and have broad implications for human health. This chapter introduces the basic principles of demography, the science that studies the size, density, and distribution of human populations; reviews global population trends and their impact on resources; and explores the ways in which these global trends link to human health.

POPULATION, RESOURCE USE, AND ENVIRONMENT

The number of people on Earth is now 6.8 billion. Despite falling fertility rates in virtually every region of the world, the population continues to grow, by about 78 million per year. At this rate the world's population will increase by 1 billion every fourteen to fifteen years. According to the United Nations Department of Economic and Social Affairs (UN-DESA), Population Division (2009), the global population is projected to reach 8 billion by 2025 and 9.1 billion by 2050 (using the midrange estimates).

About 99 percent of this growth will occur in the world's poor, developing countries. Not surprisingly, the highest growth rates are found in the poorest countries, those the United Nations (UN) categorizes as least developed. These countries are found predominantly in sub-Saharan Africa, the Middle East, and South Asia.

Even with the AIDS pandemic, population growth rates in the forty-four poorest developing countries are still above 2.5 percent per year, enough to double their populations over the next quarter century. Specifically, western Africa's population is increasing by an average of 2.7 percent per year, eastern Africa's by 2.5 percent, and middle Africa's by nearly 3 percent. Only southern Africa, which includes the relatively developed countries of South Africa, Botswana, Namibia, Lesotho, and Swaziland, has a lower collective growth rate, averaging 1 percent per year (Population Reference Bureau, 2003; World Health Organization, 2003).

In the past decade population growth has been slower than previously estimated. For example, UN-DESA, Population Division (2009), reports that the current annual growth of about 78 million people in the world's population is

Don Hinrichsen declares no competing financial interests.

about 12 million fewer than previously estimated. In fact annual world population growth fell from 2 percent in 1970 to 1.17 percent in 2005. Over the same period, average fertility fell by nearly half, from 4.5 children per woman to 2.6, while average life expectancy rose from 58 years to 67 years, and the annual death rate dropped from 11 deaths per 1,000 people to 8.6 per 1,000 (UN-DESA, Population Division, 2009). Already, sixty-five countries, of which only nine are in the developing world, have fallen below replacement-level fertility. Population growth will level off when replacement-level fertility—about 2.1 children per couple—is reached (UN-DESA, Population Division, 2009). If current trends continue, this point will be reached around the middle of the twenty-first century (UN Population Fund, 2003; UN-DESA, Population Division, 2007).

The rapid drop in fertility levels among women in the developed countries of Europe, Asia, and North America has, according to some analysts, given rise to a new demographic imperative, termed the birth dearth. Proponents argue that the population problem is over and that the world is now facing a new threat: depopulation. However, the birth dearth theory is undermined by the crucial fact that nearly half the planet's population is under the age of twenty-five. In fact, 1.2 billion people are between the ages of ten and nineteen, the largest cohort of young people in history (UN Population Fund, 2003). Because over 90 percent of them live in developing countries, their access to family planning and reproductive health, or lack of it, will to a great extent determine future human numbers. Clearly, the future demographic profile of the planet will be written by the world's poorest countries, not its richest. Moreover, although Africa's fertility rate has dropped on average across the entire continent (some countries remain exceptions), it is declining from a very high rate. A drop of half a percent—from 3 percent to 2.5 percent—will do little to stop the momentum of population growth. Poor populations will continue to grow in unsustainable fashion throughout much of Africa.

The drop in Africa's fertility levels is attributed in part to the AIDS pandemic. Currently, some 40 million people globally are HIV positive, three-quarters of them in sub-Saharan Africa. The main reason that populations are still growing in Africa is the rising numbers of young people. Even with AIDS the momentum of numbers means that populations will continue to grow, especially if couples do not have the information and means to plan their families. Moreover, according to recent studies by the Joint United Nations Programme on HIV/AIDS (UNAIDS), the pandemic appears to be leveling off in many sub-Saharan countries, a result of advocacy efforts and prevention programs (UNAIDS, UNFPA, and UNIFEM, 2004). Therefore the current trend in Africa continues to be toward a rising population.

PERSPECTIVE
Measuring Population Impact

There is no easy way to measure the impact of human activities, including population growth, on the environment nor any single agreed-upon approach. Nevertheless several approaches have been developed that demonstrate the complex relationships involved (Cohen, 1995; Ehrlich and Holdren, 1971; Goodland, 1992).

One approach to measuring the impact of human use of natural resources is to place an economic value on environmental goods and services. These include such natural resources as unpolluted freshwater, clean air, ocean life, forests, and wetlands—resources that have traditionally been regarded as free goods or common resources. A global study (Constanza and others, 1997) estimated the total value of ecosystem services and products at $33 trillion per year—an amount greater than the total value of the global economy as traditionally measured ($29 trillion in 1998).

Although there is little agreement on how to value natural resources, some economists argue that environmental goods and services should be incorporated into estimates of gross domestic product (GDP), as are manufactured assets. Unlike manufactured capital, which depreciates in value over time, environmental capital (such as forests, fisheries, and unpolluted air and water) is currently not considered to depreciate, and no charge is made against current income as these resources are used up. Robert Repetto (1989) of the World Resources Institute, in criticizing this approach, notes that a "country could exhaust its mineral resources, cut down its forests, erode its soils, pollute its aquifers, and hunt its wildlife and fisheries to extinction, but measured income would not be affected as these natural assets disappeared" (pp. 2–3).

POPULATION AND URBANIZATION

The world is also in the middle of an urban revolution. In 2008, for the first time in history, more than 50 percent of the global population lived in towns and cities. By 2030, that proportion is expected to reach the 60 percent mark (UN-DESA, Population Division, 2008). Between 2007 and 2050, the world's urban population is on course to double, from 3.3 billion to 6.4 billion (UN-DESA, 2008). The pace of urbanization in many developing countries is breathtaking. Big cities in Africa, for instance, are growing on average by around 4 percent per year, enough to double their populations in less than twenty years. (Conditions in

If natural resources were valued in the same way that manufactured assets are valued, that might help economies to use them more efficiently and to conserve them in order to ensure continued use in the future. Such valuations might help indicate the economic as well as ecological benefits of protecting the environment. In other terms, instead of drawing down their environmental capital, economies could begin to live on its interest (Goodland, 1992).

$$I = P \times A \times T$$

This equation is one way of showing how developing countries with large and rapidly growing populations affect the environment, even at low levels of affluence and technology, and how developed countries with smaller populations also have a substantial impact, because their levels of affluence and technology are so high (UN Population Fund, 1991). In this equation, I is environmental impact, P is population (including size, growth, and distribution), A is the level of affluence (consumption per capita), and T is the technology used to provide the level of consumption.

The equation also helps to show the importance of slowing population growth as part of any strategy to reduce humanity's impact on the environment. For example, even if per capita resource consumption (A) declined or technologies (T) improved enough to reduce the environmental impact (I) of humanity by 10 percent, this gain would be eroded in less than a decade if global population (P) were growing at 1.17 percent per year (UN Population Fund, 1991; UN-DESA, Population Division, 2007).

At current levels of population and technology, the impact on the environment is considerable (Vitousek, Mooney, Lubchenco, and Melillo, 1997). Because consumption levels are rising and will continue to rise, using resources more efficiently and slowing population growth are essential to ease environmental impact and protect human health (Hinrichsen and Robey, 2000; Upadhyay and Robey, 1999).

these cities and their health implications are described in Chapter Eleven.) This level of growth is unprecedented and for the most affected countries not sustainable. The infrastructure of most cities in developing countries cannot keep pace with such rapid and sustained urban population growth (Hinrichsen, Salem, and Blackburn, 2002).

The rapid urban growth in the developing world is being driven by people who are fleeing collapsing rural economies, lack of rural infrastructure and services, landlessness, and lack of rural employment opportunities. These push and pull factors will continue to drive urbanization, especially in developing countries. Young people in particular are leading the flight to the cities.

POPULATION AND ENVIRONMENT

Population increases and rising per capita consumption levels are leading to environmental degradation and resource depletion at an unsustainable pace (Kasperson, Kasperson, and Turner, 1995, 1999). In fact the world's economies are currently overshooting the Earth's capacity to regenerate natural resources by an estimated 39 percent, according to the *Ecological Footprint of Nations: 2005 Update* (Venetoulis and Talberth, 2006; see also Wackernagel and others, 1997; Venetoulis and Talberth, 2008).

Every individual has an ecological footprint—the person's effect on the surrounding environment. The aggregate impact of humanity on the environment varies in magnitude both with the number of people and with the amount of resources that they consume, waste, or pollute beyond use (Wackernagel and others, 1997). In some countries where population is growing rapidly and efficient technologies to protect the environment are lacking, there is little choice but to exploit natural resources to accommodate people's needs. In other countries, despite slower population growth and more efficient technologies, standards of living are so high that the population treads heavily upon nature.

In fact, if the entire world population were to have the same standard of living as the average American or Western European today, the equivalent of three worlds would be required to supply the needed resources at current rates of consumption and waste generation (UNDESA, 2003). In the United States, 306 million people—less than 5 percent of the world's total population—consume several times that proportion of most global resources (Brown, Gardner, and Halweil, 1999; Markham, 2006). The average person in the United States uses the energy equivalent of fifty-seven barrels of oil each year, compared to less than two barrels for the average Bangladeshi.

When consumption levels are high, even slow rates of population growth mean dramatic increases in resource use. In the United States in 1990, for example, population growth alone increased energy consumption by an estimated 110 million barrels of oil. The U.S. population was growing by around 1 percent per year in the early 1990s. That same year Bangladesh's population base was 130 million, growing by 2.5 percent per year but using only 9 million barrels of oil in total, a tiny amount compared to its size and rate of growth (UN Population Fund, 1991).

Technology plays a mitigating role. Although the 20 percent of humanity in the most affluent countries consumes close to 60 percent of the world's energy, most industrialized countries use energy more efficiently and produce less pollution than developing countries do because the latter do not have the resources to invest

PERSPECTIVE
Carrying Capacity

The term **carrying capacity** refers to the number of people the Earth can support. Estimates of carrying capacity vary a great deal, depending on what is being included and how it is being measured. In 1976, for example, ecologist Roger Revelle said that the Earth could support 40 billion people if everyone ate vegetarian diets of no more than 2,500 calories a day. Such a diet would require converting all farmland to the production of grains and vegetables (Cohen, 1995).

Another estimate is that the Earth could support up to 10 billion people eating meat diets (Cohen, 1995). Some have concluded that the Earth's carrying capacity may already have been exceeded in the sense that many people live in poverty and that if people in low-income countries were to catch up with the living standards of people in the developed world the world could support only 2 billion people (Crenson, 1999).

Making calculations of how many people could exist on the Earth under a variety of different scenarios probably is less important than determining how resources can be used wisely and managed sustainably to improve living standards without eventually destroying the natural environment that supports life itself. Environmentalists, economists, and demographers increasingly agree that efforts to protect the environment, achieve better living standards, and slow population growth tend to be "mutually reinforcing" (Roodman, 1998). The World Bank (1992) too has pointed out that reducing poverty, protecting the environment, and slowing population growth are closely linked.

in energy-saving technologies or pollution control (United Nations Development Programme [UNDP], 1997; World Health Organization, 1997). One of the greatest challenges posed by rising consumption and economic development is to use energy efficiently and to avoid pollution.

POPULATION-ENVIRONMENT SCORECARD

In 1992, concerned about worsening environmental conditions, delegates to the **United Nations Conference on Environment and Development** (UNCED), held in Rio de Janeiro, Brazil, stressed the need for action. This **Earth Summit**, as it was also called, set specific goals for making environmental improvements. Five years later, however, in 1997, a special session of the UN

General Assembly, known as the Rio Plus Five Conference, found that little progress had been made toward meeting any of the goals (United Nations Environment Programme, 2000). In each sector—arable land, freshwater, oceans, forests, biodiversity, and climate change—the 1997 UN assessment found that environmental trends either were no better than in 1992 or had worsened. The UN also found that poverty had increased, in part because of rapid population growth (UNDP, 1998).

Arable Land

Soil degradation is a widespread and growing problem, which contributes to decreased agricultural yields. Causes of soil degradation include deforestation, overexploitation for domestic uses such as fencing and fuel wood, overgrazing, unsustainable agricultural practices, and conversion of arable land to residential and industrial uses. In the late 1980s, the United Nations Environment Program (UNEP) supported the Global Assessment of Human-Induced Soil Degradation (GLASOD). This effort identified four types of soil damage—water erosion, wind erosion, chemical deterioration (including nutrient loss, acidification, salinization, and pollution), and physical deterioration (such as compaction, waterlogging, and subsidence)—corresponding to about 15 percent of total land area worldwide (Oldeman, Hakkeling, and Sombroek, 1991). Cropland was disproportionately affected; about 560 million hectares (out of a total of 1.5 billion hectares) of prime cropland worldwide were degraded. A decade later the number had risen by 10 percent to about 610 million hectares. In addition, grazing land suffering from moderate to severe degradation rose from about 1 billion hectares to about 1.2 billion hectares during the 1990s (World Resources Institute [WRI], 1998). Around the world the total amount of cropland and grazing land that suffers from soil degradation equals an area the size of the United States and Mexico combined (WRI, 1998). Fertile topsoil is being depleted between 16 and 300 times faster than it can be replenished (Kendall and Pimental, 1994). Estimates are imprecise because of marked variation across soil types and climatic conditions. Unfortunately, ongoing global assessment of soil degradation has not continued.

The Convention to Combat Desertification, negotiated at the 1992 Earth Summit, took effect in 1996 and by 2009 had been ratified by 193 countries. Nevertheless, donor countries have not committed the resources needed to tackle the problem of once productive land becoming desert, which is viewed as predominately a problem for the developing world (Agarwal, Narain, and Sharma, 1999; Adeel and others, 2007).

Population growth has contributed to land degradation throughout the least developed countries. In many countries of Africa and Asia, sons inherit equal shares of land. Thus over the generations ever-growing families have meant ever-shrinking farmsteads, forcing many people onto the less productive, marginal farmland in hilly areas, drylands, and tropical forests (Doos, 1994; Brown and Mitchell, 1997).

As the rural environment deteriorates due to land degradation and shrinking farmsteads, small-scale farmers cannot produce enough food to feed their families. Women and girls, in particular, pay the price with poorer diets; they suffer increasingly from protein energy malnutrition and lack of vitamin A. The disease burden for poor rural families unable to coax a living from shrinking farmsteads is manifested in chronic anemia and respiratory infections along with greater susceptibility to malaria, dengue fever, and cholera.

Freshwater

Growing populations place considerable pressure on freshwater supplies, as described in Chapter Fifteen. According to the World Resources Institute's Pilot Analysis of Global Ecosystems, as of 1995, 2.3 billion people, just over two of every five people worldwide, lived in water-stressed areas, with a per capita water supply of less than 1,700 m^3/year. Of these, 1.7 billion people resided in highly water-stressed areas, defined as having less than 1,000 m^3/year of water per capita. The WRI has projected that by 2025, at least 3.5 billion people—or 48 percent of the world's projected population—will live in water-stressed areas, 2.4 billion of them under highly water-stressed conditions (Revenga and others, 2000).

Chronic water shortages will be perhaps the most limiting factor on future economic development in these regions. Moreover, even though the percentage of the population without access to potable water declined during the 1990s and 2000s, rapid population growth meant that more people than before lacked clean water. As of 2007, an estimated 1.2 billion people lacked clean water, compared to about 1 billion in 1990. (The health implications of an inadequate supply of clean water are described in Chapter Fifteen.)

Oceans

During recent decades, coastal wetlands—including mangrove forests, salt ponds, marshes, and brackish water estuaries—have deteriorated (Hinrichsen, 1998), and development pressures have been a principal driver (Bryant, Rodenburg, Cox, and Nielsen, 1995). For example, the Millennium Ecosystem Assessment (2005) estimated that over half of the Earth's total mangrove area was lost over the last two decades, driven primarily by aquaculture development, deforestation, and freshwater diversion, and that about 40 percent of coral reefs were lost or degraded during the last part of the twentieth century through overexploitation, destructive fishing practices, pollution and siltation, and changes in storm frequency and intensity.

Marine fisheries have declined dramatically over recent decades. Currently, according to the Food and Agriculture Organization (FAO) of the United Nations (2009), three-quarters of the world's major commercial fish stocks are either fully exploited, overfished, depleted, or are slowly recovering; only about one-quarter of the stocks are considered underexploited. Commercial fleets, consisting of some 4 million vessels, hauled in 81.9 million tons of fish, shellfish, and marine organisms in 2006 (the last year for which data are available), a decline compared to the average of 84.1 million tons over the previous four years. The alarming state of capture fisheries has prompted FAO to warn that "the maximum wild capture fisheries potential from the world's oceans has probably been reached, and a more closely controlled approach to fisheries management is required" (FAO, 2009, pp. 7–8). Marine pollution coupled with the pressures of rising population densities and loss of coastal resources threatens the livelihood of 200 million subsistence and small-scale fishing families and indirectly affects as many as 2 billion people in coastal areas (Hinrichsen, 1998).

A number of encouraging initiatives have been launched, but so far they have had little impact. An intergovernmental agreement to combat land-based sources of pollution was adopted in 1995, but its implementation is unclear and little progress has been made. Similarly, two international initiatives launched in 1995, although well intended, have yet to make an impact: the FAO Code of Conduct for Responsible Fisheries and the UN Agreement on Straddling Fish Stocks and Highly Migratory Fish Stocks.

Meanwhile, fisheries continue to be exploited at unsustainable rates. An estimated 2 billion people, most of them in the Asia-Pacific region, depend on seafood for their protein intake. The erosion of access to seafood threatens the health of these people. Unless ways can be found to ensure access to edible fish and shellfish, the health of one-third of the planet's population is likely to deteriorate (FAO, 1995, 2009).

Forests

Since the 1992 Earth Summit, deforestation has increased in twenty countries with large forest resources. In the Amazon basin in Brazil, for instance, the deforestation rate increased by roughly 70 percent in the decade after 1992, reaching a toll of about 2.4 million hectares of tropical forest destroyed each year (Kirby and others, 2006). According to the Global Forest Resources Assessment of the FAO (2006), the net loss of global forest cover during the 1990s was estimated at 94 million hectares—an area larger than Venezuela and equivalent to 2.4 percent of the world's total forested area. Between 2000 and 2005, the world lost another 37 million hectares of forest, mostly in the tropics.

Attempts to advance an international forest convention date from 1990. But within a decade the international community shelved the idea as impractical, a move supported by many nongovernmental organizations on the grounds that a convention would only enshrine the standards of a weak consensus. The Earth Summit process did generate the Intergovernmental Panel on Forests in 1995, but in 1997, this group was transformed into the Intergovernmental Forum on Forests, with a secretariat at the UN Division for Sustainable Development, in New York. Owing to widespread opposition, no convention on forests is ever likely to get to the negotiating table. Instead, international action now centers on getting countries to enforce existing legislation and forest conservation initiatives (Kendall and Pimental, 1994; FAO, 2006).

Healthy forest ecosystems are critical for maintaining the health and well-being of approximately half a billion people who depend on forests for all or part of their daily diets. With forests gone, and biodiversity with them, subsistence cultures can no longer supplement diets dependent on one or two staples with fruits, nuts, berries, and bushmeat harvested from the forests (WRI, 1997).

Biodiversity

Population growth exerts an inexorable pressure on ecosystems as resources are depleted and as human settlements alter and fragment habitats. One result is species loss, the only truly irreversible instance of environmental damage. The Earth could be losing species at rates 100 to 1,000 times faster than natural background rates, but there is little agreement on the numbers lost over the past decade (World Conservation Union, 2007). It has been estimated, conservatively, that 27,000 plant and animal species were pushed into extinction every year during the 1990s (Eldredge, 1998).

According to the World Conservation Union (IUCN), of the 41,415 species of plants and animals on the IUCN Red List, 16,306 are threatened with extinction or listed as critically endangered, endangered, or threatened, including over 1,000 species of mammals, 1,221 species of birds (over 12 percent of the total number), 1,808 amphibians (30 percent of the total) and over 2,000 species of freshwater fish (20 percent of the total identified) (IUCN Red List, 2007). Moreover, the pace of extinction is expected to accelerate as more and more prime habitat is lost or degraded, driven by expanding populations and by rising consumer demand in the developed world for products from some of the most ecologically diverse countries (Myers, 1999). In addition, the FAO (1995) estimated that about three-quarters of the genetic diversity of domestic cultivars (cultivated crops) has been lost since 1900, with much of that destruction taking place over the past two decades.

Biodiversity has important implications for human health (Cincotta and Engelman, 2000; Grifo and Rosenthal, 1997; Chivian and Bernstein, 2008). Many medications derive from plants, and medical research depends heavily on plant and animal species. Biodiversity is essential for world food production. Species loss may result in ecological imbalances, which may in turn promote the emergence and spread of human infectious diseases. The loss of biodiversity is therefore more than an environmental concern; it is a human health concern as well (see also Chapter One).

The Convention on Biological Diversity, which was opened for signature at the 1992 UNCED in Rio, entered into force in December 1993, and 191 countries are now parties to the convention, with 168 having ratified it (as of 2008). Unfortunately, the United States has not ratified it. Without U.S. support, this convention is unlikely to fulfill its objectives (UNEP, 2008; see also Kendall and Pimental, 1994).

Climate Change

Population growth and increasing prosperity together drive energy use. As described in Chapter Thirteen, leading sources of energy such as biomass fuels and fossil fuels release carbon dioxide when burned. The atmospheric concentration of carbon dioxide has reached about 387 parts per million, up from 280 before the industrial revolution. Rising levels of atmospheric carbon dioxide, in turn, contribute to climate change (see Chapter Ten).

Climate change has become widely acknowledged as a growing global problem. Solving the problem will be more difficult than recognizing it. In 1997, delegates to the UN Framework Convention on Climate Change, in Kyoto, Japan, adopted a global framework for addressing climate change. They agreed that developed countries should achieve a 5 percent reduction from their 1990 levels in emissions of greenhouse gases by the 2008 to 2012 period. The Kyoto Protocol was designed to enter into force when at least fifty-five nations, accounting for at least 55 percent of total 1990 carbon dioxide emissions, had ratified it, a milestone that was reached in February 2005. By early 2009, 183 parties had ratified the Kyoto Protocol, but these did not include the United States, the only developed country that has not ratified the protocol. Moreover it had become clear that many signatories had not reached the goals laid out in the Kyoto Protocol.

POPULATION AND POVERTY

Rapid, unsustainable population growth is a principal contributor to poverty. Currently, between one in four and one in five of the Earth's people live in extreme poverty, defined by the World Bank as earning less than $1.25 per day (World Bank, 2008a). Each day, over a billion people in the world cannot satisfy their basic food needs. This level of poverty raises profound social justice concerns, and it has obvious health implications. Each day, 35,000 children under the age of five die from starvation or from preventable infectious diseases aggravated by malnutrition.

Although the 1992 Earth Summit did not focus directly on slowing population growth or on improving living standards, Agenda 21, the summit's blueprint for action, discussed the scope and dimension of the problems caused by population growth and poverty (United Nations Conference on Environment and Development, 1993). This document linked improvements to better resource management, identifying ecologically sensitive areas where heavy population pressures were stressing resources, and called for the empowerment of local communities to provide people with more opportunities to manage common resources on which they depend for their survival. Equally important to achieving the goal of sustainable development are improving access to basic education for both boys and girls and advancing the status of women, among other recommendations. In 1994, two years after the Earth Summit, the United Nations International Conference on Population and Development (ICPD) was held in Cairo. Although the environment was not directly on the agenda, the important links among population, development, and the environment were covered in the ICPD Programme of Action. This document specifically mentions the important interrelationships among population, resources, the environment, and development (ICPD, 1994).

Lower fertility and slower population growth, however, have not brought an improved living standard for the average person. In 1980, about 2.5 billion people lived on less than $2 a day, and that number changed little through 2005 (World Bank, 2008a). Although some of this lack of progress reflects economic downturns in 1997 (in Southeast Asia) and in 2008 and 2009 (globally), which drove millions from the lower-middle classes into poverty, it also reflects the fact that in many countries population growth has exceeded economic growth.

However, extreme poverty decreased during recent decades, from 1.9 billion in 1981 to 1.8 billion in 1990 to about 1.4 billion in 2005 (World Bank, 2008a).

Partly due to differences in population growth, the gap between rich countries and poor countries has continued to widen. Both within countries and among countries, income growth and wealth accumulation have benefited the wealthy far more than the poor (World Bank, 2008a, 2008b; International Labour

Organization, International Institute for Labour Studies, 2008). Moreover, a disproportionate number of the world's poor are women and children (Buvinic, 1997). Of particular concern is the fact that in sub-Saharan Africa and South Asia, countries with the world's highest fertility rates and fastest population growth also face the most poverty and the severest resource constraints. Chronic water shortages, widespread degradation of arable land, rampant deforestation, rapid urbanization, deteriorating health conditions, and other challenges confront these countries as they seek to develop their economies (Brown and others, 1999; UN Foundation, 2000; Munn, Whyte, and Timmerman, 1999).

Environmental Distress Syndrome

Population pressure and excessive resource use has increasingly threatened the health of the environment itself. "We are no longer talking only of an increased exposure to specific extraneous hazards as a cause of *bad* health. We are also recognizing the depletion or disruption of natural biophysical processes that are the basic source of sustained good health," in the words of Tony McMichael (1997), a professor at the Australian National University. McMichael notes the risk to ecosystems within which food production occurs, and to such global systems as the hydrologic cycle and the stratospheric ozone layer. Biologists recognize that human numbers and human actions are causing "rapid, novel, and substantial" changes to the environment (Vitousek and others, 1997). These changes include degrading soil and water supplies; altering nature's biogeochemical cycles, largely by releasing enormous amounts of carbon dioxide into the atmosphere; and destroying or altering biological resources. Chapter One discusses the links between ecosystem health and human health in detail.

The term *environmental distress syndrome* denotes deteriorating environmental conditions and concomitant threats to human health. Paul Epstein (1997), of Harvard University's Center for Health and the Global Environment, lists five symptoms of this syndrome:

1. The reemergence of infectious diseases, such as cholera, typhoid, and dengue fever, and the emergence of new diseases such as drug-resistant tuberculosis.
2. The loss of biodiversity and the consequent loss of potential sources of new drugs and crops.
3. The growing dominance of generalist species, such as crows and Canada geese.
4. The decline in pollinators such as bees, birds, bats, butterflies, and beetles, which are intrinsic to the propagation of flowering plants.

5. The proliferation of harmful algal blooms along the world's coastlines, leading to outbreaks of diseases such as ciguatera poisoning and paralytic shellfish poisoning (see also UNDP, 1998).

Such trends pose a disturbing question: At what point might the depletion of the world's ecological and biophysical capital redound against the health of humanity? There is mounting evidence that we are already witnessing profound changes in ecosystem viability and a rise in both new and old infectious diseases. For example, the World Health Organization reported that a recent epidemic of meningitis in sub-Saharan Africa coincided with an expansion of degraded agricultural and grazing land—a result of changes in land use patterns and regional climate change triggered by human activities (McMichael, 1997). Another study has linked more frequent and severe El Niño weather patterns to marked increases in diarrheal diseases in Peruvian children (Checkley and others, 2000).

Clearly, population growth plays a major role in stressing the environment, and needs to be part of the focus of those who care about environmental public health.

SUMMARY

The links among population, health, and the environment are not difficult to discern. As poverty deepens and environmental and human health conditions continue to deteriorate, scientists have been able to shed more light on the connections between the health of the environment and the health of vulnerable populations (Engelman, 1996, 2008). Good health is not just a matter of access to quality health services; it is more a matter of access to a livable and healthy environment. Clearly, people cannot be healthy without an environment conducive to good health. Maintaining healthy ecosystems, which in turn support healthy human populations, remains one of the new millennium's critical challenges.

Unfortunately, the natural environment, upon which all human development rests, continues to deteriorate at alarming rates across virtually all resource sectors. The trends do not augur well for the future. The loss of biodiversity, water shortages and pollution, deforestation, desertification, the death of coastal zones — all these major trends are moving in the wrong direction. Population growth is a major driver of this movement. These trends compel us to ask some very fundamental questions. Can the gross depletion of essential life-support systems be halted in time? If not, is the Earth headed for a sixth big extinction? Humanity's own? What will the future bring if climate change continues unabated and sea levels rise by one meter or more? What will happen as the world becomes predominantly urban? Can we learn to live within our ecological constraints or boundaries? And can we reduce our ecological footprints so as to tread more lightly on the Earth?

KEY TERMS

biodiversity

birth dearth

carrying capacity

demography

Earth Summit

ecological footprint

environmental
distress syndrome

United Nations Conference
on Environment and
Development

DISCUSSION QUESTIONS

1. Some environmental groups have focused on population control or on limits to immigration as central strategies. If you were on the board of an environmental group, would you support such an approach? Why or why not?
2. What can individuals do to reduce their ecological footprint?
3. Why is reducing fertility levels so important for poor developing countries? How does this change affect health, and how can it be done effectively?
4. Investing in and empowering women is considered one of the most cost-effective investments a country can make toward economic and social development. Why is this?

REFERENCES

Adeel, Z., and others. *Overcoming One of the Greatest Environmental Challenges of Our Times: Re-Thinking Policies to Cope with Desertification.* United Nations University and International Network on Water, Environment and Health (UNU-INWEH).http://www.inweh.unu.edu/inweh/drylands/publications/iydd_policy_brief-june_2007.pdf, 2007.

Agarwal, A., Narain, S., and Sharma, A. (eds.). *Green Politics: Global Environmental Negotiations.* New Delhi: Centre for Science and Environment, 1999.

Brown, L., Gardner, G., and Halweil, B. *Beyond Malthus: Nineteen Dimensions of the Population Challenge.* New York: Norton, 1999.

Brown, L., and Mitchell, J. *The Agricultural Link: How Environmental Deterioration Could Disrupt Economic Progress.* Worldwatch Paper No. 136. Washington, D.C.: Worldwatch Institute, Aug. 1997.

Bryant, D., Rodenburg, E., Cox, T., and Nielsen, D. *Coastlines at Risk: An Index of Potential Development-Related Threats to Coastal Ecosystems.* Washington, D.C.: World Resources Institute, 1995.

Buvinic, M. "Women in Poverty: A New Global Underclass." *Foreign Policy*, 1997, *108*, 38–53.

Checkley, W., and others. "Effects of El Niño and Ambient Temperature on Hospital Admissions for Diarrhoeal Diseases in Peruvian Children." *Lancet*, 2000, *355*, 442–450.

Chivian, E., and Bernstein, A. (eds.). *Sustaining Life: How Human Health Depends on Biodiversity.* New York: Oxford University Press, 2008.

Cincotta, R. P., and Engelman, R. *Nature's Place: Human Population and the Future of Biological Diversity*. Washington D.C.: Population Action International, 2000.

Cohen, J. *How Many People Can the Earth Support?* New York: Norton, 1995.

Constanza, R., and others. "The Value of the World's Ecosystem Services and Natural Capital." *Nature*, 1997, *387*, 253–260.

Crenson, M. "*World Population Reaches 6 Billion*." New York: Associated Press, Oct. 10, 1999.

Doos, B. "Environmental Degradation, Global Food Production and Risk for Large-Scale Migration1." *Ambio*, 1994, *23*(3), 124–130.

Ehrlich, P., and Holdren, J. "Impact of Population Growth." *Science*, 1971, *171*, 1212–1217.

Eldredge, N. *Life in the Balance: Humanity and the Biodiversity Crisis*. Princeton, N.J.: Princeton University Press, 1998.

Engelman, R. "*Population as a Scale Factor: Impacts on Environment and Development*." Paper presented at the Conference on Population, Environment and Development, Washington, D.C., Mar. 13–14, 1996.

Engelman, R. *MORE—Population, Nature and What Women Want*. Washington D.C.: Island Press, 2008.

Epstein, P. "The Threatened Plague." *People & the Planet*, 1997, *6*(3), 14–17.

Food and Agriculture Organization of the United Nations. *Dimensions of Need: An Atlas of Food and Agriculture*. Rome: Food and Agriculture Organization of the United Nations, 1995.

Food and Agriculture Organization of the United Nations. *Global Forest Resources Assessment 2005*. http://www.fao.org/forestry/fra2005/en, 2006.

Food and Agriculture Organization of the United Nations. *The State of World Fisheries and Aquaculture 2008*. http://www.fao.org/docrep/011/i0250e/i0250e00.htm, 2009.

Goodland, R. "The Case That the World Has Reached Limits." In R. Goodland, H. Daly, and S. Serafy (eds.), *Population, Technology and Lifestyle: The Transition to Sustainability*. Washington, D.C.: Island Press, 1992.

Grifo, F., and Rosenthal, J. (eds.). *Biodiversity and Human Health*. Washington, D.C.: Island Press, 1997.

Hinrichsen, D. *Coastal Waters of the World: Trends, Threats and Strategies*. Washington, D.C.: Island Press, 1998.

Hinrichsen, D., and Robey, B. Population and the Environment: The Global Challenge. Population Reports Series M, No. 15. Baltimore, Md.: Population Information Program, Center for Communication Programs, The Johns Hopkins University Bloomberg School of Public Health, 2000.

Hinrichsen, D., Salem, R., and Blackburn, R. Meeting the Urban Challenge. Population Reports Series M, No. 16. Baltimore, Md.: Population Information Program, Center for Communication Programs, The Johns Hopkins University Bloomberg School of Public Health, 2002.

International Conference on Population and Development. *Programme of Action of the International Conference on Population and Development*. United Nations Population Fund. http://www.unfpa.org/icpd/icpd_poa.htm#ch1, 1994.

International Labour Organization, International Institute for Labour Studies. *World of Work Report 2008: Income Inequalities in the Age of Financial Globalization*. Geneva: International Labour Organization, 2008.

Kasperson, J. X., Kasperson, R. E., and Turner, B. L. *Regions at Risk: Comparisons of Threatened Environments*. UNU Studies of Critical Environmental Regions. Tokyo: United Nations University Press, 1995.

Kasperson, R. E., Kasperson, J. X., and Turner, B. L. "Risk and Criticality: Trajectories of Regional Environmental Degradation." *Ambio*, 1999, *28*(6), 562–568.

Kendall, H., and Pimental, D. "Constraints on the Expansion of the Global Food Supply." *Ambio*, 1994, *23*(3), 200–206.

Kirby, K. R., and others. "The Future of Deforestation in the Brazilian Amazon Hiyya." *Futures*, 2006, *38*(4), 432–453.

Markham, V. D. *U.S. National Report on Population and the Environment*. Center for Environment and Population. http://www.cepnet.org/documents/USNatlReptFinal.pdf, 2006.

McMichael, T. "Healthy World, Healthy People." *People & the Planet*, 1997, *6*(3), 6–9.

Millennium Ecosystem Assessment. *Ecosystems and Human Well-Being: Wetlands and Water: Synthesis*. Washington, D.C.: World Resources Institute, 2005.

Munn, T., Whyte, A., and Timmerman, R. "Emerging Environmental Issues: A Global Perspective of SCOPE." *Ambio*, 1999, *28*(6), 464–471.

Myers, N. "What We Must Do to Counter the Biotic Holocaust." *International Wildlife*, 1999, *29*(2), 30–39.

Oldeman, L. R., Hakkeling, R.T.A., and Sombroek, W. G. *World Map of the Status of Human-Induced Soil Degradation: An Explanatory Note*. International Soil Reference and Information Centre and United Nations Environment Programme. http://www.isric.org/isric/webdocs/Docs/ExplanNote.pdf, 1991.

Population Reference Bureau. *2003 World Population Data Sheet*. Washington, D.C.: Population Reference Bureau, 2003.

Repetto, R., and others. *Wasting Assets: Natural Resources in the National Accounts*. Washington, D.C.: World Resources Institute, 1989.

Revenga, C., and others. *Pilot Analysis of Global Ecosystems, Freshwater Systems*. Washington, D.C.: World Resources Institute, 2000.

Roodman, D. *The Natural Wealth of Nations: Harnessing the Market for the Environment*. Worldwatch Environmental Alert Series. New York: Norton, 1998.

UNAIDS (Joint United Nations Program on HIV/AIDS), UNFPA (United Nations Population Fund), and UNIFEM (United Nations Development Fund for Women). *Women and HIV/AIDS: Confronting the Crisis*. New York: United Nations, 2004.

United Nations Conference on Environment and Development. *Agenda 21: The United Nations Programme of Action from Rio*. New York: United Nations Department of Economic and Social Affairs, Division for Sustainable Development, 1993. http://www.un.org/esa/dsd/agenda21/

United Nations Department of Economic and Social Affairs, Population Division. *World Population Prospects: The 2008 Revision*. ESA/P/WP.210. New York: United Nations, 2009. http://www.un.org/esa/population/.

United Nations Department of Economic and Social Affairs, Population Division. *World Urbanization Prospects: The 2007 Revision*. New York: United Nations, 2008.

United Nations Development Programme. *Energy After Rio: Prospects and Challenges*. New York: United Nations, 1997.

United Nations Development Programme. *Human Development Report 1998*. New York: United Nations, 1998.

United Nations Environment Programme. *Global Environmental Outlook 2000* [GEO-2]. London: Earthscan, 2000.

United Nations Environment Programme. *Convention on Biological Diversity*. http://www.cbd.int, 2008.

United Nations Foundation. "*Water: Manila Meeting Highlights Southeast Asian Woes.*" *Press Release.* Washington D.C.: UN Wire Service, Jan. 21, 2000.

United Nations Population Fund. *Population and the Environment: The Challenges Ahead.* New York: United Nations Population Fund, 1991.

United Nations Population Fund. *State of World Population 2003: Making 1 Billion Count: Investing in Adolescents' Health and Rights.* New York: United Nations Population Fund, 2003.

Upadhyay, U. D., and Robey, B. Why Family Planning Matters. Population Reports, Series J, No. 49. Baltimore, Md.1: Population Information Program, Johns Hopkins University School of Public Health, 1999.

Venetoulis, J., and Talberth, J. *Ecological Footprint of Nations: 2005 Update.* Oakland, Calif.: Redefining Progress. http://www.rprogress.org/publications/2006/Footprint%20of%20Nations%2020 05.pdf, 2006.

Venetoulis, J., and Talberth, J. "Refining the Ecological Footprint." *Environment, Development and Sustainability*, 2008, *10*, 441–469. DOI 10.1007/s10668–006–9074-z.

Vitousek, P. M., Mooney, H. A., Lubchenco, J., and Melillo, J. M. "Human Domination of Earth's Ecosystems." *Science*, 1997, *227*, 494–499.

Wackernagel, M., and others. *Ecological Footprints of Nations: How Much Nature Do They Use?* Xalapa, Mexico: Center for Sustainability Studies, Mar. 10, 1997.

World Bank. *World Development Report 1992: Development and the Environment.* New York: Oxford University Press, 1992.

World Bank. *Poverty Data: A Supplement to World Development Indicators 2008.* Washington, D.C.: International Bank for Reconstruction and Development, 2008a.

World Bank. *World Development Indicators 2008.* Washington, D.C.: International Bank for Reconstruction and Development, 2008b.

World Conservation Union. *2007 IUCN Red List of Threatened Species.* Gland, Switzerland: World Conservation Union, 2007.

World Health Organization. *Health and Environment in Sustainable Development: Five Years After the Earth Summit.* Geneva: World Health Organization, 1997.

World Health Organization. *HIV/AIDS Epidemiological Surveillance Update for the WHO African Region 2002.* http://www.who.int/hiv/pub/epidemiology/pubafro2003/en/, 2003.

World Resources Institute. *The Last Frontier Forests: Ecosystems and Economies on the Edge.* Washington, D.C.: World Resources Institute, 1997.

World Resources Institute. *World Resources 1998–99.* New York: Oxford University Press, 1998.

FOR FURTHER INFORMATION

Reports

World Resources Report. A report published biannually by the World Resources Institute, Washington, D.C. http://www.wri.org/project/world-resources.

Global Environment Outlook (GEO). An overview report published by the United Nations Environment Programme. http://www.unep.org/geo

State of the World. A report published annually by Worldwatch Institute, Washington, D.C. http://www
.worldwatch.org/taxonomy/term/37.

Organizations

Center for Environment and Population, http://www.cepnet.org. A nongovernmental organization
that addresses the relationship between human population, resource consumption, and the
environment through research, policy and public outreach.

Global Footprint Network, http://www.footprintnetwork.org. An international think tank based on
Oakland, California, that works to advance sustainability through use of the Ecological
Footprint, a resource accounting tool that measures how much nature we have, how much we
use and who uses what.

Planet 21, peopleandplanet.net, http://www.peopleandplanet.net. A Web site with information
on issues of population, poverty, health, consumption, and the environment; maintained
by Planet 21, a British nongovernmental organization, and sponsored by the United
Nations Population Fund, the World Conservation Union, the World Wide Fund for
Nature International, the International Planned Parenthood Federation, and the Swedish
Development Co-operation Agency.

Population Council, http://www.popcouncil.org. A nongovernmental organization based in
Washington, D.C., that seeks to improve the well-being and reproductive health of current
and future generations around the world and to help achieve a humane, equitable, and sustainable balance between people and resources. It focuses on HIV/AIDS, poverty, gender,
youth, and reproductive health.

Population Reference Bureau, http://www.prb.org. A nongovernmental organization based in
Washington, D.C., that serves as an information resource about the population dimensions of
important social, economic, and political issues.

Population Media Center, http://www.populationmedia.org. A nongovernmental organization based
in Vermont that addresses population issues through entertainment and the media. One of
its core issue areas is environmental preservation.

United Nations Population Fund (UNFPA), http://www.unfpa.org. An organization that provides a
number of resources on its Web site, including access to the annual *State of World Population*
reports, addressing various aspects of population, reproductive health, women's rights, and
development.

World Resources Institute, EarthTrends, http://earthtrends.wri.org. A comprehensive online database,
maintained by the World Resources Institute, that focuses on the environmental, social, and
economic trends, including population data.

CHAPTER TEN

CLIMATE CHANGE

JONATHAN A. PATZ

KEY CONCEPTS

- According to the United Nations Intergovernmental Panel on Climate Change (IPCC), by 2100 average global temperatures are projected to increase between 1.8°C and 4.0°C, sea levels will rise, and hydrologic extremes (floods and droughts) will intensify.

- Climate change is likely to have major effects on crop and livestock production, as well as on the viability of fisheries. The number of people at risk for hunger could double by midcentury.

- Climate change can threaten health more directly through heat-related morbidity and mortality; flooding and storms with associated trauma and mental health concerns; air pollution, especially from ground-level ozone and potentially from aeroallergens (for example, pollen and molds); and infectious diseases, particularly those that are water- or vector-borne.

- Weather-related health risks must be assessed in the context of concurrent environmental stressors, such as the urban health island effect and land cover–modifying weather effects on mosquito-borne diseases.

- Risk management of climate change ranges from primary mitigation of greenhouse gas emissions to a number of adaptations to a change in climate regime. Both co-benefits and unintended consequences of policy changes in the energy, transportation, agriculture, and other health-relevant sectors must be considered in any comprehensive health impact assessment of global climate change.

C LIMATE change is but one component of global environmental change that poses widespread risks to human health and well-being. Among the other aspects of global environmental change are ecosystem degradation and land use change (discussed in Chapter One), petroleum depletion (Chapter Thirteen), urban sprawl (Chapter Fourteen), and water scarcity (Chapter Fifteen). Thus, although many equate climate change alone with the broader challenge of global environmental change, this approach is too limited. In addition, climate change risks will emerge in the context of—and very likely synergistically with—these other drivers of environmental change.

Climate change, whether resulting from natural variability or from human activity, depends on the overall energy budget of the planet, the balance between incoming (solar) shortwave radiation and outgoing longwave radiation. This balance is affected by the Earth's atmosphere, in much the same way as the glass of a greenhouse (or a car's windshield on a hot day) allows sunlight to enter and then traps heat (infrared) energy inside. An atmosphere with higher levels of so-called greenhouse gases will retain more of this heat and result in higher average surface temperatures than will an atmosphere with lower levels of these gases.

A major source of information on climate change is the work of the United Nations Intergovernmental Panel on Climate Change (IPCC), which was established by the World Meteorological Organization (WMO) and the United Nations Environment Programme (UNEP) in 1988. Approximately every five years since 1990, the IPCC has conducted assessments of current scientific work on climate change, the potential impacts of this change, and various prevention options. This international body includes many outstanding scientists, representing multiple sectors, and its reports are viewed as the most authoritative assessments on the subject. Much of the information in this chapter is drawn from IPCC reports.

GREENHOUSE GASES

The composition of the Earth's atmosphere has changed since preindustrial times. These changes, which began around the mid-1700s, include increases in atmospheric levels of carbon dioxide (CO_2), methane (CH_4), and nitrous oxide (N_2O) that far exceed any changes occurring in the preceding 10,000 years. Historical levels of these **greenhouse gases** are known from analyses of air trapped in bubbles in Antarctic ice cores (Etheridge, Steele, Francey, and Langenfelds, 1998; Gulluck, Slemr, and Stauffer, 1998). For example, the concentration of CO_2, the major greenhouse gas, has risen by approximately 35 percent, from about 280 parts per million by volume (ppmv) in the late eighteenth century to

Jonathan A. Patz declares no competing financial interests.

about 380 ppmv at present. Higher greenhouse gas concentrations have contributed to warming of the Earth—an effect called positive **radiative forcing**—by absorbing and reemitting infrared radiation toward the lower atmosphere and the Earth's surface. (Figure 10.1 summarizes the principal components of radiative

FIGURE 10.1   Components of Radiative Forcing

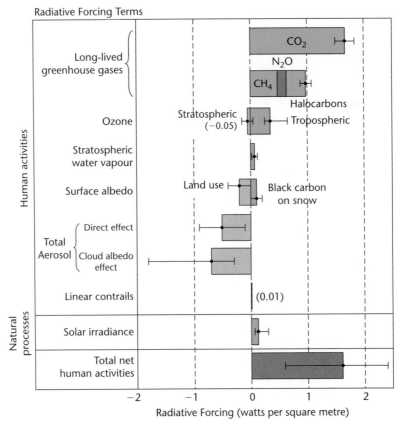

Source: Solomon and others, 2007, FAQ 2.1, fig. 2.

All these radiative forcings affect climate and are associated with human activities or natural processes discussed in the text. The values represent the forcings in 2005 relative to the start of the industrial era (about 1750). Human activities cause significant changes in long-lived gases, ozone, water vapor, surface albedo, aerosols, and contrails. The only increase in natural forcing of any significance between 1750 and 2005 occurred in solar irradiance. Positive forcings lead to warming of climate and negative forcings lead to cooling. The thick black line attached to each bar represents the range of uncertainty for the respective value.

forcing, Table 10.1 shows today's concentrations of these greenhouse gases, and Figure 10.2 shows their relative radiative forcing since 1900.)

A WARMING EARTH: FROM PAST TO FUTURE

Long-term climate change, whether from natural sources or from human activity, can be observed as a signal against a background of natural climate variability (Figure 10.2). To help detect the meaning of this signal, we need historical climate data to estimate natural variability. Because instrument records are available only for the recent past (a period of less than 150 years), previous climates must be deduced from paleoclimatic records, including tree rings, pollen series, faunal and floral abundances in deep-sea cores, isotope analyses of coral and ice cores, and diaries and other documentary evidence. Results of these analyses show that surface temperatures in the mid- to late twentieth century appear to have been warmer than they were during any similar period in the last 600 years in most regions and in at least some regions warmer than in any other century for several thousand years (Nicholls and others, 1996).

The temperature increase is accelerating rapidly. From 1906 to 2005, the global average temperature rose by 0.74°C. According to the IPCC, by 2100 average global temperature is projected to rise between 1.8°C and 4.0°C (Solomon and others, 2007). The rate of change in climate is faster now than in any period in the last thousand years.

EARTH SYSTEM CHANGES

Although the average effect across the Earth's surface is a warming, changing temperatures are only part of the story. Higher temperatures evaporate soil moisture more quickly (leading to severe droughts), but warm air can hold more moisture than cool air, resulting in heavy precipitation events; such *hydrologic extremes* (floods and droughts) are very much a part of climate change scenarios and of substantial concern to public health professionals. Additionally, Arctic and Antarctic ice caps are melting, releasing vast amounts of water into the oceans, raising ocean levels, and potentially altering the flow of ocean currents. The weather patterns that result from these and other changes vary greatly from place to place and over short periods of time, emphasizing the importance of **climate variability**. For these reasons the term **climate change** is more accurate than **global warming** and is the accepted term for this set of changes.

Accordingly, the accelerating temperature changes noted earlier have been associated with corresponding Earth system changes (see Table 10.2). Since

TABLE 10.1 The Main Greenhouse Gases

Greenhouse Gases	Chemical Formula	Preindustrial Concentration (ppbv)	Concentration in 2005 (ppbv)	Atmospheric Lifetime (years)	Anthropogenic Sources	Global Warming Potential (GWP)[a]
Carbon dioxide	CO_2	278,000	379,000	Variable[b]	Fossil fuel combustion, land use changes, cement production	1
Methane	CH_4	700	1,774	12.2 ± 3	Fossil fuel combustion, rice paddies, waste dumps, livestock	21[c]
Nitrous oxide	N_2O	275	319	120	Fertilizer, combustion, industrial processes	310
CFC-12	CCl_2F_2	0	0.538	102	Liquid coolants, foams	6,200–7,100[d]
HCFC-22	$CHClF_2$	0	0.169	12.1	Liquid coolants	1,300–1,400[d]
Perfluoromethane	CF_4	0	0.074	50,000	Aluminum production	6,500
Sulfur hexafluoride	SF_6	0	0.006	3,200	Dielectric fluid	23,900

Note: ppbv = parts per billion by volume.

[a] GWP for 100-year time horizon.

[b] No single lifetime for CO_2 can be defined because different sink processes have different rates of uptake.

[c] Includes indirect effects of tropospheric ozone water vapor production.

[d] Net global warming potential (that is, including the indirect effect due to ozone depletion).

Source: Collins and others, 2006.

**FIGURE 10.2   Temperature Changes Due to Natural and
Anthropogenic Forcings**

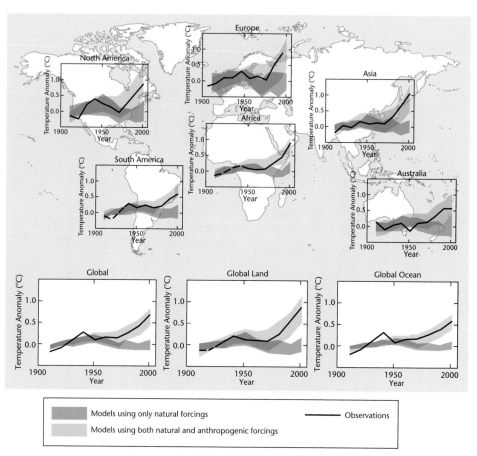

Source: Solomon and others, 2007, FAQ 9.1, fig. 1.

Temperature changes relative to the corresponding average for 1901–1950 (in degrees
Celsius) from decade to decade from 1906 to 2005 over the Earth's continents, the entire
globe, the global land area, and the global ocean. The black line indicates observed temperature change, and the shaded bands show the combined range covered by 90 percent of
recent model simulations. Dashed black lines indicate decades and continental regions for
which there are substantially fewer observations.

TABLE 10.2 Projected Earth System Changes

Phenomenon and Direction of Trend	Likelihood That Trend Occurred in Late 20th Century (typically post-1960)	Likelihood of a Human Contribution to Observed Trend	Likelihood of Future Trends (based on projections for 21st century using SRES scenarios)
Warmer and fewer cold days and nights over most land areas	Very likely[a]	Likely[b]	Virtually certain[b]
Warmer and more frequent hot days and nights over most land areas	Very likely[a]	Likely (nights)[b]	Virtually certain[b]
Warm spells/heat waves, frequency increases over most land areas	Likely	More likely than not[c]	Very likely
Heavy precipitation events, frequency (or proportion of total rainfall from heavy falls) increases over most areas	Likely	More likely than not[c]	Very likely
Area affected by droughts increases	Likely (in many regions since 1970s)	More likely than not	Likely
Intense tropical cyclone activity increases	Likely (in some regions since 1970)	More likely than not[c]	Likely
Increased incidence of extreme high sea level (excludes tsunamis)[e]	Likely	More likely than not[d,f]	Likely[g]

Note: SRES (Special Report on Emissions Scenarios) scenarios are IPCC emissions scenarios from a special report published in 2000.

[a] Decreased frequency of cold days and nights (coldest 10 percent).

[b] Warming of the most extreme days and nights each year.

[c] Increased frequency of hot days and nights (hottest 10 percent).

[d] Magnitude of anthropogenic contributions not assessed. Attribution for these phenomena based on expert judgment rather than formal attribution studies.

[e] Extreme high sea level depends on average sea level and on regional weather systems. It is defined here as the highest 1 percent of hourly values of observed sea level at a station for a given reference period.

[f] Changes in observed extreme high sea level closely follow the changes in average sea level. It is *very likely* that anthropogenic activity contributed to a rise in average sea level.

[g] In all scenarios, the projected global average sea level in 2100 is higher than in the reference period. The effect of changes in regional weather systems on sea-level extremes has not been assessed.

Source: Slightly adapted from Solomon and others, 2007, Table SPM.2.

1961, sea levels have risen on average by approximately 2 mm per year. Arctic sea ice extent has declined by 7.4 percent per decade, and snow cover and glaciers have diminished in both hemispheres. Most striking is the extent to which the Arctic ice cap has melted in the past thirty years (Figure 10.3). These trends are expected to continue. According to the IPCC, in ninety years sea level will rise between 18 and 59 centimeters. Extremes of the hydrologic cycle (such as floods and droughts) are also expected to accompany global warming trends.

Regional changes in climate, particularly increases in temperature, have already affected diverse physical and biological systems in many parts of the world. For example, river and lake ice is breaking up earlier and animal ranges are moving to higher altitudes. Alpine species, such as certain wildflowers, have been displaced to higher altitudes; when they have no further terrain to which to migrate some could go extinct. If Arctic sea ice continues to disappear at the current rapid rate, polar bears will be endangered by midcentury (Arctic Climate Impact Assessment, 2004).

The potential exists for large-scale and potentially irreversible changes in Earth systems, such as slowing of the ocean circulation that transports warm water to the North Atlantic, large-scale melting of the Greenland and west Antarctic ice sheets, and accelerated global warming due to positive feedbacks in the carbon cycle (such as the release of methane from thawing Arctic tundra). The probability of these events is unknown, but it is likely to be affected by how rapidly climate change evolves and its duration.

Ocean Temperatures and Hurricanes

Records indicate that sea surface temperatures have steadily increased over the last one hundred years, and more sharply over the last thirty-five years. The period from 1995 to 2004 saw the highest average sea surface temperature on record (Trenberth, 2005).

These trends in turn have implications for hurricane activity. Hurricanes form only in regions where sea surface temperatures are above 26°C (Gray, 1979). During the last half-decade of the twentieth century, overall hurricane activity in the North Atlantic doubled and the Caribbean experienced a fivefold increase (Goldenberg, Landsea, Mestas-Nuñez, and Gray, 2001), and hurricanes may become even more frequent with continued warming (although this point is controversial among scientists). Hurricane intensity too may be associated with warmer temperatures (Webster, Holland, Curry, and Chang, 2005; Emanuel, Sundararajan, and Williams, 2008). As Hurricane Katrina demonstrated in 2005, such events have enormous public health significance.

FIGURE 10.3   The Melting of Arctic Ice, 1980-2007

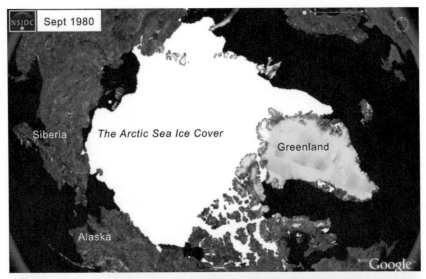

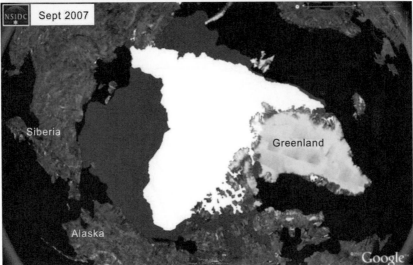

Source: Ice cap images courtesy of Don Perovich, based on data from the National Snow and Ice Data Center; graph of Arctic September sea ice extent from Stroeve and others, 2007; used with permission.

The two images on this page show the decline in Arctic Ice over twenty-seven years. The graph of the Arctic September sea ice extent on the next page displays results from observations and from thirteen climate models in the Fourth IPCC Assessment Report, together with the multi-model ensemble mean (solid black line) and standard deviation (dotted black line). Models with more than one ensemble member are indicated with an asterisk. Inset shows nine-year running means. Note that observations show more rapid loss of ice than models predicted.

FIGURE 10.3 (Continued)

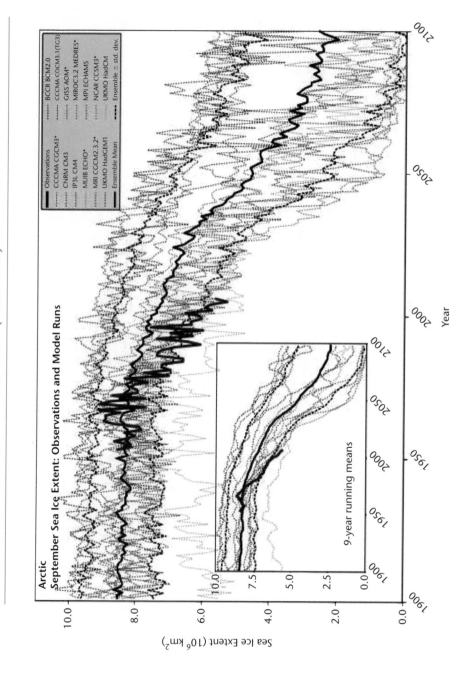

Particularly Vulnerable Regions

Certain regions and populations are more vulnerable than others to the health impacts of climate change (Hess, Malilay, and Parkinson, 2008). These vulnerable areas include

- Areas or populations within or bordering regions with a high endemicity of climate-sensitive diseases (for example, malaria)
- Areas with an observed association between epidemic disease and weather extremes (for example, El Niño–linked epidemics)
- Areas at risk from combined climate impacts relevant to health (for example, stress on food and water supplies or risk of coastal flooding)
- Areas at risk from concurrent environmental or socioeconomic stresses (for example, local stresses from land use practices or an impoverished or undeveloped health infrastructure) and with little capacity to adapt

Changes in seasonal river flows, increases in floods and droughts, decreased food security, and biodiversity loss are special concerns for parts of Africa, Latin America, and Asia. Low-lying coastal and delta regions (such as coastal China, Bangladesh, and Egypt and especially densely populated, low-lying, small island states, such as coral reef atolls throughout Polynesia) and arid regions (such as eastern Africa and central Asia, which already suffer from drought) are at risk even without climate change and at elevated risk as the global climate warms (McCarthy and others, 2001).

These Earth system changes have direct and indirect implications for human health. The sections that follow address major categories of anticipated health effects of climate change. These include malnutrition (possibly the largest problem); risks from weather extremes such as heat and cold, storms and flooding, and drought-related wildfires; air pollution and aeroallergens; and infectious diseases, particularly those that are waterborne, food-borne, or vector-borne. The last section of the chapter addresses the public health response to climate change, from preparedness to greenhouse gas mitigation. Co-benefits of mitigation are considered, as well as the ethical dimensions of climate change and health.

FOOD PRODUCTION AND MALNUTRITION

Climate change is likely to have major effects on crop and livestock production and on the viability of fisheries (Schimhuber and Tubiello, 2007; Tubiello, Soussana, Howden, and Easterling, 2007; Brown and Funk, 2008). Some changes will be positive and others negative, and the net impact on food production will likely vary from place to place. Changes in food production will depend on several key factors. First are the direct effects of temperature, precipitation, CO_2 levels (relating to, for example, the CO_2 fertilization effect), extreme climate variability, and sea-level rise (Reilly, 1996). Next are the indirect effects of climate-induced changes in soil quality, incidence of plant diseases, and weed and insect populations. Greater heat and humidity will also increase food spoilage (discussed in the infectious disease section). The last two decades have seen a continuing deterioration in food production in Africa, caused in part by persistent drought. For some foods, nutritional quality will diminish with climate change. Finally, the extent to which adaptive responses are available to farmers must be considered.

Drought and Food Production

Drought will exacerbate malnutrition, still one of the world's greatest health challenges, with 800 million people undernourished (WHO, 2002). Poorer countries already struggle with large and growing populations and malnutrition and are particularly vulnerable to changes in food production. Drought is also projected to be an increasing problem with climate change. As discussed in Chapter Fifteen, approximately 1.7 billion people, one-third of the world's population, currently live in water-stressed countries, and that number is projected to increase to 5 billion people by the year 2025.

Decreases in average annual stream flow are anticipated in central Asia and southern Africa, where the food supply may be affected. Melting of many of the glacial systems that supply dry season river flow is already occurring. Current IPCC projections suggest that glaciers of the Tibetan plateau are likely to melt entirely by year 2035; these glaciers supply water to over a billion people during the dry season (Parry and others, 2007). In addition, diarrhea and diseases such as scabies, conjunctivitis, and trachoma are associated with poor hygiene and can result from a breakdown in sanitation when water resources become depleted (Patz, 2001).

Despite technological advances such as improved crop varieties and irrigation systems, food production depends on weather conditions (National Agriculture Assessment Group, 2002). Most cultivars are already growing close to their thermal optimum. A recent study using data from twenty-three global climate models shows a high probability that by the end of the century, the average growing season temperatures will exceed the hottest temperatures on record from 1900 to 2006 (Battisi and Naylor, 2009) (Figure 10.4). Reduced yields are expected to occur throughout the tropics due to heat stress, and crops may be damaged from flooding, erosion, and wildfires. Climate change effects on global agricultural

FIGURE 10.4   Projected Summer Average Temperatures

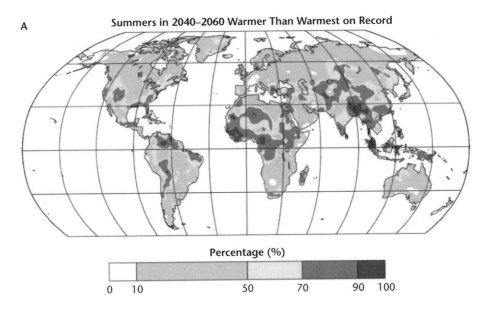

A

Summers in 2040–2060 Warmer Than Warmest on Record

Percentage (%)

0   10   50   70   90   100

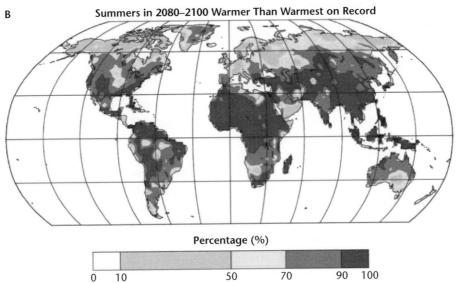

B

Summers in 2080–2100 Warmer Than Warmest on Record

Percentage (%)

0   10   50   70   90   100

Source: Battisti and Naylor, 2009; reprinted with permission from *Science*.

Likelihood (percentage) that future summer average temperatures for 2040–2060 (**A**) and for 2080–2100 (**B**) will exceed the highest summer temperature observed on record. For example, for places shown in the darkest shade there is greater than a 90% chance that the summer-averaged temperature will exceed the highest temperature on record (1900–2006).

productivity will vary regionally, with reductions especially likely in sub-Saharan Africa and South Asia (Cline, 2007). Reductions in regional productivity could destabilize food security on the global scale (Battisi and Naylor, 2009).

Although malnutrition is complex in etiology, some quantitative projections have been conducted. One analysis suggests that by the year 2060, an additional 40 to 300 million people, relative to a projected baseline of 640 million people, could be at risk of malnutrition due to anthropogenic warming (Rosenzweig, Parry, Fischer, and Frohberg, 1993). A more recent study estimates that by the 2050s, climate change will increase the proportion at risk of hunger from the current 34 percent to a level of 64 to 72 percent, unadjusted for potential adaptive interventions (Butt and others, 2005).

The nutritional value of some foods is also a concern. With higher levels of CO_2, some crops reduce their incorporation of nitrogen, resulting in lower protein levels. Studies of barley, wheat, rice, potatoes, and soybeans show reduced protein content when crops are grown under high CO_2 conditions, an effect that varies with soil conditions, air quality, and other factors (Taub and others, 2008). For populations that depend on crops for their protein, this effect could further threaten nutritional status.

Fisheries and Ocean Warming and Acidification

In addition to warming oceans, climate change is associated with the acidification of oceans, resulting from higher CO_2 levels. The threat of ocean acidification has been relatively recently recognized. Over the past 250 years the uptake of anthropogenic carbon has reduced ocean pH by 0.1 units, a trend that is continuing. IPCC scenarios predict a drop in global surface ocean pH of between 0.14 and 0.35 units over the twenty-first century. Although the effects of ocean acidification are not fully understood, this process may threaten marine shell-forming organisms (such as corals) and their dependent species (Solomon and others, 2007). Other aspects of climate change may also threaten fish populations. For example, the recent slowing of the North Atlantic Gulf Stream may reduce the abundance of plankton, a major source of food for many fish larvae (Pauly and Alder, 2005). Declining larval fish populations will affect the capacity of overexploited fish stocks to recover.

These threats to global fisheries in turn threaten coastal and island populations that rely on fish as their main source of protein. Worldwide, fish represents 16 percent of the animal protein consumed by people, with a higher proportion in some regions, for example, 26 percent in Asia. Climate change, together with other pressures such as overfishing, may seriously threaten this source of nutrition.

WEATHER EXTREMES

Extreme temperatures, severe storms, rising sea levels, and droughts all put the health of the Earth's populations at risk (National Research Council, 2001). Although slight changes in the average blood pressure or cholesterol level across a population can represent a health risk, in the case of climate it is the extremes of temperature and the water cycle that threaten human health.

Heat Waves

Extremes of both hot and cold temperatures are associated with rates of morbidity and mortality higher than the rates in the intermediate, or comfortable, temperature range (Kilbourne, 1998). The relationship between temperature and morbidity and mortality is J-shaped, with a steeper slope at higher temperatures (Curriero, Patz, Rose, and Lele, 2001). In the United States, heat waves kill more people than hurricanes, floods, and tornadoes combined.

The body's thermoregulatory mechanisms can cope with a certain amount of temperature rise through control of perspiration and vasodilation of cutaneous vessels (Horowitz and Samueloff, 1987). The ability to respond to heat stress is thus limited by the capacity to increase cardiac output as required for greater cutaneous blood flow. Over time, people can adapt to high temperatures by increasing their ability to dissipate heat through these mechanisms. Heat-related illnesses range from heat exhaustion to kidney stones (which increase with dehydration) (Brikowski, Lotan, and Pearle, 2008).

On average, about 400 Americans succumb to extremes of summer heat each year (Moore and others, 2002). An estimated 20,000 people were killed in the United States from 1936 through 1975 by the effects of heat and solar radiation (National Safety Council, Environmental Health Center, 2001), with more than 3,400 deaths occurring between 1999 and 2003. The excess deaths tend to occur during heat waves, defined by the World Meteorological Organization as periods of five or more days when temperatures exceed the average maximum (in the years from 1961 to 1990) by 5°C (9°F). The 1995 Chicago heat wave took approximately 600 lives over five days (Whitman and others, 1997), and the 2003 European heat wave is estimated to have killed more than 40,000 people in just two weeks, and more than 70,000 overall (Table 10.3) (Robine and others, 2008).

From the 1970s to the 1990s, however, heat-related mortality had declined (Davis, Knappenberger, Michaels, and Novicoff, 2003). This likely resulted from a rapid increase in the use of air-conditioning; according to the U.S. Census the proportion of the U.S. population without air-conditioning dropped from 47 percent in 1978 to 15 percent in 2005 (only 2 percent in the South). However,

TABLE 10.3   Excess Mortality from the 2003 Heat Wave in Europe
(August Only)

Countries Affected by the August 2003 Heat Wave	Excess Deaths (relative to 1998–2002 average)	
	Number	Percent Change
Belgium	438	5.31
Switzerland	469	9.81
Germany	7,295	10.97
Spain	6,461	22.86
France	15,251	36.93
Croatia	269	6.83
Italy	9,713	21.81
Luxemburg	75	25.00
Netherlands	578	5.24
Portugal	2,196	27.75
Slovenia	144	9.93
England & Wales	1,987	4.90
Total	44,878	17.34
Countries Used as Controls		
Austria	159	2.63
Czech Republic	58	0.67
Poland	−918	−3.21
Denmark	−49	−1.04
Total	−750	−1.56

Source: Robine and others, 2008.

with wide dissemination of air-conditioning, the saturation point may have been reached; a study through 2007 showed that the protective effects of air-conditioning plateaued in the mid 1990s (Kalkstein and others, 2008).

Heat waves have been well studied, and vulnerability and protection factors are well known. People who are most vulnerable include the poor, the elderly, those who are socially isolated, those who lack air-conditioning, and those with certain medical conditions that impair the ability to dissipate heat. A particular risk factor is living in cities, especially in hot parts of cities, because of the heat island effect.

An **urban heat island** is an urban area that generates and retains heat as a result of buildings, human and industrial activities, and other factors (Figure 10.5). Black asphalt and other dark surfaces (on roads, parking lots, and roofs) have a low **albedo** (reflectivity); they absorb and retain heat, reradiating it at

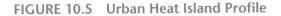

FIGURE 10.5   Urban Heat Island Profile

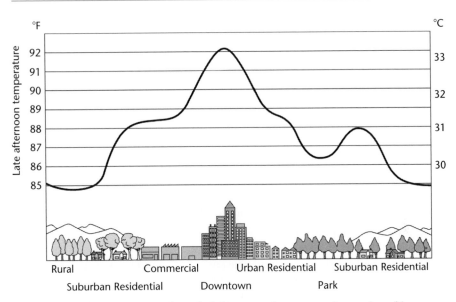

Modeling studies project that by the end of the twenty-first century, the number of heat wave days could double in Los Angeles (Hayhoe and others, 2004) and quadruple in Chicago (Vavrus and Van Dorn, forthcoming) if emissions are not reduced. A recent analysis of twenty-one U.S. cities found that the average number of deaths due to heat waves could more than double by 2050, even after controlling for acclimatization (Kalkstein and others, 2008).

night, when the area would otherwise cool down. In addition, urban areas are relatively lacking in trees, so they receive less of the cooling effect associated with evapotranspiration. Global warming is expected to increase both heat and humidity, aggravating the effects of heat islands and increasing heat stress on urban populations (Kattenberg and others, 1996). One study estimates the mean surface warming due to urban sprawl and land use change to be 0.27°C (0.49°F) for the continental United States (Kalnay and Cai, 2003). Urban areas may therefore face a compounded problem as they experience both global warming and localized warming from the heat island effect. People in cities in developing countries may be especially vulnerable to morbidity and mortality during heat waves.

Reduced Extreme Cold

In a warmer world the reduction of extreme cold could reduce the number of deaths caused by low temperatures. Because mortality rises in the winter season, one could hypothesize that potential lives saved from less extremely cold weather might offset the expected lives lost from more frequent heat waves. However, deaths in the winter season (from influenza, for example) are not necessarily linked to a temperature effect. A study of daily mortality and weather data for 6.5 million deaths in fifty U.S. cities between 1989 and 2000 showed a marked difference between mortality from hot and cold temperatures. The researchers found that on average, cold snaps increased death rates by 1.6 percent, whereas heat waves triggered a 5.7 percent increase in death rates. Relatively milder winters attributable to global warming are unlikely to offset the more severe health effects of summertime extremes (Medina-Ramon & Schwartz, 2007).

Natural Disasters

Floods, droughts, and extreme storms have claimed millions of lives during the past twenty years and have adversely affected the lives of many more millions of people and caused billions of dollars in property damage. On average, disasters killed 123,000 people worldwide each year between 1972 and 1996. Africa suffers the highest rate of disaster-related deaths (Loretti and Tegegn, 1996), although 80 percent of the people affected by natural disasters are in Asia. For every 1 person killed in a natural disaster, an estimated 1,000 people are affected (International Federation of Red Cross and Red Crescent Societies, 1998), either physically, mentally, or through loss of property or livelihood. In less developed regions, disasters can trigger large-scale dislocation of populations, often to jurisdictions ill prepared to welcome and care for them. Malnutrition and communicable diseases are pervasive in refugee populations. Displaced groups are also subjected to violence, sexual abuse, and mental illness. Overall, crude mortality rates in displaced populations may reach as high as 30 times baseline, with much of the mortality occurring in children under five (Toole and Waldman, 1997).

Mental health disorders such as posttraumatic stress disorder (PTSD) may substantially affect population well-being following disasters and displacement, depending on the unexpectedness of the impact, the intensity of the experience, the degree of personal and community disruption, and long-term exposure to the visual signs of the disaster (Green, 1982; Galea, Nandi, and Vlahov, 2005). Symptoms of PTSD have been found in as many as 75 percent of refugee children and adolescents (McCloskey and Southwick, 1996). Among survivors of Hurricane Katrina, the burden of mental illness doubled relative to that in a similar New Orleans population prior to that hurricane. Moreover, after Katrina the mental health system was ill prepared to deliver needed services (Kessler, 2006; Galea and others, 2007). Human health impacts of disasters in the United States are generally projected to be less severe than in poorer countries where the public health infrastructure is less developed. This assumes that medical and emergency relief systems in the United States will function well and that timely and effective adaptation measures will be developed and deployed. Of course, system failures were evident in the aftermath of Hurricanes Katrina and Rita. Over 2,000 Americans were killed during that hurricane season–more than double the average number of lives lost to hurricanes each year in the United States (Karl and others, 2009).

Floods   In the United States, the amount of precipitation falling in the heaviest 1 percent of rain events increased by 20 percent in the past century, and total precipitation increased by 7 percent. Over the last century, the upper Midwest experienced a 50 percent increase in the frequency of days with precipitation over four inches (Kunkel and others, 2003). Other regions, notably the South, have also seen marked increases in heavy downpours, with most of these events coming in the warm season and almost all of the increase coming in the last few decades.

Heavy rains can lead to flooding which can raise the risk of waterborne diseases such as cryptosporidium and giardia. Using 2.5 inches (6.4 cm) of daily precipitation as the threshold for initiating a combined sewer overflow (CSO) event, the frequency of such events in Chicago is expected to rise by 50 to 120 percent by the end of this century (Patz, Vavrus, Uejio, and McLellan, 2008), posing increased risks to drinking and recreational water quality. Population concentration in high-risk areas such as floodplains and coastal zones increases vulnerability. Degradation of the local environment can also contribute significantly to vulnerability. For example, Hurricane Mitch, the most deadly hurricane to strike the Western Hemisphere in the last two centuries, caused 11,000 deaths in Central America, with thousands more people still recorded as missing. Many fatalities occurred during mudslides in deforested areas (National Climatic Data Center, 1999).

Wildfires   The incidence of extensive wildfires (burning over 400 hectares each) in the Western United States rose fourfold between the 1970 to 1986 period and the 1987 to 2003 period (Westerling, Hidalgo, Cayan, and Swetnam, 2006). Several climate-related factors may have played a role in this increase: droughts that dried out forests; higher springtime temperatures that hastened spring snowmelt and thereby lowered soil moisture; and the rise of some tree pest species (Running, 2006; Westerling and others, 2006). Fire and climate change modeling for California has shown that the most severe effects of global climate change would occur in the Sierra foothills, where potentially catastrophic fires could increase by 143 percent in grassland and 121 percent in chaparral (Torn, Mills, and Fried, 1998). The same study showed that greater burn intensity resulted from predicted changes in fuel moisture and wind speeds.

Wildfires threaten health both directly and through reduced air quality. Fire smoke carries a large amount of fine particulate matter that exacerbates cardiac and respiratory problems such as asthma and chronic obstructive pulmonary disease (COPD). For example, drought-induced fires in Florida in 1998 were associated with increased hospital emergency room visits for asthma, bronchitis, and chest pain (Centers for Disease Control and Prevention, 1999).

Sea-Level Rise

Sea surface warming causes a rise in sea level due to thermal expansion of salt water. One expected effect is an increase in flooding and coastal erosion in low-lying coastal areas. This will endanger large numbers of people; fourteen of the world's nineteen current megacities are situated at sea level. Midrange estimates project a 40 cm sea-level rise by the 2080s. Under this scenario coastal regions at risk of storm surges will expand and the population at risk will increase from the current 75 million to 200 million (McCarthy and others, 2001). A greater sea level rise would be more devastating. Nicholls and Leatherman (1995) showed that the extreme case of a 1 meter rise in sea level could inundate numerous low-lying areas, affecting 18.6 million people in China, 13 million in Bangladesh (Figure 10.6), 3.5 million in Egypt, and 3.3 million in Indonesia. For Bangladesh, a 1.5 meter rise is projected to have even more catastrophic consequences (Figure 10.6). Countries such as Egypt, Vietnam, Bangladesh, and small island nations are especially vulnerable, for several reasons. Coastal Egypt is already subsiding due to extensive groundwater withdrawal, and Vietnam and Bangladesh have heavily populated, low-lying deltas along their coasts.

Rising sea levels may affect human health and well-being indirectly, in addition to directly through inundation or heightened storm surges. Rising seas, in concert with withdrawal of fresh water from coastal aquifers, could result in salt water intruding into those aquifers and could disrupt stormwater drainage and sewage disposal. These phenomena, with or without flooding, could force coastal communities to migrate (Myers and Kent, 1995). Refugees suffer substantial health burdens, overcrowding, lack of shelter, and competition for resources. Conflict may be one of the worst results emerging from such forced population migrations (Homer-Dixon, 1999; Zhang and others, 2007; Barnett and Adger, 2007).

AIR POLLUTION

Climate change may affect exposure to air pollutants in many ways because it can influence both the levels of pollutants that are formed and the ways these pollutants are dispersed. Air quality is likely to suffer with a warmer, more variable climate (Bernard and others, 2001).

FIGURE 10.6   Potential Impact of Sea-Level Rise on Bangladesh

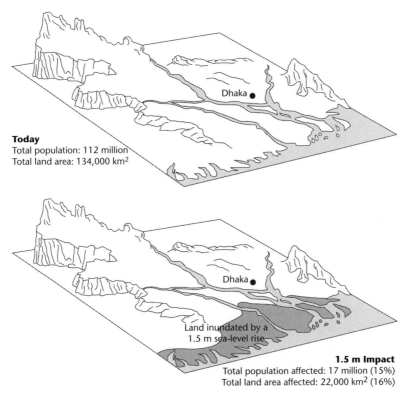

Today
Total population: 112 million
Total land area: 134,000 km^2

Dhaka ●

Land inundated by a
1.5 m sea-level rise

1.5 m Impact
Total population affected: 17 million (15%)
Total land area affected: 22,000 km^2 (16%)

Source: Adapted from United Nations Environment Programme, 2002.

Ozone

Ozone is an example of a pollutant whose concentration may increase with a warmer climate. As explained in Chapter Twelve, many species of trees emit volatile organic compounds (VOCs) such as isoprenes, which are precursors of ozone. Isoprene production is controlled primarily by leaf temperature and light. Biogenic VOC emissions are so sensitive to temperature that an increase of as little as 2°C could cause a 25 percent increase in these emissions (Guenther, 2002). Under the right circumstances, higher levels of isoprenes result in higher levels of ozone.

Moreover, higher temperatures increase ozone formation from precursors. As explained in Chapter Twelve, the ozone season in affected cities occurs during summer months, when warmer temperatures promote ozone formation. This relationship is nonlinear, with a stronger association seen at temperatures above

FIGURE 10.7   Projected Increase In Ozone Exceedance Days

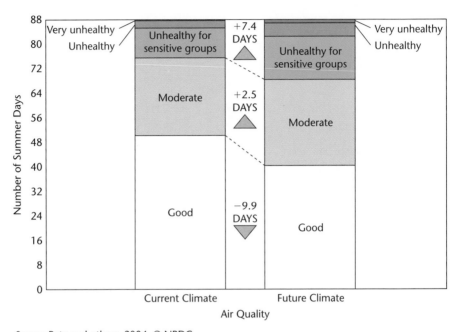

Source: Patz and others, 2004. © NRDC.

32°C. (Particulate matter formation can also increase at higher temperature, due to increased gas-phase reaction rates.) One study showed that temperature variability can change peak ozone levels and twenty-four-hour average levels of fine particulate matter ($PM_{2.5}$) by 16 percent and 25 percent, respectively, when other meteorological variables and emission patterns are held constant (Aw and Kleeman, 2003).

For fifteen cities in the eastern United States, the average number of days exceeding the health-based eight-hour ozone standard is projected to increase by 60 percent (from twelve to almost twenty days each summer) by the 2050s because of warmer temperatures (Figure 10.7) (Patz and others, 2004; Bell and others, 2007). In California higher temperatures are projected to increase the frequency, intensity, and duration of conditions conducive to air pollution formation— potentially by up to 85 percent for high-ozone days in Los Angeles and the San Joaquin Valley (Jacobson, 2008). A study from Germany also shows increases in ozone concentrations under climate change scenarios, with daily maximum ozone increasing by 6 to 10 percent and subsequent ozone exceedance days increasing by fourfold (Forkel and Knoche, 2006).

The relationship between climate change and air pollution is complex. Many feedback loops may operate, some helpful and others harmful. On the one hand, for example, some particles in the air reflect radiant energy and can help to cool the atmosphere; the best-known example is the cooling that follows major volcanic eruptions. On the other hand a warmer climate will mean more demand for energy to power air conditioners, resulting in more air pollution. Overall, for air pollution as for many other aspects of climate change, the impacts are not fully understood, but potential threats to public health deserve careful attention.

Aeroallergens

Another air contaminant that may increase with climate change is pollen. Higher levels of carbon dioxide promote growth and reproduction by some plants, including many that produce allergens. For example, ragweed plants experimentally exposed to high levels of carbon dioxide can increase their pollen production several-fold, perhaps part of the reason for rising ragweed pollen levels in recent decades (Figure 10.8) (Ziska and Caulfield, 2000; Wayne and others, 2002). In a study comparing urban and rural parts of Baltimore, ragweed grew faster, flowered earlier, and produced more pollen at urban locations than at rural locations, presumably because air temperature and CO_2 levels are significantly higher in urban areas (Ziska and others, 2003). This prompted the investigators to dub cities "harbingers of climate change." People who suffer from hay fever and seasonal allergies would be especially susceptible to these changes.

Allergens and Contact Dermatitis

Poison ivy growth and toxicity also increase greatly with higher levels of carbon dioxide. These increases exceed those of most beneficial plants. Poison ivy vines grow twice as much per year in air with doubled preindustrial carbon dioxide levels as in unaltered air—an increase five times higher than reported for tree species in other analyses (Mohan and others, 2006). Recent and projected increases in carbon dioxide have also been shown to stimulate the growth of stinging nettle and leafy spurge, two weeds that cause rashes following contact with human skin (Hunt, Hand, Hannah, and Neal, 1991; Ziska, 2003).

INFECTIOUS DISEASES

A range of infectious diseases can be influenced by climate conditions. The diseases most sensitive to influence by ambient climate conditions are those spread

FIGURE 10.8   Climate and Aeroallergens

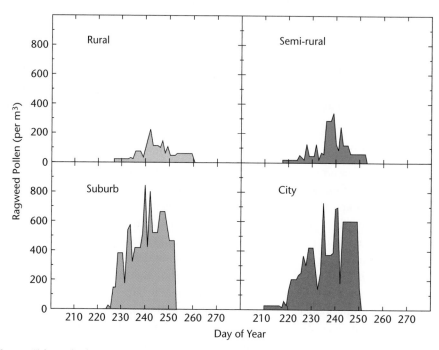

Source: Ziska and others, 2003. Reprinted with permission.

Time course of ragweed pollen production for four sites along an urban transect for 2001 as a function of day of year. Values are numbers of pollen grains per cubic meter of air.

not by person-to-person pathways but directly from the source: the water- and food-borne diseases as well as vector-borne diseases (which involve insects or rodents within the pathogen's life cycle).

Water- and Foodborne Diseases

Waterborne diseases are likely to become a greater problem as climate change continues and affects both freshwater and marine ecosystems. In freshwater systems, both water quantity and water quality can be affected by climate change. In marine waters, changes in temperature and salinity will affect coastal ecosystems in ways that may increase the risk of certain diseases.

Freshwater Ecosystems   Waterborne diseases are particularly sensitive to changes in the hydrologic cycle. As discussed in Chapter Fifteen, both water quantity and water quality play a role in waterborne disease. The impact of climate change on water *quantity* is relatively straightforward. In some regions precipitation is expected to increase, whereas in others decreased precipitation, even to the point of ongoing drought, is predicted. Water shortages contribute to poor hygiene and that in turn contributes to diarrheal disease, especially in poor countries. At the other extreme, increased precipitation, including severe rainfall events, can lead to flooding.

Climate change, and associated severe weather events, can affect water *quality* in more complex ways. Many community water systems are already overwhelmed by extreme rainfall events. Flooding can contaminate drinking water with runoff from sewage lines, containment lagoons (such as those used in animal feeding operations), or nonpoint source pollution (such as agricultural fields) across watersheds. Runoff can exceed the capacity of the sewer system or treatment plants, which then discharge the excess wastewater directly into surface water bodies (Perciasepe, 1998; Rose and Simonds, 1998). Urban watersheds sustain more than 60 percent of their annual contaminant loads during storm events (Fisher and Katz, 1988). Turbidity also increases during storm events, and studies have linked turbidity and illness in many communities (Morris and others, 1996; Schwartz, Levin, and Hodge, 1997).

Waterborne disease outbreaks in the United States are not random events. A nationwide analysis of these outbreaks from 1948 to 1994 demonstrated a distinct seasonality, a spatial clustering in key watersheds, and an association with heavy precipitation; 67 percent of reported outbreaks were preceded by unusually rainy months (defined as rainfall in the upper 80th percentile based on a fifty-year local baseline) (Curriero and others, 2001). In Walkerton, Ontario, in May 2000, heavy precipitation combined with failing infrastructure contaminated drinking water with *E. coli* 0157:H7 and *Campylobacter jejuni* resulting in an estimated 2,300 illnesses and 7 deaths (Hrudey and others, 2003). Such occurrences may become more common as severe rainfall events become more frequent.

Cryptosporidiosis, one of the most prevalent diarrheal diseases in the world, is illustrative. Cryptosporidium is a protozoan associated with domestic livestock that can contaminate drinking water during periods of heavy precipitation. The oocyst is resistant to chlorine treatment. The 1993 cryptosporidiosis outbreak in Milwaukee, in which an estimated 403,000 people were exposed to contaminated water, followed unusually heavy spring rains and runoff from melting snow (MacKenzie and others, 1994). Similarly, studies of the Delaware River have shown that giardia and cryptosporidium oocyst counts correlate with the amount of rainfall (Atherholt, LeChevallier, Norton, and Rosenothers, 1998). Certain watersheds, by virtue of associated land use patterns and the presence of human and animal fecal contaminants, are at high risk of surface water contamination after heavy rains, and this has serious implications for drinking-water purity.

Intense rainfall can also contaminate recreational waters and increase the risk of human illness (Schuster and others, 2005). For example, heavy runoff leads to higher bacterial counts in rivers in coastal areas and at beaches along the coast; this association is strongest at the beaches closest to rivers (Dwight and others, 2002). This suggests that the risk of swimming at some beaches increases with heavy rainfall, a predicted consequence of climate change. According to the 2007 report of the IPCC (Solomon and others, 2007), heavy precipitation events are expected to increase under climate change scenarios.

Marine Ecosystems   Warm water and nitrogen favor blooms of marine algae, including two groups, dinoflagellates and diatoms, that can release toxins into the marine environment. These **harmful algal blooms** (HABs)—previously called red tides—can cause acute paralytic, diarrheic, and amnesic poisoning in humans, as well as extensive die-offs of fish, shellfish, and marine mammals and birds that depend on the marine food web. Over the past three decades the frequency and global distribution of harmful algal blooms appear to have increased, and more human intoxication from algal sources has occurred (Van Dolah, 2000). For example, during the 1987 El Niño, a bloom of *Gymnodinium breve*, previously confined to the Gulf of Mexico, extended northward after warm Gulf Stream water reached far up the U.S. East Coast, resulting in human neurological poisonings from shellfish and in substantial fish kills (Tester and others, 1991). Similarly, that same year an outbreak of amnesic shellfish poisoning occurred on Prince Edward Island when warm eddies of the Gulf Stream neared the shore and heavy rains increased nutrient-rich runoff (Hallegraeff, 1993). Modeling in the Netherlands predicts that by the year 2100, a 4°C increase in summer temperatures in combination with water column stratification would double growth rates of several species of HABs in the North Sea (Peperzak, 2005).

Ciguatera, a form of poisoning caused by ingesting fish that contains toxins from several dinoflagellate species, could also expand its range. This condition has been linked to sea surface temperature in some Pacific Islands (Hales, Weinstein, and Woodward, 1999).

Some bacteria, especially *Vibrio* species, also proliferate in warm marine waters (Pascual and others, 2000). Copepods (or zooplankton), which feed on algae, can serve as reservoirs for *V. cholerae* and other enteric pathogens. For example, in Bangladesh cholera follows seasonal warming of sea surface temperatures, which can enhance plankton blooms (Colwell, 1996). Other *Vibrio* species have expanded in northern Atlantic waters in association with warm water (Thompson and others, 2004). For example, in 2004 an outbreak of *V. parahaemolyticus* shellfish poisoning was reported from Prince William Sound in Alaska. This pathogenic species of *Vibrio* had not previously been isolated from Alaskan shellfish due to the coldness of the Alaskan waters. What could have caused the species' expanded range? Water temperatures during in the 2004 shellfish harvest remained above 15°C and mean water temperatures were significantly higher than the previous six years (McLaughlin and others, 2005). Such evidence suggests the potential for warming sea surface temperatures to increase the geographic range of shellfish poisoning and *Vibrio* infections into temperate and even arctic zones.

The incidence of diarrhea from other pathogens also shows temperature sensitivity, which may in turn signal sensitivity to changing climate. During the 1997 and 1998 El Niño event, winter temperatures in Lima, Peru, increased more than 5°C above normal, and the daily hospital admission rates for diarrhea more than doubled compared to rates over the prior five years (Checkley and others, 2000) (Figure 10.9). Long-term studies of the **El Niño Southern Oscillation**, or ENSO, have confirmed this pattern. ENSO refers to natural year-to-year variations in sea surface temperatures, surface air pressure, rainfall, and atmospheric circulation across the equatorial Pacific Ocean. This cycle provides a model for

FIGURE 10.9 Time Series of Temperature and Childhood Diarrhea, Peru

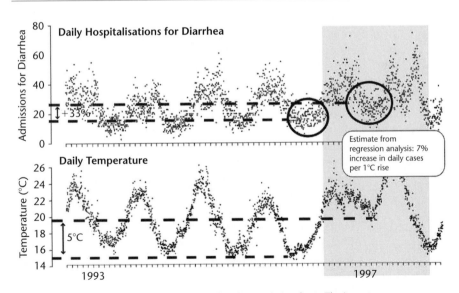

Source: Checkley and others, 2000. Reprinted with permission from *The Lancet*.

Daily time series between January 1, 1993, and November 15, 1998, for admissions for diarrhea and mean ambient temperature in Lima, Peru. Shaded area represents the 1997–1998 El Niño event.

observing climate-related changes in many ecosystems. ENSO has had an increasing role in explaining cholera outbreaks in recent years, perhaps because of concurrent climate change (Rodo, Pascual, Fuchs, and Faruque, 2002). Overall there is growing evidence that climate change can contribute to the risk of waterborne diseases in both marine and freshwater ecosystems.

Foodborne Diseases   More frequent warm days and greater humidity can change the incidence of foodborne infectious diseases. Data from Britain show a strong association between instances of food poisoning and temperatures during the preceding two to five weeks (Bentham and Langford, 1995). In Australia, Western and Central Europe, and Canada, reported cases of food poisoning increase non-linearly with each degree of increase in weekly temperature (Parry and others, 2007). Temperatures contribute to an estimated 30 percent of cases of salmonellosis in much of continental Europe, especially when they exceed a

PERSPECTIVE
Some Effects of Weather and Climate on Vector- and Rodent-Borne Diseases

Vector-borne pathogens spend part of their life cycle in cold-blooded arthropods that are subject to many environmental factors. Changes in weather and climate that can affect transmission of vector-borne diseases include variations in temperature, rainfall, wind, extreme flooding or drought, and sea-level rise. Rodent-borne pathogens can be affected indirectly by ecological determinants of food sources affecting rodent population size, and floods can displace and lead them to seek food and refuge. These effects are summarized in the following lists.

Temperature Effects on Selected Vectors and Vector-Borne Pathogens

Vector	Survival can decrease or increase depending on the species.
	Some vectors have higher survival at higher latitudes and altitudes with higher temperatures.
	Changes in susceptibility of vectors to some pathogens (for example, higher temperatures reduce size of some vectors but reduce activity of others).
	Changes in the rate of vector population growth.
	Changes in feeding rate and host contact (which may alter the survival rate).
	Changes in the seasonality of populations.
Pathogen	Decreased extrinsic incubation period in vector at higher temperatures.
	Changes in the transmission season.
	Changes in distribution.
	Changes in viral replication.

threshold of 6°C above average (Kovats and others, 2004). Other food-borne agents, such as campylobacter, are also seasonal but are not as strongly linked to temperature fluctuations. Food spoilage is temperature dependent, as pest species, especially flies, rodents, and cockroaches, have increased contact with food at higher temperatures (Goulson and others, 2005).

Vector-Borne Diseases

Vector-borne diseases, as a class, are one of the best studied health impacts of climate change. These are infectious diseases, caused by protozoa, bacteria, and viruses, that are spread by organisms such as mosquitoes and ticks. The life cycle of these pathogens involves much time outside the human host and therefore much exposure to and influence by environmental conditions. The incubation

---

Precipitation Effects on Selected Vectors and Vector-Borne Pathogens

Vector	Increased rain may increase larval habitat and vector population size by creating a new habitat.
	Excess rain or snowpack can eliminate habitat by flooding, thus decreasing the vector population size.
	Low rainfall can create habitat by causing rivers to dry into pools (dry season malaria).
	Decreased rain can increase container-breeding mosquitoes by forcing increased water storage.
	Epic rainfall events can synchronize vector host seeking and virus transmission.
	Increased humidity increases vector survival; decreased humidity decreases vector survival.
Pathogen	Few direct effects but some data on humidity effects on malarial parasite development in the anopheline mosquito host.
Vertebrate host	Increased rain can increase vegetation, food availability, and population size.
	Increased rain can also cause flooding and decrease population size but increase contact with humans.
	Decreased rain can eliminate food and force rodents into housing areas, increasing human contact, but it can also decrease population size.
Increased sea level	Can alter estuary flow and change existing salt marshes and associated mosquito species, decreasing or eliminating selected mosquito breeding sites (for example, reduced habitat for *Culiseta melanura*).

Source: Slightly adapted from Gubler and others, 2001.

time of a vector-borne infectious agent within its vector organism is typically very sensitive to changes in temperature and humidity (Patz and others, 2003) (also see the accompanying Perspective). The term *tropical diseases* is a reminder that each pathogen or vector species thrives in a limited range of climatic conditions.

Mosquito-Borne Diseases   Malaria and arboviruses are transmitted to humans by mosquitoes. Because insects are cold-blooded, climate change can shift the distribution of mosquito populations, affect mosquito biting rates and survival, and shorten or lengthen pathogen development time inside the mosquito, which ultimately determines infectivity.

Malaria is a temperature-sensitive disease. According to the World Health Organization (1996), malaria is the vector-borne disease most sensitive to long-term climate change. The incidence of malaria in highly endemic areas varies seasonally. In various regions, malaria has been shown to alter in response to weather perturbations. For example, malaria transmission has been associated with temperature anomalies in some African highland areas (Githeko and Ndegwa, 2001). Similarly, in the Punjab region of India, excessive monsoon rainfall and resultant high humidity have been recognized for years as major factors in the occurrence of malaria epidemics. In that region malaria epidemics increase approximately fivefold during the year following an El Niño year (Bouma and van der Kaay, 1996).

Malarial mosquito populations can be exquisitely sensitive to warming; an increase in temperature of just half a degree centigrade can translate into a 30 to 100 percent increase in mosquito abundance, demonstrating a *biological amplification* by temperature effects. In the African highlands, where mosquito populations are relatively small compared to those in lowland areas (Minakawa and others, 2002), such biological responses may be especially significant in determining the risk of malaria.

Arboviruses include the causative agents of dengue fever, West Nile virus, chikungunya, and Rift Valley fever. Each of these may be affected by climate.

Dengue fever is transmitted by the *Aedes aegypti* mosquito, and in laboratory studies, the rate of virus replication in the mosquito increases directly with temperature. Biologically based models have been developed to explore the influence of projected temperature change on the incidence of dengue fever. When linked to future climate change projections, these models suggest that relatively small increases in temperature in temperate regions, given viral introduction into a susceptible human population, are likely to increase the potential for epidemics (Patz, Martens, Focks, and Jetten, 1998). Modeling of *Aedes* mosquito populations in relation to climate variation suggests a strong association, and when the model is applied retrospectively, these changes are strongly correlated with historical changes in Dengue fever incidence (Hopp and Foley, 2003).

West Nile virus (WNV) had its first reported outbreak in the United States in the summer of 1999, a likely result of the virus arriving via international air transport. But July 1999 also set a high temperature record in New York City, and this new strain of West Nile virus, according to laboratory findings, was able to thrive in warmer temperatures than other strains of the virus around the world tolerated. Within five years the disease had spread across the continental United States through migration of infected birds. During the epidemic summers of 2002 to 2004, epicenters of West Nile virus occurred in locations experiencing either drought or above average temperatures (Reisen and Brault, 2007). The *Culex* genus of mosquito that carries WNV tends to breed in foul, standing water. In drought conditions, standing water pools become even more concentrated with organic material. During 2002, a more virulent strain of WNV emerged in the United States. Recent analyses indicate that this mutated strain responds strongly to higher temperatures, suggesting that greater risks from the disease may result from a future increase in the frequency of heat waves (Kilpatrick, Meola, Moudy, and Kramer, 2008).

In July 2004, during a severe drought in East Africa, an epidemic of chikungunya virus erupted in Lamu, Kenya, infecting an estimated 13,500 people (75 percent of the population) (Sergon and others, 2008). Unseasonably warm and dry conditions, especially over coastal Kenya, had occurred during May 2004 (Chretien and others, 2007). Such conditions may have led to unsafe domestic water storage practices and infrequent changing of water storage. In addition, warm dry weather may have hastened viral development in the *Aedes* mosquito. The virus spread to islands of the western Indian Ocean and then to India and most recently Italy, during the summer of 2007. Although the role of climatic conditions in Italy is not clear, southern Europe was experiencing an unusually warm and dry summer in 2007 (Rezza and others, 2007).

Rift Valley fever is usually transmitted through contact with the blood or organs of infected animals. However, it can also be transmitted by *Aedes* mosquitoes. All known Rift Valley fever virus outbreaks in East Africa from 1950 to May 1998, and probably earlier, followed periods of abnormally high rainfall. Analysis of this record and Pacific and Indian Ocean sea surface temperature anomalies, coupled with satellite-derived vegetation data, show that these East African outbreaks may be predicted up to five months in advance of their occurrence. Concurrent near-real-time monitoring with satellite data on vegetation may identify actual affected areas (Linthicum and others, 1999).

Tick-Borne Disease   Lyme disease is a prevalent tick-borne disease in North America, and new evidence suggests an association with temperature (Ogden and others, 2004) and precipitation (McCabe and Bunnell, 2004). Temperature and vapor pressure contribute to maintaining populations of the tick *Ixodes scapularis*, which, in the United States, is the microorganism's secondary host. Because tick survival requires a monthly average minimum temperature above −7°C (Brownstein, Holford, and Fish, 2003), temperature limits the northern boundary of Lyme disease. According to IPCC projections of climate change, warming temperatures could shift the range limit for this tick northward by 200 km by the 2020s and 1,000 km by the 2080s (Ogden and others, 2006).

Rodent-Borne Diseases   Hantavirus infections are transmitted largely by exposure to infectious excreta from rodents and may cause serious disease and a high fatality rate in humans. When hantavirus pulmonary syndrome newly emerged in the Southwest United States in 1993, it was associated with weather conditions, including El Niño–driven heavy rainfall, that led to a growth in rodent populations and subsequent disease transmission (Glass and others, 2000). Extreme flooding or hurricanes can lead to outbreaks of leptospirosis. An epidemic of leptospirosis in Nicaragua followed heavy flooding in 1995. In one case-control study, walking through flooded waters was associated with a fifteenfold increased risk of disease (Trevejo and others, 1998).

Plague is another climate-sensitive disease, one that is carried by fleas associated with rodents, the primary reservoir hosts of the *Yersina pestis* bacterium. In the desert southwestern United States, levels of plague bacteria in rodents have been found to increase with wet climate conditions related to El Niño and Pacific Decadal Oscillation (PDO) (Parmenter and others, 1999). Historical tree-ring data suggest that during the major plague epidemics of the Black Death period (1280 to 1350), climate conditions were becoming both warmer and wetter (Stenseth and others, 2006).

Land Use, Local Climate, and Infectious Disease   To predict climate's effect on vector-borne diseases, local landscapes need to be considered. For example, in the Amazon Basin, malaria incidence fluctuates with rainfall levels. Yet regional differences in the extent of wetlands and surface water greatly modify the effect of rainfall; in upland locations with sparse wetlands, malaria increases with rainfall, whereas in areas with abundant wetlands, malaria decreases with rainfall (Olson and other, 2009). Climate effects must be analyzed in the context of local topography and land cover data.

Intact ecosystems, which preserve landscape integrity and biodiversity, form the basis of many essential ecosystem services (see Chapter One). However, global vegetation cover is changing far more rapidly than is global climate. Land cover is disrupted by such forces as deforestation, urban sprawl, industrial development, road construction (causing linear disturbances), large water control projects (such as dams, canals, irrigation systems, and reservoirs), and climate change. Natural landscapes are being destroyed both locally and on a very large scale. A global pattern of landscape fragmentation has emerged.

These changes can affect human and wildlife health by altering both habitat and microclimate. The World Health Organization has recorded over thirty-six emerging infectious diseases since 1976; many of these are the direct result of landscape influence on plant and animal ecology. In fact it is estimated that 75 percent of all emerging diseases derive from animal zoonoses (Taylor, Latham, and Woolhouse, 2001). A similar pattern is seen with reemerging diseases such as malaria and dengue fever; landscape changes have been accompanied by the spread of pathogens into new areas (Patz, 2001). For example, the various species of anopheline mosquitoes differ in their competence to transmit malaria. Because these species occupy a variety of ecological niches, habitat alterations may favor the spread of mosquitoes more likely to transit malaria. The recognition of these apparent links gave rise to the Millennium Ecosystem Assessment, an international effort to document the effect of degraded ecosystems on human health and well-being (http://www.millenniumassessment.org).

PUBLIC HEALTH RESPONSE TO CLIMATE CHANGE

The links between human health and climate change are complex, diverse, and not always discernible, especially over short time spans. Understanding and addressing these links requires systems thinking, with consideration of many factors, ranging beyond health to such sectors as energy, transportation, agriculture, and development policy (Frumkin and McMichael, 2008). Interdisciplinary collaboration is critical. A wide range of tools is needed, including innovative public health surveillance methods, geographically based data systems, classical and scenario-based risk assessment, and integrated modeling.

Mitigation and Adaptation

Two kinds of strategies, both familiar to public health professionals, are available for responding to climate change. The first, known as **mitigation**, corresponds to primary prevention, and the second, known as **adaptation**, corresponds to secondary prevention (or preparedness).

Mitigation refers to efforts to stabilize or reduce the production of greenhouse gases (and perhaps to sequester those greenhouse gases that are produced). This goal can be achieved through policies and technologies that result in more efficient energy production and reduced energy demand. For example, sustainable energy sources, such as wind and solar energy, do not contribute to greenhouse gas emissions (see Chapter Thirteen). Similarly, transportation policies that rely on walking, bicycling, mass transit, and fuel-efficient automobiles result in fewer greenhouse gas emissions than are produced by the current U.S. reliance on large, fuel-inefficient automobiles (see Chapter Fourteen). Much energy use occurs in buildings, and green buildings that emphasize energy efficiency, together with electrical appliances that conserve energy, also play a role in reducing greenhouse gas emissions (see Chapter Nineteen). A final aspect of mitigation aims not to reduce the production of greenhouse gases, but to accelerate their removal. Carbon dioxide sinks such as forests are effective in this regard, so land use policies that preserve and expand forests are an important tool in mitigating global climate change.

An important paradigm for mitigation strategies is **stabilization wedges**. This paradigm (shown graphically in Figure 13.4 in Chapter Thirteen) was introduced by Princeton professors Stephen Pacala and Robert Socolow (2004). If carbon dioxide emissions have traced an upward trajectory for over a century, and if we wish to redirect that trend to achieve stable or decreasing emissions, then we need to employ several technologies and behavioral changes in the areas of energy efficiency, reduced transportation demand, and so on. Many of these solutions are technically feasible and available at present. According to Pacala and Socolow, each of these solutions can be viewed as a *wedge*, and combining wedges is a strategy for stabilizing climate. Health professionals have an interest not only in implementing these approaches but also in evaluating each wedge to be sure its use does not unintentionally threaten public health.

Adaptation refers to efforts to reduce the public health impact of climate change. For example, if we anticipate severe weather events such as hurricanes, then preparation by emergency management authorities and medical facilities can minimize morbidity and mortality. This presupposes rigorous efforts at **vulnerability assessment**, to identify likely events, at-risk populations, and opportunities to reduce harm (Ebi, Smith, and Burton, 2005; Kirch, Menne, and Bertollini, 2005; Menne and Ebi, 2006; Schipper and Burton, 2009). Similarly, public health surveillance systems can detect outbreaks of infectious diseases in vulnerable areas, a prerequisite to early control. Many current challenges, such as deaths from heat waves, floods, and air pollution, will be amplified by climate change. Much of preparedness thus can build on analyses of the strengths and weaknesses of current prevention efforts and a rethinking of potential thresholds that may change in the future (for example, expected change in the volume of stormwater runoff, or the frequency of heat waves).

Co-Benefits

An important theme in both mitigation and adaptation is **co-benefits**. Although the steps needed to address climate change may appear formidable, some of them—reducing greenhouse gas emissions, developing and deploying sustainable energy technologies, shifting transportation patterns, designing resiliency into cities, and others—yield multiple benefits (Corfee-Morlot and Agrawala, 2004), making them especially attractive, cost effective, and politically feasible. For example, planting trees in cities helps reduce CO_2 levels while at the same time reducing the urban heat island effect, reducing local energy demand, improving air quality, and providing an attractive venue for physical activity and social interaction (Frumkin and McMichael, 2008). Another example is reducing fossil fuel use in power plants—a principal means of reducing greenhouse gas emissions and also a strategy to reduce air pollution (Cifuentes and others, 2001). A third example is sustainable community design (Wilkinson and others, 2007). In communities designed to facilitate active transport (walking and bicycling) and transit use, vehicular travel is reduced. This reduces transportation contributions to climate change and yields other benefits as well: more physical activity, less air pollution, and reduced risk of motor vehicle injuries and fatalities (Younger, Morrow-Almeida, Vindigni, and Dannenberg, 2008). Health professionals need to be alert to such opportunities.

In planning solutions such as sustainable communities, it is essential that affected communities be involved (Adger and others, 2006). As described in Chapter Eight, poor communities and communities of color bear a disproportionate burden from many environmental health threats. These groups must be involved in planning solutions to avoid the potential for widening the already large gap in access to healthy environmental conditions. Climate solutions must also be designed with cultural sensitivity and environmental justice in mind so that all people can be afforded equitable access to health opportunities.

Unintended Consequences

Steps taken to address climate change can have unintended consequences. A leading example is biofuel production, a rapidly growing industry thanks to economic incentives and public policies. Global biofuel production may quadruple within the next fifteen to twenty years (International Energy Agency, 2004; Himmel and others, 2007; Fairless, 2007).

Biofuels are made from many sources—including animal and crop waste and food waste—but a principal source is crops such as corn and sugar cane. Critics claim that large-scale production of biofuels diverts such crops from use as food, creating scarcity and increasing food prices (Food and Agriculture Organization of the United Nations [FAO], 2008; UN-Energy, 2007). This could affect the amount of humanitarian food aid available for extremely impoverished countries, as food aid shipments from the United States are inversely correlated with commodity prices (Naylor and others, 2007). Demand for biofuels may also accelerate the conversion of forests to cropland, which could, paradoxically, increase carbon dioxide levels (Fearnside, 2001; Morton and others, 2006; Koh and Wilcove, 2008; Gibbs and others, 2008), and threaten biodiversity in sensitive areas (Keeney and Nanninga, 2008). A full life cycle analysis (LCA) for biofuels surprisingly showed slightly higher particulate matter (PM) generation from use of corn-based ethanol compared to use of gasoline and cellulosic ethanol; growing corn for ethanol involves much fertilizer and farm machinery and may simply shift air pollution to rural from urban locations (Hill and others, 2009). Critics further claim that biofuel production is economically inefficient and highly reliant on subsidies (Organisation for Economic Co-operation and Development, 2008). Each of these claims is controversial; for example, some argue that food scarcity results from maldistribution more than from absolute scarcity. Overall, the biofuel debate illustrates the potential for unintended consequences, especially for vulnerable populations, and the need for careful analysis of each major strategy taken to address climate change, to achieve what has been called *healthy solutions* for climate change (Patz and others, 2008; Epstein and others, 2008).

Climate Change Policy

International efforts to address climate change are carried out under the United Nations Framework Convention on Climate Change (UNFCCC). Adopted in 1992, the UNFCCC set out a framework that aimed to stabilize atmospheric concentrations of greenhouse gases at a level that would prevent "dangerous interference" with the climate system. The UNFCCC has carried out its business through regular meetings of the Conference of Parties (COP). Perhaps the best known was the third meeting, in 1997 in Kyoto. This resulted in the Kyoto Protocol, which committed developed countries and emerging market economies to reduce their overall emissions of six greenhouse gases by at least 5 percent below 1990 levels over the period between 2008 and 2012, with specific targets varying from country to country. Some developing nations resisted mandatory emission reductions, citing the mandate to raise living standards for their citizens and arguing that the burden of reductions ought to be borne by wealthy nations. Following the thirteenth UNFCCC COP meeting in Bali, in 2007, the United States was the only country not to ratify the treaty. Several justifications were cited, including the unwillingness of developing nations to commit to reductions and the alleged ineffectiveness of the Kyoto approach. By 2007, it was clear that many nations that had ratified the Kyoto Protocol were not on track to achieve their anticipated emission reductions, even though the protocol requires relatively modest emission reductions, far below what will be required to stabilize greenhouse gases at any level below 700 ppm (compared to a preindustrial level of 280 ppm and today's level of about 380 ppm).

After years without a clear policy response to climate change, the United States' approach is evolving rapidly following the 2008 elections. Public debate and congressional bills have centered on several policy strategies: cap-and-trade, carbon taxes, and regulatory limits on emissions (see Chapter Thirty), but none of these has matured into national policy. Either U.S. Environmental Protection Agency regulation or congressional legislation (or both) may ultimately define national policy. In the meantime, individual states and even localities have taken steps to reduce their carbon emissions.

Similarly, public health policy toward climate change has been relatively undeveloped in the United States. Some states and cities have developed climate change adaptation plans that involve the public health system. The Centers for Disease Control and Prevention has proposed a general approach to climate change, based on the essential functions of public health (Frumkin and others, 2008). State and local health departments, which bear primary responsibility for public health preparedness in the United States, are expected to address climate change increasingly in coming years.

Ethical Considerations

Climate change raises ethical concerns in several ways. First, on a global scale, the nations that are responsible for the lion's share of carbon emissions to date account for a small proportion of the world's population and are relatively resilient to the effects of climate change. In contrast the large population of the global south—the poor countries—account for a relatively small share of cumulative carbon emissions, and a very low per capita emission rate (although total emissions from developing nations are growing rapidly, with China surpassing the United States in 2006). The United States, with 5 percent of the global population, produces 25 percent of total annual greenhouse gas emissions. This discrepancy exemplifies the ethical implications posed by climate change on a global scale, shown graphically in Figure 10.10. Poor populations in the developing world have little by way of industry, transportation, or intensive agriculture; they contribute only a fraction of the greenhouse gases per capita that the developed countries produce, and their capacity to protect themselves against the adverse consequences of what are mostly others' greenhouse gases is quite limited. Of course, if developing nations do not choose energy-efficient development pathways, global climate change trends will intensify even as the imbalance of equity decreases (Patz and Kovats, 2002).

Within the United States, and within many other nations, a similar disparity exists. Poor and disadvantaged people will in many cases bear the brunt of climate change impacts, including health impacts. This was graphically demonstrated

FIGURE 10.10   Cartograms: CO_2 Emissions and Health Effects

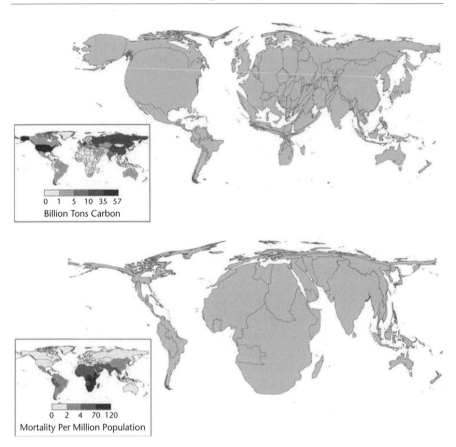

Source: Patz and others, 2007.

Note: CO_2 emissions data from Marland, Boden, and Andres, 2007, adjusted for changing boundaries between 1950 and 2000, Health impacts from McMichael and others, 2004.

Cartogram comparison of undepleted cumulative carbon dioxide (CO_2) emissions (by country) for 1950 to 2000 (upper map) versus the regional distribution of four climate-sensitive health effects (malaria, malnutrition, diarrhea, and inland flood-related fatalities) (lower map). This is only a partial list of potential health outcomes, and there are significant uncertainties in all the underlying models. These estimates should therefore be considered a conservative, approximate estimate of the health burden of climate change.

in the aftermath of Hurricane Katrina, a disaster typical of those expected to increase with climate change. The poor populations of New Orleans and the nearby Gulf region were disproportionately likely to fail to evacuate, to suffer catastrophic disruption following the storm, and to be unable to recover (Dyson, 2007; Elliott and Pais, 2006; Pastor and others, 2006).

Finally, an ethical issue arises with respect to intergenerational justice. Climate change has enormous potential impacts on the health and well-being of future generations (Page, 2007). As discussed in Chapter Seven, ethical and religious thinkers have argued that we in the present owe a moral obligation to those who will follow to reverse climate change.

SUMMARY

Climatologists now state with high certainty that global climate change is real, occurring more rapidly than expected, and caused by human activities, especially through fossil fuel combustion and deforestation. Environmental public health researchers assessing future projections for global climate have concluded that, on balance, adverse health outcomes will dominate under these changed climatic conditions.

The number of pathways through which climate change can affect the health of populations makes this environmental health threat one of the largest and most formidable of the new century. Conversely, the potential health co-benefits from moving beyond our current fossil fuel–based economy may offer some of the greatest health opportunities in over a century.

KEY TERMS

adaptation

albedo

climate change

climate variability

co-benefits

El Niño Southern
    Oscillation (ENSO)

global warming

greenhouse gases

harmful algal blooms

heat wave

mitigation

radiative forcing

stabilization wedges

urban heat island

vulnerability assessment

DISCUSSION QUESTIONS

1. Is climate change the major environmental health challenge of the twenty-first century? Explain the reasoning underlying your answer.
2. Identify a broad range of current environmental health problems likely to be exacerbated by climate change. How might existing public health practices be altered to anticipate these effects of climate change? What other key sectors (beyond health) should be engaged?
3. What are some of the major driving forces behind both the risks of climate change and our vulnerabilities to that change? Which scientific experts would be best able to assemble a comprehensive assessment of climate change risks? What types of policymakers should be involved, and at what levels (local, regional, international)?
4. What are the potential co-benefits and the potential unintended consequences of mitigating greenhouse gas emissions?

REFERENCES

Adger, W. N., Paavola, J., Huq, S., Mace, M. J., Eds. *Fairness in Adaptation to Climate Change*. Cambridge: MIT Press, 2006.

Arctic Climate Impact Assessment. *Impacts of a Warming Arctic*. New York: Cambridge University Press, 2004.

Atherholt, T. B., LeChevallier, M. W., Norton, W. D., and Rosen, J. S. "Effect of Rainfall on Giardia and Crypto." *Journal of the American Water Works Association*, 1998, *90*(9), 66–80.

Aw, J., and Kleeman, M. J. "Evaluating the First-Order Effect of Inter-Annual Temperature Variability on Urban Air Pollution." *Journal of Geophysical Research—Atmospheres*, 2003, *108*, D12.

Barnett, J., and Adger, W. N. "Climate Change, Human Security and Violent Conflict." *Political Geography*, 2007, *26*, 639–655.

Battisti, D. S., and Naylor, R. L. "Historical Warnings of Future Food Insecurity with Unprecedented Seasonal Heat." *Science*, 2009, *323*, 240–244.

Bell, M. L., and others. "Climate Change, Ambient Ozone, and Health in 50 US Cities." *Climatic Change*, 2007, *82*, 61–76.

Bentham, G., and Langford, I. H. "Climate Change and the Incidence of Food Poisoning in England and Wales." *International Journal of Biometeorology*, 1995, *39*, 81–86.

Bernard, S. M., and others. "The Potential Impacts of Climate Variability and Change on Air Pollution-Related Health Effects in the United States." *Environmental Health Perspectives*, 2001, *109*(suppl. 2), 199–209.

Bouma, M., and van der Kaay, H. "The El Niño Southern Oscillation and the Historic Malaria Epidemics on the Indian Subcontinent and Sri Lanka: An Early Warning System for Future Epidemics?" *Tropical Medicine and International Health*, 1996, *1*(1), 86–96.

Brikowski, T. H., Lotan, Y., and Pearle, M. S. "Climate-Related Increase in the Prevalence of Urolithiasis in the United States." *Proceedings of the National Academy of Sciences of the United States of America*, 2008, 105, 9841–9846.

Brown, M. E., and Funk, C. C. "Food Security Under Climate Change." *Science*, 2008, *319*, 580–581.

Brownstein, J. S., Holford, T. R., and Fish, D. "A Climate-Based Model Predicts the Spatial Distribution of Lyme Disease Vector *Ixodes Scapularis* in the United States." *Environmental Health Perspectives*, 2003, *111*, 1152–1157.

Butt, T. A., and others. "The Economic and Food Security Implications of Climate Change in Mali." *Climatic Change*, 2005, *68*(3), 355–378.

Centers for Disease Control and Prevention. "Surveillance of Morbidity During Wildfires: Central Florida, 1998." *Morbidity and Mortality Weekly Report*, 1999, *48*(4), 78–79.

Cifuentes, L., and others. "Assessing the Health Benefits of Urban Air Pollution Reductions Associated with Climate Change Mitigation (2000–2020): Santiago, São Paulo, México City, and New York City." *Environmental Health Perspectives*, 2001, *109*(3S), 419–425.

Checkley, W., and others. "Effects of El Niño and Ambient Temperature on Hospital Admissions for Diarrhoeal Diseases in Peruvian Children." *Lancet*, 2000, *355*, 442–450.

Chretien, J. P., and others. "Drought-Associated Chikungunya Emergence Along Coastal East Africa." *American Journal of Tropical Medicine and Hygiene*, 2007, *76*(3), 405–407.

Cline, W. R. *Global Warming and Agriculture Impact Estimates by Country*. Washington, D.C.: Center for Global Development and Peterson Institute for International Economics, 2007.

Collins, W. D., and others.. "Radiative Forcing by Well-Mixed Greenhouse Gases: Estimates from Climate Models in the Intergovernmental Panel on Climate Change (IPCC) Fourth Assessment Report (AR4)." *Journal of Geophysical Research—Atmospheres*, 2006, *111*, D14317, doi:10.1029/2005JD006713.

Colwell, R. R. "Global Climate and Infectious Disease: The Cholera Paradigm." *Science*, 1996, *274*, 2025–2031.

Corfee-Morlot, J., and Agrawala, S. *The Benefits of Climate Change Policies: Analytical and Framework Issues*. Paris: Organisation for Economic Co-operation and Development, 2004.

Curriero, F., Patz, J. A., Rose, J., and Lele, S. "The Association Between Extreme Precipitation and Waterborne Disease Outbreaks in the United States, 1948–1994." *American Journal of Public Health*, 2001, *91*, 1194–1199.

Davis, R. E., Knappenberger, P. C., Michaels, P. J., and Novicoff, W. M. "Changing Heat-Related Mortality in the United States." *Environmental Health Perspectives*, 2003, *111*(14), 1712–1718.

Dwight, R. H., and others. "Association of Urban Runoff with Coastal Water Quality in Orange County, California." *Water Environment Research*, 2002, *74*(1), 82–90.

Dyson, M. E. *Come Hell or High Water: Hurricane Katrina and the Color of Disaster*. New York: Basic Books, 2007.

Ebi., K. L., Smith, J., Burton, I., Eds. *Integration of Public Health with Adaptation to Climate Change: Lessons Learned and New Directions*. Abingdon, Oxford: Taylor & Francis, 2005.

Elliott, J. R., and Pais, J. "Race, Class, and Hurricane Katrina: Social Differences in Human Responses to Disaster." *Social Science Research*, 2006, *35*, 295–321.

Emanuel, K., Sundararajan, R., and Williams, J. "Hurricanes and Global Warming: Results from Downscaling IPCC AR4 Simulations." *Bulletin of the American Meteorological Society*, 2008, *89*, 347–367.

Epstein, P. R., and others. *Healthy Solutions for the Low Carbon Economy: Guidelines for Investors, Insurers and Policy Makers.* Center for Health and the Global Environment, Harvard Medical School. http://chge.med.harvard.edu/programs/ccf/documents/healthy_solutions_report.pdf, 2008.

Etheridge, D. M., Steele, L. P., Francey, R. J., and Langenfelds, R. L. "Atmospheric Methane Between 1000 a.d. and Present: Evidence of Anthropogenic Emissions and Climatic Variability." *Journal of Geophysical Research*, 1998, *103*(15), 979–993.

Fairless, D. "Biofuel: "The Little Shrub That Could—Maybe." *Nature*, 2007, *449*(7163), 652–655.

Fearnside, P. M. "Soybean Cultivation as a Threat to the Environment in Brazil." *Environmental Conservation*, 2001, *28*(1), 23–38.

Fisher, G. T., and Katz, B. G. *Urban Stormwater Runoff: Selected Background Information and Techniques for Problem Assessment with a Baltimore, Maryland, Case Study.* U.S. Geological Survey Water-Supply Paper 2347. Reston, Va.: U.S. Geological Survey, 1988.

Food and Agriculture Organization of the United Nations. *The State of Food and Agriculture 2008: Biofuels: Prospects, Risks and Opportunities.* http://www.fao.org/sof/sofa/index_en.html, 2008.

Forkel, R., and Knoche, R. "Regional Climate Change and Its Impacts on Photooxidant Concentrations in Southern Germany: Simulations with a Coupled Regional Climate-Chemistry Model." *Journal of Geophysical Research,*, 2006, *111*, D12302, doi:10.1029/2005JD006748.

Frumkin, H., and McMichael, A. J. "Climate Change and Public Health: Thinking, Communicating, Acting." *American Journal of Preventive Medicine*, 2008, *35*, 403–410.

Frumkin, H., and others. "Climate Change: The Public Health Response." *American Journal of Public Health*, 2008, *98*, 435–445.

Galea, S., Nandi, A., and Vlahov, D. "The Epidemiology of Post-Traumatic Stress Disorder After Disasters." *Epidemiologic Reviews*, 2005, *27*, 78–91.

Galea, S., and others. "Exposure to Hurricane-Related Stressors and Mental Illness After Hurricane Katrina." *Archives of General Psychiatry*, 2007, *64*, 1427–1434.

Gibbs, H. K., and others "Carbon Payback Times for Crop-Based Biofuel Expansion in the Tropics: The Effects of Changing Yield and Technology." *Environmental Research Letters*, 2008, *3*, doi:10.1088/1748–9326/3/3/034001.

Githeko, A., and Ndegwa, W. "Predicting Malaria Epidemics in the Kenyan Highlands Using Climate Data: A Tool for Decision Makers." *Global Change & Human Health*, 2001, *2*, 54–63.

Glass, G. E., and others. "Using Remotely Sensed Data to Identify Areas of Risk for Hantavirus Pulmonary Syndrome." *Emerging Infectious Diseases*, 2000, *63*(3), 238–247.

Goldenberg, S. B., Landsea, C. W., Mestas-Nuñez, A. M., and Gray, W. M. "The Recent Increase in Atlantic Hurricane Activity: Causes and Implications." *Science*, 2001, *293*, 474–479.

Goulson, D., and others. "Predicting Calyptrate Fly Populations from the Weather, and Probable Consequences of Climate Change." *Journal of Applied Ecology*, 2005, *42*, 795–804.

Gray, W. "*Hurricanes: Their Formation, Structure and Likely Role in the Tropical Circulation.*" In D. B. Shaw (ed.), *Meteorology over the Tropical Oceans.* London: Royal Meteorology Society, 1979.

Green, B. L. "Assessing Levels of Psychological Impairment Following Disaster: Consideration of Actual and Methodological Dimensions." *Journal of Nervous and Mental Disease*, 1982, *170*, 544–548.

Gubler, D. J., and others. "Climate Variability and Change in the United States: Potential Impacts on Vector- and Rodent-Borne Diseases." *Environmental Health Perspectives*, 2001, *109*(suppl. 2), 223–233.

Guenther, A. "The Contribution of Reactive Carbon Emissions from Vegetation to the Carbon Balance of Terrestrial Ecosystems." *Chemosphere*, 2002, *49*(8), 837–844.

Gulluk, T., Slemr, F., and Stauffer, B. "Simultaneous Measurements of CO_2, CH_4, and N_2O in Air Extracted by Sublimation from Antarctica Ice Cores: Confirmation of the Data Obtained Using Other Extraction Techniques." *Journal of Geophysical Research*, 1998, *103*(15), 971–978.

Hales, S., Weinstein, P., and Woodward, A. "Ciguatera Fish Poisoning, El Niño and Pacific Sea Surface Temperatures. *Ecosystem Health*, 1999, *5*, 20–25.

Hallegraeff, G. M. "A Review of Harmful Algal Blooms and Their Apparent Global Increase." *Phycologia*, 1993, *32*(2), 79–99.

Hayhoe, K., and others. "Emissions Pathways, Climate Change, and Impacts on California." *Proceedings of the National Academy of Sciences of the United States of America*, 2004, 101(34), 12422–12427.

Hess, J. J., Malilay, J. N., and Parkinson, A. J. "Climate Change: The Importance of Place." *American Journal of Preventive Medicine*, 2008, *35*, 468–478.

Hill, J., and others. "Climate Change and Health Costs of Air Emissions from Biofuels and Gasoline." *Proceedings of the National Academy of Sciences of the United States of America*, 2009, 106(6), 2077–2082.

Himmel, M. E., and others. "Biomass Recalcitrance: Engineering Plants and Enzymes for Biofuels Production." *Science*, 2007, *315*(5813), 804–807.

Homer-Dixon, T. F. *Environment, Scarcity, Violence*. Princeton: Princeton University Press, 1999.

Hopp, M. J., and Foley, J. A. "Worldwide Fluctuations in Dengue Fever Cases Related to Climate Change." *Climate Research*, 2003, *25*, 85–94.

Horowitz, M., and Samueloff, S. "*Circulation Under Extreme Heat Load*." In P. Dejours (ed.), *Comparative Physiology of Environmental Adaptations*. Vol. *2*. Basel: Karger, 1987.

Hrudey, S. E., and others. "A Fatal Waterborne Disease Epidemic in Walkerton, Ontario: Comparison with Other Waterborne Outbreaks in the Developed World." *Water Science and Technology*, 2003, *47*(3), 7–14.

Hunt, R., Hand, D. W., Hannah, M. A., and Neal, A. M. "Response to CO_2 Enrichment in 27 Herbaceous Species." *Functional Ecology*, 1991, *5*(3), 410–421.

International Energy Agency. *Biofuels for Transport: An International Perspective*. http://www.iea.org/text-base/nppdf/free/2004/biofuels2004.pdf, 2004.

International Federation of Red Cross and Red Crescent Societies. *World Disaster Report 1997*. New York: Oxford University Press, 1998.

Jacobson, M. Z. "On the Causal Link between Carbon Dioxide and Air Pollution Mortality." *Geophysical Research Letters*, 2008, *35*(3), doi:10.1029/2007GL031101.

Kalkstein, L. S., and Tan, G. "Human Health." In K. M. Strzepek and J. B. Smith (eds.), *As Climate Changes: International Impacts and Implications*. New York: Cambridge University Press, 1995.

Kalkstein, L. S., and others. "Analog European Heat Waves for U.S. Cities to Analyze Impacts on Heat-Related Mortality." *Bulletin of the American Meteorological Society*, 2008, *89*(1), 75–85.

Kalnay, E., and Cai, M. "Impact of Urbanization and Land-Use Change on Climate." *Nature*, 2003, *423*, 528–531.

Karl, T. R., Melillo, J. M., Peterson, T. C., Eds. *Global Climate Change Impacts in the United States*. New York: Cambridge University Press, 2009. http://www.globalchange.gov/us-impacts/

Kattenberg, A., and others. "Climate Models: Projections of Future Climate." In J. Houghton and others (eds.), *Climate Change 1995: The Science of Climate Change*. Contribution of Working Group I to the Second Assessment Report of the Intergovernmental Panel on Climate Change. New York: Cambridge University Press, 1996.

Keeney, D., and Nanninga, C. *Biofuel and Global Biodiversity*. Minneapolis: Institute for Agriculture and Trade Policy, 2008. http://www.agobservatory.org/library.cfm?refid=102584.

Kessler R. C. "Mental Illness and Suicidality after Hurricane Katrina." *Bulletin of the World Health Organization*, 2006, *84*, 930–993.

Kilbourne, E. M. "Illness Due to Thermal Extremes." In R. B. Wallace (ed.), *Maxcy-Rosenau-Last Public Health and Preventive Medicine*. (14th ed.) Stamford, Conn.: Appleton & Lange, 1998.

Kilpatrick, A. M., Meola, M. A., Moudy, R. M., and Kramer, L. D. "Temperature, Viral Genetics, and the Transmission of West Nile Virus by *Culex Pipiens* Mosquitoes." *PLoS Pathogens*, 2008, *4*(6), E1000092.

Kirch, W., Menne, B., Bertollini, R., Eds. *Extreme Weather Events and Public Health Responses*. New York: Springer, 2005.

Koh, L. P., and Wilcove, D. S. "Is Oil Palm Agriculture Really Destroying Tropical Biodiversity?" *Conservation Letters*, 2008, *2*(1), 1–5.

Kovats, R. S., and others. "The Effect of Temperature on Food Poisoning: A Time-Series Analysis of Salmonellosis in Ten European Countries." *Epidemiology and Infection*, 2004, *132*(3), 443–453.

Kunkel, K. E., Easterling, D. R., Redmond, K., and Hubbard, K. "Temporal Variations of Extreme Precipitation Events in the United States: 1895–2000." *Geophysical Research Letters*, 2003, *30*, 1900, doi: 10.1029/2003GL018052.

Linthicum, K. J., and others. "Climate and Satellite Indicators to Forecast Rift Valley Fever Epidemics in Kenya." *Science*, 1999, *285*, 397–400.

Loretti, A., and Tegegn, Y. "Disasters in Africa: Old and New Hazards and Growing Vulnerability." *World Health Statistics Quarterly*, 1996, *49*, 179–184.

MacKenzie, W. R., and others. "A Massive Outbreak in Milwaukee of Cryptosporidium Infection Transmitted Through the Public Water Supply." *New England Journal of Medicine*, 1994, *331*(3), 161–167.

Marland, G., Boden, T. A., and Andres, R. J. "Global, Regional, and National Fossil Fuel CO_2 Emissions." In Carbon Dioxide Information Analysis Center, *Trends: A Compendium of Data on Global Change*. Oak Ridge, Tenn.: U.S. Department of Energy, Oak Ridge National Laboratory, 2007.

McCabe, G. J., and Bunnell, J. E. "Precipitation and the Occurrence of Lyme Disease in the Northeastern United States." *Vector Borne and Zoonotic Diseases*, 2004, *4*(2), 143–148.

McCarthy, J., and others (eds.). *Climate Change 2001: Impacts, Adaptation, and Vulnerability*. Contribution of Working Group II to the Third Assessment Report of the Intergovernmental Panel on Climate Change. New York: Cambridge University Press, 2001.

McCloskey, L. A., and Southwick, K. "Psychosocial Problems in Refugee Children Exposed to War." *Pediatrics*, 1996, *97*, 394.

McLaughlin, J. B., and others. "Outbreaks of *Vibrio Parahaemolyticus* Gastroenteritis Associated with Alaskan Oysters." *New England Journal of Medicine*, 2005, *353*(14), 1463–1470.

McMichael, A., Campbell-Lendrum, D., et al. "Climate Change." In: Ezzati, M., and others, Eds. *Comparative Quantification of Health Risks: Global and Regional Burden of Disease Due to Selected Major Risk Factors*. Geneva: World Health Organization, 2004, Vol 2, pp. 1543–1649.

Medina-Ramon, M., and Schwartz, J. "Temperature, Temperature Extremes, and Mortality: A Study of Acclimatisation and Effect Modification in 50 U.S. Cities." *Occupational and Environmental Medicine*, 2007, *64*(12), 827–833.

Menne, B., Ebi, K. L., Eds. *Climate Change and Adaptation Strategies for Human Health*. Darmstadt: Steinkopff-Verlag, 2006.

Minakawa, N., and others. "The Effects of Climatic Factors on the Distribution and Abundance of Malaria Vectors in Kenya." *Journal of Medical Entomology*, 2002, *39*(6), 833–841.

Mohan, J., E., and others. "Biomass and Toxicity Responses of Poison Ivy (*Toxicodendron Radicans*) to Elevated Atmospheric CO_2. *Proceedings of the National Academy of Sciences of the United States of America*, 2006, 103(24), 9086–9089.

Moore R., Mallonee S., Garwe T., Sabogal R. I., Zanardi L., Redd J., and Malone J. "Heat-Related Deaths—Four States, July—August 2001, and United States, 1979–1999." *Morbidity and Mortality Weekly Report*, 2002, *51*(26), 567–570.

Morris R. D., and others. "Temporal Variation in Drinking Water Turbidity and Diagnosed Gastroenteritis in Milwaukee." *American Journal of Public Health*, 1996, *86*(2), 237–239.

Morton D. C., and others. "Cropland Expansion Changes Deforestation Dynamics in the Southern Brazilian Amazon." *Proceedings of the National Academy of Sciences of the United States of America*, 2006, 103(39), 14637–14641.

Myers, N., and Kent, J. *Environmental Exodus: An Emergent Crisis in the Global Arena*. Washington, D.C.: Climate Institute, 1995.

National Agriculture Assessment Group. *Agriculture: The Potential Consequences of Climate Variability and Change for the United States*. New York: Cambridge University Press, 2002.

National Climatic Data Center. "Mitch: The Deadliest Atlantic Hurricane Since 1780." http://www.ncdc.noaa.gov/ol/reports/mitch/mitch.html, 1999.

National Research Council. *Under the Weather: Climate, Ecosystems, and Infectious Disease*. Washington, D.C.: National Academies Press, 2001.

National Safety Council, Environmental Health Center. *Climate and Weather: Backgrounder Series*. http://www.nsc.org/ehc/jrn/weather.html, 2001.

Naylor, R. L., and others. "The Ripple Effect: Biofuels, Food Security, and the Environment." *Environment*, 2007, *49*(9), 30–43.

Nicholls, N., and others. "Observed Climate Variability and Change." In J. Houghton and others (eds.), *Climate Change 1995: The Science of Climate Change*. Contribution of Working Group I to the Second Assessment Report of the Intergovernmental Panel on Climate Change. New York: Cambridge University Press, 1996.

Nicholls, R., and Leatherman, S. "Global Sea-Level Rise." In K. Strzepek and J. Smith (eds.), *As Climate Changes: International Impacts and Implications* (pp. 92–123). New York: Cambridge University Press, 1995.

Ogden, N. H., and others. "Investigation of Relationships Between Temperature and Developmental Rates of Tick *Ixodes Scapularis* (Acari: Ixodidae) in the Laboratory and Field." *Journal of Medical Entomology*, 2004, 41(4), 622–633.

Ogden, N. H., and others. "Climate Change and the Potential for Range Expansion of the Lyme Disease Vector *Ixodes Scapularis* in Canada." *International Journal for Parasitology*, 2006, *36*(1), 63–70.

Olson, S. H., and others. "Surprises in the Climate-Malaria Link in the Amazon." *Journal of Emerging Infectious Diseases*, 2009, *15*(4), 659–662.

Organisation for Economic Co-operation and Development. *Biofuel Support Policies: An Economic Assessment.* http://www.oecd.org/tad/bioenergy, 2008.

Pacala, S., and Socolow, R. "Stabilization Wedges: Solving the Climate Problem for the Next 50 Years with Current Technologies." *Science*, 2004, *305*, 968–972.

Page, E. A. *Climate Change, Justice and Future Generations.* Northampton, Mass.: Elgar, 2007.

Parmenter, R. R., and others. "Incidence of Plague Associated with Increased Winter-Spring Precipitation in New Mexico." *American Journal of Tropical Medicine and Hygiene*, 1999, *61*(5), 814–821.

Parry, M. L., and others (eds.). "Summary for Policymakers." In *Climate Change 2007: Impacts, Adaptation and Vulnerability.* Contribution of Working Group II to the Fourth Assessment Report of the Intergovernmental Panel on Climate Change. New York: Cambridge University Press, 2007.

Pascual, M., and others. "Cholera Dynamics and El Niño-Southern Oscillation." *Science*, 2000, *289*, 1766–1769.

Pastor, M. and others. *In the Wake of the Storm: Environment, Disaster and Race After Katrina.* New York: Russell Sage Foundation, 2006.

Patz, J. A. "Public Health Risk Assessment Linked to Climatic and Ecological Change." *Human and Ecological Risk Assessment*, 2001, *7*(5), 1317–1327.

Patz, J., Campbell-Lendrum, D., Gibbs, H. K., and Woodruff, R. "Health Impact Assessment of Global Climate Change: Expanding upon Comparative Risk Assessment Approaches for Policy Making." *Annual Reviews of Public Health*, 2008, *29*, 27–39.

Patz, J. A., and Kovats, R. S. "Hotspots in Climate Change and Human Health." *British Medical Journal*, 2002, *325*, 1094–1098.

Patz, J. A., Vavrus, S.J., Uejio, C.K., McLellan, SL. "Climate Change and Waterborne Disease Risk in the Great Lakes Region of the U.S." *American Journal of Preventive Medicine* 2008, *35*, 451–458.;

Patz, J. A., Martens, W.J.M., Focks, D. A., and Jetten, T. H. "Dengue Fever Epidemic Potential as Projected by General Circulating Models of Global Climate Change." *Environmental Health Perspectives*, 1998, *106*, 147–153.

Patz, J. A., and others. "Climate Change and Infectious Diseases." In A. J. McMichael and others (eds.), *Climate Change and Human Health: Risks and Responses.* Geneva: World Health Organization, 2003.

Patz, J. A., and others. *Heat Advisory: How Global Warming Causes More Bad Air Days.* NRDC Report. New York: Natural Resources Defense Council, 2004.

Patz, J. A., and others. "Climate Change and Global Health: Quantifying a Growing Ethical Crisis." *EcoHealth*, 2007, *4*, 397–405.

Pauly, D., and Alder, J. "Marine Fisheries Systems." In R. Hassan, R. Scholes, and N. Ash (eds.), *Ecosystems and Human Well-being: Current State and Trends.* Vol. 1. Washington, D.C.: Island Press, 2005.

Peperzak, L. "Future Increase in Harmful Algal Blooms in the North Sea Due to Climate Change." *Water Science and Technology*, 2005, *51*(5), 31–36.

Perciasepe, R. *Combined Sewer Overflows: Where Are We Four Years After Adoption of the CSO Control Policy?* Washington, D.C.: U. S. Environmental Protection Agency, Office of Wastewater Management, 1998.

Reilly, J. "Agriculture in a Changing Climate: Impacts and Adaptations." In R. T. Watson, M. C. Zinyowera, and R. H. Moss (eds.), *Climate Change 1995: Impacts, Adaptations, and Mitigation of Climate Change: Scientific-Technical Analyses.* Contribution of Working Group II to the Second Assessment Report of the Intergovernmental Panel on Climate Change. New York: Cambridge University Press, 1996.

Reisen, W., and Brault, A. C. "West Nile Virus in North America: Perspectives on Epidemiology and Intervention." *Pest Management Science*, 2007, *63*, 641–646.

Rezza, G., and others. "Infection with Chikungunya Virus in Italy: An Outbreak in a Temperate Region." *Lancet*, 2007, *370*(9602), 1840–1846.

Robine, J.-M., and others. "Death Toll Exceeded 70,000 in Europe During the Summer of 2003." *Comptes Rendus Biologies*, 2008, *331*, 171–178.

Rodo, X., Pascual, M., Fuchs, G., and Faruque, A. S. "ENSO and Cholera: A Nonstationary Link Related to Climate Change?" *Proceedings of the National Academy of Sciences of the United States of America*, 2002, *99*(20), 12901–12906.

Rose, J. B., and Simonds, J. *King County Water Quality Assessment: Assessment of Public Health Impacts Associated with Pathogens and Combined Sewer Overflows.* Olympia: Washington State Department of Natural Resources, 1998.

Rosenzweig, C., Parry, M. L., Fischer, G., and Frohberg, K. Climate Change and World Food Supply. Research Report No. 3. Oxford, U.K.: Oxford University, Environmental Change Unit, 1993.

Running, S. W. "Is Global Warming Causing More, Larger Wildfires?" *Science*, 2006, *313*, 927–928.

Schimhuber, J., and Tubiello, F. N. "Global Food Security Under Climate Change." *Proceedings of the National Academy of Sciences of the United States of America*, 2007, *104*, 19703–19708.

Schipper, E. L., Burton, I., Eds. *The Earthscan Reader on Adaptation to Climate Change.* London: Earthscan, 2009.

Schuster, C. J., and others. "Infectious Disease Outbreaks Related to Drinking Water in Canada, 1974–2001." *Canadian Journal of Public Health*, 2005, *96*(4), 254–258.

Schwartz, J., Levin, R., and Hodge, K. "Drinking Water Turbidity and Pediatric Hospital Use for Gastrointestinal Illness in Philadelphia." *Epidemiology*, 1997, *8*(6), 615–620.

Sergon, K., and others. "Seroprevalence of Chikungunya Virus (CHIKV) Infection on Lamu Island, Kenya, October." *American Journal of Tropical Medicine and Hygiene*, 2008, *78*(2), 333–337.

Shaman, J., and others. "Using a Dynamic Hydrology Model to Predict Mosquito Abundances in Flood and Swamp Water." *Emerging Infectious Diseases*, 2002, *8*(1), 6–13.

Solomon, S, and others (eds.). *Climate Change 2007: The Physical Science Basis.* Working Group I Contribution to the Fourth Assessment Report of the Intergovernmental Panel on Climate Change. New York: Cambridge University Press, 2007.

Stenseth, N. C., and others. "Plague Dynamics Are Driven by Climate Variation." *Proceedings of the National Academy of Sciences of the United States of America*, 2006, *103*(35),13110–13115.

Stroeve, J., and others. "Arctic Sea Ice Decline: Faster Than Forecast." *Geophysical Research Letters*, 2007, *34*, L09501, doi:10.1029/2007GL029703.

Taub, D. R., Miller, B., and Allen, H. "Effects of Elevated CO_2 on the Protein Concentration of Food Crops: A Meta-Analysis." *Global Change Biology*, 2008, *14*, 565–575.

Taylor, L. H., Latham, S. M., and Woolhouse, M. E. "Risk Factors for Human Disease Emergence." *Philosophical Transactions of the Royal Society of London Part B: Biological Sciences*, 2001, *356*, 983–989.

Tester, P. A., and others. "An Expatriate Red Tide Bloom, Transport, Distribution, and Persistence." *Limnology and Oceanography*, 1991, *36*, 1053–1061.

Thompson, J. R., and others. "Diversity and Dynamics of a North Atlantic Coastal *Vibrio* Community. *Applied and Environmental Microbiology*," 2004, *70*(7), 4103–4110.

Toole, M., and Waldman, R. "The Public Health Aspects of Complex Emergencies and Refugee Situations." *Annual Review of Public Health*, 1997, *18*, 283–312.

Torn, M. S., Mills, E., and Fried, J. *Will Climate Change Spark More Wildfire Damage?* LBNL Report No. 42592. Lawrence, Calif.: Lawrence Berkeley National Laboratory, 1998.

Trenberth, K. "Uncertainty in Hurricanes and Global Warming." *Science*, 2005. *308*, 1753–1754.

Trevejo, R. T., and others. "Epidemic Leptospirosis Associated with Pulmonary Hemorrhage: Nicaragua, 1995." *Journal of Infectious Diseases*, 1998, *178*, 1457–1463.

Tubiello, F. N., Soussana, J.-F., Howden, S. M., and Easterling, W. "Crop and Pasture Response to Climate Change." *Proceedings of the National Academy of Sciences of the United States of America*, 2007, *104*, 19686–19690.

UN-Energy. *Sustainable Bioenergy: A Framework for Decision Makers*. New York: United Nations, 2007.

United Nations Environment Programme. "Potential Impact of Sea-Level Rise on Bangladesh." Vital Climate Graphics. http://www.gridano/publications/vg/climate/page/3086.aspx, 2002.

Van Dolah, F. M. "Marine Algal Toxins: Origins, Health Effects, and Their Increased Occurrence." *Environmental Health Perspectives*, 2000, *108*(suppl. 1), 133–141.

Vavrus, S., and Van Dorn, J. "Projected Future Temperature and Precipitation Extremes in Chicago." *Journal of Great Lakes Research*, forthcoming.

Wayne, P., and others. "Production of Allergenic Pollen by Ragweed (*Ambrosia Artemisiifolia L.*) Is Increased in CO_2-Enriched Atmospheres." *Annals of Allergy, Asthma & Immunology*, 2002, *88*(3), 279–282.

Webster, P. J., Holland, G. J., Curry, J. A., and Chang, H.-R. "Changes in Tropical Cyclone Number, Duration, and Intensity in a Warming Environment." *Science*, 2005, *309*, 1844–1846.

Westerling, A. L., Hidalgo, H. G., Cayan, D. R., and Swetnam, T. W. "Warming and Earlier Spring Increase Western U.S. Forest Wildfire Activity." *Science*, 2006, *313*, 940–943.

Whitman, S., and others. "Mortality in Chicago Attributed to the July 1995 Heat Wave." *American Journal of Public Health*, 1997, *87*, 1515–1518.

Wilkinson, P., and others. "Energy, Energy Efficiency, and the Built Environment." *Lancet*, 2007, *370*, 1175–1187.

World Health Organization. *World Health Report 1996: Fighting Disease, Fostering Development*. Geneva: World Health Organization, 1996.

World Health Organization. *World Health Report 2002: Reducing Risks, Promoting Healthy Life*. Geneva: World Health Organization, 2002.

Younger, M., Morrow-Almeida, H. R., Vindigni, S. M., and Dannenberg, A. L. "The Built Environment, Climate Change, and Health: Opportunities for Co-Benefits." *American Journal of Preventive Medicine*, 2008, *35*, 517–526.

Ziska, L. H. "Evaluation of the Growth Response of Six Invasive Species to Past, Present and Future Atmospheric Carbon Dioxide." *Journal of Experimental Botany*, 2003, *54*(381), 395–404.

Zhang, D. D., and others. "Global Climate Change, War, and Population Decline in Recent Human History." *Proceedings of the National Academy of Sciences*, 2007, *104*, 19214–19219, doi:10.1073/pnas.0703073104.

Ziska, L., and Caulfield, F. "The Potential Influence of Rising Atmospheric Carbon Dioxide (CO_2) on Public Health: Pollen Production of the Common Ragweed as a Test Case." *World Resources Review*, 2000, *12*, 449–457.

Ziska, L. H., and others. "Cities as Harbingers of Climate Change: Common Ragweed, Urbanization, and Public Health." *Journal of Allergy and Clinical Immunology*, 2003, *111*(2), 290–295.

FOR FURTHER INFORMATION

Review Articles

McMichael, A. J., Woodruff, R. E., and Hales, S. "Climate Change and Human Health: Present and Future Risks." *Lancet*, 2006, *367*, 859–869.

Patz, J. A., Campbell-Lendrum, D., Holloway, T., and Foley, J. A. "Impact of Regional Climate Change on Human Health." *Nature*, 2005, *438*,: 310-317.

Patz, J. A., Olson, S. H., Uejio, C. K., and Gibbs, H. K. "Disease Emergence from Climate and Land Use Change. *Medical Clinics of North America*, 2008, *92*, 1473–1491.

Reports

Intergovernmental Panel on Climate Change (IPCC), http://www.ipcc.ch. IPCC reports represent some of the most authoritative and exhaustive synthesis assessments, and following the publication of its fourth assessment report in 2007, the IPCC—along with Al Gore—received the 2007 Nobel Peace Prize. Full and summary reports and downloadable graphs and figures are available from the IPCC Web site.

U.S. Environmental Protection Agency (EPA), http://www.epa.gov/climatechange/effects/health.html. This informative EPA site covers the many sectors affected by climate change. The agency also published a new assessment on health in 2008, *Analyses of the Effects of Global Change on Human Health and Welfare and Human Systems* (http://www.climatescience.gov/Library/sap/sap4-6/final-report/sap4-6-final-front-matter.pdf), which analyzes the impacts of global change, especially those of climate variability and change, on three broad dimensions of the human condition: human health, human settlements, and human welfare.

World Health Organization (WHO), http://www.who.int/globalchange/climate/en. WHO has been assessing the health risks of climate change for nearly two decades, and this Web site contains links to WHO reports and ongoing projects.

Blogs

RealClimate, http://www.realclimate.org. A blog containing commentaries by climate scientists that sort out the often polarizing or conflicting stories in the mainstream press. Discussions are restricted to climate science topics (and not political or economic implications). Posting are signed by the author(s) so you know exactly from where the information comes.

Dot Earth, http://dotearth.blogs.nytimes.com. An interactive blog that explores trends and ideas with readers and experts. World-renowned reporter Andrew C. Revkin carefully follows and reports on climate change science and policy.

Materials for Teachers

EcoHealth, http://ecohealth101.org. A source of useful information and student exercises for middle and high school teachers and students. Topics (and lesson plans) include human health effects of climate change, ozone depletion, biodiversity and land use change, mechanized intensive agriculture, and globalization.

GRID-Arendal, http://www.grida.no. A collaborating center of UNEP. The mission of this site (which was established in 1989 by the Government of Norway) is to communicate environmental information to policymakers and facilitate environmental decision making for change.

CHAPTER ELEVEN

DEVELOPING NATIONS

JEROME NRIAGU

JAYMIE MELIKER

MARKEY JOHNSON

KEY CONCEPTS

■ The disease burden in developing countries, as measured by mortality, morbidity, and disability-adjusted life years, is elevated relative to that of wealthy countries.

■ Some of the major drivers (root causes) of these health disparities relate to environmental problems.

■ Globalization affects health in developing countries in many ways.

■ The transition to current patterns of development exposes individuals in developing countries to changing of contaminants and health risks and may aggravate health disparities.

■ Special health risks in developing countries are associated with agriculture, nutrition, water, air, motor vehicles, and disasters.

■ Rapid urban development in developing countries is associated with risks to human health.

THE health and disease patterns of societies and communities evolve in response to environmental, technological, biotic, demographic, social, economic, and cultural stimuli. The twenty-first century has dawned with the human population distributed into three distinct worlds: the **First World** (also referred to as developed countries, "Upper Earth," or developed economies), **Second World** (high-income developing countries, "Middle Earth," or developing economies) and **Third World** (low-income developing countries, "Lower Earth," or underdeveloped economies).

ONE EARTH, THREE WORLDS

The **postindustrial** countries of the First World are immersed in high technology, with glittering advances in electronics, medical research, genomic manipulation, fiber optics, synthetic materials, alloys, and fabrication processes. In this world, people's lives revolve around virtual entertainment, cash-free and Internet shopping, mobile phones, rapid transportation, and on-demand mass production. This is a culture of smart bombs and automobiles, cloned animals and human parts, space exploration, robotics, weapons of mass destruction, and an impressive computerization of most business and home life—but diminished connection to the natural environment (Meister, 2001). In this setting health statistics are dominated by degenerative and man-made diseases such as hyperlipidemias, obesity, diabetes, cardiovascular diseases, and neuropsychiatric disorders. The Second World countries are consumed by the desire to attain First World status. These countries feature rapid industrial, technological, and social change, with little concern for the attendant environmental pollution. For the Third World countries most things are going wrong. They have limited or poor management of natural resources, high infant and maternal mortality rates, low literacy and education, political instability, corrupt political leaders and governmental institutions, untrained manpower and flight of capital, vandalism by military and law enforcement officers, civil strife, famine, deteriorated educational, medical, and business infrastructures, depleted agricultural soils, and a high burden of endemic and communicable disease morbidity and mortality (Meister, 2001). How to reconcile these disparities into a cooperative framework, in which the three worlds

This document has been reviewed in accordance with U.S. Environmental Protection Agency policy and approved for publication. Mention of trade names or commercial products does not constitute endorsement or recommendation for use. In addition, Jerome Nriagu, Jaymie Meliker, and Markey Johnson declare no competing financial interests.

coexist and in which the planetary ecosystem is protected, is currently under intense discussion.

The dawn of the new millennium also reflects a major transition in the health of human populations, marked by disturbing evidence of widening gaps in health among the three worlds. During the second half of the twentieth century the global average life expectancy at birth increased by almost 20 years, from about 46.5 years in the period from 1950 to 1955 to 65.2 years in 2002. This gain is not uniformly distributed; in 2002, life expectancy ranged from 78 years for women in developed countries to less than 46 years for men in sub-Saharan Africa (World Health Organization [WHO], 2003). For millions of children in Africa, the biggest health challenge today is to survive until their fifth birthday, and their chances of doing so are less than they were a decade ago. In many Third World countries, local and regional environmental problems are major contributors to disease and death. Inadequate supplies of clean water, poor sanitation, smoky cooking fuels, waste accumulation in neighborhoods, disease-carrying pests, improper use of pesticides, foodborne illness exacerbated by poor handling and preservation techniques, and poor housing and overcrowded conditions are closely interrelated environmental processes. Virtually anyone living, working, and socializing in many Third World neighborhoods is exposed to environmental hazards, with children, women, and the elderly being particularly vulnerable (Thomas, Seager, and Mathee, 2002).

People in most countries of the Third World are disproportionately exposed to the so-called **traditional hazards** (generally associated with lack of development), which differ from the **modern hazards** (Second World) of uncontrolled industrial development and the **postmodern hazards** (First World) of sedentary lifestyles and material excess. As countries or regions shift from one economic level to another, the change in exposure patterns and in associated health risks can be described as a **risk transition** (Sims and Butter, 2000). In many countries of the Second and Third Worlds, the processes of globalization and industrialization often result in simultaneous exposure to both traditional and modern environmental hazards, a double jeopardy known as **risk overlap**. Squalid urban areas exemplify the mixed environmental hazards faced in many developing countries. In addition, **ecological risk traps** may arise, that is, major polluting industries may be located in a fairly isolated, nonadaptive traditional community. In these situations the overlay of the toxic effects of industrial emissions on the traditional risks may overwhelm a population's coping capacity, with catastrophic consequences.

The Changing Disease Burden in the Third World

Of the 57 million people who died in 2002, almost 20 percent (10.5 million) were children less than five years old. Nearly 98 percent of the child deaths occurred in the developing countries (WHO, 2003). Of the twenty countries in the world with the highest child mortality, nineteen are in Africa, the exception being Afghanistan. A baby born in Sierra Leone is 100 times more likely than a child born in Singapore or Iceland to die before the age of five. On the other end of the demographic spectrum, over 60 percent of deaths in developed countries involved people over the age of seventy, compared to 10 percent in African countries (WHO, 2003). The probability of death is remarkably different in the three worlds, with the death rates in Third World countries being much higher and occurring at younger ages.

A demographic revolution is clearly underway throughout the world (see Chapter Nine). There are now about 600 million people aged sixty years and over in the world, and this total is expected to reach 2 billion by 2050, with the vast majority being in the developing countries (WHO, 2003). It is projected that older people will make up more than 15 percent of the total population in countries like Brazil, China, and Thailand by 2025, and in Colombia, Indonesia, and Kenya their number will increase up to fourfold during the next twenty-five years (WHO, 2003). Population aging is propelled by two overlapping factors: a decline in fertility rates among the overall population, resulting in a reduction in the proportion of children, and an increase in the proportion of older people as mortality rates decline (Kinsella, 2001). The effect of the environment on this **demographic transition**, in terms of the health of the elderly population, needs more attention than it is currently getting. In developed countries aging populations have an increased prevalence of chronic diseases and disability. These health trends will likely be different in Third World countries, where a compounding of risk factors for communicable diseases and age-related chronic diseases will present an unpredictable but challenging set of health problems.

The disparity between the First and Third World countries in adult mortality risk continues to widen. Almost 75 percent of the 45 million deaths in 2002 involving adults aged fifteen years and over were caused by noncommunicable diseases. Communicable diseases and maternal, perinatal, and nutritional conditions accounted for 8.2 million adult deaths (representing about 18 percent of all deaths), whereas injuries killed 4.5 million adults in 2002 (WHO, 2003). As shown in Table 11.1, the principal attributable causes of death in developing countries are childhood and maternal undernutrition, exposure to environmental risks, and unsafe sexual practices, whereas diet-related risks are the leading cause of death in the developed countries.

Although mortality statistics are generally the simplest measure of population health status, they fail to estimate the true disease burden because they do not account for morbidity and disability. Some effort has therefore been made to derive composite measures that can better describe the health status of populations.

TABLE 11.1 Attributable Mortality by Risk Factor, Level of Development, and Gender, 2000

Risk Factor	High-Mortality Developing		Low-Mortality Developing		Developed	
	Male	Female	Male	Female	Male	Female
Total deaths (in thousands)	13,758	12,654	8,584	7,373	6,890	6,601
Childhood and maternal undernutrition						
Underweight	12.6%	13.4%	1.8%	1.9%	0.1%	0.1%
Iron deficiency	2.2	3.0	0.8	1.0	0.1	0.2
Vitamin A deficiency	2.3	3.3	0.2	0.4	<0.1	<0.1
Zinc deficiency	2.8	3.0	0.2	0.2	<0.1	<0.1
Other diet-related risks and physical inactivity						
Blood pressure	7.4	7.5	12.7	15.1	20.1	23.9
Cholesterol	5.0	5.7	5.1	5.6	14.5	17.6
Body mass index	1.1	2.0	4.2	5.6	9.6	11.5
Low fruit and vegetable intake	3.6	3.5	5.0	4.8	7.6	7.4
Physical inactivity	2.3	2.3	2.8	3.2	6.0	6.7
Sexual and reproductive health risks						
Unsafe sex	9.3	10.9	0.8	1.3	0.2	0.6
Lack of contraception	NA	1.1	NA	0.2	NA	0.0
Addictive substances						
Smoking and oral tobacco	7.5	1.5	12.2	2.9	26.3	9.3
Alcohol	2.6	0.6	8.5	1.6	8.0	20.3
Illicit drugs	0.5	0.1	0.6	0.1	0.6	0.3
Environmental risks						
Unsafe water, sanitation, and hygiene	5.8	5.9	1.1	1.1	0.2	0.2
Urban air pollution	0.9	0.8	2.5	2.9	1.1	1.2
Indoor smoke from solid fuels	3.6	4.3	1.9	5.4	0.1	0.2

(continued)

TABLE 11.1 (Continued)

Risk Factor	High-Mortality Developing		Low-Mortality Developing		Developed	
	Male	Female	Male	Female	Male	Female
Lead exposure	0.4	0.3	0.5	0.3	0.7	0.4
Climate change	**0.5**	<0.6	<0.1	<0.1	<0.1	<0.1
Occupational risks						
Risk factors for injury	1.0	0.1	1.4	0.1	0.4	0.0
Carcinogens	0.1	,0.1	0.5	0.2	0.8	0.2
Airborne particulates	0.3	,0.1	1.6	0.2	0.6	0.1
Ergonomic stressors	0.0	0.0	0.0	0.0	0.0	0.0
Noise	0.0	0.0	0.0	0.0	0.0	0.0
Other selected risks to health						
Unsafe health care injections	1.1	0.9	1.8	0.9	0.1	0.1
Childhood sexual abuse	0.1	0.2	0.1	0.2	0.1	0.1

Source: WHO, 2002.

One such approach is the **disability-adjusted life years (DALYs)** concept (Murray and Lopez, 1996), which combines **years of life lost (YLL)** through premature death with **years lived with disability (YLD)**. One DALY can be thought of as one lost year of healthy life, and the measured disease burden is the gap between the health status of a given population and that of a normative global reference population with high life expectancy lived in full health. The DALY figures for different regions of the world (Figure 11.1) provide a guide to the relative distribution of disease burdens; the higher the DALYs, the greater the burden. The leading risk factors for the global burden of disease are shown in Table 11.2. Most of these disease and disability categories have direct or indirect environmental components, although in different ways and to different degrees. Among the leading environmentally related risk factors are being underweight or having nutritional insufficiencies (undernutrition is the leading single risk factor, accounting for over 9 percent of global DALYs), having an inadequate water supply and sanitation (sixth-ranked), and being exposed to indoor air pollution, lead pollution, outdoor air pollution, and climate change. It has been estimated that 25 to 30 percent of the global disease burden is attributable to environmental factors (Smith, Corvalán, and Kjellström, 1999), and this estimate does not include environmental contributions to the etiology of other diseases.

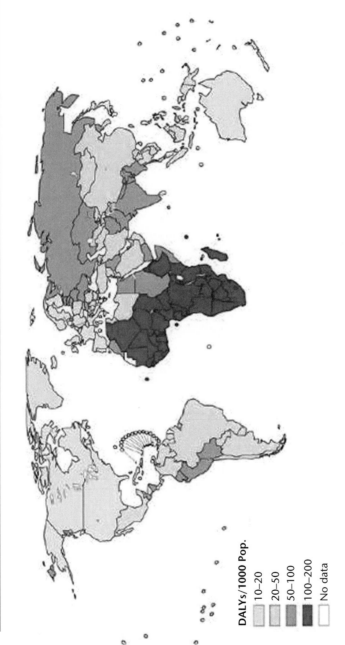

DALYs/1000 Pop.

10–20

20–50

50–100

100–200

No data

Source: Prüss-Ustün and Corvalán, 2006. Reprinted with permission of Elsevier.

TABLE 11.2   Attributable DALYs by Risk Factor, Level of Development, and Sex, 2000

Risk Factors	High-Mortality Developing		Low-Mortality Developing		Developed	
	Male	Female	Male	Female	Male	Female
Total DALYs (in thousands)	420,711	412,052	223,181	185,316	117,670	96,543
Childhood and maternal undernutrition						
Underweight	14.9%	15.0%	3.0%	3.3%	0.4%	0.4%
Iron deficiency	2.8	3.5	1.5	2.2	0.5	1.0
Vitamin A deficiency	2.6	3.5	0.3	0.4	<0.1	<0.1
Zinc deficiency	3.2	3.2	0.3	0.3	0.1	0.1
Other diet-related risks and physical inactivity						
Blood pressure	2.6	2.4	4.9	5.1	11.2	10.6
Cholesterol	1.9	1.9	2.2	2.0	8.0	7.0
Body mass index	0.6	1.0	2.3	3.2	6.9	8.1
Low fruit and vegetable intake	1.3	1.2	2.0	1.8	4.3	3.4
Physical inactivity	0.9	0.8	1.2	1.3	3.3	3.2
Sexual and reproductive health risks						
Unsafe sex	9.4	11.0	1.2	1.6	0.5	1.1
Lack of contraception	NA	1.8	NA	0.6	NA	0.1
Addictive substances						
Smoking and oral tobacco	3.4	0.6	6.2	1.3	17.1	6.2
Alcohol	2.6	0.5	9.8	2.0	14.0	3.3
Illicit drugs	0.8	0.2	1.2	0.3	2.3	1.2
Environmental risks						
Unsafe water, sanitation, and hygiene	5.5	5.6	1.7	1.8	0.4	0.4
Urban air pollution	0.4	0.3	1.0	0.9	0.6	0.5

Indoor smoke from solid fuels	3.7	3.6	1.5	2.3	0.2	0.3
Lead exposure	0.8	0.7	1.4	1.4	0.8	0.5
Climate change	0.6	0.7	0.1	0.1	<0.1	<0.1
Occupational risks						
Risk factors for injury	1.5	0.1	2.1	0.3	1.0	0.1
Carcinogens	0.1	<0.1	0.2	0.1	0.4	0.1
Airborne particulates	0.1	0.0	0.8	0.1	0.4	0.1
Ergonomic stressors	0.0	0.0	0.1	0.1	0.1	0.1
Noise	0.3	0.1	0.5	0.3	0.4	0.3
Other selected risks to health						
Unsafe health care injections	0.9	0.8	1.1	0.5	0.1	0.1
Childhood sexual abuse	0.3	0.7	0.5	0.8	0.3	1.0

Source: WHO, 2003.

Estimated DALYs for children and young adults for 2002 show a disproportionate burden of disease in Third World countries compared to the developed countries. About 40 percent of the lost years of healthy life in Third World countries in 2002 resulted from diseases in children younger than five, compared to only 6 percent for the same age group in developed countries (WHO, 2003).

There are large disparities in the environmentally related disease burden for various segments of the population. For instance, children less than five years old make up only 12 percent of the global population but account for about 43 percent of the total disease burden due to environmental risks (Smith, 2002; Smith and others, 1999). Even when the DALY is standardized with respect to age, there are still significant differences in morbidity burden between developing and developed countries. As a result of demographic trends, lifestyle transitions, and changes in the distribution of environmental risk factors (associated primarily with migration to overcrowded urban areas), there has been a rapid increase in the incidence of noncommunicable diseases (such as asthma, food-related chronic diseases, and neuropsychiatric conditions) in Third World communities. Most developing countries now face a double burden made up of both communicable and noncommunicable diseases. Furthermore, disabilities tend to be more prevalent and more severe in developing countries because risks cluster among highly vulnerable subpopulations and accumulate over time (WHO, 2003). As a result of the risk overlap, the Third World populations may confront more complex and more diverse patterns of disease than populations in developed countries do; they not only face a higher risk of premature death but also live a higher proportion of their lives with poor health.

DRIVERS OF ENVIRONMENTAL HEALTH

Factors that motivate, stimulate, or push the environmental processes that affect human health are referred to here as **environmental drivers**. These factors include population growth, technological and economic development, changing lifestyles and social attitudes, natural processes of change in the physical environment, policy interventions, and the long-term impacts of past human interventions. These drivers contribute both directly and indirectly to **health disparities** among the three worlds. With increases in population, for example, more and more people must live in limited space and in close proximity with others, and the resulting crowding contributes to health inequalities. Aggregation of people into urban areas and the resulting environmental damage and resource depletion are currently most marked in the developing countries. Unable to meet the staggering demands for basic amenities, Indian cities, for example, are characterized by teeming hovels, dirt and garbage, overcrowded and noisy lanes, and a proliferation of slums. Population growth can intensify human activities in given areas, thereby contributing to environmental damage and resource depletion. It drives the expansion of human populations into marginal areas and ecologically fragile zones and in the process makes the population vulnerable to environmental hazards.

It would be impossible within one chapter to provide a full description of all the environmental drivers of human health in developing countries. Instead, we have chosen four examples (predicated on our research interests, experience and previous work) to illustrate the complex, multidimensional phenomena that can result in health disparities between the developed and developing countries. We focus on vulnerability and coping capacity, globalization, agriculture and food security, and urbanization.

Vulnerability and Coping Capacity

The vulnerability of any human population to external stresses is a function of exposure, sensitivity, and adaptive capacity (Yohe and Tol, 2002). Adaptation includes changes in management activities, institutional settings, and infrastructure that enable effective responses to alterations in the environment. The concepts of **vulnerability**, **adaptation**, **adaptive capacity**, **coping capacity**, and **resilience** are interrelated and can provide an interesting framework for examining health disparities at the individual, local, and global levels. Working with this framework, one undeniable truth has emerged; namely that there is huge difference in the vulnerability and coping capacity of people in different parts of the world at the beginning of the twenty-first century. Factors that have increased the vulnerability of Third World countries to environmental degradation include the limited range of available technological options for adaptation; low availability and maldistribution of resources; poor institutional infrastructure; a small supply of trained human capital and security personnel; a limited stock of social capital, including community-oriented services; lack of access to information on risk-spreading processes; inability of decision makers to manage information and the low credibility of the decision makers themselves; and complacency and lack of knowledge about the sources of external stress and the significance of exposure and its local manifestations.

In sub-Saharan Africa, over 60 percent of the population lives in ecologically vulnerable areas characterized by a high degree of sensitivity and low degree of resilience to environmental change. The millions of people who depend directly on natural resources from the fragile ecosystems of Africa are therefore more vulnerable than other peoples to environmental changes. Unsustainable practices such as deforestation, loss of biodiversity, water pollution, and unsuitable agricultural practices and animal husbandry, compounded by climatic variability, contribute to reductions in environmental quality and increase the vulnerability of populations that are dependent on natural resources. Degradation of resources reduces the natural resource capital and productivity of the poor who rely primarily on such resources. Once drawn into the vicious cycle, the poor become even more susceptible to stressors such as drought, floods, economic fluctuations, and civil strife. Their poverty impedes recovery from these events and weakens social and ecological resilience, especially given that the poor are unable to invest in natural resources management. The vulnerability may be exacerbated by the affects of climate variations on biophysical support systems, thereby further reducing the coping ability of most people to live in environmentally fragile areas.

Two main elements of human vulnerability are exposure to environmental hazards (stressors, shocks, and contingencies) and coping capacity, which can offer security in the face of exposure. People who have the means and capacity to cope with the risks, shocks, stresses, and demands of environmental change tend to be better buffered, more resilient, and hence more secure against associated health consequences. Human **environmental vulnerability** occurs along a continuum ranging from highly vulnerable (undesirable) to highly secure (desirable). For any given population, the vulnerability-security continuum contains the following four categories (United Nations Environment Programme [UNEP], 2002):

1. High risk and low coping capacity
2. High risk and high coping capacity
3. Low risk and low coping capacity
4. Low risk and high coping capacity

Having low risk and high coping capacity is the desired ideal scenario. Most African countries and many developing nations in other parts of the world fall into the category of having high risk and low coping capacity. In contrast, the United States falls under the scenario of high risk and high coping capacity. This disparity is illustrated by the fact that although two to three times as many disaster events were reported in the United States as in India or Bangladesh in 1999, there were fourteen times more deaths in India and thirty-four times more deaths in Bangladesh from disasters (UNEP, 2002).

Coping strategies for environmental degradation have many dimensions, from traditional to scientific (UNEP, 2002). For millennia, traditional communities in Africa have adapted to environmental changes in various ways, from migrating to shifting livelihood activities according to seasons. They developed strategies for managing resources sustainably so as to avoid overexploitation and enhance their own food security. Recent decades, however, have been marked by high risks of disasters (earthquakes, floods, droughts, forest fires, civil strife, and wars and armed conflicts) which have increased poverty and hunger and aggravated health problems. In many African countries where exposure to natural risk is minimal, human-induced stressors have apparently increased vulnerability. The stressors (and disasters), whether natural or human-induced, have displaced populations within and across national borders and in the process increased vulnerability and insecurity. The impacts have affected the poor disproportionately because they have the least coping capacity. An emerging impact of human vulnerability to degradation of natural systems is the creation of environmental refugees by the forced movement of people. The term **environmental refugee** describes the phenomenon of large numbers of the world's least secure people being forced to seek refuge from insecure and hazardous biophysical environments. It is esti-mated that there were more than 25 million environmental refugees worldwide in 1994, with most of them in African countries (Myers, 2002). The number of environmental refugees has increased significantly since then and is projected to reach 50 million by 2010 (Conisbee and Simms, 2003), contributing to the growing health disparities between the First and Third World countries.

Globalization: Bad Medicine for Developing Countries

The twenty-first century is a time of tumultuous change in which economic inter-dependence is increasing rapidly, information technology is accelerating the spread of ideas, human influence on natural cycles and processes has become evident on a global scale, and the spread of an infectious disease around the globe is only a plane ride away. This process of interlocking economic, social, technological, political, and cultural changes emerging around the world has been called **globalization**, a phenomenon that is shrinking space and increasing the speed of interaction, changing our views of the world and of ourselves, and breaking down national and cultural barriers. An unmistakable outcome of the globalization phenomenon so far is that as the economies grow, people in the First World get richer, some in the Second World escape poverty, and disparities with the Third World widen. The wealth and health in one world are increasingly being created at the cost of development in the other two worlds, and the imbalance is marginalizing a majority of the people on the planet. This scenario has led to debate on the likely effects of globalization on the environment-health interface.

On the one hand, proponents of globalization argue that health is a crucial resource because it is linked to the stability and security that foreign investors seek. A healthy population is a critical asset for the development of a country, and businesses are more likely to invest in communities where the health risks are manageable. Proponents see globalization as providing economic, technological, and social opportunities for renewed commitments to the environment and community health. Free enterprise on a global economic playing field, leveled by international agreements to reduce market barriers, should, they argue, usher in an age of affluence for all and lift everyone to a new height of well-being. Cuts in agricultural subsidies and the opening of trade in agricultural products should increase efficiency and raise the income of farmers.

Proponents also point to the promise of technological diffusion. Agriculture, they maintain, will benefit from progress in biotechnology, which will increase yields and reduce the pressure on natural resources in many countries. Improvements in irrigation techniques will minimize the health effects of water resource developments. Advances in technology and structural changes in economies will produce social and environmental benefits by reducing production and delivery costs. The development and spread of more efficient vehicles that run on cleaner fuels will reduce the consumption of fossil fuels and the emission of pollutants from this source. Deregulation will open up micropower development, especially in rural areas of Third World countries, where the power supply has been limited by the high cost of electrical grids (UNEP, 2002). Advances in nanotechnology should improve material use efficiency, and biotechnology can have positive effects on wastewater treatment and remediation of contaminated sites. Supporters thus trust globalization and liberalization to generate corporate wealth, spur new technologies, and create new enterprises that improve people's livelihoods and help communities pay for social and health programs and abate environmental problems.

On the other hand, there is growing concern over the damaging effects of global markets on the distribution of health risks. Critics note the accumulation of wealth and power in just a few transnational corporations and countries, far removed from areas where the wastes of unbridled economic growth accumulate. They see unequal expansion of modern production methods around the world, with a disproportionate number of highly polluting industries being located in Third World countries. They worry about two-track, market-driven global development that divides humanity into privileged and excluded, North and South, and modernist and traditionalist factions. They perceive manipulative and one-sided (selfish) approaches to global negotiations and unfair international agreements on sustainable development. Too often the focus of international health agreements has been on technological fixes that originate in First World countries rather than on indigenous interventions to improve the health of local communities. Many are apprehensive that globalization's legacy to their children will be an impoverished, contaminated, and fragile world that is economically, ecologically, and socially depleted. Critics consider the emerging global consumer culture that encourages lifestyles based on individualism and greed to be a fundamental threat to the social fabric of many communities in Third World countries.

Globalization clearly produces major driving forces that can change environmental health risks on the global, regional, and local scales. The transnational forces of globalization, especially the massive movements of goods and people, alter the risk and susceptibility of local populations to ill health and disease. The movement of health hazards from the First World to the Second and Third Worlds (including the export of firearms, industrial wastes, and pollution), the heavy and inefficient use of energy, the production of greenhouse gases leading to global warming, and the plundering of natural resources and spoliation of the environment add to existing environmental risk factors. Table 11.3 shows some likely direct and indirect effects of globalization on environmental health risks in developing countries. It is clear that the effect of globalization on health involves many diffuse determinants and overlapping risks and that the critical determinants of health in many developing countries are increasingly global and cannot simply be attributed to individual nations. Many of the transnational factors noted in Table 11.3, driven by privatization-oriented policies of international institutions, seem to be at odds with the sociocultural constructs

TABLE 11.3 Effects of Globalization on the Health of People in Developing Countries

Global Transnational Factor	Consequence and Probable Impact on Health Risks in Developing Countries
Environmental degradation and unsustainable consumption patterns	
Resource depletion (arable land, freshwater, and forestry products)	Reduced standard of living leading to hunger, undernutrition, unsafe water, poor sanitation and hygiene; higher indoor pollution from burning wood substitutes; potential violence between countries
Water and air pollution	Regional and local environmental health impacts; exacerbation of existing endemic diseases
Ozone depletion and increased ultraviolet radiation	Changes in composition of local fauna and flora leading to malnutrition; toxification of human food chain; increased prevalence of systemic disorders (skin and eye)
Accumulation of greenhouse gases and global warming	Major shifts in infectious disease patterns and vector distribution; increased trauma due to frequent weather disasters (such as storms and floods) and worsening food shortages; reduced soil productivity in tropical countries; increased exposure to thermal extremes (cardiovascular and respiratory mortality)
Food security	
Increased export of cash crops to developed countries	Shortage of staple local foods as manpower and resources go into producing export crops; higher prices for locally produced foods, making them unaffordable to the poor
Increased global food trade and a decline in food aid	Food shortages in marginalized countries; increased migration and civil unrest
Overfishing to meet growing demand for seafood	Reduced supply of fish protein in coastal communities; destruction of traditional lifestyles
Increased use of pesticides and fertilizers	Exposure to toxic residues in foods; toxic metals introduced into food chain through fertilizer use
Import of protein-rich and sugared foods	Increased health problems from overnutrition (such as high blood pressure, high cholesterol, and obesity)

(continued)

TABLE 11.3   (Continued)

Global Transnational Factor	Consequence and Probable Impact on Health Risks in Developing Countries
Macroeconomics	
Structural adjustment policies and downsizing	Marginalization; poverty; inadequate social support nets
Structural and chronic unemployment	Higher morbidity and mortality; increased violence
Trade	
Marketing of tobacco	Increased morbidity and mortality due to lung cancer and to cardiovascular and chronic respiratory diseases
Dumping of unsafe and ineffective drugs by multinationals	Harmful or ineffective therapy
Import of contaminated foodstuffs and feed	Spread of infectious diseases across borders
Global redistribution of polluting industries	Increased risk of occupational and environmental exposure to toxic chemicals from disproportionate siting of these industries
Travel	
Cross-border movements of large masses for business or pleasure	Infectious disease transmission; export of harmful lifestyles (such as smoking and high-risk sexual behavior)
Migration and demographic changes	
Increased refugee population	Environmental degradation; incubation of infectious pathogens
Brain drain	Loss of trained manpower and intellectual resources, leading to poor health systems management; economic loss
Technology	
Patent protection of new technologies under trade-related intellectual property rights agreements	Benefits of new health-related technologies developed in global market unaffordable for the poor; marginalization of poor countries in research and development
Patent drugs	Traditional healing practices discouraged; new drugs from local plants unaffordable to the poor
Communications and media	
Global marketing of harmful commodities such as tobacco	Active promotion of health-damaging practices
Risk communication	Inappropriate or misunderstood in poor communities

Foreign policies	
Policies based on national self-interest, xenophobia, or protectionism	Threat to the multinationalism and global cooperation required to address shared transnational health concerns
Global security	Increased number of firearms, which can lead to increased violence; restriction on export of goods and services from some countries; reduction of investments in poor countries where health risks are unmanageable
Other selected factors	
Privatization-oriented policies	Reduced and inappropriate quality of health care for the poor; promotion of international commodification and trade in human organs
Human rights	Withholding of emergency and humanitarian assistance

Source: Adapted from Kickbusch and Buse, 2001.

and community risk-sharing traditions in many developing countries. Notions of justice, social responsibility, and human rights, key to the development of sustainable health systems, are antithetical to the continued plundering of global resources.

Despite the extraordinary advances of the twentieth century, huge disparities persist in the morbidity and mortality experienced in the First and Third Worlds, and this is due primarily to the ill effects of poverty. Environmental risks and poverty are closely interwoven. Poverty hinders the development of clean water supplies and proper sanitation, drives migration into overcrowded cities with substandard housing and high air pollution levels, is related to indoor air pollution from the burning of **biofuels** or **urban solid wastes**, increases exposure to intentional and unintentional injuries and the risk of lead poisoning, and is primarily responsible for undernutrition with far-reaching effects. Globalization has been a bad medicine for developing countries where more than half of the population still lives on less than $2 per day, and it will likely remain so for the foreseeable future.

Current environmental challenges and human vulnerabilities in sub-Saharan Africa show the limitations and difficulties of globalizing health in Third World regions (Thomas and others, 2002). Both the poverty of most sub-Saharan African countries and their total dependence on natural resources for people's livelihoods increase their vulnerability to environmental change and risk overlaps.

The changes that began in the 1960s seem to have deepened their poverty, and their environments and human capital have continued on a downward spiral, making the population more susceptible to environmental health risks. Rapid population growth and overexploitation of natural resources, deepening poverty, and increasing food insecurity have brought about environmental changes that have taken a toll on the public's health. Mismanagement of natural resources, the impacts of disasters and civil strife, and response to external pressures (such as economic adjustment plans) have exacerbated environmental health risks in the region. Other factors such as weak institutional and legal frameworks, corruption, and poor economic performance have left most sub-Saharan countries with limited choices and low coping capacity. It is easy to see why the distinction between globalization and exploitation is blurred for many people in this part of our Earth.

Agriculture

Agriculture, forestry, and fishing not only furnish the food and natural resources on which societies depend but also provide the livelihood of about half the world's population. In many Third World countries, subsistence farming accounts for over 75 percent of the gross domestic product. The output of the world's food-producing systems has greatly increased and changed over recent decades to meet the rising demand of a rapidly growing population. In spite of degradation of land and water resources, there is as yet no global shortage of food or of the capacity to produce it. However, due to social, political, and economic constraints and lack of education, undernutrition remains a leading risk factor for ill health and premature death in most Third World countries.

As agriculture is integrated into the global economy, agricultural systems must be intensified, marginal lands brought into use, and new crops and farming practices developed. At the same time, arable land is being threatened by soil erosion, overgrazing, soil depletion in clear-cut areas, salinization, and other types of land degradation and also by the expansion of urban, industrial, and other developments. The development of the agro-ecosystems needed to feed the local population and grow cash crops for the export market invariably involves environmental changes. Health and its environmental determinants are closely related to land use and land tenure, and the phenomenon of the **green revolution** in the developing countries has been accompanied by significant shifts in environmental health risk factors, a matter that has not received much scientific enquiry. An important element of the green revolution, for example, is an increasing reliance on pesticides, which has led to untold numbers of poisonings in many developing countries.

PERSPECTIVE
Pesticide Hazards in Developing Countries

Chemical pesticides are used throughout the world to protect crops, forests, and plantations (for example, cotton plantations) from pests and to combat insect-borne endemic diseases such as malaria. In developing countries hundreds of thousands of tons of pesticides are applied annually, with applications increasing each year. Access to expensive, safer pesticides is limited in developing countries, whereas less expensive, more acutely toxic pesticides are widely available. Although the use of many of these pesticides has been banned or curtailed in more developed countries, they remain widely available on the world market.

In addition, more than 500,000 tons of obsolete pesticides are stockpiled in developing countries. These stockpiles accumulated when the governments of developing countries prohibited the use of some pesticides after quantities of them had been imported. The list of banned pesticides includes the persistent organic pollutants (POPs) aldrin, chlordane, DDT, dieldrin, endrin, and heptachlor. Many of these stockpiles receive no attention, even though over time pesticides deteriorate and form by-products; occasionally these by-products are more toxic than the original substances. Pesticides and their by-products frequently volatilize into the air or leak into soil, contaminating groundwater. Reliable estimates of pesticide exposures and poisonings are rare because of inadequate surveillance systems. However, surveys suggest that pesticides poison approximately 25 million agricultural workers in developing countries each year—affecting, for example, about 7 percent of agricultural workers in Malaysia, 4.5 percent in Costa Rica, and 3 percent in Sri Lanka. Aside from acute poisonings, the long-term effects of persistent exposure to pesticides include reproductive dysfunction, neurological disease, and cancer.

Pesticide poisoning in developing countries is frequently attributed to lack of personal protective equipment or protective clothing suitable for tropical climates, poor knowledge and understanding of safety procedures, application of pesticides in concentrations exceeding guidelines, and poor maintenance facilities for spray equipment and container disposal. For instance, training programs for agricultural workers to learn how to apply, store, and dispose of pesticides are rarely available. Similarly, legislation to manage pesticide use is patchy and seldom enforced. Enforcement of legislation and implementation of training programs could prevent numerous pesticide poisonings and result in immediate health benefits.

Source: London and others, 2002; Ecobichon, 2001; Koh and Jeyaratnam, 1996.

Expected shifts in environmental determinants of health related to agricultural development programs are shown in Table 11.4. The impacts of the risk factors may be moderated by simultaneous demographic and socioeconomic shifts. All agricultural developments must be contextualized, however—that is, considered in terms of their local ecological and human impacts. For instance, changes in land use patterns can have varying impacts on environmental health in different parts of the world (WHO, 1997). The expansion of irrigation in Senegal following the construction of the Diama Dam at the mouth of the Senegal River caused a massive epidemic of intestinal schistosomiasis. However, deforestation in Southeast Asia destroyed the habitat of the most important local malaria vector, *Anopheles dirus*, and caused a sharp decline in malarial transmission. Subsequent afforestation (commercial tree planting, usually on grasslands), reforestation, and the development of plantation agro-ecosystems (with fruit, rubber, and palm trees) are reversing this trend and sometimes leading to higher malarial transmission rates than occurred in the primary forest environment (WHO, 1997). Another example may be found in irrigation projects in Sri Lanka that have led to major biodiversity loss, leaving the malarial vector, *Anopheles culicifacies*, as the sole representative of a previously rich mosquito fauna. Insect disease-vector densities, biting patterns, and associated transmission risks can also be influenced by the presence or absence of livestock in agro-ecosystems. The risk burden attributable to the change in agrobusiness from simple agrarian to modern methods has not been quantified. However, the potential for adverse impacts is enormous; a recent report (Mascie-Taylor and Karim, 2003) showed that helminthic infections and schistosomiasis (both of which can be aggravated by large-scale agricultural development) account for 43.5 million DALYs, second only to tuberculosis (46.5 million) and well ahead of malaria (34.5 million).

Food Security   Traditional lifestyles remain part of the ancient heritage of peoples in most Third World countries. Methods of gathering, preparing, and using native foods and medicines evolved in ways that promote health. Unlike practices in the developed countries, every element of traditional meals is intertwined with the environment through medicinal, religious, educational, or social customs and beliefs. Traditional duties in the provision and service of meals, and associated exposure patterns, are often gender and age specific. Although many factors are involved in what and how people choose to eat, people generally prefer the foods they grow up eating. Every region in the world has its own staple crops and sources of animal protein, and local communities have developed their own ways of combining foods to make meals.

Environmental factors, including water availability, the physical and chemical properties of soils, and prevailing climatic conditions, control local food patterns. These factors also determine the bioavailable forms of essential microelements

TABLE 11.4   Changes in Environmental Health Risk Factors Associated
with Agricultural Development

Development Program	Direct Environmental Changes	Secondary Environmental Changes	Environmental Health Risk Factors
Irrigation projects	Waterlogging	Increased weed densities; possible biodiversity loss	Introduction of new vector species
	Hydrologic changes		Increased vector densities
	Salinization	Increased insect populations	
	Increased water surface area	Greater chemical inputs	Chemical poisoning
	Increased relative humidity		Changed composition of vector population
		Magnet for urban and industrial development	Prolonged transmission season
		Increased erosion	Exposure of villagers to new pathogens
Land use changes	Reduced biodiversity or habitat	Changed composition of flora and fauna	Changed vector longevity
		Increased erosion and loss of soil fertility	Changed composition of vector population
Cropping patterns	High-yield varieties	Greater chemical inputs	Chemical poisoning
	Shift from subsistence to cash crops	Greater densities of insect populations	Reduced predator insect densities
	Accelerated cropping cycle	Spread of opportunistic and invasive species	Increased pests and disease-vector densities
	Plantation agriculture	Increased water pollution	Mycotoxins
Livestock management	Changes in livestock densities and distribution	Changed densities of blood-sucking pests	Changed disease transmission potential
	New breeds of livestock	Soil pollution	Hormones, antibiotics, and pesticides used in animal husbandry
	Contaminated animal wastes		

(continued)

TABLE 11.4   (Continued)

Development Program	Direct Environmental Changes	Secondary Environmental Changes	Environmental Health Risk Factors
Mechanization	Changes in livestock densities	Changed densities of blood-sucking insects	Changed disease transmission potential
	Loss of ecological features	Reduced refuge areas for predator insects	
	Increased loss of soil quality	Air and water pollution	
Chemical inputs	Increased levels of herbicides, pesticides, and fungicides	Chemical contamination	Chemical poisoning
		Eutrophication of water bodies	Introduction of new vector species
	Increased fertilizer application	Expansion of aquatic weeds	Development of pesticide resistance in vector populations
		Soil contamination with toxic metals (for example, cadmium)	

Source: Adapted from Bradley and Narayan, 1987.

in soils and hence their concentrations in foods. Under wet tropical conditions, weathering processes preferentially leach out key essential micronutrients (such as zinc, copper, cobalt, and selenium) from the characteristic pisolitic, bauxitic, and "red" soils found in many developing countries. Foods in many developing countries thus tend to be naturally deficient in some essential microelements, as exemplified by the epidemic of Keshan-Beck disease due to selenium deficiency in some regions of China. Undernutrition, often driven by deficiencies of essential micronutrients, involves a complex interplay between the physical environment and social, political, cultural, and economic elements. Because work on hunger and malnutrition has been dominated by social and political scientists, the underlying environmental determinants of the problem have often been overlooked.

The Impact of Undernutrition   Hunger and **undernutrition** remain the most pervasive risk factors for human morbidity and mortality, especially in the developing countries (Tables 11.1 and 11.2). Many people associate food shortages and malnutrition with famines caused by wars and political upheavals, by environmental disasters (such as floods and earthquakes), and by environmental catastrophes (such as overgrazing). However, the problem in developing countries often relates to complex ongoing socioecological factors such as poor resource management and economic adjustment plans; these limit food choices, increase local food prices, and reduce people's buying power. Factors that can influence the availability and equitable distribution of safe, nutritious, and affordable foods in developing countries include

- Traditions and beliefs that constrain an individual's food choices. In many African cultures, pregnant and postpartum women are limited to certain foods, and other foods (including eggs, onions, certain seafood, and many green, leafy vegetables) are strictly forbidden. Restriction of food choices increases the risk of inadequate consumption of essential microelements.
- Reduced capacity for local food production, owing to unfavorable land titles that debar a majority of the population from owning land.
- Declining investments in agricultural research, irrigation, and rural infrastructure.
- Uneducated farmers who cannot adopt advanced technologies and crop management techniques to achieve higher rates of return on their lands.
- Conversion of forests to cropping and grazing lands, leading to loss of hunting grounds (game is an important source of animal protein in traditional diets) and reducing the availability of wild fruits and vegetables that used to be traditional food staples.
- Urbanization and associated roadways that destroy arable lands and suck away the able-bodied workers while placing excessive demand on the food supply from rural communities.
- Inadequate food-handling and distribution systems, which result in massive preharvest and postharvest losses.
- Lack of food storage and preservation capacity, making some critical dietary sources of essential microelements seasonal commodities.

These changes in land use and agriculture in developing nations have had a major impact on health and its environmental determinants. Over generations, many small farmers had developed sophisticated knowledge of how to sustain yields from their farms under difficult circumstances. In recent years, drivers of environmental degradation have left large numbers of poor farmers with only poor-quality land. The impact of the impoverishment of peasant farmers on the disease burden is dramatic.

It is estimated that undernutrition (and especially underweight) caused 3.7 million deaths, about 1 in 15 deaths globally, in 2000 (Table 11.1). Almost 1.8 million deaths from this cause occurred in Africa and accounted for about 20 percent of deaths in that region (Table 11.1). About 138 million DALYs (9.5 percent of the global total) were attributed to underweight in 2002; the high loss of healthy life years reflecting the fact that undernutrition results in high mortality among young children (WHO, 2002). Underweight accounts for about 15 percent of the DALYs in sub-Saharan Africa, compared to about 1 percent in many developed countries. The synergy between undernutrition and infectious diseases is well documented. Diarrhea, pneumonia, acute upper respiratory infections, measles, and other infections are more severe in undernourished children and carry a higher risk of mortality (Pelletier, 1994). At the same time, some of the most common infectious diseases in children (including diarrhea, respiratory infections, measles, intestinal helminth infections, and malaria) have long been recognized to influence rates of physical growth and of malnutrition (West, Caballero, and Black, 2001). Analyses of underweight-morbidity relationships suggest that 50 to 70 percent of the burden of diarrheal diseases, measles, malaria, and lower respiratory infections in children is attributable to undernutrition (WHO, 2002). An estimated 56 percent of all childhood deaths may be explained by the potentiating effects of undernutrition on the burden of infectious diseases (Pelletier, 1994). Complications accompanying malnutrition are believed to claim nearly half of the 10 million annual deaths among children under the age of five in the developing countries (West and others, 2001).

Elderly people must be considered to be at high risk of undernutrition, especially those living in impoverished settings in developing countries. Results from a limited number of surveys suggest that 25 to 35 percent of older people in low-income populations may be in a chronic state of acute undernutrition (Chilima and Ismail, 1998). This is not surprising because poverty is a strong risk factor for undernutrition. Specific age-related disorders that may be potentiated by undernutrition include sarcopenia with attendant muscle weakness and impaired mobility and body function, various dementias likely of nutritional origin, and osteoporosis with resultant bone fracture (West and others, 2001). The aging-environment-disease interface remains unexplored, but a number of perspectives can be mentioned. Higher susceptibility of the elderly to indoor air pollution from biofuels has been reported (Mishra, 2003). Aging brings to the fore the cumulative environmental insults, which gradually reduce the resiliency of cellular and body functions below the threshold for diseases. Aging is an inevitable and programmed cellular degradation process that can be potentiated by exposure to environmental and nutritional stressors. Irrespective of the exact mechanisms of aging-environment interactions, undernutrition among the elderly population is an immense and growing public health problem in the developing countries that needs considerably more attention than it is currently getting.

The Risk Transition to Overnutrition   On the other end of the nutrition spectrum in developing countries lies the problem of **overnutrition**. The globalization of production and marketing, along with changes in the social and economic status of the upper and middle classes, are rapidly increasing the consumption of alcohol, tobacco, and processed and fast foods in developing countries. Policies regarding local production and processing, import regulations, and subsidies have also altered the relative balance between the kinds and costs of imported foods and the kinds and costs of locally grown foods. Diets are shifting toward a higher fat content (meats and fat-rich foods are considered status symbols of economic advancement), more refined carbohydrates, less fiber, more salt, and more diversity. This Westernization process also involves changes in living and working patterns as people shift to less physical activity and less labor and also to smoking cigarettes. This changing pattern in dietary habits and physical inactivity has given rise to overnutrition, with attendant hypertension, hyperlipidemias, overweight, and obesity, which are in turn risk factors for chronic diseases such as cancers, heart disease, stroke, diabetes, and mental illness, especially in rapidly growing urban populations. At the same time, parasitic infections associated with diarrhea, impaired growth and development, bladder cancers, micronutrient deficiency anemia, decreased physical fitness and work capacity, and impaired cognitive function remain pandemic in most of these urban and rural communities. The arrival of a whole group of noncommunicable diseases on top of persistent communicable diseases has resulted in a dramatic increase in the burden of disease in Third World countries, the so-called double jeopardy phenomenon.

Cardiovascular diseases (CVDs) (including heart disease and stroke), often caused by tobacco use, overnutrition, and physical inactivity, have recently emerged as a major public health problem in most Third World countries (WHO, 2003). CVDs have become the first and second causes of adult death in many developing countries, accounting for about one-third of all deaths. Twice as many deaths from CVDs occur in developing countries as in developed countries. For example, stroke mortality rates in rural and urban areas of Tanzania are higher than those for England and Wales. In terms of DALYs, CVDs rank third in disease burden (after injuries and neuropsychiatric disorders) in developing countries (WHO, 2003) and have reached epidemic proportion.

Urbanization

The global issue of urbanization today is unprecedented in terms of the number and size of the world's largest cities and the concentration of urban growth in developing countries (Montgomery, 2008). At the beginning of the twentieth century, only 16 cities in the world contained a million people or more, and most of these cities were located in the developed countries. By the beginning of the twenty-first century, about 400 cities had a million inhabitants or more, and about 70 percent of these cities were in developing countries. In the 1980s, 22 of the 35 largest metropolitan areas, containing about 45 percent of the world's metropolitan population, were in developing countries. In 1950, there was only 1 city in the world with a population of over 10 million inhabitants (New York), and only 8 with over 5 million inhabitants. By 2000, there were 42 cities above the 5 million mark, 30 of them in developing world. It is projected that by 2015, there will be 23 cities with populations over 10 million, 19 of them in developing countries (Vlahov and others, 2007). Today, for the first time in human history, the number of people living in towns and cities exceeds the number living in rural areas.

Urbanicity and Urbanization   There is a distinction between **urbanicity**—the extent of urban population concentration—and **urbanization**—the process over time of urban growth. In wealthy countries, there is typically a high degree of urbanicity, including the presence of megacities, but with slowly expanding or stable populations. In contrast, rapid urbanization is more common among cities in developing world. The rate of urbanization may be a more important predictor of health in urban populations than the population size. As Vlahov, Galea, Gibble, and Freudenberg (2005) point out, with rapid urbanization, population growth may outstrip available resources. Moreover, although the current literature focuses on the impact in megacities, the effects of urbanization may be greater in small to midsized cities (Montgomery, 2008), where urbanization is occurring more rapidly than in megacities. Growth in megacities is expected to level further in the coming decade (Vlahov and others, 2007). Smaller cities typically have fewer resources and less infrastructure with which to provide basic services, such as sanitation and water distribution. Growth in these areas is often driven by policies that are aimed at preventing growth in megacities, and that encourage rural migrants to move to smaller cities instead.

Among Third World regions, Asia leads with the largest number of urban dwellers and the most rapid rates of urbanization, followed by Latin America and Africa (Ooi and Phua, 2007; Montgomery, 2008). Africa's urban population is growing particularly rapidly, almost twice as fast as in any other major region of the world. Africa's total population will increase from around from 794 million in 2000 to about 1.5 billion in 2030 (Cohen, 2006), and most (70 percent) of this growth will occur in towns and cities, which will expand from 295 million to 748 million, reaching a larger urban population than in North America, Europe, or Latin America. An unusual feature of current urbanization in Africa is that the growth is decoupled from economic development (Cohen, 2006). Most African cities are economically marginalized and continue to grow despite poor planning, poor economic management and limited foreign investment. A World Bank (2000) report aptly observed that "cities in Africa are not serving as engines of growth and structural transformation. Instead, they are part of the cause and a major symptom of the economic and social crisis that have enveloped the continent."

The rapid growth of urban areas is the result of two factors: natural increase in population (excess of births over deaths) and migration to urban areas. *Migration* refers to the relocation of a person, household, or group to a new location outside the original community. Internal, rural-to-urban migration in developing countries is a rapidly growing phenomenon. International migration is also increasing but at a lower rate. Internal migration is often explained in terms of either *push factors*—conditions in the place of origin that are perceived by migrants as detrimental to their well-being or economic security—or *pull factors*—the circumstances in new places that attract people to move there. Examples of push factors include high unemployment and political persecution; examples of pull factors include job opportunities or a better climate (Population Reference Bureau, 2008).

Globalization and the so-called structural adjustment plans (SAPs) are well-known drivers of rural migration in many developing countries. In their effort to pay foreign debt, gain foreign exchange, and compete in international markets, national governments tend to encourage the export of natural resources and agricultural products at giveaway prices. Natural resource capital, including agricultural products (such as fruits and vegetables, coffee, flowers, and sugar) and primary-sector goods (such as land, minerals, timber, and fish), is traded to bolster the national economy. In an effort to improve agricultural practices to produce export cash crops cheaply and quickly, national governments displace the local small farmers in favor of balkanized production and resource extraction by large enterprises with capital-intensive facilities and lower per unit cost of production. This process turns land into a commodity that can be bought and sold and is viewed purely in terms of its productive capabilities. Free-market economics promotes economic efficiency that can deliver goods at the lowest possible price, and its advocates maintain that any government intervention diminishes this efficiency. Consequently, they seek to eliminate farm programs such as farm subsidies, cheap credit policies, and the like, intended to help the farmer and to maintain stable prices. Farmers face a stark choice: to continue to eke out a living by traditional farming practices or to sell their land to a foreign investor or a domestic-owned enterprise and move to the cities with the hope for a better life. Other government policies serve to reinforce this scenario. To constrain civil unrest and reduce the cost of urban labor and urban life, governments strive to maintain artificially low food prices (well below the market levels) in urban areas. This policy of not compensating rural farmers adequately for locally produced foods tends to aggravate rural poverty and drive internal migration (Population Reference Bureau, 2008).

The Growth of Slums   The high rate of urban growth with consequent increase in demand for basic housing and services, as well as skewed distribution of investment toward affluent suburban developments, has resulted in rapid expansion of illegal or unplanned and unserviced settlements with unhealthy living conditions and extreme overcrowding (Ooi and Phua, 2007). Only 60 percent of urban dwellings in Africa are considered permanent, and nearly half fall short of compliance with regulations (UNEP, 2002). About 55 percent of the population of Nairobi lived in informal settlements in 1993, and nearly half of the population of South Africa did not have adequate housing in the late 1990s. Over 40 percent of the population of Monrovia, Liberia, was reportedly living in squatter camps in 1998. The average person in African cities has a mere 8 m^2 of space, indicative of extreme overcrowding conditions; the average in Asian cities is 9.5 m^2. By comparison, the average floor space in the developed countries is 34.5 m^2 and the global average is 13.6 m^2 (UNEP, 2002). Overcrowding is a risk factor for communicable diseases such as gastrointestinal infections and respiratory diseases such as tuberculosis, which is commonly associated with poor ventilation and air pollution. In unplanned settlements, where space is usually at a premium, shelters are erected in fragile environments such as delicate slopes, wetlands, and flood zones. These ecosystems are vulnerable to pollution and physical degradation, and shelters located in them expose the residents to risks of flooding, subsidence, and mud slides.

Inadequate revenue streams in African municipalities reduce development spending and infrastructure maintenance. This situation has been exacerbated by slow economic growth during the last three decades and increasing bias among donor agencies in favor of development projects in rural areas. Another collateral environmental health concern is that the poor often pay relatively higher prices for housing and associated services such electricity and water. It is estimated that in African cities, people spend about 40 percent of their incomes on rent, a proportion that is twice that by urban residents in the developed countries (UNEP, 2002). The high cost of accommodation is indirectly linked to the problem of undernutrition, described in a previous section.

Urban Health in Developing Nations   Environmental health in cities is affected both by the rate of urbanization and by the social and physical environments associated with urbanicity. Although many of the health impacts of urbanicity are similar across the middle classes in both developed and developing countries, the rate of urbanization in Third World cities creates vastly different environmental and health impacts for the urban poor.

The health impacts of urbanization and urbanicity result from two critical factors: physiological responses to physical aspects of the environment and behavioral responses to the urban environment. In developing countries, urban residents, especially those in unplanned or unserviced settlements (squatter camps and slums), often lack access to adequate housing and basic amenities including sanitation, piped water, waste disposal, and electricity. The physical environment includes many stressors such as chemical and biological agents, natural disasters, noise pollution, and extreme heat. Chemical agents include industrial, mobile, and indoor air pollution, as well as chemical pollution of drinking water, and hazardous wastes. Biological agents include bacterial, viral, and fungal diseases that may be influenced or propagated by urban ecology. Many of these issues are discussed in depth elsewhere in the chapter; this section focuses on environmental health impacts specific to urbanization.

Ambient Air Pollution   Urban areas in developing countries are burdened with high levels of ambient air pollution generated by industrial and transportation-related sources, as well as combustion by-products from domestic cooking and heating. Transportation contributes a majority of the ambient air pollution in Third World cities. It has been estimated that over 50 percent of the ambient air pollution in Third World megacities, such as Beijing, Delhi, and Mumbai, is produced by the transport sector (Goyal, Ghatge, Nema, and Tamhane, 2006). According to the World Health Organization, over 800,000 deaths per year are caused by urban air pollution (Duh, Shandas, Chang, and George, 2008).

Indoor Air Pollution   In the numerous megaslums that have formed in the outskirts of Third World cities, access to electricity is unreliable, and people depend on dirty-burning fuels for cooking. Even among urban residents with access to electricity, many continue to rely on coal, kerosene, and biomass for heating and cooking. In a study of fuel smoke pollution and health in Hanoi, 96 percent of respondents were connected to the electrical grid, but only 35 percent used electricity for cooking (Ellegard, 1996). A similar study in Maputo found that although 30 percent were connected, less than a third of that number used electricity in cooking (Ellegard, 1996). Overcrowding in urban areas, especially in conditions of extreme poverty, can intensify exposure to indoor pollutants and environmental transmission of infectious agents. For example, crowding may require household members to sleep in close proximity to indoor pollution sources such as the stove or fireplace.

Water   Urban areas affect water security and water quality in several ways. Urban development introduces changes in hydrologic patterns (Duh and others, 2008). Urban populations create an enormous demand for potable water, which may outstrip available supply and infrastructure for water sanitation and delivery in Third World nations. Urban conditions may also provide increased opportunities for biological and chemical contamination. WHO estimates that half of the world's population does not have access to basic sanitation, with the result that water quality–related mortality is the third leading cause of child death in developing countries (Duh and others, 2008).

Infectious Diseases   Infectious diseases flourish in the low-income urban settlements common in developing countries. High population density, crowded conditions, and concentration of commerce facilitate the emergence and reemergence of infectious diseases by increasing the probability of transmission (Vlahov and others, 2005; WHO, 2005). Changes in urban ecology, including factors such as stagnant water, inadequate drainage or flooding, and improper waste disposal, can increase outbreaks of vector-borne diseases such as dengue, malaria, yellow fever, plague, leishmaniasis, filariasis, Lyme disease, and schistomaniasis (Vlahov and others, 2005; WHO, 2005).

Crowded conditions in urban slums produce high volumes of human waste, and the unplanned land use development typical in Third World slums may lead to contamination of water and food supplies with biological wastes and interfere with personal hygiene practices. In some crowded cities people may also keep livestock, a practice that contributes to microbial pollution, contamination of food and water, and transmission of pathogens from animals to humans (zoonoses). These conditions foster communicable disease transmission among the urban poor.

Waste Disposal   Another factor contributing to disease is deficient waste management practices: illegal dumping and burning of solid wastes and sewage in the informal settlements, and the tendency for polluting industries, waste dumps, and waste management facilities to be located near low-income neighborhoods, with no clear demarcation between residential and industrial areas. Bad sanitation may lead to contaminated water supplies and human wastes finding their way into the local food chain. Solid wastes may clog drains, resulting in accumulation of water in which mosquitoes breed; use of mosquito coils and pesticides to combat these pests may add to air pollution and chemical hazards. Flies and other vectors that thrive on wastes may contaminate food with pathogens, and lack of education on food safety can lead to a high incidence of food poisoning. In African cities, inadequate waste management has been called a monster. It has resisted most governmental and private efforts, and as these cities continue to discharge ever increasing amounts of wastes into the air, water and soils, a major crisis looms that will be beyond the financial capacity of the cities themselves to solve.

Disaster Vulnerability   Colonial practices in developing countries resulted in many cities, including national capitals, being located on the coast, that is, in defensible positions that could be used to maximize access to trade routes, international travel, and development. These costal cities are now at increased risk of sea-level rise, extreme weather events, and flooding, (Montgomery, 2008), a sobering thought considering that 14 of the world's 19 megacities (those with over 10 million inhabitants) are located in coastal areas (UN Habitat, 2008). Furthermore, construction patterns and lack of planning in many developing cities generally result in the degradation of natural protection (through deforestation and building on floodplains, for instance), the building of poor-quality and extemporaneous housing, often on exposed slopes, and the extensive paving of surfaces without providing adequate drainage. Hurricanes, tornadoes, and heavy rains can therefore result in intense and massive destruction of buildings, properties, and lives by storm surges and flash floods. Developing countries are equally vulnerable to other natural disasters, including earthquakes, landslides, fires, and coastal storms (Vlahov and others, 2005). Anthropogenic disasters such as warfare and industrial mishaps and spills may also affect population health in developing countries. Increased population density found in urban areas, particularly in megacities, increases the potential devastation to human life and welfare resulting from these events. In addition, urbanization may accelerate global climate change, increasing the frequency and intensity of extreme weather events burdening Third World cities (Duh and others, 2008). Urbanization can also concentrate population growth in geographic areas vulnerable to natural disasters, such as the earthquake belt stretching from the Mediterranean through the Middle East and extending into Asia. In this region the devastation caused by earthquakes has increased as a result of urban development (Jackson, 2006).

Social and Behavioral Factors   Rural-urban migration in the Third World changes the social environment and lifestyle of the newly urbanized population. Reduced activity and increased consumption of sugars and fats have produced an epidemic of obesity and related health problems in Third World cities. The permissive social environment, relative anonymity, and erosion of traditional mores in the cities are conducive to sexual promiscuity, smoking, drinking, and drug use. The crowding and relative anonymity in the city also give rise to increased violence and unintentional injuries. The relaxation of formerly strict sexual taboos among young city dwellers can have many negative consequences, ranging from unwanted pregnancies to the spread of sexually transmitted diseases such as AIDS. The anonymity and lack of social support, along with the appalling conditions faced by many urban dwellers, have also given rise to an epidemic of mental health problems among these men, women, and children.

Rapid urbanization and slum formation also contribute to disparities in social determinants that affect health, such as wealth and health care access. In the low-income settlements common in the developing world, health impacts are exacerbated by the absence of adequate resources and infrastructure. In addition, slum dwellers often have little or no legal claim to municipal resources and assistance that may be available to wealthier city dwellers. In low-income settlements local environmental problems are generally major contributors to disease and death.

PERSPECTIVE
Urbanization and Asthma in Developing Countries

The increasing asthma burden among urban residents in the developing countries demonstrates the joint impact of behavioral and traditional environmental risk factors in these populations. The prevalence of asthma is currently highest in the wealthier countries of Western Europe and North America, which are loosely referred to as *Westernized* in the literature (Beasley, Crane, Lai, and Pearce, 2000, Wong and Chow, 2008). However, the prevalence of asthma is increasing among populations that have become increasingly Westernized, a process closely linked with urbanization (Wong and Chow, 2008). Immigrant populations tend to acquire the asthma prevalence of their destination countries, as suggested by data from the United States and Australia (Johnson and others, 2005; Powell and others, 1999), suggesting that relocation to Westernized countries confers increased risk of asthma (Leung, Carlin, Burdon, and Czarny, 1994). Comparisons of urban and rural communities in the developed world consistently report higher asthma prevalence among urban populations. Epidemiological studies have reported that people who grow up on a farm have a lower risk of developing asthma, suggesting that agrarian exposures may be a protective aspect of a traditional lifestyle (Alm and others, 1999; Wong and Chow, 2008).

Obesity, an emblematic disease of Westernization, is another risk factor for asthma in the developed countries. An association between high dietary fat and asthma has also been found in the developing countries (Huang and Pan, 2001), suggesting that changes in traditional diet and lifestyle such as increased fast-food consumption and reduced exercise may contribute to asthma risk, in addition to risks for other chronic diseases, among transitioning populations. The level of ambient air pollution is an obvious difference between urban and rural communities; however, it is unclear whether ambient air pollution plays a causal or exacerbatory role in asthma etiology. It has also been suggested that the disparity between urban and rural asthma prevalence can be explained by characteristics of urban lifestyle such as carpets, indoor pets, and crowding, which increase indoor allergen concentrations in urban environments (Ng'ang'a and others, 1998; Woodcock and others, 2001). The explanation for the increase in asthma in transitioning populations remains elusive and likely involves a complex interaction between behavioral and environmental risk factors.

Protecting Public Health in Third World Cities   With few exceptions, urban growth in many Third World cities has outstripped the capacity of municipal and local governments to provide even basic services. Policy and decision makers in developing countries often lack the experts, assessment tools, and surveillance systems needed to address urban health challenges (Chow and others, 2004; Ooi and Phua, 2007). However, they may benefit from the ability to use lessons, strategies, and decision-making tools from developed countries, thus reducing the cost of generating these resources through trial and error (Chow, 2004).

In developing countries with burgeoning economies, environmental cost must also be weighed against economic advancement. In a global economy, loose regulations on industrial pollution may entice foreign corporations and allow domestic business to produce competitive exports.

Urban health is more than an aggregate of individual risk factors (Vlahov and others, 2005). Urban health is influenced by the interaction of multiple systems and predictors, making simple interventions less effective. Mitigation of health impacts associated with urbanization requires an understanding of the time-dependent factors, interactions, and feedback present in an urban landscape. Finally, more research has been conducted in established megacities than in rapidly urbanizing areas (Duh and others, 2008). This lack of information about the ongoing urbanization in developing countries hampers planning and other decision making that could improve urban health in these areas.

The remainder of this chapter deals with recent trends in environmental risk factors that have contributed to health disparities across the three worlds. It addresses three domains: air quality, water and sanitation, and injuries. Each is a primary domain of environmental health, and each poses particular health challenges to the people of developing nations.

AIR POLLUTION

The global perspective reveals a clear dichotomy in air pollution trends. In First World countries levels of many pollutants have declined markedly, the combined result of technical, legislative, and community interventions. In most developing countries, in contrast, levels of air pollution continue to rise, reflecting growing fossil fuel consumption and intensification of manufacturing activities (Krzyzanowski and Schwela, 1999). Third World cities now boast some of the highest levels of air pollution in the world. Combustion processes generate a complex mixture of substances that may be primary pollutants (such as particulates) or that may form in subsequent atmospheric reactions (as ozone and sulfate aerosols do). Although attention is generally focused on a few **priority pollutants**—sulfur oxides (SO_x), nitrogen oxides (NO_x), particulate matter (PM), ozone, carbon monoxide (CO), and lead—thousands of additional toxic substances are released to the atmosphere. Our knowledge of the chemical composition, speciation, and toxicity of many air pollutants has serious gaps. (The origins and effects of ambient air pollutants in Third World cities differ only in magnitude from those in wealthy nations, and a detailed discussion of these issues appears in Chapter Twelve.)

It is estimated that as many as 1.4 billion urban residents, many of them in developing countries, breathe air with contaminant levels that exceed WHO air quality guidelines. Ambient air pollution has been linked to a variety of chronic and acute health effects. For instance, as described in Chapter Twelve, exposure to fine particulate matter is associated with respiratory and cardiovascular disease and lung cancer (Samet and Cohen, 1999; WHO, 2002). Pollutants such as ozone and lead are associated with other serious health effects, and the bioaerosols may be a vector for a number of infectious pathogens. Urban air pollution plays a major role in childhood respiratory infections (Romieu, Samet, Smith, and Bruce, 2002). It has been estimated that fine particulate matter is responsible for 5 percent of global lung cancer incidence as well as 2 percent of cardiovascular deaths and 1 percent of mortality from respiratory infections, corresponding to about 800,000 deaths (1.4 percent of the total) and 7.9 million DALYs (0.8 percent of the total) annually (Lopez and others, 2006). This burden occurs predominantly in developing countries, especially in the Western Pacific and Southeast Asian regions. Reliable air pollution morbidity estimates are not available; when a proper assessment is done, the burden of disease attributed to ambient air pollution will likely be very high.

Indoor Air Pollution

Biomass Burning   Anthropogenic air pollution began when humans discovered and tamed the wildfire. Combustion is a "dirty" process that releases a variety of pollutants that threaten human health. Indoor air pollution in developing countries results from the use of biomass (such as crop waste and animal dung) and coal for cooking and heating and of liquid fuel (heating oil and kerosene or paraffin) for heating and lighting. Even woodsmoke—sometimes considered benign because it is a "natural" product—poses a range of toxic exposures (Naeher and others, 2007). An estimated 75 percent of homes in developing countries still rely on biofuels for cooking and heating, and among rural populations in developing countries, biofuels supply 90 percent of domestic energy (Torres-Dosal and others, 2008). These fuels typically are burned indoors in simple household devices, such as a pit, three-stone hearth, or U-shaped brick enclosure, and in small rooms without adequate ventilation. These highly inefficient burners result in incomplete combustion. Under these conditions high volumes of harmful air pollutants are generated, including SO_x (primarily from coal), NO_x, PM, CO, polycyclic aromatic hydrocarbons (PAHs), heavy metals, and dozens of other organic compounds. Specific cooking styles release other types of toxic fumes to the indoor environment. Stir-frying, deep-frying in oil, and preheating oil before food is added often release cooking oil fumes, a complex mixture of compounds including aldehydes (malonyldialdehyde, 4-hydroxy-2,3-nonenal, and 4-hydroxy-2,3-alkenals of different chain lengths), PAHs, aromatic amines, and nitro-PAHs, which are also common in tobacco smoke (Wu and others, 2004). Because cooking occurs for several hours each day and at times when people are present indoors, the potential exposure to cookfire emissions is high. Recent studies show that typical indoor concentrations of PM, CO, and PAHs often exceed WHO-recommended safe levels (Ezzati and Kammen, 2002), with fine PM concentrations in excess of 2,000 $\mu g/m^3$ reported in some biofuel-using households (Balakrishnan and others, 2002). Indoor use of biofuels is also responsible for some of the highest levels of ambient air pollution recorded in rural communities (Smith, 1987; Roy, Bruce, and Dalgado, 2002). In cities in China the burning of biomass (mostly coal) in individual homes contributes about 30 percent of the outdoor particulate and sulfur dioxide pollution (Moore, Gould, and Keary, 2003). In China it has been estimated that 80 to 90 percent of exposure to PM_{10} in rural populations and 50 to 60 percent of exposure in urban populations is due to indoor biofuel combustion (Mestl and others, 2007). It has also been estimated that developing countries produce 76 percent of total particulate matter pollution (Figure 11.2).

Exposure to indoor air pollution from biofuel combustion has been linked, with varying degrees of robustness, to a number of health outcomes, including acute respiratory infection (ARI), middle ear infection (otitis media), chronic obstructive pulmonary disease (COPD), lung cancer (mainly from coal smoke), asthma, cancer of the nasopharynx and larynx, tuberculosis, perinatal conditions, low birthweight, undernutrition and anemia, and diseases of the eye such as cataract and blindness (Bruce, Perez-Padilla, and Albalak, 2000; Roy and others, 2002; Ezzati and Kammen, 2002; Balakrishnan and others, 2002; Pokhrel and others, 2005; Emmelin and Wall, 2007; Mishra and Retherford, 2007; Fullerton and others, 2008). There is also some evidence that indoor biofuel combustion exacerbates respiratory infections among those with HIV/AIDs (Fullerton and others, 2008). Cooking oil fumes have been associated with lung cancer among nonsmoking women in some areas of China (Tung and others, 2001) and are known to be genotoxic (Wu and others, 2004). Indoor smoke from biofuels accounts for an estimated 36 percent of lower respiratory infections, 22 percent of the COPD, and 1.5 percent of trachea, bronchus, and lung cancer worldwide

FIGURE 11.2   Total Global Exposure to Particulate Matter
Air Pollution

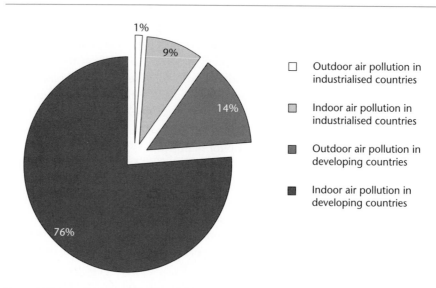

Source: Fullerton, Bruce, and Gordon, 2008.

(WHO, 2002). About 5 percent of the disease burden in developing countries and
2.7 percent of DALYs worldwide have been attributed to indoor air pollution; in
comparison, outdoor air pollution accounts for 0.8 percent of DALYs, and unsafe
water and poor sanitation and hygiene account for 3.7 percent (Smith, Mehta,
and Maeusezahl-Feuz, 2004), with 32 percent of this DALY burden occurring in
Africa and 37 percent in Southeast Asia. Global mortality due to indoor air pollution from biofuels is estimated to range from 1.5 to 2 million, about 4 to 5 percent of total deaths worldwide (Ezzati and Kammen, 2002). It is estimated that
acute respiratory infections account for one-fifth to one-third of mortality among
children under five years of age globally. Moreover, acute respiratory infection
incidence and mortality in developing countries exceed those in the developed
world (Emmelin and Wall, 2007; Rudan and others, 2008). For example, 45 percent of global pneumonia deaths in children younger than five occur in Africa,
although Africa accounts for only about 20 percent of the children in this age
group (Rudan and others, 2008).

In most developing countries women are mainly responsible for gathering
and carrying fuel wood and cooking with it (Golshan, Faghihi, and Marandi,
2002; Sims and Butter, 2000) and thus are disproportionately exposed to risk

from these sources. Each element of the biofuel cycle (gathering, carrying, burning) carries its own health risks for women. Besides exposure to heat, sun, and rain, women wood gatherers can suffer falls, bruises, cuts, fractures, and insect and snake bites and are exposed to infectious disease pathogens (such as mosquito and tsetse fly bites) and even to land mines. Fuel wood typically is transported by headloading, which can result in fatigue, headaches, joint and chest pain, musculoskeletal disorders, increased risk of prolapsed uterus, and weakened resistance to infections (Smith, 1987). The risks of exposure to biofuel emissions were noted earlier. Children, especially girls, usually stay with their mothers while food is being prepared and thus also experience extended exposure to biofuel emissions.

Cooking Emissions in Food   Smoking and drying are common, age-old food preservation techniques in developing countries. In most cases the foods (fish, meat, or vegetables) are dried or smoked indoors by placing them above the biofuel-burning, nonvented cookstoves. During this drying or smoking the toxic chemicals in the biofuel emissions (especially PAHs, aldehydes, and toxic metals) coat and permeate the foods being processed. The health risks of the dried fish and meats sold widely in African countries have not been well studied. The black, smoky exterior of these foods likely contains carcinogens and may represent a human health hazard. A recent study found high concentrations of arsenic (30 to 70 percent higher than those in normal food) in chili peppers and corn dried over coal-burning cookstoves; consumption of these dried foods was responsible for widespread chronic arsenic poisoning in the Guizhou Province of China (Liu and others, 2002). In urban areas the food-drying smoke may be generated by burning plastic, newspapers, wrapping papers, preserved wood, and other types of household wastes, which would change the concentrations and types of toxic substances in the dried foods.

Other Sources of Indoor Air Pollution   Although the bulk of indoor air pollution in developing countries results from burning biofuels, significant contributions also derive from environmental tobacco smoke, pesticide sprays and mosquito coils, and household furnishings and products (Smith and Mehta, 2003; Schmidt, 2007). These sources emit a host of pollutants, including PM, CO, PAHs, and volatile organic compounds (VOCs). Indoor air quality is also affected by outdoor pollution sources. A significant fraction of the load of indoor pollutants is deposited as house dust or trapped by rugs, furniture, furry pets, and stuffed animals. Contaminated house dust is a major health hazard to children, who readily ingest it through hand-to-mouth activities, and thus it must be included in any discussion of indoor risk factors. Finally, poor housing quality and water damage in developing countries can contribute to high levels of bioaerosols, such as mold and fungal spores, and biological contaminants, such as dust mites (Chaudhuri, 2004).

Lead Poisoning

Lead poisoning remains one of the most preventable diseases of environmental origin in the world today. The sources of lead in the environments of developing countries are legion: base metal and secondary smelters, iron and steel production, leaded house paints, lead pipes in water distribution systems, automobile parts (from solder to wheel-balancing weights), ammunition, batteries, cable shields, pigments, laboratory chemicals, and various alloys (Agency for Toxic Substances and Disease Registry, 2000). The environmental lead source of greatest concern has been the automobile tailpipe, although this source is now coming under control. By 2002, over 100 countries representing about 90 percent of global gasoline sales had phased lead out of their gasoline, leading to substantial decreases in population blood lead levels (Meyer, McGeehin, and Falk, 2003). The 25 sub-Saharan countries came later to this action, but following the Declaration of Dakar in 2001 (Regional Conference on the Phasing-Out of Leaded Gasoline in Sub-Saharan Africa, 2001), all have reportedly completed the phaseout of lead from motor fuel. Only a few nations continue to use leaded gasoline, including several in north Africa, central Europe, and Asia (Partnership for Clean Fuels and Vehicles and United Nations Environment Programme, 2008). The continued sale of leaded gasoline by multinational corporations despite mounting evidence that millions of children in urban areas of developing countries are poisoned by lead raises compelling ethical questions.

Emission of lead from smelting operations in developing countries is an ongoing concern. These smelters generally employ outdated technology and are equipped with inefficient pollution control devices. Secondary smelters, involved in recycling the lead in car batteries, are being disproportionately sited in developing countries because they cannot meet pollution control regulations in the developed countries. Cottage industries, including such service and repair businesses as appliance repair, battery repair or reprocessing, welding, paint finishing, auto bodywork, carburetor repair, oil change services, and processing of metal scraps, are also a well-recognized source of lead pollution in developing countries. Environmental risks from cottage industries are highest in the home environment, where children live and play. Deteriorating lead paint on walls of older buildings, improperly glazed pottery and ceremonial glasses, traditional and herbal medicines, and cosmetics (such as kohl, also known as surma or kajal, in parts of Asia, Africa, and the Middle East) can become significant sources of lead exposure in some countries as well.

Worldwide, about 120 million people have levels of blood lead (PbB) in the range of 5 to 10 µg/dL, and levels for 50 to 100 million people are believed to exceed 10 µg/dL. About 10 to 30 percent of all children have PbB levels above 5 µg/dL, with over 90 percent of the affected children living in developing countries (WHO, 2002). Most countries in the world currently define a PbB value above 10 µg/dL to be a level of concern. About 234,000 deaths worldwide and 12.9 million (0.9 percent) DALYs are attributable to lead poisoning (WHO, 2002). Young children in developing countries are particularly susceptible to lead poisoning. They accompany their mothers, often tied to their mothers' backs, when their mothers go to crowded marketplaces or vend foods or small goods at roadside stalls. Many of the common endemic diseases (including malaria, schistosomiasis, and dengue fever) can affect the absorption of lead or development of systemic lead poisoning. More important, significant inverse associations have been demonstrated between blood lead levels and the dietary intake of a number of micronutrients, including iron, zinc, calcium, and vitamins C and D (Gallicchio, Scherer, and Sexton, 2002). In addition, total fat and caloric intakes have been positively associated with blood lead levels. The fact that nutrient deficiency in young children is a risk factor for elevated blood lead levels is of concern in view of the epidemic of undernutrition and underweight in developing countries. The health effects of lead at various exposure doses are summarized in the Perspective on the following page).

SANITATION AND WATER QUALITY AND QUANTITY

Access to clean water has been designated a human right by the United Nations Committee on Economic, Cultural and Social Rights. Nevertheless, approximately 900 million people in developing countries live without continuous access to safe drinking water. In low-income developing countries, close to 50 percent of the population has access to safe drinking water, as compared to 75 to 90 percent in high-income developing countries and more than 90 percent in developed countries. Rural populations in low-income developing countries have considerably less access to safe drinking water than do those living in urban areas (Table 11.5). In parts of sub-Saharan Africa and Oceania, less than 54 percent of the rural population has access to safe drinking water. Furthermore, the availability of safe drinking water in rural areas often depends on the labor of women, who spend hours each day fetching water for the home.

Safe drinking water generally refers to water that is free of disease-causing microbes, including bacteria, viruses, protozoa, and small animals such as worms.

PERSPECTIVE
Health Effects of Environmental Lead Exposure

The literature on human lead toxicity is voluminous. At high doses no human organ is immune to lead toxicity, and the domino effect may progress to coma and even death. At the moderately elevated and low levels of exposure typical in environmental media, lead can damage the central nervous, renal, cardiovascular, hematological, and reproductive systems. Infants are particularly susceptible to lead poisoning because they absorb lead more readily than adults and their developing nervous and immune systems are more vulnerable than adults' systems to the effects of lead. Epidemiological studies have found that childhood lead exposure is associated with neuropsychiatric disorders including lowered IQ, impaired mental and physical development, hyperactivity, hearing loss, reduced attention span, aggression, somatic complaints, and antisocial and delinquent behavior. A significant association between elevated blood lead at relatively low levels and delayed pubertal development in girls has recently been reported (Wu, Buck, and Mendola, 2003). There does not appear to be a safe threshold of lead exposure. Even exposures to picomolar concentrations of lead have been shown to stimulate kinase C, a calcium- and phospholipid-dependent enzyme that can mediate cellular proliferation, differentiation, and function and is critical to signal transduction. The effects of such cellular change on the viability of organ systems and the wellness of an individual are unknown.

A weak association between long-term, low-level exposure to lead and development of hypertension has been reported for men and women. Past exposure to lead may result in decreased reserve capacity of the brain and detrimental effects on neuropsychological functions, which may become manifest in old age. More than 90 percent of the body burden of lead is located in the bone, where it has an average half-life of about ten years. During periods of increased bone turnover, such as during pregnancy, lactation, and menopause, these skeletal bone stores can be mobilized, long after the external exposure, posing a hazard to the fetus at critical times in its organ development and to the nursing child. The bone loss during menopause, mediated by decreased estrogen production, may release enough lead to constitute a hazard to women in old age. Lead exerts both direct and indirect effects on bone turnover and has been implicated as a risk factor for osteoporosis, which is increasing rapidly in developing countries, especially among women (Vahter, Berglund, Akesson, and Linden, 2002).

These organisms can be considered *traditional* health hazards in drinking-water supplies. In addition to traditional hazards, water may carry high concentrations of chemical contaminants that can threaten health. In developing countries, concentrations of anthropogenic chemical contaminants are on the rise and can be designated *modern* health hazards. Examples are pesticides, nitrates, industrial

TABLE 11.5 Proportion of Population with Access to Safe Drinking Water, 2006

Region	Urban Population with Access (%)	Rural Population with Access (%)
Commonwealth of Independent States	99	86
Eastern Asia	98	81
Latin America & Caribbean	97	73
Northern Africa	96	87
Western Asia	95	80
Southern Asia	95	84
Southeastern Asia	92	81
Oceania	91	37
Sub-Saharan Africa	81	46
Developing regions	94	76
Developed regions	100	97
World	96	78

Source: WHO, 2008a.

pollutants, and disinfection by-products. In addition to anthropogenic contaminants, elevated concentrations of natural environmental contaminants may be found in drinking-water supplies. Though these natural contaminants are difficult to categorize in a traditional-modern framework, the presence in drinking water of naturally occurring contaminants, such as arsenic and fluoride, causes unwanted health effects. Natural contaminants are most prevalent in groundwater supplies and are a growing concern in developing countries, due to their increasing reliance on groundwater. A detailed overview of water and health is provided in Chapter Fifteen; this chapter focuses on water-related hazards of particular concern in Third World countries.

Effective prevention of waterborne microbial pathogen exposure requires sanitation. Effective (or *improved*) sanitation facilities prevent human fecal pollution of the environment, thereby ensuring hygienic separation of excreta from human contact. Examples of improved sanitation facilities include the flush or pour-flush toilet or latrine connected to a piped sewer, septic tank, or pit latrine; the ventilated improved pit latrine; the pit latrine with a slab; and the composting toilet. Sanitation is widely considered one of the most important health advances in the past two hundred years; however, only 62 percent of the world's population has access to improved sanitation facilities (WHO, 2008a). In sub-Saharan Africa, only 31 percent of the population has access to improved sanitation facilities; the corresponding figures are 33 percent in Southern Asia and 52 percent in Oceania. In contrast, 99 percent of the population in developed regions has access to improved sanitation facilities. Progress toward improved sanitation has been slow, with a skip from 41 percent to only 53 percent coverage in developing countries between 1990 and 2006. As further testament to the dire need for sanitation facilities, 31 percent of rural populations in developing countries defecate in the open, with as many as 63 percent practicing open defecation in Southern Asia (WHO, 2008a).

Microbial contamination of source water, lack of sanitation services, and inadequate personal hygiene form a triad that gives rise to communicable diseases. Volumes have been written on communicable diseases transmitted through unsafe drinking water (Hunter, Waite, and Ronchi, 2002; WHO and UNICEF Joint Monitoring Programme for Water Supply and Sanitation, 2000). Because these diseases are detailed in Chapter Fifteen, they are discussed only briefly here. Approximately 3.5 million people, mostly children, die annually from water-related communicable diseases in developing countries. In contrast just 73,000 deaths from this cause befall citizens of developed countries (WHO, 2008b). *Shigella*, a bacterium species that causes dysentery, or bloody diarrhea, is responsible for approximately 1.5 million deaths each year. Intestinal worms infect about 33 percent of the world's population, leading to malnutrition, anemia, and retarded growth. Trachoma, caused by the bacterium *Chlamydia trachomatis*, is the leading cause of preventable blindness, leading to 5 million cases worldwide. These microbial diseases can largely be prevented by providing access to microbe-free drinking water, adequate disposal systems for human excrement, and information about appropriate personal hygiene. An estimated 3.5 million deaths and 9 percent of all DALYs could be prevented through improvements in safe drinking water and sanitation (WHO, 2008b).

Concerted efforts have been made during recent decades to increase access to safe drinking water in Third World countries. They have resulted in increased distribution of disinfected surface water in many urban areas and in more access to groundwater supplies through the drilling of community wells in rural communities. More recently, increasing attention is being given to inexpensive point-of-use disinfection systems for household water treatment, especially in rural areas where groundwater is not available. One such device, known as the Safe Water System (SWS), consists of locally produced and bottled sodium hypochlorite solution, a 5 to 10 mL measuring cap on each bottle to monitor dosage, a plastic container in which to store disinfected water and prevent recontamination, and educational and social marketing materials to encourage changes in personal hygiene. The inexpensive SWS has been shown to be effective in reducing rates of diarrhea in periurban and rural communities of Bolivia and Zambia, and some effort is being made to export it to other countries (Suk and others, 2003). Point-of-use solar disinfection also shows promise (Fisher, Keenan, Nelson, and Voelker, 2008). Few countries in the Third World can afford the capital investment needed to pipe safe water to most citizens, and inexpensive household-level interventions are increasingly being viewed as worthwhile alternatives.

Modern health hazards from anthropogenic contaminants are also beginning to receive attention in developing countries. Centralized chlorination of drinking water leads to the formation of disinfection by-products that may be carcinogenic to humans (International Agency for Research on Cancer, 1987). Industrial discharges of toxic chemicals taint groundwater and surface water supplies. Estimates suggest that approximately 60 percent of smelting and 50 percent of lead mining operations are located in developing countries (Yáñez and others, 2002), causing trace metal pollution (for example, cadmium, nickel, and lead) in aquatic systems (Nriagu and Pacyna, 1988). In most cases water is consumed without effective treatment for these contaminants. Millions of people in developing countries drink rainwater collected from rooftops, stem flows, or other systems. In many urban areas this source of drinking water becomes contaminated through scavenging of airborne pollutants and leaching of air toxics deposited on the roof surfaces.

Non–point source water pollution from agricultural activity is also a concern in developing countries. Pesticides and nitrates are applied heavily to farmland in developing countries and infiltrate well water supplies. For instance, in the Philippines, concentrations of nitrates and pesticides (DDT, butachlor, endosulfan, and carbofuran) exceeding safe drinking-water standards have been detected in shallow groundwater supplies (Bouman, Castaneda, and Bhuiyan, 2002). Exposure to elevated nitrate levels in well water supplies can cause methemoglobinemia, a disease characterized by insufficient oxygen reaching the brain, turning babies, who are especially vulnerable, a faint bluish color. A wide variety of diseases, from cancer to neurodegenerative disorders, are associated with exposure to nitrates and pesticides, but the contribution of this exposure pathway to the disease burden in developing countries has yet to be assessed.

Finally, elevated concentrations of natural elements also cause numerous health problems for populations around the world. Specific elements of concern in water include arsenic, fluoride, radon, sodium, and uranium. Excessive levels of these natural contaminants are commonly detected in groundwater supplies. For example, high fluoride concentrations have been documented in groundwater in large parts of Africa, the Middle East, China, and Southern and Western Asia. Low concentrations of fluoride (for example, 0.8 to 1.2 mg/L) can prevent tooth decay and strengthen bones. At slightly higher concentrations, however, dental and skeletal fluorosis can result, with attrition of tooth enamel and fluoride deposits in bone, respectively. The total number of people drinking water with fluoride concentrations above WHO's guideline (1.5 mg/L) is not known. However, estimates suggest that tens of millions of individuals are suffering from fluorosis, with high prevalences in China and India.

Elevated levels of arsenic have been reported in groundwater in many parts of the world. To date, high levels of arsenic have been identified in groundwater from twenty-seven countries on six continents, and additional contaminated aquifers are continually being discovered. Globally, at least 55 million people are estimated to be exposed to levels of arsenic in drinking water exceeding 50 μg/L, the maximum contaminant limit (MCL) allowable in many countries (Table 11.6). More than 100 million people are exposed to levels of arsenic exceeding the WHO's MCL of 10 μg/L.

Health effects associated with ingestion of groundwater high in arsenic include peripheral vascular diseases (such as blackfoot disease, which presents with numbness of one or more extremities, progressing to black discoloration, ulceration, and gangrene), skin lesions, diabetes mellitus, cerebrovascular disease, and cancer. More recent studies have linked high levels of arsenic in drinking water with health

TABLE 11.6   Estimated Population Exposed to Arsenic in Drinking Water
at Concentrations > 50 μg/L

Country	Population Exposed
Bangladesh	30,000,000
West Bengal, India	6,000,000
Taiwan	900,000
Mainland China	5,600,000
Vietnam	6,000,000
Cambodia	5,000,000
Argentina	270,000
Chile	500,000
Mexico	400,000
USA	350,000
Hungary	29,000
Total	55,000,000

Source: Adapted from Smedley and Kinniburgh, 2002.

effects ranging from infant mortality to cancers of the skin, lungs, bladder, and kidney. Arsenic poisoning has become an epidemic and a major public health problem in some developing countries, and investigators continue to explore affordable methods to reduce arsenic concentrations in water to safe levels.

People in developing countries face triple and sometimes quadruple jeopardy when attempting to manage environmental risks from unsafe water

PERSPECTIVE
Arsenic Poisoning in Bangladesh

Historically, surface water in Bangladesh has been contaminated with microorganisms, causing significant morbidity in infants and children. In the 1970s and '80s, the United Nations Children's Fund (UNICEF), working with the Bangladesh Department of Public Health Engineering, installed tube wells as a putative source of safe drinking water for the Bangladeshi people. A tube well is constructed from a pipe about 5 cm in diameter, which is inserted into the ground at shallow depths less than 50 m and capped with a cast-iron or steel hand pump. It is estimated that more than 11 million tube wells have been installed in Bangladesh. In the early 1990s, the well water, which had seemingly provided a solution to the country's water problems, was discovered to have high concentrations of arsenic in many parts of the country. Standard water-testing procedures did not check for arsenic during initial well installation.

The maximum concentration of arsenic permitted in drinking water in Bangladesh is 50 μg/L, whereas the WHO recommended standard is 10 μg/L. The scale of the arsenic contamination has not been fully documented, and precise estimates of the population at risk are unavailable. However, an estimated 25 to 35 million people are exposed to arsenic in drinking water at levels exceeding 50 μg/L, and 50 to 60 million people are exposed to concentrations exceeding 10 μg/L. The effects mentioned earlier—skin lesions, peripheral vascular diseases, diabetes mellitus, cerebrovascular disease, and cancer—have been linked to this arsenic exposure and are estimated to affect more than 100,000 people in Bangladesh. Arsenic contamination of water in Bangladesh is one of the worst environmental health disasters in history, and more health problems are expected in coming years.

Despite the unimaginable scale of arsenic-related health problems in Bangladesh, there is hope. More than 50 percent of the tube wells in Bangladesh have arsenic concentrations below 10 μ/L. Efforts are ongoing to identify tube wells that have water with low arsenic content and to discover simple, inexpensive, effective arsenic treatment strategies for tube wells with high arsenic concentrations (see, for example, Massachusetts Institute of Technology, 2001). (For further information on chronic arsenic poisoning, see Arsenic Project, 2005.)

supplies. Traditional health hazards of microbial contamination, modern hazards of anthropogenic pollutants, and hazards of natural environmental contaminants have been discussed. In addition, *postmodern* water quality hazards, such as endocrine disruptors, are a growing problem around the world. Endocrine disruptors are widespread in water supplies in developed countries due to extensive use of human and veterinary pharmaceuticals and reproductive hormones. Endocrine disruptors are likely to be a concern in water supplies of developing countries in the future, as personal care products and industrial pharmaceuticals are more broadly adopted. In addition, heavy use of bottled water may be a source of exposure to endocrine disruptors leaching from the plastic bottles; this is only beginning to be investigated (Le, Carlson, Chua, and Belcher, 2008).

INJURIES

Most injuries are associated directly or indirectly with environmental risk factors and are thus preventable. Examples of environmental factors that drive injuries include poorly designed cookstoves that carry a risk of burns (especially to children) and house fires; poorly designed roadways; substandard housing at risk of collapse, especially in slum areas; inadequate land use planning that places people in the path of flooding and landslides; accidental poisonings by pesticides needed to deal with effects of newly created breeding grounds or of building next to pest-infested habitat such as a stream; and festering domestic and interpersonal violence, especially in urban slums. It is estimated that about 30 percent of the global burden of unintentional injuries is attributable to environmental risk factors (WHO, 1997). A general review of injuries as an environmental health problem is presented in Chapter Twenty-Two. This chapter focuses on the effects on injuries of the environmental risk transition in developing countries, with special emphasis on roadway injuries.

Although injuries are major contributors to global morbidity and mortality in both developing and developed countries, a clear transition in injury risks occurs with a change in level of development. Injuries from fires, agricultural injuries, drownings, wood-acquisition injuries, and war-related violence dominate the early stages of development, whereas road traffic, intentional, and industrial injuries appear to increase with economic development (WHO, 1997). Because injuries disproportionately affect young adults, their economic impact can be profound; the resulting long-term disability affects productivity, especially among low-income groups, whose earning capacity is often based on physical ability. Injuries can be divided into two broad categories: **intentional injuries** (such as rape, battery, child and spousal abuse, suicide, police or military brutality, and war-related violence) and **unintentional injuries** (such as road traffic injuries, harm from fires, drownings, falls, poisonings, injuries resulting from natural disasters, and workplace injuries). Together, injuries from these sources constitute a hidden epidemic among young adults in the developing countries. They have been among the major causes of healthy life years lost, accounting for 182.6 million DALYs in 2002, or 12.2 percent of the global total (15.5 percent among men and 8.7 percent among women) (Table 11.7). In Africa, injuries accounted for 31 million DALYs, or 8.5 percent of the total. In parts of South America, Eastern Europe, and the eastern Mediterranean, more than 30 percent of the disease burden among male adults fourteen to forty-four years old can be attributed to injuries (WHO, 2003). Worldwide, intentional injuries accounted for 3.3 percent of DALYs, and unintentional injuries for 8.9 percent (Table 11.7).

Road traffic injuries are among the leading causes of disease burden, especially in the fourteen- to forty-four-year-old age group. Traffic crashes kill or severely

TABLE 11.7 DALYs Due to Injuries, Globally, by Gender, and in Africa, 2002

	Global %	Male %	Female %	Africa %	Africa (% all injuries)[b]
All injuries[a]	12.2 (182.6)	15.5 (120.4)	8.7 (62.2)	8.5 (31.0)	
Unintentional injuries[a]	8.9 (133.5)	10.9 (84.4)	6.8 (49.0)	5.9 (21.5)	69.5
Road traffic accidents	2.6	3.5	1.6	2.0	23.2
Poisonings	0.5	0.6	0.4	0.3	3.4
Falls	1.1	1.3	0.9	0.3	0.0
Fires	0.8	0.6	1.0	0.5	6.4
Drownings	0.7	1.0	0.5	0.5	6.2
Other	3.3	3.9	2.6	2.3	26.8
Intentional injuries[a]	3.3 (49.1)	4.6 (36.0)	1 (13.1)	2.6 (9.5)	30.5
Self-inflicted	1.4	1.6	1.2	0.2	2.9
Violence	1.4	2.3	0.5	1.5	17.1
War	0.4	0.7	0.1	0.9	10.6
Other	0.0	0.0	0.0	0.0	0.0

[a] The number of DALYs (in millions) is shown in parentheses.

[b] The contribution (as a percentage) of each risk factor to the total injury burden for Africa.

Source: WHO, 2003.

injure more than 20 million drivers, passengers, and pedestrians each year, with the burden falling most heavily on developing countries (WHO, 2003). Developing countries bear 90 percent of the DALYs lost to traffic injuries and death, and this epidemic is rising rapidly, especially in Asia. It is projected that by 2020, vehicular deaths will increase by nearly 150 percent in China and by 80 percent or more in many developing countries (Kopits and Cropper, 2003). Injuries due mostly to traffic crashes account for up to one-third of the acute patient cases in many Third World hospitals and 30 to 86 percent of trauma admissions (Odero, Garner, and Zwi, 1997). Besides the human toll, the economic cost of road crashes in developing countries has been estimated at about $65 billion, a heavy burden on economic development and a financial drain on national health care systems (WHO, 2003).

Road infrastructure in developing countries rarely keeps pace with the sharp rise in the number of vehicles on the roads, resulting in unsafe driving conditions, massive traffic jams, road rage, vehicular crashes, and harm to pedestrians. Vehicles in developing countries are more likely to be involved in fatal crashes (by as much as 200-fold in some cases) than are vehicles in more developed countries (Jacobs, Aaron-Thomas, and Astrop, 2000). The face of traffic death is different in the three worlds. In developed countries, driver and passenger deaths generally account for 50 to 60 percent of traffic fatalities, with the majority of deaths occurring on rural roads (WHO, 2003). In developing countries, in contrast, a large fraction of the fatalities occur among vulnerable road users in urban areas (including pedestrians, bicyclists, people using carts or rickshaws, motorcyclists, and moped and scooter riders) and among passengers on trucks and buses (WHO, 2003). The urban poor in developing countries are disproportionately exposed to vehicular injuries because they tend to live in overcrowded areas with narrow streets and no speed controls, to operate businesses from roadside stalls, to walk on the streets to get to their destinations, and to have their children play on streets. A substantial proportion of vehicular mortality and morbidity can be prevented by environmental intervention strategies.

SUMMARY

Environmental health exists against a complex backdrop of environmental, technological, demographic, political, economic, and cultural factors. For much of the world's population, living in Third World countries, these factors seem to conspire to threaten health. People are exposed to traditional environmental hazards, such as contaminated water and biofuel smoke, and at the same time to modern environmental hazards, such as chemical toxins. Globalization has accelerated change throughout the world; one result has been migration of hazards from developed nations to developing nations, concentrating hazardous environmental exposures and creating a risk overlap by superimposing modern on traditional exposures. In combination with poverty, undernutrition, and rapid urbanization, the toll on health can be enormous.

This chapter has discussed major drivers of environmental health challenges in developing nations, including vulnerability and coping capacity, globalization, agriculture and food security, and urbanization, and three domains of environmental risk factors that affect health and help account for global disparities: air quality, sanitation and water, and injuries. (Another such domain, occupational health, also has special relevance in developing nations and is discussed in Chapter Twenty; also see Frumkin, 1999.) Much of the discussion in this chapter reprises material presented elsewhere in this book, but with a focus on developing nation settings, where exposure levels are often higher, populations more susceptible, and public health responses less effective than they are in developed nations. As the twenty-first century proceeds, achieving environmental health for all remains a pressing challenge and a moral necessity.

KEY TERMS

adaptation

adaptive capacity

biofuels

coping capacity

demographic transition

disability-adjusted life years (DALYs)

ecological risk trap

environmental drivers

environmental refugee

environmental vulnerability

First World

globalization

green revolution

health disparities

intentional injuries

modern hazards

overnutrition

postindustrial

postmodern hazards

priority pollutants

resilience

risk overlap

risk transition

Second World

Third World

traditional hazards

undernutrition

unintentional injuries

urban solid wastes

urbanicity

urbanization

vulnerability

years of life lost (YLLs)

years lived with disability (YLDs)

DISCUSSION QUESTIONS

1. What is the environmental risk transition? What are the impacts of this phenomenon on the health of people in Third World countries?

2. What are the risks and benefits of globalization on the health of people in (a) developed countries and (b) developing countries? What are the effects of environmental risk transition for Third World countries?

3. What diseases are commonly associated with (a) traditional lifestyles and (b) Westernized lifestyles?

4. How can a safe drinking-water supply, sanitary disposal of human waste, and good behavioral hygiene practices limit water-based microbial diseases?

5. Despite tremendous efforts by WHO and UNICEF, billions of people currently live without safe drinking-water or sanitation services. Why does this situation continue?

6. Although two to three times as many disaster events were reported in the United States as were reported in India or in Bangladesh in 2000, there were fifteen times more deaths in India and thirty times more deaths in Bangladesh from disasters. What are the likely reasons for this disparity?

7. What might account for the rising incidence of asthma in developing countries?

8. Pick an environmental health problem (other than asthma) that is influenced by urbanization in developing countries. What is the impact of urbanization on community and individual risk factors for that health problem? What is the net influence of urbanization on that health problem?

REFERENCES

Agency for Toxic Substances and Disease Registry. *Toxicological Profile for Lead (Update)*. Atlanta, Ga.: Agency for Toxic Substances and Disease Registry, 2000.

Alm, J., and others. "Atopy in Children of Families with an Anthroposophic Lifestyle." *Lancet*, 1999, *353*, 1485–1488.

Arsenic Project. "Introduction." http://phys4.harvard.edu/~wilson/arsenic/arsenic_project_introduction.html. 2005.

Balakrishnan, K., and others. "Daily Average Exposures to Respiratory Particulate Matter from Combustion of Biomass Fuels in Rural Households of Southern India." *Environmental Health Perspectives*, 2002, *110*, 1069–1075.

Beasley, R., Crane, J., Lai, C., and Pearce, N. "Prevalence and Etiology of Asthma." *Journal of Allergy and Clinical Immunology*, 2000, *105*(2), 466–472.

Bouman, B.A.M., Castaneda, A. R., and Bhuiyan, S. I. "Nitrate and Pesticide Contamination of Groundwater Under Rice-Based Cropping Systems: Past and Current Evidence from the Philippines." *Agriculture, Ecosystems and Environment*, 2002, *92*, 185–199.

Bradley, D. J., and Narayan, R. "Epidemiological Patterns Associated with Agricultural Activities in the Tropics with Special Reference to Vector-Borne Diseases." In *Effects of Agricultural Development on Vector-Borne Diseases*. Rome: Food and Agriculture Organization of the United Nations, 1987.

Bruce, N., Perez-Padilla, R., and Albalak, R. "Indoor Air Pollution in Developing Countries: A Major Environmental Health Challenge." *Bulletin of the World Health Organization*, 2000, *78*, 1080–1092.

Chaudhuri, N. "Interventions to Improve Children's Health by Improving the Housing Environment." *Reviews on Environmental Health*, 2004, *19*, 197–221.

Chilima, D. M., and Ismail, S. J. "Anthropometric Characteristics of Older People in Malawi." *European Journal of Clinical Nutrition*, 1998, *52*, 643–649.

Chow, J. C. "Introduction to the A&WMA 2004 Critical Review 'Megacities and Atmospheric Pollution.'" *Journal of the Air and Waste Management Association*, 2004, *54*, 642–643.

Chow, J. C., and others. "Megacities and Atmospheric Pollution." *Journal of the Air and Waste Management Association*, 2004, *54*(10), 1226–1235.

Cohen, B. "Urbanization in Developing Countries: Current Trends, Future Projections, and Key Challenges for Sustainability." *Technology in Society*, 2006, *28*, 63–80.

Conisbee, M., and Simms, A. *Environmental Refugees: The Case for Recognition*. New Economics Foundation. http://www.neweconomics.org/gen/z_sys_PublicationDetail.aspx?PID=159, 2003.

Duh, J. D., Shandas, V., Chang, H., and George, L. A. "Rates of Urbanisation and the Resiliency of Air and Water Quality." *Science of the Total Environment*, 2008, doi:10.1016/j.scitotenv.2008.05.002.

Ecobichon, D. J. "Pesticide Use in Developing Countries." *Toxicology*, 2001, *160*, 27–33.

Ellegard, A. "Cooking Fuel Smoke and Respiratory Symptoms Among Women in Low-Income Areas in Maputo." *Environmental Health Perspectives*, 1996, *104*, 980–985.

Emmelin, A., and Wall, S. "Indoor Air Pollution: A Poverty-Related Cause of Mortality Among the Children of the World." *Chest*, 2007, *132*(5), 1615–1623.

Ezzati, M., and Kammen, D. M. "The Health Impacts of Exposure to Indoor Air Pollution from Solid Fuels in Developing Countries: Knowledge, Gaps and Data Needs." *Environmental Health Perspectives*, 2002, *110*, 1057–1066.

Fisher, M. B., Keenan, C. R., Nelson, K. L., and Voelker, B. M. "Speeding Up Solar Disinfection (SODIS): Effects of Hydrogen Peroxide, Temperature, pH, and Copper Plus Ascorbate on the Photoinactivation of E-Coli." *Journal of Water and Health*, 2008, *6*, 35–51.

Frumkin, H. "Across the Water and Down the Ladder: Occupational Health in the Global Economy." *Occupational Medicine*, 1999, *14*(3), 637–663.

Fullerton, D. G., Bruce, N., and Gordon, S. B. "Indoor Air Pollution from Biomass Fuel Smoke Is a Major Health Concern in the Developing World." *Transactions of the Royal Society of Tropical Medicine and Hygiene*, 2008, *102*(9), 843–851.

Gallicchio, L., Scherer, R., and Sexton, M. "Influence of Nutrition Intake on Blood Lead Levels of Young Children at Risk for Lead Poisoning." *Environmental Health Perspectives*, 2002, *110*, A767–A771.

Golshan, M., Faghihi, M., and Marandi, M. "Indoor Women Jobs and Pulmonary Risks in Rural Areas of Isfahan, Iran, 2000." *Respiratory Medicine*, 2002, *96*(6), 382–388.

Goyal, S. K., Ghatge, S. V., Nema, P. M., and Tamhane, S. "Understanding Urban Vehicular Pollution Problem Vis-a-Vis Ambient Air Quality—Case Study of a Megacity (Delhi, India). *Environmental Monitoring and Assessment*, 2006, *119*(1–3), 557–569.

Huang, S., and Pan, W. "Dietary Fats and Asthma in Teenagers: Analyses of the First Nutrition and Health Survey in Taiwan (NAHSIT)." *Clinical and Experimental Allergy*, 2001, *31*, 1875–1880.

Hunter, P. R., Waite, M., and Ronchi, E. (eds.). *Drinking Water and Infectious Disease: Establishing the Links.* London: IWA, 2002.

International Agency for Research on Cancer. *Overall Evaluations of Carcinogenicity: An Updating of IARC Monographs, Volumes 1 to 42.* IARC Monographs on the Evaluation of Carcinogenic Risk to Humans. Lyon, France: International Agency for Research on Cancer, 1987.

Jacobs, G., Aaron-Thomas, A., and Astrop, A. *Estimating Global Road Fatalities.* Report No. 445. London: Transport Research Laboratory, 2000.

Jackson, J. "Fatal Attraction: Living with Earthquakes, the Growth of Villages into Megacities, and Earthquake Vulnerability in the Modern World." *Philosophical Transactions of the Royal Society A: Mathematical, Physical and Engineering Sciences*, 2006, *364*(1845), 1911–1925.

Johnson, M., and others. "Asthma Prevalence and Severity in Arab American Communities in the Detroit Area, Michigan." *Journal of Immigrant Health*, 2005, *7*(3), 165–178.

Kickbusch, I., and Buse, K. "Global Influences and Global Responses: International Health at the Turn of the Twenty-First Century." In M. H. Merson, R. E. Black, and A. J. Mills (eds.), *International Public Health.* Gaithersburg, Md.: Aspen, 2001.

Kinsella, K. "Urban and Rural Dimensions of Global Population Aging: An Overview." *Journal of Rural Health*, 2001, *17*, 314–322.

Koh, D., and Jeyaratnam, J. "Pesticide Hazards in Developing Countries." *Science of the Total Environment*, 1996, *188*(suppl. 1), S78–S85.

Kopits, E., and Cropper, M. "Traffic Fatalities and Economic Growth." Policy Research Working Paper No. 3035. Washington, D.C.: World Bank, 2003.

Krzyzanowski, M., and Schwela, D. "Patterns of Air Pollution in Developing Countries." In S. T. Holgate, H. S. Koren, J. M. Samet, and R. L. Maynard (eds.), *Air Pollution and Health.* San Diego: Academic Press, 1999.

Le, H. H., Carlson, E. M., Chua, J. P., and Belcher, S. M. "Bisphenol A Is Released from Polycarbonate Drinking Bottles and Mimics the Neurotoxic Actions of Estrogen in Developing Cerebellar Neurons." *Toxicology Letters*, 2008, *176*, 149–156.

Leung, R. C., Carlin, J. B., Burdon, J. G., and Czarny, D. "Asthma, Allergy and Atopy in Asian Immigrants in Melbourne." *Medical Journal of Australia*, 1994, *161*(7), 418–425.

Liu, J., and others. "Chronic Arsenic Poisoning from Burning of High-Arsenic-Containing Coal in Guizhou, China." *Environmental Health Perspectives*, 2002, *110*, 119–122.

London, L., and others. "Pesticide Usage and Health Consequences for Women in Developing Countries: Out of Sight, Out of Mind?" *International Journal of Occupational and Environmental Health*, 2002, *8*, 46–59.

Lopez, A. D., and others (eds.), *Global Burden of Disease and Risk Factors.* New York: World Bank and Oxford University Press, 2006.

Mascie-Taylor, C. G. N., and Karim, E. "The Burden of Chronic Disease." *Science*, 2003, *302*, 192 1–1922.

Massachusetts Institute of Technology. *Arsenic Remediation Technologies: Online Informational Database.* http://web.mit.edu/murcott/www/arsenic, 2001.

Meister, E. A. "Global Environmental Health." In R. W. Buckingham (ed.), *A Primer on International Health.* Needham Heights, Mass.: Allyn & Bacon, 2001.

Mestl, H. E., and others. "Urban and Rural Exposure to Indoor Air Pollution from Domestic Biomass and Coal Burning Across China." *Science of the Total Environment*, 2007, *377*(1), 12–26.

Meyer, P. A., McGeehin, M. A., and Falk, H. "A Global Approach to Childhood Lead Poisoning Prevention." *International Journal of Hygiene and Environmental Health*, 2003, *206*, 363–369.

Mishra, V. "Effect of Indoor Air Pollution from Biomass Combustion on Prevalence of Asthma in the Elderly." *Environmental Health Perspectives*, 2003, *111*, 71–76.

Mishra, V., and Retherford, R. D. "Does Biofuel Smoke Contribute to Anaemia and Stunting in Early Childhood?" *International Journal of Epidemiology*, 2007, *36*(1), 117–129.

Montgomery, M. R. "The Urban Transformation of the Developing World." *Science*, 2008, *319*(5864), 761–764.

Moore, M., Gould, P., and Keary, B. S. "Global Urbanization and Impact on Health." *International Journal of Hygiene and Environmental Health*, 2003, *206*, 269–278.

Murray, C. J. L., and Lopez, A. D. (eds.). *The Global Burden of Disease, Global Health Statistics: A Compendium of Incidence, Prevalence and Mortality Estimates for over 200 conditions.* Global Burden of Disease and Injury Series, Vol. *2*. Cambridge, Mass.: Harvard School of Public Health on behalf of the World Health Organization and the World Bank, 1996.

Myers, N. "Environmental Refugees: A Growing Phenomenon of the 21st Century." *Philosophical Transactions: Biological Sciences*, 2002, *357*, 609–613.

Naeher, L. P., and others. "Woodsmoke Health Effects: A Review." *Inhalation Toxicology*, 2007, *19*(1), 67–106.

Ng'ang'a, L. W., and others. "Prevalence of Exercise Induced Bronchospasm in Kenyan School Children: An Urban-Rural Comparison." *Thorax*, 1998, *53*(11), 919–926.

Nriagu, J. O., and Pacyna, J. M. "Quantitative Assessment of Worldwide Contamination of Air, Water and Soils by Trace Metals." *Nature*, 1988, *333*, 134–140.

Odero, W., Garner, P., and Zwi, A. "Road Traffic Injuries in Developing Countries: A Comprehensive Review of Epidemiological Studies." *Tropical Medicine and International Health*, 1997, *2*, 445–460.

Ooi, G. L., and Phua, K. H. "Urbanization and Slum Formation." *Journal of Urban Health*, 2007, *84*(suppl. 3), i27–34.

Partnership for Clean Fuels and Vehicles and United Nations Environment Programme. *Leaded Petrol Phase-Out: Global Status August 2008.* http://www.unep.org/pcfv/PDF/MapWorldLead-August2008.pdf, 2008.

Pelletier, D. L. "The Potentiating Effects of Malnutrition on Child Mortality: Epidemiologic Evidence and Policy Implications." *Nutrition Reviews*, 1994, *52*, 409–415.

Pokhrel, A. K., and Others. "Case-Control Study of Indoor Cooking Smoke Exposure and Cataract in Nepal and India." *International Journal of Epidemiology*, 2005, *34*(3), 702–708.

Population Reference Bureau. *Urbanization and Global Change.* http://www.globalchange.umich.edu/globalchange2/current/lectures/urban_gc, 2008.

Powell, C. V., and others. "Respiratory Symptoms and Duration of Residence in Immigrant Teenagers Living in Melbourne, Australia." *Archives of Disease in Childhood*, 1999, *81*(2), 159–162.

Prüss-Üstün, A., and Corvalán, C. *Preventing Disease Through Healthy Environments.* Geneva: World Health Organization, 2006.

Regional Conference on the Phasing-Out of Leaded Gasoline in Sub-Saharan Africa. *Declaration of Dakar.* http://www.unep.org/pcfv/pdf/DataDakarDecl.pdf, 2001.

Romieu, I., Samet, J. M., Smith, K. R., and Bruce, N. "Outdoor Air Pollution and Acute Respiratory Infections Among Children in Developing Countries." *Journal of Occupational and Environmental Medicine*, 2002, *44*, 640–649.

Roy, E., Bruce, N., and Dalgado, H. "Birth Weight and Exposure to Kitchen Wood Smoke During Pregnancy in Rural Guatemala." *Environmental Health Perspectives*, 2002, *110*, 109–114.

Rudan, I., and others. "Epidemiology and Etiology of Childhood Pneumonia." *Bulletin of the World Health Organization*, 2008, *86*(5), 408–416.

Samet, J. M., and Cohen, A. J. "Air Pollution and Lung Cancer." In S. T. Holgate, H. S. Koren, J. M. Samet, and R. L. Maynard (eds.), *Air Pollution and Health*. San Diego: Academic Press, 1999.

Schmidt, C. W. "Spheres of Influence: A Change in the Air." *Environmental Health Perspectives*, 2007, *115*(8), 413–415.

Sims, J., and Butter, M. E. *Gender Equity and Environmental Health*. Harvard Center for Population and Development Studies, Working Paper Series Vol. 10, No. 5. http://www.hsph.Harvard.edu/ organizatons/healthnet/HUpapers/gender/simsbutter.html, 2000.

Smedley, P. L., and Kinniburgh, D. G. "A Review of the Source, Behavior and Distribution of Arsenic in Natural Waters." *Applied Geochemistry*, 2002, *17*, 517–568.

Smith, K. R. *Biomass Fuels, Air Pollution and Health: A Global Perspective*. New York: Plenum, 1987.

Smith, K. R. "Indoor Air Pollution in Developing Countries: Recommendations for Research." *Indoor Air*, 2002, *12*, 198–207.

Smith, K. R., Corvalán, C., and Kjellstrom, T. "How Much Global Ill Health Is Attributable to Environmental Factors?" *Epidemiology*, 1999, *10*, 573–574.

Smith, K. R., and Mehta, S. "The Burden of Disease from Indoor Air Pollution in Developing Countries: Comparison of Estimates." *International Journal of Hygiene and Environmental Health*, 2003, 206, 279–289.

Smith, K. R., Mehta, S. and Maeusezahl-Feuz, M. "Indoor Air Pollution from Household Use of Solid Fuels." In Ezzati, M., Lopez, A.D., Rodgers, A. and Murray, C,J.L., Eds. *Comparative Quantification of Health Risks: Global and Regional Burden of Disease Attrbutable to Selected Major Risk Factors*. Geneva: WHO, 2004, pp 1435–1493.

Suk, W. A., and others. "Environmental Threats to Children's Health in Southeast Asia and the Western Pacific." *Environmental Health Perspectives*, 2003, 111, 1340–1347.

Thomas, E. P., Seager, J. R., and Mathee, A. "Environmental Health Challenges in South Africa: Policy Lessons from Case Studies." *Health & Place*, 2002, 8, 251–261.

Torres-Dosal, A., and others. "Indoor Air Pollution in a Mexican Indigenous Community: Evaluation of Risk Reduction Program Using Biomarkers of Exposure and Effect." *Science of the Total Environment*, 2008, *390*(2–3), 362–368.

Tung, Y. H., and others. "Cooking Oil Fume-Induced Cytokine Expression and Oxidative Stress in Human Lung Epithelial Cells." *Environmental Research*, 2001, *87*(1), 47–54.

United Nations Environment Programme. *Africa Environment Outlook: Past, Present and Future Perspectives*. Nairobi: United Nations Environment Programme, 2002. http://www.unep.org/dewa/ Africa/publications/AEO-1/.

United Nations Habitat. *State of the World's Cities 2008/2009 - Harmonious Cities*. London: Earthscan, 2008.

Vahter, M., Berglund, M., Akesson, A., and Linden, C. "Metals and Women's Health." *Environmental Research*, 2002, *A88*, 145–155.

Vlahov, D., Galea, S., Gibble, E., and Freudenberg, N. "Perspectives on Urban Conditions and Population Health." *Cadernos de Saúde Pública/Reports in Public Health*, 2005, *21*(3), 949–957.

Vlahov, D., and others. "Urban as a Determinant of Health." *Journal of Urban Health*, 2007, *84*(suppl. 3), i16–26.

West, K. P., Caballero, B., and Black, R. E. "Nutrition." In M. H. Merson, R. E. Black, and A. J. Mills (eds.), *International Public Health*. Gaithersburg, Md.: Aspen, 2001.

WHO and UNICEF Joint Monitoring Programme for Water Supply and Sanitation. *Global Water Supply and Sanitation Assessment 2000 Report*. Geneva: World Health Organization, 2000.

Wong, G. W., and Chow, C. M. "Childhood Asthma Epidemiology: Insights from Comparative Studies of Rural and Urban Populations." *Pediatric Pulmonology*, 2008, *43*(2), 107–116.

Woodcock, A., and others. "Pet Allergen Levels in Homes in Ghana and the United Kingdom." *Journal of Clinical Immunology*, 2001, *108*(3), 463–465.

World Bank. *World Development Report 1999/2000: Entering the 21st Century*. New York: Oxford University Press, 2000.

World Health Organization. *Health and Environment in Sustainable Development: Five Years After the Earth Summit*. Geneva: World Health Organization, 1997.

World Health Organization. *The World Health Report 2001: Mental Health: New Understanding, New Hope*. Geneva: World Health Organization, 2001.

World Health Organization. *The World Health Report 2002: Reducing Risks, Promoting Healthy Life*. Geneva: World Health Organization, 2002.

World Health Organization. *The World Health Report 2003: Shaping the Future*. Geneva: World Health Organization, 2003.

World Health Organization. *A Billion Voices: Listening and Responding to the Health Needs of Slum Dwellers and Informal Settlers in New Urban Settings*. http://www.who.intsocial_determinantsresourcesurban_settings.pdf, 2005.

World Health Organization. *Progress on Drinking Water and Sanitation*. Geneva: World Health Organization, 2008a.

World Health Organization. *Safer Water, Better Health*. Geneva: World Health Organization, 2008b.

Wu, T., Buck, G. M., and Mendola, P. "Blood Lead Levels and Sexual Maturation in U.S. Girls: The Third National Health and Nutrition Examination Survey, 1988–1994." *Environmental Health Perspectives*, 2003, *111*(7), 37–740.

Wu, M. T., and others. "Environmental Exposure to Cooking Oil Fumes and Cervical Intraepithelial Neoplasm." *Environmental Research*, 2004, *94*, 25–32.

Yáñez, L., and others. "Overview of Human Health and Chemical Mixtures: Problems Facing Developing Countries." *Environmental Health Perspectives*, 2002, *110*(suppl. 6), 901–909.

Yohe, G., and Tol, R.S.J. "Indicators for Social and Economic Coping Capacity: Moving Toward a Working Definition of Adaptive Capacity." *Global Environmental Change*, 2002, *12*, 25–40.

FOR FURTHER INFORMATION

Aron, J. L., and Patz, J. A. (eds.). *Ecosystem Change and Public Health: A Global Perspective*. Baltimore, Md.:
    Johns Hopkins University Press, 2001.
IRC International Water and Sanitation Centre. *World Water Day Report, 2001*. http://www.worldwaterday.org/
    2001/report/index.html, 2001.
Kasperson, J. X., and Kasperson, R. E. (eds.). *The Global Environmental Risk*. Tokyo: United Nations
    University Press, 2001.
Merson, M. H., Black, R. E., and Mills, A. J. (eds.). *International Public Health*. Gaithersburg, Md.: Aspen,
    2001.
United Nations. *Johannesburg Summit 2002: World Summit on Sustainable Development*. http://www
    .johannesburgsummit.org, 2002.
United Nations Health and Development Section, Emerging Social Issues Division (UNESCAP).
    Urbanization and Health. http://www.unescap.org/esid/hds/issues/UrbanizationHealth.pdf, n.d.

PART THREE

ENVIRONMENTAL HEALTH ON THE REGIONAL SCALE

CHAPTER TWELVE

AIR POLLUTION

Michelle L. Bell

Jonathan M. Samet

KEY CONCEPTS

- Air pollution is a major contributor to adverse human health conditions, from asthma to cardiovascular disease to premature death.

- Air pollution is not just a modern phenomenon; it has been recognized as a problem for thousands of years.

- Air pollution is not a single entity; it consists of distinct, identifiable components (such as ozone and particulate matter), each with its own sources, chemistry, and toxic effects.

- Air pollution emissions come from many sources; these can be natural sources or human activities.

- The ambient concentration of an air pollutant in a particular location depends on many factors, including emissions sources, weather, and land patterns.

- Air quality management strategies include controlling emissions at the source, reducing the volume of emissions, and decreasing population exposure.

THIS chapter discusses the relationship between outdoor air pollutants and human health. This set of environmental contaminants differs from many others in that exposure is unavoidable and affects all segments of the population. For example, when point source water contamination occurs, the natural resource needed (water) can be retrieved from another location or treated, but outdoor air pollution affects everyone because we all need that air.

The discussion begins with a brief history of air pollution, which has been recognized to some extent as a human health problem for centuries. Various study designs used to assess health effects are discussed, as each has key strengths and weaknesses in studying the adverse effects of air pollution. Our understanding of how air pollution affects human health is based on a synthesis of research over a variety of disciplines and research designs. This chapter reviews the general sources and health effects of major outdoor air pollutants (particulate matter, sulfur dioxide, nitrogen oxides, volatile organic compounds, tropospheric ozone, carbon monoxide, lead, mercury, and air toxics). It concludes with a discussion of the links between air pollution and other environmental health concerns.

HISTORY OF AIR POLLUTION

Air pollution has long been a contributor to ill health. With the discovery of fire, humans began to pollute the air, both the air in the places they lived and the outside air. As urban areas developed, pollution sources, such as chimneys and industrial processes, were concentrated, leading to visible and damaging pollution dominated by smoke. The harmful effects of air pollution were recognized early. In "Air, Water, and Places," written nearly 2,500 years ago, Hippocrates noted that people's health could be affected by the air they breathe and that the quality of the air differed by area (Hippocrates, 1849). In thirteenth-century London air pollution was so severe that a commission was established to address the problem and abatement strategies followed (Brimblecombe, 1986). At that time, air pollution was generally a local issue, generated from kilns, hearths, and furnaces; since then the nature of air pollution has changed along with growing populations, industrialization, and fossil-fuel based transportation. High-volume production and transport of pollution across large distances mean that the damaging effects of air pollution often occur far from their source. Air pollution problems now range geographically from the local to the global scale and occur on a variety of timescales. Chapters Ten and Nineteen address climate change and indoor

Michelle L. Bell and Jonathan M. Samet declare no competing financial interests.

air pollution, respectively. This chapter focuses on major ambient or outdoor air pollutants, which today generally cause harm to health and the environment on local, regional, and global scales.

Modern-day recognition of the dangers of ambient air pollution can be traced to several extreme episodes during the last century. In 1930, in the Meuse Valley in Belgium, more than sixty people died during such an episode, over ten times the underlying mortality rate (Firket, 1936; Nemery, Hoet, and Nemmar, 2001). In describing the event the original investigators warned that should such an air pollution episode occur in a city with a larger population, such as London, thousands would die. In late October 1948, industrial pollution settled on Donora, a small town in southwestern Pennsylvania (Davis, 2002; Schrenk and others, 1949). Twenty people died during and shortly after the event, or about six times the typical mortality rate. Perhaps the most severe such event took place in London in December 1952 (see Figure 12.1 and the Perspective titled "London 1952"). In these and similar episodes, pollution levels and subsequent health effects were so severe that the connection between air pollution and health was readily apparent.

In response to severe air pollution episodes such as those in Donora and London, many governments, particularly those of the United States and the United Kingdom, enacted legislation to improve air quality and initiated research to increase understanding of risks to health. Today most of the industrialized world rarely experiences air pollution concentrations on the scale of the London fog of 1952, yet exceedingly high levels still exist in many developing regions (see Chapter Eleven). Despite regulatory control measures that have lowered concentrations, air pollution continues to harm health in the industrialized world as well. The World Health Organization's Global Burden of Disease Initiative recently estimated that each year ambient air pollution causes 800,000 premature deaths (Ezzati and others, 2002).

TYPES OF AMBIENT AIR POLLUTION

The ambient concentration of an air pollutant in a particular location depends on many factors, including emissions sources, weather (for example, temperature, wind speed and direction, and precipitation), and land patterns. During weather conditions of stagnant winds and a temperature inversion, pollution does not disperse, leading to higher air pollutant concentrations; this is a relatively common occurrence in valleys and areas lacking open spaces. A temperature inversion occurs when temperature increases with altitude, contrary to normal conditions, creating a layer of warmer air above a layer of cooler air on the Earth's surface. This typically occurs in the morning or when air descends from higher altitudes.

PERSPECTIVE
London 1952: One of the World's Worst Air Pollution Disasters

By the 1950s high concentrations of air pollutants in London were common, with levels far above modern-day regulatory standards. In fact, dirty air and London's characteristic "pea souper" fogs were long known as *London particulars*, noted by tourists, authors such as Charles Dickens, and painters such as Claude Monet. However from December 5 to 9, 1952, an unprecedented air pollution event took place, so severe that it warranted attention from the general public, scientists, the media, and the government.

Several factors contributed to the high pollution levels in London. Coal was a primary method of home heating at the time. A particularly cold winter meant that even more coal was burned. Stagnant atmospheric conditions prevented pollution from dispersing, in effect allowing pollution to accumulate in the city. Levels of sulfur dioxide and total particulate matter reached dangerous levels, far above the prevailing British standards. Pollution became so thick that visibility was reduced to near zero. Even some longtime residents became lost, finding their homes by feeling their way along the sides of buildings. A theater performance was closed because pollution seeped into the auditorium and the audience could not see the stage. Traffic came to a near standstill.

The association between health and air pollution during the episode was evident as the strong rise in air pollution was immediately followed by a sharp increase in sickness and death. Mortality rates rose to three times their normal levels. As the death toll mounted, mortuaries did not have enough room for the bodies, undertakers ran out of coffins, and florists ran out of flowers. Hospital admissions and insurance claims also rose. Applications to the Emergency Bed Service, which occurred when a patient could not be admitted to a particular hospital, reached a record high. The rates of these indicators of morbidity followed patterns similar to the air pollution concentrations. Later analysis of archived autopsy lung tissue found soot and an excess of other particles (Hunt, Abraham, Judson, and Berry, 2003).

Mortality rates did not return to normal levels until several months after the fog. The initial government report on this episode (U.K. Ministry of Health, 1954)

Pollutant concentrations for a given area can vary on a seasonal or daily basis depending on weather and source emissions, such as traffic patterns and wood burning. Some pollutants, such as tropospheric ozone (O_3) and small particles that have long residence times in the atmosphere, can travel large distances, so their damaging effects are not localized to people living near the pollution sources.

Air pollutants can be categorized by their source or by their physical and chemical characteristics. Table 12.1 describes the characteristics of several major air pollutants, provides examples of their sources and health effects, and summa-

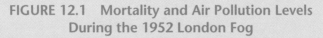

FIGURE 12.1   Mortality and Air Pollution Levels During the 1952 London Fog

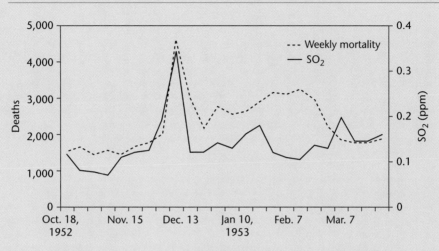

Source: Adapted from Bell and Davis, 2001.

hypothesized that an influenza epidemic accounted for the extra deaths during these months. However, more recent analysis showed that only a fraction of the excess mortality could be attributed to influenza (Bell and Davis, 2001; Bell and others, 2004), which indicates that the true death toll from this pollution event was 10,000 to 12,000 rather than the 3,000 to 4,000 typically reported.

This air pollution disaster, along with others, including the incident in Donora, Pennsylvania, in 1948 (Davis, 2002), acted as a catalyst for the study of air pollution epidemiology and for government intervention. The U.K.'s Clean Air Act was enacted in 1956, followed by the Clean Air Act in the United States in 1963. This and similar episodes serve as a reminder of the dangers of air pollution.

rizes the relevant regulations and guidelines from National Ambient Air Quality Standards (NAAQS), which were established under the U.S. Clean Air Act, and from the World Health Organization (WHO) (2006). An air pollutant may be either directly emitted (a **primary pollutant**) or formed in the atmosphere through the physical and chemical conversion of precursors (a **secondary pollutant**). For example, car tailpipe emissions of carbon monoxide (CO) are primary emissions; however, ozone, a secondary pollutant, is formed in the atmosphere when sunlight chemically converts other pollutants into ozone and other oxidant species. (These

TABLE 12.1 Major Ambient Air Pollutants: Sources, Health Effects, and Regulations

	Source Types and Major Sources	Health Effects	Regulations and Guidelines
Lead	Primary Anthropogenic Leaded fuel (phased out in some locations such as the United States), lead batteries, metal processing.	Accumulates in organs and tissues. Learning disabilities, cancer, damage to the nervous system.	*U.S. NAAQS* Quarterly average: 1.5 µg/m^3 *WHO guidelines* Annual: 0.50 µg/m^3
Sulfur dioxide	Primary Anthropogenic Combustion of fossil fuel (power plants), industrial boilers, household coal use, oil refineries. Biogenic Decomposition of organic matter, sea spray, volcanic eruptions.	Lung impairment, respiratory symptoms. Precursor to PM. Contributes to acid precipitation.	*U.S. NAAQS* Annual arithmetic mean: 0.03 ppm (80 µg/m^3) 24-hour average: 0.14 ppm (365 ug/m^3) *WHO guidelines* 10-minute average: 500 µg/m^3 Annual: 20 µg/m^3
Carbon monoxide	Primary Anthropogenic Combustion of fossil fuels (motor vehicles, boilers, furnaces). Biogenic Forest fires.	Interferes with delivery of oxygen. Fatigue, headache, neurological damage, dizziness.	*U.S. NAAQS* 1-hour average: 35 ppm (40 mg/m^3) 8-hour average: 9 ppm (10 mg/m^3) *WHO guidelines* 15-minute average: 100 mg/m^3 30-minute average: 60 mg/m^3 1-hour average: 30 mg/m^3
Particulate matter[a]	Primary and secondary Anthropogenic Burning of fossil fuel, wood burning, natural sources (for example, pollen), conversion of precursors (NO_x, SO_x, VOCs). Biogenic Dust storms, forest fires, dirt roads.	Respiratory symptoms, decline in lung function, exacerbation of respiratory and cardiovascular disease (for example, asthma), mortality.	*U.S. NAAQS* PM_{10} 24-hour average 150 µg/m^3 $PM_{2.5}$ Annual arithmetic mean: 15 µg/m^3 24-hour average: 35 µg/m^3 *WHO guidelines* PM_{10} Annual: 20 µg/m^3 24-hour average: 50 µg/m^3 $PM_{2.5}$ Annual: 10 µg/m^3 24-hour average: 25 µg/m^3

Pollutant	Sources[a]	Health effects	Standards and regulations
Nitrogen oxides	Primary and secondary Anthropogenic Fossil fuel combustion (vehicles, electric utilities, industry), kerosene heaters. Biogenic Biological processes in soil, lightning.	Decreased lung function, increased respiratory infection. Precursor to ozone. Contributes to PM and acid precipitation.	*U.S. NAAQS* Annual arithmetic mean: 0.053 ppm (100 μg/m³) Related to compliance with NAAQS for ozone *WHO guidelines* 1-hour average: 200 μg/m³ Annual: 40 μg/m³
Tropospheric ozone	Secondary Formed through chemical reactions of anthropogenic and biogenic precursors (VOCs and NO_x) in the presence of sunlight.	Decreased lung function, increased respiratory symptoms, eye irritation, bronchoconstriction.	*U.S. NAAQS* 1-hour average: 0.12 ppm (235 μg/m³); applies in limited areas 8-hour average: 0.075 ppm (147 μg/m³) *WHO guidelines* 8-hour average: 100 μg/m³
"Toxic" pollutants ("hazardous" pollutants) (for example, asbestos, mercury, dioxin, some VOCs)	Primary and secondary Anthropogenic Industrial processes, solvents, paint thinners, fuel.	Cancer, reproductive effects, neurological damage, respiratory effects.	EPA rules on emissions for more than 80 industrial source categories (for example, dry cleaners, oil refineries, chemical plants) EPA and state rules on vehicle emissions
Volatile organic compounds (for example, benzene, terpenes, toluene)	Primary and secondary Anthropogenic Solvents, glues, smoking, fuel combustion. Biogenic Vegetation, forest fires.	Range of effects, depending on the compound. Irritation of respiratory tract, nausea, cancer. Precursor to ozone. Contributes to PM.	EPA limits on emissions EPA toxic air pollutant rules Related to compliance with NAAQS for ozone
Biological pollutants (for example, pollen, mold, mildew)	Primary Anthropogenic Systems, such as central air conditioning, can create conditions that encourage production of biological pollutants. Biogenic Trees, grasses, ragweed, animals, debris.	Allergic reactions, respiratory symptoms, fatigue, asthma.	

Note: This table lists only a sample of the sources and health effects associated with each pollutant. Additionally, health effects may be the result of characteristics of a pollutant mixture rather than of a single pollutant. Additional legal requirements often apply, such as state regulations.

[a] Sources and effects of PM can differ by particulate size.

terms should not be confused with the regulatory definitions of "primary" and "secondary" standards, which refer to health-based and welfare-based standards, respectively, without regard to how the pollutant is formed.)

Another important feature of air pollution sources is whether the emissions are natural (*biogenic*) or the result of human activity (*anthropogenic*). Naturally occurring pollutants include volatile organic compounds (VOCs) from vegetation, pollens, volcanic gases, and dust from deserts.

Air pollutants differ in their physical form; they can be either gases or particles. Pollutants that are *aerosols* consist of small solid or liquid particles suspended in air. A pollutant's physical form and chemical composition and characteristics (for example, its solubility if it is a gas) affect the pollutant's ability to penetrate the respiratory system. Other factors that affect respiratory penetration are the pollutant's ambient concentration and the exposed individual's ventilation rate that is, number of breaths per minute). For example, exercise increases the depth and rate of ventilation, as well as the amount of oral breathing, which enables pollutants to bypass the nasal passages, where they might be prevented from entering the lungs. Gaseous pollutants that are highly soluble in water, such as sulfur dioxide (SO_2), are largely removed by the upper airway, whereas less water-soluble gases, such as O_3, and particles can penetrate deeper into the lungs (Figure 12.2).

A final way of classifying air pollutants relates to the way they are legally regulated. A commonly used term in the United States is **criteria pollutants**, a regulatory category of key outdoor air pollutants defined by the Clean Air Act. This category includes the major pollutants (carbon monoxide, lead, nitrogen dioxide, ozone, particulates, and sulfur oxides) for which the U.S. Environmental Protection Agency (EPA) promulgates National Ambient Air Quality Standards (NAAQS), under the Clean Air Act, in order to protect human health and welfare. (Welfare in this context includes such public goods as agricultural crops and livestock, property, air and ground transportation; and even views.) A second regulatory category is **hazardous air pollutants**. This category, established by the Clean Air Act Amendments of 1990, includes a number of volatile organic chemicals, pesticides, herbicides, and radionuclides. The name is somewhat confusing because this category does not include all known hazardous air pollutants (for example, it does not include carbon monoxide), and it does include some pollutants for which the hazard level is unknown.

STUDIES OF AIR POLLUTION AND HEALTH

The health effects of air pollution have been extensively studied through diverse research methods including epidemiological, human exposure, and animal and

FIGURE 12.2   Respiratory System

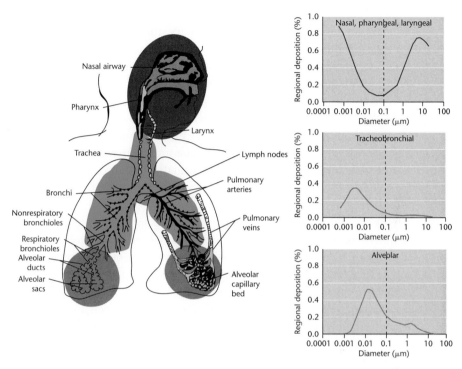

Source: Oberdörster, Oberdörster, and Oberdörster, 2005. Reproduced with permission from *Environmental Health Perspectives*. Drawing courtesy of J. Harkema.

The figure shows the lung structure as well as the fraction of particles of different sizes deposited in the various parts of the lung. Very large particles are stopped at the nose while very small particles reach the alveoli and deposit there.

other toxicological studies. Each approach has strengths and weakness, and results from complementary research designs are needed to paint a complete picture of how air pollution affects health.

Epidemiological studies investigate the relationship between air pollutant concentrations and health outcomes under the real-world conditions of exposure, typically in large populations in community settings (Gordis, 2004). Data on pollutant concentrations obtained by air monitoring are often used as surrogates for individual exposure. That is, one or more monitors placed in a city are assumed to represent the exposures of all people in the city. This assumption simplifies the actual ways in which people are exposed; in reality, people's activity patterns (the ways they spend their time in different environments, such as work and home) also determine their individual exposures. Adverse health effects or outcomes are generally assessed through public health databases, questionnaires, or tests of pulmonary functions. For example, a landmark study of air pollution and mortality in six U.S. cities enrolled both schoolchildren and adults. Outdoor monitors in each city were used to estimate exposure to air pollution. On follow-up, people in the city with the highest air pollution had a 26 percent higher mortality rate than those in the least polluted city did (Dockery and others, 1993). Another epidemiological study, the American Cancer Society's Cancer Prevention Study II (CPSII), tracked about 500,000 adults in 151 U.S. metropolitan areas. This work also used aggregate level exposure data (that is, monitor measurements) and individual-level health information. The investigators found that participants in the most polluted areas had a 17 percent higher mortality rate than those in the least polluted areas did (Pope and others, 1995, 2002).

A key advantage of epidemiological studies is the investigation of real-world populations and air pollution exposures. However, epidemiological studies can potentially be limited by the inability to control for other factors, referred to as *confounding factors*, such as temperature, weather, population characteristics, and pollutants other than those being investigated, and by the difficulty of accurately estimating personal exposure (see Chapter Three). In general, random error in the estimation of exposure tends to reduce the sensitivity of epidemiological studies in detecting effects. Confounding by other factors may falsely increase or decrease the apparent effect of air pollution. In carrying out epidemiological studies, investigators try to understand any inaccuracies in their exposure measures and the consequences of such inaccuracies and they also attempt to control for any confounding.

Controlled human exposure studies involve exposure of volunteers to a specified concentration of a particular air pollutant or pollutant mixture in a laboratory setting and then measurements of their health responses (Sandstrom, 1995). Unlike epidemiological research, exposure studies can control for potential confounding factors, deliver a carefully characterized exposure, and incorporate relatively invasive and complex methods for outcome assessment. To protect participants' safety, such research examines health effects that are mild, acute, and reversible. For example, human exposure studies can investigate heart rate variability and lung function changes (Devlin and others, 2003) and the fraction of particles deposited in the lung (Daigle and others, 2003). Exposures are typically of short duration and at low concentrations. Human exposure studies cannot ethically be used for research on chronic health effects or more severe health outcomes. Those that can ethically be done, however, are particularly useful for characterizing mechanisms of injury in order to bridge from animal to human studies and for assessing threshold concentrations for short-term effects. They have been particularly important for studying gaseous pollutants (including carbon monoxide, sulfur dioxide, and nitrogen dioxide).

Animal studies involve exposures on a short- or long-term basis to a pollutant or to a pollutant mixture under well-characterized conditions. Animals are sometimes exposed to outdoor pollution and even placed at sites of particular interest, such as along roadways. Generally rodents are used for such experiments, but dogs and primates have also been studied. Like human exposure studies, animal studies in the laboratory have the strength of well-defined pollution exposures; thus exposure-response relationships can be addressed. For example, animal exposure studies of air pollution have been used to research respiratory and heart rates in rats (Nadziejko and others, 2002), DNA damage in mice (Soares and others, 2003), brain damage in dogs (Calderón-Garcidueñas and others, 2002), and myocardial ischemia in dogs (Wellenius and others, 2003).

Animal studies sometimes incorporate invasive assessment procedures, such as lung biopsies. Biological samples can be collected for detailed studies of mechanism of injury. Various animal models are used that mimic human diseases, such as asthma, coronary heart disease, and congestive heart failure. However, evidence from animal studies may be subject to uncertainty when extended to exposures for people, and responses to a particular pollutant sometimes vary even among animal species.

Cellular and molecular studies are increasingly important, particularly for investigating mechanisms of disease. Elegant mechanistic studies may assess gene expression in response to air pollution exposure. Emerging technologies (so-called -omics approaches, as discussed in Chapter Six) are expected to deepen mechanistic understanding and to provide useful biomarkers of exposure.

SOURCES AND EFFECTS OF OUTDOOR POLLUTANTS

The health consequences of air pollution are wide-ranging, extending from effects on comfort and well-being to respiratory symptoms and even to premature death.

This section reviews the sources and health impacts of the common outdoor air pollutants; they are summarized in Table 12.1. Much human health research aims to investigate a particular pollutant, while controlling for potential confounding by other pollutants, and Table 12.1 presents information in this way. Indeed, some pollutants, such as CO, appear to have individual, specific health effects. However, air pollution is actually a complex mixture of multiple pollutants, such as sulfur dioxide and tropospheric ozone, which may not act independently.

Damage from air pollution may result from the combined effects of several pollutants (interaction). Synergistic interactions may produce effects that are larger than anticipated from studies of the individual pollutants. Programs for air pollution control generally provide individual standards for each pollutant, although the adverse health effects of different pollutants may be related and a number of pollutants have common sources.

Particulate Matter

Particulate matter (PM) refers to a generic class of pollution rather than to a particular, individual pollutant with a specified chemical structure, such as SO_2. PM includes solid or liquid particles suspended in air, regardless of their chemical composition. PM can be either primary (directly emitted) or secondary (formed in the atmosphere through physical and chemical conversion of gaseous precursors such as nitrogen oxides [NO_x], sulfur oxides [SO_x], and VOCs). PM results from the burning of fuel (for example, emissions from power plants), driving on unpaved roads, industrial activity, and wood-burning stoves, and from natural sources such as pollen, dust, salt spray, erosion, and mold. PM concentrations can vary within a region or even a city (for example, concentrations will be higher near major highways).

The composition of PM differs by geographic area and can vary with season, source, and meteorology (Bell and others, 2007). In the Eastern United States, PM often has a substantial sulfate component, reflecting the contributions of emissions from power plants. In the Western United States, transportation emissions contribute a larger fraction of PM, creating a substantial nitrate component. In the Northwestern United States, wood burning may be a dominant source of PM during colder seasons. Windblown dust can be an important source of PM in desert climates, such as the Southwestern United States. Variation can also exist at the subregional level.

Particles are generally categorized according to their size, using a measure called **aerodynamic diameter**. This is the diameter of a uniform sphere of unit density that would attain the same terminal settling velocity as the particle of interest. Aerodynamic diameter is determined by a particle's shape and density, and this measure permits comparison of particles having irregular shapes and different sizes and densities. **PM$_{10}$** refers to particles with an aerodynamic diameter of 10 microns or less, whereas **PM$_{2.5}$**, or **fine PM**, has an aerodynamic diameter up to 2.5 microns, and **ultrafine PM** particles have an aerodynamic diameter up to 0.1 microns. **Coarse PM** (PM$_{10-2.5}$) refers to particles with an aerodynamic diameter between 2.5 and 10 microns. **Total suspended particles** (TSP) refers to almost all particles in the air and is typically measured as PM mass of particles up to about 45 microns in aerodynamic diameter. Figure 12.3 depicts the typical mass distribution of particles in an urban area, showing two modes, one of fine particles, which tend to be of secondary origin, and the other of coarse particles, which are more likely to be primary. There is often a third mode of very small particles in the nano size range (below 0.1 μm) that are generated freshly by combustion.

A particle's size is related to its source and determines how it is transported in the atmosphere, where it is deposited in the environment, and where it is deposited in the respiratory system. Smaller particles are of special health concern because they penetrate more deeply into the lung. Such particles are typically generated through combustion processes. Diesel exhaust, a combination of gases and particles, is of particular concern because of widespread diesel use and because the resulting particles are extremely small (<1 μm) (Kagawa, 2002). In addition to particles, the gas phase of diesel contains numerous hazardous air pollutants such as benzene, formaldehyde, and polycyclic aromatic hydrocarbons.

Ambient levels of PM, as indicated by PM_{10}, $PM_{2.5}$, or other measures, have been associated with health effects including increased hospital and emergency

FIGURE 12.3   Particulate Matter Mass Distribution

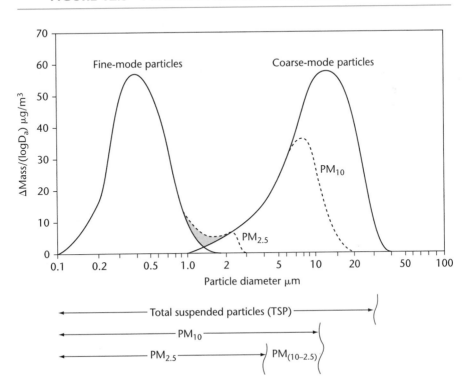

room admissions, respiratory symptoms, decline in pulmonary function, exacerbation of chronic respiratory and cardiovascular diseases, and premature mortality (U.S. EPA, 2003; Pope and Dockery, 2006). Laboratory animals exposed to PM experienced a range of responses including inflammation and pulmonary injury (Broeckaert and others, 1997; Dye and others, 2001). Time series studies—tracking day-to-day variation in PM levels and in health outcomes—have shown that acute PM exposure is associated with higher risk of mortality, reminiscent of the London and Donora episodes but occurring even at modern levels of PM exposure (see, for example, Health Effects Institute, 2003; Samet and others, 2000a, 2000b; Schwartz, 2000). Longitudinal studies, such as the Six Cities study and CPSII (described above), also demonstrate a link between long-term PM exposure and mortality (for example, Dockery and others, 1993; Krewski and others, 2000; Laden, Schwartz, Speizer, and Dockery, 2006; Pope and others, 1995, 2002). The status of this evidence was reviewed in 2004 by a committee of the National Research Council (NRC) and in 2006 by Pope and Dockery.

Regulations for controlling PM have evolved in response to a greater understanding of how PM affects human health. The first U.S. NAAQS was established for TSP, in 1971, but this standard was replaced with one for PM_{10} when it became clear that these smaller particles were more closely associated with health effects. Later evidence demonstrated that even smaller particles, $PM_{2.5}$, were responsible for adverse health effects and a $PM_{2.5}$ standard was added in 1997. The World Health Organization (WHO) concluded that the scientific literature provides strong evidence that airborne particles harm health and, as a result, set air quality guidelines of $20\ \mu g/m^3$ for PM_{10} and $10\ \mu g/m^3$ for $PM_{2.5}$ (WHO, 2006).

Although the health risks of PM have been studied extensively, much remains unknown. For example, the health risk of PM exposure may depend on characteristics such as the particulates' content of metals, acidity, organics, sulfates, or particular combinations of these (Health Effects Institute, 2002). Identifying the aspects of PM that are harmful is a critical research need (NRC, 2004). Similarly, the biological mechanisms by which PM causes premature mortality are not well understood. Leading hypotheses focus on reflexes in the lung that lead to autonomic nervous systems changes, perhaps predisposing to arrhythmias, and on inflammation that in turn predisposes to thrombosis or related changes (Brook and others, 2004). Further research will help to clarify the effects of PM and will likely have an impact on regulation as well.

Sulfur Dioxide

Sulfur dioxide, SO_2, is a water-soluble gas that was a primary component of the 1952 London fog. Sulfur oxides are produced from the combustion of sulfur-containing fuels and materials, such as coal and metal ores. Some coal, such as that from the Eastern United States, has particularly high sulfur content. Power plants are the main source of SO_2 emissions in the United States. Other sources are industrial boilers, trains, ships, and metal-processing facilities. Household use of coal can contribute significant amounts of SO_2 as well. In some areas, such as parts of China, coal is the primary fuel for cooking and heating and causes high levels of SO_2 indoors (see Chapters Eleven and Nineteen). Natural sources of SO_2 include volcanoes.

SO_2 can be converted to sulfuric acid (Seinfeld and Pandis, 1998), and therefore contributes to acid deposition, which harms vegetation, other materials, and wildlife. SO_2 also contributes to the formation of particulate matter. Sulfate aerosols, a major component of fine particulate matter, can travel far from their sources. Tall stacks of power plants often release pollution above the inversion layer, which reduces local pollution but allows pollutants to migrate long distances and undergo chemical transformation.

Because SO_2 is highly soluble in water, most inhaled SO_2 is absorbed by the mucous membranes of the upper airways with little reaching the lung; however, increased ventilation and oral breathing, such as from exercise, can raise the dose delivered to the lung (Schlesinger, 1999). SO_2 exposure has been associated with reduced lung function, bronchoconstriction (increased airway resistance), respiratory symptoms, hospitalizations from cardiovascular and respiratory causes, eye irritation, adverse pregnancy outcomes, and mortality. However, it is difficult to attribute these reported associations to SO_2 itself, because it is a precursor to particulate matter and generally exists as a component of a complex, combustion-related pollutant mixture. Experimental studies suggest that some persons with asthma may be particularly sensitive to SO_2 itself. Controlled exposure studies have shown that effects can occur with very short-term exposure (for example, ten minutes) in some people with asthma, whereas epidemiological research has shown effects associated with long-term exposure (for example, yearly levels).

Nitrogen Oxides

Nitrogen oxides, NO_x, make up a category of highly reactive gases containing nitrogen and oxygen, such as nitrogen dioxide (NO_2) and nitrogen oxide (NO). NO_x are produced through combustion, including fossil fuel combustion, when the nitrogen that constitutes almost 80 percent of air is oxidized. The sources of NO_x therefore include car and truck engines, electric utilities, and industries. Indoor sources can also contribute to NO_2 through kerosene heaters, nonvented gas stoves and heaters, and tobacco smoke. NO_x have natural sources such as stratospheric intrusion (when NO_x enter the troposphere from the stratosphere) and biological processes in soil, forest fires, and lightning, but the principal sources are power plants and motor vehicles. In the United States, motor vehicles currently account for half of all NO_x emissions.

Like ozone, NO_2 is nearly insoluble in water and can reach the lower respiratory tract. Health effects of NO_2 include irritation of the eyes, nose, and throat at higher concentrations; short-term decreases in lung function; and possibly increased respiratory infections and symptoms for children. It is difficult to separate the effects of NO_2 from the effects of related air pollution components such as ozone and particulate matter (Ackermann-Liebrich and Rapp, 1999). Both NO and NO_2 are toxic gases, and NO_2 is regulated in the United States as a criteria pollutant under the Clean Air Act. Nitrogen oxides also have indirect but important roles as precursors. They are precursors of tropospheric ozone and secondary particulate matter and play a crucial role in the formation of acid precipitation. NO is a greenhouse gas, which contributes to global warming (see Chapter Ten). NO_x and the pollutant species formed as it undergoes chemical reactions can travel long distances, so that health effects may take place far from the source. Emissions have declined in recent decades, approximately 30 percent between 1990 and 2006 (U.S. EPA, 2008).

Volatile Organic Compounds

Volatile organic compounds (VOCs) are a category of organic chemicals with a high vapor pressure, which readily evaporate at normal temperature and pressure. They include benzene, chloroform, formaldehyde, isoprene, methanol, monoterpenes, and hundreds of additional compounds. VOCs originate from natural sources (primarily vegetation such as oak and maple trees); industrial processes involving such things as chemical processing, use of solvents, and power generation; and transportation, including motor vehicles and off-road transportation sources such as aircraft, construction equipment, and lawn mowers. Motor vehicle emissions account for about 75 percent of transportation-related VOC emissions, with most of these emissions originating from the approximately 20 percent of vehicles that are older and poorly maintained (U.S. EPA, 1996). In many locations biogenic sources contribute more to VOCs than anthropogenic emissions do. For example, in 1990, 77 percent of VOC emissions in the Mid-Atlantic region were biogenic (Mid-Atlantic Regional Air Management Association, 1997). In fact, the natural appearance that gives the Blue Ridge mountains and the Great Smoky Mountains their names results from biogenic VOCs (mostly isoprene) that form aerosols. VOCs are precursors of ozone but also have independent health effects, including irritation of the respiratory tract, headaches, and carcinogenicity.

Tropospheric Ozone

Ozone (O_3), a gas, is present in the troposphere, the lowest atmospheric layer, which extends from the Earth's surface to the stratosphere, a distance of approximately 10 to 15 km, and in the stratosphere, which extends from the troposphere to about 45 to 55 km above the earth's surface. Stratospheric ozone forms the naturally occurring **ozone layer** that protects us from ultraviolet radiation, whereas tropospheric ozone, sometimes called **ground-level ozone**, is a harmful pollutant. To communicate the difference between stratospheric and **tropospheric ozone**, the U.S. Environmental Protection Agency has introduced the slogan "Good up high—bad nearby."

Tropospheric ozone is a colorless gas and a photochemical oxidant formed through complex, nonlinear chemical reactions involving the precursors VOCs and NO_x in the presence of sunlight. As a result, pollution involving ozone is sometimes referred to as *photochemical smog*. Stratospheric ozone can also intrude into the troposphere. The basic photochemical cycle of NO_x and O_3, which is driven by solar radiation, is shown in the following formulas, although ozone formation involves numerous other chemical reactions (Seinfeld and Pandis, 1998):

$$NO_2 + hv \rightarrow NO + O$$
$$O + O_2 + M \rightarrow O_3 + M$$
$$O_3 + NO \rightarrow NO_2 + O_2$$

where hv represents light energy and M represents N_2, O_2, or another molecule that absorbs excess energy, which stabilizes O_3.

Due to ozone's complex chemistry, controlling ozone levels is a difficult challenge. Decreased emissions of either NO_x or VOCs could potentially result in higher ozone levels, depending on the initial concentrations of the two main categories of precursors, among other factors (Seinfeld and Pandis, 1998). In some areas, referred to as *NO_x-limited*, reductions of NO_x may be the most effective way to reduce ozone levels, whereas in VOC-limited areas, reducing VOC emissions may be more effective.

Concentrations of ozone are highly seasonal, with higher levels during the hotter months, and also show strong diurnal patterns, following sunlight and transportation emissions patterns. Urban areas tend to have higher ozone concentrations because of the proximity to emissions of ozone precursors. After ozone precursors are emitted they can travel downwind in an expanding plume and contribute to the formation of ozone, which can itself travel with wind patterns. Thus, elevated concentrations can result from the transport of ozone and its precursors up to hundreds of miles away. Ozone problems tend to be more regional than localized. Ozone levels are lower indoors than outdoors, because ozone adsorbs to indoor surfaces and rapidly breaks down.

Ozone is not highly soluble in water and can thus reach the lower respiratory tract. Because of its oxidant properties, ozone can break molecular bonds and rapidly damage human tissue. Short-term exposure to ozone for healthy adults has been associated with temporarily decreased lung function, increased airway resistance, and increased respiratory symptoms, such as coughing and wheezing. These changes are reflected by increases in clinic visits, emergency room visits, school absenteeism, and hospitalizations following high-ozone days. Short-term variations in ozone concentrations have also been associated with daily mortality (Bell and others, 2004).

People with asthma are especially susceptible to the effects of ozone, because ozone inflames the airway linings and can trigger asthmatic attacks. However, healthy people can also be affected (U.S. EPA, 1996; Lippmann, 1989). Children, with their narrow caliber airways, are also especially susceptible (see Chapter Twenty-Five). People who spend time outdoors, such as outdoor exercisers or workers, are susceptible because of their greater ozone exposure. Long-term ozone exposure may contribute to the development of chronic lung diseases, such as asthma and bronchitis, and accelerate aging of the lungs. Ozone concentrations have also been associated with impaired lung development in children (Gauderman and others, 2002) and with onset of asthma (McConnell and others, 2002).

Carbon Monoxide

Carbon monoxide (CO) is a colorless, odorless gas formed by incomplete combustion of carbonaceous material, such as gasoline, natural gas, oil, coal, tobacco, and other organic materials. Motor vehicles contribute the majority of CO emissions to outdoor air, and consequently CO concentrations tend to be higher in areas with high traffic density and during times of high traffic volume. Carbon monoxide levels may also be high in congested urban areas with slow-moving traffic. Automobiles emit more CO during periods of colder temperature and while idling or moving slowly. Other sources include off-road vehicles and wildfires.

PERSPECTIVE
Leaded Gasoline and Blood Lead Levels in the United States

The phasing out of lead from gasoline is one of the most important and successful environmental health initiatives of the twentieth century and illustrates the successful motivation of regulation and policy by epidemiological evidence in order to improve human health (Needleman, 2000). In December 1921, three General Motors engineers

Wood burning also produces significant CO emissions in some areas. Elevated CO levels typically occur during colder periods because of increased vehicular emissions and inversion conditions that prevent pollution from dispersing.

When CO is inhaled, it binds to hemoglobin, with over 200 times the affinity of oxygen, to form carboxyhemoglobin (COHb). An increased level of COHb reduces the transport of oxygen to tissues and inhibits the release of oxygen (U.S. EPA, 2000). The brain and heart are sensitive to low oxygen conditions and are especially vulnerable to the effects of COHb on oxygen transport and delivery to tissues. Thus persons with cardiovascular and respiratory disease are particularly susceptible to CO. Health responses to CO include visual impairment, fatigue, decreased dexterity, dizziness, and nausea. Mortality and severe neurological damage can result from extremely high CO levels, as can occur in cases of CO poisoning from exposures indoors.

Lead

Lead (Pb) has been used in pipes, paint, solder in food cans, and batteries; however, historically, lead in ambient air came largely from leaded fuel, that is, fuel with lead added as an antiknocking agent. The rise and fall of leaded gasoline use in the United States coincided with a rise and fall in population blood lead levels, demonstrating the effectiveness of air pollutants at reaching much of the population. In 1994, the United Nations Commission on Sustainable Development called for elimination of leaded gasoline worldwide. Blood levels of lead have been shown to decline with the elimination of lead additives in fuel. Most countries have already phased out leaded gasoline or have plans to do so. In these areas, nonairborne sources of lead, such as ingestion of leaded paint, are a larger health concern than airborne lead. However, lead additives are still used elsewhere, such as in some African countries. Metal processing, lead smelters, waste incineration, and the manufacture and reclamation of lead batteries are also sources of atmospheric lead.

reported that the addition of tetraethyl lead (TEL) to motor vehicle fuel both enhanced the performance of internal combustion engines and reduced engine knock, and gasoline spiked with TEL was introduced into the American fuel market in 1923. Within a year of the widespread use of leaded gasoline, the lethal potential of TEL surfaced when workers involved in production of the additive at several refineries in New Jersey and Ohio fell sick and died. This epidemic of lead poisoning prompted the U.S. surgeon general to temporarily suspend the production and sale of leaded gasoline in 1925; he then appointed a panel of experts to investigate the recent fatalities and to assess the possible danger that might arise from the widespread distribution of lead via its sale as a gasoline additive. The panel ruled that there was no justification for the prohibition of leaded gasoline, provided that its distribution and use were regulated. However, the development of such regulations was not of the highest priority during the ensuing decades of depression, war, and postwar boom. It was not until the implementation of the Clean Air Act in the early 1970s that the U.S. EPA moved to lower lead levels in U.S. gasoline in order to accommodate catalytic converters, which were fouled by the lead. By this time, evidence had been growing on the adverse health effects of chronic, low-level lead exposure as well.

The Clean Air Act of 1970 required that the EPA establish National Ambient Air Quality Standards (NAAQS) to reduce ambient air levels of several major air pollutants, including airborne lead. Further, the law specifically required that leaded gasoline be phased out by the mid-1980s. Although these mandatory reductions were controversial, their issuance coincided with General Motors' introduction of the catalytic converter, a device designed to reduce exhaust emissions of NO_x, CO, and hydrocarbons. The converters themselves would not lower lead emissions, but they could not be used with leaded gasoline because the lead would deactivate the main catalytic element, platinum. After the implementation of the Clean Air Act and the introduction of the catalytic converter, steps were quickly taken to shift the country's vehicle fleet to unleaded gasoline, which was introduced in the United States in 1975. The total market share of unleaded gasoline increased over the following decades as lead additives were phased out; on January 1, 1996, leaded gasoline was prohibited for use in highway vehicles in the United States. The consequent reduction in air lead particulate concentrations, measured at monitoring sites across the United States from 1977 to 1996, is presented in Figure 12.4.

As the use of leaded gasoline decreased, so did human exposure to inhaled lead, a result that has been documented though the analysis of human blood samples collected across the United States. The second National Health and Nutrition Examination

FIGURE 12.4   Maximum Quarterly Observed Lead Particulate Concentration at U.S. Monitoring Sites, 1977 to 1996

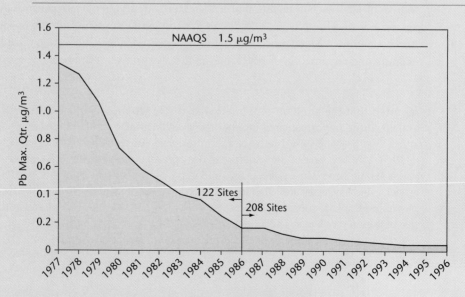

Survey (NHANES II) began in 1976, just after the introduction of unleaded gasoline in the United States, and the blood lead levels of 9,832 participants aged one to seventy-four years were measured. The mean blood lead level of all participants from 1976 to 1980 was 12.8 to 13.9 μg/dL (geometric mean 12.8 μg/dL). When these results were published in 1982, 1.9 percent of the study population met the definition of the Centers for Disease Control and Prevention (CDC) for "elevated" blood lead levels, which at the time was ≥30 μg/dL, and 77.8 percent of the participants had blood lead levels ≥10 μg/dL (Mahaffey and others, 1982). During the first phase of NHANES III, blood samples of 12,119 participants were collected from 1988 to 1991. The geometric mean blood lead level had dropped 78 percent, to 2.8 μg/dL, in NHANES III participants, and the decrease was observed across all age and racial and ethnic groups. Further, the proportion of the study population with blood lead levels ≥30 μg/dL decreased to 0.2 percent, and the proportion with a concentration ≥10 μg/dL (the new CDC definition of an "elevated" blood lead level) was 4.3 percent. Pirkle and colleagues attributed the observed decline in blood lead levels to the removal of lead from gasoline and also the removal of lead from soldered cans (Pirkle and others, 1994). In 1997, the CDC updated this information with data from the second phase of NHANES III (covering the years 1991 to 1994), reporting a further drop in the overall mean blood level to 2.3 μg/dL (CDC, 1997). Preliminary data on blood lead levels obtained from the subsequent NHANES IV study in the period from 1999 to 2000 revealed that blood lead levels continued to decline; the mean blood lead concentration of the study participants greater than one year of age was 1.66 μg/dL (CDC, 2003). This followed the 1996 ban on leaded gasoline sales in the United States. Figure 12.5 illustrates the change in young children's blood lead (PbB) levels in the United States from 1997 to 2006.

FIGURE 12.5 Tested and Confirmed Elevated PbB Levels by Year and Group for Children Less Than 72 Months Old

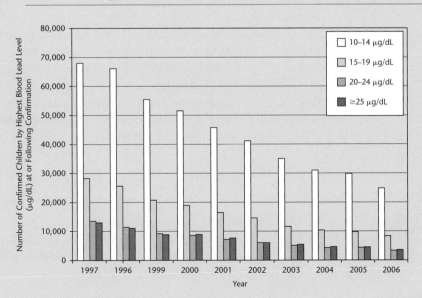

Lead can be harmful even at low doses because it accumulates in the body, mostly in the bones, which continue to function as an internal source of exposures. The absorption of lead depends on physiological characteristics, including health, age, and nutritional status. The health effects of lead have been studied extensively. Exposure to lead can cause damage to the nervous system and kidneys and can interfere with red blood cell formation, reproductive function, and gastrointestinal function. Children and pregnant women are particularly vulnerable, because the developing nervous system is a target of lead toxicity.

Mercury

Mercury is naturally occurring, but can be released into the atmosphere, soil, or water through human activities. Because mercury commonly contaminates coal, coal-fired power plants are the largest source of airborne mercury in the United States, contributing approximately 40 percent of the mercury in the atmosphere. Mercury exposure can occur through inhalation, skin contact, or ingestion. The health effects of mercury depend on its chemical form. For example, elemental mercury is more toxic to the kidney, whereas methylmercury is more toxic to the brain (National Research Council and Commission on Life Sciences, 2000).

Elemental mercury in the atmosphere can be deposited into water bodies, converted into methylmercury by microorganisms, and then consumed by fish. Because mercury bioaccumulates in tissues, fish can have high concentrations of mercury, especially those higher in the food chain, such as shark, swordfish, and king mackerel; this can then be passed on to people when they eat mercury-contaminated fish. The U.S. Food and Drug Administration (FDA) has issued an advisory recommending that nursing women, pregnant women, and women of childbearing age who may become pregnant avoid eating shark, swordfish, king mackerel, and tilefish and that they eat no more than an average of twelve ounces a week of other types of fish (U.S. FDA, 2001). The health dangers of consuming mercury are at odds with the nutritional benefits of seafood (Egeland and Middaugh, 1997). Mercury targets the nervous system, causing impaired vision and coordination, memory loss, personality disturbances, and occasionally death, and targets the kidneys as well. Children and fetuses are at special risk for mercury poisoning.

Air Toxics

Hundreds of other ambient air pollutants exist besides those just described. They include hydrochloric acid, captan, parathion, naphthalene, biphenyl, vinyl bromide, methyl bromide, dioxin, and cadmium, to name a few. Exposure to these pollutants can occur through inhalation, but they also enter other environmental media such as water and food. Therefore exposure can occur through eating foods, drinking water, or coming into contact with soil contaminated by atmospheric deposition. Health effects of these air toxics include damage to the neurological, immune, respiratory, and reproductive (for example, reduced fertility) systems, as well as developmental problems and some cancers. Like humans, animals may experience health problems if exposed to sufficient quantities of air toxics. Some air toxics bioaccumulate in tissues, so that the concentrations in aquatic or marine animals can rise to levels far above those in the surrounding air and water. The concentrations increase higher in the food chain, for example, as larger fish eat contaminated smaller fish. This can result in humans being exposed to elevated levels through eating seafood. Polychlorinated biphenyls (PCBs) are one example of such a pollutant.

AIR POLLUTION PREVENTION AND CONTROL

There are many approaches to improving air quality. Air quality management is a topic that is too diverse for full treatment here, but we note that air quality management strategies are based on a foundation of evidence that builds from sources of air pollution to patterns of population exposure and then to associated health risks. Approaches include controlling emissions at the source, by such means as scrubbers at coal-fired power plants; reducing the volume of emissions, by such means as increased use of public transportation to lower vehicular air pollutants or emissions controls for automobiles; and decreasing population exposure by such means as the EPA's Air Quality Index, which provides a health warning on high air pollution days to encourage sensitive individuals to avoid the outdoors. These strategies reflect the preventive approaches described in Chapter Twenty-Six.

Reduction of the health effects of air pollution comes from actions at multiple spatial and institutional levels, ranging from personal decisions by individuals, to community and state plans, and to multigovernment agreements. Due to the transport of pollution across state boundaries, many pollutants such as ozone are addressed through multistate consortiums, such as the Ozone Transport Commission, which aims to address ozone levels in the Northeastern and Mid-Atlantic regions of the United States. Because air pollution crosses national boundaries, agreements between national governments may be needed. Actions by individuals may also contribute to improved air quality; use of mass transit instead of private automobiles and lessened use of wood-burning fireplaces may enhance air quality locally.

LARGER EFFECTS OF REGIONAL AIR POLLUTION

Many atmospheric pollutants affect air quality and human health through multiple pathways. For example, NO_2 affects health directly but also contributes to the formation of ozone, and SO_2 contributes to the formation of particulate matter. Ambient air pollutants also figure into many other environmental problems. NO_x and SO_x are the primary causes of acid precipitation. Indoor air pollution levels are related to indoor sources and the penetration of outdoor air. PM and ozone both reduce visibility. The same fossil fuel–burning processes that generate the ambient air pollutants also produce greenhouse gases, such as CO_2 and methane (CH_4), which contribute to global warming. Many technologies and policies to mitigate ambient air pollution could also reduce production of greenhouse gases, and vice versa (Cifuentes and others, 2001). Thus the control of regional air pollution and the related health consequences are intertwined with ecological health and climate change.

SUMMARY

Although the link between air pollution and human health has been known for centuries, research in recent decades has shown the full scope of the continued serious threat posed to public health. Findings from a broad range of research, including epidemiological and toxicological studies, provide scientific evidence on the association between air pollution and health. Collectively, these complementary research approaches, each having particular strengths and weaknesses, provide a more complete understanding than previously possible of the health risk posed by air pollution.

Ambient air pollution results from a variety of natural and anthropogenic sources and has a wide range of health impacts.

Particulate matter pollution is unique in that it is defined without regard to chemical composition, whereas other air pollutants are defined based on chemical structure (for example, ozone as O_3, carbon monoxide as CO). Health responses to ambient air pollution range from an increased risk in respiratory symptoms such as coughing and wheezing to an increased risk of hospitalizations and mortality. Many air pollutants have common sources, and some primary pollutants contribute to the formation of other secondary pollutants. Many of the same sources that produce pollution of local concern are also contributors to the greenhouse gases that are causing global climate change.

KEY TERMS

aerodynamic diameter

coarse PM ($PM_{10-2.5}$)

criteria pollutants

fine PM

ground-level ozone

hazardous air pollutant

nitrogen oxides

ozone layer

particulate matter

PM_{10}

$PM_{2.5}$

primary pollutant

secondary pollutant

sulfur dioxide

total suspended particles (TSP)

tropospheric ozone

ultrafine PM

volatile organic compounds

DISCUSSION QUESTIONS

1. What are the primary air pollution problems in your community? What are the main sources?
2. How do your everyday activities contribute to air pollution?
3. How is regional air pollution related to other health and environmental issues?
4. Air pollution is a complex mixture of multiple contaminants, however air pollutants are often regulated and studied individually. Why is this the case? What are the consequences of this separation? How can this be addressed?
5. What actions can be taken to lower air pollution emissions? Consider possibilities at multiple levels: the individual, community, government, etc.

REFERENCES

Ackermann-Liebrich, U., and Rapp, R. "Epidemiological Effects of Oxides of Nitrogen, Especially NO₂." In S. T. Holgate, H. S. Koren, J. M. Samet, and R. L. Maynard (eds.), *Air Pollution and Health* (pp. 559–584). San Diego: Academic Press, 1999.

Bell, M. L., and Davis D. L. "Reassessment of the Lethal London Fog of 1952: Novel Indicators of Acute and Chronic Consequences of Acute Exposure to Air Pollution." *Environmental Health Perspectives*, 2001, *19*(suppl. 3), 389–394.

Bell, M. L., Davis D. L., and Fletcher T. "A Retrospective Assessment of Mortality from the London Smog Episode of 1952: The Role of Influenza and Pollution." *Environmental Health Perspectives*, 2004, *112*, 6–8.

Bell, M. L., and others. "Ozone and Short-Term Mortality in 95 US Urban Communities, 1987–2000." *JAMA*, 2004, *292*, 2372–2378.

Bell, M. L., and others. "Spatial and Temporal Variation in $PM_{2.5}$ Chemical Composition in the United States for Health Effects Studies." *Environmental Health Perspectives*, 2007, *115*, 989–995.

Brimblecombe, P. *The Big Smoke: A History of Air Pollution in London Since Medieval Times.* New York: Methuen, 1986.

Broeckaert, F., and others. "Reduction of the Ex Vivo Production of Tumor Necrosis Factor Alpha by Alveolar Phagocytes After Administration of Coal Fly Ash and Copper Smelter Dust." *Journal of Toxicology and Environmental Health*, 1997, *51*, 189–202.

Brook, R. D., and others. "Air Pollution and Cardiovascular Disease. A Statement for Healthcare Professionals from the Expert Panel on Population and Prevention Science of the American Heart Association." *Circulation*, 2004, *109*, 2655–2671.

Calderón-Garcidueñas, L, and others. "Air Pollution and Brain Damage." *Toxicologic Pathology*, 2002, *30*, 373–389.

Centers for Disease Control and Prevention. "Update: Blood Lead Levels—United States, 1991–1994." *Morbidity and Mortality Weekly Report*, 1997, *46*, 141–146.

Centers for Disease Control and Prevention. *Second National Report on Human Exposure to Environmental Chemicals.* Atlanta: Centers for Disease Control and Prevention, 2003.

Cifuentes, L., and others. "Climate Change: Hidden Health Benefits of Greenhouse Gas Mitigation." *Science*, 2001, *293*, 1257–1259.

Daigle, C. C., and others. "Ultrafine Particle Deposition in Humans During Rest and Exercise." *Inhalation Toxicology*, 2003, *15*, 539–552.

Davis, D. L. *When Smoke Ran Like Water: Tales of Environmental Deception and the Battle Against Pollution.* New York: Basic Books, 2002.

Devlin, R. B., and others. "Elderly Humans Exposed to Concentrated Air Pollution Particles Have Decreased Heart Rate Variability." *European Respiratory Journal*, 2003, *40*(suppl.) 76s–80s.

Dockery D. W., and others. "An Association between Air Pollution and Mortality in Six U.S. Cities." *New England Journal of Medicine*, 1993, *329*, 1753–1759.

Dye, J. A., and others. "Acute Pulmonary Toxicity of Particulate Matter Filter Extracts in Rats: Coherence with Epidemiological Studies in Utah Valley Residents." *Environmental Health Perspectives*, 2001, *109*(suppl. 3), 395–403.

Egeland, G. M., and Middaugh, J. P. "Balancing Fish Consumption Benefits with Mercury Exposure." *Science*, 1997, *278*, 1904–1905.

Ezzati, M., and others (Comparative Risk Assessment Collaborating Group). "Selected Major Risk Factors and Global and Regional Burden of Disease." *Lancet*, 2002, *360*, 1347–1360.

Firket, J. "Fog Along the Meuse Valley." *Transactions of the Faraday Society*, 1936, *32*, 11927.

Gauderman, W. J., and others. "Association Between Air Pollution and Lung Function Growth in Southern California Children: Results from a Second Cohort." *American Journal of Respiratory and Critical Care Medicine*, 2002, *166*, 76–84.

Gordis, L. *Epidemiology.* (3rd ed.) Philadelphia: Saunders, 2004.

Health Effects Institute. *Understanding the Health Effects of Components of the Particulate Matter Mix: Progress and Next Steps.* Cambridge, Mass.: Health Effects Institute, 2002.

Health Effects Institute. *Revised Analyses of Time-Series Studies of Air Pollution and Health: Revised Analyses of the National Morbidity, Mortality, and Air Pollution Study, Part II: Revised Analyses of Selected Time-Series Studies.* Cambridge, Mass.: Health Effects Institute, 2003.

Hippocrates. *The Genuine Works of Hippocrates* (F. Adams, trans.). London: Sydenham Society, 1849.

Hunt A., Abraham, J. L., Judson, B., and Berry, C. L. "Toxicologic and Epidemiologic Clues from the Characterization of the 1952 London Smog Fine Particulate Matter in Archival Autopsy Lung Tissues." *Environmental Health Perspectives*, 2003, *111*, 1209–1214.

Kagawa, J. "Health Effects of Diesel Exhaust Emissions: A Mixture of Air Pollutants of Worldwide Concern." *Toxicology*, 2002, *27*, 349–353.

Krewski, D., and others. *Reanalysis of the Harvard Six Cities Study and the American Cancer Society Study of Particulate Air Pollution and Mortality.* Special Report of the Institute's Particle Epidemiology Reanalysis Project. Cambridge, Mass.: Health Effects Institute, 2000.

Laden, F., Schwartz, J., Speizer, F. E., and Dockery, D. W. "Reduction in Fine Particulate Air Pollution and Mortality: Extended Follow-Up of the Harvard Six Cities Study." *American Journal of Respiratory and Critical Care Medicine*, 2006, *173*, 667–672.

Lippmann, M. "Health Effects of Ozone: A Critical Review." *Journal of the Air Pollution Control Association*, 1989, *39*, 672–695.

Mahaffey, K. R., Annest, J. L., Roberts, J., and Murphy, R. S. "National Estimates of Blood Lead Levels, United States, 1976–1980: Association with Selected Demographic and Socioeconomic Factors." *New England Journal of Medicine*, 1982, *307*, 573–579.

McConnell, R., and others. "Asthma in Exercising Children Exposed to Ozone: A Cohort Study." *Lancet*, 2002, *359*, 386–391.

Mid-Atlantic Regional Air Management Association. *1995 Ozone Atlas for the Mid-Atlantic Region.* Baltimore, Md.: Mid-Atlantic Regional Air Management Association, 1997.

Nadziejko, C., and others. "Immediate Effects of Particulate Air Pollutants on Heart Rate and Respiratory Rate in Hypertensive Rats." *Cardiovascular Toxicology*, 2002, *2*, 245–252.

National Research Council and Commission on Life Sciences. *Toxicological Effects of Methylmercury.* Washington, D.C.: National Academies Press, 2000.

National Research Council, Committee on Research Priorities for Airborne Particulate Matter. *Research Priorities for Airborne Particulate Matter, IV: Continuing Research Progress.* Washington, D.C.: National Academies Press, 2004.

Needleman, H. L. "The Removal of Lead from Gasoline: Historical and Personal Reflections." *Environmental Research*, 2000, *84*, 20–35.

Nemery, B., Hoet, P.H.M., and Nemmar, A. "The Meuse Valley Fog of 1930: An Air Pollution Disaster." *Lancet*, 2001, *357*, 704–708.

Oberdörster, G., Oberdörster, E., and Oberdörster, J. "Nanotoxicology: An Emerging Discipline Evolving from Studies of Ultrafine Particles." *Environmental Health Perspectives*, 2005, *113*, 823–839.

Pirkle, J. L., and others. "The Decline in Blood Lead Levels in the United States: The National Health and Nutrition Examination Surveys (NHANES)." *JAMA*, 1994, *272*, 284–291.

Pope, C. A., 3rd and Dockery, D. W. "Health Effects of Fine Particulate Air Pollution: Lines That Connect." *Journal of the Air and Waste Management Association*, 2006, *56*, 709–742.

Pope, C. A., 3rd and others. "Particulate Air Pollution as a Predictor of Mortality in a Prospective Study of U.S. Adults." *American Journal of Respiratory and Critical Care Medicine*, 1995, *151*, 669–674.

Pope, C. A., 3rd and others. "Lung Cancer, Cardiopulmonary Mortality, and Long-Term Exposure to Fine Particulate Air Pollution." *JAMA*, 2002, *287*, 1132–1141.

Samet, J. M., and others. *The National Morbidity, Mortality, and Air Pollution Study, Part I: Methods and Methodologic Issues*. Cambridge, Mass.: Health Effects Institute, 2000a.

Samet, J. M., and others. *The National Morbidity, Mortality, and Air Pollution Study, Part II: Morbidity and Mortality from Air Pollution in the United States*. Cambridge, Mass.: Health Effects Institute, 2000b.

Sandstrom, T. "Respiratory Effects of Air Pollutants: Experimental Studies in Humans." *European Respiratory Journal*, 1995, *8*, 976–995.

Schlesinger, R. B. "Toxicology of Sulfur Oxides." In S. T. Holgate, H. S. Koren, J. M. Samet, and R. L. Maynard (eds.), *Air Pollution and Health* (pp. 585–602). San Diego: Academic Press, 1999.

Schrenk, H. H., and others. *Air Pollution in Donora, PA: Epidemiology of the Unusual Smog Episode of October 1948, Preliminary Report*. Public Health Bulletin No. 306. Washington, D.C.: U.S. Public Health Service, 1949.

Schwartz, J. "The Distributed Lag Between Air Pollution and Daily Deaths." *Epidemiology*, 2000, *11*, 320–326.

Seinfeld, J. H., and Pandis, S. N. *Atmospheric Chemistry and Physics: From Air Pollution to Climate Change*. Hoboken, N.J.: Wiley, 1998.

Soares, S. R., and others. "Urban Air Pollution Induces Micronuclei in Peripheral Erythrocytes of Mice in Vivo." *Environmental Research*, 2003, *92*, 191–196.

U.K. Ministry of Health. *Mortality and Morbidity During the London Fog of December 1952*. Report on Public Health and Medical Subjects No. 95. London: U.K. Ministry of Health, 1954.

U.S. Environmental Protection Agency. *Air Quality Criteria for Ozone and Related Photochemical Oxidants*. EPA/600/P-93/004a-CF. Washington, D.C.: U.S. Environmental Protection Agency, Office of Research and Development, National Center for Environmental Assessment, 1996.

U.S. Environmental Protection Agency. *Air Quality Criteria for Carbon Monoxide*. EPA 600/P-99/001F. Washington, D.C.: U.S. Environmental Protection Agency, Office of Research and Development, 2000.

U.S. Environmental Protection Agency. *Fourth External Review Draft of Air Quality Criteria for Particulate Matter (June 2003)*. EPA/600/P-99/002aD. Research Triangle Park, N.C.: National Center for Environmental Assessment, RTP Office, Office of Research and Development, 2003.

U.S. Environmental Protection Agency. *Latest Findings on National Air Quality: Status and Trends Through 2006*. EPA 454/R-07-007. Research Triangle Park, N.C.: U.S. Environmental Protection Agency, Office of Air Quality Planning and Standards, Emissions, Monitoring, and Analysis Division, 2008.

U.S. Food and Drug Administration. *"An Important Message for Pregnant Women and Women of Childbearing Age Who May Become Pregnant About the Risks of Mercury in Fish."* Consumer Advisory. College Park, Md.: U.S. FDA Center for Food Safety and Applied Nutrition, 2001.

Wellenius, G. A., and others. "Inhalation of Concentrated Ambient Particles Exacerbates Myocardial Ischemia in Conscious Dogs." *Environmental Health Perspectives*, 2003, *111*, 402–408.

World Health Organization. *Air Quality Guidelines: Global Update 2005—Particulate Matter, Ozone, Nitrogen Dioxide and Sulfur Dioxide*. Copenhagen: World Health Organization, 2006.

FOR FURTHER INFORMATION

Books

Ayres, J., Maynard, R.L., and Richards, R. *Air Pollution and Health*. Hackensack, N.J.: World Scientific, 2006.

Jacobson, M. Z. *Atmospheric Pollution: History, Science and Regulation*. New York: Cambridge University Press, 2002.

National Research Council, Committee on Air Quality Management in the United States. *Air Quality Management in the United States*. Washington, D.C.: National Academies Press, 2004.

Vallero, D. *Fundamentals of Air Pollution*, (4th ed.) San Diego: Academic Press, 2008.

Agencies and Organizations

American Lung Association (ALA), http://www.lungusa.org (click on "air quality). Information on both indoor and outdoor air quality and a link to the periodic ALA report *State of the Air*, summarizing recent research, are available at this agency Web site.

Centers for Disease Control and Prevention (CDC), http://www.cdc.gov/nceh/airpollution. General information on air pollution and health, information on asthma epidemiology, and information on specific subtopics such as carbon monoxide can be found on this Web site.

U.S. Environmental Protection Agency (EPA), http://www.epa.gov/ebtpages/air.html. A wide range of articles on air quality, addressing various pollutants, their sources and effects, and how to monitor and control them and including information on the Air Quality Index, is available from this Web site.

In addition, most state environment departments provide information on current air quality levels on their Web sites.

CHAPTER THIRTEEN

ENERGY PRODUCTION

JEREMY J. HESS

KEY CONCEPTS

- There are several energy sources on Earth. The sun is primary among them, as direct sunlight, as energy for plant growth, and as stored solar energy in fossil fuels. Other energy sources include geothermal, hydro, and nuclear.

- A society's energy use varies with its level of socioeconomic development.

- A nation's development is associated with increased energy use, cleaner energy sources, greater distance between energy production and end use, and deferment of health impacts over time.

- Each source of energy has a profile of health impacts.

- Life cycle analysis—from "harvesting" and transporting raw materials, to fuel production, to energy transmission and consumption, to waste generation and management—clarifies the full health impacts.

- Major changes in energy patterns may be imminent, driven by such forces as petroleum depletion and global climate change. These changes will have important health consequences.

- Energy policy is health policy. Rigorous analysis, using scientific evidence and tools such as health impact assessments, can help nations reach the most health-protective energy policies.

ENERGY is fundamental to life and central to the health and function of all ecosystems. It is a major, and remarkably little studied, influence on human health. As an environmental health concern, energy production offers a unique lens through which a host of issues can be viewed. Close study of the environmental health effects of energy production also deepens our understanding of upstream determinants of some of our most pressing global health concerns.

The term **energy** itself has a range of definitions and meanings in technical and vernacular speech. In physics, energy is defined as the ability to do work, such as lifting a weight from one height to another, cooling a warm space, slowing a moving vehicle, organizing atoms into proteins, or boiling water. **Power** is work done over time. As Joule illustrated in using gravity to power a paddlewheel in an insulated barrel, warming the water slightly via conversion of gravitational to thermal energy, work involves the conversion of one type of energy into another. The amount of energy required to heat one pound of water by 1°F is now termed the British thermal unit (BTU). In thermodynamics the total energy of a closed system is conserved, and the use of energy to do work does not change the system's total energy endowment. Ecosystems on Earth, however, are not closed, and some energy used to do work is often "lost" in the form of heat. The sun continuously introduces energy into the Earth's ecosystem, as well, contributing to the flux.

Human activity, both individual and collective, depends on the ready availability of energy. The planet boasts abundant energy stores, but ultimately they trace back to a small number of sources. The sun is the major source; sunlight, converted to chemical energy through photosynthesis, is the origin of **coal** and **petroleum** (which formed millions of years ago), of wood (which grew over decades), and of **biodiesel** and ethanol (manufactured from this year's crops). Wind and wave activity also result primarily from solar radiation heating the Earth's surface. Other energy sources derive their potential from other forces such as gravity (hydroelectric); thermal energy stored in the Earth's mantle (geothermal); or nuclear reactions, primarily fission (nuclear power).

As energy is a fundamental input for human activity, it is also important for human health. As individuals, we extract the potential energy from chemical bonds in food to support our metabolic and homeostatic processes. Large-scale industrial and agricultural processes require similar energy inputs. Health care is a particularly energy-intensive sector of the economy, and public health too

Jeremy J. Hess declares no competing financial interests.

depends on energy inputs, particularly petroleum, to carry out many of its basic functions. On a population basis, there is a clear association between energy consumption and health; greater energy availability is associated with longer life spans and improved health (Woods, 2000; Deaton, 2004), although at the upper end of the spectrum, increased energy use generates only marginal health gains (Wilkinson, Smith, Joffe, and Haines, 2007) (Figure 13.1).

Energy production, transmission, and consumption are also associated with a range of potential harms, both direct and indirect. The direct harms depend on the energy source, the method of production, and the point in the production life cycle. Indirect harms range from environmental degradation and climate perturbations to income inequality within and between nations and geopolitical destabilization. As with most environmental hazards, the potential harms associated with energy production are not equally distributed, and marginalized groups often bear disproportionate risk.

The study of energy and health is global in scope, interdisciplinary, and dynamic. Current concerns—constraints on petroleum supply and concerns over **climate change**—are tremors that signal a seismic shift in the energy sector. Energy use patterns will change in coming years, and as with previous energy revolutions, there will likely be significant consequences for population growth and human health. Focusing on clean energy production and judicious energy use, and on maximizing the health benefits of each, offers the opportunity to ensure social and health benefits now and for generations to come.

This chapter introduces the study of energy production and health. It begins by reviewing patterns of energy use to provide historical context and highlight the importance of technical innovation. Next, it provides a **life cycle analysis** of specific energy sources and their health effects. Finally, it closes with a discussion of both proximate and distant health impacts of energy use and the suggestion that energy policy is health policy.

TECHNOLOGY AND PATTERNS OF ENERGY USE

Humans have long used technology to harness potential energy sources, from draft animals to nuclear reactors. The level of technological development determines the primary sources of energy that people employ, the efficiency with which they convert energy to productive work, and the extent to which they limit or control potentially harmful by-products. This can be roughly illustrated by the **energy ladder** (Figure 13.2); as prosperity increases, societies tend to substitute cleaner, more efficient, and more convenient energy sources for the less costly but more polluting sources at the ladder's base. The energy ladder captures only

FIGURE 13.1   Infant Mortality and Life Expectancy as a Function of
Energy Consumption, by Country

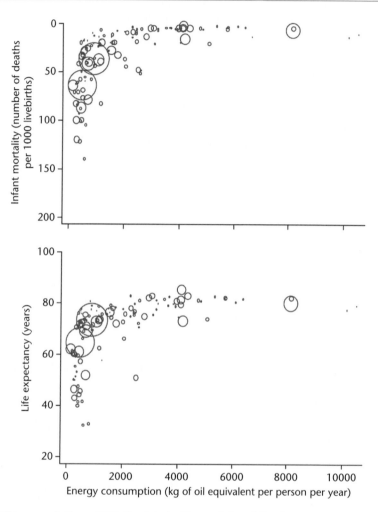

Source: Wilkinson and others, 2007. Reprinted with permission of Elsevier.

The upper panel shows infant mortality and the lower panel shows life expectancy. Symbol
sizes are proportional to country population, and "kg of oil equivalent" refers to energy
equivalent to that produced by combustion of 1 kg of oil.

FIGURE 13.2   The Energy Ladder

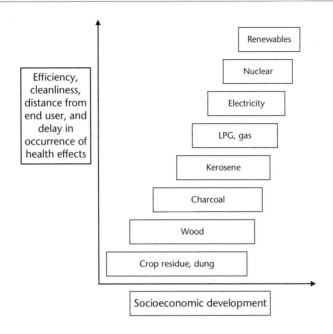

two dimensions of the relationship, however; as development increases, so does the physical distance between energy generation and the end user, as does the time between energy use and occurrence of health effects on a generational scale (Holdren and Smith, 2000).

Prior to the 1700s, humans used several forms of energy to cook, keep warm, and produce goods, and there was relatively little variation across the globe. Manual and animal labor were the primary means of production, and the energy sources depended on availability: solar energy was important for farming and animal husbandry, and **biomass**—including dung, wood, brush, peat, and other fuels—was often used for cooking, lighting, and other purposes, given relative ease of access to these fuels with basic tools. Coal that could be scavenged from the Earth's surface was also used in several areas; Roman historians note that it was a significant heating fuel source in Bronze Age Brittania (Freese, 2003), and there is evidence of a coal trade beginning in A.D. 200 when coal was burned to dry grain (Salway, 2001). There is archeological evidence of more sophisticated coal mining in China around 1000 A.D., when smelting caused deforestation and a replacement fuel was needed (Ebrey, Walthall, and Palais, 2006). This illustrates the tendency to employ the most readily available energy sources first.

In the late 1700s, during the industrial revolution, technology transformed the energy landscape. The means of production shifted from manual labor, draft animals, and water power to machines as a result of innovations in the textile industry, the widespread use of the steam engine, and production of **coke** (a residue made from the reductive combustion of carbonaceous fuel) from coal. Industrial production grew dramatically. Coal became a primary fuel; in fact the availability of coal has been cited as a necessary prerequisite to the innovation that spawned the industrial revolution (Pomeranz, 2000). Coal powered the steam engines that defined the new economy and was a raw material and energy source for coke production, which in turn enabled the production of refined metals and machine tools (Ashton, 1998). Toward the end of the industrial revolution, **coal gasification** began, producing coal gas, or *town gas*, from coal for use in lighting. Coal gas replaced tallow and oil, and improved lighting allowed increased urban security and economic activity (Thomson, 2003).

Great Britain spawned the industrial revolution, but its innovations quickly spread to the rest of Europe and North America and then, more slowly, to other parts of the world. The industrial revolution marked a turning point not only in economic development but also in the global distribution of energy production and utilization. Previously, productivity and growth had been limited by energy input from the sun and what could be gathered, harvested, or otherwise forced into production. With the industrial revolution, humans began to capitalize on the Earth's energy stores, uncoupling productivity from immediate inputs and, in the process, spawning the global energy trade. The term *seacoal* for coal shipped to the United Kingdom from distant shores dates from the industrial revolution and reflected the new importance of transboundary energy trade in the country's development.

Although coal powered the industrial revolution, two inventions ushered in the modern era in terms of energy usage. One was the gasoline-powered internal combustion engine, which was perfected through a series of progressive refinements in the late 1800s. This led to the production of motor cars in the late 1880s and a relentless increase in the demand for petroleum-based fuels, resulting in major incentives to identify and exploit oil deposits the world over. At roughly the same time, the electromechanical generator was perfected, enabling centralized production and distribution of electrical energy from various substrates. Electricity was widely and quickly adopted in the developing world. Although various energy sources are used to convert mechanical or thermal energy into electrical energy, the primary source to this day is coal.

PERSPECTIVE
Health Impacts of the Dublin Coal Ban

In 1990, Dublin banned the sale of bituminous coal, which had long been a primary source of energy for household heating. Hypothesizing that this natural experiment would provide evidence of coal combustion's health effects on a regional scale, Clancy and colleagues compared measures of air pollution and several health outcomes for six years before and after the ban. Adjusting their time series data for weather, respiratory epidemics, and death rates in the rest of Ireland, they evaluated the effect of the ban on age-standardized death rates in Dublin. The results were dramatic. Pollution, as indicated by average black smoke concentrations, declined by 35.6 mg/m³ after the ban, and adjusted nontrauma death rates decreased by 5.7 percent (95% CI 4–7, $p < 0.0001$). The standardized rates for both respiratory and cardiovascular deaths fell when the ban was instituted. Dublin experienced an annual reduction of approximately 116 respiratory and 243 cardiovascular deaths after the ban, an even more dramatic drop than expected from prior time series studies (Clancy, Goodman, Sinclair, and Dockery, 2002). A second, follow-up study examined rates of lung cancer deaths in association with the ban, and found that reduced particulate emissions as a result of the ban were associated with a modest reduction (Kabir, Bennett, and Clancy, 2007).

Current patterns of energy use exhibit four characteristics that date from the industrial revolution:

1. More developed areas of the world have higher per capita energy consumption (and higher associated emissions per capita as well).
2. More developed areas rely disproportionately on cleaner forms of energy production that are higher on the energy ladder.
3. More developed regions rely more heavily on electricity, a more efficient mode of energy production. This translates to greater economic output per unit of energy input than countries in the developing world achieve (Grubler, Nakicenovic, and Jefferson, 1996).
4. Higher levels of development are associated with increased capacity and willingness to distribute health impacts both onto distant populations and to future generations (Holdren and Smith, 2000).

Some of these energy use patterns are presented in Tables 13.1 and 13.2. Figure 13.3 depicts world trends in energy sources since 1970.

TABLE 13.1   Energy Use by Sector and Region, 2001

Region	Energy Use (million metric TOE)	Sector (% of Total)				
		Industry	Transport	Agriculture	Service	Residential
World	7,585	31.9	25.2	2.5	7.8	27.5
Asia	2,175	34.7	16.7	2.9	5.9	35.3
Europe	1,858	32.2	25.0	2.7	8.7	27.5
Middle East and North Africa	408	32.4	24.9	2.1	4.3	20.4
Sub-Saharan Africa	259	19.4	12.5	1.6	2.2	56.2
North America	1,725	27.2	38.9	1.1	16.3	16.5
Central America and Caribbean	138	34.7	34.9	2.7	3.6	22.1
South America	304	38.9	31.9	4.3	5.1	16.5
Oceania	86	36.2	38.4	2.3	6.9	12.3
Developed	4,184	30.6	30.8	2.0	10.7	21.3
Developing	2,791	33.3	18.6	2.9	3.9	35.7

Note: TOE = tons of oil equivalent.

Source: Adapted from World Resources Institute, 2005.

Future patterns of energy use are difficult to determine, but a major energy transition, comparable to the energy revolutions of the late nineteenth and early twentieth centuries, may be underway (Carr, 2008). The future energy constellation will be shaped by several emerging concerns, including greenhouse gas emissions and petroleum depletion, as well as by health impacts and global equity concerns. The energy challenges posed by climate change in particular are stark, likely requiring a massive research and development effort (Hoffert and others, 1998). Pacala and Socolow have devised a prescription for multisector energy transition and climate stabilization involving stabilization wedges, activities subdivided by sector, such as increasing global wind-power generation 400-fold over fifty years. Here is a list of these wedges (adapted from Pacala and Socolow, 2004).

TABLE 13.2 Energy Use Per Capita, by Source, Electrification, and Electricity Consumption, 2001

Region	Energy Use Per Capita (KGOE)	Consumption by Source (%)					Electrification	
		Fossil Fuels	Solid Biomass	Nuclear	Hydroelectric	Other Renewables	% with Electricity	Use Per Capita (kWh)
World	1,631	79.5	10.4	6.9	2.2	0.7	73	2,326
Asia	890	75.3	18.2	4.2	1.6	0.5	70	1,087
Europe	3,621	84.2	2.0	10.5	2.4	0.3	100	5,598
Middle East and North Africa	1,487	96.9	1.8	0.0	0.8	0.3	87	1,848
Sub-Saharan Africa	NA	NA	NA	NA	NA	NA	24	NA
North America	7,921	85.3	2.5	9.1	1.8	0.8	100	13,416
Central America and Caribbean	1,265	82.7	11.1	1.1	1.7	3.2	85	1,409
South America	1,089	70.9	14.9	1.5	11.3	1.6	90	1,639
Oceania	NA	NA	NA	NA	NA	NA	NA	NA
Developed	4,600	83.9	2.4	10.4	2	0.7	100	7,578
Developing	828	73.6	21.7	1.4	2	0.7	67	896

Note: KGOE = kilograms of oil equivalent; kWh = kilowatt-hours.
Source: Adapted from World Resources Institute, 2005.

FIGURE 13.3   Global Total Primary Energy Supply, 1971–2005

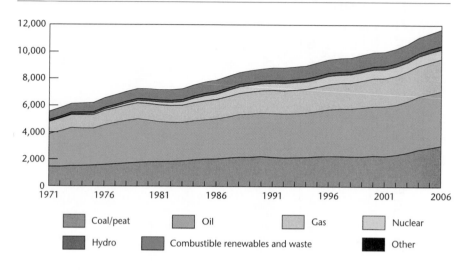

Source: International Energy Agency, 2007a. © OECD/IEA.

Pacala and Socolow's Stabilization Wedges

Energy efficiency and conservation
   1. Increase vehicle efficiency.
   2. Reduce use of vehicles.
   3. Increase building efficiency.
   4. Increase efficiency of baseload coal plants.

Fuel shift
   5. Substitute gas for coal for baseload power.

Carbon dioxide (CO_2) capture and geological storage
   6. Capture CO_2 at baseload power plant.
   7. Capture CO_2 at H_2 plant.
   8. Capture CO_2 at coal-to-synfuels plant.

Nuclear fission
   9. Substitute nuclear power for coal power.

Renewable electricity and fuels
   10. Substitute wind power for coal power.
   11. Substitute solar energy (using photovoltaic cells) for coal power.

12. Substitute H_2 in fuel-cells (using wind energy) for gasoline in cars.
13. Substitute biomass fuel for fossil fuel.

Forests and agricultural soils
14. Reduce deforestation and increase planting.
15. Implement conservation tillage.

When summed, a sufficient number of wedges (see Figure 13.4) could keep atmospheric CO_2 levels at 450 parts per million (ppm), arguably low enough to stave off further dangerous climate change (Pacala and Socolow, 2004). The number of stabilization wedges required has been debated (Meisel, 2008). Pacala and Socolow did revise their initial estimates, but the conceptual power of the

FIGURE 13.4   The Concept of Climate Stabilization Wedges

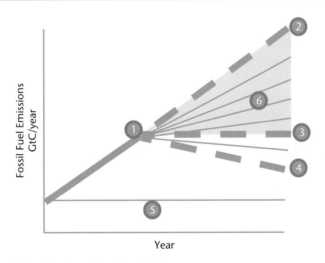

Source: Adapted from Pacala and Socolow, 2004.

The Y-axis shows fossil fuel–based emissions of CO_2 in gigatons (billions of tons) of carbon (GtC) per year. The line that contains points 1 and 2 shows *business as usual*, with steadily increasing emissions (the dashed portion represents projected future emissions). The line from point 1 to point 3 shows *stabilization*, with emissions no longer increasing. The line from point 1 to point 4 is even more ambitious; it represents a decline in emissions over time, starting at point 1. The horizontal line (5) represents some baseline, sustainable level of emissions. The triangle between business as usual and the reduced emissions scenarios represents the emissions that need to be avoided. This mitigation can be accomplished through *wedges* (collectively, area 6). Each wedge is a specific intervention such as reduced vehicular travel, more efficient vehicles, or carbon capture and sequestration.

argument stands (Socolow and Pacala, 2006). (Climate change is discussed in detail in Chapter Ten.)

HEALTH EFFECTS BY ENERGY SOURCE

This section takes a life cycle approach, considering energy production at all stages, including raw material "harvesting" and transporting, fuel production, energy transmission and consumption, and waste generation and management. Energy production throughout this life cycle has health effects, some of them quite distant from the energy use itself. Higher up on the energy ladder, energy production tends to occur further from the end user, and the health effects of production are thus removed from higher-income consumers. Lower-income users, in contrast, are subject to more immediate and severe health effects.

Fossil Fuels

Fossil fuels were formed over millions of years as organic material deposited on the Earth's surface was buried and then subjected to pressure and temperature in the Earth's crust. Fossil fuels derive their energy from the chemical bonds created during photosynthesis. Depending on where the organic matter was deposited and the geological forces to which it was subject, it became coal, oil, **natural gas**, or one of a variety of other less common materials.

Fossil fuels constitute the world's dominant energy source; the developed world derives approximately 84 percent of its energy from fossil fuels, and the developing world 74 percent (World Resources Institute, 2005). Oil is the most commonly used fossil fuel, and accounts for 35 percent of the world's energy consumption; coal accounts for 23 percent and natural gas 21 percent (International Energy Agency [IEA], 2007a). As noted previously, fossil fuels are also very important to other industrial processes, such as chemical synthesis, fertilizer and plastics production, and textiles manufacture. For example, approximately 85 percent of plastics are derived from petroleum, underscoring its importance in the modern world (Goodstein, 2004).

Petroleum   Petroleum (also called *oil* here) has several attributes that make it an ideal transport fuel, and it is a versatile input for a wide array of industrial processes. Oil fuels over 95 percent of global transport (Fulton, 2004). Oil is energy dense, light, relatively stable, and abundant, though, the petroleum supply is limited and the point of peak petroleum production is near. One forty-two-gallon barrel of oil has a wide variety of uses (see Figure 13.5), but the majority of oil is used to produce transport fuels, including gasoline, diesel, and jet fuel. Globally, approximately 60 percent of petroleum was used for transportation in 2005; other uses included home heating and other domestic uses, agricultural operations, and industrial needs (International Energy Agency [IEA], 2007a). By 2030, approximately 58 percent of liquid fuel production is anticipated to go to transportation worldwide (EIA, 2008).

Crude oil is pumped from underground stores under both land and sea; it is then transported to refineries, where it is distilled into a variety of fuels and other products. There are direct and indirect health effects from petroleum production, transport, and refinement. Oil exploration and drilling are associated with several occupational hazards, particularly injuries at the well (Valentić, Stojanović, Mićović, and Vukelić, 2005) and during transport by sea and land. The U.S. petroleum drilling industry has higher nonfatal occupational injury rates than the overall industry average (Centers for Disease Control and Prevention [CDC], 1993), and the occupational fatality rate for the U.S. oil and gas extraction industry was seven times the national average for occupational fatalities for the period from 2003 to 2006 (CDC, 2008). Oil production exposes workers to a host of potential carcinogens (Steinsvåg, Bråtveit, and Moen, 2007). Exposure to crude oil and its constituents, particularly benzene, is associated with increased risk of hematological malignancies such as acute myelogenous leukemia and multiple myeloma in petroleum workers (Kirkeleit, Riise, Bråtveit, and Moen, 2008). Communities near petroleum extraction activities may also suffer increased risk of such malignancies (Gazdek, Strnad, Mustajbegovic, and Nemet-Lojan, 2007). In contrast, several studies have demonstrated no significant health effects from working in petroleum refineries (Wong and others, 1986; Dagg and others, 1992; Wong and others, 2001; Tsai, and others, 2004; Gun, Pratt, Ryan, and Roder, 2006).

Petroleum transport, particularly international transport of crude oil in seaborne tankers, carries some risk as well. Mishaps involving tankers or pipelines can result in large spills. Following spills, those intensely exposed during cleanup and those who rely on the ecosystem services damaged by oil spills may be affected. Cleanup workers show reversible declines in lung function after spill exposure (Meo and others, 2008) and a host of other health concerns, including injuries and ill-defined respiratory and mucus membrane irritation syndromes (Suarez and others, 2005). These symptoms are also in evidence for people living near spills (Lyons and others, 1999; Janjua and others, 2006). The mental health effects of spills on local residents are dramatic, resulting from significant impacts on fisheries and other ecosystem services (Surís-Regueiro, Garza-Gil, and Varela-Lafuente, 2007), displacement and other issues (Palinkas, Petterson, Russell, and Downs, 1993).

Significant indirect health effects result from the ways in which petroleum is used and from dependence on petroleum exports. For instance, in some developing

PERSPECTIVE
Peak Petroleum and Public Health

Petroleum is of paramount importance to the current world economy and has a central role as a fuel, particularly in the transportation sector; it is also a key ingredient in a wide range of synthetic processes, such as the production of fertilizers, plastics, resins, textiles, pesticides, and pharmaceuticals, Approximately 84 percent of petroleum, by volume, is converted to fuel. Petroleum has important roles in public health and medicine both as a transportation fuel for patients, health workers, and supplies and as a synthetic precursor for a wide range of medical devices and pharmaceuticals.

A fossil fuel, petroleum began as prehistoric algae and zooplankton that were deposited on lake or ocean floors, buried, and subjected to particular temperature and pressure conditions. There are many different types of deposits. Conventional sources are more easily accessible, can be refined more economically, and serve as the primary source of petroleum today. Nonconventional sources, including bitumen, tar sands, and oil shale, are more costly to recover. The world's oil deposits are limited resources; they were formed over millennia and are not being replenished on any meaningful human time scale. Production must at some point be limited by resource depletion and fall short of demand. **Peak petroleum** is the point of maximum production, after which production inexorably falls.

M. King Hubbert, an American oil geologist, introduced the peak petroleum concept and term in the 1950s (Hubbert, 1956). He hypothesized that as with any limited resource, the date of peak petroleum production could be accurately predicted if the total endowment and production rates were known. Using formulas originally developed for bacterial colony growth, he accurately predicted peak production for the oil fields in the contiguous United States in the early 1970s. His methods have since been used to predict the point of peak production in several other oil fields around the globe, as well as the point of global peak production.

countries, lead is added to gasoline to improve combustion efficiency. Lead has significant effects on neurological development, and removing lead from gasoline has led to dramatic declines in blood lead levels (Luo, Zhang and Li, 2003; Hwang and others, 2004; Pino and others, 2004; Nichani and others, 2006). Also, as noted, petroleum is used in the vast majority of motorized transportation. Much motorized transport involves significant kinetic energy and is associated with significant morbidity and mortality; the World Health Organization estimates that road traffic injuries resulted in 1.2 million fatalities and 50 million injuries globally in 2002 (Peden and others 2004) (see Chapter Twenty-Two).

Analyses have been complicated, however, by uncertainties in reserves estimates, differing reporting protocols, and incentives for oil-producing nations to skew estimates of total reserves (Deffeyes, 2003). Hubbert placed the global peak between 1996 and 2006. Most current experts place the global peak sometime before 2030, many before 2010, and some assert that it is already occurring (Hirsch, Bezdek, and Wendling, 2005).

Regardless of the precise date, global peak oil production is looming, and the transition to a postpeak world is likely to be fraught with difficulty. Various scenarios have been proposed. With no comparably economical, portable, and energy-dense transport fuel, demand for petroleum will continue to rise as populations grow and become more prosperous. Prices for petroleum-based fuels and products made from oil precursors are likely to rise steadily in the long run, though the period of the peak may show significant price fluctuations as high prices reduce demand.

The effects of this transition on health care and public health are likely to be considerable and will be felt in at least four areas: medical supplies and equipment, including pharmaceuticals; medical transport; food production; and energy generation (Frumkin, Hess, and Vindigni, 2008). Other possible health effects include a persistent economic downturn, with associated social disruption, mental health effects (Miller, 1972), and possibly armed conflict (Klare, 2004).

The health sector has only just begun to confront this challenge. Important activities include scenario building and contingency planning, addressing the areas noted earlier that are most likely to be affected. Although public health functions and health services will face considerable challenge, there will also likely be health benefits, such as improvements in cardiovascular health from reduced vehicular travel and increased walking and bicycling, increased efficiency, less consumption of meat (whose production is highly petroleum intensive), and localization (Frumkin, Hess, and Vindigni, 2008). As with any public health preparedness activity, anticipation and planning will help in managing health impacts.

Finally, in countries that rely heavily on petroleum exports, economic and social arrangements seem to distort development, resulting in associated health deficits (Sachs and Warner, 2001). Such countries are frequently unstable, and suffer resource wars more frequently (Christian Aid, 2003; Klare, 2004); these conflicts significantly threaten public health.

As petroleum is the world's premier fossil fuel, its combustion contributes significantly to greenhouse gas emissions and thus to the health effects of climate change. Coal produces more CO_2 emissions (950g CO_2/kWh) than other fossil fuels (Department of Energy and Environmental Protection Agency, 2000) and is

FIGURE 13.5   Products Derived from a 42-Gallon Barrel of Oil

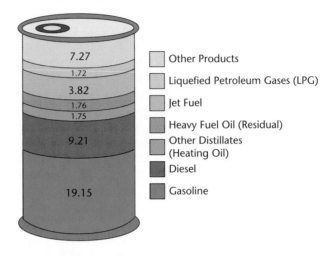

7.27   Other Products

1.72   Liquefied Petroleum Gases (LPG)

3.82   Jet Fuel

1.76   Heavy Fuel Oil (Residual)

1.75   Other Distillates (Heating Oil)

9.21   Diesel

19.15   Gasoline

Source: EIA, 2009.

responsible for the majority of cumulative atmospheric CO_2 above preindustrial levels, but petroleum is now responsible for more emissions in absolute terms. As discussed in Chapter Ten, climate change will have several significant health effects, including more heat-related illness; exacerbations of climate-sensitive cardiovascular and respiratory disease; increased incidence of waterborne, food-borne, and allergic disease; and morbidity and mortality from extreme weather and floods. Indirectly, climate change may result in population displacement, worsening malnutrition, and conflict over scarce resources. (These health impacts and other concerns are discussed further in Chapter Ten.)

Coal   Coal is a combustible sedimentary rock composed of the fossilized remains of prehistoric vegetable matter preserved from biodegradation by water and mud. Peat is its precursor. It is composed primarily of carbon and hydrogen but includes small amounts of other elements, most importantly sulfur. The primary source for electricity generation worldwide, coal is extracted using various mining methods, including pit and underground mines. Total world production equaled approximately 6.2 billion tons in 2006, of which approximately 75 percent is used for electricity generation; in 2006, 40 percent of the world's electricity production and 25 percent of the total primary energy production was from coal (Hetherington and others, 2008). Like petroleum, the world's coal endowment is finite and subject to similar production constraints, though estimates as to the date of peak coal vary more widely than those for peak petroleum, secondary to difficulties in estimating the total world endowment. The EIA (2007) estimates the world's total recoverable coal endowment to be 997,748 million short tons or 905 gigatonnes. There are abundant coal stores in the United States, Russia, Europe, South Africa, and Australia. China was the world's leading producer in 2006 with 2.4 billion tons (Hetherington and others, 2008).

Coal is produced in pit, underground, strip, and other types of mines. Mining is a hazardous occupation. Underground mining in the United States is associated with increased mortality from injuries, nonmalignant respiratory disease (coal workers pneumoconiosis, or *black lung*) and other causes (Attfield and Kuempel, 2008). In other regions, such as Turkey, miners experience high mortality rates from asphyxiation after shaft collapses, from underground railway crashes, and from gas poisoning (Kucuker, 2006).

Mining also causes significant environmental disruption, as does industrial coal processing (Freese, 2003; Yilmaz, Inac, Dikici, and Reyhanli, 2004). Coal mines, particularly open pit mines, can contaminate nearby aquatic environments as well as aquifers that humans access for drinking water.

Coal combustion is also associated with significant health effects at the point of use. The majority of China's households rely on coal and biomass fuels for cooking, heating, and other household activities, and **indoor air pollution** from these fuels is estimated to cause 420,000 premature deaths annually from respiratory illnesses, lung cancer, chronic obstructive pulmonary disease, weakening of the immune system, and compromise in lung function (Zhangand Smith, 2007). Different types of coal are associated with different cancer risks (Lan and others, 2008). Arsenic and selenium poisoning and fluorosis have also been observed (Guijian and others, 2007). Preliminary research suggests that biomass burning may pose more of a risk to health from indoor air pollution than coal (Zhang and others, 2007). Several strategies have been proposed for limiting indoor air pollution from coal combustion, and widespread adoption would likely have dramatic effects on the burden of disease in the developing world (Mestl, Aunan, and Seip, 2007).

Coal combustion at centralized power plants also has significant health impacts, through formation of nitrogen and sulfur oxides and particulates and of the greenhouse gases CO_2 and methane. The oxides are associated with an array of health effects, including respiratory and eye irritation, asthma, cardiopulmonary disease, and cancer. Particulates have significant cardiovascular health effects, including increased risk for atherosclerosis, dysrhythmias, deep vein thrombosis, and sudden cardiac death (Brook, 2007; Baccarelli and others, 2008). Respiratory effects, including decreased lung function and increased incidence of chronic obstructive pulmonary disease, are also associated with particulate exposure (Alfaro-Moreno, Nawrot, Nemmar, and Nemery, 2007. These effects are discussed in greater detail in Chapter 12. Greenhouse gas emissions from coal combustion have significant health effects as noted previously.

In the future coal use is likely to exhibit several patterns. First, as other energy sources become more scarce and expensive, coal demand is likely to increase disproportionately. Technological improvements are likely to result in increased efficiency for coal combustion and may result in enhancements such as carbon sequestration. Rising fuel costs may make it cost effective to use coal-to-liquid technologies, in which coal is used as a substrate to generate liquid fuels such as diesel and gasoline; these technologies liberate significantly more CO_2 than petroleum extraction and refinement, and this carbon would have to be captured and sequestered in order to limit the environmental and health impacts of coal-to-liquid technologies.

Natural Gas   Natural gas, another of the fossil fuels, is often found with oil deposits; its prehistoric organic matter was subject to higher temperatures than those that produced the adjacent oil. It is also found in coal beds (coal-bed methane) and in isolated natural gas fields. Natural gas is a mixture of several different gases, primarily methane but also ethane, propane, butane, and pentane and several inorganic gases, such as CO_2, nitrogen, helium, and hydrogen sulfide. It has a wide range of uses, including electricity generation, hydrogen production, fertilizer manufacture, transport, aviation, and household cooking and heating. Natural gas has several advantages over other fossil fuels; it has fewer impurities so it is less polluting, and it produces more energy per unit than petroleum or coal. Per unit of heat produced, natural gas generates about 30 percent less CO_2 than petroleum and 45 percent less than coal (EIA, 1999). Its main disadvantages are difficulties of transport and storage, given its volatility and low density.

Like other fossil fuels, natural gas is a limited resource, and geological stores are not being replenished. (Methane can be readily produced through anaerobic degradation of organic matter; this biogas is currently a minor energy source.) Total world stores are estimated at just over 6,300 trillion cubic feet, and world consumption is just over 100 trillion cubic feet annually (EIA, 2008c). This estimate may increase as new sources, such as shale, are developed (Krauss, 2009). As with peak oil, peak natural gas is anticipated within the next twenty years. Different from peak oil, however, peak natural gas is likely to be a regional phenomenon to at least some degree, owing to the difficulty of efficiently and safely transporting large volumes of natural gas.

As with oil extraction, natural gas extraction comes with significant occupational hazards, particularly for injuries, and there is a small but significant risk of hydrogen sulfide toxicity (Hendrickson, Chang, and Hamilton, 2004). Extraction work is also associated with certain types of cancers (Mills and others, 1984). Natural gas processing, in which water and various organic and inorganic impurities are removed, is not associated with health risks in the medical literature. Occupational exposure to natural gas combustion products does carry a small increased risk of bladder cancer (Siemiatycki, Dewar, Nadon, and Gèrin, 1994; Siemiatycki and others, 1988).

Overall, given its cleaner emissions profile and more efficient combustion, natural gas produces fewer health hazards per joule produced than other fossil fuels do. However, natural gas combustion does produce substantial CO_2 emissions, and its contribution is expected to increase significantly in coming years. In 2004, natural gas combustion contributed 5,300 megatonnes (Mt) of CO_2 to the atmosphere (compared with 10,600 from coal and 10,200 from petroleum); by 2030, projections suggest natural gas may be responsible for 11,000 Mt, coal 8,400, and petroleum 17,200 (Metz and others, 2007).

Biomass

Biomass fuels are a heterogenous group of organic materials generated by plants through photosynthesis. In contrast to fossil fuels, biomass fuels are produced on a human time scale, ranging from months to decades. Biomass includes wood, corn husks, coconut shells, peat, and animal dung. Important to the discussion of impact is that the carbon in biomass fuels is part of the carbon cycle; when it is released into the atmosphere on combustion, it is often reincorporated into organic matter through plant respiration and photosynthesis. Any carbon released into the atmosphere reenters the carbon cycle, but combustion of fossil fuels releases carbon that has been sequestered for millennia, overwhelming the cycle's current capacities.

Depending on how biomass fuels are planted, cultivated, harvested, and used, their health effects and energy efficiency vary widely. Poorly ventilated household combustion in the developing world causes indoor air pollution that has significant health effects, whereas industrial combustion can occur at higher temperatures with fewer ill effects. Conversion of biomass fuels to fuels such as ethanol, methanol, and methane is also an emerging strategy for biomass use. The energy inputs and net energy balance of these strategies, as well as their health effects, are still much debated.

Household Biomass Combustion Over 3 billion people, particularly in Africa and Asia, use biomass for their primary household energy needs (Rehfuess, 2006), and biomass energy sources constitute 7 percent of the world's primary energy production (IEA, 2007a). In rural areas of the developing world, biomass fuels include wood, crop residues, and animal dung, whereas charcoal is often used in more urban areas. Biomass fuel collection often requires long trips on foot and, as a result, exposes women and children, who are the primary gatherers, to injuries, malnutrition, vector-borne diseases, sexual violence, and other hazards.

There is also an opportunity cost in that time spent gathering fuel could be used productively in other areas, including education. Once biomass for fuel is secured, burning it has other health effects. As noted in Table 13.3, these include respiratory tract infections, lung cancer, and tuberculosis. Injuries, particularly burns, are also associated with biomass burning and are a significant burden of disease in the developing world (as discussed in Chapter Twenty-Two).

The World Health Organization estimates that approximately 1.5 million people died from indoor air pollution in 2002 (Rehfuess, 2006). As energy prices rise, biomass fuels are expected to be a significant, ongoing energy source in decades to come; the developing world's use may increase disproportionately (IEA, 2007b). Although not a significant source of deforestation (Mathews, Payne, Rohweder, and Murray, 2000), biomass fuel collection can nevertheless devastate local ecosystems where it is practiced intensively and population density is high.

There are several effective strategies for reducing the health effects of reliance on biomass. Sustainable forestry management and woodlots can minimize the burden of gathering fuel. Increased ventilation, chimneys, and improved stove design are important engineering controls.

Controlled Biomass Combustion   Biomass can also be burned in ways that are more technologically intensive but that are also more efficient, generate less air pollution, and produce fewer greenhouse gas emissions than open combustion. Centralized, controlled biomass combustion for electricity generation is more commonly employed in the developed than developing world, and will be

TABLE 13.3   Health Effects of Household Biomass Combustion

Health Outcome	Population	Relative Risk (95% CI)	Evidence
Acute lower respiratory infection	Children 0–4 years	2.3 (1.9–2.7)	Strong
Chronic obstructive pulmonary disease	Women 30+	3.2 (2.3–4.8)	Strong
	Men 30+	1.8 (1.0–3.2)	Moderate
Lung cancer	Women 30+	1.5 (1.0–2.1)	Moderate
Asthma	Children 5–14	1.6 (1.0–2.5)	Moderate
	Adults 15+	1.2 (1.0–1.5)	Moderate
Tuberculosis	Adults 15+	1.5 (1.0–2.4)	Moderate
Cataracts	Adults 15+	1.3 (1.0–1.7)	Moderate

Source: Adapted from Rehfuess, 2006.

increasingly important in coming years. Biomass is converted to energy via several different processes, but in the United States it is primarily either burned to produce steam and electricity in industry or to power turbines and generate electricity for domestic use, or used as a substrate to produce liquid fuels for transport.

Controlled biomass combustion is a growing energy source in the United States. In 2007, biomass constituted 53 percent of renewable energy sources (although renewables are only 7 percent of the total U.S. energy budget) (EIA, 2008b). The paper and pulp industries are by far the largest biomass consumers in the United States (EIA, 2003). Biomass has several advantages over coal and natural gas as a fuel: it has dramatically lower CO_2 emissions when part of a closed-loop process in which fuel stocks are grown specifically for energy production and emissions are sequestered during the planting cycle; considerably fewer sulfur and nitrogen oxides are produced during combustion than with coal; and it is renewable on a human time scale. Biomass supply is a significant concern for the United States, which has only recently started wide-scale energy crop production, and there are several uncertainties, including the ways in which mass diversion of biomass for energy production will affect other industries that currently rely on a cheap biomass supply, will affect soil quality, might alter forest fire prevention programs in order to increase supply, and might leverage municipal waste streams by diverting biomass from landfills to energy production (EIA, 2003). Worldwide, there is significant potential for economical biofuel production, particularly if energy crop management can be maximized (Johnston and Holloway, 2007).

Biofuels   Biomass is also used to produce liquid **biofuels** (primarily ethanol and biodiesel), which are used principally in the transport sector. In comparison with fossil fuels for transport, biofuels have several of the same advantages and concerns as biomass. There are some important differences, however: the energy crops used currently for biofuels overlap more significantly with food crops than do energy crops for electricity production. In the United States, corn is the primary input for ethanol and soybeans for biodiesel (though any source of free fatty acids can be used, including waste animal fats and recycled grease from restaurants), and a percentage of these crops is diverted from the food supply. Corn is a particularly important food crop in the United States and is used in a variety of agricultural products, including animal feed, sweeteners, and processed foods (Pollan, 2006). Although the ultimate significance of this substitution is debated, there is considerable concern over food price inflation resulting from ethanol subsidies and crop substitution (Daschle, 2007; and Senauer, 2007, 2008).

In addition, the two principal biofuels have different energy, efficiency, and emissions profiles and, further complicating comparisons, are used in different percentage blends. Currently, ethanol is added to gasoline as an oxidizing agent (this fuel is known as E10, as it contains 10 percent ethanol); it is also used as a primary fuel (E85). However, ethanol is less energy dense than gasoline, with 67 percent of gasoline's energy per unit volume, which leads to lower mileage, and there is a question over ethanol's true degree of energy efficiency when all energy inputs are accounted for. Comparison using a life cycle approach suggests that biodiesel has a much greater net energy gain (energy released during combustion minus energy put into production) than does ethanol from corn (93 percent versus 25 percent), pollutes at a much lower rate, and reduces greenhouse gas emissions 41 percent compared with petroleum, versus a 12 percent reduction for ethanol (Hill and others, 2006). Biodiesel thus comes out significantly ahead of corn ethanol in terms of this set of comparisons. Other candidates with favorable profiles may be waiting in the wings: biofuels from nonfood crops, such as cellulosic ethanol and synfuel, could potentially be produced in much greater supply without affecting food prices significantly (Hill and others, 2006).

The possible health effects of biofuel combustion products are not well known and are under active investigation (Swanson, Madden, and Ghio, 2007). Although there is evidence of reduced emissions and thus health benefits from using ethanol as a fuel oxidizer (Schifter and others, 2001; see also Gaffney and Marley, 2001), there is also a concern that large-scale conversion from gasoline to E85 will result in greater ozone production and acetaldehyde emissions, with potential overall net negative health impacts (Jacobson, 2007; also see Engelhaupt, 2007). The effect may depend on the fuel ethanol is replacing; another study shows net positive health effects if diesel is replaced partially with ethanol (Miraglia, 2007). A blend of 20 percent biodiesel tends to reduce emissions of several harmful chemical species, including particulate matter, carbon monoxide, and total hydrocarbons, among others (McCormick, 2007). Other studies have examined different biodiesel blends and found fuel mixes with even more favorable emissions profiles, although this work is preliminary (Yuan and others, 2007). More work is needed to characterize the emissions profiles of specific fuel mixtures, their health effects in biological systems, and the public health effects of fuel substitution.

Hydropower

Hydroelectric power transforms gravitational energy in falling water into electrical energy. Globally, hydroelectric energy generation is the most widely used form of renewable energy, and it has been growing; the most recent figures show that in 2005 the world generated 29 quadrillion BTUs using hydroelectric power (EIA, 2005). In 2006, **hydropower** generated 15 percent of the world's electricity and roughly 46 percent of the electricity from renewable sources (Martinot, 2008).

There is significant heterogeneity in the world's hydroelectric generating power, with South and Central America and Asia producing the most in absolute terms.

The advantages and disadvantages of hydropower have come under some scrutiny of late. The principal, and substantial, advantage of hydroelectric power generation is its low apparent cost. Although up-front costs (for example, dam construction) can be significant, these are often quickly recouped from sale of electricity. Until recently, conventional wisdom also held that hydropower generated very low greenhouse gas emissions compared with fossil fuel combustion. However, recent investigations show that dams and their associated reservoirs result in the accumulation and release of significant amounts of methane, a potent greenhouse gas. Although research is preliminary, it seems that the total estimate of global methane emissions may need to be adjusted upward by as much as 20 percent (Giles, 2006). This emerging concern is in addition to the established costs and disadvantages of hydropower, including displacement of human settlements, local ecosystem destruction damage, and increased incidence of malaria and other vector-borne diseases (Johnson, Kastenberg, and Griesmeyer, 1981; Joyce, 1997). Overall, hydropower seems not to be the completely clean, sustainable energy source once thought.

Nuclear

Nuclear power, also referred to as **nuclear energy**, is generated through fission of uranium 235, which heats water to do mechanical work, primarily electricity generation. Nuclear engines are also used to propel some ships. Nuclear energy is a relative newcomer and has a reputation of being hazardous, resulting from several high-profile nuclear accidents, including those at Three Mile Island and Chernobyl. The Earth's uranium supply is finite, so nuclear energy is not considered renewable. However, nuclear energy production does not emit greenhouse gases, so in climate change terms nuclear energy is quite favorable and has enjoyed renewed attention in recent years. As of 2005, nuclear energy constituted 6.3 percent of the world's total energy supply, and 15.2 percent of electricity generation; 84.7 percent of nuclear power is generated in Organisation for Economic Co-operation and Development countries (IEA, 2007a).

There are potential direct and indirect health effects upstream of the end user secondary to uranium mining, refinement, and transport. Apart from the usual injuries associated with mining and an association with nonmalignant pulmonary disease such as silicosis, uranium mining is associated with several cancers, including lung cancer, lymphoma, and leukemia, resulting from exposure to radioactive uranium and radon (Archer, 1981; Samet, 1991; Hornung, 2001; Grosche, and others, 2006; Rericha and others, 2006; see also Möhner, 2006). Uranium mining and milling are not associated with significant health effects in surrounding communities (Boice, Mumma, Schweitzer, and Blot, 2003; Boice, Mumma, and Blot, 2007). Occupational exposures in nuclear power plants are associated with increased cancer rates, as well (Cardis and others, 2007; Richardson and Wing, 2007), and there is preliminary evidence of a small increase in risk of circulatory disease in nuclear power plant workers (McGeoghegan and others, 2008; see also McGale and Darby, 2008). There is a small risk of childhood blood cancers in areas around nuclear facilities, but the results are difficult to interpret and may not be related to radiation exposure (Morris, 1994). As uranium is also used as a primary material for nuclear weapons and other weapons of mass destruction such as dirty bombs, security is a concern, and nuclear terrorism is a recognized public health threat (Barnett and others, 2006). To the extent that nuclear energy production increases uranium availability, there are potential health effects from terrorism and armed conflict.

Downstream health effects of nuclear energy production are primarily from nuclear accidents and potential exposure to radiation from contaminated sites and during transport and storage of spent fuel. The reactor explosion at Chernobyl was the largest nuclear accident to date and resulted in significant acute and chronic health effects. The most dramatic impacts were from acute radiation sickness (Mettler, Guskova, and Gusev, 2007) and pediatric thyroid cancers (Demidchik, Saenko, and Yamashita, 2007); acute and chronic mental health effects were also quite significant (Bromet and Havenaar, 2007). Although increased incidence of other cancers has not yet been detected, the possibility remains that there will be a long-term effect (Cardis and others, 2006; Howe, 2007) (see also Chapter Twenty-One). The disaster spawned many novel protections, and the nuclear industry is significantly safer as a result (Gonzalez, 2007).

Even with significant safeguards, there will be concern over site contamination and radiation exposure during transport and storage of spent nuclear fuel (McBeth and Oakes, 1996; Wolbarst and others, 1999). The dialogue around nuclear waste handling hinges on fundamental questions relevant to energy production generally, including how to frame the dialogue about risk management (Kemp, Bennett, and White, 2006) and how to distribute risk both among populations presently and between contemporary and future generations (Okrent, 1999).

Other Renewables

There are several other **renewable** sources of energy, including solar, geothermal, wind, and wave energy. Renewables are increasing as a proportion of the world's total energy budget, and they have several distinct advantages over fossil fuels, including lower long-term cost and minimal greenhouse gas emissions.

In many cases, debate over renewables concerns site location and aesthetic concerns, although some initiatives also raise ecological concerns. There are occupational health concerns related to hazardous materials involved in production for certain renewables, such as solar, that can be minimized through innovations and meticulous waste stream management. From a human health perspective, however, renewables offer great potential for improvement over fossil fuels.

SUMMARY

Energy is fundamental to a range of human activities, including transportation (Woodcock and others, 2007), electricity generation (Markandya and Wilkinson, 2007), and food production (McMichael, Powles, Butler, and Uauy, 2007). Many approaches to supplying energy for these activities are available. The choices made about how energy is generated and used have broad implications for health, including implications for health equity. Energy policy is health policy, on both a local and global scale.

Energy decision making occurs at several levels simultaneously. Individuals make choices about the types of energy they will employ many times a day; households and communities make collective energy choices; and states, regions, and countries make crucial energy decisions that determine the options available to smaller entities and individuals. In addition to health concerns, important considerations include financial costs, security, and environmental impacts. Some costs (and, less commonly, benefits) remain as *externalities*—impacts that are not included directly in financial analysis.

When health impacts are overlooked, decision makers at every level may reach suboptimal decisions and forfeit opportunities to protect health. Health externalities borne by the general public or by particular regions of the world constitute an implied subsidy of the underlying activity that may not have been intended. Conversely, when health concerns are methodically addressed, unexpected findings may emerge and inform policymaking. For example, health impact assessments of energy projects have examined social dynamics and other complex downstream effects sometimes not intuitively associated with energy policy, such as the increased incidence of HIV infection associated with a dam project in South Africa (Lerer and Scudder, 1999).

An important role for public health is to determine the health burdens of these externalities so policymakers can account for them in their decision making. There are many strategies for addressing the market failure of externalities, including regulation (such as limits on particulate emissions), taxes (such as a direct tax on CO_2 emissions), and direct subsidies to industries with fewer externalities (such as subsidies for biodiesel production). Health impact assessments (described in Exhibit 14.4) will allow some energy sources to emerge as clearly healthier than others. The challenge for the coming century will be to pursue energy choices that result in ethical, economic, sustainable patterns of development.

KEY TERMS

biodiesel

biofuels

biomass

climate change

coal

coal gasification

coke

energy

energy ladder

fossil fuels

hydropower

indoor air pollution

life cycle analysis

natural gas

nuclear energy

nuclear power

peak petroleum

petroleum

power

renewable energy sources

DISCUSSION QUESTIONS

1. List all the different types of energy you use over the course of a typical day. Create a table that lists each activity and describes the energy type and source, the alternatives available to you for each activity, where the energy is produced (at the point of consumption or more remotely), and the health effects of the energy source. Be sure to consider energy embedded in food as well.

2. Calculate your carbon footprint. Online calculators are available at these sites:

    http://www.carbonfootprint.com/calculator.aspx

    http://www.climatecrisis.net/takeaction/carboncalculator

    http://www.nature.org/initiatives/climatechange/calculator

3. Pick a technical innovation that reduces work and thus improves energy efficiency, such as a smaller, more fuel-efficient car or a well-insulated building with little air circulation. Write a paragraph that outlines the resulting co-benefits to energy and health and the potential trade-offs (such as the increased risk of injuries from driving a smaller car or increased exposure to respiratory pathogens in a building with little ventilation). How might a health impact assessment determine the ultimate value of the innovation?

4. Externalities signal a form of market failure. List several strategies that could address these market failures, including those that will result in proper pricing (for greenhouse gas emissions, for instance), and those that will allow redress for adverse impacts on vulnerable populations. Which is more effective, proper pricing to minimize externalities or redress after the fact? Which is more just?

REFERENCES

Alfaro-Moreno, E., Nawrot, T.S., Nemmar, A., and Nemery, B. "Particulate Matter in the Environment: Pulmonary and Cardiovascular Effects." *Current Opinion in Pulmonary Medicine*, 2007, *13*(2), 98–106.

Archer, V. E. "Health Concerns in Uranium Mining and Milling." *Journal of Occupational Medicine*, 1981, *23*(7), 502–505.

Ashton, T. *The Industrial Revolution: 1780–1830*. New York: Oxford University Press, 1998.

Attfield, M. D., and Kuempel, E. D. "Mortality Among U.S. Underground Coal Miners: A 23-Year Follow-Up." *American Journal of Industrial Medicine*, 2008, *51*(4), 231–245.

Baccarelli, A., and others. "Exposure to Particulate Air Pollution and Risk of Deep Vein Thrombosis." [Comment]. *Archives of Internal Medicine*, 2008, *168*(9), 920–927.

Barnett, D. J., and others. "Understanding Radiologic and Nuclear Terrorism as Public Health Threats: Preparedness and Response Perspectives." *Journal of Nuclear Medicine*, 2006, *47*(10), 1653–1661.

Boice, J. D., Jr., Mumma, M. T., and Blot, W. J. "Cancer and Noncancer Mortality in Populations Living Near Uranium and Vanadium Mining and Milling Operations in Montrose County, Colorado, 1950–2000." *Radiation Research*, 2007, *167*(6), 711–726.

Boice, J. D., Jr., Mumma, M., Schweitzer, S., and Blot, W. J. "Cancer Mortality in a Texas County with Prior Uranium Mining and Milling Activities, 1950–2001." *Journal of Radiological Protection*, 2003, *23*(3), 247–262.

Bromet, E. J., and Havenaar, J. M. "Psychological and Perceived Health Effects of the Chernobyl Disaster: A 20-Year Review." *Health Physics*, 2007, *93*(5), 516–521.

Brook, R. D. "Is Air Pollution a Cause of Cardiovascular Disease? Updated Review and Controversies." *Reviews on Environmental Health*, 2007, *22*(2), 115–137.

Cardis, E., and others. "Cancer Consequences of the Chernobyl Accident: 20 Years On." *Journal of Radiological Protection*, 2006, *26*(2), 127–140.

Cardis, E., and others. "The 15-Country Collaborative Study of Cancer Risk Among Radiation Workers in the Nuclear Industry: Estimates of Radiation-Related Cancer Risks." *Radiation Research*, 2007, *167*(4), 396–416.

Carr, G. "The Power and the Glory: A Special Report on Energy." *The Economist*, 2008, *389*, S1–S14.

Centers for Disease Control and Prevention. "Injuries to International Petroleum Drilling Workers, 1988–1990." *Morbidity and Mortality Weekly Report*, 1993, *42*(7), 128–131.

Centers for Disease Control and Prevention. "Fatalities Among Oil and Gas Extraction Workers— United States, 2003–2006." *Morbidity and Mortality Weekly Report*, 2008, *57*(16), 429–431.

Christian Aid. *Fuelling Poverty: Oil, War and Corruption. Why the Oil Industry Is Bad for Poor Countries*. London: Christian Aid, 2003.

Clancy, L., Goodman, P., Sinclair, H., and Dockery, D.W. "Effect of Air-Pollution Control on Death Rates in Dublin, Ireland: An Intervention Study." *Lancet*, 2002, *360*, 1210–1214.

Dagg, T. G., and others. "An Updated Cause Specific Mortality Study of Petroleum Refinery Workers." *British Journal of Industrial Medicine*, 1992, *49*(3), 203–212

Daschle, T., "Food for Fuel?" *Foreign Affairs*, 2007, *86*(5), 157–160.

Deaton, A. *Health in an Age of Globalization*. Research Program in Development Studies. Princeton, N.J.: Princeton University, 2004.

Deffeyes KS. *Hubbert's Peak: The Impending World Oil Shortage*. Princeton: Princeton University Press, 2003.

Demidchik, Y. E., Saenko, V. A., and Yamashita, S. "Childhood Thyroid Cancer in Belarus, Russia, and Ukraine after Chernobyl and at Present." *Arquivos Brasileiros de Endocrinologia e Metabologia*, 2007, *51*(5), 748–762.

Ebrey, P., Walthall, A., and Palais, J. B. *East Asia: A Cultural, Social, and Political History*. Boston: Houghton Mifflin, 2006.

Energy Information Administration. *Natural Gas 1998: Issues and Trends*. Washington, D.C.: Energy Information Administration, 1999.

Energy Information Administration. *Biomass for Electricity Generation*. http://www.eia.doe.gov/oiaf/analysispaper/biomass, 2003.

Energy Information Administration. *International Energy Annual 2005*. http://www.eia.doe.gov/emeu/iea/elec.html, 2005.

Energy Information Administration. *World Estimated Recoverable Coal*. Washington, D.C.: Energy Information Administration, 2007.

Energy Information Administration. *International Energy Annual 2006: World Dry Natural Gas Consumption*. Washington, D.C.: Energy Information Administration, 2008a.

Energy Information Administration. *Renewable Energy Consumption and Electricity Preliminary 2007 Statistics*. http://www.eia.doe.gov/cneaf/alternate/page/renew_energy_consump/rea_prereport.html, 2008b.

Energy Information Administration. *World Proved Reserves of Oil and Natural Gas: Most Recent Estimates*. http://www.eia.doe.gov/emeu/international/reserves.html, 2008c.

Energy Information Administration. "Products Made from a Barrel of Crude Oil." http://www.eia.doe.gov/kids/energyfacts/sources/non-renewable/oil.html, 2009.

Engelhaupt, E. "Clearing the Air on Ethanol." [Comment.] *Environmental Science & Technology*, *41*(11), 3788, 2007.

Freese, B. *Coal: A Human History*. Cambridge, Mass.: De Capo Press, 2003.

Frumkin, H., Hess, J., and Vindigni, S.. "Peak Petroleum and Public Health." *JAMA*, 2008, *298*(14), 1688–1690.

Fulton, L. *Reducing Oil Consumption in Transport: Combining Three Approaches*. Paris: International Energy Agency, 2004.

Gaffney, J. S., and Marley, N. A. *Environmental Science & Technology*, 2001, *35*(24), 4957–4960.

Gazdek, D., Strnad, M., Mustajbegovic, J., and Nemet-Lojan, Z. "Lymphohematopoietic Malignancies and Oil Exploitation in Koprivnica-Krizevci County, Croatia." *International Journal of Occupational and Environmental Health*, *2007*, *13*(3), 258–267.

Giles, J. "Methane Quashes Green Credentials of Hydropower." *Nature*, 2006, *444*, 524–525.

Gonzalez, A. J. "Chernobyl Vis-à-Vis the Nuclear Future: An International Perspective." *Health Physics*, 2007, *93*(5), 571–592.

Goodstein, D. *Out of Gas: The End of the Age of Oil*. New York: Norton, 2004.

Grosche, B., and others. "Lung Cancer Risk Among German Male Uranium Miners: A Cohort Study, 1946–1998." *British Journal of Cancer*, 2006, *95*(9), 1280–1287.

Grubler, A., Nakicenovic, N., and Jefferson, M. "Global Energy Perspectives: A Summary of the Joint Study by the International Institute for Applied Systems Analysis and World Energy Council." *Technological Forecasting and Social Change*, 1996, *51*, 237–264.

Guijian, L., and others. "Health Effects of Arsenic, Fluorine, and Selenium from Indoor Burning of Chinese Coal." *Reviews of Environmental Contamination and Toxicology*, 2007, *189*, 89–106.

Gun, R. T., Pratt, N., Ryan, P., and Roder, D. and others. "Update of Mortality and Cancer Incidence in the Australian Petroleum Industry Cohort." Occupational and Environmental Medicine, 2006, *63*(7), 476–481.

Hendrickson, R. G., Chang, A., and Hamilton, R.J. "Co-Worker Fatalities from Hydrogen Sulfide." *American Journal of Industrial Medicine*, 2004, *45*(4), 346–350.

Hetherington, L., and others. *World Mineral Production 2002–2006*. Keyworth, U.K.: British Geological Survey, 2008.

Hill, J., and others. "Environmental, Economic, and Energetic Costs and Benefits of Biodiesel and Ethanol Biofuels." *Proceedings of the National Academy of Sciences of the United States of America*, 2006, *103*(30), 11206–11210.

Hirsch, R.L., Bezdek, R., and Wendling, R. *Peaking of World Oil Production: Impacts, Mitigation, & Risk Management.* Science Applications International Corporation Report for the U.S. Department of Energy, 2005. http://www.netl.doe.gov/publications/others/pdf/Oil_Peaking_NETL.pdf

Hoffert, M., and others. "Energy Implications of Future Stabilization of Atmospheric CO_2 Content." *Nature*, 1998, *395*(675), 881–884.

Holdren, J., and Smith, K. "Energy, the Environment, and Health." In J. Goldemberg and others (eds.), *World Energy Assessment: Energy and the Challenge of Sustainability.* New York: United Nations Development Programme, 2000.

Hornung, R. W. "Health Effects in Underground Uranium Miners." *Occupational Medicine*, 2001, *16*(2), 331–344.

Howe, G. R. "Leukemia Following the Chernobyl Accident." *Health Physics*, 2007, *93*(5), 512–515.

Hubbert MK. *Nuclear Energy and the Fossil Fuels.* American Petroleum Institute Drilling and Production Practice Proceedings. Spring 1956: 5–75. http://www.hubbertpeak.com/hubbert/1956/1956.pdf.

Hwang, Y. H., and others. "Transition of Cord Blood Lead Level, 1985–2002, in the Taipei Area and Its Determinants After the Cease of Leaded Gasoline Use." *Environmental Research*, 2004, *96*(3), 274–282.

International Energy Agency. *Key World Energy Statistics 2007.* http://www.iea.org/textbase/nppdf/free/2007/key_stats_2007.pdf, 2007a.

International Energy Agency. *World Energy Outlook 2006.* Paris: International Energy Agency, 2007b.

Jacobson, M. Z. "Effects of Ethanol (E85) Versus Gasoline Vehicles on Cancer and Mortality in the United States." *Environmental Science & Technology*, 2007, *41*(11), 4150–4157.

Janjua, N. Z., and others. "Acute Health Effects of the Tasman Spirit Oil Spill on Residents of Karachi, Pakistan." *BMC Public Health*, 2006, *6*, 84.

Johnson, D. H., Kastenberg, W. E., and Griesmeyer, J. M. "Prospectives on the Risks of Alternative Fuel Cycles." *American Journal of Public Health*, 1981, *71*(9), 1050–1057.

Johnston, M., and Holloway, T. "A Global Comparison of National Biodiesel Production Potentials." *Environmental Science & Technology*, 2007, *41*(23), 7967–7973.

Joyce, S. "Is It Worth a Dam?" *Environmental Health Perspectives*, 1997, *105*(10), 1050–1055.

Kabir Z, Bennett K, and Clancy L. "Lung Cancer and Urban Air-Pollution in Dublin: A Temporal Association?" *Irish Medical Journal*, 2007, *100*, 367–369.

Kemp, R. V., Bennett, D.G., and White, M.J. "Recent Trends and Developments in Dialogue on Radioactive Waste Management: Experience from the UK." *Environment International*, 2006, *32*(8), 1021–1032.

Kirkeleit, J., Riise, T., Bråtveit, M., and Moen, B. E. "Increased Risk of Acute Myelogenous Leukemia and Multiple Myeloma in a Historical Cohort of Upstream Petroleum Workers Exposed to Crude Oil." *Cancer Causes & Control*, 2008, *19*(1), 13–23.

Klare, M. *Blood and Oil: The Dangers and Consequences of America's Growing Dependency on Imported Petroleum.* New York: Metropolitan Books, 2004.

Krauss, C. "New Way to Tap Gas May Expand Global Supplies." *New York Times*, 9 October 2009, p. 1

Kucuker, H. "Occupational Fatalities Among Coal Mine Workers in Zonguldak, Turkey, 1994–2003." *Occupational Medicine* (Oxford, England), 2006, *56*(2), 144–146.

Lan, Q., and others. "Variation in Lung Cancer Risk by Smoky Coal Subtype in Xuanwei, China." *International Journal of Cancer*, 2008, *123*(9), 2164–2169.

Lerer, L., and Scudder, T. "Health Impacts of Large Dams." *Environmental Impact Assessment Review*, 1999, *19*, 113–123.

Luo, W., Zhang, Y., and Li, H.. "Children's Blood Lead Levels After the Phasing Out of Leaded Gasoline in Shantou, China." *Archives of Environmental Health*, 2003, *58*(3), 184–187.

Lyons, R. A., and others. "Acute Health Effects of the Sea Empress Oil Spill." *Journal of Epidemiology and Community Health*, 1999, *53*(5), 306–310.

Markandya, A., and Wilkinson, P. "Electricity Generation and Health." *Lancet*, 2007, *370*, 979–990.

Martinot, E. *Renewables 2007 Global Status Report*. Paris: Renewable Energy Policy Network for the 21st Century, 2008.

Mathews, E., Payne, R., Rohweder, M., and Murray, S. *Pilot Analysis of Global Ecosystems: Forest Ecosystems*. Washington, D.C.: World Resources Institute, 2000.

McBeth, M. K., and Oakes, A. S. "Citizen Perceptions of Risks Associated with Moving Radiological Waste." *Risk Analysis*, 1996, *16*(3), 421–427.

McCormick, R. L. "The Impact of Biodiesel on Pollutant Emissions and Public Health." *Inhalation Toxicology*, 2007, *19*(12), 1033–1039.

McGale, P., and Darby, S. C. "Commentary: A Dose-Response Relationship for Radiation-Induced Heart Disease—Current Issues and Future Prospects." *International Journal of Epidemiology*, 2008, *37*(3), 518–523.

McGeoghegan, D., and others. "The Non-Cancer Mortality Experience of Male Workers at British Nuclear Fuels PLC, 1946–2005." *International Journal of Epidemiology*, 2008, *37*(3), 506–518.

McMichael, A., Powles, J.W., Butler, C.D., and Uauy, R.. "Food, Livestock Production, Energy, Climate Change, and Health." *Lancet*, 2007, *370*, 1253–1263.

Meisel, L. "The Technology Challenge: An Interview with Physicist Marty Hoffert." http://www.thebreakthrough.org/blog/2008/04/post_1.shtml, 2008.

Meo, S. A., and others. "Lung Function in Subjects Exposed to Crude Oil Spill into Sea Water." *Marine Pollution Bulletin*, 2008, *56*(1), 88–94.

Mestl, H.E.S., Aunan, K., Seip, H.M. "Health Benefits from Reducing Indoor Air Pollution from Household Solid Fuel Use in China—Three Abatement Scenarios." *Environment International*, 2007, *33*(6), 831–840.

Mettler, F. A., Jr., Guskova, A.K., and Gusev, I. "Health Effects in Those with Acute Radiation Sickness from the Chernobyl Accident." *Health Physics*, 2007, *93*(5), 462–469.

Metz, B., and others (eds.). *Climate Change 2007: Mitigation of Climate Change.* Contribution of Working Group III to the Fourth Assessment Report of the Intergovernmental Panel on Climate Change. New York: Cambridge University Press, 2007.

Miller L, Ed. *Mental Health in Rapid Social Change.* Jerusalem: Jerusalem Academic Press, 1972.

Mills, P. K., and others. "Testicular Cancer Associated with Employment in Agriculture and Oil and Natural Gas Extraction." *Lancet*, 1984, *1*(8370), 207–210.

Miraglia, S. G. "Health, Environmental, and Economic Costs from the Use of a Stabilized Diesel/Ethanol Mixture in the City of Sao Paulo, Brazil." *Cadernos De Saúde Pública/Reports in Public Health*, 2007, *23*(suppl. 4), S559–S569.

Müohner, M. "Risk of Lymphohematopoietic Malignancies in Uranium Miners." *Environmental Health Perspectives*, 2007, *115*(4), A184.

Morris, J. A. "Childhood Cancer Around Nuclear Installations." *European Journal of Cancer Prevention*, 1994, *3*(1), 15–21.

Nichani, V., and others. "Blood Lead Levels in Children After Phase-out of Leaded Gasoline in Bombay, India." *Science of the Total Environment*, 2006, *363*(1–3), 95–106.

Okrent, D. "On Intergenerational Equity and Its Clash with Intragenerational Equity and on the Need for Policies to Guide the Regulation of Disposal of Wastes and Other Activities Posing Very Long-Term Risks." *Risk Analysis*, 1999, *19*(5), 877–901.

Pacala, S., and Socolow, R. "Stabilization Wedges: Solving the Climate Problem for the Next 50 Years with Current Technologies." *Science*, 2004, *305*, 968–972.

Palinkas, L.A., Petterson, J.S., Russell, J., and Downs, M.A.. "Community Patterns of Psychiatric Disorders After the Exxon Valdez Oil Spill." *American Journal of Psychiatry*, 1993, *150*(10), 1517–1523.

Peden, M., and others (eds.). *World Report on Road Traffic Injury Prevention.* Geneva: World Health Organization, 2004.

Pino, P., and others. "Rapid Drop in Infant Blood Lead Levels During the Transition to Unleaded Gasoline Use in Santiago, Chile." *Archives of Environmental Health*, 2004, *59*(4), 182–187.

Pollan, M. *The Omnivore's Dilemma: A Natural History of Four Meals.* New York: Penguin Press, 2006.

Pomeranz, K. *The Great Divergence: China, Europe, and the Making of the Modern World Economy.* Princeton, N.J.: Princeton University Press, 2000.

Rehfuess, E. *Fuel for Life: Household Energy and Health.* Geneva: World Health Organization, 2006.

Rericha, V., and others. "Incidence of Leukemia, Lymphoma, and Multiple Myeloma in Czech Uranium Miners: A Case-Cohort Study." *Environmental Health Perspectives*, 2006, *114*(6), 818–822.

Richardson, D. B., and Wing, S. "Leukemia Mortality Among Workers at the Savannah River Site." *American Journal of Epidemiology*, 2007, *166*(9), 1015–1022.

Runge, C., and Senauer, B. "How Biofuels Could Starve the Poor." *Foreign Affairs*, 2007, *86*(3), 41–53.

Runge, C., and Senauer, B. "How Ethanol Fuels the Food Crisis." http://www.foreignaffairs.org/20080528faupdate87376/c-ford-runge-benjamin-senauer/how-ethanol-fuels-the-food-crisis.html, 2008.

Sachs, J., and Warner A. "Natural Resources and Economic Development: The Curse of Natural Resources." *European Economic Review*, 2001, *45*, 827–838.

Salway, P. *A History of Roman Britian*. New York: Oxford University Press, 2001.

Samet, J. M. "Diseases of Uranium Miners and Other Underground Miners Exposed to Radon." *Occupational Medicine*, 1991, *6*(4), 629–639.

Schifter, I., and others. "Environmental Implications on the Oxygenation of Gasoline with Ethanol in the Metropolitan Area of Mexico City." *Environmental Science & Technology*, 2001, *35*(10), 1893–1901.

Siemiatycki, J., Dewar, R. Nadon, L., and Gèrin, M. "Occupational Risk Factors for Bladder Cancer: Results from a Case-Control Study in Montreal, Quebec, Canada." *American Journal of Epidemiology*, 1994, *140*(12), 1061–1080.

Siemiatycki, J., and others. "Associations Between Several Sites of Cancer and Ten Types of Exhaust and Combustion Products. Results from a Case-Referent Study in Montreal." *Scandinavian Journal of Work, Environment & Health*, 1988, *14*(2), 79–90.

Socolow, R., and Pacala, S. "A Plan to Keep Carbon in Check." *Scientific American*, 2006, *295*, 50–57.

Steinsvåg, K., Bråtveit, M., and Moen, B. E. "Exposure to Carcinogens for Defined Job Categories in Norway's Offshore Petroleum Industry, 1970 to 2005." *Occupational and Environmental Medicine*, 2007, *64*(4), 250–258.

Suarez, B., and others. "Acute Health Problems Among Subjects Involved in the Cleanup Operation Following the Prestige Oil Spill in Asturias and Cantabria (Spain)." *Environmental Research*, 2005, *99*(3), 413–424.

Surís-Regueiro, J.C., Garza-Gil, M.D., and Varela-Lafuente, M.M. "The Prestige Oil Spill and Its Economic Impact on the Galician Fishing Sector." *Disasters*, 2007, *31*(2), 201–215.

Swanson, K.J., Madden, M.C., and Ghio, A.J.. "Biodiesel Exhaust: The Need for Health Effects Research." *Environmental Health Perspectives*, 2007, *115*(4), 496–499.

Thomson, J. *The Scot Who Lit the World, The Story of William Murdoch, Inventor of Gas Lighting*. Glasgow: Janet Thomson, 2003.

Tsai, S. P., and others. "Cancer Incidence Among Refinery and Petrochemical Employees in Louisiana, 1983–1999." *Annals of Epidemiology*, 2004, *14*(9), 722–730.

U.S. Department of Energy and U.S. Environmental Protection Agency. *Carbon Dioxide Emissions from the Generation of Electric Power in the United States*. Washington, D.C.: Department of Energy and Environmental Protection Agency, 2000.

Valentić, D., Stojanović, D., Mićović, V., and Vukelić, M. "Work Related Diseases and Injuries on an Oil Rig." *International Maritime Health*, 2005, *56*(1–4), 56–66.

Wilkinson, P., Smith, K., Joffe, M., and Haines, A. "A Global Perspective on Energy: Health Effects and Injustices." *Lancet*, 2007, *370*, 965–978.

Wolbarst, A. B., and others. "Sites in the United States Contaminated with Radioactivity." *Health Physics*, 1999, *77*(3), 247–260.

Wong, O., and others. "An Epidemiological Study of Petroleum Refinery Employees." *British Journal of Industrial Medicine*, 1986, *43*(1), 6–17.

Wong, O., and others. "Updated Mortality Study of Workers at a Petroleum Refinery in Torrance, California, 1959 to 1997." *Journal of Occupational & Environmental Medicine*, 2001, *43*(12), 1089–1102.

Woodcock, J., and others. "Energy and Transport." *Lancet*, 2007, *370*, 1078–1088.

Woods, R. *The Demography of Victorian England and Wales*. New York: Cambridge University Press, 2000.

World Resources Institute. *Energy and Resources: Data Tables*. http://earthtrends.wri.org/datatables/ index.php?theme=6, 2005.

Yilmaz, K., Inac, S., Dikici, H., and Reyhanli, A.C. "The Effects of a Coal Power Plant on the Environment and Wildlife in Southeastern Turkey." *Journal of Environmental Biology*, 2004, *25*(4), 423–429.

Yuan, C. S., and others. "A New Alternative Fuel for Reduction of Polycyclic Aromatic Hydrocarbon and Particulate Matter Emissions from Diesel Engines." *Journal of the Air & Waste Management Association*, 2007, *57*(4), 465–471.

Zhang, J. J., and Smith, K.R.. "Household Air Pollution from Coal and Biomass Fuels in China: Measurements, Health Impacts, and Interventions." *Environmental Health Perspectives*, 2007, *115*(6), 848–855.

FOR FURTHER INFORMATION

Books and Papers

Hirsch, R. L., Bezdek, R., and Wendling, R. *Peaking of World Oil Production: Impacts, Mitigation, & Risk Management*. DOE NETL. http://www.mnforsustain.org/oil_peaking_of_world_oil_ production_study_hirsch.htm, Feb. 2005. A source of additional information about peak petroleum and how the United States may fare during the transition to other energy sources.

The Lancet. This eminent medical journal ran an excellent series on energy and health in 2007. The series was introduced by a short article by Professor Andy Haines, called Energy and Health (*Lancet* 2007, 370, 922). The remaining papers in the series can easily be found through that article.

In addition, for an engaging treatise on food; embedded energy and food miles; and the intersection between health policy, energy policy, and food policy, see Pollan (2006), and for a cogent discussion of peak oil and energy at the turn of the twentieth century, see Goodstein (2004); both works are listed in the References.

Agencies and Organizations

The following Web sites of agencies and organizations provide useful information on energy, including production and consumption statistics, reports, and forecasts.

Energy Information Administration (EIA), http://www.eia.doe.gov.

International Energy Agency (IEA), http://www.iea.org.

World Resources Institute (WRI), http://www.wri.org.

CHAPTER FOURTEEN

HEALTHY COMMUNITIES

SARAH K. HEATON

JOHN M. BALBUS

JAMES W. KECK

ANDREW L. DANNENBERG

KEY CONCEPTS

- The design of neighborhoods, towns, and cities can affect people's health.

- Modern public health is historically tied to urban planning and land use policy.

- Land use and transportation decisions can either support or undermine routine physical activity, air quality, safety, social interaction, mental well-being, social equity, and other determinants of health.

- Smart Growth principles support sustainable community design and offer both environmental and human health benefits.

- Health impact assessment (HIA) is a tool that can assist decision makers in considering the potential impacts of proposed plans, projects, and policies on the health of populations.

- Emerging research and trends in both community development and public health are conducive to increasing collaboration between land use planners and public health professionals.

HEALTH AND THE BUILT ENVIRONMENT

In the fifth century B.C., Hippocrates offered this advice to the readers of his treatise "On Airs, Waters, and Places": "When one comes into a city to which he
is a stranger, he ought to consider its situation, how it lies as to the winds and
the rising of the sun; for its influence is not the same whether it lies to the north
or the south, to the rising or to the setting sun" (Hippocrates, n.d.). What did
Hippocrates mean when he warned his readers to consider a city's "situation"?
He was pointing out that to understand a community's health, the wise physician
must consider the environment in which its people live: the place, the city, the
town. He recognized that environment affects health.

Twenty-five hundred years later, Frederick Law Olmsted (1916) echoed this
idea in his advice to city planners: "We are learning how, in the complex organism of a city, anything we decide to do or leave undone may have important and
inevitable consequences wholly foreign to the motives immediately controlling
the decision but seriously affecting the welfare of the future city; and with our
recognition of this is growing a sense of social responsibility for estimating these
remoter consequences and giving them due weight in reaching every decision"
(p. 1). Manipulation of the urban environment, Olmsted recognized, could have
far-reaching, sometimes unexpected human impacts.

Buildings, streets, parks, plazas, and transportation systems all constitute the
built environment, which affects health through a variety of means: by making access to healthy food and jobs easier or harder, by facilitating or impeding
physical activity, by influencing air quality for better or worse, by promoting social
interaction or social isolation, and more. This chapter examines how features of
the built environment affect public health.

Community design poses different sets of issues in wealthy nations and in
developing nations. The rapid pace and chaotic nature of urbanization in developing nations—from São Paulo to Bangkok to Lagos—have a wide range of
health impacts, which are discussed in Chapter Eleven. This chapter focuses on
community design in wealthy nations, and particularly in the United States, with
special attention to the predominant pattern of the last half-century, sometimes
called **urban sprawl**.

Portions of this chapter are adapted from H. Frumkin, L. Frank, and R. Jackson, *Urban Sprawl
and Public Health: Designing, Planning, and Building for Healthy Communities* (Washington, D.C.: Island
Press, 2004), and H. Frumkin and A. L. Dannenberg, "Health and the Built Environment," in
L. Cohen, V. Chavez, and S. Chehimi (eds.), *Prevention Is Primary: Strategies for Community Well-Being*
(San Francisco: Jossey-Bass, 2007), pp. 257–286. In addition, Sarah K. Heaton, John M. Balbus,
James W. Keck, and Andrew L. Dannenberg declare no competing financial interests. John Balbus
reports previous employment with the Environmental Defense Fund, a nonprofit organization.

From Micro to Macro: Scale in the Built Environment

When we consider how community design affects people's health, we must consider the spectrum of scales within the built environment. A person's chair is a component of the built environment, on a very small (or micro) scale. Chair design can affect well-being; consider how a poorly designed chair can cause back pain. Ergonomic issues are discussed in Chapter Twenty. Building scale is also important, because people spend most of their time in buildings; this is discussed in Chapter Nineteen. This chapter looks more toward the macro end of the spectrum: the neighborhood, the town, the city, and the region.

Components of Community Design

Community design is an amalgam of many decisions, made by people in many different disciplines and professions. **Land use** refers to decisions about what functions—homes, factories, schools, stores, parks, and so on—are placed where. **Transportation** refers to systems for moving people and goods from place to place, including roads, sidewalks, bicycle paths, buses, subways, and rail lines. Land use and transportation are intimately connected. On the one hand, for example, homes that are located far from workplaces (a land use decision) boost **travel demand** because employees need to get to work (a transportation requirement). On the other hand, if schools are located within residential neighborhoods, then students can walk or bicycle to school, reducing the need for automobile and bus transportation. Community design also addresses **landscape architecture**, the design and management of such settings as streetscapes and public spaces; **land conservation**, efforts to preserve land in its natural state; **parks and recreation**; and **historic preservation**. Many other upstream forces—energy policy, economic development policy, housing policy, food policy, and environmental policy, to name a few—play a role in determining how communities are designed and built.

CITIES: THE BIRTHPLACE OF MODERN PUBLIC HEALTH

Early cities were established along trade routes or at points where the movement of goods shifted from one mode of transportation to another, such as at river and ocean ports. Early population hubs often developed around a central public plaza. The main form of travel was walking, so people needed to live near where they worked, traded, and prayed; compact, high-density settlement was the norm. The need to move goods and people locally led to the development of street networks for use by wagons and carriages.

Industrialization in the nineteenth century brought an influx of manufacturing jobs, and therefore people, into cities. Before long, crowded, squalid conditions and inadequate infrastructure facilitated the spread of diseases such as tuberculosis and typhoid. Later in the nineteenth century, a growing understanding of the spread of infectious diseases led public health professionals to intervene in **urban planning**, public infrastructure, and housing quality (Duffy, 1990; Melosi, 2000).

Accordingly, much of modern public health developed in cities. Public health professionals helped develop enforceable standards for potable water supplies, sewage systems, and waste management. The interplay between the built environment and health was a basis of the sanitary movement spearheaded by Edwin Chadwick and promoted by Charles Dickens in mid-nineteenth-century London (Litsios, 2003). An architect and an urban housing specialist were among the founding members of the American Public Health Association in 1873, further evidence of the historical relationship between public health and cities (Glasser, 2002).

Technological developments during the 1800s and 1900s enabled profound changes in urban form (Jackson, 1985). With the advent of electrification in the late nineteenth and early twentieth centuries, railroads and streetcars, could be extended into the surrounding countryside. Automobile ownership became widespread during the 1920s. Construction techniques changed as well; for example, the balloon frame house (dating to the 1830s) enabled rapid, inexpensive construction of large numbers of private homes. Houses outside the city went from being second homes for the wealthy to being permanent, residential alternatives to the gritty urban center for middle- and upper-class citizens who could now easily commute greater distances to their jobs in the urban core.

THE MODERN METROPOLIS: URBAN SPRAWL

The American Dream

For many, the American Dream has much to do with community design. In the years after World War II, for many Americans, this ideal consisted of a family, a house, a yard, a car in the garage, and a white picket fence. With a booming birthrate, home loan guarantee programs for veterans, the rise of the personal automobile, and the construction of the interstate highway system, a new form of development began to characterize much of the nation's landscape: *suburbanization*. This American Dream became a reality for tens of millions of people during the second half of the twentieth century.

Land use and transportation practices evolved rapidly. As farmland and forest at the urban edge were converted to residential use, standard housing densities declined to one or two households per acre, a departure from traditional city and town densities of five to ten or more per acre. **Land use mix** declined; instead of admixing residential, commercial, recreational, educational, and other uses, planners began separating distinct uses, often to comply with local zoning laws (Figure 14.1). As a result, long distances between destinations such as home, school, work, and the store became the norm. With longer trip distances, nonmotorized travel (walking and bicycling) became less practical. Mass transit could not

FIGURE 14.1   Schematic Comparison of Street Networks and Land Use in a Traditional Neighborhood and in an Area of Sprawl

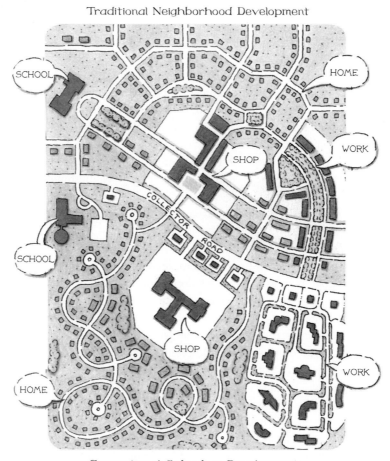

Source: Courtesy of Thomas E. Low, DPZ Charlotte.

The traditional town and city design in the upper panel features a gridlike arrangement of streets, high connectivity, placement of different land uses near each other, and high density. In the "loop and lollipop" arrangement of streets shown in the lower panel, different parcels of land are developed independently and not linked to each other, resulting in low connectivity, low density land use, and separation of different land uses.

be supported in low-density communities because too few people were clustered near trip origins and destinations to justify transit stations. Transportation planners estimate a housing density of at least twelve dwelling units per acre is needed to support rapid rail service and 7 units per acre to support local bus service every half hour (Booth, Leonard, and Pawlukiewicz, 2002).

Modern Community Design

The features of sprawling communities, reflecting both land use and transportation decisions, are familiar. Key features are described in the following paragraphs.

Separation of land uses through zoning. When planners make zoning decisions, they determine how specific parcels of land and areas within a community are used. Initially intended to protect people from harmful industrial exposures, zoning decisions now often separate communities from sources of employment and services and can encourage social isolation through the segregation of populations by age, family size, or income.

Low density development. Planners in the nineteenth-century city responded to disease epidemics associated with crowding by establishing limits on the number of residences and buildings per unit area. Limiting the **density** of development has become standard in suburban and rural land use planning, contributing to urban sprawl.

Dispersion of activity centers. In contrast to the compact downtown areas of traditional cities and towns, commercial and recreational activities in sprawling metropolitan areas are arrayed along long stretches of busy roads, in strip malls, big box stores, and office parks. Traditional gathering places such as parks, plazas, and sidewalks are often absent.

Automobile-oriented transportation systems. Sprawling metropolitan areas have extensive roadway systems. Multilane freeways, divided highways, vast parking lots, drive-through services for everything from food to weddings, and a relative absence of sidewalks and bicycle paths define a *mode share* (the distribution of different modes of travel) that emphasizes the automobile over other modes of transportation, such as walking or bicycling.

Disinvestment in central cities. A key feature of urban history during the second half of the twentieth century was the flight of middle- and upper-class people, investments, and economic opportunities from central cities. In many cities the result was large swaths of concentrated poverty, with high rates of unemployment, substandard housing, social breakdown, and poor health—so much so that in public health, the term *urban health* became synonymous with "the health of poor people." This pattern raises profound questions of equity and social justice (International City/County Management Association, 2005; Kennedy and Leonard, 2001).

PERSPECTIVE
Policies That Regulate Land Use

Development regulations are largely the domain of local governments. They range from local building codes to larger scale zoning and subdivision regulations. All types of development regulations can either help or hinder the development of healthy places depending on what is required, permitted, or prohibited. For example, a regulation that limits the number of alcohol outlets may enhance the quality of community life (Aboelata, 2004), whereas one that requires a minimum number of parking spaces may encourage local automobile use and reduce the walkability of a development.

Building codes prescribe the bulk, scale, massing, and style of structures. For example, codes that require uniform setbacks of buildings from streets, and retail space on the first floors of urban buildings, contribute to a pedestrian-friendly realm at the street level. (Smart Growth, an approach to better community design, is discussed later in this chapter.) Appropriate scaling of buildings, continuity of building materials, and a coherent design "vocabulary" all help establish a sense of place for a community, creating environments where people like to live, work, play, and travel.

Zoning codes prescribe certain locations as appropriate for specific uses, such as residential, commercial, industrial, recreational, or open space uses, and regulate such parameters as density, lot coverage, and building setbacks. Zoning began in the early 1900s to protect public health, safety, and welfare and to enforce social norms (Schilling and Linton, 2005). Although zoning has helped communities to separate incompatible land uses such as noxious industries and homes, it has not always delivered high-quality, livable environments. In fact, the attractive old neighborhoods of Charleston, Annapolis, and Georgetown would fail to meet the current zoning codes of many cities because of their narrow streets, mixed land uses, and other design features. Innovative zoning codes, such as the model codes developed by the American Planning Association (2006), can be used to promote smart growth and healthy community design.

Subdivision regulations operate on a larger scale than zoning, governing the layout and form of entire communities. When a large parcel of land is being developed, it is typically subdivided into smaller parcels. The process of subdividing, or *platting*, land and laying out streets, lots, and other land uses, is controlled by subdivision regulations. Subdivision regulations are particularly critical to community design, because they govern street network arrangements, open space placement, and connectivity both within the development and to adjacent developments.

Source: Adapted from Frumkin, Frank, and Jackson, 2004, pp. 207–209.

COMMUNITY DESIGN AND HEALTH

The design of neighborhoods, towns, cities, and transportation systems can have wide-ranging effects on health. These effects operate through the physical activity people get, the air they breathe, their risk of injuries, their access to healthy food, the noise they endure, and their contact with each other, which affects social capital and mental health. Each of these is discussed in the following sections.

Physical Activity and Obesity

There is growing evidence that land use and transportation practices of the last century have had major impacts on individuals' physical activity levels. In 2005, the Transportation Research Board (TRB) and the Institute of Medicine (IOM) examined this evidence in a special report, *Does the Built Environment Influence Physical Activity?* (TRB and IOM, 2005). Their answer was a qualified yes, but they concluded that more research is needed.

Sedentary lifestyles have become the norm in the United States. More than half of American adults are physically inactive on a regular basis, and over one-quarter of Americans report no regular leisure-time physical activity (Macera and others, 2003). A sedentary lifestyle increases the risk of cardiovascular disease, stroke, and all-cause mortality, whereas physical activity prolongs life (Lee and Paffenbarger, 2000; Wannamethee, Shaper, and Walker, 1998; Wannamethee, Shaper, Walker, and Ebrahim, 1998). Low physical fitness elevates cardiovascular risk as hypertension, high cholesterol, diabetes, and smoking do and to a similar degree (Blair and others, 1996; Wei and others, 1999). Physical activity appears to protect against cancers of the breast, colon, and other organs (Bauman, 2004; Kampert, Blair, Barlow, and Kohl, 1996; Lee, 2003).

Beyond its direct effects on health, physical inactivity is a risk factor for weight gain. Overweight and obesity are defined by **body mass index** (BMI), a measure calculated by dividing a person's weight (in kilograms) by height (in meters squared). A BMI between 25 and 30 indicates overweight and a BMI of 30 or more signals obesity. Overweight and obesity have rapidly become one of the most pressing and costly public health crises in the United States (Figure 14.2). In 1960, one in four American adults was overweight (Kuczmarski, Flegal, Campbell, and Johnson, 1994); in the 2003 and 2004 period that proportion had increased to two in three (Ogden and others, 2006). The prevalence of obesity has followed a similar trajectory, reaching one in three by 2003–2004 (Ogden and others, 2006). These trends have occurred in children as well as in adults and disproportionately in poor and minority communities. Obesity is a risk factor for overall mortality, cardiovascular mortality, diabetes, hypertension, depression, and gall bladder disease. An analysis of

FIGURE 14.2   Percentage of Obese Adults in the United States, by State, 2007

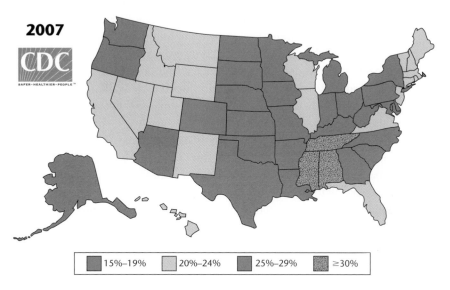

| 15%–19% | 20%–24% | 25%–29% | ≥30% |

Source: Centers for Disease Control and Prevention (CDC), 2008.

Percentage of adults who were obese by state.

overweight- and obesity-related medical costs found that 9.1 percent of health care dollars in the United States are spent on these largely preventable conditions (Finkelstein, Fiebelkorn, and Wang, 2003). Unforeseen societal costs of rising obesity have ranged from increased fuel costs for airlines as the average weight of their passengers has increased (Dannenberg, Burton, and Jackson, 2004) to a need for larger beds in hospitals (Rundle, 2002) and increased load capacity for consumer automobiles (Woodyard, 2007).

Design for Physical Activity   Land use mix, density, and design play a significant role in physical activity levels in communities (Cervero and Kockelman, 1997), and a greater mix of land uses in an area is associated with more physical activity (TRB and IOM, 2005). Co-location of different land uses (for example, residential, offices, retail, and schools) brings destinations closer, and enables people to travel from place to place on foot or bicycle. Just as important, this physical activity becomes a part of the daily routine, in contrast to recreational physical activity, and thus more sustainable over the long term.

Higher density development is also associated with increased walking and bicycling (TRB and IOM, 2005). Many modern employment centers, schools, and shopping malls are located in low-density exurban enclaves, far from urban centers or residential subdivisions. Such locations are accessible primarily by automobile rather than by walking, bicycling or using public transit.

Certain features of street design, such as a highly connected grid or network of streets and the presence of sidewalks or paths, are associated with increased physical activity through walking and bicycling (TRB and IOM, 2005). Rather than the gridlike street network, many suburban neighborhoods feature low connectivity, with design features such as cul-de-sacs and long block lengths. By increasing trip distances these features discourage walking and bicycling. Urban planners typically use a quarter- or a half-mile as the longest distance people are willing to walk to a destination.

Other community design features such as shade, scenery, and safety are also associated with increased walking trips (TRB and IOM, 2005). In addition, perceptions of neighborhood safety and crime affect decisions about outdoor activity, including walking (Frank and Engelke, 2000). High local temperatures and poor air quality also discourage outdoor physical activity (see Chapter Twelve).

Parks and Green Space   Public parks provide places in which people can be physically active, enjoy contact with nature (see Chapter Twenty-Four) and with other people, and relax (Cohen and others, 2007). Parks add substantially to the quality of life of a city's residents. Many great city parks, such as New York's Central Park or San Francisco's Golden Gate Park, were designed and built early in those cities' growth, while large tracts of land was still available. Other, often smaller, parks have been added to cities during urban redevelopment efforts, to make these cities more attractive and livable. A commonly used benchmark for city planners recommends 10 acres of parkland per 1,000 individuals (Cohen and others, 2007). People use parks more when the parks are conveniently located, especially within safe walking distance of their homes. Although there is no established standard, urban planners try to create a mix of accessible, small, local parks, distributed throughout a city, and a few larger parks with space for a wider range of recreational facilities, such as ball fields and longer walking and biking trails.

Air Quality

For thousands of years humans have recognized that air quality affects health. In the essay cited at the beginning of this chapter, Hippocrates noted that air quality varies from place to place, with implications for health. In modern times, patterns of urbanization and transportation—features of community design—have emerged as primary determinants of both local and global air pollution.

Air pollutants from the transportation sector fall into three broad categories: greenhouse gases (primarily carbon dioxide) that contribute to climate change (see Chapter Ten), criteria air pollutants (particulate matter, ozone, oxides of nitrogen and sulfur, carbon monoxide, and lead) and air toxics (more than 100 types of hazardous air pollutants) (see Chapter Twelve). The transportation sector accounts for about 29 percent of greenhouse gas emissions (U.S. Environmental Protection Agency [EPA], Office of Transportation and Air Quality, 2006).

Human exposures to air pollution can increase the risk of premature death, asthma, cardiovascular disease, cancer, and other conditions, as described in Chapter Twelve. The risk varies with duration of exposure and proximity to pollution sources. Pollution from cars and trucks is most marked near transportation corridors with high traffic density, leading to **pollution hot spots**, or small areas with particularly high air pollution levels. Accordingly, people at higher risk include those living, working, or attending school within 150 meters of a busy road (Venn and others, 2001; Schikowski and others, 2005; Kim and others, 2008). The association between traffic-related air pollution and childhood asthma is particularly well documented and may account for some of the dramatic increase in asthma over the last two decades (Delfino and others, 2008; McConnell and others, 2006; Brauer and others, 2002). Transportation-related air toxics and diesel particulates appear to contribute to the development of lung cancer among people who live near roadways, increasing their risk up to 40 percent (Nyberg and others, 2000; Vineis and others, 2006). Exposure to traffic-related air pollutants is also associated with premature mortality, particularly from cardiovascular causes (Hoek and others, 2002; Finkelstein, Jerrett, and Sears, 2004; Maynard, Coull, Gryparis, and Schwartz, 2007). Many of these hot spots are in low-income neighborhoods that also face other environmental and social threats to health (see Chapter Eight).

In cities the evolution of larger roads and escalating levels of traffic, secondary to regional land use patterns, explains why the roadways themselves seem to represent the source of air pollutants. California first officially recognized this issue in the 1950s by instigating motor vehicle emission regulations. Technological advances since then have reduced vehicle pollutant emissions by over 90 percent per mile driven, although increasing **vehicle miles traveled** (VMT) have partially offset these gains (U.S. Department of Transportation [USDOT], 2002). Reducing VMT in single-occupancy vehicles is a primary way to reduce air pollution and the resulting health consequences in both the local and global environments. This underscores the need for alternative modes of dependable and safe transportation as a goal for community design and **transportation planning**.

Injury Risk

Community design has considerable influence on the risk of injuries, especially those related to transportation. Since the first recorded motor vehicle collision in 1896 in New York City (USDOT, 2007), motor vehicle crashes and fatalities increased, peaking in the 1970s and 1980s. They are a major contributor to the toll of unintentional injuries, which represent one of the top five causes of premature mortality in the United States (Foege, 2006). Public health approaches to reducing fatal and nonfatal motor vehicle injuries, such as interventions in vehicle design, driver behavior, and the environment, have grown in effectiveness, helping to reduce motor vehicle fatality rates by 75 percent over the last forty years (USDOT, 2008a).

Motor Vehicle Injuries   The burden of fatal and nonfatal injuries from motor vehicle crashes is enormous. In 2007 in the United States, 41,059 people were killed and another 2,491,000 were injured in motor vehicle crashes. Motor vehicle collisions continue to be a leading cause of death in children and young adults three through thirty-four years of age (USDOT, 2008b). Drivers, passengers, pedestrians, or bicyclists can be killed or injured in motor vehicle collisions. Even though fatalities have decreased per mile traveled, traffic fatalities have remained level over the last twenty years because the exposure, measured by total VMT, continues to grow. American vehicles traveled 3 trillion miles in 2007 (USDOT, 2008a).

The form of the built environment plays a considerable role in the number and severity of motor vehicle collisions. The sprawling communities that characterize American cities encourage automobile use and higher speed roadways. States with lower population densities experience higher rates of traffic fatalities per VMT (Clark and Cushing, 2004), as do communities with greater urban sprawl, likely due to the higher "exposure" to vehicle miles traveled in these communities (Ewing, Schieber, and Zegeer, 2003). One approach to prevention, therefore, would be decreasing travel demand.

Another approach to prevention focuses on the design of roadways. Interstate highways incorporate design features such as limited access interchanges and center medians that give them a relatively low rate of fatalities per VMT. Local roadway design uses traffic-calming techniques such as roundabouts, one-way streets, and speed bumps to alter driver behavior and reduce crash likelihood and severity. On average these measures reduce traffic crashes by 15 percent and related injuries by 11 percent (Bunn and others, 2003; Elvik, 2001). Modern roundabouts reduce injury crashes at intersections by 76 percent and fatal or incapacitating crashes by 90 percent (Retting, Persaud, Garder, and Lord, 2001).

Pedestrian and Bicyclist Injuries   More than 10 percent of those killed in motor vehicle crashes are pedestrians (USDOT, 2008a), and bicyclists account for roughly 2 percent of fatal and nonfatal motor vehicle crash injuries (USDOT, 2008c). Fatal and nonfatal pedestrian injury rates per unit of population have declined steadily over the past thirty years, but this is due at least in part to reduced rates of walking (Surface Transportation Policy Project [STPP], 2004)—a Pyrrhic victory in a society suffering from sedentary lifestyles and the associated health consequences. Community design can influence both how much people walk and their risk of pedestrian injury. When pedestrian fatality rates are compared across cities, after adjusting for walking rates, a pattern emerges: sprawling cities such as Orlando, Houston, and Phoenix, which have lower walking rates and less pedestrian infrastructure, have the highest pedestrian fatality rates. Older cities with higher walking rates and more compact designs, such as New York and Boston, have far lower pedestrian fatality rates (Ewing and others, 2003; STPP, 2004). Cross-national comparisons reveal the same pattern: in nations such as Holland and Germany, where walking and bicycling are far more common than in the United States, pedestrian and bicyclist injury rates are far lower. This finding is attributed to design decisions in Europe that have resulted in, for example, improved pedestrian and bicyclist infrastructure and traffic calming in residential neighborhoods (Pucher and Dijkstra, 2003).

Pedestrian-friendly street designs that include crosswalks and sidewalks reduce injury risk. Forty percent of fatalities occur in locations with no crosswalks. Risk factors for bicyclist fatalities are also well characterized; they are more likely in nonintersection locations, in urban areas, and between the hours of 6 and 9 P.M. (USDOT, 2008c).

Walking and bicycling are known as **active transportation** because they entail physical exertion; for this reason, promoting these forms of travel is a public health goal. Healthy community design both facilitates these forms of travel, and reduces the associated risk of injuries. At present, building and improving infrastructure for pedestrians and bicyclists appears to be a low priority in U.S. transportation policy. Although pedestrians account for over 10 percent of roadway fatalities and 9 percent of all trips made, pedestrian infrastructure receives less than 1 percent of federal transportation spending (STPP, 2004; USDOT, 2008c).

The concept of **complete streets** addresses this issue with a focus on multimodal accessibility and safety for all users, including pedestrians and bicyclists (McCann, 2005). Salt Lake City, for example, has implemented several measures consistent with complete streets principles, and pedestrian fatalities have decreased by more than 40 percent since 2001 (STTP, 2004). Research also shows that increasing the number of pedestrians and bicyclists can contribute to safety, possibly because drivers become more aware of and more careful around pedestrians and bicyclists as their numbers increase. Doubling the number of pedestrians and bicyclists appears to reduce an individual's risk of being struck by a car or truck by approximately 66 percent (Jacobsen, 2003).

Healthy Food

Healthy eating is a central strategy in reducing obesity and chronic diseases. However, changes in diet require access to healthy foods in addition to education and motivation. The retail food environment, both at the community level (for example, the presence and location of food stores or retail outlets) and at the consumer level (for example, the availability of healthful, affordable foods at these locations) affects dietary choices (Glanz, Sallis, Saelens, and Frank, 2005) (Figure 14.3). Low-income and predominately minority communities often have limited access to grocery and retail stores that sell high-quality fruits and vegetables (Zenk and others, 2006; Powell and others, 2007; Horowitz, Colson, Hebert, and Lancaster, 2004), and they have a disproportionate number of unhealthful fast-food outlets (Block, Scribner, and DeSalvo, 2004).

FIGURE 14.3   Access to Healthy Food Options

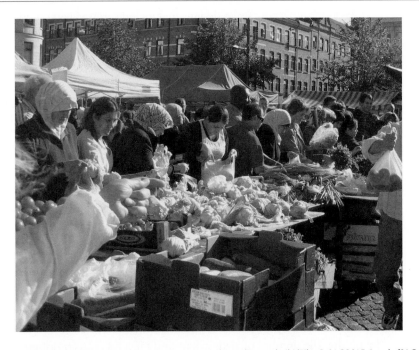

Source: Wikimedia Commons, http://commons.wikimedia.org/wiki/File:Gr%C3%B6nsaksf%C3%B6rs%C3%A4ljning,_M%C3%B6llev%C3%A5ngstorget,_Malm%C3%B6.jpg. Permission granted under the terms of the GNU Free Documentation License, Version 1.2 or any later version published by the Free Software Foundation.

Zoning, transportation decisions, public infrastructure development, and other land use decisions may encourage or discourage development of a healthy food environment and therefore have an impact on health outcomes in affected communities. Examples of strategies to improve the food environment include providing incentives for grocery store and supermarket development, restricting fast-food retail store density (Mair, Pierce, and Teret, 2005), and encouraging community-supported agricultural programs, farmers markets, street carts with fruit and vegetables, and community gardens. Land use policy and environmental changes are emerging as important and potentially modifiable loci for public health interventions to improve the food environment (Story, Kaphingst, Robinson-O'Brien, and Glanz, 2008).

Noise

City dwellers have long been forced to tolerate unwanted noise from neighbors, industrial and commercial activities, vehicles, and aircraft. Noise exposure contributes to hearing loss, increased blood pressure, heart disease, changes in hormonal levels, and circulatory problems (Passchier-Vermeer and Passchier, 2000). Noise-induced hearing loss begins to occur with prolonged exposure to noise levels over 70 decibels (dB) (World Health Organization, n.d.). Although few communities face these levels of exposure, residents and workers in close proximity to urban traffic experience varying degrees of hearing loss (Barbosa and Cardoso, 2005; Leong and Laortanakul, 2003).

Evidence also supports a relationship between transportation-related noise exposure and cardiovascular health effects, from hypertension to myocardial infarction (Spreng, 2000). Studies have shown a dose-response relationship between road traffic noise above a threshold of 60 dB and myocardial infarctions (Babisch, 2008) and consistent associations between aircraft noise and hypertension are also seen (Babisch, 2006; Jarup and others, 2008). Noise exposure has been associated with adverse psychological, performance, and sleep impacts as well (Jakovljević, Belojević, Paunović, and Stojanov, 2006; Stansfeld and Matheson, 2003). Schoolchildren exposed to aircraft noise exhibited poorer reading comprehension, decreased recognition memory, and heightened annoyance (Matheson, Stansfeld, and Haines, 2003; Stansfeld and others, 2005). Students near airports achieved higher average standardized test scores and lower test failure rates after abrupt noise reduction (Federal Interagency Committee on Aviation Noise, 2007).

There are several ways to reduce community exposure to transportation noise: reduce the amount of noise produced per vehicle; reduce the number or speed, or both, of vehicles driving past communities; construct sound barriers around large highways and other major noise sources; and route new or expanded highways through less densely populated areas (Federal Highway Administration, 2006). Aircraft noise in surrounding communities can similarly be reduced by changes in runway use or flight path location, compatible land use zoning, and sound insulation of buildings (Federal Aviation Administration, 1999). Efforts at aircraft noise reduction since 1970 have reduced the number of people exposed to excessive aircraft noise (>65 dB day-night weighted average) from 7 million in 1975 to 500,000 in 2006, while air traffic increased twofold (U.S. Congress, House of Representatives, Subcommittee on Aviation, 2007).

Social Capital

Social capital refers to the social networks and resources within a community and also the norms of reciprocity and social benefit that arise from them. The strength of these resources and networks reflects the level of community involvement in such local organizations as community centers, churches, and locally focused philanthropic organizations and also the existence of support systems that ensure disadvantaged community members have access to food, shelter, and health care (Campbell, 2006; Minkler and Wallerstein, 2005). Social capital is associated with a wide range of health benefits, and indicators of low social capital, such as social isolation and income inequality, are associated with higher mortality (Kawachi, Kennedy, Lochner, and Prothrow-Stith, 1997; Kawachi, 1999; Lynch, Smith, Kaplan, and House, 2000; House, Landis, and Umberson, 1988).

Community design may affect social capital in several ways. Long commute times may reduce social capital, perhaps by reducing the time or the will to become involved in social activities (Besser, Marcus, and Frumkin, 2008). According to Robert Putnam (2000), "each 10 additional minutes in daily commuting time cuts involvement in community affairs by 10 percent." Another feature of community design relevant to social capital is the presence of "great good places"—the "cafés, coffee shops, bookstores, bars, hair salons, and other hangouts at the heart of a community" where people gather to socialize (Oldenburg, 1989). Communities with an ample stock of such places may provide more opportunities for social interchange. A third feature of community design that may affect social capital is the mix of housing types. Neighborhoods suitable for young families may not include housing suitable for "empty nesters" or for elders who can no longer drive. Without such options, people are obliged to move from their communities as they age, which deprives them of the opportunity for "aging in place" and disrupts community networks formed over many years (Fried, Freedman, Endres, and Wasik, 1997; Alley and others, 2007). This realization has given rise to a field called *environmental gerontology*, reflecting the recognition that community design has a great impact on the well-being of elders (Wahl and Weisman, 2003).

Mental Health

Mental health can be affected by a variety of factors in the social, natural, and built environments, some of them related to community design (Halpern, 1995; Evans, 2003). Several examples are illustrative. First, as noted earlier, noise from roadways and other sources can be a long-term stressor for nearby neighborhoods, contributing to sleeplessness, anxiety, and other mental health disorders. Second, it has been suggested that sprawling suburbs can be isolating and may contribute to depression (Kunstler, 1993). Third, automobile commuting in heavy traffic has been linked to increased blood pressure, back pain, cardiovascular disease, and self-reported stress (Koslowsky, Kluger, and Reich, 1995; Novaco, Stokols, Campbell, and Stokols, 1979. Stokols, Novaco, Stokols, and Campbell, 1978). Fourth, aggressive driving and the impulsive behavior known as *road rage* may be associated with the stresses of long commutes on crowded roads (Joint, 1997; Rathbone and Huckabee, 1999). Fifth, and on a more positive note, parks and green space can provide opportunities for relaxation, attention restoration, and reduced stress, as discussed in Chapter Twenty-Four. These examples illustrate the many aspects of community design that may promote or threaten mental health, and the many pathways through which they may operate.

DESIGN FOR HEALTHY COMMUNITIES

In a landmark 1926 decision (*Village of Euclid* v. *Ambler Realty*), the U.S. Supreme Court upheld local governments' authority to regulate land use through zoning, citing the protection of public health as part of the justification for this ruling. In recent years urban planners, transportation engineers, and related professionals have rediscovered their professional links to public health, and public health professionals have rediscovered the importance of community design in promoting health (Hoehner and others, 2003; Corburn, 2004; Malizia, 2006; Kochtitzky and others, 2006). From these efforts have arisen many insights into the unintended health consequences of contemporary land use and transportation decisions, and many strategies for promoting health through community design.

Many of these strategies are found in an approach known as **smart growth**. The nonprofit Smart Growth Network (SGN) is made up of environmental, historic preservation, and real estate groups; developers; and Federal, state and local government entities. The Smart Growth Principles (Exhibit 14.1) established

EXHIBIT 14.1
Smart Growth Principles

- *Mix land uses.* Smart growth supports the integration of mixed land uses into communities as a critical component of achieving better places to live.
- *Create walkable neighborhoods.* Walkable communities are desirable places to live, work, learn, worship and play, and therefore a key component of smart growth.
- *Provide a variety of transportation choices.* Providing people with more choices in housing, shopping, communities, and transportation is a key aim of smart growth.
- *Preserve open space, farmland, natural beauty, and critical environmental areas.* Open space preservation supports smart growth goals by bolstering local economies, preserving critical environmental areas, improving our communities' quality of life, and guiding new growth into existing communities.
- *Create range of housing opportunities and choices.* Providing quality housing for people of all income levels is an integral component in any smart growth strategy.
- *Foster distinctive, attractive communities with a strong sense of place.* Smart growth encourages communities to craft a vision and set standards for development and construction which respond to community values of architectural beauty and distinctiveness, as well as expanded choices in housing and transportation.
- *Encourage community and stakeholder collaboration.* Growth can create great places to live, work and play—if it responds to a community's own sense of how and where it wants to grow.
- *Strengthen and direct development toward existing communities.* Smart growth directs development towards existing communities already served by infrastructure, seeking to utilize the resources that existing neighborhoods offer, and conserve open space and irreplaceable natural resources on the urban fringe.
- *Take advantage of compact building design.* Smart growth provides a means for communities to incorporate more compact building design as an alternative to conventional, land consumptive development.
- *Make development decisions predictable, fair, and cost effective.* For a community to be successful in implementing smart growth, it must be embraced by the private sector.

Source: Smart Growth Network, 2009.

by the SGN did not arise primarily as a public health strategy; proponents cited economic, environmental, and aesthetic benefits. The fortunate fact that health also improves is an example of a **co-benefit**. Features of smart growth include higher density than is typical in most suburban development; mixed land use; co-location of diverse housing types; transportation choices that balance automobile use with walking, bicycling, and public transit (including good pedestrian infrastructure and a high degree of connectivity between places); activity centers such as traditional downtown areas; and an emphasis on parks, green space, and public spaces (Geller, 2003). Smart growth typically incorporates strategies familiar to public health as well. For example, it can emphasize community and stakeholder involvement in planning, and it can focus on **universal design** (Exhibit 14.2) to ensure access to community facilities regardless of ability (Center for Universal Design, 1997). Smart growth principles are implemented through a combination of market forces, social marketing, and deliberate policymaking, often with the active participation of public health professionals (Perdue, Stone, and Gostin, 2003; Bragg, Galloway, Spohn, and Trotter, 2003; De Ville and Sparrow, 2008).

Other terms overlap to some extent with smart growth. **New urbanism** is an architectural and planning movement whose principles similarly include walkable neighborhoods, a range of housing choices, mixed land uses, participatory planning, and revitalization of urban neighborhoods (http://www.cnu .org). A **traditional neighborhood development** (TND) is a compact, mixed-use, transit-oriented, pedestrian-friendly community of the sort common before World War II. A **transit-oriented development** (TOD) follows similar principles while creating easy access to public transit. A **brownfield redevelopment** often incorporates a mixed-use, walkable community while focusing on cleaning up and reusing a contaminated urban area fallen into decay (http://www.epa.gov/brownfields).

The elements of smart growth are mutually reinforcing. For example, land use strategies such as more compact development and mixed use create the density needed to make mass transit economically feasible. Selecting sites for schools near children's homes and providing safe walking routes to such schools encourages child physical activity, reduces automobile trips, and offers benefits for the larger community (EPA, 2003; Boarnet and others, 2005; Watson and Dannenberg, 2008). Infrastructure investments in sidewalks and bicycle paths, combined with policy initiatives such as bicycle parking and showers at workplaces and more costly automobile parking, can lead to changes in travel behavior. For example, Portland, Oregon, experienced a dramatic increase

EXHIBIT 14.2
Principles of Universal Design

Universal design: The design of products and environments to be usable by all people, to the greatest extent possible, without the need for adaptation or specialized design.

1. *Equitable use.* The design is useful and marketable to people with diverse abilities.
2. *Flexibility in use.* The design accommodates a wide range of individual preferences and abilities.
3. *Simple and intuitive use.* Use of the design is easy to understand, regardless of the user's experience, knowledge, language skills, or current concentration level.
4. *Perceptible information.* The design communicates necessary information effectively to the user, regardless of ambient conditions or the user's sensory abilities.
5. *Tolerance for error.* The design minimizes hazards and the adverse consequences of accidental or unintended actions.
6. *Low physical effort.* The design can be used efficiently and comfortably and with a minimum of fatigue.
7. *Size and space for approach and use.* Appropriate size and space are provided for approach, reach, manipulation, and use regardless of user's body size, posture, or mobility.

Source: Center for Universal Design, 1997.

in bicycle usage by expanding its bicycle infrastructure (Figure 14.4). Other solutions that reduce congestion are collectively known as **transportation demand management** (TDM). These measures include transit, employer, and ride-sharing incentives; special highway lanes for high occupancy vehicles; car insurance rates based on number of miles driven per year; increased charges for or reduced availability of parking spaces; and promotion of telecommuting.

A number of tools are available to facilitate community designs that incorporate Smart Growth Principles and health-promoting attributes. Created by the U.S. Green Building Council, LEED for Neighborhood Development (LEED-ND) is a set of prerequisites and credits based on energy efficiency, sustainability,

FIGURE 14.4   Go by Cycle in Portland, Oregon

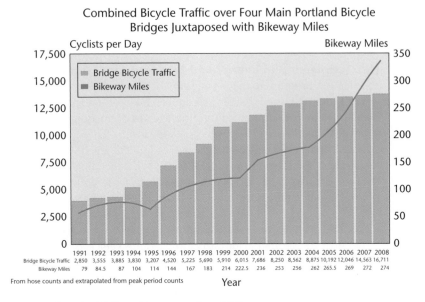

Combined Bicycle Traffic over Four Main Portland Bicycle
Bridges Juxtaposed with Bikeway Miles

Year	1991	1992	1993	1994	1995	1996	1997	1998	1999	2000	2001	2002	2003	2004	2005	2006	2007	2008
Bridge Bicycle Traffic	2,850	3,555	3,885	3,830	3,207	4,520	5,225	5,690	5,910	6,015	7,686	8,250	8,562	8,875	10,192	12,046	14,563	16,711
Bikeway Miles	79	84.5	87	104	114	144	167	183	214	222.5	236	253	256	262	265.5	269	272	274

From hose counts and extrapolated from peak period counts

Source: City of Portland Office of Transportation, 2008.

Between 1991 and 2008, the City of Portland increased its established bikeways from 79 to 274 miles, and otherwise improved bicycle-related infrastructure. The number of daily bicycle trips across Portland's four main bridges increased from 2850 trips in 1991 to 16,711 trips in 2008, and the bicycle mode-share as a percentage of all vehicles on those bridges increased from 2 percent in 1991 to 13 percent in 2008. There was no increase in the number of automobiles traveling over these bridges during this time, despite a 40 percent increase in the Portland metropolitan population since 1990.

and health promotion characteristics (Exhibit 14.3). **Health impact assessment** is a tool that can be used by public health professionals and others to examine the health consequences of a proposed project or policy prospectively and then yield recommendations that promote the positive health impacts and mitigate the adverse health consequences of the proposal (Exhibit 14.4). Many public health organizations, such as the National Association of County and City Health Officials (NACCHO), National Association of Local Boards of Health (NALBOH), and National Environmental Health Association (NEHA), provide guidance to their members on incorporating health into community planning. (Some of these resources are shown in the For Further Information section at the end of this chapter.)

EXHIBIT 14.3
LEED for Neighborhood Development Certification Program

LEED (**Leadership in Energy and Environmental Design**) is a third-party certification program managed by the U.S. Green Building Council (USGBC). Under the LEED system, building designers, builders, owners, and operators can benchmark their performance through a series of measurable indicators in five areas: sustainable site development, water savings, energy efficiency, materials selection, and indoor environmental quality. In 2008, the USGBC introduced LEED for Neighborhood Development (LEED-ND), in collaboration with the Congress for the New Urbanism and the Natural Resources Defense Council.

The current version of LEED-ND includes 13 prerequisites. For example:

- *Smart location.* Encourages development within and near existing communities or public transportation infrastructure. Reduces vehicle trips and miles traveled and supports walking as a transportation choice.
- *Compact development.* Conserves land, promotes livability, walkability and transportation efficiency, including reduced vehicle miles traveled.
- *Minimum building energy efficiency.* Encourages the design and construction of energy efficient buildings to reduce air, water, and land pollution and environmental impacts from energy production and consumption.

The current version of LEED-ND offers up to 110 credits; the number of credits determines the level of LEED-ND certification achieved (silver, gold, or platinum). Credits are given for design features such as these:

- *Neighborhood schools.* Promotes community interaction and engagement and reduced risk of chronic diseases by encouraging daily physical activity associated with alternative modes of transportation, such as walking or biking.
- *Bicycle networks.* Encourages use of bicycles for transportation and decreased automobile dependency, thereby encouraging regular physical activity and reduced risk of chronic diseases.
- *Mixed-income diverse communities.* Promotes socially equitable and socially engaging communities by enabling citizens from a wide range of economic levels, household sizes, and age groups to live within a community.
- *Access to public spaces.* Provides a variety of open spaces close to home and work to encourage walking and other physical activities and time spent outdoors.

Source: U.S. Green Building Council, 2008.

SUSTAINABLE DEVELOPMENT AND HUMAN HEALTH

"Treat the earth well. It was not given to you by your parents. It was loaned to you by your children."

—Kenyan proverb

The World Commission on Environment and Development (1987) defined *sustainability* as "meeting the needs of the present without compromising the ability of future generations to meet their own needs." **Sustainable development** initiatives are emerging as cities and nations contend with the impacts of depleting natural resources, surging populations, and global climate change. Sustainability programs focus on community-planning and land use actions that support long-term environmental, social, and economic vitality in communities (ICLEI—Local Governments for Sustainability, 2008). Key targets for sustainable development approaches are air quality, energy efficiency, water resources management, waste stream management, and increased active transportation (walking and bicycling). Sustainable development practices offer co-benefits for improved natural environments and for human health promotion and protection. Like other principles for development, sustainable development initiatives must be designed to be appropriate for specific localities.

Organizations such as ICLEI–Local Governments for Sustainability are creating tools and measures to increase the capacity of cities to implement sustainable development practices. One such project is the STAR Community Index project, now under development in the United States, which will offer cities around the country a standardized rating system to verify and promote local sustainability policies and practices (ICLEI USA–Local Governments for Sustainability, 2008). Other organizations and programs, such as UN-Habitat and the Sustainable Cities Network, are also working with cities around the globe to facilitate sustainable development through such means as infrastructure development and technical assistance. (See the For Further Information section at end of this chapter for more sustainable development resources.)

Consistent with the sustainable development approach, the **Healthy Cities** program, begun by the World Health Organization (WHO) in 1986, was the first widespread, community-level application of an ecological health promotion model that highlights the links between people's behavior and their environment (Flynn, 1996). The 11 initial European cities now anchor a global movement that numbers over 4,000 cities (de Leeuw, 2001). Healthy Cities has also inspired the creation of WHO's Healthy Settings program, which brings health promotion not only to cities but also to villages, workplaces, universities, marketplaces, and prisons, among other places. Healthy Cities uses a set of guiding principles (WHO,

EXHIBIT 14.4
Health Impact Assessment: A Tool for Land Use and Transportation Decision Making

Health impact assessment (HIA) is a tool that focuses on the health consequences of decisions in nonhealth sectors, including community design (CDC, n.d.). An HIA can be used to evaluate the potential health effects of a project or policy *before* it is built or implemented. It can provide recommendations to increase positive and minimize adverse health outcomes. A major benefit of the HIA process is that it brings public health issues to the attention of people who make decisions in areas such as transportation or land use, that is, areas outside the traditional public health concerns. An HIA is defined as "a combination of procedures, methods, and tools by which a policy, program, or project may be judged as to its potential effects on the health of a population and the distribution of those effects within the population" (European Centre for Health Policy, 1999). For example, if planners are considering whether to invest in a highway-widening project, bicycle trail network, or a trolley system, the local health department might carry out an HIA to clarify the health consequences of each option.

The major steps in conducting an HIA include

- *Screening*. Identify proposed projects or policies for which an HIA would be useful.
- *Scoping*. Identify which health effects to consider.

Regional Office for Europe, 1997) that have a focus on the creation of healthy communities and individuals as a central goal.

SUMMARY

For the last two or three generations, cities and towns in the United States and in other wealthy nations have evolved in a historically unprecedented way featuring geographic expansion over large areas, low-density development, separation of different land uses, low connectivity among places, and heavy reliance on the automobile for travel. This pattern is sometimes referred to as urban sprawl. In recent years the health consequences of urban sprawl have become better understood. They include reduced opportunities for routine physical activity; increased air pollution, from large amounts of traffic, with effects on cardiovascular and respiratory health; and greater injury risks. In contrast, some forms of community design promote health and environmental sustainability. Some of the health-promoting features of

- *Assessing risks and benefits.* Identify which people may be affected and how they may be affected.
- *Developing recommendations.* Suggest changes to proposal to promote positive or mitigate adverse health effects.
- *Reporting.* Present the results to decision makers.
- *Evaluating and monitoring.* Determine the affect of the HIA on the decision process.

HIAs are similar in some ways to environmental impact assessments (EIAs), which are mandated analyses of environmental outcomes such as air and water quality. EIAs can incorporate health impacts under existing laws but seldom do (Bhatia and Wernham, 2008). Unlike EIAs, HIAs can be voluntary or regulatory processes that focus on health outcomes such as obesity, physical inactivity, asthma, injuries, and social equity. An HIA encompasses a wide array of qualitative and quantitative methods and tools. HIAs can be completed in a few days or may take many months, depending on availability of time and resources.

Numerous HIAs have been performed in Europe, Canada, and elsewhere. Some countries have mandated HIAs as part of a regulatory process; others have used them on a voluntary basis. In the United States, interest in the topic is growing, with HIA work being performed by the University of California, Los Angeles, San Francisco Department of Public Health, Centers for Disease Control and Prevention, and other agencies and organizations (Dannenberg and others, 2008).

such communities are a balance of transportation options including a walking and bicycling infrastructure and mass transit, ample parks and green space, mixed land use, and increased density. Those who design and build communities—urban planners, transportation engineers, and others—are increasingly working with health professionals to achieve healthy, safe communities.

KEY TERMS

active transportation

body mass index

brownfield redevelopment

building codes

built environment

co-benefit

complete streets

density

health impact assessment

Healthy Cities

historic preservation

land conservation

land use

land use mix

landscape architecture

leadership in energy and environmental design for neighborhood development (LEED-ND) new urbanism

parks and recreation

pollution hot spots

smart growth

social capital

subdivision regulations

suburbanization

sustainable development

traditional neighborhood
    development

transit-oriented
    development

transportation

transportation demand
    management

transportation planning

travel demand

universal design

urban planning

urban sprawl

vehicle miles traveled
    (VMT)

zoning codes

DISCUSSION QUESTIONS

1. When and why did public health initially become involved with urban planning?

2. What kind of roles could a public health professional undertake if hired to work in a city planning or transportation department? What kind of roles could an urban planner or a transportation planner undertake if hired to work in a local or state health department?

3. Given unlimited resources, what interventions would you implement to improve the health of urban populations in wealthy countries? In less wealthy countries?

4. You have been asked to perform a health impact assessment for a highway expansion project. What information about the community and about the project would you request? What kinds of recommendations might you consider to mitigate the adverse impacts and promote the healthy aspects of the proposed project?

5. Consider this statement: *transportation policy is health policy*. Do you agree or disagree? Justify your answer.

6. You have been asked by local officials to increase the number of children who walk to school in your community. How would you undertake this project?

REFERENCES

Aboelata, M. *The Built Environment and Health: 11 Profiles of Neighborhood Transformation.* Prevention Institute. http://www.preventioninstitute.org/pdf/BE_South_Los_Angeles_CA.pdf, 2004.

Alley, D., and others. "Creating Elder-Friendly Communities: Preparations for an Aging Society." *Journal of Gerontological Social Work,* 2007, *49,* 1–18.

American Planning Association. *Smart Growth Codes*. http://www.planning.org/research/smartgrowth, 2006.

Babisch, W. "Transportation Noise and Cardiovascular Risk: Updated Review and Synthesis of Epidemiological Studies Indicate That the Evidence Has Increased." *Noise & Health*, 2006, *8*(30), 1–29.

Babisch, W. "Road Traffic Noise and Cardiovascular Risk." *Noise & Health*, 2008, *10*(38), 27–33.

Barbosa, A.S.M., and Cardoso, M.R.A. "Hearing Loss Among Workers Exposed to Road Traffic Noise in the City of São Paulo in Brazil." *Auris, Nasus, Larynx*, 2005, *32*, 17–21.

Bauman, A. E. "Updating the Evidence That Physical Activity Is Good for Health: An Epidemiological Review 2000–2003." *Journal of Science and Medicine in Sport*, 2004, *7*(1 suppl.), 6–19.

Besser, L. M., Marcus, M., and Frumkin, H. "Commute Time and Social Capital in the U.S." *American Journal of Public Health*, 2008, *34*(3), 207–211.

Bhatia, R., and Wernham, A. "Integrating Human Health into Environmental Impact Assessment: An Unrealized Opportunity for Environmental Health and Justice." *Environmental Health Perspectives*, 2008, *116*(8), 991–1000.

Blair, S. N., and others. "Physical Activity, Nutrition, and Chronic Disease." *Medicine & Science in Sports & Exercise*, 1996, *28*(3), 335–349.

Block, J. P., Scribner, R. A., and DeSalvo, K. B. "Fast Food, Race/Ethnicity, and Income: A Geographic Analysis." *American Journal of Preventive Medicine*, 2004, *27*(3), 211–217.

Boarnet, M. G., and others. "Evaluation of the California Safe Routes to School Legislation: Urban Form Changes and Children's Active Transportation to School." *American Journal of Preventive Medicine*, 2005, *28*(2, suppl. 2), 134–140.

Booth, G., Leonard, B., and Pawlukiewicz, M. *Ten Principles for Reinventing America's Suburban Business Districts*. Urban Land Institute. http://www.smartgrowth.org/pdf/uli_Ten_Principles.pdf, 2002.

Bragg, B., Galloway, T., Spohn, D. B., and Trotter, D. E. "Land Use and Zoning for the Public's Health." *Journal of Law, Medicine & Ethics*, 2003, *31*(4), 78–80.

Brauer, M., and others. "Air Pollution from Traffic and the Development of Respiratory Infections and Asthmatic and Allergic Symptoms in Children." *American Journal of Respiratory and Critical Care Medicine*, 2002, *166*(8), 1092–1098.

Bunn, F., and others. "Traffic Calming for the Prevention of Road Traffic Injuries: Systematic Review and Meta-Analysis." *Injury Prevention*, 2003, *9*, 200–204.

Campbell, J. M. "Renewing Social Capital: the Role of Civil Dialogue." In S. Schuman (ed.), *Creating a Culture of Collaboration*. San Francisco: Jossey-Bass, 2006.

Center for Universal Design. *The Principles of Universal Design, Version 2.0*. North Carolina State University. http://design.ncsu.edu/cud/about_ud/udprinciplestext.htm, 1997.

Centers for Disease Control and Prevention. *Overweight and Obesity: U.S. Obesity Trends*. http://www.cdc.gov/obesity/data/trends.html, 2008.

Centers for Disease Control and Prevention. *Healthy Places: Health Impact Assessment*. http://www.cdc.gov/healthyplaces/hia.htm, n.d.

Cervero, R., and Kockelman, K. "Travel Demand and the Three Ds: Density, Diversity, and Design." *Transportation Research Record*, 1997, *2*, 199–219.

City of Portland Office of Transportation. "Portland Bicycle Counts 2008." http://www.portlandonline.com/shared/cfm/image.cfm?id=217489, 2008.

Clark, D. E., and Cushing, B. M. "Rural and Urban Traffic Fatalities, Vehicle Miles, and Population Density." *Accident Analysis and Prevention*, 2004, *36*, 967–972.

Cohen, D. A., and others. "Contribution of Public Parks to Physical Activity." *American Journal of Public Health*, 2007, *97*, 509–514.

Corburn, J. "Confronting the Challenges in Reconnecting Urban Planning and Public Health." *American Journal of Public Health*, 2004, *94*, 541–546.

Dannenberg, A. L., Burton, D. C., and Jackson, R. J. "Economic and Environmental Costs of Obesity: The Impact on Airlines." [Letter.] *American Journal of Preventive Medicine*, 2004, *27*, 264.

Dannenberg, A. L., and others. "Use of Health Impact Assessment in the U.S.: 27 Case Studies, 1999–2007." *American Journal of Preventive Medicine*, 2008, *34*(3), 241–256,

de Leeuw, E. "Global and Local (Glocal) Health: The WHO Healthy Cities Programme." *Global Change & Human Health*, 2001, *2*(1), 34–45.

De Ville, K. A., and Sparrow, S. E. "Zoning, Urban Planning, and the Public Health Practitioner." *Journal of Public Health Management and Practice*, 2008, *14*, 313–316.

Delfino, R. J., and others. "Personal and Ambient Air Pollution Exposures and Lung Function Decrements in Children with Asthma." *Environmental Health Perspectives*, 2008, *116*(4), 550–558.

Duffy, J. *The Sanitarians: A History of American Public Health*. Urbana: University of Illinois Press, 1990.

Elvik, R. "Area-Wide Urban Traffic Calming Schemes: A Meta-Analysis of Safety Effects." *Accident Analysis and Prevention*, 2001, *33*, 327–336.

European Centre for Health Policy. *Health Impact Assessment: Main Concepts and Suggested Approach.* Gothenburg Consensus Paper. http://www.euro.who.int/document/PAE/Gothenburgpaper.pdf, 1999.

Evans, G. W. "The Built Environment and Mental Health." *Journal of Urban Health*, 2003, *80*, 536–555.

Ewing, R., Schieber, R.A., and Zegeer, C.V. "Urban Sprawl as a Risk Factor in Motor Vehicle Occupant and Pedestrian Fatalities." *American Journal of Public Health*, 2003, *93*(9), 1541–1549.

Federal Aviation Administration. *Land Use Compatibility and Airports: A Guide for Effective Land Use Planning.* http://www.faa.gov/about/office_org/headquarters_offices/aep/planning_toolkit, 1999.

Federal Highway Administration. *Highway Traffic Noise in the United States: Problem and Response.* FHWA-HEP-06-020. U.S. Department of Transportation. http://www.fhwa.dot.gov/environment/probresp.htm, 2006.

Federal Interagency Committee on Aviation Noise. *Findings of the FICAN Pilot Study on the Relationship Between Aircraft Noise Reduction and Changes in Standardized Test Scores.* http://www.fican.org/pages/findings.html, 2007.

Finkelstein, E. A., Fiebelkorn, I. C., and Wang, G. "National Medical Spending Attributable to Overweight and Obesity: How Much, and Who's Paying?" *Health Affairs*. Web Exclusive. http://content.healthaffairs.org/cgi/content/full/hlthaff.w3.219v1/DC1, May 14, 2003.

Finkelstein, M. M., Jerrett, M., and Sears, M. R. "Traffic Air Pollution and Mortality Rate Advancement Periods." *American Journal of Epidemiology*, 2004, *160*(2), 173–177.

Flynn, B. C. "Healthy Cities: Toward Worldwide Health Promotion." *Annual Review of Public Health*, 1996, *17*, 299–309.

Foege, W. H. "CDC's 60th Anniversary: Director's Perspective—William H. Foege, MD, MPH, 1977–1983." *Morbidity and Mortality Weekly Report*, 2006, *55*(39), 1071–1074.

Frank, L., and Engelke, P. *How Land Use and Transportation Systems Impact Public Health*. Centers for Disease Control and Prevention. http://www.cdc.gov/nccdphp/dnpa/pdf/aces-workingpaper1.pdf, 2000.

Fried, L. P., Freedman, M., Endres, T. E., and Wasik, B. "Building Communities That Promote Successful Aging." *Western Journal of Medicine*, 1997, *167*, 216–219.

Frumkin, H., Frank, L., and Jackson, R. *Urban Sprawl and Public Health: Designing, Planning, and Building for Healthy Communities*. Washington, D.C.: Island Press, 2004.

Geller, A. L. "Smart Growth: A Prescription for Livable Cities." *American Journal of Public Health*, 2003, *93*(9), 1410–1415.

Glanz, K., Sallis, J. F., Saelens, B. E., and Frank, L. D. "Healthy Nutrition Environments: Concepts and Measures." *American Journal of Health Promotion*, 2005, *19*(5), 330–333, ii.

Glasser, J. "Back to the Future." [Transcript.] Presentation at the Annual Meeting of the Hawai'i Public Health Association, *Global Public Health: Issues and Strategies for Hawai'i and the Pacific*. http://www.hawaii.edu/global/projects_activities/Past/GlasserXscript2.pdf, June 12–13, 2002.

Halpern, D. *Mental Health and the Built Environment*. London: Taylor & Francis, 1995.

Hippocrates. *On Airs, Waters and Places*. Whitefish, MT: Kessinger Publishing, n.d.

Hoehner, C. M., and others. "Opportunities for Integrating Public Health and Urban Planning Approaches to Promote Active Community Environments." *American Journal of Health Promotion*, 2003, *18*, 14–20.

Hoek, G., and others. "Association Between Mortality and Indicators of Traffic-Related Air Pollution in the Netherlands: A Cohort Study." *Lancet*, 2002, *360*(9341), 1203–1209.

Horowitz, C. R., Colson, K. A., Hebert, P. L., and Lancaster, K. "Barriers to Buying Healthy Foods for People with Diabetes: Evidence of Environmental Disparities." *American Journal of Public Health*, 2004, *94*, 1549–1554.

House, J. S., Landis, K. R., and Umberson, D. "Social Relationships and Health." *Science*, 1988, *241*, 540–545.

ICLEI–Local Governments for Sustainability. *Building Sustainable Cities*. http://www.iclei.org/index.php?id=801, 2008.

ICLEI USA–Local Governments for Sustainability. *STAR Community Index*. http://www.icleiusa.org/programs/sustainability/star-community-index, 2008.

International City/County Management Association. *Active Living and Social Equity: Creating Healthy Communities for All Residents: A Guide for Local Governments*. http://www.icma.org/upload/library/2005-02/{16565E96-721D-467D-9521-3694F918E5CE}.pdf, 2005.

Jackson, K. T. *Crabgrass Frontier: The Suburbanization of the United States*. New York: Oxford University Press, 1985.

Jacobsen, P. L. "Safety in Numbers: More Walkers and Bicyclists, Safer Walking and Bicycling." *Injury Prevention*, 2003, *9*, 205–209.

Jakovljević, B., Belojević, G., Paunović, K., and Stojanov, V. "Road Traffic Noise and Sleep Disturbances in an Urban Population: Cross-Sectional Study." *Croatian Medical Journal*, 2006, *47*, 125–133.

Jarup, L., and others. "Hypertension and Exposure to Noise Near Airports: The HYENA Study." *Environmental Health Perspectives*, 2008, *116*(3), 329–333.

Joint, M. "Road Rage." In AAA Foundation for Traffic Safety, *Aggressive Driving: Three Studies*. http://www.aaafoundation.org/pdf/agdr3study.pdf, Mar. 1997.

Kampert, J. B., Blair, S. N., Barlow, C. E., and Kohl, H. W. "Physical Activity, Physical Fitness, and All-Cause and Cancer Mortality: A Prospective Study of Men and Women." *Annals of Epidemiology*, 1996, *6*(5), 452–457.

Kawachi, I. "Social Capital and Community Effects on Population and Individual Health." *Annals of the New York Academy of Sciences*, 1999, *896*, 120–130.

Kawachi, I., Kennedy, B. P., Lochner, K., and Prothrow-Stith, D. "Social Capital, Income Inequality, and Mortality." *American Journal of Public Health*, 1997, *87*, 1491–1498.

Kennedy, M., and Leonard, P. *Dealing with Neighborhood Change: A Primer on Gentrification and Policy Choices.* Discussion paper prepared for the Brookings Institution Center on Urban and Metropolitan Policy and PolicyLink. http://www.policylink.org/pdfs/BrookingsGentrification.pdf, 2001.

Kim, J. J., and others. "Residential Traffic and Children's Respiratory Health." *Environmental Health Perspectives*, 2008, *116*(9), 1274–1279.

Kochtitzky, C. S., and others. "Urban Planning and Public Health at CDC." *Morbidity and Mortality Weekly Report*, 2006, *55*(suppl. 2), 34–38.

Koslowsky, M., Kluger, A. N., and Reich, M. *Commuting Stress: Causes, Effects, and Methods of Coping.* New York: Plenum, 1995.

Kuczmarski, R. J., Flegal, K. M., Campbell, S. M., and Johnson, C. L. "Increasing Prevalence of Overweight Among US Adults: The National Health and Nutrition Examination Surveys, 1960 to 1991." *JAMA*, 1994, *272*(3), 205–211.

Kunstler, J. H. *The Geography of Nowhere: The Rise and Decline of America's Man-Made Landscape.* New York: Simon & Schuster, 1993.

Lee, I. M. "Physical Activity and Cancer Prevention—Data from Epidemiologic Studies." *Medicine & Science in Sports & Exercise*, 2003, *35*(11), 1823–1827.

Lee, I. M., and Paffenbarger, R. S., Jr. "Associations of Light, Moderate, and Vigorous Intensity Physical Activity with Longevity: The Harvard Alumni Health Study." *American Journal of Epidemiology*, 2000, *151*(3), 293–299.

Leong, S. T., and Laortanakul, P. "Monitoring and Assessment of Daily Exposure of Roadside Workers to Traffic Noise Levels in an Asian City: A Case Study of Bangkok Streets." *Environmental Monitoring and Assessment*, 2003, *85*(1), 69–85.

Litsios, S. "Charles Dickens and the Movement for Sanitary Reform." *Perspectives in Biology & Medicine*, 2003, *46*(2), 183–199.

Lynch, J. W., Smith, G. D., Kaplan, G. A., and House, J. S. "Income Inequality and Mortality: Importance to Health of Individual Income, Psychosocial Environment, or Material Conditions." *British Medical Journal*, 2000, *320*, 1200–1204.

Macera, C. A., and others. "Prevalence of Physical Activity, Including Lifestyle Physical Activities Among Adults—United States, 2000–2001." *Morbidity and Mortality Weekly Report*, 2003, *52*, 764–779.

Mair, J. S., Pierce, M. W., and Teret, S. P. "The Use of Zoning to Restrict Fast Food Outlets: A Potential Strategy to Combat Obesity." Center for Law and the Public's Health at Johns Hopkins and Georgetown Universities. http://www.publichealthlaw.net/Zoning%20Fast%20Food%20Outlets.pdf, 2005.

Malizia, E. E. "Planning and Public Health: Research Options for an Emerging Field." *Journal of Planning Education and Research*, 2006, *25*, 428–432.

Matheson, M. P., Stansfeld, S. A., and Haines, M. M. "The Effects of Chronic Aircraft Noise Exposure on Children's Cognition and Health: 3 Field Studies." *Noise & Health*, 2003, *5*(19), 31–40.

Maynard, D., Coull, B. A., Gryparis, A., and Schwartz, J. "Mortality Risk Associated with Short-Term Exposure to Traffic Particles and Sulfates." *Environmental Health Perspectives*, 2007, *115*(5), 751–755.

McCann, B. "Complete the Streets!" *Planning*, May 2005, pp. 18–23.

McConnell, R., and others. "Traffic, Susceptibility and Childhood Asthma." *Environmental Health Perspectives*, 2006, *114*(5), 766–772.

Melosi, M. V. *The Sanitary City: Urban Infrastructure in American from Colonial Times to the Present*. Baltimore, Md.: Johns Hopkins University Press, 2000.

Minkler, M., and Wallerstein, N. "Improving Health Through Community Organization and Community Building: A Health Education Perspective." In M. Minkler (ed.), *Community Organizing and Community Building for Health*. (2nd ed.) Piscataway, N.J.: Rutgers University Press, 2005.

Novaco, R., Stokols, D., Campbell, J., and Stokols, J. "Transportation, Stress, and Community Psychology." *American Journal of Community Psychology*, 1979, *7*, 361–380.

Nyberg, F., and others. "Urban Air Pollution and Lung Cancer in Stockholm." *Epidemiology*, 2000, *11*(5), 487–495.

Ogden, C. L., and others. "Prevalence of Overweight and Obesity in the United States, 1999–2004." *JAMA*, 2006, *295*, 1549–1555.

Oldenburg, R. *The Great Good Place: Cafés, Coffee Shops, Community Centers, Beauty Parlors, General Stores, Bars, Hangouts, and How They Get You Through the Day*. New York: Paragon House, 1989.

Olmsted, F. L. "Basic Principles of City Planning." In J. Nolen (ed.), *City Planning: A Series of Papers Presenting the Essential Elements of a City Plan* (pp. 1–18). New York: Appleton, 1916.

Passchier-Vermeer, W, and Passchier, W. F. "Noise Exposure and Public Health." *Environmental Health Perspectives*, 2000, *108*(suppl. 1), 123–131.

Perdue, W. C., Stone, L. A., and Gostin, L. O. "The Built Environment and Its Relationship to the Public's Health: The Legal Framework." *American Journal of Public Health*, 2003, *93*, 1390–1394.

Powell, L. M., and others. "Associations Between Access to Food Stores and Adolescent Body Mass Index." *American Journal of Preventive Medicine*, 2007, *33*(suppl. 4), S301–S307.

Pucher, J., and Dijkstra, L. "Promoting Safe Walking and Cycling to Improve Public Health: Lessons from the Netherlands and Germany." *American Journal of Public Health*, 2003, *93*(9), 1509–1516.

Putnam, R. D. *Bowling Alone: The Collapse and Revival of American Community*. New York: Simon & Schuster, 2000.

Rathbone, D. B., and Huckabee, J. C. *Controlling Road Rage: A Literature Review and Pilot Study*. Washington, D.C.: AAA Foundation for Traffic Safety, June 1999.

Retting, R. A., Persaud, B. N., Garder, P. E., and Lord, D. "Crash and Injury Reduction Following Installation of Roundabouts in the United States." *American Journal of Public Health*, 2001, *91*, 628–631.

Rundle, R. L. "U.S.'s Obesity Woes Put a Strain on Hospitals in Unexpected Ways." *Wall Street Journal*. May 1, 2002.

Schikowski, T., and others. "Long-Term Air Pollution Exposure and Living Close to Busy Roads Are Associated with COPD in Women." *Respiratory Research*, 2005, *6*, 152.

Schilling, J., and Linton, L. "The Public Health Roots of Zoning: In Search of Active Living's Legal Genealogy." *American Journal of Preventive Medicine*, 2005, *28*(2, suppl. 2), 96–104.

Smart Growth Network. "Principles of Smart Growth." http://www.smartgrowth.org/about/principles/default.asp, 2009.

Spreng, M. "Possible Health Effects of Noise Induced Cortisol Increase." *Noise & Health*, 2000, *2*(7), 59–64.

Stansfeld, S. A., and Matheson, M. P. "Noise Pollution: Non-Auditory Effects on Health." *British Medical Bulletin*, 2003, *68*, 243–257.

Stansfeld, S. A., and others. "Aircraft and Road Traffic Noise and Children's Cognition and Health: A Cross-National Study." *Lancet*, 2005, *365*, 1942–1949.

Stokols, D., Novaco, R., Stokols, J., and Campbell, J. "Traffic Congestion, Type A Behavior, and Stress." *Journal of Applied Psychology*, 1978, *63*, 467–480.

Story, M., Kaphingst, K.M., Robinson-O'Brien, R., and Glanz, K. "Creating Healthy Food and Eating Environments: Policy and Environmental Approaches." *Annual Review of Public Health*. 2008, *29*, 253–272.

Surface Transportation Policy Project. *Mean Streets 2004*. http://www.transact.org/library/reports_html/ms2004/pdf/final_mean_streets_2004_4.pdf, 2004.

Transportation Research Board and Institute of Medicine. *Does the Built Environment Influence Physical Activity? Examining the Evidence*. TRB Special Report 282. Washington D.C.: National Academy of Sciences, 2005.

U.S. Congress, House of Representatives, Subcommittee on Aviation. *Aviation and the Environment: Impact of Aviation Noise on Communities Presents Challenges for Airport Operations and Future Growth of the National Airspace System: Testimony Before the Subcommittee on Aviation, Committee on Transportation and Infrastructure*. Testimony of Gerald L. Dillingham. 110th Cong. (2007). http://www.gao.gov/new.items/d08216t.pdf.

U.S. Department of Transportation. *Vehicle Miles Traveled (VMT) and Vehicle Emissions*. http://www.fhwa.dot.gov/environment/vmtems.htm, 2002.

U.S. Department of Transportation. "Bicyclists and Other Cyclists." *Traffic Safety Facts*. (2006 data.) http://www.nhtsa.dot.gov/portal/nhtsa_static_file_downloader.jsp?file=/staticfiles/DOT/NHTSA/Traffic%20Injury%20Control/Articles/Associated%20Files/TSF2006_810802.pdf, 2007.

U.S. Department of Transportation. "2007 Traffic Safety Annual Assessment—Highlights." *Traffic Safety Facts*. http://www-nrd.nhtsa.dot.gov/Pubs/811017.pdf, 2008a.

U.S. Department of Transportation. "Motor Vehicle Traffic Crashes as a Leading Cause of Death in the United States, 2005." *Traffic Safety Facts*. http://www-nrd.nhtsa.dot.gov/Pubs/810936.pdf, 2008b.

U.S. Department of Transportation. *Traffic Safety Facts 2006: A Compilation of Motor Vehicle Crash Data from the Fatality Analysis Reporting System and the General Estimates System*. http://www-nrd.nhtsa.dot.gov/Pubs/TSF2006FE.pdf, 2008c.

U.S. Environmental Protection Agency. *Travel and Environmental Implications of School Siting*. EPA 231-R-03-004. http://www.epa.gov/dced/pdf/school_travel.pdf, 2003.

U.S. Environmental Protection Agency, Office of Transportation and Air Quality. *Greenhouse Gas Emissions from the U.S. Transportation Sector, 1990–2003*. EPA 420-R-06-003. http://www.epa.gov/oms/climate/420r06003.pdf, Mar. 2006.

U.S. Green Building Council. *LEED for Neighborhood Development*. http://www.usgbc.org/DisplayPage.aspx?CMSPageID=148, 2008.

Venn, A. J., and others. "Living Near a Main Road and the Risk of Wheezing Illness in Children." *American Journal of Respiratory and Critical Care Medicine.* 2001, *164*(12), 2177–2180.

Vineis, P., and others. "Air Pollution and Risk of Lung Cancer in a Prospective Study in Europe." *International Journal of Cancer*, 2006, *119*(1), 169–174.

Wahl, H. W., and Weisman, G. D. "Environmental Gerontology at the Beginning of the New Millennium: Reflections on Its Historical, Empirical, and Theoretical Development." *Gerontologist*, 2003, *43*, 616–627.

Wannamethee, S. G., Shaper, A. G., and Walker, M. "Changes in Physical Activity, Mortality, and Incidence of Coronary Heart Disease in Older Men." *Lancet*, 1998, *351*(9116), 1603–1608.

Wannamethee, S. G., Shaper, G., Walker, M., and Ebrahim, S. "Lifestyle and 15-Year Survival Free of Heart Attack, Stroke, and Diabetes in Middle-aged British Men." *Archives of Internal Medicine*, 1998, *158*, 2433–2440.

Watson, M., and Dannenberg, A. L. "Investment in Safe Routes to School Projects: Public Health Benefits for the Larger Community." *Preventing Chronic Disease.* http://www.cdc.gov/pcd/issues/2008/jul/07_0087.htm, 2008.

Wei, M., and others. "Relationship Between Low Cardiorespiratory Fitness and Mortality in Normal-Weight, Overweight, and Obese Men." *JAMA*, 1999, *282*, 1547–1553.

Woodyard, C. "Car Weight Limits Are a Big, Fat Problem." *USA Today*. http://www.usatoday.com/money/autos/2007–09–13-overloaded-cars_N.htm?imw=Y, Sept. 13, 2007.

World Commission on Environment and Development. *Our Common Future*. New York: Oxford University Press, 1987.

World Health Organization. *Guidelines for Community Noise: Adverse Health Effects of Noise*. http://www.who.int/docstore/peh/noise/Comnoise3.htm, n.d.

World Health Organization, Regional Office for Europe. *Twenty Steps for Developing a Healthy Cities Project*. http://www.euro.who.int/document/e56270.pdf, 1997.

Zenk, S. N., and others. "Fruit and Vegetable Access Differs by Community Racial Composition and Socioeconomic Position in Detroit, Michigan." *Ethnicity & Disease*, 2006, *16*(1), 275–280.

FOR FURTHER INFORMATION

Books and Articles

Bullard, R. D., and Johnson, G. S. (eds.). *Just Transportation: Dismantling Race and Class Barriers to Mobility*. Gabriola Island, B.C.: New Society Publishers. 1997.

Corburn, J. *Toward the Healthy City: People, Places and the Politics of Urban Planning*. Cambridge: MIT Press, 2009.

Frank, L. D., Engelke, P. O., and Schmid, T. L. *Health and Community Design: The Impact of the Built Environment on Physical Activity*. Washington, D.C.: Island Press, 2003.

Frumkin, H. "Urban Sprawl and Public Health." *Public Health Reports.* 2002, *117*, 201–217.

Kemm, J., Parry, J., and Palmer, S. (eds.). *Health Impact Assessment Concepts, Theory, Techniques, and Applications.* New York: Oxford University Press, 2004.

Malizia, E. E. "City and Regional Planning: A Primer for Public Health Officials." *American Journal of Health Promotion,* 2005, *19*(5, suppl.) 1–13.

Younger, M., Morrow-Almeida, H. R., Vindigni, S., and Dannenberg, A. L. "The Built Environment, Climate Change, and Health: Opportunities for Co-Benefits." *American Journal of Preventive Medicine.* 2008, *35*(5), 517–526.

Reports and Tools

Centers for Disease Control and Prevention. *LEED-ND and Healthy Neighborhoods: An Expert Panel Review.* http://www.cdc.gov/healthyplaces/publications/LEED-ND_tabloidFINAL2.pdf, Oct. 2008.

National Association of County and City Health Officials (NACCHO). *Community Revitalization and Public Health: Issues, Roles, and Relationships for Local Public Health Agencies.* (Binder, for purchase.) http://www.naccho.org/publications, 2000.

National Association of County and City Health Officials (NACCHO). *Public Health and Planning (Community Design) 101.* (CD, for purchase.) http://www.naccho.org/publications, 2005.

National Association of Local Boards of Health (NALBOH). *Land Use Planning for Public Health: The Role of Local Boards of Health in Community Design and Development.* (For purchase.) http://www.nalboh.org/PDF/RO_Catalog.pdf, n.d.

U.S.-Based Agencies and Organizations

American Planning Association (APA) and National Association of County and City Health Officials (NACCHO), Planning for Healthy Places with Health Impact Assessment, http://professional.captus.com/Planning/hia/default.aspx. These two professional associations offer an on-line training course on the basics of using health impact assessment in planning.

Association of State and Territorial Health Officers (ASTHO), http://www.astho.org/index.php?template=built_synthetic_environment.html. A professional association with a Web site that provides information on health and the built and synthetic environment that is relevant to state-level policies and projects.

Centers for Disease Control and Prevention, http://www.cdc.gov/healthyplaces. The CDC's Healthy Places Web site offers information and key resources about the major health issues related to land use.

Congress for the New Urbanism (CNU), http://www.cnu.org. This organization's efforts encourage the restoration of existing urban centers, reconfiguration of suburbs, conservation of natural environments, and preservation of the built legacy.

ICLEI–Local Governments for Sustainability USA (ICLEI-USA), http://www.icleiusa.org. This network of 500 cities, towns, and counties strives to reduce greenhouse gas emissions and create more sustainable communities.

Local Government Commission (LGC), Center for Livable Communities, http://www.lgc.org/clc/ center.html. This organization helps local governments and community leaders adopt programs and policies that lead to more livable and resource-efficient land use patterns. LGC sponsors the annual Smart Growth conference (http://www.newpartners.org).

National Association of County and City Health Officials (NACCHO), http://www.naccho.org/ topics/environmental/landuseplanning/index.cfm. NACCHO's Web site provides information on health and the built environment relevant to local-level policies and projects.

National Association of Local Boards of Health (NALBOH), http://www.nalboh.org. NALBOH supports local boards of health on many issues, including improving the built environment.

Robert Wood Johnson Foundation, Active Living Research program, http://www.activelivingresearch. org. The Active Living Research program focuses on preventing childhood obesity nationwide by many means, including making improvements in the built environment to encourage physical activity.

Safe Routes to Schools (SRTS) National Partnership, http://www.saferoutespartnership.org. This network of nonprofit organizations, governmental agencies, schools, and professionals works to advance the SRTS movement in the United States.

San Francisco Department of Public Health, Health, Equity, and Sustainability Program, http://www .sfphes.org. This health department Web site provides tools, training, research, and other useful information for health impact assessment (HIA) practitioners.

Smart Growth Network, http://www.smartgrowth.org. This site offers a catalogue of Smart Growth–related news, events, information, and resources.

Thunderhead Alliance for Biking and Walking, http://www.thunderheadalliance.org. This national coalition of state and local bicycle and pedestrian advocacy organizations works to promote bicycling and walking in North America.

UCLA School of Public Health, Health Impact Assessment (HIA) Project, http://www.ph.ucla.edu/ hs/health-impact. This project conducts research on HIA and is developing a database of completed HIAs. The Web site provides links to many HIA resources.

Urban Land Institute (ULI), http://www.uli.org. The mission of this nonprofit research and educational institute is to provide responsible leadership in the use of land in order to enhance the total environment. ULI members span the entire spectrum of the land use and development disciplines.

U.S. Department of Transportation, Federal Highway Administration (FHWA), National Center for Safe Routes to School (SRTS), http://www.saferoutesinfo.org. The FHWA provides funding and guidance for the SRTS program.

U.S. Environmental Protection Agency, http://www.epa.gov/smartgrowth. This agency's Web site provides smart growth information and key resources.

Global Organizations

Association of Public Health Observatories (APHO), HIA Gateway, http://www.hiagateway.org.uk. This U.K.-based organization's Web site offers the largest single collection of health impact assessment information, resources, and links.

ICLEI—Local Governments for Sustainability, http://www.iclei.org/index.php?id=801. This organization is an international association of local governments and national and regional local government organizations that have made a commitment to sustainable development.

International Healthy Cities Foundation, http://www.healthycities.org. People interested in health and quality of life issues in their communities can share information on this foundation's Web site.

Sustainable Cities Network, http://www.rec.org/REC/Programs/Sustainablecities. This network facilitates communication among world's leading sustainable development organizations.

United Nations Human Settlements Programme (UN-Habitat), http://www.unhabitat.org/categories.asp?catid=540. UN-Habitat works to promote socially and environmentally sustainable towns and cities, with the goal of providing adequate shelter for all.

World Health Organization (WHO), http://www.who.int/hia/en. WHO supports health impact assessment because it can beneficially influence policies, programs, and projects. This WHO Web site provides HIA resources and tools.

World Health Organization, Healthy Cities Programme, http://www.euro.who.int/healthy-cities. The WHO Healthy Cities Programme engages local governments in health development through a process of political commitment, institutional change, capacity building, partnership-based planning, and innovative projects. It also strives to include health considerations in economic regeneration and urban development efforts.

CHAPTER FIFTEEN

WATER AND HEALTH

TIM FORD

KEY CONCEPTS

- Water is critical to all forms of life on this planet.

- There are many ways in which we directly threaten both the quality and quantity of this resource and thus our health and the planet's health.

- To protect our health and our environment we must conserve water, reduce wastewater production, and begin to recycle.

- A regulatory framework exists in the United States to ensure the provision of safe drinking water to the public.

- We need to begin to think about future risks to our water resources and potential mitigation activities, both in the developed and the developing worlds.

THE ROLE OF WATER IN LIFE

The existence of life, whether human, animal, avian, reptilian, amphibian, plant, or microbe, depends on water. The search for life (as we understand it) on other planets is always predicated on the search for evidence of water. We humans are approximately 60 percent water, and we cannot survive for more than a few days without it. It is therefore not surprising that human culture has been defined by water over the centuries. One has only to look at development along the major river systems of the world to realize how the water environment has dominated, and continues to dominate, human cultures.

The Hydrologic Cycle

Our planet would appear to have a surfeit of water, but most of this water is unavailable for human use. Over 97 percent of the world's water is salty, found in the oceans and (to a much lower extent) in inland seas and salt water lakes. What remains is freshwater, but over two-thirds of this is locked in the Antarctic and Arctic ice caps. The freshwater that remains, in rivers and lakes, in the atmosphere, and in the ground, makes up less than 1 percent of the world's water. This is the supply potentially available for drinking, irrigating crops, and other uses.

Water is in continuous motion between these various locations, in a so-called **hydrologic cycle** that dominates the health of the planet. Without continuous evaporation from the oceans, precipitation on land, and runoff back to the oceans, no surface or groundwater recharge can take place, and we would eventually exhaust our available freshwater supplies. Figure 15.1 provides a diagrammatic overview of the hydrologic cycle, the dominant flows, or fluxes, and the critical reservoirs, or pools.

The hydrologic cycle teaches us to view water and health with a holistic perspective. The compartments of the hydrologic cycle are either directly or indirectly connected, and perturbation of one compartment is likely to affect all other compartments and therefore both human and ecological health. These interconnections are diagrammatically illustrated in Figure 15.2.

This chapter explores these interconnections. It describes several processes that are crucially important to humans, including water consumption, waste production, waste treatment and discharge, and treatment for reuse, and outlines the multitude of health concerns at each step.

Tim Ford declares no competing financial interests.

FIGURE 15.1   The Hydrologic Cycle

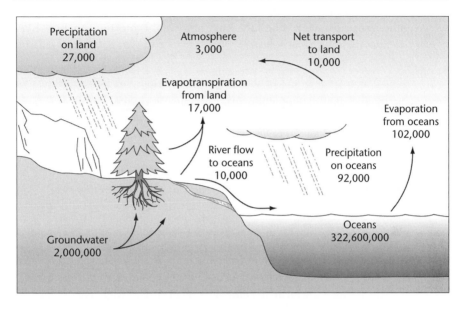

Note: Pools are in cubic miles; fluxes are in cubic miles per year.

Source: Redrawn from Winter, Harvey, Franke, and Alley, 1998. Originally modified from W. H. Schlesinger, *Biogeochemistry—An Analysis of Global Change* (Academic Press, 1991), with permission from Elsevier.

FIGURE 15.2   Schematic of the Interconnections Between Water and Health

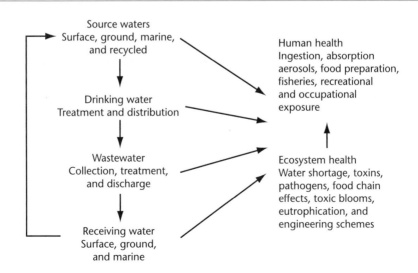

Important Definitions

Available freshwater supplies are often conceptually divided into **surface water** and **groundwater**. The U.S. Environmental Protection Agency (EPA) (2007b) defines these terms as follows:

> *Surface water*: all water naturally open to the atmosphere (rivers, lakes, reservoirs, ponds, streams, impoundments, seas, estuaries, and so forth)
> *Groundwater*: the supply of fresh water found beneath the Earth's surface, usually in aquifers, which supplies wells and springs

Because surface water and groundwater are not independent of each other, an overlap category is also recognized. The EPA defines this as

> *Groundwater under the direct influence of surface water*: any water beneath the surface of the ground with: (1) significant occurrence of insects or other microorganisms, algae, or large-diameter pathogens; (2) significant and relatively rapid shifts in water characteristics such as turbidity, temperature, conductivity, or pH which closely correlate to climatological or surface water conditions

These distinctions are important because they directly affect how we view the quality of a water resource and how we manage that resource. Ideally, water used as a drinking water source (often called **source water**) should be of the highest quality, reducing the cost of **water treatment** and the risk of **contamination**. Groundwater has traditionally been considered a high-quality resource, because as rainfall and other surface waters percolate through soil into groundwater, they are cleaned by physical, chemical, and microbiological processes in the soil. However, the traditional confidence in groundwater may not always be well placed, as human activities such as land management practices can influence even relatively deep aquifers. Surface water, and **groundwater under the direct influence of surface water** (GWUDI), have traditionally been less favored as sources for drinking water. However, groundwater is not always available, and municipalities may have no choice but to implement extensive and costly surface water treatment. At present, just over half of Americans get their drinking water from surface sources.

Surface and GWUDI water may be considered suitable for agricultural, industrial, or recreational uses with no or limited treatment. Different criteria are therefore developed and applied to source waters depending on their ultimate use. Surface waters that are used as drinking-water sources are regulated by far stricter criteria, for example, than waters used to irrigate crops. (A fuller discussion of water regulations appears later in this chapter.)

Water Use and Water Scarcity

Water scarcity may be one of the most critical health threats to human society today. In the long term, societies must be able to survive on renewable resources. When a resource is nonrenewable then it is available only in finite quantities, and when a resource is extracted faster than it can be renewed then eventually supplies will not meet demand. This pattern of use is nonsustainable. The most familiar examples of finite resources are fossil fuels. As explained in Chapter Thirteen, fossil fuel use is nonsustainable in the long term, leading to considerable pressure to develop alternative energy sources. Just as fossil fuels are mined, so is water. Technology has allowed us to extract more and more of the water trapped within the Earth's crust. This has allowed human habitation, and its ensuing agricultural and industrial development, to spread to arid areas of the planet that are poorly suited to sustain human life. In arid regions **aquifer recharge** rates are low, and the deep aquifers laid down by countless ice ages are gradually being depleted. (Several authors provide informative discussions of water use and water scarcity; see, for example, Gleick, 1993, 1998, 2000, 2002; Clarke, 1993; Postel, 1997.)

Figure 15.3 shows the Ogallala Aquifer, a groundwater resource so well known that it has been highlighted in *National Geographic* magazine (Zwingle, 1993). This vast aquifer underlies 175,000 square miles in parts of eight states; stretching from South Dakota to Texas, it provides an estimated 30 percent of all groundwater used for irrigation in the United States (U.S. Geological Survey [USGS], 2007). It was water from the Ogallala that helped farmers convert the central plains of North America from a dustbowl to an agriculturally rich region. However, the Ogallala is a finite resource. It consists of **fossil water**, water sequestered underground for thousands of years, and the current rate of water extraction far exceeds the rate at which it is replenished. In some states, groundwater supplies are expected to be depleted in the next twenty to thirty years. Already, farmers in the region are having to drill much deeper wells or rely on surface water instead, which has lowered farm yield in the region substantially. In addition to the problem of water scarcity, water quality in parts of the aquifer may have been compromised by agricultural practices.

Population and Water Scarcity

Whether or not a water supply is adequate depends on the balance that exists among **water availability**, population, and the ways in which people use water. In many parts of the world, as described in Chapter Nine, population pressure places a severe strain on water resources. According to the U.S.-based research and advocacy organization Population Action International, by 2025 27 percent of nations will face **water stress**, which is defined as a water supply at or below

FIGURE 15.3   The Ogallala Aquifer

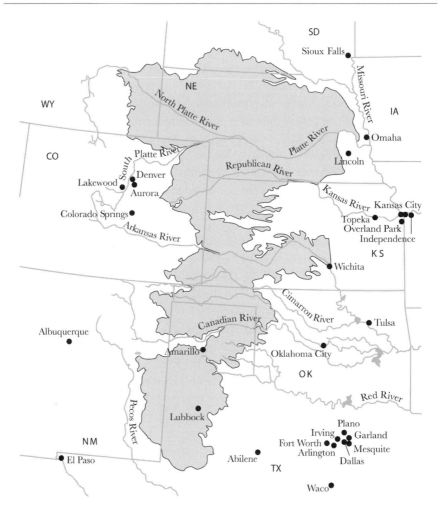

Source: USGS High Plains Regional Ground-Water Quality Study.

1,700 m³ per person per year, and an additional 11 percent of nations will face **water scarcity**, defined as a water supply at or below 1,000 m³ per person per year (using medium projections for population growth) (Engelman and others, 2006). These numbers take into account all domestic, industrial, and agricultural water use for a region. If population growth is higher than anticipated, then water will be relatively more scarce. Although some countries have enormous supplies of water (Greenland, the world's leader, has more than 10 million m³ per capita per year), others are arid. At the extreme limit of water availability, the West Bank and the Seychelles have zero per capita water availability and are entirely dependent on other countries for their water supply.

Water use varies not only with population but with the level of development and affluence. At one extreme, people in wealthy countries with ample water supplies are relatively profligate users of water. In the United States, for example, where the supply of renewable freshwater is estimated to be 10,527 m^3 per person per year, the estimated annual per capita withdrawal is 1,654 m^3. Of this, 13 percent is used in homes, 46 percent in industry, and 41 percent in agriculture (Food and Agriculture Organization of the United Nations [FAO], 2008). The 13 percent used in homes represents 590 liters per person per day, of which less than 0.2 percent is required for drinking (based on the EPA's estimated daily ingestion of community water of 926 mL per person per day; EPA, 2004). Advanced sanitation (including flush toilets) is the norm in the United States and requires large amounts of domestic water use.

In contrast, Somalia's supply of renewable freshwater is far lower, an estimated 1,787 m^3 per person per year. The per capita withdrawal is also far lower than that in the United States, an estimated 401 m^3 per year, of which <0.5 percent is used in homes, a negligible amount is used in industry, and 99.5 percent is used for agriculture (FAO, 2008). In this case, domestic water use represents 5.5 liters per person per day, of which close to 20 percent is required for consumption. There is little margin of safety in this situation, and a temporary disruption of the water supply, such as a drought, can be devastating.

Agriculture and Water Scarcity

The division of water use in Somalia is typical for many less developed countries and reflects the enormous amount of water needed to grow food. In fact, on a global scale, agriculture accounts for 70 percent of water withdrawal (United Nations Educational, Scientific and Cultural Organization [UNESCO], 2003). Many environmentally oriented Web sites list water-related facts, and one much quoted figure, taken from the Web site of National Wild and Scenic Rivers (NWSR) System (2008), is that approximately 6,800 gallons of water are required to grow a day's food for a family of four. Another oft-quoted figure is that 1,000 tons of water are required to produce 1 ton of wheat (Postel, 1999). Nonedible crops, such as cotton, also require large amounts of water; the reduction of the surface area of the Aral Sea by about 90 percent is attributed to cotton irrigation (Micklin, 2007). As a result, it is not surprising that agricultural uses of water are the greatest global contributors to water scarcity and aquifer depletion. Considerable efforts have been made over the past decade to replace conventional irrigation with methods that minimize water wastage, such as drip or other micro-irrigation techniques. (The irrigation "crisis" is described in detail in Postel, 1999.)

Political Implications

The dependence of food production on **irrigation** links freshwater use with food security and therefore with human nutrition and well-being. Accordingly, the political implications of water scarcity are enormous. Most of the major rivers and aquifers of the world cross international or at least state borders. Any use of water by one nation or state affects all downstream users. Impoundments (dams) are particularly damaging to downstream users, as they dramatically reduce water flow for these communities, particularly during dry seasons. There are numerous examples of national and international crises emerging from shared water resources, as shown in Table 15.1. In extreme instances these crises may erupt

TABLE 15.1   Hot Spots: Past and Potential Water Resource Conflicts

River Basin	Length (km)	Countries	Sources of Conflict
Nile	6,693	Tanzania, Kenya, Zaire, Burundi, Rwanda, Ethiopia, Uganda, the Sudan, Egypt	Irrigation
Tigris/Euphrates	1,840/2,700	Turkey, Syria, Iraq, (Iran)	Hydroelectric projects, irrigation
Indus/Beas/Sutlej/Ravi	2,896 (Indus)	India, Pakistan, Tibet	Diversions, Sikh versus Hindu
Ganges/Brahmaputra	2,414/2,896	India, Bangladesh, Nepal, Bhutan	Deforestation and siltation, diversions
Jordan	93	Israel, Jordan, Lebanon, Syria	Diversions (arguably an underlying cause of Arab-Israeli conflicts)
Paraná/Paraguay	3,998 (Paraná)	Brazil, Paraguay, Bolivia, Argentina, Uruguay	Dams (for hydroelectric power)
Rio Grande	3,057	United States, Mexico	Development, irrigation
Colorado	2,336	United States, Mexico	Development, irrigation

into what have been called **resource wars** (Klare, 2001). (More detailed discussion can be found in Clarke, 1993; Gleick, 1993, 1998.)

Climate Change and Water

Global climate change is discussed in detail in Chapter Ten. Here, we consider the effects of climate change on water. Warming global temperatures will result in increased evaporation from the oceans, an increase in water vapor in the atmosphere, and increasing **precipitation**, including, as Easterling and others (2000) discuss, more severe weather events. There is a positive feedback loop involved in these effects, because more water vapor in the atmosphere will exacerbate the greenhouse effect. Weather changes are expected to be complex, with precipitation increasing in some regions and decreasing in others. The burden of water scarcity may shift. For example, arid regions may benefit from increased rainfall while mountainous regions that depend primarily on snowpack for their water may experience shortages if warmer temperatures prevent snow accumulation. Although climate models are filled with uncertainty and predictions must be viewed with extreme caution, it appears likely that the hydrologic cycle as we now know it will change in coming decades and that in some regions water scarcity may substantially worsen.

Human Impacts on Aquatic Systems

Not only do water quantity and quality affect human health but human activities affect every aspect of aquatic ecosystems. **Hydrodynamics**—the way water moves—is dramatically altered by such construction projects as dams, levies, and canals and by such activities as channelization, concretization, and extraction. In turn, fundamental nutrient cycles are altered in ways that completely change the biology and chemistry of a system. In extreme cases this can lead to **eutrophication** (when high nutrient loads stimulate blooms of algae in the water, in turn stimulating microbial activity). Oxygen is depleted and massive fish kills may result. As shown in Table 15.2, changes such as these can directly affect health, completing a cycle of humans to water to humans.

Water contaminants fall into two general categories, chemical and biological. Chemical contaminants, such as arsenic, may occur naturally or may be discharged into water through industrial, agricultural, municipal, or recreational activity. Biological contaminants include **bacteria, viruses,** and **protozoa;** these originate from many sources, including human and animal wastes. The next two sections of this chapter present information on these two categories of contaminants.

TABLE 15.2   Examples of Health Consequences of Engineering Schemes

Engineering Scheme	Examples	Environmental Consequence	Health Effect
Dams and irrigation projects	Aswan High Dam, Egypt; Sennâr Dam, Sudan; Akosombo Dam, West Africa	Created habitat for snails that carry the schistosome parasite.	Dramatic increases in schistosomiasis
Hydroelectric projects	James Bay, Canada	Created conditions for methylation of mercury in sediments and its subsequent accumulation in upper levels of the food chain.	Levels of mercury in Inuit that exceed World Health Organization health guidelines
Channelization	Mississippi River	Exacerbated extreme Midwest flooding events.	Huge economic consequences, loss of property and livestock, and increase in depression
Channelization, intensive draining, diking, and developing	Florida's Kissimmee River, Lake Okeechobee, and the Everglades	Destroyed habitat for wildfowl and fish nurseries; caused lake eutrophication, algal blooms, and fish kills; reduced groundwater recharge; and dramatically changed the Everglades ecosystem.	Primarily ecological and economic consequences; long-term effects on human health of changes in Florida's hydrologic cycle as yet unknown

CHEMICAL CONTAMINANTS

A wide variety of chemicals can contaminate water, as shown in Table 15.3. A contaminant may originate from either a **point source** or a **nonpoint source**, which the EPA (2007b) defines as follows:

Point source: a stationary location or fixed facility from which pollutants are discharged; any single identifiable source of pollution; for example, a pipe, ditch, ship, ore pit, factory smokestack.

TABLE 15.3   Classes of Chemical Contaminants in Water

	Classes	Examples
Petroleum and coal hydrocarbons	Crude oil	Alkanes, heterocyclics, aromatics
	Refined oil	Gasoline, diesel, heating fuels
	Combustion or conversion products	Polycyclic aromatic hydrocarbons (PAHs), synfuels and by-products
Synthetic organics	Halogenated hydrocarbons	Polychlorinated biphenyls (PCBs), chlorofluorocarbons (CFCs), pesticides, solvents
	Plasticizers, phthalic acid esters	Polyvinyl chloride (PVC), DEHP
	Others	Surfactants, organophosphate pesticides, synthetic pyrethroids, fuel additives (MTBE)
Metals	Cadmium (Cd), mercury (Hg), lead (Pb), silver (Ag), zinc (Zn), copper (Cu), chromium (Cr), nickel (Ni), arsenic (As)	
Radionuclides	Transuranics	Plutonium (Pt), americium (Am), curium (Cm)
	Fission products	Cesium-137 (^{137}Cs), strontium-90 (^{90}Sr)
	Activation products	Cobalt-60 (^{60}Co), manganese-54 (^{54}Mn), zinc-65 (^{65}Zn), chromium-51 (^{51}Cr)
	Natural	U-Th decay series
Disinfection by-products	Chlorination, chloramination and ozonation by-products	Chloroform, trichloroacetic acids, chlorinated furanones, bromate
Industrial wastes	Process by-products, including mining, dredging, and other resource extraction processes	Many of the above chemicals plus acids, ash, desalination brines, heat (from cooling water), anticorrosion chemicals, cyanide, and so forth
Municipal and agricultural wastes (not including pathogens)	Nutrients, range of household and agricultural chemicals, including those suspected to cause endocrine disruption	Phosphorus, nitrogen, carbon, silicon, antibiotics, disinfectants, pesticides, fluoride, nonylphenol ethoxylates, and so forth

Source: Adapted in part from Capone and Bauer, 1992.

Nonpoint sources: diffuse pollution sources (that is, the pollutants do not have a single point of origin or are not introduced into a receiving stream from a specific outlet; for example, they are generally carried off the land by storm water). Common nonpoint sources are agriculture, forestry, urban, mining, construction, dams, channels, land disposal, saltwater intrusion, and city streets.

Examples of point source chemical releases include discharges of mercury, solvents, or **polychlorinated biphenyls** (PCBs) from industrial drainpipes and leakages of MTBE and petrochemicals from corroding underground gasoline tanks. A major example of nonpoint sources is agricultural runoff containing pesticides and nutrients. City streets and parking lots are important nonpoint sources; they can result in massive contamination of surface and groundwaters, as the impermeable surfaces accumulate high concentrations of street contaminants such as oils and household wastes that run off during heavy rainfall. Some contaminants, such as toxic metals and acidic drainage from mines, can arise from both point and nonpoint sources. Other sources of anthropogenic contaminants include deep injection of wastes into groundwater, lead leaching from old drinking-water distribution pipes, and the vast quantities of pharmaceuticals and personal care products (PPCPs) that are released into water from human sewage and from agricultural and aquacultural activities.

Naturally Occurring Chemical Contaminants

Many naturally occurring chemicals are toxic to humans. In most cases these result from nonpoint sources. Chemicals that naturally occur in the Earth's soils and rocks, for example, can readily diffuse into ground or surface waters. As a result, water may be naturally enriched with fluoride, selenium, arsenic and a variety of other chemicals, including salt. Here are three examples.

Nitrate   Nitrogen contamination of ground and surface waters is often attributed to wastewater discharge or excessive addition of fertilizers. However, leguminous plants, such as soybeans and alfalfa, which have a symbiotic relationship with bacteria that fix atmospheric nitrogen, may also contribute to nitrate enrichment of ground and surface waters (Cox and Kahle, 1999). Nitrate is of particular concern because of the connection between high levels of nitrate in drinking water and *blue baby* syndrome, or methemoglobinemia (Manassaram, Backer, and Moll, 2006). Nitrate is converted into nitrite by bacteria in an infant's gastrointestinal tract; the nitrite in turn reacts with hemoglobin to form methemoglobin, which does not carry oxygen. The decrease in oxygen circulating in the infant's blood can result in cyanosis and, if untreated, death. As the infant's digestive system

PERSPECTIVE
Salt as a Contaminant

Residents of coastal areas that depend on shallow groundwater for drinking water are all too familiar with the problem of saltwater intrusion. Overdevelopment of these coastal areas results in a drawdown of the aquifer, reduction in freshwater pressure, and consequent intrusion of seawater, which eventually reaches the well. Coal bed methane (CBM) exploration is now raising concerns about saline water intrusion into groundwaters in inland areas. The constant search for new energy sources has made extraction of CBM seem an economically viable option, particularly in the mountainous U.S. West, where extensive underlying coal beds and a long history of extractive industries have made a number of states easy targets for development. However, there appears to be a cost to the environment and potentially to human health in that the water that overlies these coal beds needs to be pumped out before the methane is released. This *produced water* is often saline, and its use in irrigation has been implicated in crop destruction. A major argument against further development is that both ground and surface waters will become contaminated with salt and other minerals present in produced water. As a result there is now a strong movement to ensure that CBM companies treat their produced water, increasing the cost of extraction and potentially decreasing the competitiveness of CBM as an energy source.

matures, the pH in the upper digestive tract decreases and the nitrate-reducing bacterial population declines.

Fluoride Fluoride can be both healthy and unhealthy. Many wealthy nations add fluoride to drinking water to protect against tooth decay. However, in other parts of the world fluoride poisoning, or fluorosis, is epidemic due to exposure to high levels of both waterborne and airborne fluoride, in groundwater and from the combustion of coal, for example. Fluoride can interfere with tooth- and bone-forming cells (ameloblasts and osteoblasts), with health effects ranging from mottling of teeth to dental and skeletal fluorosis with extreme bone deformation and fracture risk (see, for example, Yadav, Lata, Kataria, and Kumar, 2008). In India, 60 to 65 million people are thought to drink water with elevated fluoride (Rao, 2008). The toxicity of fluoride drives an ongoing debate about the fluoridation of drinking water. To many, this is an ethical debate around the topic of "forced" mass medication (see, for example, Murphy, 2008). However, the overwhelming consensus is that fluoride does prevent tooth decay but that the range of concentrations that are protective is very narrow. A recent review of the literature on this topic concluded that "fluoridation of drinking water remains the most effective and socially equitable means of achieving community-wide exposure to the caries prevention effects of fluoride." The article also recommended that "water be fluoridated in the target range of 0.6 to 1.1 mg/l, depending on the climate to balance reduction of dental caries and occurrence of dental fluorosis" (Yeung, 2008).

Arsenic   Arsenic is an important example of a naturally occurring toxic contaminant of water. Very high levels of arsenic exist in groundwater in Bangladesh and West Bengal. To reduce risks of epidemic cholera and other diarrheal diseases, the United Nations Children's Fund (UNICEF) began a program in the 1970s to install tube wells throughout these regions. The consequent exposure to arsenic in drinking water (described in greater detail in Chapter Eleven) is considered one of the greatest mass chemical poisonings in history. However, even lower levels of arsenic contamination, as occur in many parts of the United States, are cause for concern, as there is strong evidence linking these exposures to skin disease and cancer. Stricter regulations have met political barriers due to the fact that arsenic is a naturally occurring compound that is expensive to remove from drinking water. Many medium, small, and very small water systems (defined as serving 3,301 to 10,000, 501 to 3,300, and 25 to 500 people, respectively) use source water contaminated with arsenic, at concentrations that barely met the old standard of 50 µg/L To meet the new recommended standard of 10 µg/L, many of these systems require technologies far beyond their limited operating budgets (Ford, Rupp, Butterfield, and Camper, 2005). For some water systems, meeting these standards may result in generation of large volumes of arsenic-contaminated wastes. This in itself could present an environmental health risk, as disposal practices have not yet been fully established or their safety tested.

In addition, an increasingly recognized natural source of chemical contaminants of water is toxins produced primarily by algae and cyanobacteria. Human activity can promote the production of these toxins through nutrient loading and resulting eutrophication. From the perspective of drinking water and recreational use of freshwaters, cyanobacterial blooms are of particular concern.

Cyanobacteria, sometimes imprecisely called *blue-green algae*, are simple photosynthetic organisms closely related to bacteria and found in water bodies throughout the world. Water bodies that are rich in nutrients, such as eutrophic lakes, agricultural ponds, or catch basins, may support proliferation of cyanobacteria. In some cases a body of clear water can become turbid, discolored (green, blue-green, or reddish-brown), and covered with a film, or scum, in just a few days. Several genera of cyanobacteria, including *Microcystis*, *Anabaena*, and

Aphanizomenon, release a wide range of low molecular weight chemicals that include neurotoxins, hepatotoxins, skin and gastrointestinal irritants, enzyme inhibitors, and compounds that create taste and odor problems, such as geosmin. People who drink or swim in contaminated waters may be at risk, as may livestock and wildlife. Numerous fatalities have been reported (Chorus and Bartram, 1999; Metcalf and Codd, 2004).

In addition to the cyanobacteria, many species of planktonic algae produce toxins that accumulate in shellfish or finfish and result in poisonings. These include paralytic shellfish poisoning (PSP, caused by saxitoxins), diarrheic shellfish poisoning (DSP, caused by okadaic acid), amnesic shellfish poisoning (ASP, caused by domoic acid), neurotoxic shellfish poisoning (NSP, caused by brevetoxins), and ciguatera fish poisoning (CFP, caused by ciguatoxin or maitotoxin). A number of these poisonings are life threatening and constitute major public health threats worldwide, with enormous economic implications due to fisheries closures. (Many resources on this topic are available through the Woods Hole Oceanographic Institution, 2008.)

Anthropogenic Chemical Contaminants

Industrialization has left an enormous legacy of contamination. Exploitation of the Earth's resources has resulted in ground and surface waters contaminated with heavy metals and hydrocarbons. Uncontrolled industrial discharges, military activities, landfills, leaking underground storage tanks, agricultural activities, and many other human activities have contaminated and continue to contaminate ground and surface waters.

Anthropogenic chemicals can be divided into a number of classes, as described in Table 15.3. However, in terms of broad categories, they can be thought of as organic or inorganic or as a combination of these two, as in the case of methylmercury. The environmental fate and transport of a contaminant chemical is a direct function of its chemistry (discussed later in this section). For example, the organic contaminants popularly known as **persistent organic pollutants** (POPs) are so named because their chemistry dictates that they are degraded at negligible or only very slow rates by naturally occurring microbes, are rapidly partitioned into soils or sediments, and consequently are present in the environment for very long periods of time. PCBs, the classic example of a POP, persist for decades at multiple hazardous waste sites throughout the United States and globally (see the section on environmental reservoirs later in this chapter).

It is sobering to think about the number of chemicals that are dispersed into the environment. The U.S. Environmental Protection Agency (EPA, 2007a) estimates that more than 1.2 billion pounds of *traditional* pesticides are used in the United States every year. If wood preservatives, specialty biocides, and chlorine and hypochlorites are included in this estimate, the total number jumps to nearly 5 billion pounds. As part of its National Water Quality Assessment Program (NAWQA), the USGS is conducting the Pesticide National Synthesis Project to obtain an assessment of pesticides in the streams, rivers, and groundwater of the United States. (For a wealth of information on pesticide contamination and a variety of other water quality issues in the United States, see USGS, 2008.) Very few of the pesticides discharged to the environment have been rigorously tested for aquatic toxicity but may be considered POPs that will remain in sediments and soils for many years, decades, or even centuries (see the section on storage later in this chapter).

PPCPs deserve special mention as they have attracted considerable interest since the World Wildlife Fund and others began to investigate the toxic effects of many commonly used, and readily discarded, household products (Colborn, Dumanoski, and Meyers, 1996). The EPA (2008a) refers to PPCPs as "any product used by individuals for personal health or cosmetic reasons or used by agribusiness to enhance growth or health of livestock. PPCPs comprise a diverse collection of thousands of chemical substances, including prescription and over-the-counter therapeutic drugs, veterinary drugs, fragrances, and cosmetics." In terms of household products, although the science remains relatively weak, accruing evidence directly links many of these chemicals to developmental anomalies in wildlife, and therefore they may pose the risk of health effects in humans. Although thousands of chemicals in household products could potentially affect ecological and human health, the nonylphenol group of chemicals, whose members are common ingredients in plastics and surfactants, has received the most attention. This is due, in part, to the endocrine-disrupting effects of these nonionic surfactants in animal models (see, for example, Nagao and others, 2000).

In contrast to the debate on personal care products, few scientists today would argue that widespread contamination of the environment with pharmaceuticals is a good idea, yet we continue to discharge these chemicals to receiving waters in vast quantities, through wastewater discharge and agricultural and aquacultural practices. The likely consequence of these discharges is increased antibiotic resistance among naturally occurring microbes, with the potential for transfer of resistance factors to human pathogens (Levy, 1998). It is highly likely that these environmental reservoirs of antibiotics (and genes for antibiotic resistance) have contributed to our current epidemic (and pandemic) of antibiotic resistant infections (Spellberg and others, 2008).

Transformations

Once contaminants are released into the aquatic environment, they have considerable potential for either chemical or biological transformation to more or less toxic forms, analogous to the human biotransformation described in Chapter Two. As a result, although water may contain parent compounds such as pesticides and herbicides, a range of their degradation products may also be present. Remediation, whether chemical or biological, attempts to replicate some of these changes, reducing toxic chemicals to nontoxic degradation products such as CO_2, CH_4, H_2O, or in the case of metals, insoluble or otherwise nonbioavailable forms. Unfortunately, transformations in the natural environment frequently result in more toxic or increasingly bioavailable forms. For example, in the presence of oxygen (aerobic conditions), many groups of organisms are capable of breaking down trichloroethylene, a commonly used solvent that frequently ends up in groundwater. One end product is vinyl chloride, a known carcinogen that cannot be further degraded under aerobic conditions.

Biological Transformations   For almost every organic contaminant released to the aquatic environment, there appears to be a microbe that can employ the compound as an energy or carbon source or simply assists in its degradation through the process of cometabolism, where enzymes that evolved for another substrate fortuitously degrade the contaminant with no benefit to the microbe. As with organic contaminants, reduced forms of certain metals can be used as energy sources (electron donors) and oxidized forms can be used as energy sinks (electron acceptors). (Many textbooks discuss microbial metabolism and pollutant interactions; see, for example, Young and Cerniglia, 1995; Díaz, 2008.)

The methylation of mercury is an important example, although the specific benefits of this process to the microbe are currently unknown. The case of the James Bay poisonings mentioned in Table 15.2 provides a good example of the process. Impoundments built for hydroelectricity in the James Bay region of Quebec resulted in extensive flooding of forested lands. Organic matter degradation by microbes resulted in consumption of oxygen, anoxic conditions at the sediment-water interface, and ideal conditions for growth of anaerobic, sulfate-reducing bacteria (SRB). SRB are known to convert inorganic mercury, either naturally occurring in soils or from atmospheric deposition, to methylmercury, which is highly lipid soluble and rapidly accumulates through the food chain. Contaminated fish were then eaten by the Inuit communities, resulting in concentrations of mercury in people that exceed World Health Organization (WHO) guidelines (Callow and Petts, 1992).

Chemical Transformations   A leading example of chemical transformations is the formation of **disinfection by-products** (DBPs). When chlorine is added to drinking water as part of the disinfection process, it reacts with naturally occurring organic compounds present in source and distributed waters. The result is potentially toxic chlorinated by-products. Examples of these compounds include halomethanes such as chloroform, bromoform, dichloromethane, and dibromomethane. Similarly, ozone reacts with naturally occurring bromine to form toxic bromates. DBPs are discussed in more detail later in this chapter. An unanticipated consequence of water treatment practices designed to reduce DBP formation occurred in Washington, D.C. Disinfection practices were changed in 2002 to accommodate anticipated DBP rules being developed by the EPA. Chlorination was changed to chloramination, resulting in lower concentrations of free chlorine available to react with organic compounds. However, the resulting changes in redox chemistry are thought to have resulted in release of previously stable lead from service pipes supplying the many older homes in the District of Columbia area. Lead in drinking water rose to concentrations that in some homes were twenty times higher than EPA action levels. Lead is a potent neurotoxin (see Chapters Eleven, Twelve, and Twenty-Five) that is particularly dangerous for the developing child, hence release of this information caused widespread concern and a rapid (and effective) public health response (Guidotti and others, 2007). However, it is important to note that any event of this magnitude has both economic and political ramifications and, at least over the short term, can cause considerable damage to the reputation of the responsible water and sewer authority.

Deposition, Storage, and Bioconcentration

For many years, it was thought that chemicals discharged into receiving waters would simply be diluted to the point where they could be ignored. In recent years it has become abundantly clear that dilution is no solution. Chapter Two described how chemicals move through the body in predictable ways, a keystone of toxicology; the same is true for chemicals in ecosystems, including hydrologic cycles, as demonstrated in Figure 15.4.

The fate of a given chemical in receiving waters is a function of both its physical and chemical nature. The degree to which a chemical may partition into sediments or into the biota depends to some degree on its partition coefficient, a measure of its relative affinity for an organic solvent (octanol) and water. This in turn depends to some degree on measures of solubility and hydrophobicity. In turn, each of these parameters affects the bioavailability and subsequent toxicity of a given chemical.

Bioavailability   An insoluble metal salt such as cadmium, lead, or copper sulfide or an organic contaminant that is tightly adsorbed to sediment particles is unlikely to be taken up by an organism. Conversely, other substances are physically and chemically available to be taken up, and they are known as **bioavailable**. This concept requires careful definition. Although contaminants resting in undisturbed

FIGURE 15.4   Pesticide Movement in the Hydrologic Cycle,
Including to and from Sediment and Aquatic Biota in the Stream

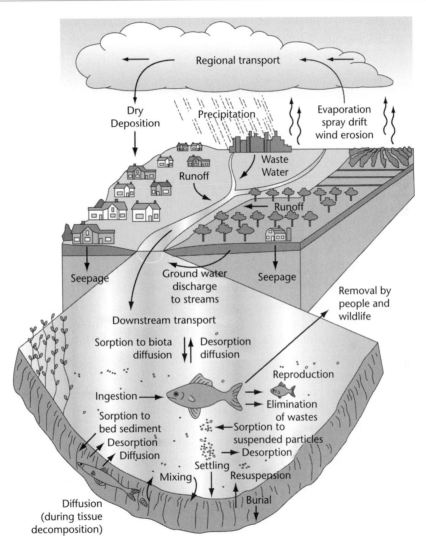

Source: USGS, 2008, as modified from Majewski and Capel, 1995.

sediments may not pose an immediate health threat, their chemical characteristics
may predispose them to accumulate in biological tissues. Such organic or organo-
metallic compounds are generally nonpolar (**hydrophobic**, or "water fearing")
as opposed to polar (**hydrophilic**, or "water loving"). They are relatively insoluble

in water, but once ingested (for example, by benthic invertebrates that burrow in the sediments) they may accumulate through the food chain, as they are readily soluble in lipids. (Excellent textbooks are available to further an understanding of the complexities of chemical partitioning in sediments, water, and the biota; see, for example Schwarzenbach, Gschwend, and Imboden, 1993; Morel and Hering, 1993; Stumm and Morgan, 1996.)

Environmental Reservoirs   Many environments therefore represent potential reservoirs of contaminants. The group of organic compounds that degrade slowly in the environment (the POPs described earlier) includes many of the synthetic organic chemicals mentioned in Table 15.3. Because they generally have low solubility, they tend to partition to sediments, particulate material, or the biota in aquatic systems, where they have been considered no longer bioavailable. One group of POPs that has received attention over the last two decades has been the PCBs. Originally considered inert, PCBs were used extensively in the electronics industry as dielectric material in capacitors and transformers and as binding or insulating materials for a wide range of applications, including building materials. As a result of past disposal practices, numerous sites now exist in the United States and globally where concentrations of PCBs reach levels in the tens of thousands of parts per million. The Hudson River in New York and New Bedford Harbor in Massachusetts are two of the better-known PCB-contaminated Superfund sites in the United States.

Now, however, evidence is accruing that PCBs cause cancer and other health effects in animals (Agency for Toxic Substances and Disease Registry, 2000) and are therefore of concern to human health. PCBs are broken down at extremely slow rates by sediment bacteria. Anaerobic organisms can initially remove chlorine atoms from highly chlorinated PCBs, but the resulting molecules resist further degradation unless exposed to aerobic conditions where other groups of bacteria continue the degradation process. Although considerable research has been undertaken to find ways to accelerate biodegradation in situ, to date these biological processes are so slow that several decades to centuries may be needed to demonstrate substantial levels of degradation. Short of extensive dredging, sediments remain reservoirs of PCBs and sources of exposure through the food chain for the foreseeable future.

Health Effects

A vast number of potentially toxic chemicals have been discharged into or formed in waterways and can potentially end up in surface water and groundwater. Evidence suggests multiple health effects, ranging from birth defects to cancer (Table 15.4). However, the links between waterborne chemical exposures

TABLE 15.4 Examples of Research on Links Between Chemicals in Drinking Water and Increased Health Risk

Place	Contaminant	Source	Health Effect	Certainty	Useful reference
Cape Cod, Massachusetts	Tetrachloroethylene (PCE or perc)	Leachate from vinyl lining of water pipes	Breast cancer	Small to moderate increased risk	Aschengrau, Rogers, and Ozonoff, 2003
Churchill County, Nevada	Tungsten and arsenic	Unknown	Leukemia	Speculative	Centers for Disease Control and Prevention, 2003
Woburn, Massachusetts	Solvents including trichloroethylene (TCE)	Chemical manufacturing wastes	Childhood leukemia	Probable, with caution	Costas, Knorr, and Condon, 2002
Bergen, Essex, Morris, and Passaic Counties, New Jersey	TCE and PCE	Not specified	Leukemia and non-Hodgkins lymphoma	Link with exposure suggested	Cohn and others, 1994
Gassim Region, Saudi Arabia	Petroleum oils	Refineries?	Carcinoma of the esophagus	Speculative	Amer, El-Yazigi, Hannan, and Mohamed, 1990
Northwestern Illinois	TCE, PCE, and other solvents	Landfill?	Bladder cancer	Speculative	Mallin, 1990

and health outcomes have been difficult to prove conclusively. Epidemiological studies face several challenges: exposures that are relatively low and difficult to measure, exposures to the chemicals of concern through other routes than water, the synergistic and antagonistic effects of mixtures of chemicals, and confounding by competing causes of diseases of interest. (These challenges are more fully explained in Chapter Three.)

MICROBIOLOGICAL CONTAMINANTS

After considering sources of microbiological contaminants and how they may be used to indicate water quality, this section describes some specific environmental pathogens of concern and the transformation, deposition, storage, and bioconcentration of microbiological contaminants in the water supply.

Sources

Since ancient times, people have recognized that human and animal wastes can contaminate water and threaten health. A great many pathogenic organisms can be found in water. Many of these are shown in Table 15.5, together with their infectious dose and the diseases they cause. Like chemicals, biological contaminants can come from point sources, such as leaking septic systems, or nonpoint sources, such as runoff from city streets.

Because most (but not all) biological contaminants result from human or animal wastes, waste treatment practices play a major role in water contamination. Sewage is managed in many ways, from the primitive to the highly technical, as illustrated in Figure 15.5. Human waste can be discharged directly to receiving waters through surface water runoff from open defecation sites, a common occurrence in many developing countries, or processed in ways ranging from a simple shallow pit to a larger community sewage system. These latter systems require large volumes of water for efficient operation, so large amounts of wastewater are generated, requiring subsequent treatment before release to receiving waters. **Wastewater treatment** and discharge can place a heavy burden on receiving waters in terms of pathogens, nutrients, and toxic chemicals. For some river systems, wastewater makes up the primary flow during dry seasons. Groundwater can also be contaminated with human pathogens from leaking septic systems, contaminated runoff infiltrating wellheads, and seepage from animal feedlots.

An idealized wastewater treatment process is shown in Figure 15.6, which is loosely based on Boston's Deer Island treatment plant (Massachusetts Water

TABLE 15.5 Pathogens in Drinking Water: Infectious Doses, Diseases, and Additional Comments

	Infectious Dose[a]	Diseases	Comments
Bacteria			
Vibrio cholerae	10^8	Cholera	New toxigenic serogroups with antibiotic resistance
Salmonella spp.	10^{6-7}	Typhoid; salmonellosis	Antibiotic resistance
Shigella spp.	10^2	Shigellosis	Antibiotic resistance
Toxigenic E. coli, for example, E. coli O157	10^{1-9}	Diarrheal diseases Hemolytic-uremic syndrome	Major identified cause of diarrheal disease. Enteropathogenic, enterotoxigenic, and enterohemorrhagic strains identified—include multiple antibiotic resistant strains
Campylobacter spp.	10^6	Campylobacteriosis	Antibiotic resistance
Leptospira spp.	3	Leptospirosis	Increases with flooding events
Francisella tularensis	10	Tularemia	Significance in drinking water unknown
Yersinia enterocolitica	10^9	Yersiniosis	Significance in drinking water unknown
Aeromonas spp.	10^8	Skin and respiratory infections	Gastritis?
Helicobacter pylori	?	Gastric ulcers/cancer	Essentially, exposure route unknown
Legionella pneumophila	>10	Legionellosis Pontiac fever	Underestimated cause of pneumonia
Mycobacterium avium	?	Disseminated infections	Increasing in healthy populations
Burkholderia pseudomallei	~10	Melioidosis	Major cause of water- and soil-borne disease in tropical countries.

(continued)

TABLE 15.5 (Continued)

	Infectious Dose[a]	Diseases	Comments
Protozoa			
Giardia lamblia	1-10	Giardiasis	Underdiagnosed
Cryprosporidium parvum	$1-10^3$	Cryptosporidiosis	Underdiagnosed, extreme chlorine resistance
Naegleria fowleri	High?	Primary amoebic meningoencephalitis	Disease very rare, yet exposures common
Acanthamoeba spp.	?	Encephalitis and others	Transmission of bacterial pathogens?
Entamoeba histolytica	10–100	Dysentery	High rates of infection and associated mortality
Cyclospora cayetanensis	?	Cyclosporidiosis	Most outbreaks associated with contaminated produce
Isospora belli	?		Significance in drinking water unknown
Microsporidia	?	Microsporidiosis	May be widespread
Ballantidium coli	25–100		Significance in drinking water unknown
Toxoplasma gondii	?	Toxoplasmosis	Significance in drinking water unknown
Viruses[b]	1–10	Diarrheal disease, meningitis, heart disease, liver disease, and so forth.	Incidence probably dramatically underestimated; many viruses may remain to be discovered

Note: Data compiled from WHO, 1993; Hazen and Toranzos, 1990; Geldreich, 1996.

[a] Infectious dose is the number of infectious agents that produce infection (asymptomatic or symptomatic) in 50 percent of tested volunteers and is therefore not useful for risk estimates for disease.

[b] Viruses include caliciviruses (especially Norovirus), Poliovirus, Coxsackievirus, Echovirus, Reovirus, Adenovirus, hepatitis A virus, hepatitis E virus, Rotavirus, Astrovirus, Coronavirus, and others to be identified.

Source: Adapted from Ford, 2004.

FIGURE 15.5 Sanitation Options

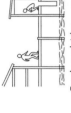

Open defecation — obvious health risks, particularly in built-up areas.

Pit latrine. There are many versions of the pit latrine: simple, borehole, ventilated (shown here), double-pit, pour-flush and off-set pour-flush (both have water traps to prevent flies and odor); each has its own set of advantages, detailed in Franceys, Pockford, and Reed, 1992.

air flow

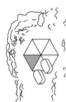

Shallow pit — flies and hookworm problems.

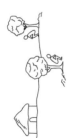

Septic tank — the septic tank (and its smaller version the Aqua-privy) relies on separation of solids (sludge), liquid, and scum. The liquid and scum flow out to an absorption field, and the sludge requires regular mechanical removal. A major concern is the soil type and siting of the absorption field, particularly in relation to drinking-water wells.

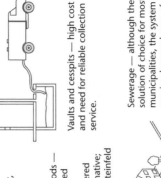

Bucket latrine — door flies, excreta disposal (known as "nightsoil")

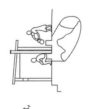

Composting latrine — needs careful operation and separate urine collection. However, composting toilet systems and other similar wastewater management methods — where waste is turned into humus — are increasingly considered the ecological alternative; see Del Porto and Steinfeld 2000.

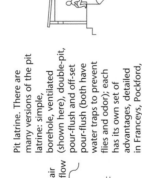

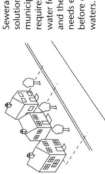

Overhung latrine — severe health risks, particularly for downstream users.

Vaults and cesspits — high cost and need for reliable collection service.

Sewerage — although the solution of choice for most municipalities, the system requires large volumes of water for efficient operation and the collected wastewater needs extensive treatment before discharge to receiving waters.

Source: Diagrams from Franceys and others, 1992. © World Health Organization.

FIGURE 15.6   An Idealized Wastewater Treatment System, Based on Boston's Deer Island System

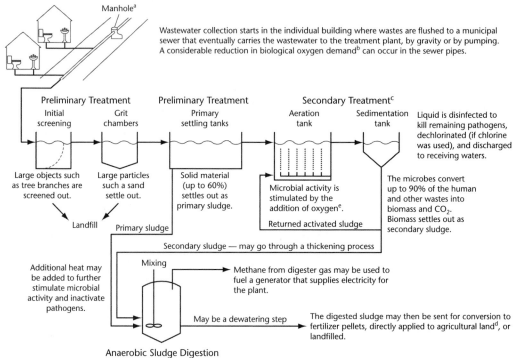

Manhole[a]

Wastewater collection starts in the individual building where wastes are flushed to a municipal sewer that eventually carries the wastewater to the treatment plant, by gravity or by pumping. A considerable reduction in biological oxygen demand[b] can occur in the sewer pipes.

Preliminary Treatment
Initial screening

Preliminary Treatment
Grit chambers

Preliminary Treatment
Primary settling tanks

Secondary Treatment[c]
Aeration tank

Sedimentation tank

Liquid is disinfected to kill remaining pathogens, dechlorinated (if chlorine was used), and discharged to receiving waters.

Large objects such as tree branches are screened out.

Large particles such a sand settle out.

Solid material (up to 60%) settles out as primary sludge.

Microbial activity is stimulated by the addition of oxygen[e].

Returned activated sludge

The microbes convert up to 90% of the human and other wastes into biomass and CO_2. Biomass settles out as secondary sludge.

Landfill

Primary sludge

Secondary sludge — may go through a thickening process

Additional heat may be added to further stimulate microbial activity and inactivate pathogens.

Mixing

Methane from digester gas may be used to fuel a generator that supplies electricity for the plant.

May be a dewatering step

The digested sludge may then be sent for conversion to fertilizer pellets, directly applied to agricultural land[d], or landfilled.

Anaerobic Sludge Digestion
Anaerobic microbes transform sludge primarily to CO_2 and CH_4. Because of the slow growth rate of these microbes relatively little biomass isformed.

Note: Most municipal wastewater can be treated using this or a similar treatment train. However, if industrial or other sources of toxic chemicals are present, wastes may need to undergo far more technologically sophisticated and expensive tertiary treatment. Further discussion of wastewater treatment is beyond the scope of this chapter and many excellent texts are availabl to the reader (for example, Bitton, 1999).

[a] Manholes give access from the street to the main sewer for maintenance. However, there may also be direct connections to street drains in the case of a combined sewer system. This may dramatically increase the volume of wastewater that the treatment plant has to process, often overwhelming the system and allowing untreated wastewater to be released to receiving waters.

[b] **Biological oxygen demand**, or BOD, is a measure of the readily assimilable organic carbon present in wastewater. BOD is defined as the amount of oxygen used by microorganisms in the aerobic degradation of organic wastes over a set time period and temperature (usually five days at 20°C).

[c] Secondary treatment can range from an energy-intensive activated sludge system, where oxygen is added to accelerate microbial activity, to simple aeration ponds, which rely on the action of wind, algae, and macrophytes to facilitate oxygen transfer.

[d] Land application of sewage sludge is facing increasingly stringent regulations due to concerns about pathogens and toxic chemicals in the food chain and about potential contamination of ground and surface waters.

Resources Authority, 2008). Systems such as this are expensive to build and maintain, and in general only the wealthiest municipalities can afford such extensive systems.

In recent years **waterborne disease outbreaks** in North America have been linked to exceptionally heavy rainfall and resultant flooding. This is not surprising given the increased emphasis on high-density farming practices and their proximity to water supplies. Two outbreaks are illustrative: the outbreak of cryptosporidiosis in Milwaukee in 1993 and the outbreak of *Escherichia coli* O157 in Walkerton, Ontario, in 2000. (These and other outbreaks are discussed in detail by Hrudey and Hrudey, 2004.)

The Milwaukee outbreak was the largest documented waterborne disease outbreak in the United States. An estimated 400,000 people became ill, and there were more than 50 associated deaths. At the time of this outbreak, the city's water routinely underwent complete treatment (coagulation, sedimentation, rapid sand filtration, and chlorination), disinfection (1.5 mg/L chlorine) was not deficient or interrupted, and met standards for coliforms (<1/100 mL) and turbidity (<1 NTU [nephelometric turbidity unit]) were met. Afterward, operational lapses were identified, including poor mixing during coagulation and restarting of dirty filters without backwashing. However, the root cause was presumably massive numbers of *Cryptosporidium parvum* oocysts being washed into Milwaukee's source water, Lake Michigan, close to the city's water intakes. A number of sources of contamination were suspected, including runoff from farms, sewage treatment, or other unidentified sources during the heavy rainfalls that preceded the outbreak (Mac Kenzie and others, 1994). Archived stool samples subsequently showed that the *C. parvum* were all the human genotype (type 1), strongly suggesting that human sewage was in fact the source (Sulaiman and others, 1998).

The 2000 outbreak of *E. coli* O157 in Walkerton, Ontario, sickened hundreds of people and caused seven deaths. In this case the indicator organism, *E. coli*, was measured in drinking water, but no action was immediately taken. The root cause was presumably *E. coli* O157 and other pathogens, such as *Campylobacter*, contaminating a shallow well that was sited inappropriately close to an adjacent cattle farm. Retrospective studies established *E. coli* O157:H7 and *Campylobacter* as the primary agents of the outbreak, with strains matched between stool samples, water samples, and manure samples by molecular typing methods (discussed in Hrudey and Hrudey, 2004). The accompanying Perspective provides a chronology of the outbreak. However, the reader is also referred to the *Report of the Walkerton Inquiry* (O'Connor, 2002) for fascinating insights into this tragic event, the lessons learned, and the political ramifications from waterborne disease deaths that few would think could happen in developed countries.

PERSPECTIVE
Chronology of Events During the Walkerton, Ontario, *E. Coli* O157 Outbreak in 2000

The town of Walkerton, Ontario, was taking part of its source water from a well adjacent to a local farming operation. Problems began around May 2000.

May 12	Heavy rains sustained for several days are thought to have caused pathogens in cattle manure either to infiltrate the well-head or to contaminate the aquifer through seepage.
May 17	Tests of the drinking water indicated the presence of Coliforms and *E. coli*, in samples taken on May 15. However, the general manager of the Public Utilities Commission failed to notify appropriate health official.
May 18	Walkerton residents begin to report symptoms of gastrointestinal illness; two children with bloody diarrhea are hospitalized.
May 19	Health officials contact the Public Utilities Commission and are assured that the water is safe.
May 20–21	The number of illnesses continues to rise. The government health officer orders a "boil water" advisory, despite continued assurances from the utility personnel.
May 22	First person dies.
May 23	Independent tests show that *E. coli* O157:H7 is present in the drinking water. Hundreds of people complain of symptoms, more than 150 people seek hospital treatment, and a two-year-old girl dies.
May 24	Two more deaths.
May 25	Fifth death, and four children listed as critical.
May 29	Sixth death.
May 30	Seventh death.
May 31	Public inquiry ordered.

Outcome. The utility had been falsifying records for some time, and the chlorination system had not been working properly. The utility operator "did not like the taste of chlorine." Class action suits and criminal investigations have followed, but the real outcome of this tragedy is the implementation of far stricter regulations for Ontario's drinking water—and the realization that proper operator training is critical.

Source: Adapted from Ford and others, 2005.

The Indicator Concept

Monitoring the microbiological quality of water requires measurable **indicators**. Although many microbial species could be chosen for this purpose (see Table 15.6), the traditional indicator has been the coliform group. The premise has been that the concentration of coliform organisms reflects the overall microbial quality of water. Methods to detect and quantify coliform counts have become increasingly sophisticated. In the early 1900s, growth of bacteria on a nutrient agar plate at 37°C was thought to be indicative of possible contamination by enteric organisms (reviewed in Payment, Sartory, and Reasoner, 2003). In more recent decades, coliform bacteria were enumerated in selective liquid culture media, using a technique known as the *most probable number* method. More recently the *membrane filtration* technique has gained in popularity, and currently *enzyme specific assays*, which are accurate and can be easily conducted by water utility personnel, have gained favor. (Geldreich, 1996, provides a good discussion of these tests.)

However, the indicator concept with its reliance on total coliform counts has recently been challenged. Once human pathogens have contaminated ground and surface waters, their fate is very much organism specific. In fact the coliform group is inactivated relatively rapidly, whereas other human pathogens can survive for extended periods. This is particularly true for the pathogenic protozoa that form highly resistant cysts or oocysts and the viruses that appear to survive adsorbed to particulate material. As a result, a reassuringly low coliform count could belie a dangerous level of other organisms. Alternative approaches to monitoring water quality might include using direct measurements of *E. coli*, perhaps using molecular tools, rather than of total coliforms as the primary indicator of fecal contamination and also using indicators of viral and protozoan contamination. (The advantages and shortcomings of the indicator approach have been discussed extensively in the literature; useful references are available on the American Academy for Microbiology Web site; Ford and Colwell, 1995; Rose and Grimes, 2001.)

Environmental Pathogens

There is also a wide range of environmental pathogens—organisms that although they may be discharged in human sewage are distinguished by their ability not only to persist in the environment but also to grow and proliferate. Two of the better-known examples of this type of pathogen are *Legionella pneumophila* and the environmental mycobacteria.

As with exposure to chemicals, exposure to **waterborne pathogens** can occur through multiple transmission routes. Some are obvious, such as ingestion

TABLE 15.6   The Indicator Approach

Indicator	What does it indicate	Limitations
Coliforms	Presence of the coliform group of bacteria, many of which are present in human or animal fecal material.	Certain coliforms grow naturally in drinking-water biofilms, particularly at warmer temperatures. Not indicative of protozoa or viruses.
E. coli	Presence of E. coli; strong indication of fecal contamination.	Inactivated more rapidly than other pathogens. Not indicative of protozoa or viruses.
Coliphage	Presence of viruses specific to E. coli.	May or may not be indicative of viral pathogens. Not indicative of protozoa or bacteria.
Enterococci	May be indicative of presence of animal wastes as well as human waste.	Not indicative of protozoa or viruses.
Clostridium	Presence of spore-forming bacteria; anaerobes; protozoa.	Not indicative of viruses.
Pseudomonas	Survives in drinking-water biofilms; may indicate presence of bacterial pathogens that are more persistent than the coliforms.	Not indicative of protozoa or viruses.
Aeromonads	Survives in drinking-water biofilms; may indicate presence of bacterial pathogens that are more persistent than the coliforms.	Not indicative of protozoa or viruses.
Human-specific Bacteroides fragilis bacteriophage	Presence of viruses specific to B. fragilis; may be present when coliphage is absent.	May or may not be indicative of viral pathogens. Not indicative of protozoa or bacteria.
Turbidity	May indicate that the water exceeds turbidity regulations. Some studies show increased risk for waterborne disease at high turbidity (pathogens adhere to particles).	Only measures turbidity; cannot be directly correlated to pathogen loading.
Residual chlorine	Measures the disinfectant residual at the tap. Absence of residual chlorine has been shown in some studies to be consistent with waterborne disease.	Only measures residual chlorine; cannot be directly correlated to pathogen loading.

of contaminated water or exposure through recreational use, either through unintended ingestion or through skin abrasions or alternative *portals of entry* (eye, ear, anal, urogenital). Other, perhaps less obvious, routes of exposure include breathing contaminated aerosols arising from showers, toilet flushing, dish washing, garden hoses, fountains, waterfalls, and cooling towers and from air conditioner, humidifier, and refrigerator drip pans. Many infectious agents are also transmitted through use of hot tubs and whirlpool spas.

PERSPECTIVE
The Hidden Hazards of Hot Tubs

When you next decide to bathe in a hot tub, indoor swimming pool, or even your shower, you will not be alone! Many bacteria find these environments ideal for survival and proliferation. In particular the environmental mycobacteria have been implicated in a number of outbreaks of the pulmonary disease known as *hot tub lung*. *Legionella pneumophila* has caused outbreaks of legionellosis and Pontiac fever and *Pseudomonas aeruginosa* has been implicated in outbreaks of folliculitis. In addition, *lifeguard lung*, a form of hypersensitivity pneumonitis, is associated with frequent exposure to pool aerosols containing endotoxin, a cell-wall component of gram-negative bacteria. In fact bacteria thrive in these environments, particularly in piping systems where water remains stagnant for much of the time, and are probably associated with biofilms (discussed in the section on storage).

Transformations

Like chemical contaminants, microbial contaminants can be transformed once they are discharged into receiving waters. Often these changes result in less risk to humans. Environmental stress can rapidly inactivate a number of pathogenic organisms, or at least create a viable but nonculturable (Colwell and others, 1985) or *injured* (Singh and McFeters, 1990) state. However, those same stress factors might also increase an organism's virulence. One way in which this may occur is through adaptation to intracellular survival and growth. Research suggests that some pathogens can survive, resist chlorine, and even grow within protozoan hosts. Examples include species of *Escherichia, Citrobacter, Enterobacter, Klebsiella, Salmonella, Yersinia, Shigella, Legionella,* and *Campylobacter* (King, Shotts, Wooley, and Porter, 1988). More recently, some environmental mycobacteria have been shown to survive in protozoan hosts (reviewed in Pedley and others, 2004). At least in the case of *Legionella* and the mycobacteria, adaptation to the protozoan host may be a mechanism that allows the pathogens to elude the human immune system through intracellular survival and growth in macrophages (reviewed in Samrakandi, Ridenour, Yan, and Cirillo, 2002).

Vibrio cholerae, the organism that causes cholera, presents a special case of an interaction between a pathogen and plankton, one that can be viewed as an environmental transformation. The *Vibrio* associates with plankton, particularly zooplankton such as copepods, a strategy that appears to allow it to multiply and concentrate to infectious doses. Although this may not directly increase virulence, it seems to play a role in initiating the cycle of epidemic cholera transmission (Colwell, 1996).

Deposition, Storage and Bioconcentration

Just as chemicals may accumulate in higher organisms, a number of different pathogens can become concentrated in organisms. The best-known examples of such organisms are filter feeding shellfish, such as oysters and clams. Outbreaks of food poisoning often occur as the result of consumption of shellfish that have concentrated planktonic algae, viruses, bacteria, or even protozoa. Infectious disease outcomes from eating contaminated shellfish, crustacea, and fish that contain concentrated fecal wastes include hepatitis A, norovirus, campylobacteriosis, salmonellosis, cryptosporidiosis, and *Vibrio*-related diseases including cholera. In fact any infectious disease agent transmissible by water could potentially be concentrated in aquatic organisms.

What about storage reservoirs for pathogens? Early studies showed that the fecal coliform indicator organisms (Table 15.6) were concentrated 100- to 1,000-fold more in bottom sediments compared with overlying waters (Van Donsel and Geldreich, 1971). Similarly, salmonella and other pathogens have been shown to survive in sediments for extended periods. Recent research suggests that salmonella may even be transmitted from contaminated sediments via chironomid (midge) larvae (Moore, Martinez, Gay, and Rice, 2003).

Biofilms   An important *storage area* is the **biofilm**, or slime, that forms on any surface in contact with water but is of particular concern in drinking-water pipes. Biofilms provide protective environments that may allow microbes to survive chemical stressors such as disinfectants in the overlying water and may even allow certain pathogens (for example, *Legionella*, the mycobacteria, and others) to proliferate. Biofilms are also known to contribute to pipeline degradation, "dirty water," odor, and blockage (Ford, 1993). They are also nutrient-rich environments that potentially provide ideal conditions for gene transfer (including virulence factors or antibiotic resistance factors) between microbes in close proximity.

Wildlife and Wildfowl   The other major environmental reservoir for pathogens consists of wildlife and wildfowl. Many enteric pathogens, such as *Salmonella* species, are natural inhabitants of the intestinal tracts of both warm- and cold-blooded animals. Others may be fortuitously carried through the intestinal tracts of wildlife and wildfowl due to their presence in human and animal garbage. Wildfowl have emerged as a particular concern for protected watersheds. However well the perimeter of a body of surface water is fenced, only the smallest areas can be effectively covered. Scavenger birds such as gulls may be a particular problem, as they are attracted to human garbage. A USGS report (Converse, Woolcott, Dockerty, and Cole, 2001) reviewed studies that showed that *Campylobacter, Listeria, Salmonella, Escherichi coli, Cryptosporidium, Chlamydia,* Rotavirus, and other potentially pathogenic genera of microbes have been isolated from feces of wildfowl, including gulls, Canada geese, and ducks.

THE GLOBAL BURDEN OF WATERBORNE DISEASE

The primary source of information on the **global burden of disease** is the World Health Organization (2008b). The most recent statistics available, for 2002, report both mortality and morbidity (reported as disability-adjusted life years, or **DALYs**), to express both the years lost through premature death and the severity of disease. This information is obtained through national registries that are estimated to represent about 30 percent of the global burden of disease. Although waterborne disease is not specifically identified, the category of **diarrheal disease** is included, as are malaria and a number of other tropical diseases related to water. From these data, WHO estimates that diarrheal disease amounts to an estimated 4.1 percent of the total DALY global burden of disease (61.1 million DALYs) and is responsible for the deaths of 1.8 million people every year. This burden is comparable to the mortality and morbidity figures for other leading infectious diseases: 2.8 million deaths and 86.1 million DALYs for HIV/AIDS; 1.6 million deaths and 35.4 million DALYs for tuberculosis; and 1.2 million deaths and 44.7 million DALYs for malaria.

In the case of diarrheal disease, multiple routes of exposure to infectious (and chemical) causes exist, including water, food, and person-to-person transmission. However, it is virtually impossible to distinguish these routes clearly, as the spread of diarrheal disease within a population can be dominated by **secondary transmission**. An initial infection may be caused by consumption of contaminated drinking water but may then rapidly spread through person-to-person transmission or through food contaminated by the water itself or by the infected individual. Since 2002, WHO has identified risk factors for the global burden of disease (Lopez and others, 2006). Building on this information, the most recent publication from WHO suggests that on a global scale, 88 percent of cases of diarrhea are the result of poor hygiene and sanitation, including unsafe water (Prüss-Üstün, Bos, Gore, and Bartram, 2008). WHO also estimates that these cases of diarrheal disease result in 1.5 million deaths per year, primarily among children. The report's analysis suggests that approximately 10 percent of the global burden of all diseases is related to water and is therefore preventable.

When examining the global burden of waterborne disease, several considerations are important:

1. WHO figures are based on numbers reported by individual member states and undoubtedly underestimate the burden of diarrheal disease. Questionnaire-based studies to examine community incidence of gastrointestinal disease suggest that officially reported figures may underestimate actual incidence by several hundredfold (reviewed in Ford, 1999).
2. *The World Health Report for 1996* suggests that 70 percent of diarrheal episodes are caused by contaminated foods (WHO, 1996). However, water may play a role in this pathway, as contaminated water may have been used in food preparation.
3. Diarrheal disease is not the only disease outcome from waterborne contaminants (discussed in Ford and Colwell, 1995).
4. WHO figures may understate the importance of waterborne diseases. Patients with HIV/AIDs often die of opportunistic infections, including waterborne diseases such as cryptosporidiosis and disseminated infections from environmental mycobacteria. Therefore some deaths attributed to HIV/AIDS may also be attributable to waterborne diseases.
5. Malaria is considered a water-related disease, and anthropogenic changes to the watershed may increase the habitat for mosquitoes that carry the protozoan pathogen.

Vector-Borne Diseases

Some of the most prevalent and deadly infectious diseases in the world are transmitted by vectors related to water (see Table 15.7). In fact water plays a critical role in **vector-borne disease** transmission. The mortality and morbidity figures for malaria show increasing counts since 2000 (WHO, 2008c). Clearly, the global burden of suffering from malaria remains vast. Other major vector-borne diseases whose life cycles are associated with water include those caused by blood, liver, lung, and gastrointestinal flukes; hemorrhagic viruses; hemoflagellate protozoa; blood and tissue nematodes; and tapeworms. Their vectors include mosquitoes, blackflies, crustacea, and fish.

TABLE 15.7   Examples of Vector-Borne Diseases with Risk Factors Associated with Water

Disease	Pathogen	Vector	Risk factors	Control strategies
Malaria	*Plasmodium falciparum, P. vivax, P. malariae,* and *P. ovale* (protozoa)	Anopheles mosquitoes	Standing water (mosquito breeding sites); being outdoors in malaria endemic areas, particularly in the evenings; no prior exposures	Removal of standing water; use of chemoprophylaxis, bed nets, behavior modification, insecticide sprays
Onchocerciasis (river blindness)	*Onchocerca volvulus* (nematode)	*Simulium* spp. (blackflies)	Flowing streams with vegetation	Avoiding endemic areas
Schistosomiasis	*Schistosoma mansoni, S. japonicum,* and *S. haematobium* (trematodes)	Snails	Flooding; damming; creation of irrigation ditches	Destruction of snails or habitat; avoiding contact with water in endemic areas; proper disposal of human waste
Dracunculiasis	*Dracunculus medinensis* (guinea worm— nematode)	Copepod	Contaminated drinking water	Provision of disinfected drinking water; prevention of source water contamination
West Nile encephalitis	West Nile virus (Flavivirus)	Culex mosquitoes	Standing water; vegetation; discarded tires (when holding stagnant water)	Removal of standing water; use of screens, behavior modification, insecticide sprays
Lymphatic filariasis (elephantiasis)	*Wuchereria* spp. and *Brugia* spp.	Culex, anopheles, and aedes mosquitoes	Standing water, and so forth	Mass drug administration; use of insecticides
Fish tapeworm	*Diphyllobothrium* spp. (cestoda)	Copepods and fish	Ingestion of undercooked or raw fish	Thorough cooking

Waterborne diseases may be controlled, and in some cases eliminated, through changes in water sources, water quality, and human behavior, offering enormous prospects for public health advances. The effort to control dracunculiasis is perhaps the best example of a successful eradication program (aside from the program that eradicated smallpox). **Dracunculiasis** is an extremely debilitating disease caused by ingestion of copepods carrying the guinea worm. The disease causes extraordinary suffering to people in the poorer nations who depend on low-quality water sources. Essentially through hygiene education and water source protection, a disease that previously infected millions of people every year has been reduced to about 10,000 cases in 2008, localized to Sudan, Ghana, Nigeria, Niger, and Mali (Carter Center, 2008). (See the Perspective "Dracunculiasis Eradication" for a description of the rapid decline in dracunculiasis cases and the measures currently being undertaken.)

PERSPECTIVE
Dracunculiasis Eradication

In the 1980s, millions of people were infected with dracunculiasis (guinea worm disease), and hundreds of millions were considered at risk from contaminated water. The guinea worm's larvae live in copepods in water. When a person drinks the contaminated water, the ingested larvae begin to burrow into surrounding tissues and mate. The males die, but the females may grow to a meter in length and contain millions of embryos. The female eventually migrates to the skin surface and breaks through, causing intense pain with severe risks of secondary infections of the ulcerated tissue. Before the female breaks through the skin, approximately one year after initial infection, the victim may be unaware of the infection. He or she typically bathes the infected ulcer in water, and this releases the larvae, which subsequently mature in the copepod host to complete the cycle. In 1986 and again in 1991, the World Health Organization established the Dracunculiasis Eradication Program, effectively reducing incidence of the disease by 95 percent (WHO data are reported in Spearman, 1998). Since then, progress is continuing and each year new countries report the successful elimination of the disease. Today, dracunculiasis remains in the poorest countries which lack access to clean water. The Sudan has clearly been one of the major problem areas.

Eradication of the disease is relatively straightforward—stopping the transmission cycle. Because there is no treatment for the disease once acquired, programs focus,

Waterborne Diseases

Although a wide range of diseases is caused by waterborne pathogens (Table 15.5), the most common outcome, and the one that most frequently remains undiagnosed, is **acute gastrointestinal infection** (AGI). AGI can be caused by viruses, bacteria, or protozoa. In addition, symptoms similar to AGI may be caused by chemical contaminants. The etiology of waterborne disease is strongly affected by the sources of the infectious agents. For example, *Shigella* species are primarily human pathogens, and shigellosis outbreaks can usually be associated with contamination from human sewage. *E. coli, Campylobacter, Salmonella,* and many of the protozoan and viral pathogens are zoonotic. In other words, they are also associated with livestock, wildlife, and wildfowl. Hence, fecal contamination of water from any of these sources can result in a waterborne disease outbreak, which is why there is increasing concern about high-density animal

first, on identifying infected individuals and preventing them from recontaminating water sources and, second, on educating people to filter or boil drinking water (relatively coarse filtration material can remove the copepods) and on treating selected water sources to kill the copepods.

Together with UNICEF, the Centers for Disease Control and Prevention (CDC), and the Carter Center, WHO has adopted the following strategy (WHO, 2008a).

- Implement effective case containment measures in all endemic villages.
- Establish community-based surveillance systems in every known endemic village with monthly reporting of cases, supervision, and integration of surveillance for other major preventable diseases.
- Target the implementation of specific interventions including the provision of safe water, health education, community mobilization, filter distribution, and treatment of infected water sources with temephos insecticide (Abate®).
- Map all endemic villages and maintain global and national dracunculiasis databases for monitoring of the epidemiological situation using HealthMap software.
- Sustain and strengthen advocacy for eradication of the disease
- Manage the certification process for dracunculiasis eradication country by country world-wide.

husbandry practices, particularly in areas prone to flooding (Wing, Freedman, and Band, 2002).

Viral Diseases Viruses are increasingly implicated as major causative agents of AGI. In the United States alone, it has been estimated that 80 percent of the 38.6 million annual cases of gastroenteritis are caused by viruses (Mead and others, 1999). Of well over 100 known viruses that can potentially be transmitted in drinking water, the caliciviruses and rotaviruses are most commonly diagnosed. However, types of Poliovirus, Coxsackievirus, Echovirus, Reovirus, Adenovirus, hepatitis A, Astrovirus, Coronavirus, and hepatitis E have been implicated in waterborne outbreaks and there may be many further, as yet uncharacterized, groups of viruses that could cause AGI and other disease manifestations.

Scientific understanding of the role of viruses in waterborne diarrhea has been limited by the difficulties inherent both in their specific diagnosis and in measurement of the agents in drinking water and food. For example, the caliciviruses are now thought to be the major causes of both food and waterborne illness worldwide, but research has been limited by the fact that until 2007, no research groups had successfully cultured the caliciviruses involved in human infections. This fascinating family of viruses first came to light in 1972 after electron microscopists identified small round particles in samples from an outbreak of AGI that had occurred in Norwalk, Ohio, four years earlier, sickening 50 percent of children and teachers at an elementary school. Analysis of surveillance data between 1995 and 2000 in Europe suggested that this specific group of caliciviruses (one of potentially four different *Calicivirus* genera), now known as noroviruses, accounts for more than 85 percent of all nonbacterial outbreaks of gastroenteritis (Lopman and others, 2003). In the United States, Mead and others (1999) have estimated that noroviruses cause 23 million cases of gastroenteritis each year.

Three distinct groups pathogenic to humans have now been identified using molecular epidemiology techniques (reviewed in Lopman, Brown, and Koopmans, 2002). This approach amplifies and "fingerprints" genetic material (in this case RNA), so researchers can compare potential sources of infection with clinical samples. Using these techniques, it has been shown that caliciviruses are transmitted through drinking water, shellfish, uncooked foods such as salads and fruits, food handling, environmental exposures (bathing, using contaminated surfaces, and so forth), and person to person. In fact, person-to-person transmission is thought to be the major route of infection, including infection through aerosol formation caused by the *projectile vomiting* characteristic of these infections. Further advances in molecular epidemiology may also show that animals are a source of infection, as they have been shown to be infected by strains of calicivirus that are quite similar to the three human pathogen groups. The clinical and public health significance of human caliciviruses is considerable, particularly as there appears to be no long-term immunity to these agents in humans. In early 2007, Straub and coworkers reported successfully infecting and replicating human norovirus in a cell culture model (Straub and others, 2007). Although it is currently unclear whether this work has been repeated to date, this opens the door to a far better understanding of the pathogenesis of this important virus.

Bacterial Diseases   Of the bacterial diseases, campylobacteriosis remains the most common form of bacterial dysentery, followed by pathogenic *E. coli* infection, salmonellosis, and shigellosis. The global incidence of these diseases is difficult to estimate. In the United States, Morris and Levin (1995) estimated that bacteria in water cause 35,000 case of shigellosis, 59,000 cases of salmonellosis, 150,000 cases of *E. coli* infection, and 320,000 cases of campylobacteriosis each year. These diseases are of course prevalent worldwide, but many other infectious agents that are relatively under control in developed countries remain epidemic in other countries. Cholera (caused by *Vibrio cholerae*) and typhoid (caused by *Salmonella typhi*) are perhaps the best-known examples of waterborne disease that have caused global pandemics in the past. Typhoid tends to emerge in less developed countries in epidemic proportions where sanitation is compromised. This happened in Chile during the 1980s and was attributed, at least in part, to irrigation of vegetables with wastewater, increased rainfall, inadequate water treatment, and a deteriorating economy (Cabello and Springer, 1997).

On a global basis, morbidity and mortality from *E. coli* infections are today thought to exceed those of cholera and other identified waterborne disease. The *E. coli* strains that produce enterotoxin (**enterotoxigenic *E. coli,* or ETEC**), can also be enteropathogenic (causing intestinal disease) or enterohemorrhagic (causing intestinal bleeding), as in the notorious *E. coli* O157-H7 outbreak in Walkerton, Ontario, described earlier. Estimates of morbidity and mortality from cholera are in the tens of thousands per year. In contrast, ETEC are estimated to cause approximately 400 million diarrheal episodes, with 700,000 deaths each year among children younger than five (reported in Chakraborty and others, 2001).

Many opportunistic pathogens can also be transmitted through water. These include species of *Aeromonas, Pseudomonas, Klebsiella,* and others. It is extremely difficult to estimate the contributions of these agents to morbidity and mortality through consumption of drinking water. Certainly they are a major cause of hospital-acquired infections with high associated mortality risks. Other opportunistic pathogens of interest include *Legionella,* the nontuberculous mycobacteria and *Helicobacter pylori. Legionella* and the nontuberculous mycobacteria occupy a unique niche in their ability to proliferate in hot water systems, their environmental ubiquity, and their resistance to disinfection. In the case of *Legionella,* the global burden of disease is thought to exceed reported numbers by a wide margin. In the United States it has been estimated that *Legionella* causes at least 13,000 cases of bacterial pneumonia per year (Breiman and Butler, 1998). Researchers are divided on whether water is a significant route for dissemination of *Helicobacter pylori*.

Cholera remains both **epidemic** and **pandemic** (affecting multiple countries) due in part to its ability to survive and multiply in the environment associated with plankton and other aquatic organisms (Colwell, 1996). There have now been seven pandemics of cholera since 1817, the most recent of which reached South America in 1991 and reportedly caused more than a million cases and 10,000 deaths by 1994 (Pan American Health Organization, 1995). Several possible theories have been offered to account for cholera's arrival in South America, including transport in a ship's bilge water (associated with plankton), transport in infected individuals, and transport in imported foods. Alternatively, the disease could have been endemic, surviving in the environment and only emerging at a time of compromised sanitation, after the continent had been free of epidemic cholera for more than 100 years. The truth may never be known, but it seems increasingly likely that the aquatic environment provided a niche for *V. cholerae* (Salazar-Lindo, Seas, and Gutierrez, 2008). Blooms of aquatic organisms have been associated with cholera outbreaks in Bangladesh (Colwell and Huq, 1994) and may have contributed to the rapid spread of cholera in South America. The ecological linkages are fascinating and the reader is encouraged to examine the growing literature on this topic. The correlations between environmental factors such as sea surface temperature, salinity, chlorophyll, and cholera outbreaks have led to an exciting new area of epidemic disease prediction using satellite imaging (Gil and others, 2004).

Cholera is of particular interest because there is evidence that it is beginning to change. The causative agent of the past seven pandemics has been *V. cholerae* serogroup O1. In the early 1990s, *V. cholerae* serogroup O139 emerged in India in epidemic form, the first time that a non-O1 serogroup of *V. cholerae* was shown to cause epidemic cholera. There is now molecular evidence that O139 strains were derived from O1 strains through genetic modification (Faruque, Albert, and Mekalanos, 1998). It is important to learn more about the conditions that resulted in emergence of the toxigenic O139 serogroups, and could therefore result in many more, perhaps environmentally hardier, serogroups of this pathogen. The emergence of epidemic strains could occur through mutation of existing strains or through gene transfer. This is diagramatically represented in Figure 15.7. Although the example is *V. cholerae*, this principle could equally apply to other pathogens, such as the toxigenic *E. coli*. In the case of gene transfer, virulence factors could also be transferred between species. Both mutation and gene transfer would appear possible within the drinking-water distribution system, where

FIGURE 15.7 Emergence of New Epidemic Serogroups of *Vibrio Cholerae*

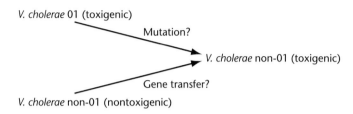

V. cholerae 01 (toxigenic)

Mutation?

V. cholerae non-01 (toxigenic)

Gene transfer?

V. cholerae non-01 (nontoxigenic)

Source: Ford, 2004.

organisms are likely to be exposed to a variety of stressors, such as chlorine and metal ions (Ford, 1993).

Protozoal Diseases Protozoa receive considerable media attention due to the size of recent outbreaks, which are partially due to low infectious doses and high resistance to water treatment. *Cryptosporidium parvum* has attracted most attention, with *C. parvum* replacing *Giardia lamblia* as the most common cause of waterborne disease outbreaks in the United Kingdom and the second most common cause in the United States In the case of cryptosporidia, global distribution is far broader than reported, due in part to misdiagnosis. For example, in Russia, where monitoring for the pathogen has been introduced only in the last few years, recent seroprevalence studies (studies that examine whether or not antibodies to a specific pathogen are present in blood samples) suggested that almost 90 percent of the population sampled had been exposed to cryptosporidium infection (Egorov and others, 2004). Studies by the same authors found cryptosporidium oocysts in most source waters tested and in stool samples of approximately 7 percent of people with diarrhea (Egorov and others, 2002).

Additional protozoa of current interest include cyclospora and toxoplasma, although a waterborne route of transmission is far from proven. A third group of protozoa, the microsporidia, are smaller than other protozoa and are increasingly recognized as causative agents of both human and animal diseases. They are also more likely to penetrate filtration systems than the larger protozoa are, so it is reasonable to suspect a waterborne route of exposure. (A number of publications provide useful in-depth reviews of the protozoan pathogens; see, for example, Marshall, Naumovitz, Ortega, and Sterling, 1997; Hunter, 1997.)

Fungal Diseases Studies have suggested that fungal species including *Aspergillus* spp., *Cladosporium* spp., *Epicoccum* spp., *Penicillium* spp., and *Trichoderma* spp. can be frequently isolated from treated drinking water (Arvanitidou, Kanellou, Constantinides, and Katsouyannopoulos, 1999). *Candida* yeasts are also occasionally isolated from drinking water and apparently correlate with levels of the indicator organisms total and fecal coliforms. A number of fungi and yeasts isolated from drinking water are potential pathogens or at least can produce toxic metabolites and readily spoil foods.

Viroids and Prions   To date there is no direct evidence of transmission of viroids through water. Viroids, consisting of single-stranded RNA, are thought to cause only plant diseases. Like similar infectious agents known as satellite RNAs which are dependent on a helper virus for replication, these agents are unlikely to pose a serious threat to human health through drinking water. Of course the absence of any information linking these agents to human disease does not mean that in future linkages will not emerge. For example, the hepatitis Delta agent is essentially a viroid encapsulated in a hepatitis B coat.

In contrast, prions, infectious proteinaceous material, have risen to prominence following the devastating economic threat and perceived human health threat from the bovine spongiform encephalopathy (BSE) outbreak in the United Kingdom (The BSE Inquiry, 2000). Although prions have not been isolated from drinking waters, it is reasonable to consider the risks of contamination of water from, for example, rendering wastes, abattoirs, and landfills.

SAFE DRINKING WATER

For most developing countries, **hygiene** and **sanitation** remain the cornerstones of public health. The simplest interventions, such as educating people to avoid defecation near drinking-water sources, use cloth filtration, and put up bed nets (to reduce exposure to mosquitoes), can dramatically reduce the burden of disease (reviewed in Ford and Hamner, 2009). In more developed nations, a **multibarrier approach** is more economically feasible, so that the process of making drinking water safe extends from the source to the faucet, with protection of water sources from contamination, water treatment to remove contamination, and protection of water from recontamination during distribution.

Source Protection

Probably the most important consideration for the protection of human health in relation to potable water supplies is provision of high-quality source water. **Watershed protection** is critical to this process but often comes into direct conflict with development and with recreational uses of watersheds. In many metropolitan areas development has dramatically outstripped the availability of high-quality source water. Inevitably, many municipalities are dependent today on surface waters that receive wastewaters, both treated and untreated. Protection of source water involves maintaining generous buffers, limiting access for recreational purposes, and preventing agricultural and industrial uses. Many would argue that all wildlife and wildfowl should be prevented from accessing source water, however impractical this may be. New York City has gone to extraordinary lengths to protect upstate source water, as described in the accompanying Perspective. This approach turned out to be more cost effective than treating water arriving from contaminated sources.

Water Treatment

Given that many source waters are of poor quality and that even high-quality source water can become contaminated, some level of water treatment is considered essential. Arguably, the water treatment process begins with conveyance of water from the source to the plant. Prevention of contamination during conveyance, which in certain cases could be hundreds of miles of pipeline, aqueduct, or even open ditches, is clearly important.

Water treatment consists of several sequential steps (Figure 15.9). Water entering the treatment plant may undergo coarse filtration to remove vegetation, trash, dead animals, and other large solids. Chemicals may be added for specific purposes; for example, potassium permanganate may be added to oxidize soluble iron and manganese, making them easier to remove. (These metals, when present, discolor water and stain clothing and plumbing fixtures.) The next step is coagulation and precipitation. In this step a chemical such as aluminum sulfate is added, together with lime and sodium bicarbonate, which causes suspended solids, bacteria, and other particles to clump together into *floc*. The floc is allowed to settle out, removing these materials from the water. Filtration comes next, although in some plants a disinfecting step, such as ozonation, is added to reduce microbial counts and prevent excessive microbial growth on filter materials. Filtration methods range from simple, time-honored techniques such as slow sand filtration to sophisticated technologies such as nanofiltration, depending on the resources available and the size of population served.

The final step is postfiltration disinfection. Since the early twentieth century, chlorination has been the most widely used form of disinfection. Chlorine and chlorine compounds are thought to act as disinfectants by denaturing enzymes. Chlorine has the advantage of forming a residual in water as it flows from the treatment plant through the pipes of the distribution system to faucets. This helps prevent regrowth of microorganisms in the distribution system (although biofilms

PERSPECTIVE
Protecting Source Water for New York City

Early settlers in what is now New York obtained water from shallow wells. The chronology of subsequent water source development for New York City, adapted from a history of the New York City Water System (New York City Department of Environmental Protection, 2008), is presented in the following list:

1677	The first public well is dug.
1776	A local reservoir is constructed to serve a population of approximately 22,000. Water is distributed through hollow logs.
Early 1800s	Local wells and reservoirs become polluted and supply is insufficient. The decision is made to extract water from the Croton River through construction of a reservoir and aqueduct (see Figure 15.8).
1842	The "Old Croton Reservoir" and the "Old Croton Aqueduct" (as they are now informally called) are put in service. Water is conveyed to storage reservoirs in the city prior to distribution, primarily through cast iron pipes.
1890	A second aqueduct (the "New Croton Aqueduct") is put in service to convey more water from the Croton watershed.
1905	The Board of Water Supply is created and the decision is taken to develop the Catskill Watershed.
1915	The Ashokan Reservoir and Catskill Aqueduct are completed.
1928	Development of the Catskill system is completed, including the Schoharie Reservoir and the Shandaken Tunnel.
1927	Plans are submitted to develop the Rondout watershed and Delaware River Tributaries within the State of New York.
1937	In spite of legal action brought by the State of New Jersey, construction of the "Delaware system" is begun.
1944	The Delaware Aqueduct is completed, followed in 1950 by the completion of the Rondout Reservoir; 1954, completion of the Neversink Reservoir; 1955, completion of the Pepacton Reservoir; and 1964, completion of the Cannonsville Reservoir.

New York City's water supply is specifically designed so that reservoirs have interconnections that allow flexibility and virtually ensure that effects of localized droughts are minimized. The system delivers water to the city primarily by gravity and is therefore relatively economical. However, development of these watersheds is not without political implications. The Delaware River Basin includes parts of Delaware, New Jersey, New York, and Pennsylvania. Each state relies in part on the basin for water for drinking or industrial uses. However, as the upstream user, New York's development of this water supply can potentially affect the three downstream users. The Croton, Catskill, and Delaware watersheds include prime recreational and agricultural lands. In addition, the many upstream communities that have developed in these watersheds resent the fact that they cannot fully use these resources that must be protected to serve a population some 100 miles downstream.

For New York City, as for other major municipalities in the United States without filtration (including Boston, Portland, and Seattle), the rules changed in 1989. Under the provisions of the Safe Drinking Water Act passed in this year, the EPA promulgated the Surface Water Treatment Rule (SWTR). The SWTR requires filtration of all public water supply systems supplied by unfiltered surface water unless a series of criteria, referred to as the *filtration avoidance criteria*, are met. New York City has published these criteria on its Web site (New York City Department of Environmental Protection 2008):

- Objective Water Quality Criteria—the water supply must meet certain levels for specified constituents including coliforms, turbidity and disinfection by-products.
- Operational Criteria—a system must demonstrate compliance with certain disinfection requirements for inactivation of *Giardia* and viruses; maintain a minimum chlorine residual entering and throughout the distribution system; provide uninterrupted disinfection with redundancy; and undergo an annual on-site inspection by the primacy agency to review the condition of disinfection equipment.
- Watershed Control Criteria—a system must establish and maintain an effective watershed control program to minimize the potential for contamination of source waters by *Giardia* and viruses.

The City of New York faces billions of dollars in costs to implement filtration of its drinking water and hence has gone to exceptional lengths to prove that it can meet these criteria. In addition to programs to purchase land in the watersheds, the New York City Department of Environmental Protection publishes annual and other reports describing its extensive efforts to avoid filtration. These reports cover watershed protection efforts, water quality, and waterborne disease assessments (New York City Department of Environmental Protection, 2008).

FIGURE 15.8   New York City's Water Supply System

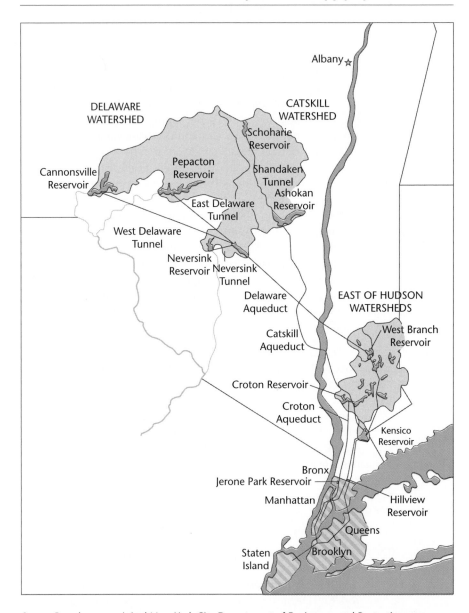

Source: Based on an original New York City Department of Environmental Protection map: "New York City's Water Supply System," as modified by The Catskill Center for Conservation and Development (http://www.nyc.gov/html/dep/html/drinking_water/wsmaps_wide.shtml).

FIGURE 15.9   A Multibarrier Approach to Maximize Microbiological Quality of Water

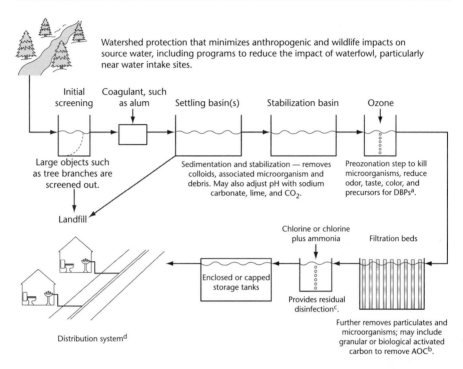

Note: This presumes a treatment system that has sufficient capacity to maintain adequate pressure throughout the distribution system for twenty-four hours per day and that minimizes opportunities for microbial colonization of the pipelines.

[a] Disinfection by-products (DBPs) are formed by ozonation of source waters, including aldehydes and brominated by-products (discussed in Boorman and others 1999). UV disinfection, used extensively in wastewater treatment, is rapidly gaining acceptance as an alternative to ozonation.

[b] AOC = assimilable organic carbon—carbon that can be readily utilized by microorganisms and that therefore stimulates their growth.

[c] Residual disinfection requires a chemical that will not be rapidly broken down in the distribution system so that it retains some disinfecting activity at point of use (the tap). To date the only practical chemicals appear to be chlorine or chloramines. Chloramination may be preferable to chlorination, as it is believed that chloramines penetrate biofilms more effectively than chlorine alone. They also reduce DBP formation and are more effective at a high pH (a high pH is often necessary for corrosion control). Where chloramination is used, intermittent chlorination and system flushing are recommended, as chlorine is a more powerful oxidizing agent.

[d] A rigorous program is necessary to upgrade distribution system networks and to prevent undesirable interconnections through leakage, backflushing, improper hydrant use, and so forth.

impede this goal). More recently, with concerns about potential toxicity of chlorination by-products, alternative forms of disinfection such as ozonation and pulsed UV have been gaining popularity. Table 15.8 compares alternative forms of disinfection and chlorination.

Disinfection Resistance   One reason for exploring alternatives to chlorination is the growing realization that a number of microbes are apparently capable of surviving at the "safe" chlorination levels typically maintained in drinking water. Mechanisms of survival vary from a relatively resistant cell wall to intracellular survival. One of the most resistant microorganisms is the protozoan *Cryptosporidium parvum*, mentioned earlier. *C. parvum* forms extremely environmentally resistant oocysts that allow the organism to resist chlorine concentrations at levels that far exceed those considered safe for drinking-water treatment. Ozonation is thought

TABLE 15.8   Approaches to Disinfection

Disinfectant	Benefits	Concerns	Cost
Chlorine	Retains a residual; strong disinfectant	Taste and odor; toxicity of by-products; some microbes are resistant; not effective at high pH	Moderate
Chloramination	Retains a residual; used for a wider range of pHs; may penetrate biofilms more effectively than free chlorine	Weaker disinfectant; some by-products formed but less than with free chlorine; may leach lead from pipes	Moderate
Chlorine dioxide	Powerful disinfectant; no by-products formed	Toxic; chemically unstable and cannot be stored; no residual	Expensive
Ozone	Powerful disinfectant; can be effective against chlorine-resistant microbes	Must be generated on site; can increase assimilable organic carbon; forms bromates	Expensive, but can be economical with a large operation
UV (pulsed)	Short contact time; no toxic by-products; not influenced by pH or temperature	No residual; not effective with high turbidity water	Increasingly competitive and gaining in popularity

to be marginally more effective against *C. parvum* but does tend to be more expensive and does not provide a residual in the distribution system. There appears to be no alternative to chlorination for maintaining a residual, although addition of ammonia with chlorine to form chloramines is an alternative, particularly if a high pH is maintained as part of a corrosion control strategy. (However, be aware that changing chemical conditions can have unintended consequences as happened in the Washington, D.C., lead exposure case discussed earlier.)

Strategies organisms use to resist disinfection can be summarized as follows (in part from Ford, 1999):

- Biochemical changes, for example, synthesis of stress proteins
- Cyst formation (protozoa); spore formation (for example, *Bacillus* spp.)
- Resistant cell wall (for example, mycobacteria)
- Viable but nonculturable (many bacterial species); injured (for example, indicator species); dwarf forms (for example, *Vibrio* spp.)
- Biofilm association (for example, *Legionella pneumophila*, *Pseudomonas aeruginosa*, and many others); particle association (for example, viruses)
- Intracellular survival (for example, *Legionella pneumophila*, *Mycobacterium avium*, and so forth)

Disinfection By-Product Toxicity   Given the necessity for residual disinfection in distributed water, a quantity of chlorine (or chloramines) must be added posttreatment. However, chlorine compounds react with naturally occurring organic matter to form **disinfection by-products** (DBPs). The best recognized DBPs are trihalomethanes such as chloroform and trichloroacetic acid. However, the range of disinfection by-products is enormous, given the range of chemical precursors that can occur in source water. Some recent research has focused on a chlorinated furanone, 3-chloro-4-(dichloromethyl)-5-hydroxy-2(5H)-furanone, also known as mutagen X. A laboratory in Finland has estimated that this compound may be more than one 100-fold more mutagenic than chloroform. However, it is also present at much lower concentrations than chloroform (Boorman and others, 1999).

The evidence is accumulating that many chlorinated organic compounds are carcinogenic. Much of this evidence comes from animal experiments and is based on high-dose exposures. Human exposures through drinking water are typically orders of magnitude lower, and the extent of risk to humans has been difficult to quantify. Moreover, although toxicological data are available for the trihalomethanes and haloacetates, little information is available on other DBPs. Hence, there is great uncertainty about the overall risk of DBPs. One estimate is that DBPs are responsible for 4,200 cases of bladder cancer and 6,500 cases of rectal cancer in the United States each year (Morris and others, 1992), and

DBPs have been estimated to cause approximately 3 additional cancer deaths per 10,000 population in Taiwan (Yang, Chiu, Cheng, and Tsai, 1998).

The risk levels associated with DBPs are of concern, but they are substantially lower than the risks associated with contaminated water, especially in developing nations. In Africa, infant mortality rates from inadequate and unsafe water are between 2 and 5 percent annually (Taylor, 1993). In Latin America in 1990, several million cases of diarrheal disease were reported, with an estimated 300,000 deaths (de Macedo, 1993). And in the United States, 5,000 deaths are attributed to foodborne illness each year (Mead and others, 1999), of which some proportion is very likely due to preparation of food with contaminated water.

In many settings, then, the risk of microbiological contamination of water eclipses the risk of DBPs. Many water experts conclude that the microbiological quality of drinking water should never be compromised for ill-defined health risks from DBPs. However, once tap water is confirmed to be free of infectious doses of pathogens, it is reasonable to explore ways to reduce the potential toxicity from DBPs. In the United States and other developed countries, this has involved examination of alternative forms of disinfection (Clark and Boutin, 2001). However, for many countries, economic reality makes these technologies and their continued maintenance an unrealistic solution, and chlorine remains the most practical effective way to reduce waterborne disease.

Water Distribution

Water distribution is a critical step, and its failure has been implicated in many cases of drinking-water contamination and waterborne disease outbreaks. Water, generally containing a disinfectant residual, may be distributed through hundreds of miles of pipeline throughout a major city. In addition to the major distribution lines, the water also flows through building pipelines. All of these pipes are potential sites for **cross-contamination** through a variety of processes. Metal pipes are susceptible to corrosion and through time can develop holes that may allow external sources of water to enter during periods of low pressure. This happens, for example, when hydrants are extensively used during firefighting. Low pressure in the drinking-water system can also cause back siphonage from pipes or tubing left hanging in sinks or other water or waste storage. This is a particular issue in high-rise buildings, where distribution system pressure may be insufficient to maintain supply to top floors throughout a twenty-four-hour period. Where this is the case, there is a tendency for residents to fill bath tubs and other vessels to provide a reserve. In the absence of external contamination, regrowth of microorganisms in distribution lines is a very real problem. This is particularly true at dead-end sites such as fire hydrants. Water remains essentially stagnant at these sites, and any residual chlorine in the system is rapidly combined with organic matter, allowing microbes to grow and proliferate (Ford, 1993).

Point-of-Use Treatment and Bottled Water

Alternatives to direct consumption of tap water that consumers increasingly consider for their potable water supply are **point-of-use treatment** and **bottled water**. Point-of-use treatment refers to simple techniques used in homes to disinfect water, such as filtering the water or adding bleach to plastic water storage vessels. These are certainly viable options, but it is necessary to maintain a point-of-use device properly to avoid exacerbating water quality problems by, in effect, providing a "biofilm reactor" that encourages microbial growth. Bottled water places the consumer at the mercy of the manufacturer, as bottled water is not currently as rigorously regulated as municipal water. In addition, there is a compelling argument that if the money people are willing to pay for point-of-use filters or bottled water were invested in municipal treatment and distribution, many current health risks (real and perceived) could be mitigated.

REGULATORY FRAMEWORK

Water quality monitoring regulations are well developed for a vast suite of chemicals, driven primarily by the increasingly sensitive technologies that can be used for measuring trace levels of contaminants. Unfortunately, the same is not true for microbial contaminants. The indicator approach (Table 15.6) remains the primary method for assessing microbiological quality of drinking water, despite the fact that many pathogens survive for extended periods in drinking water in the absence of these indicators. Indeed, a number of environmental pathogens may be present in drinking water in the complete absence of any contamination source.

The Safe Drinking Water Act

In the **Safe Drinking Water Act** (SDWA) (EPA, 2008b), passed in 1974 and amended in 1986 and 1996, the U.S. Congress mandated the Environmental Protection Agency to regulate contaminants in drinking water that might pose a risk to human health. This complex piece of legislation has a number of important provisions.

A central strategy of the SDWA is to set permissible levels of contaminants in drinking water provided by public drinking-water utilities. (Private wells and systems with fewer than fifteen connections or serving fewer than twenty-five people are not regulated by the SDWA.) The EPA establishes two sets of benchmarks, one based on ideal health goals and the other based on feasibility. In the first set, known as *maximum contaminant level goals* (MCLGs), a goal is defined as the "level of a contaminant in drinking water below which there is no known or expected risk to health" after drinking two liters of water each day for seventy years. These goals are set to include a margin of safety. For many contaminants, such as carcinogens, lead, and some pathogens, MCLGs are set at zero. MCLGs are public health goals, not enforceable standards. In contrast, **maximum contaminant levels** (MCLs) are legal limits. They are set as close to MCLGs as possible, taking into account both technological feasibility and cost.

The **National Primary Drinking Water Regulations** (NPDWR) promulgated by the EPA are based on these benchmarks. These regulations extend to fifty-three organic compounds, sixteen inorganic compounds, four classes of radionuclides, four types of disinfection by-products, and three disinfectants. In terms of microbial contaminants, *Cryptosporidium, Giardia lamblia, Legionella*, and viruses are regulated, but only in terms of percentage of removal or inactivation by treatment. Heterotrophic plate counts (a measure of microbial load), turbidity, and total coliform levels (including fecal coliform and *E. coli*) are also regulated and can be directly measured, but as discussed earlier, these indicators are imperfect markers of the presence of pathogens. The EPA also publishes National Secondary Drinking Water Regulations (NSDWR), which are nonenforceable guidelines for contaminants that cause cosmetic or aesthetic problems in drinking water.

The SDWA includes additional regulatory requirements. For example, the EPA has established monitoring schedules, monitoring methods, and acceptable treatment technologies. Also the Surface Water Treatment Rule governs filtration of public water supply systems.

As a requirement of the 1996 amendment to the SDWA, the EPA is required to publish, every five years, a list of contaminants that are not subject to regulation at the time of publication but that are anticipated to occur in drinking water and may require future regulation. Known as the **Contaminant Candidate List** (CCL), the latest iteration, CCL 3, includes ninety-three chemical and eleven microbiological contaminants. The CCL helps guide the EPA's research agenda. Chemicals on the list undergo extensive toxicity assessments, and risks of exposure through drinking water are characterized to the degree our current methodologies allow. The CCL 3 includes the following microbiological contaminants:

- Viruses: caliciviruses, hepatitis A virus
- Bacteria: *Campylobacter jejuni, Escherichia coli* (0157), *Helicobacter pylori, Legionella pneumophila, Salmonella enterica, Shigella sonnei, Vibrio cholerae*
- Protozoa: *Entamoeba histolytica, Naegleria fowleri*

The CCL provides an important indication of contaminants that will receive growing public health attention.

Total Coliform Rule

In 1989, the EPA finalized the **Total Coliform Rule**. This rule is currently the driving force behind drinking-water safety and frequently serves as the first indication (other than turbidity) of potential contamination. The rule requires a water system to establish a regular coliform sampling plan, with sample sites that accurately represent water quality throughout the distribution system. Any sample that is positive for total coliforms requires repeat samples and must be tested for fecal coliforms or *E. coli*. Specific requirements vary somewhat depending on population served; however, for a large municipality, having more than 5 percent of samples test positive for total coliforms in a month constitutes a monthly maximum contaminant level violation that must be reported to the municipality's respective state by the end of the next business day and the public must be notified within thirty days. Acute MCL violations result from any repeat fecal coliform or *E. coli* positive sample, or any routine fecal coliform or *E. coli* positive sample followed by a repeat total coliform sample. In the case of an acute violation, the state must be notified by the end of the next business day and the public must be notified within twenty-four hours.

An additional component of the total coliform rule that is designed to protect smaller public water systems is the *sanitary survey*. Every system collecting fewer than five samples per month is required to have regular sanitary surveys, usually every five years. This survey is designed to evaluate the entire water system, its operations, and its maintenance in order to ensure public health. (The EPA Web site provides numerous resources for conducting sanitary surveys; see EPA, 2008c.)

Consumer Confidence Reports

An important outcome from the 1996 amendment of the SDWA has been the requirement for utilities to provide **consumer confidence reports** (EPA, 2006). The requirement was finalized in 1998 and is designed to "enable Americans to make practical, knowledgeable decisions about their health and their environment." In addition to carrying out rapid notification when coliform counts are high, water systems are required, at a minimum, to inform consumers annually of

- The lake, river, aquifer, or other source of the drinking water
- A brief summary of the susceptibility to contamination of the local drinking-water source, based on the source water assessments by states
- How to get a copy of the water system's complete source water assessment

- The level (or range of levels) of any contaminant found in local drinking water, as well as the EPA's health-based standard (maximum contaminant level) for comparison
- The likely source of that contaminant in the local drinking-water supply
- The potential health effects of any contaminant detected in violation of an EPA health standard, and an accounting of the system's actions to restore safe drinking water
- The water system's compliance with other drinking water–related rules
- An educational statement for vulnerable populations about avoiding *Cryptosporidium*
- Educational information on nitrate, arsenic, or lead in areas where these contaminant may be a concern; and phone numbers of additional sources of information, including the water system and EPA's Safe Drinking Water Hotline (800-426-4791) (EPA, 2008d).

Recreational Water Standards

The EPA and state agencies also regulate recreational waters. For example, **swimming advisories** are posted where indicator organisms exceed recommended levels. For freshwater, current standards are 126 *E. coli* per 100 mL or 33 enterococci per 100 mL. Regulations state that only one of these two indicator organisms should be used. For seawater, the standard is set at 35 enterococci per 100 mL. (For further information on recreational water safety and on the rationale for standards, see EPA, 2003; Bartram and Rees, 2000; WHO, 2003a.)

RISK CHARACTERIZATION FOR WATER CONTAMINANTS

Risk assessment is the process used to prioritize interventions and to reduce human exposure to environmental sources of chemicals and pathogens, as described in Chapter Twenty-Nine. However, **microbiological risk assessment** raises some additional considerations. These involve exposure assessment, variability, and complexity.

To identify microbial hazards, *spot samples* are generally taken from finished water at the treatment plant and occasionally at conveniently accessible sites in the distribution system. However, distribution of pathogens is extremely heterogeneous in drinking water. Most consumers will not ingest an infectious dose of a pathogen, and measurements of water samples will frequently be zero. However, a few individuals may consume a large number of infectious microbes. Moreover, as previously discussed, most pathogens are poorly indicated by the presence of the routinely monitored coliform group. Utilities expect that major contamination events in a watershed will be recognized from turbidity spikes; however, this is not always the case. Turbidity spikes were not excessive for the contamination event in Milwaukee in 1993 (Mac Kenzie and others, 1994). An event of far smaller magnitude may not result in elevated turbidity, or minor spikes may be missed. Although a rare event, a *plug* of infectious oocysts, cysts, or viruses could enter the distribution system and be very easily missed by a spot sampling program yet contain sufficient numbers to virtually ensure that ingestion will result in infection (Gale, 2001). Exposure assessment therefore remains a challenge in microbial risk assessment.

Similarly, variability is a key challenge. People vary in the doses of pathogens they sustain, an outcome related both to variation across the drinking-water system and to variation in individuals' consumption of water. People also vary in their responses to a specific infectious dose, depending on individual susceptibility (age, health, and other factors), prior exposure (immunity), and the degree of virulence of the pathogen itself (affected by numerous environmental factors). Infectious agents themselves vary. Organisms may lose virulence and even infectivity in the distribution system or after exposure to disinfection. Conversely, organisms may increase or change in virulence and in their ability to resist antibiotics following environmental exposures.

Complexity arises in numerous ways. To begin with, water is a complex environment. It may be contaminated by both chemicals and microbes, and these two classes of contaminants interact. Some chemicals of concern are actually bacterial, fungal, or algal toxins. Some may be produced within the distribution system pipeline by the action of certain groups of organisms; the sulfate-reducing bacteria produce sulfides and other sulfur containing chemicals, nitrifying bacteria produce nitrites and nitrates from ammonia compounds (either in source water or from chloramination). And some chemicals—the disinfection by-products—result from water treatment practices to minimize microbial contamination.

Partly for these reasons, the health risks associated with drinking water are still not fully defined and quantified. The World Health Organization publishes drinking-water quality standards that are internationally recognized (WHO, 2006). In some cases, such as the WHO's current standard for arsenic, these standards are more stringent than those of the U.S. EPA. It is likely that health risks are minimal for individuals without predisposing factors—in developed nations individuals with predisposing factors would be the very young, the elderly, the pregnant and those with compromised immune function. However, on the global scale, susceptible individuals may be as common as the nonsusceptible. Malnutrition, stress, concomitant diseases, and socioeconomic deprivation increase susceptibility. The global risk from contaminated water may be enormous.

Despite this risk, people in areas with contaminated water may, paradoxically, be protected by immunity resulting from multiple prior exposures. By all the criteria just mentioned, these populations are highly susceptible, yet immunity results in lower than expected incidence of many waterborne diseases. This immunity must come at some cost to the individual, but there is not yet a robust approach for estimating the burden of disease from exposure to multiple infectious agents (and toxins). This complexity—like the complexity within water itself—continues to challenge microbial risk assessment efforts (Gale, 2001; Fewtrell and Bartram, 2001).

EMERGING ISSUES

Public health issues related to water are highly dynamic. Emerging issues include new and shifting diseases, new techniques for assessing water quality, and new approaches to managing water quality.

The Phenomenon of New Disease

Many factors can promote the real or apparent emergence of a new disease. New ecological niches, such as the hot-water systems that support growth of *Legionella*, may contribute. Factors such as population density and increasing numbers of susceptible individuals (the very young, the elderly, pregnant women, and the immunocompromised) could provide an extensive human reservoir for opportunistic pathogens and promote changes in virulence patterns, even in developed countries. Increased adaptation to the human host might be responsible for increased infection rates (of mycobacterial diseases, for example) in populations with no underlying susceptibility.

Legionella pneumophila, *E. coli* O157, *Vibrio cholerae* O139, *Helicobacter pylori*, *Cryptosporidium parvum*, and hepatitis E virus, are all examples of microorganisms categorized as *new* or *newly recognized* pathogens. Well-established pathogens should arguably be added to this list as they develop antibiotic resistance and change virulence patterns (Ford, 1999). Research is clearly needed to understand better the ecology of the water environment that may promote new disease emergence. One research priority is biofilms, the microbial films that form on the surfaces of pipe material, which may provide an opportunity for horizontal gene transfer both within and between species. The biofilm environment may also promote expression of plasmids through exposure to chemical stressors such as metals. An increasing body of research links metal resistance with multiple antibiotic resistance determinants, presumably expressed on the same plasmids (discussed in Ford, 1993).

Molecular Epidemiology

Gene chips are tiny devices whose surfaces contain arrays of DNA or RNA fragments. When water comes into contact with the gene chip, biological materials in the sample could potentially be identified by fluorescent labeling. This emerging technology may one day play a role in monitoring water quality. A recent American Academy for Microbiology report begins with the imagined scenario that a gene chip placed in the flow of water will one day detect each pathogen, with the fluorescence response triggering an alarm that prompts an appropriate treatment response (Rose and Grimes, 2001).

At present, however, the role of gene chip technology is limited by the inability to analyze and interpret accurately the vast amounts of data generated. There are also at least two major technical challenges. First, in order for a gene chip to be developed and its results understood, the target organisms must be characterized and a highly specific gene segment recognized. However, most organisms in drinking water have yet to be characterized. Second, the organism's genetic material must come in contact with the chip surface in order to hybridize to the probe. However, the heterogeneous distribution of microbes in drinking water and the need to lyse the cell are barriers that dramatically reduce the potential sensitivity of the technique. Nevertheless, gene chip technology is likely to play an increasing role in identifying water contaminants.

Wastewater Reuse

This discussion would not be complete without returning to the topic of wastewater. A vital step in providing adequate, safe drinking water is to understand that wastewater is a valuable resource. Today, **wastewater reuse** programs are increasingly encouraged in the more arid states in the United States, primarily for nonpotable use. This involves separate collection of **black water** (primarily toilet wastes, although it may also include other wastewater rich in organics, such as the effluent from a garbage disposal system) and **gray water** (other sources of wastewater such as bath and shower water). The gray water can then be used to irrigate nonedible plants and in some cases can also be used for toilet flushing.

The simplest use of gray water is direct discharge from the house to the landscape. However, there are understandable health concerns as bath and shower water may contain potential pathogens. A wide range of gray water treatment systems is available. These systems may be sufficiently sophisticated (and expensive) to remove both chemical and biological contaminants and essentially to mimic the water treatment process on a small scale. The use of recycled wastewater to augment diminishing supplies of drinking water is just beginning. The barriers to wastewater recycling are probably issues of public perception more than cost. Just as many arid nations increasingly rely on desalination to supply drinking water, treatment technologies are more than capable of recycling wastewater to a potable quality. The predicted increase in the number of water-scarce countries during the 21st makes education in this area critical. However, water recycling alone will not be sufficient without a concerted effort to conserve the available remaining resources. Figure 15.10 shows an idealized scheme for future provision

FIGURE 15.10   Idealized Scheme for Future Provision of Safe Drinking Water

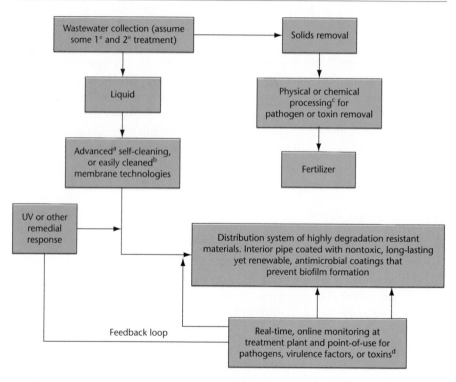

[a] Many companies now invest heavily in microfiltration, ultrafiltration, nanofiltration, and reverse osmosis membrane technologies. Hollow-fiber filtration technologies, for example, are allowing filtration capacities adequate for municipal water systems.

[b] For example, the patented gas backwash systems for USFilter's Memcor® microfiltration systems.

[c] There is currently considerable debate on appropriate criteria for land application of sewage sludges, known as *biosolids*. Treatment produces biosolids that range from Class B biosolids, with a consequent risk to surface waters, to Class A biosolids, which are essentially pathogen free.

[d] The ideal monitoring tool depicted in an American Academy of Microbiology report (Rose and Grimes, 2001).

Source: Ford, 2004.

of safe drinking water. Although this process would be expensive, it is increasingly recognized that water is dramatically undervalued and should be appropriately priced. It is often stated that water is a human right (WHO, 2003b). Certainly, like food, it is a human necessity. However, as mentioned earlier, people are willing to purchase bottled water at considerable expense because of their real and perceived concerns for the quality of water at the tap. There is no question that the true cost of water should be subsidized for those who cannot afford it, but realistic pricing for those who can afford to pay could dramatically improve the safety of drinking water for everyone.

However, a word of caution is necessary. How safe should our drinking water be? Arguably, for the immunocompromised it can never be too safe. Filtration technologies may one day provide water, at least at the level of the treatment plant, that is 100 percent free not only of infectious agents but also of all microorganisms. Perhaps distribution pipes will eventually be lined with materials that effectively prevent biofilm buildup. However, is this in fact optimal for the immunocompetent? Some waterborne exposure to microorganisms may be important in developing and maintaining healthy immune systems.

SUMMARY

Water is critical to all forms of life on this planet, yet we would appear to have been systematically threatening this precious resource through agricultural, municipal, and industrial development. This development has happened with little regard for the amount of water we squander, the wastes we produce, or the engineering schemes that degrade this resource. The key messages to be learned from a careful evaluation of the critical role that water plays in human and ecological health are that we must conserve the resource, we must reduce our waste production, and we must recycle what we use. We must also educate communities on how to reduce their burden of waterborne disease. Finally, we must improve our abilities to predict future waterborne disease outbreaks, and be ready to provide public health intervention on a global scale to prevent future pandemic disease.

KEY TERMS

acute gastrointestinal
   infection (AGI)

aquifer recharge

bacteria

bioavailable

biofilm

biological oxygen demand
   (BOD)

black water

bottled water

cholera

consumer confidence
  reports

Contaminant Candidate
  List

contamination

cross contamination

cyanobacteria

DALYs

diarrheal disease

disinfection by-products

dracunculiasis

enterotoxigenic E. coli
  (ETEC)

epidemic

ETEC

eutrophication

fossil water

global burden of
  disease

global climate change

gray water

groundwater

groundwater under the
  direct influence of
  surface water

hydrodynamics

hydrologic cycle

hydrophilic

hydrophobic

hygiene

indicator concept

irrigation

maximum contaminant
  level

microbiological risk
  assessment

multibarrier approach

National Primary
  Drinking Water
  Regulations

nonpoint source

pandemic

persistent organic
  pollutants

point source

point-of-use treatment

polychlorinated biphenyls
  (PCBs)

precipitation

protozoa

resource wars

Safe Drinking Water Act

sanitation

secondary transmission

source water

surface water

swimming advisories

total coliform rule

vector-borne disease

viruses

wastewater reuse

wastewater treatment

water availability

water distribution

water scarcity

water stress

water treatment

waterborne disease
  outbreaks

waterborne pathogens

watershed protection

DISCUSSION QUESTIONS

1. Global warming may bring increasing temperatures over the next twenty years. What might be the potential consequences for waterborne and water-related diseases? Choose a specific disease, and discuss how it may be affected.

2. Almost every city has a deteriorating water distribution system. As a result, municipalities lose between 30 and 50 percent of distributed water. Imagine yourself to be the manager of a municipal water facility, and discuss options for reducing water loss. What are the alternatives, if any, to distributed water, and what would be the health risks associated with each alternative?

3. Given the number of options for water treatment available today, what would your recommendations need to take into account if you were involved in installing a new water treatment plant in a developing country with high rates of enteric diseases?

4. *The coliform group has been used for most of the past century as an indicator of fecal pollution. However, directly monitoring for pathogens such as* Vibrio cholerae *would be far more protective of public health.* Please agree or disagree with this statement, and give your reasons.

5. Research and describe the Aral Sea disaster. Discuss health consequences to the local communities and the long-term fate of this ecosystem.

6. *The answer to a waterborne disease outbreak is to "shock" chlorinate.* Explore this statement and the health risks that would be mitigated. What new health risks might emerge from the application of large doses of chlorine?

7. What health concerns arise from reuse of wastewater? What exposure pathways to pathogens might occur from land application of sewage sludge and reuse of wastewater for irrigation of garden plants and toilet flushing?

8. *Relative to the situation in developing countries, waterborne disease in the United States is a nonissue. The CDC reports very few deaths from waterborne disease outbreaks, and we therefore have no reason to worry.* Identify and discuss some of the potential fallacies in this statement.

REFERENCES

Agency for Toxic Substances and Disease Registry. "Toxicological Profile for Polychlorinated Biphenyls (PCBs)." http://www.atsdr.cdc.gov/toxprofiles/tp17.html, 2000.

Amer, M. H., El-Yazigi, A., Hannan, M. A., and Mohamed, M. E. "Water Contamination and Esophageal Cancer at Gassim Region, Saudi Arabia." *Gastroenterology*, 1990, *98*, 1141–1147.

Arvanitidou, M., Kanellou, K., Constantinides, T. C. and Katsouyannopoulos, V. "The Occurrence of Fungi in Hospital and Community Potable Waters. *Letters in Applied Microbiology*, 1999, *29*, 81–84.

Aschengrau, A., Rogers, S., and Ozonoff, D. "Perchloroethylene-Contaminated Drinking Water and the Risk of Breast Cancer: Additional Results from Cape Cod, Massachusetts, USA." *Environmental Health Perspectives*, 2003, *111*, 167–173.

Bartram, J., and Rees, G. (eds.). *Monitoring Bathing Waters: A Practical Guide to the Design and Implementation of Assessments and Monitoring Programmes*. World Health Organization. http://www.who.int/water_sanitation_health/bathing/bathing3/en, 2000.

Bitton, G. *Wastewater Microbiology.* (2nd ed.) Hoboken, N.J.: Wiley-Liss, 1999.

Boorman, G. A., and others. "Drinking Water Disinfection Byproducts: Review and Approach to Toxicity Evaluation." *Environmental Health Perspectives,* 1999, *107,* 207–217.

Breiman, R. F., and Butler, J. C. "Legionnaires' Disease: Clinical, Epidemiological, and Public Health Perspectives." *Seminars in Respiratory Infections,* 1998, *13,* 84–89.

The BSE Inquiry. *The BSE Inquiry Report.* http://www.bseinquiry.gov.uk/report, 2000.

Cabello, F., and Springer, A. D. "Typhoid Fever in Chile 1977–1990: An Emergent Disease." *Revista medica de Chili,* 1997, *125,* 474–482.

Callow, P., and Petts, G. (eds.). *The Rivers Handbook: Hydrological and Ecological Principles.* Vol. *1.* Oxford, U.K.: Blackwell Scientific, 1992.

Capone, D. G., and Bauer, J. E. "Microbial Processes in Coastal Pollution." In R. Mitchell (ed.), *Environmental Microbiology.* Hoboken, N.J.: Wiley, 1992.

Carter Center. "Guinea Worm Eradication Program." http://www.cartercenter.org/health/guinea_worm/index.html, 2008.

Centers for Disease Control and Prevention. *Cross-Sectional Exposure Assessment of Environmental Contaminants in Churchill County, Nevada.* http://www.cdc.gov/nceh/clusters/Fallon/study.htm, 2003.

"Chakraborty, S., and others." Concomitant Infection of Enterotoxigenic *Escherichia Coli* in an Outbreak of Cholera Caused by *Vibrio Cholerae* O1 and O139 in Ahmedabad, India." *Journal of Clinical Microbiology,* 2001, *39,* 3241–3246.

Chorus, I., and Bartram, J. (eds.). *Toxic Cyanobacteria in Water: A Guide to Their Public Health Consequences, Monitoring and Management.* World Health Organization. (http://www.who.int/water_sanitation_health/resourcesquality/toxicyanbact/en, 1999.

Clark, R. M., and Boutin, B. K. (eds.). *Controlling Disinfection By-Products and Microbial Contaminants in Drinking Water.* EPA/600/R-01/110. http://www.epa.gov/ORD/NRMRL/Pubs/600R01110/600R01110.htm, 2001.

Clarke, R. *Water: The International Crisis.* Cambridge, Mass.: MIT Press, 1993.

Cohn, P., and others. "Drinking Water Contamination and the Incidence of Leukemia and Non-Hodgkin's Lymphoma. *Environmental Health Perspectives,* 1994, *102,* 556–561.

Colborn, T., Dumanoski, D., and Meyers, J. P. *Our Stolen Future: Are We Threatening Our Fertility, Intelligence, and Survival? A Scientific Detective Story.* New York: Dutton, 1996.

Colwell, R. R. "Global Climate and Infectious Disease: The Cholera Paradigm." *Science,* 1996, *274,* 2025–2031.

Colwell, R. R., and Huq, A. "Vibrios in the Environment: Viable but Nonculturable *Vibrio Cholerae.*" In I. K. Wachsmuth, O., Olsvik, and P. A. Blake (eds.), *Vibrio Cholerae and Cholera: Molecular to Global Perspectives.* Washington, D.C: ASM Press, 1994.

Colwell, R. R., and others. "Viable but Nonculturable *Vibrio Cholerae* and Related Pathogens in the Environment: Implications for Release of Genetically Engineered Microorganisms. *Biotechnology,* 1985, *3,* 817–820.

Converse, K., Wolcott, M., Docherty, D., and Cole, R. *Screening for Potential Human Pathogens in Fecal Material Deposited by Resident Canada Geese on Areas of Public Utility.* Madison, Wis.: U.S. Geological Service, National Animal Health Center, 2001.

Costas, K., Knorr, R. S., and Condon, S. K. "A Case-Control Study of Childhood Leukemia in Woburn, Massachusetts: The Relationship Between Leukemia Incidence and Exposure to Public Drinking Water." *Science of the Total Environment,* 2002, *300,* 23–35.

Cox, S. E., and Kahle, S. C. *Hydrogeology, Ground-Water Quality, and Sources of Nitrate in Lowland Glacial Aquifers of Whatcom County, Washington and British Columbia Canada.* USGS Water-Resources Investigations Report 98–4195. Washington, D.C.: U.S. Geological Survey, 1999.

de Macedo, C. G. "Balancing Microbial and Chemical Risks in Disinfection of Drinking Water: The Pan American Perspective." In G. F. Craun (ed.), *Safety of Water Disinfection: Balancing Chemical and Microbial Risks.* Washington, D.C.: ILSI Press, 1993.

Del Porto, D., and Steinfeld, C. *The Composting Toilet System Book: A Practical Guide to Choosing, Planning and Maintaining Composting Toilet Systems, a Water-Saving, Pollution-Preventing Alternative.* Concord, Mass.: Center for Ecological Pollution Prevention, 2000.

Díaz, E. (ed.). *Microbial Biodegradation: Genomics and Molecular Biology.* Norfolk, U.K.: Caister Academic Press, 2008.

Easterling, D. R., and others "Climate Extremes: Observations, Modeling, and Impacts." *Science*, 2000, *289*, 2068–2074.

Egorov, A. I., and others. "Contamination of Water Supplies with *Cryptosporidium* and *Giardia Lamblia* and Diarrheal Illness in Selected Russian Cities." *International Journal of Hygiene and Environmental Health*, 2002, *205*, 281–289.

Egorov, A. I., and others. "Serological Evidence of *Cryptosporidium* Infections in a Russian City and Evaluation of Risk Factors for Infection." *Annals of Epidemiology*, 2004, *14*, 129–136.

Micklin, P. "The Aral Sea Disaster." *Annual Review of Earth and Planetary Sciences*, 2007, *35*(4), 47–72.

Engelman, R., and others. *People in the Balance: Update 2006.* Population Action International. http://216.146.209.72/Publications/Reports/People_in_the_Balance/Interactive/peopleinthebalance/pages/index.php, 2006.

Faruque, S. M., Albert, M. J., and Mekalanos, J. J. "Epidemiology, Genetics, and Ecology of Toxigenic *Vibrio Cholerae*." *Microbiology and Molecular Biology Review*, 1998, *62*, 1301–1314.

Fewtrell, L., and Bartram, J. (eds.). *Water Quality—Guidelines, Standards and Health: Assessment of Risk and Risk Management for Water-Related Infectious Disease.* http://www.who.int/water_sanitation_health/dwq/whoiwa/en, 2001.

Food and Agriculture Organization of the United Nations. *AQUASTAT.* http://www.fao.org/nr/water/aquastat/main/index.stm, 2008.

Ford, T. E. "The Microbial Ecology of Water Distribution and Outfall Systems." In T. E. Ford (ed.), *Aquatic Microbiology: An Ecological Approach.* Malden, Mass.: Blackwell, 1993.

Ford, T. E. "Microbiological Safety of Drinking Water: United States and Global Perspectives." *Environmental Health Perspectives*, 1999, *107*, 191–206.

Ford, T. E. "Future Needs and Priorities." In T. E. Cloete, J. Rose, L. H. Nel, and T. E. Ford (eds.), *Microbial Waterborne Pathogens.* London: IWA, 2004.

Ford, T. E., and Colwell, R. R. "A Global Decline in Microbiological Safety of Water: A Call for Action." http://www.asm.org/academy/index.asp?bid=2202, 1995.

Ford, T. E., and Hamner, S. "Control of Water-Borne Pathogens in Developing Countries." In R. Mitchell and J.-D. Gu (eds.), *Environmental Microbiology*, Second Edition. Hoboken, N.J.: Wiley, 2009.

Ford, T. E., Rupp, G., Butterfield, P., and Camper, A. "Protecting Public Health in Small Water Systems: Report of an International Colloquium." Montana Water Center. http://water.montana.edu/colloquium, 2005.

Franceys, R., Pickford, J., and Reed, R. *Guide to the Development of On-site Sanitation.* World Health Organization. http://www.who.int/water_sanitation_health/hygiene/envsan/onsitesan/en/, 1992.

Gale, P. "Developments in Microbiological Risk Assessment for Drinking Water." *Journal of Applied Microbiology*, 2001, *91*, 191–205.

Geldreich, E. E. *Microbial Quality of Water Supply in Distribution Systems.* Boca Raton, Fla.: CRC Press, 1996.

Gil, A. I., and others. "Occurrence and Distribution of *Vibrio Cholerae* in the Coastal Environment of Peru." *Environmental Microbiology*, 2004, *6*, 699–706.

Gleick, P. H. (ed.). *Water in Crisis: A Guide to the World's Fresh Water Resources.* New York: Oxford University Press, 1993.

Gleick, P. H. (ed.). *The World's Water: The Biennial Report on Freshwater Resources*, Washington, D.C.: Island Press, 1998, 2000, 2002.

Guidotti, T. L., and others. "Elevated Lead in Drinking Water in Washington, DC, 2003–2004: The Public Health Response." *Environmental Health Perspectives*, 2007, *115*, 695–701.

Hazen, T. C., and Toranzos, G. A. "Tropical Source Waters." In G. A. McFeters (ed.), *Drinking Water Microbiology.* New York: Springer, 1990.

Hrudey, S. E., and Hrudey, E. J. *Safe Drinking Water: Lessons from Recent Outbreaks in Affluent Nations.* London: IWA, 2004.

Hunter, P. R. *Waterborne Disease: Epidemiology and Ecology.* Hoboken, N.J.: Wiley, 1997.

King, C. H., Shotts, E. B., Wooley, R. E., and Porter, K. G. "Survival of Coliforms and Bacterial Pathogens Within Protozoa During Chlorination." *Applied and Environmental Microbiology*, 1988, *54*, 3023–3033.

Klare, M. T. *Resource Wars: The New Landscape of Global Conflict.* New York: Henry Holt, 2001.

Levy, S. B. "The Challenge of Antibiotic Resistance." *Scientific American*, Mar. 1998, pp. 46–53.

Lopez, A. D., and others (eds.). *Global Burden of Disease and Risk Factors.* New York: Oxford University Press, 2006.

Lopman, B. A., Brown, D. W., and Koopmans, M. "Human Caliciviruses in Europe." *Journal of Clinical Virology*, 2002, *24*, 137–160.

Lopman, B. A., and others "Viral Gastroenteritis Outbreaks in Europe, 1995–2000." *Emerging Infectious Diseases*, 2003, *9*, 90–96.

Mac Kenzie, W. R., and others. "A Massive Outbreak in Milwaukee of *Cryptosporidium* Infection Transmitted Through the Public Water Supply." *New England Journal of Medicine*, 1994. *331*, 161–167.

Majewski, M. S., and Capel, P. D. *Pesticides in the Atmosphere: Distribution, Trends, and Governing Factors.* Chelsea, Mich.: Ann Arbor Press, 1995.

Mallin, K. "Investigation of a Bladder Cancer Cluster in Northwestern Illinois." *American Journal of Epidemiology*, 1990, *132*, 96–106.

Manassaram, D. M., Backer, L. C., and Moll, D. M. "A Review of Nitrates in Drinking Water: Maternal Exposure and Adverse Reproductive and Developmental Outcomes." *Environmental Health Perspectives*, 2006, *114*, 320–327.

Marshall, M. M., Naumovitz, D., Ortega, Y., and Sterling, C. R. "Waterborne Protozoan Pathogens." *Clinical Microbiology Reviews*, 1997, *10*, 67–85.

Massachusetts Water Resources Authority. "The Deer Island Sewage Treatment Plant." http://www.mwra.state.ma.us/03sewer/html/sew.htm, 2008.

Mead, P. S., and others. "Food-Related Illness and Death in the United States." *Emerging Infectious Diseases*, 1999, *5*, 607–625.

Metcalf, J. S., and Codd, G. A. *Cyanobacterial Toxins in the Water Environment: A Review of Current Knowledge.* http://www.fwr.org/cyanotox.pdf, 2004.

Moore, B. C., Martinez, E., Gay, J. M., and Rice, D. H. "Survival of *Salmonella Enterica* in Freshwater and Sediments and Transmission by the Aquatic Midge *Chironomus Tentans (Chironomidae: Diptera)." Applied and Environmental Microbiology*, 2003, *69*, 4556–4560.

Morel, F.M.M., and Hering, J. G. *Principles and Applications of Aquatic Chemistry.* (2nd ed.) Hoboken, N.J.: Wiley, 1993.

Morris, R. D., and Levin, R. "Estimating the Incidence of Waterborne Infectious Disease Related to Drinking Water in the United States." In E. G. Reichard and G. A. Zapponi (eds.), *Assessing and Managing Health Risks from Contamination: Approaches and Applications.* Wallingford, U.K.: IAHS, 1995.

Morris, R. D., and others. "Chlorination, Chlorination By-Products, and Cancer: A Meta-Analysis." *American Journal of Public Health*, 1992, *82*, 955–963.

Murphy, C. "Should Fluoride Be Forced Upon Us?" http://news.bbc.co.uk/1/hi/health/7226655 .stm, 2008.

Nagao, T., and others. "Disruption of the Reproductive System and Reproductive Performance by Administration of Nonylphenol to Newborn Rats." *Human & Experimental Toxicology*, 2000, *19*, 284–296.

National Wild and Scenic Rivers System. *River & Water Facts.* http://www.rivers.gov/waterfacts. html, 2008.

New York City Department of Environmental Protection. *NYC Water Supply Watersheds—Watershed Protection.* http://www.nyc.gov/html/dep/html/watershed_protection/home.html, 2008.

O'Connor, D. R. *Report of the Walkerton Inquiry.* Parts 1 and 2. http://www.attorneygeneral.jus.gov. on.ca/english/about/pubs/walkerton, 2002.

Pan American Health Organization. "Cholera in the Americas." *Epidemiological Bulletin*, 1995, *16*, 11–13.

Payment, P., Sartory, D. P., and Reasoner, D. J. "The History and Use of HPC in Drinking-Water Quality Management." In J. Bartram, and others (eds.), *Heterotrophic Plate Counts and Drinking-Water Safety: The Significance of HPCs for Water Quality and the Human Health.* http://www.who.int/ water_sanitation_health/dwq/hpc/en, 2003.

Pedley, S., and others (eds.). *Pathogenic Mycobacteria in Water: A Guide to Public Health Consequences, Monitoring and Management.* London: IWA, 2004.

Postel, S. *Last Oasis: Facing Water Scarcity.* (2nd ed.) New York: Norton, 1997.

Postel, S. *Pillar of Sand: Can the Irrigation Miracle Last?* New York: Norton, 1999.

Prüss-Üstün, A., Bos, R., Gore, F., and Bartram, J. *Safer Water, Better Health: Costs, Benefits and Sustainability of Interventions to Protect and Promote Health.* Geneva: World Health Organization, 2008.

Rao, N. S. "Fluoride in Groundwater, Varaha River Basin, Visakhapatnam District, Andhra Pradesh, India." *Environmental Monitoring and Assessment*, May 29, 2008. (Epub ahead of print.)

Rose, J. B., and Grimes, D. J. *Reevaluation of Microbial Water Quality: Powerful New Tools for Detection and Risk Assessment.* http://www.asm.org/academy/index.asp?bid=2156, 2001.

Salazar-Lindo, E., Seas, C., and Gutierrez, D. "ENSO and Cholera in South America: What Can We Learn About It from the 1991 Cholera Outbreak?" *International Journal of Environment and Health*, 2008, *2*, 30–36.

Samrakandi, M. M., Ridenour, D. A., Yan, L., and Cirillo, J. D. "Entry into Host Cells by *Legionella*." *Frontiers in Bioscience*, 2002, *7*, 1–11.

Schwarzenbach, R. P., Gschwend, P. M., and Imboden, D. M. *Environmental Organic Chemistry*. Hoboken, N.J.: Wiley-Interscience, 1993.

Singh, A., and McFeters, G. A. "Injury of Enteropathogenic Bacteria in Drinking Water." In G. A. McFeters (ed.), *Drinking Water Microbiology*. New York: Springer, 1990.

Spearman, P. "Imported Dracunculiasis—United States, 1995 and 1997." *Morbidity and Mortality Weekly Report*, 1998, *47*, 209–211.

Spellberg, B., and others. "The Epidemic of Antibiotic-Resistant Infections: A Call to Action for the Medical Community from the Infectious Diseases Society of America." *Clinical Infectious Diseases*, 2008, *46*, 155–164.

Straub, T. M., and others. "In Vitro Cell Culture Infectivity Assay for Human Noroviruses." *Emerging Infectious Diseases*, 2007, *13*, 396–403.

Stumm, W., and Morgan, J. J. *Aquatic Chemistry*. (3rd ed.) Hoboken, N.J.: Wiley, 1996.

Sulaiman, I. M., and others. "Differentiating Human from Animal Isolates of *Cryptosporidium Parvum*." *Emerging Infectious Diseases*, 1998, *4*, 681–685.

Taylor, P. "Global Perspectives on Drinking Water: Water Supplies in Africa." In G. F. Craun (ed.), *Safety of Water Disinfection: Balancing Chemical and Microbial Risks*. Washington, D.C.: ILSI Press, 1993.

United Nations Educational, Cultural and Scientific Organization, World Water Assessment Program. *Water for People, Water for Life: The UN World Water Development Report*. http://unesdoc.unesco.org/images/0012/001295/129556e.pdf, 2003.

U.S. Environmental Protection Agency. *Bacterial Water Quality Standards for Recreational Waters (Freshwater and Marine Waters), Status Report*. EPA-823-R-03-008. http://www.epa.gov/waterscience/beaches/local/statrept.pdf, 2003.

U.S. Environmental Protection Agency. *Estimated Per Capita Water Ingestion and Body Weight in the United States—An Update*. EPA-822-R-00-001. http://www.epa.gov/waterscience/criteria/drinking/percapita/2004.pdf, 2004.

U.S. Environmental Protection Agency. "Consumer Confidence Reports (CCR)." http://www.epa.gov/safewater/ccr/index.html, 2006.

U.S. Environmental Protection Agency. "2000–2001 Pesticide Market Estimates: Usage." http://www.epa.gov/oppbead1/pestsales/01pestsales/usage2001.htm#3_1, 2007a.

U.S. Environmental Protection Agency. "Terms of the Environment." http://www.epa.gov/OCEPAterms, 2007b.

U.S. Environmental Protection Agency. "Pharmaceuticals and Personal Care Products (PPCPs)." http://www.epa.gov/ppcp, 2008a.

U.S. Environmental Protection Agency. "Safe Drinking Water Act." http://www.epa.gov/safewater/sdwa/index.html, 2008b.

U.S. Environmental Protection Agency. "Sanitary Survey Resources." http://www.epa.gov/OGWDW/dwa/resources.html, 2008c.

U.S. Environmental Protection Agency. "Safe Drinking Water Hotline 1–800–426–4791." http://www.epa.gov/safewater/hotline, 2008d.

U.S. Geological Survey. *High Plains Regional Ground-Water (HPGW) Study.* http://co.water.usgs.gov/nawqa/hpgw, 2007.

U.S. Geological Survey. *National Water-Quality Assessment (NAWQA) Program.* http://water.usgs.gov/nawqa, 2008.

Van Donsel, D. J., and Geldreich, E. E. "Relationships of Salmonellae to Fecal Coliforms in Bottom Sediments." *Water Research,* 1971, *5,* 1079–1087.

Wing, S., Freedman, S., and Band, L. "The Potential Impact of Flooding on Confined Animal Feeding Operations in Eastern North Carolina." *Environmental Health Perspectives,* 2002, *110,* 387–391.

Winter, T. C., Harvey, J. W., Franke, O. L., and Alley, W. M. *Ground Water and Surface Water—A Single Resource.* U.S. Geological Survey Circular 1139. http://pubs.usgs.gov/circ/circ1139, 1998.

Woods Hole Oceanographic Institution. "Red Tide." http://www.whoi.edu/redtide, 2008.

World Health Organization. *Guidelines for Drinking Water Quality,* Vol. *1: Recommendations.* (2nd ed.) Geneva: World Health Organization, 1993.

World Health Organization. *World Health Report 1996: Fighting Disease, Fostering Development.* http://www.who.int/whr/1996/en, 1996.

World Health Organization. *Guidelines for Safe Recreational Waters,* Vol. *1: Coastal and Fresh Waters.* http://www.who.int/water_sanitation_health/bathing/en, 2003a.

World Health Organization. *The Right to Water.* http://www.who.int/water_sanitation_health/en/rtwintro.pdf, 2003b.

World Health Organization. *World Health Report 2003: Shaping the Future.* http://www.who.int/whr/2003/en, 2003c.

World Health Organization. *Guidelines for Drinking Water Quality,* Vol. 1: *Recommendations.* (3rd ed.) http://www.who.int/water_sanitation_health/dwq/gdwq3rev/en, 2006.

World Health Organization. *Dracunculiasis eradication initiative,* http://www.who.int/dracunculiasis/eradication/en, 2008a.

World Health Organization. *Global Burden of Disease.* http://www.who.int/topics/global_burden_of_disease/en, 2008b.

World Health Organization. *World Malaria Report 2008.* http://apps.who.int/malaria/wmr2008/, 2008c.

Yadav, J. P., Lata, S., Kataria, S. K., and Kumar, S. "Fluoride Distribution in Groundwater and Survey of Dental Fluorosis Among School Children in the Villages of the Jhajjar District of Haryana, India." *Environmental Geochemistry and Health,* July 24, 2008. (Epub ahead of print.)

Yang, C. Y., Chiu, H. F., Cheng, M. F., and Tsai, S. S. "Chlorination of Drinking Water and Cancer Mortality in Taiwan." *Environmental Research,* 1998, *78,* 1–6.

Yeung, C. A. "A Systematic Review of the Efficacy and Safety of Fluoridation." *Evidence-Based Dentistry,* 2008, *9,* 39–43.

Young, L. Y., and Cerniglia, C. E. *Microbial Transformation and Degradation of Toxic Organic Chemicals.* Hoboken, N.J.: Wiley, 1995.

Zwingle, E. "Ogallala Aquifer: Wellspring of the High Plains." *National Geographic,* Mar. 1993, pp. 80–109.

FOR FURTHER INFORMATION

American Water Works Association (AWWA). [Home page.] http://www.awwa.org, 2008. This asso-
    ciation of water professionals provides consumer information on drinking water and many
    other water-related topics, and its home page contains many useful links, including a link to
    an online reference guide for physicians, sponsored by the American College of Preventive
    Medicine and titled, "Recognizing Waterborne Disease and The Health Effects of Water
    Pollution" (http://www.waterhealthconnection.org/index.asp, 2008).

British Geological Survey. "Arsenic Contamination of Groundwater." http://www.bgs.ac.uk/arsenic,
    2008. This organization's Web site provides information on the greatest mass poisoning from
    contaminated water ever recorded, the arsenic crisis in Bangladesh.

Centers for Disease Control and Prevention (CDC). *Morbidity and Mortality Weekly Report.* http://www
    .cdc.gov/mmwr. *MMWR* is the authoritative source on outbreaks of infectious disease in
    the United States. However, at least for waterborne disease, reports likely underestimate by
    orders of magnitude the actual incidence. The CDC's Division of Parasitic Diseases also
    offers the useful Web site "Parasitic Disease Information: Waterborne Illnesses," with infor-
    mation on drinking water, diarrheal disease, and recreational water quality (http://www.cdc
    .gov/ncidod/dpd/parasites/waterborne/default.htm, 2000).

U.S. Environmental Protection Agency (EPA). [Home page.] http://www.epa.gov. The EPA's Web site
    offers numerous useful resources related to water and health. In addition to the EPA Web
    sites in the References, see, for example, "Ground Water and Drinking Water" (http://www
    .epa.gov/safewater, 2008); "List of Contaminants and Their MCLs" (http://www.epa.gov/
    safewater/contaminants, 2008); and "Superfund Program" (http://www.epa.gov/superfund,
    2008). The publications of the EPA's National Risk Management Research Laboratory
    (NRMRL) are also of interest (http://www.epa.gov/nrmrl/publications.html, 2008).

Pacific Institute. [Home page.] http://www.pacinst.org. 2008. This "nonpartisan research institute . . .
    works to advance environmental protection, economic development, and social equity." Its
    Web site has links to a selection of publications that form a considerable database on, for
    example, global water availability and water use, as well as many other critical water issues.

United Nations. [Home page.] http://www.un.org. 2008. UN agencies offer a number of water-related
    Web sites, see, for example:

  United Nations Children's Fund (UNICEF). "Water, Environment and Sanitation." http://www.
      unicef.org/wes, 2008.

  United Nations Development Programme (UNDP). "Water Governance." http://www.undp.org/
      water, 2008.

  United Nations Educational, Scientific and Cultural Organization (UNESCO). "Water." http://
      www.unesco.org/water, 2008.

  United Nations Environmental Programme (UNEP). "Freshwater." http://www.unep.org/themes/
      freshwater, 2008.

U.S. Geological Survey (USGS). "National Water Quality Assessment Program." http://water.usgs.
    gov/nawqa, 2008. The USGS maintains an extremely useful online resource with current
    assessments of ground and surface water quality in many U.S. river basins and aquifers.

Water and Sanitation Program (WSP). [Home page.] http://www.wsp.org, 2007. The WSP describes itself as "an international partnership to help the poor gain sustained access to improved water and sanitation services."

Water Environment Federation (WEF). [Home page.] http://www.wef.org, 2008. The WEF describes itself as a "technical and educational organization" with members from varied disciplines who work toward the WEF vision of "preserving and enhancing the global water environment."

Water Environment Research Foundation. [Home page.] http://www.werf.org//AM/Template.cfm?Section=Home, 2008. This foundation is "America's leading independent scientific research organization dedicated to wastewater and stormwater issues," with information on its reports and research available from its Web site.

World Bank. [Home page.] http://www.worldbank.org, 2008. The World Bank Web site provides links to major World Bank-funded projects; see, for example, "Water Resources Management" (http://web.worldbank.org/WBSITE/EXTERNAL/TOPICS/EXTWAT/0,,contentMDK:21630583~menuPK:4602445~pagePK:148956~piPK:216618~theSitePK:4602123,00.html, 2008), and "Water Supply and Sanitation" (http://web.worldbank.org/WBSITE/EXTERNAL/TOPICS/EXTWAT/0,,contentMDK:21706928~menuPK:4602430~pagePK:148956~piPK:216618~theSitePK:4602123,00.html, 2008).

Woods Hole Oceanographic Institution (WHOI). "Harmful Algae." http://www.whoi.edu/redtide, 2007. In this Web site, WHOI offers probably the best maintained source of online information on toxic algal blooms.

World Health Organization (WHO). [Home page.] http://www.who.int/en, 2008. WHO publishes the Weekly *Epidemiological Record* (http://www.who.int/wer/en) and the annual World Health Report (http://www.who.int/whr/en)and is arguably the leading source of information for internationally accepted statistics on human health, including water and health, see, for example, "Health Topics," a Web site with links to pages on diarrheal disease, cholera, dracunculiasis, malaria, and so forth (http://www.who.int/topics/en, 2008); "WHO Guidelines for Drinking Water Quality" (http://www.who.int/water_sanitation_health/dwq/guidelines/en, 2008); and "Water, Sanitation and Health" (http://www.who.int/water_sanitation_health/en, 2008).

World Water Council. [Home page.] http://www.worldwatercouncil.org, 2005. The World Water Council, an "international multi-stakeholder platform for a water secure world," offers many articles on water policies and the barriers to and solutions for effective management of the world's water resources.

PART FOUR

ENVIRONMENTAL HEALTH ON THE LOCAL SCALE

CHAPTER SIXTEEN

SOLID AND HAZARDOUS WASTE

SVEN RODENBECK

KENNETH ORLOFF

HENRY FALK

KEY CONCEPTS

- Waste is an important by-product of human activities. It can be divided into several categories, including solid waste, hazardous waste, and specialized waste such as medical waste.

- Each kind of waste may have potential effects on human health.

- Various laws and policies govern the management of waste.

- The preferred approach to waste is to minimize waste generation.

- Waste can be managed in a variety of ways, such as incineration and landfilling. Each has potential health consequences, and each must be carried out in ways that maximally protect health.

HISTORICAL PERSPECTIVE

As are all animal species, humans are producers of wastes. It is significant, however, that as humankind has evolved, the character of the waste produced has changed markedly. No other species in the animal kingdom shares this trait. Like the animal's, the waste of early humans was highly organic, and consisted of such materials as excreta, bedding materials, crude clothing, and implements. As humans evolved, however, refined and inorganic materials such as paper, cloth, ceramics, and metals were added to their wastes.

For many centuries, human waste products reflected a fundamentally agrarian lifestyle. As human endeavors evolved to include more technology and industry, the mix of wastes produced by society changed radically and irrevocably. Mining spoils, ashes and slag from metal processing, and other industrial wastes became commonplace. As industry grew in complexity through the nineteenth and twentieth centuries, the waste mix became more varied and complex to manage. Waste management has emerged as a significant challenge because of the growing variety of wastes and the trend throughout the twentieth century toward more packaging and disposal features.

Finally, along with the industrialization and modernization of society, the steady trend toward urbanization of much of the population has challenged waste management. As cities became more crowded, a shortage of space to accommodate all the waste developed. Open dumping and backyard burn barrels were no longer acceptable means of waste disposal. This chapter describes the types of wastes produced by modern society, the significance of those wastes with respect to human health and the environment, and some of the ways in which wastes are managed.

SOLID WASTE

Determining whether something is **solid waste** is not a trivial matter. People have debated for years about what solid waste is and how it should be managed. In fact some material that is managed as solid waste is not a solid at room temperature but is rather a liquid or gas (for example, gasses in cylinders). A fundamental premise is that a material is *waste* if it no longer has value—a judgment that may be subjective and may vary over time. There have been situations where material designated as waste was later found to have value. For example, using new technology former mining wastes have been reextracted to recover residual metals. Cultural norms also influence the value judgment. Western industrial

Sven Rodenbeck, Kenneth Orloff, and Henry Falk declare no competing financial interests.

societies often throw away material with little thought of reuse or repair alternatives. However, as a starting point, the fundamental premise that it lacks value is probably adequate to characterize solid waste.

In the United States and in most modern industrial countries, waste material is typically divided into three broad categories:

1. Municipal solid waste
2. Special waste
3. Hazardous waste

Complex laws and regulations govern how these materials are identified, stored, collected, transported, treated, and finally disposed.

PERSPECTIVE
U.S. Solid and Hazardous Waste Laws

Prior to 1965, there were no federal laws to govern the management and disposal of solid and hazardous waste. Each state and territory had its own set of laws and regulations, and these rules were not always consistent. The Solid Waste Disposal Act of 1965 brought about, for the first time, a national focus on the management of these wastes. That Act granted limited authority to the U.S. Public Health Service to provide money to assist in the development of statewide solid waste management plans; provide technical assistance to state and local waste management authorities, and conduct applied and basic research.

In 1976, Congress amended the Solid Waste Disposal Act of 1965 and granted the U.S. Environmental Protection Agency (EPA) regulatory and enforcement authority over the management of solid and hazardous waste. That Act, called the Resource Conservation and Recovery Act of 1976 (RCRA), provided, for the first time, a national regulatory framework for solid and hazardous waste management. The most significant change brought about by the RCRA regulations was the requirement that hazardous waste be tracked from its point of generation to its final disposal or treatment. The regulations also required that all future solid waste landfills be designed and constructed to meet minimum standards, including having liners to prevent the movement of water through the waste into the underlying aquifer.

Another important federal law is the Comprehensive Environmental Response, Compensation and Liability Act of 1980 (CERCLA), commonly known as Superfund. This law gave the EPA the authority to clean up old hazardous waste sites that endanger the health of people and the environment.

Over the years, the U.S. Congress has amended RCRA and CERCLA to expand the authority of the EPA and to improve that agency's ability to protect the environment and health of the U.S. population (Hickman, 1999).

Municipal Solid Waste

Municipal solid waste consists of everyday items that are commonly generated from homes. Over half of the U.S. municipal solid waste generated in 2006
consisted of containers, packaging, and nondurable goods such as newspapers
and magazines (Figure 16.1). Other major components of municipal solid waste
include yard trimmings, food wastes, and durable goods such as appliances, tires,
and batteries. Local laws and regulations may prohibit the disposal of some of
these materials (such as tires) as municipal solid waste. More and more frequently,
municipal and county governments are also prohibiting the disposal of yard clippings with municipal solid waste, requiring that the clippings be composted or
disposed of in some other, more environmentally friendly manner.

In the United States the per capita generation of municipal solid waste has
steadily increased over recent decades. In 2006, the average American generated

**FIGURE 16.1   Composition of the 251 Million Tons of Municipal
Solid Waste Produced in the United States (Before Recycling),
May 2006**

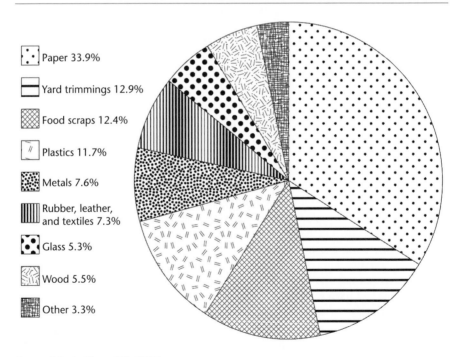

Paper 33.9%

Yard trimmings 12.9%

Food scraps 12.4%

Plastics 11.7%

Metals 7.6%

Rubber, leather,
and textiles 7.3%

Glass 5.3%

Wood 5.5%

Other 3.3%

Source: Adapted from EPA, 2006a.

approximately 4.6 pounds of waste each day, a 70 percent increase from the 1960 average of 2.7 pounds per person per day (Figure 16.2).

Municipal solid waste from nonresidential sources, such as office buildings, is usually handled along with residential waste unless specifically regulated. For example, companies that discard large quantities of spent dry cell batteries may be required to manage them as hazardous waste.

Special Waste

Special waste is a catch-all category. However, if a waste is neither municipal solid waste nor a designated hazardous waste; it likely has a special designation and associated laws or regulations. Some commonly identified special wastes are

- Medical waste
- Construction debris
- Asbestos
- Mining waste
- Agricultural waste

FIGURE 16.2   Total Amount and Per Capita Generation Rate of Municipal Solid Waste Produced in the United States (Before Recycling), 1960–2006

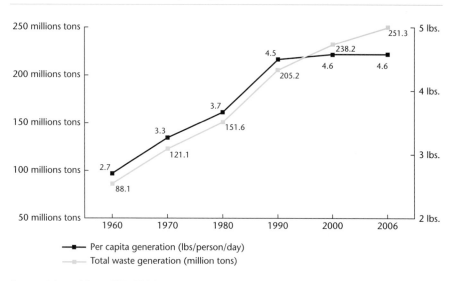

Source: Adapted from EPA, 2006a.

- Radioactive waste
- Sewage sludge
- Electronic waste

Medical Waste **Medical waste** includes items that are generated from health care treatment or research facilities (human and nonhuman) and that have come into contact with body fluids (for example, blood) or other materials that may contain infectious agents and may cause disease. Some examples of medical waste are

- Soiled or blood-soaked bandages
- Culture dishes and other associated glassware
- Items such as gloves, gowns, and scalpels used during surgery
- Needles used to give injections or draw blood
- Body fluids and tissues

One of the reasons medical waste is handled separately from municipal solid waste is to protect sanitation workers from infectious agents in the waste materials.

Construction Debris Unless the material is regulated separately (as asbestos is, for example), the **construction debris** waste stream consists of material generated from the construction and demolition of buildings and other facilities. Typically this rubble is disposed of in specific construction debris landfills or in municipal solid waste landfills. Recent research has found that construction debris is not as innocuous as previously thought. If water is allowed to infiltrate through the waste drywall in a landfill, hydrogen sulfide can be formed and the surrounding population could be exposed to hydrogen sulfide levels of health concern (Agency for Toxic Substances and Disease Registry [ATSDR], 2006).

Asbestos In the United States, **asbestos** is designated as a special waste, with its own rules and regulations. In the past this class of fibrous minerals was used extensively in such consumer products as car brake linings and construction materials. Most uses of asbestos have been banned in the United States because of its demonstrated capacity to cause disease in workers and other exposed people. To prevent the airborne release of asbestos fibers, federal regulations provide detailed guidance on the removal, packaging, and disposal of materials containing asbestos.

Mining Waste The extraction of metals, coal, and oil from the Earth's crust generates huge quantities of **mining waste** materials. The volume of wastes from mining operations exceeds the volume of wastes from all other categories combined (EPA, 1985). The disposal of this leftover rubble and liquid material is

PERSPECTIVE
Health Risks of Medical Waste

Concerns about the proper management and disposal of waste material generated during health care activities have been a topic of discussion for several years (Lichtveld, Rodenbeck, and Lybarger, 1992). The U.S. public's concerns about medical waste heightened after medical care debris washed up on East coast beaches during the summers of 1987 and 1988. In addition to aesthetic concerns, fear of AIDS (acquired immunodeficiency syndrome) contributed heavily to the public's anxiety regarding medical waste.

The predominant health risk associated with medical waste is the presence of infectious organisms (parasites, bacteria, and viruses). It is important to remember that infectious disease can occur only when all of the following are present: an infectious agent, a sufficient quantity of this agent to cause infection, a susceptible host, and an appropriate portal of entry into that susceptible host. If any one of these factors is missing, then disease will not occur. Because many infectious agents do not remain viable for an extended period of time outside a host, the potential for transmitting disease is greatest at the point where the waste is generated, usually in a hospital, clinic, or medical office. People who provide medical care at home may also be exposed to infectious wastes. Studies have documented that the greatest risk of disease transmission from medical waste is associated with accidental skin punctures from hypodermic needles and other *sharps*. This is particularly true for sharps contaminated with blood-borne pathogens (specifically hepatitis B or C viruses, and, to a much lesser extent, HIV).

Owing to aesthetic concerns and studies demonstrating that health care workers have a higher risk than the rest of the population of being infected with hepatitis B or C and HIV from medical waste, medical waste is separated at the source from municipal solid waste. Separate containers are located in or near medical treatment areas in the health care facility. In particular, sharps are placed in penetration-resistant containers. The containers are then sealed and, usually, shipped to specifically designed and managed medical waste incinerators. In some situations the waste material is treated in large autoclaves and then shipped to a secure landfill.

regulated both by solid waste laws and regulations and by water pollution control and land use and reuse laws and regulations.

Agricultural Waste   In technologically advanced countries the production of food has become highly industrialized. A common arrangement for raising animals on a large scale is the concentrated animal feed operation (CAFO). CAFOs can bring thousands of poultry, swine, or cattle together in confined spaces. These facilities can become large-scale sources of **agricultural waste** in the form of air emissions (such as ammonia, hydrogen sulfide, odors, and particles contaminated with a wide range of microorganisms) (Heederik and others, 2007) and **animal waste**. The animal waste in turn contains nutrients, microbes, and veterinary chemicals. For example, antibiotics are used in raising animals; these can be discharged into the environment, where they may contribute to the development of antibiotic resistant pathogens (Gilchrist and others, 2007; Silbergeld, Graham, and Price, 2008). The waste stream may also contain other veterinary chemicals, such as arsenic (Silbergeld and Nachman, 2008). The EPA's clean water protection program regulates the management of the liquid waste and the sludge, or manure, from animal feed lots and CAFOs. Those waste materials not regulated by federal laws are managed either by local authorities or in accordance with best practices developed by the industry. There is concern, however, that these protective strategies may not suffice to protect the public's health (Burkholder and others, 2007).

Radioactive Waste   **Radioactive waste** contains radioactive chemical elements. Generally it is divided into two subcategories: low-level waste and high-level waste. Low-level waste consists of used protective clothing and other items that contain low levels of radioactivity per mass or volume. It is typically disposed of in specifically designated landfills. High-level radioactive waste consists of spent nuclear fuel and waste materials left after spent fuel is reprocessed. The disposal of this nuclear waste is very controversial. The United States has been trying for years to establish a permanent high-level radioactive waste repository inside Yucca Mountain, Nevada. Currently, most of the high-level radioactive waste in the United States is stored temporarily in spent fuel pools and in dry cask storage facilities.

Sewage Sludge   Before waste water is discharged back into the environment, it undergoes a series of treatments (mostly biological and chemical) to remove or break down any hazardous biological or chemical constituents. One of the main by-products of this treatment processes is **sewage sludge**; which is made up primarily of concentrated solid materials. The disposal of sewage sludge is regulated, and the methods allowed are based on whether any hazardous materials are present. Some sewage sludge is safe enough after it has been disinfected to be applied to cropland.

Electronic Waste   More commonly called *e-waste*, **electronic waste** includes unwanted, obsolete, or unusable electronic equipment such as computers, computer display monitors, televisions, VCRs, DVD players, cell phones, and electronic games. This waste stream is described in the accompanying Perspective.

PERSPECTIVE
E-Waste

The volume of e-waste is growing rapidly as technology advances (Schmidt, 2002). In 2007, the EPA estimated that e-waste totaled 2.5 million tons or about 2 percent of the municipal waste steam. About 82 percent of e-waste was discarded, primarily in landfills, and the rest was recycled (EPA, 2008a).

Improper disposal of e-waste is of concern because electronic components contain hazardous metals, such as lead, cadmium, and mercury, and the plastic housings and cables contain brominated flame retardants, such as polybrominated diphenyl ethers (PBDEs) and polybrominated biphenyls (PBBs). Cathode ray tubes (CRTs), or *picture tubes*, are of particular concern because they contain, on average, about 4 pounds of lead. If disposed in an unlined landfill, this lead could leach into groundwater. Under RCRA regulations, households and small-volume generators can dispose of CRTs in municipal trash. However large-volume generators (more than 100 kilograms of hazardous wastes per month) must dispose of the e-waste in a hazardous waste landfill. Some states, such as California and Massachusetts, regulate all CRTs as hazardous waste and ban their disposal in municipal landfills (Schmidt, 2006; Osibanjo and Nnorom, 2007).

As with other waste materials, the preferred strategies for e-waste management are (in order of preference) to

1. Reuse the equipment
2. Recycle the materials
3. Properly dispose of the equipment in an approved landfill

In the United States the EPA is working with stakeholders in the private and public sectors to promote greater electronic products stewardship. Efforts are being made to reduce the amounts of toxic substances in electronic equipment and to increase the reuse and recycling of used electronics. To encourage recycling some states have imposed fees on new computers and televisions, which will be used to establish a statewide electronics recycling system, and several electronics manufactures have implemented take-back programs. In the United States the high costs of labor and equipment, and strict environmental regulations are obstacles to economically viable recycling of e-waste. Consequently, the United States and other industrialized nations ship large quantities of e-waste to Asia and more recently to Africa for recycling (Schmidt, 2006). This practice has been characterized as international trafficking in hazardous wastes, as discussed later in this chapter.

Hazardous Waste

Hazardous waste can be defined simply as waste with properties that make it capable of harming human health or the environment. However, for regulatory purposes this simple definition is not sufficient. In the United States the Environmental Protection Agency, in order to carry out the provisions of the Resource Conservation and Recovery Act, has developed specific criteria for defining hazardous waste. Two different mechanisms are applied. The first is to include the materials from approximately 500 specific **industrial waste** streams. These listed wastes include spent solvents, electroplating wastes, and wood-preserving wastes. The second mechanism relates to the waste's characteristics. The EPA has developed standardized test criteria to determine a waste's ignitability, corrosiveness, reactivity, and toxicity. If a waste possesses defined levels of any of these characteristics, it is classified as hazardous. At the same time, under the terms of the Act many waste materials (such as petroleum-related materials) are specifically excluded from the hazardous waste definition and regulations.

In 2005, approximately 38 million tons of hazardous waste was generated in the United States (EPA, 2006b). The states that generated the most hazardous waste tended to be those with a large petrochemical industry.

In general, other industrialized countries designate hazardous waste much as the United States does, although they may use different coding or terminology.

SOLID WASTE MANAGEMENT STRATEGIES

Because solid and hazardous wastes may affect human health, **waste management** is a fundamental part of environmental public health. Waste management is best accomplished through a multitiered approach. The first tier is primary waste stream reduction. Materials recycling, substitution of materials, and changes in consumer habits, among other methods, can help industries, communities, and other groups achieve waste stream reduction. All sectors of a modern society, when approached with effective informational campaigns and incentives, can practice waste reduction.

The second tier of solid waste management involves proper handling and disposal of waste, that is, in a manner that protects the public health and the environment. Although complete avoidance of solid waste generation is the ideal, it is likely that there will always be some residual of mankind's activities requiring disposal.

In the United States, landfilling is the means of disposal for 55 percent of municipal waste. Approximately 50 percent of U.S. hazardous waste is disposed

PERSPECTIVE
Community Right to Know

In the United States, effort has been given to providing local communities with ample information regarding the release of hazardous materials into the environment. In 1986, Congress passed the Emergency Planning and Community Right-to-Know Act (EPCRA). This Act establishes planning and reporting requirements for federal, state, and local governments; Indian tribes; and industry and requires the involvement of the local community (Schierow, 2007).

One of the centerpieces of the Act concerns preplanning for the accidental release of hazardous materials. Community emergency response plans, developed with the public, should, as described in Section 303 of the Act:

- Identify facilities and transportation routes of extremely hazardous substances;
- Describe emergency response procedures, on-site and off-site;
- Designate a community coordinator and facility coordinator(s) to implement the plan;
- Outline emergency notification procedures;
- Describe how to determine the probable area and population affected by releases;
- Describe local emergency equipment and facilities and the persons responsible for them;
- Outline evacuation plans;
- Provide a training program for emergency responders (including schedules); and,
- Provide methods and schedules for exercising emergency response plans.

Another centerpiece of EPCRA is the requirement that certain industrial facilities and operations annually report an estimate of what types of hazardous materials and how much of these materials are stored on-site, treated on-site, and released to the environment. With this information the EPA maintains the National Toxics Release Inventory, or TRI (www.epa.gov/tri).

The EPCRA requirements and the additional sources information available (from discharge permits for waste water and air releases, for example) provide the public with a substantial amount of information to help communities plan for growth and environmental protection. The public can also better understand the potential for contact with and exposure to hazardous materials.

of via underground injection (EPA, 2006b). Each of these approaches has public health implications.

The next two sections of this chapter explore each of these two tiers of solid waste management in greater detail.

PRIMARY PREVENTION OF WASTE

The ideal waste management strategy is not to produce the waste in the first place. This goal can be approached in several ways, that is, through efforts to **reduce, reuse, and recycle**. In an industrial setting this goal might be achieved by altering production processes to avoid or reduce the use of a hazardous chemical. For example, in some electroplating operations, less toxic alternatives can replace highly toxic cyanide salts. In office settings, converting to electronic commerce and records management can reduce waste paper production.

Waste reduction also applies to municipal wastes. The quantity of raw materials in food and beverage containers is being reduced because of economic pressures. In the past few decades, manufacturers have reduced the amount of steel and aluminum in cans and the amount of plastic in milk jugs and plastic bags. These efforts have reduced the cost of these containers and decreased the amount of wastes to be disposed. Further reductions in packaging could be achieved if consumers carried reusable canvas shopping bags instead of expecting plastic or paper bags with each purchase.

If the generation of waste cannot be abated or reduced, then the next best alternative is to recycle the waste. Recycling can refer to using waste material to produce more of the original product or to using waste material in something else. Examples of the first kind of recycling include making glass or paper from used glass or paper and making new lead batteries from old lead batteries. An example of the second kind of recycling is using mining wastes as aggregate for asphalt and concrete production. In recent years, increased efforts to reduce the amount of trash dumped into landfills have led municipalities to encourage recycling of paper, plastic, aluminum, and glass. In some communities homeowners are also encouraged to compost yard waste to recycle it into a useful soil amendment. Recycling of municipal solid waste has steadily increased in the United States; today about 32.5 percent of waste is recycled (Figure 16.3). Other industrialized nations tend to have a higher rate of recycling (Figure 16.4).

The importance of waste minimization has led to the emerging field of industrial ecology. **Industrial ecology** is the study of the physical, chemical, and biological interactions and interrelationships both within and between industrial and ecological systems (Garner and Keoleian, 1995). A primary goal of industrial ecology

FIGURE 16.3   Total Amount and Percentage of Municipal Solid
Waste Recycled in the United States, 1960–2006

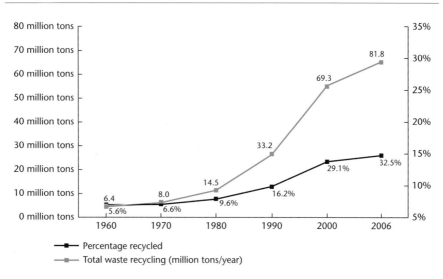

- Percentage recycled
- Total waste recycling (million tons/year)

Source: Adapted from EPA, 2006a.

FIGURE 16.4   Glass and Paper Recycling in Industrial Nations

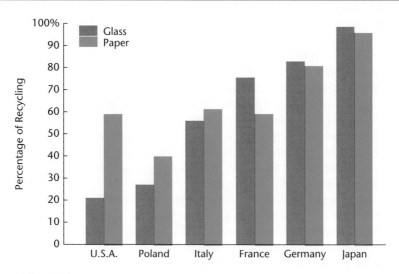

Source: Zeller, 2008.

is to change the linear nature of our industrial systems, in which raw materials are used and products and wastes are discarded, into a cyclical system where the wastes are used as raw materials or energy for another product.

A famous example of an eco-industrial park is the Kalunborg industrial park in Denmark (Ehrenfeld and Gertler, 1997). In this park the companies reuse each other's wastes in the production of their own products. For example, Asnævæket, a coal-fired power plant, captures sulfur dioxide from its flue stack gas and converts it to calcium sulfate (gypsum), which is sold to a plaster board plant. Another example is Novo Nordisk, a biotechnology company that produces insulin and industrial enzymes and then supplies biosludge waste to a nearby farm that uses it for fertilizer. These examples illustrate an industrial symbiosis in which energy and wastes are recycled and reused by another process within the system.

PERSPECTIVE
Tire Reuse and Recycling

Some types of wastes have evolved to pose unique challenges and opportunities. Just over 100 years ago, waste from transportation operations consisted mainly of horse manure and also ash and clinker produced from burning coal in steam engines. One century later these transportation wastes have been replaced with, among other things, an estimated yearly production of a quarter of a billion waste rubber tires in the United States alone.

Waste tires are problematic for both storage and disposal (Figure 16.5). They are hard to bury in landfills. Landfill operators report that tires tend to work their way up to the surface of the fill and disrupt the integrity of the cover. Tires also serve as mosquito-breeding sites when stored outdoors. And, when stored in large piles, tires are vulnerable to fire. Tire fires are very difficult to extinguish and can cause substantial pollution of both the air and underlying soil and water environment.

Approximately 20 percent of all used tires are recycled directly, through the retreading process, leading to interest in identifying additional ways of reusing or recycling waste tires (Rubber Manufacturers Association, 2004). After being broken into chunks of rubber, used tires are being used in truck bed liners, antifatigue mats, soaker hoses, shoe soles, swings and civil engineering material (for leachate drainage material and for an alternative daily cover at solid waste landfills). Ground, or crumb, rubber has been added to asphalt for paving, and research has been done on adding crumb rubber to concrete. When crumb rubber is blended with plastic, the resultant material can be processed like plastic but retains some of the elasticity of rubber. Pallets and railroad ties have been made from plastic and rubber blends.

WASTE TREATMENT AND DISPOSAL

As discussed earlier, it would be ideal if all solid and hazardous or special waste could be recycled, reused, or avoided. Unfortunately, this ideal goal may not be attained. As a result, society should strive to dispose of all such wastes in a manner that minimizes harm to human health and the environment. Both budgetary limitations and the need to comply with applicable regulations influence selection of the most practical option.

In years past it was common to burn wastes in backyard barrels, open dumps, and crude incinerators. All these methods had undesirable environmental and health impacts. During the second half of the twentieth century, public demand

As with any material recycling, economic factors enter into the ultimate fate of a particular waste stream, such as used tires. One potential use of waste tires is as tire derived fuel (TDF), which is blended with coal as a fuel supplement. Cement kilns have been considered good candidates for such fuel blends because the resultant ash can be incorporated directly into the final product and the air pollution impacts from the blended fuel are less than from burning coal alone. As energy costs continue to escalate, the prospects of using more TDF seem favorable.

FIGURE 16.5   Waste Tires

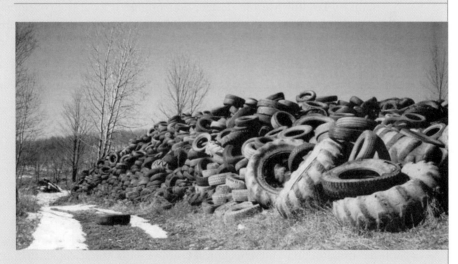

Source: CDC/ATSDR, 2002.

and governmental regulations led to improved waste treatment and disposal methods. Controlled or sanitary landfills replaced dumps. More sophisticated and controlled combustion systems replace crude incinerators. Newer incinerators were specifically designed for the type of wastes burned, such as medical waste, industrial waste, or municipal solid waste. Some industrial wastes, such as liquid brines, were discharged far beneath the Earth's surface, through deep well injection. Potentially harmful industrial wastes that had been previously discarded haphazardly in dumps or burial pits were also treated with remedial technologies designed to reduce or limit harmful impacts.

Sanitary Landfill

Open-burning municipal waste dumps, which were once prevalent throughout the United States, were the source of many environmental and public health problems. These problems included air pollution; groundwater pollution; and rats, flies and other disease-carrying vectors, as well as nuisance odors and unsightly conditions. The creation of the EPA in 1970 prompted a major move in the United States to eliminate open dumps and replace them with the improved **sanitary landfill**. Careful site selection and preparation, the application of a daily covering of earth for each day's accumulation of waste, and other procedural provisions eliminated most of the problems with open dumping. Between 1996 and 2006, the number of operating municipal sanitary landfills in the United States decreased from about 3,100 to 1,754 (EPA, 2006a).

Sanitary landfills vary in design, depending on local site considerations. However, by definition, all sanitary landfills share certain design features and operating principles, as discussed here.

Site Selection and Preparation   Many technical and social factors go into selecting a site for a municipal sanitary landfill. Technical considerations include the cost of the land and ensuring

- An adequate area to provide waste disposal capacity for a reasonable time period
- An adequate elevation or separation to protect regional ground water
- Available or appropriate soil for daily soil cover requirements
- An adequate buffer from surrounding populations

Normally, several candidate sites will be identified and evaluated using these criteria. In addition to these technical requirements, the selected site must also meet with community acceptance or, at least, attempt to minimize community outrage. Solid waste treatment or disposal sites of any kind are generally perceived as bad neighbors; consequently, community and political pressures and concerns often influence site selection.

Once a landfill site has been selected, site preparation can begin. In addition to grading and installing sediment and erosion controls to protect local surface waters, provisions must also be made to protect groundwater from leachate. **Leachate,** a liquid, organic waste decomposition product sometimes contaminated with chemicals, can migrate down and into the local aquifer. In the absence of a natural barrier, installing an underlying man-made impervious barrier can provide protection. Where significant amounts of leachate are anticipated, some landfills have systems to collect and treat the leachate. Similarly, provisions are often made for collecting and controlling gaseous products of waste decomposition, consisting mainly of methane. In some cases the methane is cleaned and used as fuel for local energy production. Other site preparations can include aesthetic screening of the site, scales for weighing incoming trash trucks, maintenance facilities, flares or gas vents, security arrangements, and monitoring wells to sample leachate. Figure 16.6 provides a generalized depiction of a modern sanitary landfill.

Site Operations   Sanitary landfills are operated in a manner intended to contain and control waste. Each day's accumulation of waste is placed in the cell, compacted, and covered with earth. Usually waste is spread and compacted by heavy equipment on a sloped working face within the cell. This compaction reduces the waste volume, thereby extending the life of the landfill, and it also reduces the potential for fires. At the end of the day the working face and entire cell are covered with approximately six inches of compacted soil. This minimizes litter problems, helps control odors, and largely eliminates problems from animal and insect vectors. Some municipalities use precompacted, baled solid waste so landfill operators can stack the waste like building blocks each day and thereby maximize site life.

Other operating features also minimize nuisance and health threats associated with landfills. For example, movable fence sections control blowing litter during particularly windy conditions. A supply of appropriate cover material may be stockpiled for cold or wet weather when daily excavation for cover soil would not be suitable. Odor and bird control provisions are sometimes made. Portions of the landfill may be dedicated to the disposal of hard-to-handle wastes such as bulky demolition debris or large appliances. And lastly, the sanitary landfill may be designed so that after it is closed, the land can be converted to a community asset, such as a golf course or park.

Industrial and hazardous waste landfills share many of the containment and control features of sanitary landfills; however, they are much more heavily regulated.

FIGURE 16.6   Generalized Depiction of a State-of-the-Art Sanitary Landfill

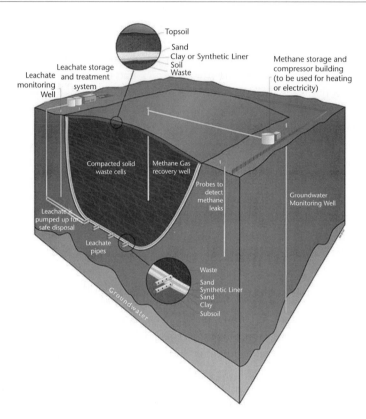

Source: CDC/ATSDR, 2002.

The type of waste allowed in a given landfill is strictly defined in the operating permit. In some cases certain hazardous wastes must be specially treated, packaged, or stabilized before being placed in the landfill. Periodic analysis of the wastes may be required to ensure that adequate characterization of the fill is maintained.

Incineration

Broadly defined, **incineration** is the controlled combustion of a waste. Incineration has been used for all types of wastes, including municipal solid wastes, sewage sludge, industrial and hazardous waste, and medical wastes. Some large municipal and industrial incinerators are designed to capture energy for reuse.

The goal of incineration is to reduce the volume of the waste being processed or to reduce the hazardous characteristics of a particular waste stream, or both. All incineration attempts to control several variables in an effort to maximize the completeness of combustion. The classic 3 T's of combustion are

1. Time: the length of time that solids and combustion gases are in the ignition and burn zones of the incinerator
2. Temperature: an indication of the amount of heat energy in the combustion chambers available to break molecular bonds and facilitate oxidation toward the desired end products of combustion (carbon dioxide, water vapor, inorganic ash)
3. Turbulence: the agitation of both solids and the combustible by-products needed to provide opportunity for complete oxidation to take place.

The other major factor in fundamental combustion control is the provision of adequate oxygen, usually in the form of combustion air, to complete all oxidation reactions. The theoretically required amount of air for complete combustion of a given waste stream is known as the *stoichiometric air requirement*. In actual incineration systems, air in excess of this requirement is provided to force the reaction toward complete oxidation of the organic wastes. This excess air is usually reported as a percentage of stoichiometric air.

Specific incineration designs vary widely in the ways that wastes are introduced into the units and in the ways that air control and mixing is achieved. Some incinerators have multiple chambers for combustion. Ignition and preliminary combustion take place in a *primary* chamber. The volatile products from the primary chamber are oxidized to completion in a *secondary* chamber, or afterburner. Some incinerators, sometimes known as starved air or pyrolytic combustors, seek to minimize entrainment of particulate in the primary chamber by keeping combustion air below the stoichiometric amount. Another way to reduce gas volume flow in the primary chamber is to use pure oxygen, rather than ambient air, for combustion.

Early incinerators were noted for smoke, odors, and sometimes even live embers coming out of the exhaust stacks. Because of these unacceptable conditions, regulations now require strict air pollution control technology. Now, devices such as wet or caustic scrubbers control acid gas. Electrostatic precipitators, venturi scrubbers, and baghouses capture fine particulates. Some of the newest hazardous waste incinerators have a final activated-carbon filtration system. This polishing device minimizes emission of low-level products of incomplete combustion (PICs), such as dioxins and polycyclic aromatic hydrocarbons (PAHs). Inorganic waste contaminants, such as heavy metals (mercury, lead, and chromium, for example) can be difficult to control and can require special pollution control systems or elimination from the waste being fed to the incinerator (Figure 16.7). Because of increased traffic from trucks hauling in wastes and also because of odors and aesthetic objections, communities rarely welcome incinerators or waste landfills.

Deep Well Injection

Deep well injection is a liquid waste disposal technology that uses deep injection wells to force treated or untreated liquid waste into geological formations that do not allow migration of contaminants into potential potable water aquifers. These wells, typically several thousand feet deep, extend into a permeable injection zone containing highly saline brines that render the water nonpotable. Impermeable rock or soil layers confine the injection zone vertically. The wastes injected can be radioactive wastes, hydrocarbon wastes, oil and gas drilling brines, hazardous wastes, and other wastes not suitable for landfill. In the United

FIGURE 16.7   Generalized Diagram of Incineration Material and Process Flow

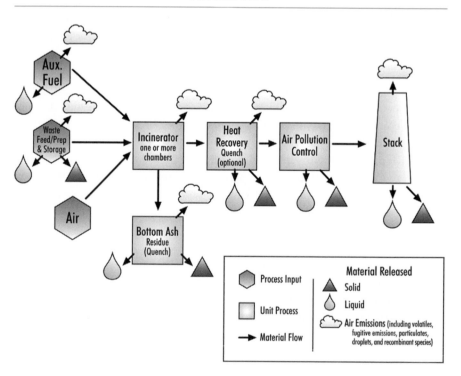

Source: CDC/ATSDR, 2002.

States' injection wells are regulated and classified under an EPA definition that addresses uses and characteristics of such wells.

Injection wells can only be located in areas free of faults and other geological features that could allow wastes to migrate into potable water aquifers. Liquid wastes high in suspended solids, iron content, or organic substrates that could serve as food for microbial growth should not be disposed of in such wells because of their potential to foul or clog the well. Injection wells are double sleeved to allow monitoring for system integrity and to provide dual boundaries for protecting intervening geological layers.

Other Technologies

The previous discussion touches on some of the most prevalent methods for treating and disposing wastes, but many other waste treatment techniques are in practice or evolving. Treatment methods such as supercritical water oxidation, molten metals and molten salt oxidation, glass melt and vitrification processes, and waste-specific biological treatment systems and composting are a few such technologies. Dedicated treatment technologies, such as thermal desorption, have been developed for in situ and extractive remediation of old industrial waste disposal sites. Waste disposal technology has undergone tremendous technological evolution to keep pace with the changing character of society's waste products.

HEALTH CONCERNS

Exposure to solid and hazardous wastes can adversely affect human health in several ways. The aesthetic impact of poor waste management—trash piling up in streets and vacant lots—can undermine the livability and even the safety of a community. At least five kinds of health hazards are well recognized:

1. Infectious disease risks from poorly managed solid waste
2. Contamination of drinking water and soil by biological, chemical, and mining wastes
3. Gas migration and leachate discharges from landfills
4. Emissions of air pollutants from incinerators
5. Contamination of food by waste chemicals that escape into the environment

Poorly operated landfills can be havens for flies, mosquitoes, rats, and mice. Uncovered garbage and trash provide them with food, shelter, and a breeding ground. These insects and animals can be vectors for disease by carrying pathogenic

PERSPECTIVE
Waste Management During National Disasters

National emergencies tend to cause a significant increase in waste material over what would normally be generated. In addition, the waste streams will likely not be compatible with the normal management methods, because various types of waste will be mixed together. These factors and others must be carefully considered by the emergency recovery managers.

The 2001 attack on and collapse of the twin towers of the World Trade Center resulted in the generation of over 1.2 million tons of waste (U.S. Army Corps of Engineers, 2002). Recovery operations required that this waste be removed from lower Manhattan Island across the Hudson River to the Fresh Kills Landfill on Staten Island, New York. A new barge-loading area was constructed near ground zero specifically for this purpose, and for ten months the World Trade Center waste was transported to the landfill (on average 10,000 tons per day). Because asbestos-containing material and other hazardous substances were intermixed with the debris, specific management and worker safety procedures were employed. In addition, the waste was searched so that any identifiable human remains could be separated from the waste. Over 50,000 tons of World Trade Center steel was recycled, with approximately 7 tons of that steel being used to manufacture the bow stem of the new U.S. Navy amphibious transport dock ship USS *New York* (LPD-21) (U.S. Navy, 2007).

In the summer of 2005, Hurricanes Katrina and Rita caused damage across a 90,000-square-mile area in Alabama, Mississippi, Louisiana, and Texas. It has been estimated that over 63 million tons of debris was generated because of these storms (Luther, 2007). The intermixed debris found in Louisiana included

microbes into the surrounding community. Rats and mice can spread thirty-five diseases to humans, including leptospirosis, hantavirus pulmonary syndrome, and lymphocytic choriomeningitis virus (Centers for Disease Control and Prevention, 2008). Furthermore, rats can carry many kinds of mites, lice, fleas, and ticks that act as disease vectors. Modern landfills, which require wastes to be covered daily with clean soil, have greatly reduced the spread of disease by these vectors.

Improper disposal of solid and hazardous wastes can contaminate drinking water. Both groundwater and surface water can be affected. Most old landfills or dumps lack liners, which allows chemicals buried in the landfill to leach down into the underlying aquifer. Volatile organic compounds (VOCs), such as trichloroethylene and tetrachloroethylene, and petroleum distillates are common contaminants in municipal and industrial landfills. These organic solvents are widely used as degreasers, dry cleaning fluids, and components of paints, varnishes,

- Normal municipal solid waste
- Vegetative debris—bushes and trees
- Construction debris—from damaged homes and commercial buildings
- Asbestos—household insulation, tile, and siding
- Household hazardous waste—oil, pesticides, paints, cleaning agents
- Over 891,900 white goods—refrigerators, freezers, washers, dryers, stoves, water heaters, dishwashers, and air conditioners
- Over 602,700 electronic waste items
- Over 350,000 cars and 60,000 fishing and pleasure boats

In the New Orleans area alone, over 19,000 tons of rotten meat and other food from commercial cold storage facilities had to be managed. Similar types and quantities of intermixed debris were found in the other affected areas.

To manage the complex, hurricane-generated waste stream, the recovery officials undertook a multiple-prong approach that emphasized separation of the intermixed wastes when possible and recycling. As is true across the United States, landfill space was at a premium in the hurricane-damaged area. Therefore volume reduction was also a key part of the waste management recovery plan. Vegetative debris was either shredded or ground up by industrial shredders or grinders or it was incinerated. At several locations industrial grinders were also used in the management of municipal solid waste. Unfortunately, some situations dictated that the waste could not be separated. For example, it was not safe for recovery workers to enter structurally unsound homes to separate out asbestos-containing materials. Therefore, the whole structure and its contents had to be managed and disposed of as asbestos-containing materials. This required that special handling procedures be used and that the whole home and its contents be disposed of in those landfills authorized to receive asbestos-containing materials.

and adhesives. Because these chemicals are highly mobile, they readily migrate through unlined landfills into the underlying groundwater. Heavy metals in landfills, such as lead, cadmium, mercury, and chromium, can also be a source of groundwater contamination. Moreover, microbial degradation of garbage and vegetative wastes in a landfill can produce organic acids that lower the pH of the milieu, making buried metals more soluble. Old industrial sites where waste chemicals were sometimes dumped into open pits or onto the ground have also been known to contaminate nearby groundwater. If the contaminated groundwater migrates off site, it can affect people who drink from down-gradient private and public water wells. In Hardeman County, Tennessee, for example, leachate from a hazardous waste landfill contaminated private drinking-water wells with carbon tetrachloride and other VOCs (Clark and others, 1982). People who drank from these wells experienced headaches, nausea, and visual disturbances.

Physicians who examined the victims reported that several of them had enlarged livers. In addition, clinical laboratory tests documented the presence of elevated levels of liver enzymes and altered serum chemistries, evidence of liver toxicity. Fortunately, these abnormalities resolved several months after the people stopped drinking the contaminated water.

Most old landfills also lack adequate leachate collection systems for above-ground discharges. As a result, leachate from these landfills can be carried by surface water runoff into nearby lakes and streams, introducing chemical contaminants. People who use these bodies of water for recreation or fishing can be exposed to this contamination. The Kin-Buc landfill in Edison, New Jersey, is an example of this scenario (Figure 16.8). Municipal, industrial, and hazardous wastes, including liquids and oily wastes, were buried at the landfill during its thirty years of operation. Large quantities of oily liquids containing polychlorinated biphenyls (PCBs) leached out of the landfill into the adjacent wetlands. The PCBs contaminated a creek, which discharged into the Raritan River. Because PCBs resist biological metabolism and are lipophilic, they bioaccumulated in fish and shellfish in the river.

FIGURE 16.8   Leachate Collection Ponds at the Kin-Buc Landfill in Edison, New Jersey

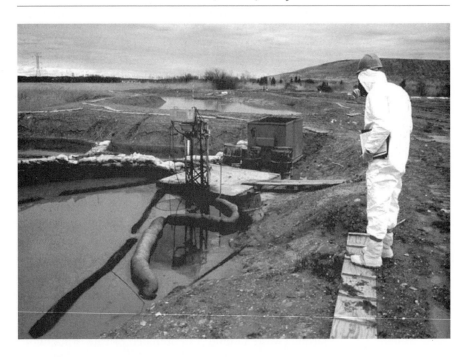

Source: Photo supplied by Ken Orloff.

State environmental officials tested striped bass, white perch, and blue crabs from the river and detected elevated concentrations of PCBs. This finding prompted local health officials to issue a health advisory against eating fish and shellfish from the river, depriving people of recreation and a valuable food source.

Municipal landfills can also be a source of air pollutants such as methane, hydrogen sulfide, and VOCs. Anaerobic microbial digestion of organic matter buried in landfills generates large quantities of methane gas. In 1969, in Winston-Salem, North Carolina, methane gas from a landfill migrated underground through the soil into the basement of an armory building adjacent to the landfill. The methane built up to an explosive level in the basement, and a lit cigarette triggered an explosion that killed three men and injured five others. Methane and carbon dioxide released to the atmosphere from landfills can also have ecological effects, given that these gases may contribute to global warming (see Chapter Ten). It has been estimated that landfills accounted for about 23 percent of total U.S. methane emissions to the atmosphere from anthropogenic sources in 2006 (EPA, 2008b).

Landfills can also be a source of odiferous gases such as hydrogen sulphide, mercaptans, and ammonia. The decay of organic material and some construction materials, such as gypsum wallboard, produce these gases. The concentrations of these gases in ambient air in neighbourhoods near a landfill are usually not high enough to cause adverse health effects. However, their objectionable odor can adversely affect quality of life, and they may provoke respiratory irritation in sensitive individuals.

As mentioned, wastes from mining and petroleum production are the largest category of solid wastes produced in the United States. Huge piles of mine tailings, left behind after the extraction of metals, are a potential source of environmental contamination (Figure 16.9). In the past, inefficient metal extraction processes left behind mine tailings with residual concentrations of lead and other metals as high as 20,000 parts per million, or 2 percent. Fine particulates from these tailings can be transported by wind action and surface water runoff into residential areas. In some instances, mine tailings were used to construct driveways and to fill in low-lying areas in yards, resulting in high concentrations of lead and other metals in residential soils. Smelters are often located near the mining areas and release additional metal-contaminated particulates to the ambient air and soil. At several mining and smelting sites, it has been demonstrated that children's exposure to lead-contaminated soil has contributed to increased blood lead concentrations (Gulson and others, 1994; Murgueytio and others, 1998). Such exposures are of health concern because there is no clear threshold for lead-induced neurotoxicity in children.

Residual metals can leach out of the tailings and contaminate groundwater and surface water resources. In Hunan Province in China, mining wastes containing arsenic were placed in an open-air dump. During the rainy season, leachate

FIGURE 16.9   Mine Tailings Pile: The Legacy of Sixty Years of Lead
and Zinc Mining in Ottawa County, Oklahoma

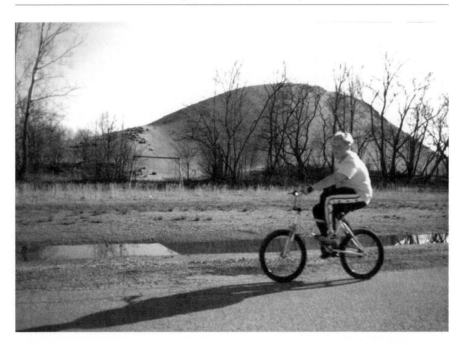

Source: Photo supplied by Ken Orloff.

from the waste piles infiltrated groundwater that was being used as a drinking-water source. Use of the contaminated groundwater caused acute arsenic poisoning in hundreds of people, and six people died (Gongli, 1994).

Municipal and hazardous waste incinerators that release particulates, vapors, and gases to the ambient air are also of potential health concern. Burning even nontoxic materials, such as wood and paper, produces particulate matter, carbon monoxide, aldehydes, and polycyclic aromatic hydrocarbons. In addition, burning commonplace materials, such as paints, solvents, insecticides, and plastics, can form chlorinated dibenzodioxins and chlorinated dibenzofurans, collectively known as dioxins. Small amounts of dioxins are released from hazardous waste incinerators, which operate under strict environmental regulations. Backyard burning of household trash in open barrels can also be a significant source of atmospheric dioxin emissions. It has been estimated that backyard trash burning by only two to forty households can generate as much dioxin as a municipal waste incinerator (Lemieux, Lutes, Abbott, and Aldous, 2000).

Although inhalation of dioxins in ambient air is a potential source of exposure, the major source of exposure to dioxins is through food consumption. Once dioxins are released to the environment, they resist chemical, physical, and biological degradation, and they can bioaccumulate in aquatic and terrestrial animals. More than 90 percent of the dioxin exposure in the general population is derived from background, low-level dioxin contamination in dairy products, meats, fish, eggs, and other foodstuffs (ATSDR, 1998).

The improper disposal or treatment of waste materials can lead to releases of other environmentally stable chemicals, such as PCBs, polybrominated diphenyl ethers (flame retardants), and plasticizers, as well as heavy metals, such as mercury, cadmium, and lead. Migration of these chemicals into waterways and agricultural fields can result in contamination of food sources. A classic example of food contamination occurred in Minamata Bay in Japan in the 1950s (Weiss, 1996). Inorganic mercury, used as a catalyst by a chemical company, was discharged into the bay. Bacteria in the sediment converted the inorganic mercury into methylmercury, which bioaccumulated in fish. Residents who ate the local fish developed classic neurological symptoms of methylmercury toxicity that included paresthesia, ataxia, loss of hearing and vision, and tremors. Children born to methylmercury-exposed mothers developed a cerebral palsy-like syndrome that was often fatal.

Some metals found in waste streams, such as cadmium, can bioaccumulate in edible plants. In Japan, zinc mining in the Jinzu River basin contaminated the river with cadmium and other metals. Farmers used cadmium-contaminated water from the river to irrigate their rice fields, resulting in cadmium contamination of their rice crops (Nogawa and Ishizaki, 1979). After years of exposure to high doses of cadmium from the rice they ate, many farmers developed kidney disease, which led to a loss of calcium from their bones. Postmenopausal women who had borne several children were especially prone to developing fragile, painful bones that spontaneously fractured, which gave the condition its name, *itai-itai byo*, or "ouch-ouch disease."

In spite of this historical experience, instances of human health affects due to food contamination from improper handling or disposal of chemical wastes continue to occur. In 1999 in Belgium, waste transformer oil containing PCBs was mixed into recycled animal fat that was added to animal feed (van Larebeke and others, 2001). The contaminated feed was distributed to poultry farms in Belgium and resulted in widespread contamination of chickens and eggs with PCBs and dioxins. This contamination prompted the Belgian government to remove all poultry products, eggs, and derived products from the market and led to the destruction of 2 million chickens.

Public health practice emphasizes prevention over treatment. This principle is especially relevant in the field of environmental health because preventing environmental contamination is easier and less costly than cleaning it up after it has occurred. Therefore both industrialized and developing countries should learn from the mistakes of the past and strive to manage and treat wastes in a manner that protects public health.

PERSPECTIVE
International Trafficking in Hazardous Wastes

As industrialized countries' environmental laws for disposing of hazardous wastes became more stringent and expensive to comply with, some generators began shipping wastes to other countries for disposal (Orloff and Falk, 2003). The United Nations Environmental Programme estimates that about 10 percent of hazardous waste produced worldwide is shipped across international borders. In some cases the recipient country is ill-prepared to safely handle the hazardous wastes. Hazardous waste workers often lack adequate personal protective equipment and training, which puts their health and safety at risk. Furthermore, if the wastes are not adequately treated and disposed of, they can create a potentially dangerous environmental legacy for the recipient country.

Concern over the international shipping of hazardous wastes led to the establishment in 1989 of a treaty known as the Basel Convention. The convention's goal is to regulate the international movement of hazardous materials and to ensure that these wastes are managed and disposed of in an environmentally sound manner. One of the key provisions of the convention is that transboundary movement of hazardous wastes can take place only upon prior written notification by the state of export to competent authorities of the state of import.

As of June 2008, 167 countries and the European Union had ratified the Basel Convention. The United States signed the convention in 1992 but has not ratified it, which would require Congressional action. One factor preventing the United States from ratifying the convention is that its acceptance would require changes in Resource Conservation and Recovery Act regulations that specify how hazardous wastes are defined and how those wastes are managed.

One of the challenges facing the convention is how to deal with trafficking in recyclable materials, such as spent lead-acid batteries and other nonferrous scrap metal. These wastes are valuable commodities on the world market, and recycling these materials provides jobs and generates income in countries with struggling economies. Under a proposed amendment to the convention, the transfer of such materials from industrialized to developing countries would be banned.

In recent years, the practice of ship breaking has attracted the attention of the environmental community. Some environmental groups have characterized this practice as being a covert form of international trafficking in hazardous wastes. The term *ship breaking* refers to sending decommissioned ships to other countries where they are dismantled to recover steel and other recyclables. Concerns have been raised because workers may not be protected from exposure to lead, asbestos, polychlorinated biphenyls, mercury, and other hazardous materials during ship dismantling operations. India is the world's leader in ship breaking (38 percent), followed by China (25 percent), Bangladesh (19 percent), Pakistan (7 percent), and other countries (11 percent).

SUMMARY

Human activities produce a huge volume and variety of waste materials that are regulated by federal, state, and local laws and regulations. Waste management strategies emphasize the importance of reducing, reusing, and recycling waste materials. When this is not possible, proper disposal and treatment of wastes is important. Selection of the best means for waste disposal or treatment requires consideration of factors such as technological feasibility, compliance with regulatory requirements, long-term effectiveness, community acceptance, and cost. Proper handling and disposal of wastes is necessary to prevent environmental contamination and potential adverse impacts on public health and ecological systems.

KEY TERMS

agricultural waste	incineration	radioactive waste
animal waste	industrial ecology	reduce, reuse, and recycle
asbestos	industrial waste	sanitary landfill
construction debris	leachate	sewage sludge
deep well injection	medical waste	solid waste
electronic waste	mining waste	special waste
hazardous waste	municipal solid waste	waste management

DISCUSSION QUESTIONS

1. What are the different approaches to solid waste management? Discuss their advantages and disadvantages.
2. What are the different types of solid wastes, and how are they identified?
3. How can you reduce the amount of waste you produce? Name each way and discuss it.
4. Select one of the waste treatment or disposal technologies discussed in this chapter. How could this technology be effectively used in a solid waste management program? Specify the type of solid waste, and discuss how using the technology would protect the health of people and the environment.
5. What are the ways in which people can be exposed to toxic substances in solid waste and hazardous waste?

REFERENCES

Agency for Toxic Substances and Disease Registry. *Toxicological Profile for Dibenzo-p-Dioxins (Update)*. Atlanta: Public Health Service, Agency for Toxic Substances and Disease Registry, 1998.

Agency for Toxic Substances and Disease Registry. *Health Consultation: Exposure Investigation Report, Air Sampling for Sulfur Gases, Warren Township, Trumball County, Ohio*. Atlanta: Public Health Service, Agency for Toxic Substances and Disease Registry, 2006.

Burkholder, J., and others. "Impacts of Waste from Concentrated Animal Feeding Operations on Water Quality." *Environmental Health Perspectives*, 2007, *115*, 308–312.

Centers for Disease Control and Prevention. "Got Mice? Seal, Trap, and Clean Up to Control Rodents." http://www.cdc.gov/Features/Rodents, 2008.

Clark, C. S., and others. "An Environmental Health Survey of Drinking Water Contamination by Leachate from a Pesticide Waste Dump in Hardeman County, Tennessee." *Archives of Environmental Health*, 1982, *37*(1), 9–18.

Comprehensive Environmental Response, Compensation and Liability Act of 1980. PL 95-510, codified at *U.S. Code* 42, §6901 et seq.

Ehrenfeld, J., and Gertler, N. "Industrial Ecology in Practice: The Evolution of Interdependence at Kalundborg." *Journal of Industrial Ecology*, 1997, *1*, 67–79.

Emergency Planning and Community Right-to-Know Act of 1986. PL 99-499, codified at *U.S. Code* 42, §6901 et seq.

Garner, A., and Keoleian, G. A. *Industrial Ecology: An Introduction*. University of Michigan, National Pollution Prevention Center for Higher Education. http://www.umich.edu/~nppcpub/resources/compendia/INDEpdfs/INDEintro.pdf, Nov. 1995.

Gilchrist, M. J., and others. "The Potential Role of Concentrated Animal Feeding Operations in Infectious Disease Epidemics and Antibiotic Resistance." *Environmental Health Perspectives*, 2007, *115*, 313–316.

Gongli, H. "*Environmental and Health Effects of Hazardous Wastes in China*." In J. S. Andrews and others (eds.), *Hazardous Waste and Public Health: International Congress on the Health Effects of Hazardous Waste*. Princeton, N.J.: Princeton Scientific, 1994.

Gulson, B. L., and others. "Lead Bioavailability in the Environment of Children: Blood Lead Levels in Children Can Be Elevated in a Mining Community." *Archives of Environmental Health*, 1994, *49*(5), 326–331.

Heederik, D., and others. "Health Effects of Airborne Exposures from Concentrated Animal Feeding Operations." *Environmental Health Perspectives*, 2007, *115*, 298–302.

Hickman, H. L. *Principles of Integrated Solid Waste Management*. Annapolis, Md.: American Academy of Environmental Engineers, 1999.

Lemieux, P. M., Lutes, C. C., Abbott, J. A., and Aldous, K. M. "Emissions of Polychlorinated Dibenzo-*p*-Dioxins and Polychlorinated Dibenzofurans from the Open Burning of Household Waste in Barrels." *Environmental Science & Technology*, 2000, *34*, 377–384.

Lichtveld, M. Y., Rodenbeck S. E., and Lybarger J. A. "The Findings of the Agency for Toxic Substances and Disease Registry Medical Waste Tracking Act Report." *Environmental Health Perspectives*, 1992, *98*, 243–250.

Luther, L. *Congressional Research Service Report for Congress: Disaster Debris Removal After Hurricane Katrina: Status and Associated Issues*. Washington, D.C.: Congressional Research Service, 2007.

Murgueytio, A. M., and others. "Relationship Between Lead Mining and Blood Lead Levels in Children." *Archives of Environmental Health*, 1998, *53*(6), 414–423.

Nogawa, K., and Ishizaki, A. "A Comparison Between Cadmium in Rice and Renal Effects Among Inhabitants of the Jinzu River Basin." *Environmental Research*, 1979, *18*, 410–420.

Orloff, K., and Falk, H. "An International Perspective on Hazardous Waste Practices." *International Journal of Hygiene and Environmental Health*, 2003, *206*, 291–302.

Osibanjo, O., and Nnorom, I. C. "The Challenge of Electronic Waste (e-Waste) Management in Developing Countries." *Waste Management & Research*, 2007, *25*(6), 489–501.

Resource Conservation and Recovery Act of 1976. PL 94-580, codified at *U.S. Code* 42, § 6901 et seq.

Rubber Manufacturers Association. *U.S. Scrap Tire Markets: 2003 Edition*. Washington, D.C.: Rubber Manufacturers Association, 2004.

Schierow, L. J. *CRS Report to Congress: The Emergency Planning and Community Right-to-Know Act (EPCRA), A Summary*. Washington, D.C.: Congressional Research Service, 2007.

Schmidt, C. W. "e-Junk Explosion." *Environmental Health Perspectives*, 2002, *110*(4), A188–A194.

Schmidt, C. W. "Unfair Trade: e-Waste in Africa." *Environmental Health Perspectives*, 2006, *114*(4), A232–A235.

Silbergeld, E. K., Graham, J., and Price, L. B. "Industrial Food Animal Production, Antimicrobial Resistance, and Human Health." *Annual Review of Public Health*, 2008, *29*, 151–169.

Silbergeld E. K., and Nachman, K. "The Environmental and Public Health Risks Associated with Arsenical Use in Animal Feeds." *Annals of the New York Academy of Sciences*, Oct. 2008, *1140*, 346–357.

Solid Waste Disposal Act of 1965. PL 89-272, codified at *U.S. Code* 42, §6901 et seq.

U.S. Army Corps of Engineers. "USACE Team on Site at WTC from First Minutes." http://www.hq.usace.army.mil/cepa/pubs/sep02/story10.htm, 2002.

U.S. Environmental Protection Agency. *Report to Congress: Wastes from the Extraction and Beneficiation of Metallic Ores, Phosphate Rock, Asbestos, Overburden from Uranium Mining, and Oil Shale*. Washington, D.C.: U.S. Environmental Protection Agency, 1985.

U.S. Environmental Protection Agency. *Municipal Solid Waste Generation, Recycling, and Disposal in the United States: Facts and Figures for 2006*. Washington, D.C.: U.S. Environmental Protection Agency, 2006a.

U.S. Environmental Protection Agency. *The National Biennial RCRA Hazardous Waste Report (Based on 2005 Data)*. Washington, D.C.: U.S. Environmental Protection Agency, 2006b.

U.S. Environmental Protection Agency. "eCycling: Frequent Questions." http://www.epa.gov/epawaste/conserve/materials/ecycling/faq.htm, 2008a.

U.S. Environmental Protection Agency. *Inventory of U.S. Greenhouse Gas Emissions and Sinks: 1990–2006*. http://epa.gov/climatechange/emissions/downloads/08_ES.pdf, Apr. 15, 2008b.

U.S. Navy. "USS New York LPD-21: Forged from the Steel of the World Trade Center." http://www.ussnewyork.com/ussny_construction.html, Jan. 11, 2007.

van Larebeke, N., and others. "The Belgian PCB and Dioxin Incident of January-June 1999: Exposure Data and Potential Impact on Health." *Environmental Health Perspectives*, 2001, *109*(3), 265–273.

Weiss, B. "Long ago and Far Away: A Retrospective on the Implications of Minamata." *Neurotoxicology*, 1996, *17*(1), 257–264.

Zeller, T. "Recycling: The Big Picture." *National Geographic*, Jan. 2008, 82–87.

FOR FURTHER INFORMATION

Books and Articles

Carroll, C. "High-Tech Trash: Will Your Discarded TV or Computer End Up in a Ditch in Ghana?" *National Geographic*, Jan. 2008, 64–87.

Chang, H. O. *Hazardous and Radioactive Waste Treatment Technologies Handbook*. Boca Raton, Fla.: CRC Press, 2000.

Gorner, I. K. "Waste Incineration: European State of the Art and New Developments." *IFRF Combustion Journal*, July 2003, article no. 200303.

Johnson, B. L. *Impact of Hazardous Waste on Human Health: Hazard, Health Effects, Equity, and Communications Issues*. New York: Lewis, 1999.

Manuel, J. S. "Unbuilding for the Environment." *Environmental Health Perspectives*, 2003, *111*(16), A881–A887.

National Research Council. *Environmental Epidemiology: Public Health and Hazardous Wastes*. Washington, D.C.: National Academies Press, 1991.

Rathje, W. L., and Murphy, C. *Rubbish! The Archaeology of Garbage*. Tucson: University of Arizona Press, 2001.

Schneider, A., and McCumber, D. *An Air That Kills*. New York: Putnam, 2004.

Taylor, D. "Talking Trash: The Economic and Environmental Issues of Landfills." *Environmental Health Perspectives*, 1999, *108*(7), A404–A409.

Tchobanoglous, G., and Kreith, F. *Handbook of Solid Waste Management*. (2nd ed.) New York: McGraw-Hill, 2002.

Willis, B. C., Howie, M. M., and Williams, R. C. *Public Health Reviews of Hazardous Waste Thermal Treatment Technologies: A Guidance Manual for Public Health Assessors*. Atlanta: Agency for Toxic Substances and Disease Registry, Division of Health Assessment and Consultation, 2002.

Agencies

Because federal governmental agencies frequently revise and update the information and data posted on their Web sites, specific Web pages are not provided. However, each of these home page Web sites has a search engine that will assist you in locating appropriate information.

Agency for Toxic Substances and Disease Registry, http://www.atsdr.cdc.gov.

Centers for Disease Control and Prevention, http://www.cdc.gov.

U.S. Environmental Protection Agency, http://www.epa.gov.

CHAPTER SEVENTEEN

PEST CONTROL AND PESTICIDES

MARK G. ROBSON

GEORGE C. HAMILTON

WATTASIT SIRIWONG

KEY CONCEPTS

- Pests are plants, animals, or microorganisms that threaten human health or well-being. Humans have contended with pests since ancient times.

- Each pest has specific biological and ecological characteristics.

- Modern pest control has come to rely heavily on chemical agents—pesticides. Many of these are toxic.

- There are discrete classes of pesticides, each with its own toxicity profile.

- People can sustain pesticide exposures in a wide range of settings (home, workplace, and so forth) and through a wide range of pathways (ingestion, inhalation, and skin absorption).

- Pesticide regulation is complex, relying on several federal laws.

- Integrated pest management is a strategy that combines chemical and nonchemical approaches to pest control.

PESTS have plagued humankind since the beginning of time, as recorded in the ancient writings of the Chinese, Egyptian, and Hebrew peoples. For example, there is a vivid description of a serious pest invasion in the book of Exodus (10:14–15): " . . . and the locusts came up over all the land of Egypt and settled on the whole country of Egypt. They covered the face of the whole land so that the land was darkened and they ate all the plants in the land and all the fruit of the trees. Not a green thing remained, neither tree nor plant of the field, through all the land of Egypt." Diseases such as plague and malaria—both propagated by pests—have changed the course of human history (Zinsser, 1963; McNeill, 1976; Sullivan, 2004).

Efforts to control pests are also as old as history. Early control measures used chalk, plant extracts, mercury, arsenic, lead, and other compounds. Over time, people also have attempted to control pests through sacrifices, prayers, rituals, dancing, and other approaches. Some appear quite humorous to us today; during an outbreak of cutworms in Switzerland in 1476, "Several of the offending insects were hauled into court, proclaimed guilty, excommunicated by the archbishop, and banished from the land" (Nadakavukaren, 1995).

Over the last century or two, chemicals have come to dominate human efforts at pest control. As with medications, the ideal pesticide is both safe in terms of human and ecosystem health and effective at controlling the target species. Historically, although many compounds were recommended to control pests, almost none were empirically tested and most turned out to be ineffective (Keifer, Wesseling, and McConnell, 2005). Paris green (copper acetoarsenite) was among the first compounds to be used on a large scale in agricultural production. In the 1860s, it was shown to have insecticidal properties and was used to control the Colorado potato beetle, *Leptinotarsa decemlineata*. Paris green was also an effective fungicide. Later in the nineteenth century lead arsenate became a popular pesticide and was widely used in agriculture. Chemical pest control changed dramatically in 1939. Paul Müller, a chemist with the Geigy Corporation in Switzerland, found that a compound synthesized more than half a century earlier was an effective insecticide while boasting low mammalian toxicity. This compound was dichlorodiphenyltrichloroethane, or DDT. DDT was widely used during World War II to control a number of insect problems that plagued the war effort, including body lice, the carriers of typhus, and mosquitoes, the carriers of yellow fever, malaria, and dengue. DDT is still used in many parts of the world for vector control, particularly for malaria and other mosquito-borne diseases. Müller received the Nobel Prize in Physiology or Medicine in 1948 for his work on DDT.

After the war DDT and similar chlorinated pesticides made their way into the agricultural marketplace. (Figures 17.1 and 17.2 display modes of applying

Mark G. Robson, George C. Hamilton, and Wattasit Siriwong declare no competing financial interests.

FIGURE 17.1   Application of Lead Arsenate in the Early 1900s

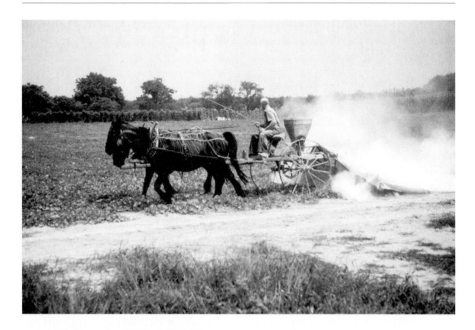

Source: Photo supplied by E. G. Christ.

FIGURE 17.2   Modern Pesticide Application Equipment

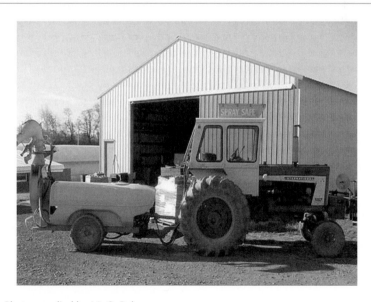

Source: Photo supplied by M. G. Robson.

PERSPECTIVE
Effects of Persistent Organochlorine Pesticides on Ecosystems

People have been concerned with the effects of organochlorine pesticides since Rachel Carson wrote *Silent Spring* in 1962. Organochlorine pesticides have the potential to accumulate through the food chain and can eventually lead to adverse health effects in the human population. Evidence shows that persistent environmental residues are still detected globally (Ritter and others, 1995). To protect human health and the environment from chemicals that remain intact in the environment for long periods, the Stockholm Convention on Persistent Organic Pollutants (POPs) was adopted in 2001 and entered into force in 2004. The agreement prohibits the use of eight organochlorine pesticides: aldrin, chlordane, DDT, dieldrin, endrin, heptachlor, hexachlorobenzene (HCB), and toxaphene.

In agricultural countries, such as Thailand, and other countries in Southeast Asia, DDT and its derivatives have been banned since the 1980s. However, in 2002, DDE, a derivative of DDT, was detected in the egg of the little egret, *Egretta garzetta*, whose habitat is located in the paddy ecosystem of Central Thailand. DDE levels ranged from 33.4 to 116.0 ng/g wet weight (Keithmaleesatti and others, 2007). A recent investigation by Siriwong (2006) indicated that DDT derivatives exist in the aquatic ecosystem and are currently playing an important role in nontarget aquatic species such as fish, shrimp, snail, plankton, and so forth, via bioaccumulation, bioconcentration, and biomagnification through the food web (Figure 17.3). This evidence underlines new scientific concern about the critical linkage between environmental contaminants and potential human health risks.

DDT and its derivatives are well-known endocrine disrupting compounds (EDCs). EDCs are generally present in low concentrations but are ubiquitous and persistent in the environment. Although environmental concentrations are low, EDCs appear to exert a range of adverse effects on animals of many species, including humans. These compounds can disrupt reproductive functions and the immune system and can be carcinogenic (Rhind, 2002). A number of species in Figure 17.3 may be exposed to comparatively high concentrations of EDCs due to bioaccumulation. The EDC that persist in aquatic systems are absorbed and ingested by these species, which can concentrate in fat tissue.

Rachel Carson's message was straightforward: if pesticide use continues as usual, there might someday come a spring with no birds—and with ominous impacts on humans as well. Today DDT and its derivatives are no longer used in many countries, but their persistent residues can still have an impact on human health in the future.

FIGURE 17.3 Bioaccumulation Factor (BAF), Bioconcentration Factor (BCF), and Biomagnification Factor (BMF) of Low Concentrations of DDT and Derivatives in the Aquatic Food Web of Rangsit Agricultural Area, Central Thailand

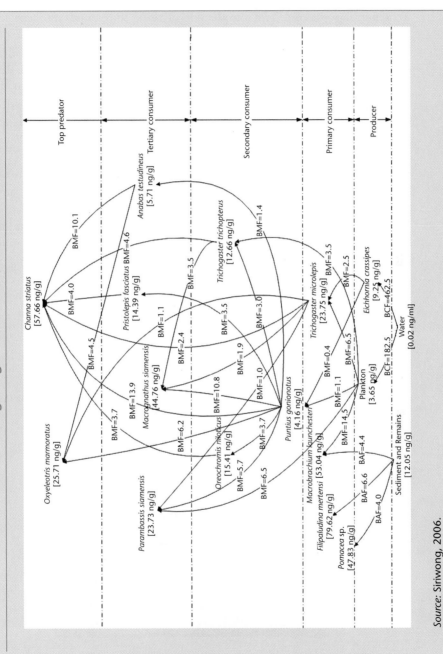

Source: Siriwong, 2006.

agricultural pesticides.) The introduction of these compounds into agriculture changed pest control and food production worldwide. However, public health and ecological research has increasingly revealed problems with pesticides, ranging from human toxicity to wildlife toxicity to ecosystem disruption. Rachel Carson's *Silent Spring*, published in 1962, was a powerful wake-up call, alerting the public and policymakers to the downsides of widespread pesticide use. Modern pest control has therefore sought to move beyond exclusive reliance on pesticides, using combinations of chemical and nonchemical methods (Ware and Whitacre, 2004).

A **pest** can be any species of plant, animal, or microorganism that threatens human health and well-being (Figure 17.4). However, most pests fill specific ecological niches and have functions that are important to ecosystem integrity (even if not directly useful to humans). Bees sting but pollinate plants and make honey; ants interrupt picnics and may sting but play an essential role in nutrient cycles; termites destroy homes but are essential in processing fallen trees in forests. It is a rare pest that is *only* a pest.

The U.S. Environmental Protection Agency (EPA) defines seven categories of public health pests:

1. *Cockroaches.* Cockroaches are controlled to reduce asthma, allergies, and food contamination.

FIGURE 17.4   A Corn Borer, an Example of an Insect Pest, Causing Damage in the Stalk of a Corn Plant

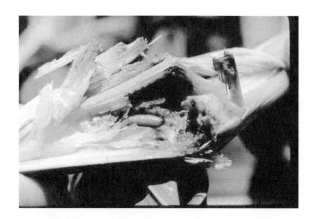

Note: The borers cause the stalks to lodge (fall over), making the corn difficult to harvest. One-fourth to one-third of the global corn harvest is lost to pests.

Source: Photo supplied by M. G. Robson.

2. *Body, head, and crab lice.* These lice are controlled to prevent the spread of skin irritations and rashes and to prevent the occurrence of louse-borne diseases, such as epidemic typhus, trench fever, and epidemic relapsing fever.

3. *Mosquitoes.* Mosquitoes are controlled to prevent the spread of mosquito-borne diseases such as malaria, yellow fever, dengue fever, and certain encephalitides (for example, St. Louis, Eastern, Western, West Nile, and LaCrosse).

4. *Various rats and mice.* Rats and mice are controlled to prevent the spread of rodent-borne diseases and the contamination of food for human consumption.

5. *Various microorganisms, including bacteria, viruses, and protozoa.* Microorganisms listed as public health pests are controlled by public health agencies and hospitals for the purpose of preventing the spread of numerous diseases.

6. *Reptiles and birds.* Certain reptiles and birds are controlled to prevent the spread of disease and to prevent direct injury.

7. *Various mammals.* Certain mammals have the potential to inflict direct human injury and can act as disease reservoirs (for rabies, for example).

This chapter describes various categories of pests and specific examples in these categories in some detail, including their physical characteristics, habitats, and impacts on human health. It begins with insects and moves next to vertebrate pests. It then turns to pest control, a traditional and still important function of environmental health, beginning with pesticides and concluding with the broader set of strategies known as integrated pest management (IPM).

INSECT PESTS

Insects belong to the class Insecta or Hexapoda and have three body regions (head, thorax, and abdomen), six legs that are connected to the thorax, and in the adults of most species, thoracic wings (Triplehorn and Johnson, 2005). Insects can have either chewing or sucking mouthparts. Those with chewing mouthparts, such as grasshoppers, termites and fleas, tear and crush plant material, insects, or other materials. Insects with sucking mouthparts, such as aphids, head lice, and mosquitoes, pierce their food and then extract fluids in order to feed.

All insects go through one of two types of development, or metamorphosis: *gradual* (egg, nymph, and adult) or *complete* (egg, larva, pupa, and adult). Among insects that undergo gradual metamorphosis, juveniles look identical to adults and feed on the same food resources; as they mature they expand in size through a series of molts. Each time they molt, they develop external wing pads; during their final molt, to the adult form, fully functional wings and reproductive structures appear. Among insects that undergo complete metamorphosis, juveniles look dramatically different from the adults and feed on different food resources; caterpillars and butterflies are an example. These insects go through a series of larvae molts, culminating in a resting stage called the pupa. During this stage, the body tissues of the insect reorient themselves to produce the adult. When the final molt occurs, the insect breaks its way out of the pupal skin as a fully functional adult.

Here are eight examples of common insect pests.

Bedbugs

Bedbugs are human *ectoparasites* (that is, they live on external surfaces) that are universal pests. They belong to the order Hemiptera and are flightless as nymphs and adults (Triplehorn and Johnson, 2005). They undergo gradual metamorphosis and must feed on blood in order to survive. Common names for the bedbug include mahogany flat, chinch, and red coat (Truman, Bennet, and Butts, 1982). The adult common bedbug, *Cimex lectularius*, is about 0.2 inches long, 0.1 inch wide, and oval. Its extremely flat body allows it to get in cracks and crevices, making it more difficult to detect. Bedbugs have piercing-sucking mouthparts that are used to penetrate the host's skin in order to feed on blood. Eggs are laid away from hosts and attached to surfaces and can hatch in six to seventeen days under normal room temperatures. Once the eggs hatch the small, colorless nymphs undergo gradual metamorphosis, taking blood meals as they develop. Humans are the preferred host of bedbugs, but bedbugs feed on canaries, cats, dogs, mice, poultry, and rats when humans are not available. Normally, they feed at night and hide in areas such as cracks and crevices, the folds of mattresses, the upholstery of chairs and sofas, and bedsprings. Bedbugs give off a distinctive odor from thoracic glands; the odor can be quite strong during heavy infestations. In the laboratory, bedbugs are capable of transmitting anthrax, plague, tularemia, yellow fever, relapsing fever, and typhus, but there is little evidence that they transmit these diseases under normal conditions. Accordingly, they are not considered an important vector species.

Cockroaches

Cockroaches belong to the order Blattodea (Triplehorn and Johnson, 2005). Most cockroaches are tropical, and they are very common in the southern areas of the United States. In northern areas, those most commonly encountered are the ones that live indoors, in houses, restaurants, and other buildings. Cockroaches are not known to transmit any serious diseases. However, they contaminate food, produce an unpleasant odor, can become a serious nuisance, and exposure to cockroach antigen is an important risk factor for developing asthma. The four most common problem species in the United States are the German, brown-banded, Oriental, and American cockroaches.

Cockroaches undergo gradual metamorphosis (Truman and others, 1982) and have egg, nymph, and adult stages. Adult females produce egg cases, called *ootheca*. These protect the eggs from desiccation and, depending on species, may be carried around by the female until hatching or deposition in protected areas. The wings of adult cockroaches may be long and fully functional or short and almost nonexistent. In some species only the males have functional wings and may or may not fly. Most cockroaches are nocturnal but may be seen during the day when population numbers are high.

The German cockroach, *Blattella germanica*, is the most common cockroach in homes in the United States. Adults are about 1.3 cm in length, pale brown, and have two dark stripes on the pronotum, or back, of the insect. Females carry their ootheca until the eggs are ready to hatch and are the only common house-infesting cockroach to do so. German cockroaches are generalist feeders but prefer fermented food, and if water is present, adults can live for about a month.

The American cockroach, *Periplaneta americana*, or water bug, Bombay canary, or flying water bug, is the largest of the house-dwelling cockroaches (4 cm or more). It is reddish-brown, and males and females are fully winged but seldom fly. Females drop or secure ootheca in areas where food may be present, along baseboards or outdoors in damp, decaying wood (southern United States). They prefer dark, moist areas and are common in basements. American cockroaches feed on a variety of food sources, including book bindings, manuscripts, and other starchy substances and also syrup and other types of sweets.

The Oriental cockroach, *Blattella orientalis*, or water bug, black beetle, or shad roach, is a cosmopolitan pest, found throughout the world. These roaches are black in color and about 3 cm in length. Females have rudimentary wings; male wings cover about three-quarters of the abdomen. Females drop their eggs or attach them to protected surface near a food supply. Oriental cockroaches feed on filth and rubbish and are especially fond of garbage. They also like high-moisture areas and must have water to survive.

The brown-banded cockroach, *Supella longipalpa*, is a small cockroach (less than 1.5 cm), with two lighter transverse bands across the base of the wings and abdomen. Females carry ootheca for one or two days and then attach them to a protected surface. This species is found high on ceilings, hiding behind picture frames, and near motors and electrical devices that generate heat. They require less water than other cockroaches and are rarely found in kitchens and bathrooms. Brown-banded cockroaches prefer to feed on starchy substances but can be found feeding on just about anything.

PERSPECTIVE
Insect Repellants

Insect repellants are designed not to kill insects but to deter them from settling on skin and clothes. These are popular products, used both to avoid the discomfort of bites by mosquitoes and other insects and to prevent disease transmission. The public health benefit of reducing insect bites is considerable. For instance, mosquitoes alone transmit disease to more than 700 million persons annually. Malaria remains a common disease in poor and middle-income countries (as discussed later), and in the United States, mosquitoes transmit eastern equine encephalitis, western equine encephalitis, St. Louis encephalitis, and La Crosse encephalitis, and since 1999, West Nile virus, serving as a reminder that no part of the world is immune from mosquito-borne diseases (Fradin and Day, 2002).

A variety of insect repellants is commercially available, some derived from plants and others consisting of synthetic chemicals. Many factors determine the effectiveness of a repellant, including the species of biting organism; the user's age, sex, level of activity, biochemical attractiveness to biting arthropods; and the ambient temperature, humidity, and wind speed (Fradin and Day, 2002). As a result, any given repellent is not equally protective for all users.

The major component of nearly all consumer insect repellants is N,N-diethyl-m-toluamide (now called N,N-diethyl-3-methylbenzamide), or DEET (Bell, Veltri, and Page, 2002). Discovered by scientists at the U.S. Department of Agriculture and patented by the U.S. Army in 1946, DEET has been used in commercial repellants since the late 1950s (DEET Is Hard to Beat, 2003). It is a broad-spectrum repellent, effective against many species of mosquitoes, biting flies, chiggers, fleas, and ticks (Fradin and Day, 2002). When compared to alternatives, including such synthetic chemicals as IR3535 and such natural repellants as citronella, soybean oil, peppermint oil, eucalyptus oil, and prickly pear cactus, DEET has generally been shown to be far superior in repelling insects.

Is DEET safe? Once applied to the skin it is absorbed, in quantities that have ranged between 5 percent and 15 percent in different studies (Sudakin and Trevathan, 2003). It is metabolized and excreted in the urine in twelve to twenty-four hours.

Fleas

Fleas are small ectoparasites (2 to 4 mm long) belonging to the order Siphonaptera (Triplehorn and Johnson, 2005). As juveniles they have chewing mouthparts, and as adults they have piercing-sucking mouthparts, which are used to feed on blood (Truman and others, 1982), Fleas go through complete metamorphosis. Eggs are laid on the host animal but fall off into carpets, upholstery, and pet bedding

Acute toxicity is extremely rare. Fewer than fifty cases of serious toxic effects have been documented in the medical literature since 1960; most of these followed extremely large exposures and resolved without lasting effects (Fradin and Day, 2002). However, some animal testing has suggested that DEET may cause neurological effects (Sudakin and Trevathan, 2003; Abdel-Rahman and others, 2004). It is therefore prudent to use DEET in moderation. Guidelines for use include the following:

- Do not use concentrations above 50 percent, as efficacy plateaus at that level (Buescher, Rutledge, Wirtz, and Nelson, 1983). Concentrations of 20 to 30 percent are generally sufficient.
- Apply DEET on or near all exposed skin surfaces; it is not effective more than about two inches from the point of application. To minimize skin absorption, DEET may be applied to clothing, but it is a plasticizer, capable of dissolving some synthetic fabrics.
- DEET is efficacious for a matter of hours (approximately five hours in one careful study; Fradin and Day, 2002) so periodic reapplication may be necessary.
- The efficacy of DEET decreases at higher temperatures.
- DEET is readily washed off by perspiration, rain, or other water sources, so reapplication is necessary after wetting.

Permethrin- and DEET-impregnated clothing is often issued to military personnel for the control of insect pests. Efficacy studies on these pesticides have shown a significant reduction of pest bites when the impregnated clothing has been used. There have been reports of serious health problems associated with military personnel being exposed to these compounds; these symptoms include headaches, fatigue, muscle and joint pain, skin rashes, respiratory difficulties, and other health problems (Punareewattana and others, 2000).

It is important to remember that DEET is only one aspect of protection from arthropod bites. People should also avoid infested habitats, avoid outdoor exposure at times of the day when biting is most active, and wear protective clothing. (For further information see Fradin, 1998; Pollack, Kiszewski, and Spielman, 2002; Roberts and Reigart, 2004.)

material. The eggs hatch into legless, wormlike larvae. Larvae feed on debris and other organic material, including the feces of adult fleas and bits of dried blood. Larvae go through three stages (*instars*) until they spin cocoons and enter the pupal stage. When the adults emerge (in seven to fourteen days) they are ready to feed and mate. Fleas are of great importance because they are carriers of diseases such as plague and murine typhus.

There are several species of fleas, including those that feed on humans and pets. The cat flea, *Ctenocephalides felis*, and the dog flea, *C. canis*, are common throughout the United States and prefer to feed on dogs, cats, and humans and sometimes rats. They prefer areas with high amounts of organic material and are common in houses, under buildings, and in yards. Both species are intermediate hosts for dog tapeworm *Dipylidium caninum*, which can be transmitted to children who accidentally ingest infested fleas while playing with pets. The human flea, *Pulex irritans*, is common through the United States, especially in the Pacific coast region. It feeds almost exclusively on humans but can be found on swine and occasionally dogs. It can carry plague under laboratory conditions but is not normally a carrier of this disease. The oriental rat flea, *Xenopsylla cheopis*, is commonly found on Norway and roof rats and has become distributed throughout the United States. It is the chief carrier of bubonic plague in rats. Rats are its preferred host, but it will occasionally feed on humans. The northern rat flea, *Nosopsyllus fasciatus*, is also found throughout the United States, feeding on rats and mice. Although it is a known carrier of the plague organism it rarely bites humans. The sticktight flea, *Echidnophaga gallinacea*, is primarily a pest of poultry in the southern and southwestern United States; however, it will attack other animals including man. This flea can be infected with plague and murine typhus; however, because females tend to feed on only one host, its importance as a vector is reduced. The mouse flea, *Leptopsylla segnis*, is commonly found on rats in the Gulf states and California, and to a lesser extent on house mice, and is not known to transmit disease.

Lice

Lice that attack humans are flightless, ectoparasitic insects that belong to the order Phthiraptera. Sucking lice belong to the suborder Anoplura, and chewing lice belong to several suborders (Rhynchophthirina, Amblycera, and Ischnocera) (Triplehorn and Johnson, 2005). They are small insects (2 to 3 mm long) that exhibit gradual metamorphosis. Sucking lice insert their mouthparts into their host in order to feed on blood (Truman and others, 1982). Chewing lice feed on host skin scales and secretions. Sucking lice can be differentiated from chewing lice by the relationship between head and thorax; sucking lice have heads that are conical and narrower than their thoraxes, whereas chewing lice have heads that are shield shaped and wider than the thorax. Both groups spend their entire life on their host.

There are approximately 500 species of sucking lice that feed on mammals. Only two species attack humans: *Pediculus humanus*, which includes the body louse (*P. humanus humanus*) and the head louse (*P. humanus capitis*), and the crab or pubic louse (*Phthirus pubis*). Eggs are laid on the host, connected to body hair. They hatch into nymphs that immediately begin feeding on the host. Body lice are known to spread typhus and relapsing fever. Head lice and pubic lice do not transmit disease but are rapidly transferred between hosts in settings such as schools and day-care centers and can be a serious nuisance. There are roughly 2,600 species of chewing lice. All are parasitic on either birds or mammals but do not attack humans.

Mosquitoes

Mosquitoes belong to the order Diptera (Triplehorn and Johnson, 2005). Mosquitoes are a large (169 species in North America), well-known, and important group of biting flies that spend their larval life living in water and their adult life above the water's surface. Mosquitoes are the vector for numerous human diseases, including malaria, dengue fever, yellow fever, and several encephalitis viruses.

Mosquitoes undergo complete metamorphosis (Hamilton and Racz, 1998). Female mosquitoes lay their eggs either as rafts on the surface of water or singly in or near water. In the latter situation the eggs remain dormant until the presence of water stimulates their development. Upon hatching, larvae, or wrigglers, feed on algae and other organic debris. All mosquitoes need air to breathe and must periodically stop feeding to do so. How this occurs depends on the species. Larval culicine mosquitoes, except *Anopheles* species, insert an air tube, or siphon, on the tip of the abdomen through the water's surface like a snorkel in order to breathe. Anopheline mosquitoes do not have an air tube and must position themselves horizontal to the water surface to breathe. Other mosquito species can insert their breathing apparatus into the roots of aquatic plants in order to breathe. Under optimal conditions, larvae pupate within seven days. The small, comma-shaped pupae hang in the tension of the water surface, so that their breathing tubes maintain contact with air. When the adults emerge, both females and males feed on plant juices, such as nectar, in order to survive. Females, however, must also feed on blood in order to develop their eggs. Depending on the species, they may obtain blood from birds, mammals, reptiles, or amphibians. Only the species that feed on humans are directly associated with the transmission of disease.

Several species of mosquitoes are responsible for transmitting the most serious diseases. For example, malaria is transmitted by *Anopheles* species. *Aedes aegypti* transmits both yellow fever and dengue fever (Triplehorn and Johnson, 2005). The Asian tiger mosquito, *Aedes albopictus*, is a vector of dengue fever, eastern equine encephalitis, West Nile virus, and chikungunya virus (Gratz, 2004; Paramasivan and others, 2006). Filariasis, which is caused by a filarial worm, is transmitted by *Culex* species. West Nile virus is spread by a variety of species, primarily in the genus *Culex*, that have fed on birds. Eastern equine encephalitis is known to be circulated by *Culiseta melanura* in birds, but *Aedes sollicitans*, *Aedes vexans*, and *Coquillettidia perturbans* are suspected as major vectors of the disease in humans (Hamilton and Racz, 1998). *Culex pipiens*, the common house mosquito, transmits St. Louis encephalitis. Because *C. pipiens* is an urban mosquito, St. Louis encephalitis is prevalent in urban centers when it occurs.

Sand Flies

Sand flies belong to the order Diptera, family Psychodidae, subfamily Phlebotominae (Triplehorn and Johnson, 2005). Females of this small group (thirteen species in North America) are bloodsucking as adults and occur in the southern United States and tropical areas. Larvae undergo complete metamorphosis and, depending on the species, live in decaying vegetable matter, mud, moss, or water. Females vector several diseases including pappataci fever (Mediterranean region and southern Asia), leishmaniasis (South America, Central America, southwestern United States, northern Africa and southern Asia, and Oroya fever (South America).

Termites

Termites are insects that belong to the order Isoptera and are responsible for millions of dollars of damage to wood and wooden structures throughout the world (Triplehorn and Johnson, 2005). Worldwide there are about 1,900 species of termites. There are four families of termites: Kalotermitidae (seventeen U.S. species), Termopsidae (three U.S. species), Rhinotermitidae (nine U.S. species) and Termitidae (fifteen U.S. species). Termites have moniliform (beadlike) or filiform (filament-like) antennae, a broad connection between the thorax and abdomen, and when front and hind wings are present, they are equal in shape and size—characteristics that distinguish termites from ants (which have elbowed antennae; a thin connection, called a petiole, between the thorax and abdomen; and front wings that are larger than the hind wings).

Termites live in highly organized societies with three distinct castes: reproductive females and males, workers, and soldiers. Reproductive termites may have wings, and as mentioned, when present there are four wings. Termites undergo gradual metamorphosis and feed on cast skins, feces of other termites, dead individuals, and plant materials such as wood and wood products. The cellulose in the wood and wood products that termites eat is digested by a myriad of flagellate protists that live in the termite's digestive system.

Without these organisms termites would starve to death. Termites are not born with these organisms but obtain them from feeding on the anal fluids of other termites.

Termites are important to humans for several reasons. First, because of their affinity for wood, they are very destructive to wooden portions of buildings, furniture, books, utility poles, fence posts, and other structures. Worldwide they also produce large amounts of atmospheric methane. Termites are also important because they help convert dead trees and other plant substances into decayed matter that can be used by other organisms.

Three main groups of destructive termites are of concern in the United States: subterranean termites, drywood termites, and dampwood termites. Subterranean termites live in wood that is either buried in the soil or is in contact with the soil. They may also enter wood not in contact with soil but must maintain contact in some way with soil. These termites are serious pests in the eastern United States. One introduced member of this group is the Formosan termite, *Coptotermes formosanus*. This termite is native to China and Taiwan and is one of the most destructive termites in the world. It has been introduced into several countries, including Japan, Guam, and the United States. It was first introduced into Texas in 1965 and has since spread to Alabama, Louisiana, Mississippi, Georgia, Florida, Tennessee, and North and South Carolina. It attacks living trees as well as dead stumps and wooden structures. Drywood termites live aboveground in wooden posts, tree stumps, trees, and buildings made of wood and do not need to be in contact with soil. Dampwood termites live in moist, dead wood, tree roots, and similar structures. They occur in Florida and southern, western, and Pacific coast areas of the United States.

Ticks

Ticks belong to the class Arachnida, order Acarina, and are relatives of insects. Ticks have piercing-sucking mouthparts and undergo a development cycle similar to that of insects with gradual metamorphosis. Mating occurs while the females and males are on the host. Females then drop to the ground to lay eggs (Truman and others, 1982). When they hatch, the resultant larvae, or seed ticks, have six legs. They then seek out a host on which to feed. After ingesting a blood meal, they drop to the ground and molt to the next stage, called the nymph. The larvae of some ticks that feed on only one host will remain on the host to molt. Nymphs have eight legs and resemble adults but have no genital pore. Like larvae, nymphs must find a host in order to receive a blood meal to survive. When they do, they molt to the adult stage. Adult male and female ticks may feed for several days before being able to reproduce. Most ticks can feed on a wide variety of hosts, including birds, reptiles, and mammals. In some species, such as the black-legged *Ixodes scapularis*, immature ticks and adult ticks feed on different hosts. Ticks can be divided into two categories: hard ticks (for example, the brown dog tick, American dog tick, and black-legged tick) and soft ticks (for example, the common fowl tick and relapsing fever tick). Ticks are responsible for at least nine human diseases in the United States, including Lyme disease, Rocky Mountain spotted fever, relapsing fever, babesiosis, and more recently, ehrlichiosis (American Lyme Disease Foundation [ALDF], 2005).

The brown dog tick, *Rhipicephalus sanguineus*, feeds on a wide range of hosts (Truman and others, 1982). Its most common host is dogs. Brown dog ticks are generally associated with structures that house dogs, such as kennels, veterinary hospitals, and homes. In the United States, *R. sanguineus* is a vector of canine ehrlichiosis (*Ehrlichia canis*) and canine babesiosis (*Babesia canis*) (Lord, 2001). These rarely cause disease in humans; only a few cases are known. In dogs, symptoms of canine ehrlichiosis include lameness and fever; babesiosis causes fever, anorexia, and anemia. In parts of Europe, Asia, and Africa, *R. sanguineus* is a vector of *Rickettsia conorii*, known locally as Mediterranean spotted fever, boutonneuse fever, or tick typhus. *Rhipicephalus sanguineus* has not been shown to transmit the bacteria that cause Lyme disease. Adult American dog ticks, *Dermacentor variabilis*, also prefer to feed on dogs but will feed on other larger mammals (Truman and others, 1982). Larvae and nymphs feed on small wild rodents such as mice. They may be found both indoors and outdoors and are the most widely distributed tick in the United States. American dog ticks are vectors for Rocky Mountain spotted fever and tick paralysis. All stages of the lone star tick, *Amblyomma americanum*, attack humans and other animals, such as cattle, sheep, horses, hogs, dogs, deer, and birds (North Carolina Agricultural Extension Service, 2005). The lone star tick is also a vector for Rocky Mountain spotted fever and tick paralysis and is a secondary vector for Lyme disease. The black-legged tick is a known vector for Lyme disease (ALDF, 2005). The black-legged tick larvae feed on small mammals found in leaf litter. Nymphs feed on small mammals and birds and, if not already infected, usually acquire Lyme disease during this stage. Adults feed on larger mammals, such as deer. Nymphs and adults also feed on humans and, if infected, can transmit Lyme disease to humans. Black-legged ticks can also transmit babesiosis. The western deer tick, *Ixodes pacificus*, which is common in the midwestern and western United States, is also a carrier of Lyme disease and babesiosis.

Vertebrate Pests

Vertebrate pests include rats, mice, and birds.

Rats

Rats are relatively large rodents that are important pests (Truman and others, 1982). They contaminate grain, destroy food in processing and storage plants, and can bite sleeping children and adults. Rats, over time, have caused more human death, misery, and economic hardship than any other vertebrate pest. Rats are known carriers of insects (lice, fleas, and mites) that transit plague and murine typhus, and as such they helped cause the outbreaks of plague in the fourteenth century that killed an estimated 25 million people (Cantor, 2001). Rats can also transmit Weil's disease, or leptospirosis; trichinosis and acute food poisoning can occur from food contaminated with rat feces. Rats also harbor organisms that cause typhoid, dysentery, and rabies.

Rats are very adaptable and can change their habits to match different environments. The roof rat, *Rattus rattus*, is an excellent climber and is commonly found in higher levels of buildings but can also be found in sewers. The Norway rat, *Rattus norvegicus*, lives in burrows but can be found in conditions favoring roof rats.

Rats live in well-protected areas and make nests out of soft material that is chewed or separated into small pieces. Outdoors, nests may be in the ground or tangled in tree limbs, trash dumps, or piles of rubbish. Indoors, nests can be found in wall voids, underneath floors next to the ground, and in undisturbed rubbish or stored materials. Rats have poor vision but excellent hearing and senses of smell and touch. Rats need a supply of water in order to survive and can squeeze through holes as small as a quarter.

The Norway rat (house rat, brown rat, wharf rat, sewer rat, or water rat) weighs between 10 and 17 ounces and is 31.2 to 49 cm in length (tip of nose to tip of tail). These rats have a blunt muzzle and a thick, heavy body. The tail is shorter than the head and body together, and is light colored underneath. Their ears are small, close set, and appear half buried in fur. Norway rat fur is coarse and generally red-brown to gray-brown. Norway rats are well distributed and are adept at displacing other species. They prefer traveling over flat surfaces to climbing but will climb pipes, wires, and rough walls when necessary. They prefer food with a high carbohydrate and protein content but will eat almost anything, including their own young.

The roof rat (black rat, ship rat, or gray-bellied rat) weighs between 8 and 12 ounces and is 34.9 to 45.1 cm in length (tip of nose to tip of tail). These rats have a pointed muzzle and a slender body. The tail is longer than the head and body together and uniformly colored. Their ears are large, prominent, and stand out from their fur. Roof rat fur is black to slate-gray or tawny above and gray-white below, or tawny above with a white to lemon belly. These rats are common at seaports. They are excellent climbers and frequently build nests in tree holes, in underground burrows, inside buildings, and under rubbish piles. Roof rats prefer to eat seeds, fresh vegetables and fruits, potatoes, wheat, corn, and other related foods. Like Norway rats, however, they will eat just about anything to survive.

Mice

Several species of **mice**, including field mice and house mice, can invade homes and other structures. The house mouse, *Mus musculus*, is the species most often encountered (Truman and others, 1982). House mice are considerably smaller than rats, generally weighing between 0.5 and 0.75 ounces and being 15.2 to 19.1 cm in length (tip of nose to tip of tail). House mice have small heads and bodies. Their tails are equal in length to their heads and bodies together. Their ears are prominent and appear large for the size of the body. Their fur is silky and dusky gray in color. House mice can enter structures using holes the size of dimes.

House mice have a keen sense of smell, touch, and hearing and can run, jump, and swim very well. Their nests can be made up of any soft material. House mice can occasionally be found in large colonies in which several females communally raise their young. They prefer human foods and will eat cereals, seeds, fruit, vegetables, and especially sweet liquids. House mice do not need a source of free water to survive, as rats do, and can get all the water they need directly from their food.

Mice can transmit diseases to humans and can be a vector for rat-bite fever and Weil's disease. In addition, their droppings can carry organisms that cause food poisoning. House mice can also carry fleas that transmit murine typhus, and they harbor mites that transmit rickettsialpox.

Hantavirus pulmonary syndrome (HPS) is another disease transmitted by infected rodents, through urine, droppings, or saliva (Centers for Disease Control and Prevention, 2005). Humans can contract the disease when they inhale aerosolized virus. HPS was first recognized in 1993 and has since been identified throughout the United States. Although rare, HPS is potentially deadly. Rodent control in and around the home remains the primary strategy for preventing hantavirus infection. The deer mouse, *Peromyscus maniculatus*, is the primary reservoir of the hantavirus that causes HPS in the United States.

Birds

Many birds are common inhabitants of urban areas (Truman and others, 1982). Species such as pigeons (*Columba livia*), European starlings (*Sturnus vulgaris*), and English house sparrows (*Passer domesticus*) are common sights in parks, along sidewalks, and at feeders in our own yards. Most of the general public, however, is unaware that birds are associated with several diseases of humans and that a number of parasites they carry may irritate or bite humans and play a role in food contamination. The close association between birds and humans presents potential epidemiological problems, because birds harbor several serious diseases.

One of the best-recognized diseases is ornithosis in pigeons (psittacosis in parrotlike birds). This disease is similar to viral pneumonia and is transmitted to man though infected droppings or respiratory droplets; it may infect 30 to 75 percent of the pigeons in a given area without being noticed. Several species of birds, including pigeons, have been shown to be reservoirs for encephalitides. These diseases of the nervous system include West Nile virus, equine encephalitis, and St. Louis encephalitis, and are transmitted to man by bird-biting mosquitoes. More recently, outbreaks of avian flu in Asia have called attention to the potential of both free-living birds and domestic poultry to spread diseases. Systemic fungal diseases such as histoplasmosis (*Histoplasma capsulatum*) and cryptococcosis (*Cryptococcus neoformans*) have been traced to pigeon and European starling manure. Pigeons have also been shown to harbor *Salmonella typhimurium*, which causes food poisoning, and the protozoan *Toxoplasma gondii*, which is responsible for toxoplasmosis and can appear in humans. Diseases carried by birds that are of lesser importance to humans include Newcastle disease, aspergillosis, pseudotuberculosis, pigeon coccidiosis, swine erysipelas, and trichomoniasis.

Pesticides

Pesticides, materials that are used to kill, repel, or change the behavior of an unwanted organism, are a mainstay of pest control. They are sprayed on crops and alongside residential streets, poured in gardens, squirted along baseboards and in basements, and impregnated into clothing and bed nets. Over 900 active ingredients are in commercial use, and these are formulated into more than 35,000 commercial products. The EPA (2005a) estimates that in 1999, over 1 billion pounds of pesticides were applied in the United States and over 5.6 billion pounds were applied worldwide. It is common for an active ingredient to have several different formulations—a spray, a wettable powder, and a liquid concentrate, for example—each of which can be formulated at several different concentrations.

Pesticides are often classified according to the type of pest they control. For examples, insecticides control insects, herbicides control vegetation, fungicides control fungi, and so forth. Exhibit 17.1 displays various categories of pesticides.

EXHIBIT 17.1
Pesticides Classified by Target

Algicides	Substances that control algae in lakes, canals, swimming pools, water tanks, and other sites
Antifouling agents	Substances that kill or repel organisms that attach to underwater surfaces, such as boat bottoms
Antimicrobials	Substances that kill microorganisms (such as bacteria and viruses)
Attractants	Substances that attract pests (for example, to lure an insect or rodent to a trap; food, however, is not considered a pesticide when used as an attractant)
Biopesticides	Pesticides that are derived from such natural materials as animals, plants, bacteria, and certain minerals
Biocides	Substances that kill microorganisms
Disinfectants and sanitizers	Substances that kill or inactivate disease-producing microorganisms on inanimate objects
Fumigants	Substances that produce gas or vapor intended to destroy pests in buildings or soil
Fungicides	Substances that kill fungi (including blights, mildews, molds, and rusts)
Herbicides	Substances that kill weeds and other plants that grow where they are not wanted
Insecticides	Substances that kill insects and other arthropods

Pesticides may also be classified according to chemical structure. Although many categories of chemicals have some action against insects or other pests, four categories account for most pesticides in use: organophosphates, carbamates, organochlorines, and pyrethroids. A fifth important category, defined not so much by chemical structure as by origin, consists of the biopesticides.

Organophosphates were developed during the early nineteenth century, but their effects on insects, which are similar to their effects on humans, were not discovered until 1932. These pesticides are nervous system toxins. They function by phosphorylating, and therefore inactivating, molecules of acetylcholinesterase,

Microbial pesticides	Microorganisms that kill, inhibit, or outcompete pests, including insects and other microorganisms
Miticides (also called acaricides)	Substances that kill mites that feed on plants and animals
Molluscicides	Substances that kill snails and slugs
Nematicides	Substances that kill nematodes (microscopic, wormlike organisms that feed on plant roots)
Ovicides	Substances that kill the eggs of insects and mites
Pheromones	Biochemicals that disrupt the mating behaviors of insects
Repellents	Substances that repel pests, including insects (such as mosquitoes) and birds
Rodenticides	Substances that control mice and other rodents

The term *pesticide* also includes these substances:

Defoliants	Substances that cause leaves or other foliage to drop from a plant, usually to facilitate harvest
Desiccants	Substances that promote drying of living tissues, such as unwanted plant tops
Insect growth regulators	Substances that disrupt the molting, maturing from pupal to adult stage, or other life processes of insects
Plant growth regulators	Substances (excluding fertilizers and other plant nutrients) that alter the expected growth, flowering, or reproduction rate of plants

the enzyme that regulates the neurotransmitter acetylcholine. Many species, from insects to humans, use this neurotransmitter, so many species are potentially susceptible to the effects of the organophosphates. In fact some of the more toxic organophosphates have been used as nerve gases, and one, sarin, was used in the infamous Tokyo subway attacks in 1995 (Ohbu and others, 1997). Some examples of organophosphates in common use are chlorpyrifos, diazinon, malathion, and azinphos-methyl. The organophosphates vary in toxicity and are usually are not persistent in the environment.

Carbamates function through a mechanism similar to that of the organophosphates—binding to and inactivating acetylcholinesterase. However, carbamates have lower affinity for acetylcholinesterase than do organophosphates, which reduces their toxicity to humans. Carbamate insecticides are widely used in homes, gardens, and agriculture. Examples include carbaryl and methomyl. Carbamates are also nonpersistent in the environment.

Organochlorine insecticides, which are also nerve poisons, were commonly used in the past. However, with growing recognition of their role as persistent organic pollutants (POPs)—chemicals that persist for many years, can bioaccumulate, and may harm ecosystems and human health—many of them have been removed from use, including DDT, aldrin, dieldrin, chlordane, and heptachlor.

Pyrethroid pesticides were developed as a synthetic version of the naturally occurring pesticide pyrethrin, which is found in certain chrysanthemum flowers. They have been modified to increase their stability in the environment. Examples include allethrin, permethrin, fenvalerate, and resmethrin. All synthetic pyrethroids are toxic to the nervous system.

Biopesticides are pesticides of biological origin, derived from such natural materials as animals, plants, bacteria, and certain minerals. For example, canola oil and baking soda have pesticidal applications and are considered biopesticides. At the end of 2001, there were approximately 195 registered biopesticide active ingredients and 780 products. Biopesticides fall into four major classes:

- **Microbial pesticides** have a microorganism (for example, a bacterium, fungus, virus, or protozoan) as the active ingredient. Microbial pesticides can control many different kinds of pests, although each separate active ingredient is relatively specific for its target pest(s). For example, there are fungi that control certain weeds and other fungi that kill specific insects. The most widely used microbial pesticides are subspecies and strains of *Bacillus thuringiensis*, or Bt. Each strain of this bacterium produces a different mix of proteins, many of which are toxic to one or a few related species of insect larvae.

- **Plant-incorporated-protectants** (PIPs) are pesticidal substances that plants produce from genetic material that has been added to the plant. For example, scientists can introduce the gene for the Bt pesticidal protein into a plant's own genetic material, enabling the plant to manufacture the substance that destroys the pest that preys on that plant. The protein and its genetic material, but not the plant itself, are regulated by EPA.

- **Biochemical pesticides** are naturally occurring substances that control pests by nontoxic mechanisms. Conventional pesticides, in contrast, are generally synthetic materials that directly kill or inactivate the pest. Among the biochemical pesticides are substances, such as insect sex pheromones, which interfere with mating, and also various scented plant extracts that attract insect pests to traps.

- **Botanical pesticides** are those derived from plants or plant parts. Botanicals are popular pest control compounds because, in general, they are safe for nontarget organisms and natural enemies. Because botanicals do not affect natural enemies they are well suited to be part of integrated pest control programs. In general botanicals have low mammalian toxicity and are often less expensive than their synthetic counterparts.

Patterns of Pesticide Use and Human Exposure

People encounter pesticides in many ways: by inhalation of sprayed pesticides near farms or in offices, by ingestion of pesticides on foods, and by skin contact with recently applied pesticides.

Residential exposure is common. Eighty percent of U.S. households use pesticides more than once a year in and around their homes (Davis, Brownson, and Garcia, 1992; Whitmore and others, 1994). Many of the pesticides applied indoors are semivolatile (Dalaker and Naifeh, 1997). Once applied, semivolatile pesticides can vaporize from treated surfaces and can distribute in and on targeted and nontargeted surfaces and objects (Gurunathan and others, 1998; Lewis, Fortune, Blanchard, and Camann, 2001; Hore and others, 2005). This raises concern about exposures because U.S. householders, including children, may spend up to 90 percent of their time indoors, within or around treated areas (Savage and others, 1981). Children in pesticide-treated homes may be exposed to pesticides via multiple routes and from multiple media. Given their inherent biological vulnerabilities and characteristic behaviors, which are different from those of adults, children can be particularly susceptible to the effects of pesticides (Freeman, Ettinger, Barry, and Rhoads, 1997; also see Chapter Twenty-Five). Work by many researchers has indicated that pesticides can persist in the home for long periods of time. They can also accumulate on surfaces that pose a particular risk to children. The plush toys that small children often carry and sleep with, for example, can act as sinks for pesticides applied in the home.

Occupational exposure is also common among farmworkers and other high-risk occupations. Workers who directly handle pesticides, including mixers and loaders, are at highest risk (Figure 17.5), followed by those who apply pesticides in agricultural or commercial settings. Finally, farmworkers who enter fields where pesticides have been applied and perform allowed tasks there, such as weeding, irrigating, or picking crops, are also at risk.

PERSPECTIVE
Who Is Responsible for Applying Pesticides?

Humans and insects prefer many of the same ecosystems, so they encounter each other in many settings—on agricultural fields, in gardens, in homes, and elsewhere. As a result, efforts at pest control, including pesticide use, take many forms. Who actually applies pesticides?

Pesticides are divided into two categories: general use and restricted use. The difference between them is analogous to the difference between over-the-counter medications and prescription medications.

Homeowners can buy a variety of general use pesticides at garden centers, hardware stores, and grocery stores to combat day-to-day pests. These pesticides are usually less toxic and less concentrated than restricted use pesticides. Many are in ready-to-use formulations, such as household sprays and garden sprays. Some substances defined as pesticides may seem surprising. For instance, common household bleach, because it claims germicidal properties, must be registered as a pesticide, and it has an EPA registration number under the Federal Insecticide, Fungicide, and Rodenticide Act.

Commercial pesticide use is more tightly regulated. It is generally carried out by private firms, which may be small local businesses or large national franchises. These firms must be registered as pest control businesses with the appropriate state agency, typically the state department of agriculture or the state department of environmental protection. They must have certified applicators on staff, and they must show proof of liability insurance, in case a misapplication should occur. Most specialize in a particular type of pest control, such as structural or turf and ornamental.

The people who apply pesticides for pest control firms are known as commercial applicators. State laws define the scope of their work in terms such as these: the application of pesticides (including general use and restricted use pesticides) to land, plants, seeds, animals, water, structures, or vehicles, using aerial, ground, or hand equipment, on a contractual or for-hire basis. Commercial applicators must pass a series of EPA-approved tests, which are administered by the state agency. They must demonstrate general knowledge about pesticides plus specific knowledge and training in their area of specialty. In most states, any commercial application of a pesticide, even a general use pesticide, requires that the applicator be licensed and certified or

Pesticide Toxicity

Pesticides are toxic. This is a desired property, responsible for the ability of pesticides to kill unwanted species. However, pesticide toxicity may also affect humans, making this a public health issue. Pesticide damage to unintended species, and therefore to entire ecosystems, is also a serious concern in some circumstances.

work under the supervision of a licensed and certified applicator. To maintain a commercial license the applicator must undergo a recertification program every three to five years (the period varies from state to state). This usually entails participating in educational programs and earning a required number of continuing education units.

Despite the requirement that commercial pesticide application be carried out by licensed and trained professionals or people under their supervision, pesticides are sometimes applied by untrained individuals. For example, building superintendents and school custodians commonly apply "structural and household pest control" compounds without the necessary training and background. This can result in serious health and environmental problems.

Farmers are one of the largest users of pesticide products. Although some hire commercial applicators, some qualify as private applicators in order to apply pesticides to their own land. If they do, they must be trained and certified to perform this task, as commercial applicators are, and they must apply specified pesticides to specified crops in accordance with the notations on the pesticide labels. Pesticides registered for agricultural use may not be used for residential or interior needs.

Most mosquito and public health pest control is handled by county and state agencies. In many states it is the local mosquito control commission that sprays for a variety of mosquito species.

Aquatic weed control is usually carried out by the application of herbicides. This too is a specialty task that should be performed only by individuals with appropriate training and working for either private firms or governmental agencies. This is a sensitive job because misapplication can have serious effects on humans, on fish and other marine animals, and on beneficial plants.

Other uses of pesticides are frequent as well. Veterinarians apply flea and tick insecticides to control these pests on cats and dogs. Physicians apply pesticides to patients suffering from body lice and head lice. Federal agencies apply pesticides to cargo ships and airplanes importing or exporting food and fiber products.

Overall, pesticides are applied by a wide variety of people and organizations in a wide variety of situations. Although federal and state regulations have gone a long way toward ensuring safety, unapproved or sloppy procedures can still result in potential hazards to people and the environment.

The EPA has estimated that between 10,000 and 20,000 medically treated pesticide poisonings occurred each year in the United States during the 1990s (Blondell, 1997), including suicides, attempted suicides, and unintentional poisonings. In the United States in 1983, the mortality rate from unintentional acute pesticide poisoning was estimated to be 2.7 per 10 million among men and 0.5

FIGURE 17.5   Workers in Ghana Mixing and Loading an
Organophosphate Insecticide Without Adequate Personal Protective
Equipment

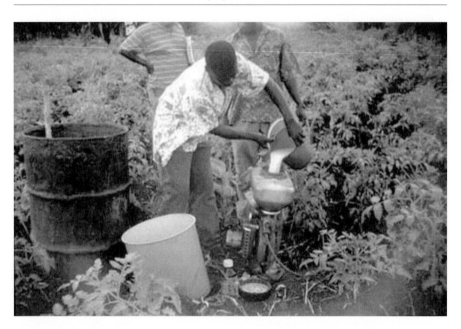

Source: Photo supplied by M. G. Robson.

among women (Keifer and others, 2005). This burden may have declined in
recent years (Blondell, 2007).

Acute toxicity is most associated with the organophosphates and the
carbamates. These compounds block the action of acetylcholinesterase at
peripheral nerves and in the central nervous system. The early symptoms of poisoning include headache, hypersecretion, muscle twitching, nausea, and diarrhea.
(Health care providers remember this syndrome with the mnemonic SLUDGE,
for Salivation, Lacrimation, Urination, Diarrhea, GI upset, and pulmonary
Edema, or DUMBELS, for Diarrhea, Urination, Miosis, Bronchospasm, Emesis,
Lacrimation, and Salivation.) More severe poisoning can feature respiratory
depression, loss of consciousness, and death. Victims who survive may develop
weakness or paralysis of the arms and legs, known as **organophosphate-
induced delayed neuropathy** (OPIDN), or they may exhibit an intermediate
syndrome characterized by respiratory depression and muscular weakness.

Pesticides are required to carry warning statements on their labels; these
warnings are based mostly on acute toxicity. They reflect oral LD_{50} (lethal dose

for 50 percent; see Chapter Two), inhalation LD_{50}, dermal LD_{50}, and what is known about eye effects and skin effects. The toxicity warning categories are shown in Exhibit 17.2.

Chronic toxicity is also a growing concern as epidemiological and toxicological evidence accumulates. A review of epidemiological evidence reveals that pesticide exposure is associated with increases in the risk of several cancers, including non-Hodgkin's lymphoma (relative risk 2), leukemia (relative risk 1.5), multiple myeloma (an excess risk exists, although the specific exposure link is weak), soft-tissue sarcoma (inconsistent patterns have been observed), prostate

EXHIBIT 17.2
Pesticide Toxicity Categories and Labeling Requirements

Toxicity Category I—All pesticide products meeting the criteria of Toxicity Category I shall bear on the front panel the signal word "Danger." In addition if the product was assigned to Toxicity Category I on the basis of its oral, inhalation or dermal toxicity (as distinct from skin and eye local effects) the word "Poison" shall appear in red on a background of distinctly contrasting color and the skull and crossbones shall appear in immediate proximity to the word "Poison."

Toxicity Category II—All pesticide products meeting the criteria of Toxicity Category II shall bear on the front panel the signal word "Warning."

Toxicity Category III—All pesticide products meeting the criteria of Toxicity Category III shall bear on the front panel the signal word "Caution."

Toxicity Category IV—All pesticide products meeting the criteria of Toxicity Category IV shall bear on the front panel the signal word "Caution."

Child hazard warning—Every pesticide product label shall bear on the front panel the statement "keep out of reach of children." Only in cases where the likelihood of contact with children during distribution, marketing, storage, or use is demonstrated by the applicant to be extremely remote, or if the nature of the pesticide is such that it is approved for use on infants or small children, may the Administrator waive this requirement.

Further information on these criteria and labeling requirements is published in the *Code of Federal Regulations* (40 CFR 156.10).

Source: EPA, 2005b.

cancer (relative risk 1.5), pancreatic cancer (increased risk found in some studies), lung cancer (causally associated with arsenical compounds), ovarian cancer (an association with triazine use has been found), breast cancer (possible estrogenic activity of chlorinated compounds), testicular cancer (antiandrogenic activity of chlorinated compounds), and Hodgkin's disease (small but significant excess risk found) (Alavanja, Hoppin, and Kamel, 2004).

In addition to acute neurotoxicity, pesticide exposure may have chronic effects on the nervous system, manifested by a range of symptoms, deficits in neurobehavioral performance, and abnormalities in nerve function. Neurotoxicity can result from high-level exposure to most types of pesticides, including organophosphates, carbamates, organochlorines, fungicides, and fumigants (Alavanja and others, 2004). There is also evidence linking pesticide exposure with chronic neurodegenerative diseases, especially Parkinson's disease (Priyadarshi, Khuder, Schaub, and Priyadarshi, 2001).

Pesticides may also have developmental, endocrine, and reproductive effects. This has been recognized for several decades; in fact Rachel Carson's landmark book *Silent Spring* took its title from the loss of songbirds that followed DDT-induced thinning of eggshells. Recent work has shown similar endocrine effects in other animals. Research at Lake Apopka, Florida, following contamination of the lake by organochlorine pesticides, dibromochloropropane, and ethylene dibromide, has shown marked changes in the alligator population, including decreased testosterone levels, smaller genitalia, and altered gender ratios in newborns, findings attributed to the effects of pesticides (Guillette and others, 1996; Semenza and others, 1997). Similarly, recent observations of demasculinization of atrazine-exposed frogs suggest that triazine compounds may have endocrine-disrupting effects (Hayes and others, 2002).

Pesticides also have direct and indirect effects on animal habitats. In the 1960s, the development of so-called no-till agriculture—a technique that involves heavy applications of chemicals, rather than tilling the soil, to control pests and weeds—caused widespread habitat destruction for many animals.

Pesticide Regulation

The EPA is the agency responsible for pesticide regulation, under the authority of two federal statutes: the Federal Insecticide, Fungicide, and Rodenticide Act and the Federal Food, Drug, and Cosmetic Act. Here is the EPA's summary of important features of these Acts (EPA, 2005c):

> The Federal Insecticide, Fungicide, and Rodenticide Act (FIFRA) provides the basis for regulation, sale, distribution and use of pesticides in the U.S. This law authorizes EPA to review and register pesticides for specified uses. EPA also has

the authority to suspend or cancel the registration of a pesticide if subsequent information shows that continued use would pose unreasonable risks. Some key elements of FIFRA include:

- is a product licensing statute; pesticide products must obtain an EPA registration before manufacture, transport, and sale
- registration based on a risk/benefit standard
- strong authority to require data—authority to issue Data Call-ins
- ability to regulate pesticide use through labeling, packaging, composition, and disposal
- emergency exemption authority—permits approval of unregistered uses of registered products on a time limited basis
- ability to suspend or cancel a product's registration: appeals process, adjudicatory functions, etc.

The Federal Food, Drug, and Cosmetic Act (FFDCA) authorizes EPA to set maximum residue levels, or **tolerances,** for pesticides used in or on foods or animal feed. Features of FFDCA include:

- mandates strong provisions to protect infants and children
- provides the authority to set tolerances in foods and feeds (pesticide levels)
- also provides authority to exempt a pesticide from the requirement of a tolerance
- rule-making process required to set tolerances or exemptions
- before a registration can be granted for a food use pesticide, a tolerance or tolerance exemption must be in place
- mandates a primarily health-based standard for setting the tolerance— "reasonable certainty of no harm"
- benefits may be considered only in limited extreme circumstances
- pesticide residues in foods are monitored and the tolerances enforced by FDA (fruits and vegetables, seafood) and USDA (meat, milk, poultry, eggs, and aquacultural foods)

The Food Quality Protection Act of 1996 (FQPA) amended FIFRA and FFDCA setting tougher safety standards for new and old pesticides and calling for uniform requirements regarding processed and unprocessed foods. Major provisions of this law include:

- amended both FIFRA and FFDCA, significantly changing the way EPA regulates pesticides

- establishes a single safety standard for setting tolerances under FFDCA—not a risk/benefit standard (with some exceptions)
- assessment must include aggregate exposures including all dietary exposures, drinking water, and non-occupational (e.g., residential) exposures
- when assessing a tolerance, EPA must also consider cumulative effects and common mode of toxicity among related pesticides, the potential for endocrine disruption effects, and appropriate safety factor to incorporate
- requires a special finding for the protection of infants and children
- must incorporate a 10-fold safety factor to protect infants and children further unless reliable information in the database indicates that it can be reduced or removed
- establishes a tolerance reassessment program and lays out a schedule whereby EPA must reevaluate all tolerances that were in place as of August 1996 within 10 years
- requires a minor use program and provides that special considerations be afforded minor use actions
- requires review of antimicrobial actions within prescribed timeframes
- EPA must now periodically review every pesticide registration every 15 years
- now required to set tolerances for use of pesticides under emergency exemptions (FIFRA Section 18)

Two other pieces of legislation are also relevant. The Pesticide Registration Improvement Act (PRIA) of 2003 "establishes pesticide registration service fees for registration actions in three pesticide program divisions: Antimicrobials, Biopesticides and Pollution Prevention, and Registration" (EPA, 2005c). The Endangered Species Act (ESA) of 1973 "prohibits any action that can adversely affect an endangered or threatened species or its habitat. In compliance with this law, EPA must ensure that use of the pesticides it registers will not harm these species" (EPA, 2005c).

Pesticide labeling was discussed in Exhibit 17.2. Another important aspect of pesticide regulation is restrictions on use. In the United States and in many other countries, pesticides are sold either for general use or for restricted use. As mentioned earlier, the best analogy for the difference between these uses is the difference between over-the-counter medications and those requiring a prescription from a physician. **General use** pesticides are lower in toxicity, require few special precautions other than the standard safety measures, and are sold in lower concentrations. **Restricted use** pesticides are limited to sale to and use by a licensed pesticide applicator. Some compounds are general use at a low concentration or formulation and restricted use at a higher concentration. The licensed pesticide applicator will have received proper training for the use of these compounds and will have demonstrated to the state regulatory agency adequate knowledge for the safe and efficacious use of the product. Most states require examination and certification of the applicator, followed by continuing education and recertification. In most states commercial pest control can be carried out only by a licensed applicator.

Pesticide regulations have focused specifically on two high-risk groups: children and workers. Children are especially vulnerable to pesticide exposure. In 1996, the Food Quality Protection Act mandated that contributions from all routes of exposure and from all possible sources be considered when setting food tolerance levels for pesticides, paying particular attention to the potential risks to infants and small children. The EPA subsequently undertook several actions to protect children:

- It set tougher standards to protect infants and children from pesticide risks, including an additional safety factor to account for developmental risks, incomplete data, and any special sensitivity and exposure to pesticide chemicals that infants and children may have.
- It restricted some uses of pesticides; for example, in 1999, the EPA disallowed major uses of the organophosphate methyl parathion in children's food and placed significant restrictions on the use of another organophosphate, azinphos-methyl.
- It required additional studies on pesticides to clarify specific effects (such as developmental neurotoxicity and acute and subchronic neurotoxicity) in children.
- It developed new tests and risk assessment methods to target risk factors unique to infants and children.
- It increased consumer education; for example, a consumer information brochure was distributed to grocery stores nationwide and an interactive Web site (http://www.epa.gov/pesticides/food) was targeted to consumers.

Agricultural workers' risks of pesticide exposure are addressed by the EPA's **Worker Protection Standard** (WPS) that specifically protects agricultural workers. The WPS applies to over 3.5 million people who work with pesticides at over 560,000 workplaces. The WPS contains requirements for

- Pesticide safety training
- Notification of pesticide applications
- Use of personal protective equipment
- Restricted entry intervals following pesticide application

- Decontamination supplies
- Emergency medical assistance

International Pesticide Use

Pesticides continue to be an important tool in the control of insects, diseases, and weeds in areas such as agriculture, forestry, and horticulture. The EPA (2009) recently reported that in 2000 and 2001, world pesticide use exceeded 5 billion pounds. Insecticides accounted for the largest portion of total use, followed by herbicides and fungicides.

Currently, pesticide use is highest in developing countries, particularly those in tropical regions, that are seeking to enter the world economy by providing rice and also fresh fruits and vegetables that are out of season in other countries. Without the use of pesticides, growers and farmers face the risk of losing significant proportions of their production and subsequently their incomes.

Although there are clearly benefits to pesticide use, it is important to manage any associated risks. In some agricultural countries, the tendency is to still use the "older," nonpatented, less expensive, more acutely toxic, and more environmentally persistent agents that can be manufactured in-country or formulated from active ingredients imported from regional sources having chemical synthesizing capabilities. Many of these chemicals have been banned or severely restricted in the Western nations. However, these chemicals are still obtainable in the world market (Ecobichon, 2001). There should be increased concern in countries that still use banned or restricted pesticides, due to pesticide residue contamination of local, fresh produce and potential long-term and adverse health effects on consumers.

INTEGRATED PEST MANAGEMENT

Integrated pest management, or IPM, is an approach that uses multiple control techniques to maintain, or *manage*, pest populations below economically damaging levels while maintaining environmental quality. The IPM concept was first developed for use in agriculture in the 1960s, in response to environmental and developing pest-resistance issues caused by the use of various pesticides (Carson, 1962; Pedigo, 2002). In agriculture, IPM is defined as "a comprehensive approach to pest control that uses combined means to reduce the status of pests to tolerant levels while maintaining a quality environment" (Pedigo, 2002).

Since the 1960s, the IPM concept has been applied in numerous other settings, including turf and ornamental landscapes, homes, workplaces, and facilities such as schools, malls, restaurants, and hospitals. IPM is defined slightly differently for each of these applications. For turf and ornamental landscapes, for example, IPM definitions address maintaining aesthetic quality. For buildings, homes, and schools, IPM definitions usually address sanitation, the preference for low-impact or reduced-risk chemicals, and the use of chemicals as a last resort. Finally, some states have also developed their own definitions of IPM and require the use of IPM in various situations (see, for example, New Jersey Department of Environmental Protection, 2005; Pesticide Control Regulations, 2009). This complexity makes IPM difficult for the lay public to understand.

Common to all IPM definitions, however, are the goals of using more than one tool to control pests, keeping pest populations below damaging levels, maintaining environmental quality, and protecting human health. A useful overall definition of IPM is the following: A sustainable approach to managing pests by using all appropriate technology and management practices in a way that minimizes health, environmental and economic risks. In addition, IPM employs pest monitoring, consumer education, and cultural management techniques; sanitation and solid waste management; structural maintenance; and physical, mechanical, biological, and chemical controls.

Monitoring

Monitoring is the key to any good IPM program. Monitoring provides information on pest populations so that targeted, data-based control decisions can be made. The alternative to monitoring is to spray for pests whether they are present or not, which in today's society is unacceptable. Monitoring can also reveal how well a program is working and can identify problem areas that need more attention. A wide variety of species-specific monitoring methods are available, including the use of traps baited with various attractants.

Cultural Management Techniques

Cultural management techniques modify the environment to make it unattractive to pests. Practices such as covering garbage bins can eliminate a food source that rodents need to survive. Keeping dry food goods such as flour and sugar in sealed containers can keep storage pests from contaminating these products. Avoiding the placement of plants close to buildings can reduce the likelihood that carpenter ants will enter the structure. Removing or modifying areas that can hold water (gutters, empty cans, tires, low areas in the landscape) can remove potential breeding areas for mosquitoes. In the landscape the use of cultural management techniques can make plants better able to withstand pest attack. Proper site selection and proper fertilization and watering, for example, reduce stress on plants, making them more vigorous and able to withstand attack. Another tactic is proper pruning. Pruning can remove diseased or insect-infested plant parts and can keep the pests from spreading to healthy tissue or further damaging the plant, providing control without the use of a pesticide.

Sanitation and Solid Waste Management

Sanitation and solid waste management can be important steps toward controlling certain pests. It is especially important in food service and storage areas. Not leaving food out overnight, cleaning under and behind kitchen appliances, and having regular refuse pickups are examples of practices that can keep pests such as cockroaches from gaining a foothold.

Structural Maintenance

Structural maintenance can keep pests from entering structures. Removing or repairing openings on a structure's facade can eliminate entry points for rodents. Placing screens over attic vents can keep insects from entering. Structural maintenance can also remove places where pests might obtain vital resources. Simple actions like fixing leaky faucets can remove water sources that are vital to rats and several cockroach species. Fixing water leaks and reducing the subsequent decay of water-soaked wood also reduces the potential for carpenter ant infestations.

Control Measures

When pest-monitoring procedures indicate a pest problem and when measures such as sanitation and cultural management are either not available or not completely effective, use of a control measure may be warranted. Depending on the pest and the situation, several measures may be available: physical and mechanical interventions, biological control agents, or chemical pesticide applications. The optimal control measure is the one that is least harmful to the environment and human health while still providing effective control. The discussion in the following Perspective of the pros and cons of using DDT as a control measure against malaria illustrates general considerations to apply when selecting among various control tactics.

Physical and mechanical controls include the use of techniques or materials that will keep pests from becoming a problem. These controls may include such simple measures as painting building foundations white and creating light-colored borders around foundations to help prevent rats and mice from entering buildings, or raising dumpsters and other outdoor refuse containers off the ground to reduce hiding places for rats. Other possibilities include installing bug zappers at doors leading to the outside to help prevent flying insects from entering a building, caulking doors and windows to remove access points for insects and rodents, and using door sweeps or sealing voids around pipes to prevent the entry of pests. What can or should be used depends on the pest involved and the situation at hand. What is appropriate for one pest may not be appropriate for another. For example, window screens keep flying insects such as mosquitoes from entering a structure but have little impact on mice. Bug zappers used at the entrances to food preparation areas and warehouses help prevent flying insects from entering the structure but do not prevent termites from entering. Termite guards help prevent termite infestations but have little or no impact on other pest species. Bug zappers used outdoors do little more than attract insects into the areas, and sonic devices to repel pests have little or no effect. One should be careful to choose an appropriate, effective control measure.

Biological control involves the use, manipulation, and conservation of living organisms that feed on insects and weeds for the purpose of controlling a pest. By definition, biological control agents (natural enemies) are beneficial organisms that create or re-create a natural balance to control pests. Although biological control is used primarily in agriculture, this method, when feasible, can also provide effective control in an environmentally friendly manner in many other situations. For example, nematodes, living organisms that attack certain insects, can be used in place of chemicals to control fungus gnats in houseplant pots or white grubs in turf. Given the right conditions, gambusia (mosquito fish) released into ponds can control mosquito larvae. Using biological control also means avoiding management tactics that might be detrimental to beneficial organisms. Using environmentally friendly chemicals or alternative control measures can avoid reductions in natural enemy populations. Outdoors, certain measures can encourage natural enemies in an area and keep them there once they are present. Using plant species that are attractive to beneficial organisms and that provide alternative or supplemental food sources, such as nectar and pollen, will help control ornamental and garden pests and reduce the need to use pesticides.

The use of chemical pesticides to control pests should be seen as a last resort; they should be used only when other tactics are not available, practical, or effective. Many state universities and extension services provide information on pesticides. These recommendations can be used in deciding which chemicals are

PERSPECTIVE
DDT in Antimalaria Campaigns: An Example of Public Health Trade-Offs

Up through the first part of the twentieth century, malaria control relied on environmental approaches such as drainage and landfills to eliminate the larval mosquito habitat and on biological controls such as larvivorous fish in ponds and larvicidal applications of oil and Paris green (Mabaso, Sharp, and Lengeler, 2004; Najera, 2001). These methods were effective, especially in Europe and North America, but malaria continued to be a problem in many poor nations.

DDT, or dichlorodiphenyltrichloroethane, was introduced as an agricultural pesticide during the 1930s, and during World War II military forces used it for typhus control (Gahan, Travis, Morton, and Lindquist, 1945). During the 1950s and 1960s, as part of malaria control campaigns worldwide, DDT played an important role in reducing mosquito populations and reducing the burden of disease.

However, DDT belongs to a category of chemicals known as **persistent organic pollutants (POPs)**; it persists for years in the environment, it is bioconcentrated as it moves up the food chain, and it may harm wildlife and even humans. Rachel Carson's *Silent Spring* alerted the public that chemicals such as DDT could have catastrophic ecosystem effects, killing not only insects but birds and other species. In addition, although DDT has low acute toxicity in humans, there is some evidence that it may disrupt reproductive and endocrine functions. Because of these concerns, Sweden banned the use of DDT in 1970, the United States did so in 1972, and many other countries have followed suit. The Stockholm Convention on Persistent Organic Pollutants, an international treaty that requires the elimination of DDT and other POPs, was signed in 2001 and took effect in 2004, when the fiftieth nation ratified it (Kapp, 2004b; Stockholm Convention on Persistent Organic Pollutants, 2001).

Malaria remains a common and deadly disease in much of the developing world. It kills 3 million people each year, including one child every thirty seconds, despite decades of research on vaccines, new drugs, and alternative control strategies. If DDT is effective in controlling malaria, should it continue to be used? In 2006, the World Health Organization (WHO) announced increased support for the use of DDT in combating malaria. Limited application, such as impregnating mosquito netting or spraying on interior walls, was felt to be less dangerous than widespread fumigation.

This is a classic example of a trade-off in public health, a dilemma in which one public health goal—the elimination of a persistent chemical pollutant—collides with another public health goal—the control of a killer disease. Strong arguments have been advanced on both sides of the debate.

Arguments Against Continued DDT Use

- DDT accumulates in ecosystems, persists for years or even decades, bioconcentrates, and has been shown to cause reproductive failure and other adverse

outcomes in fish, birds, and other species beyond target insect species (Turusov, Rakitsky, and Tomatis, 2002).
- DDT accumulates in the adipose tissue of humans and other organisms (WHO, 1989).
- Although the acute toxicity of DDT is low, there is some evidence that DDT may disrupt reproductive and endocrine functions and neurological development (Longnecker, Klebanoff, Zhou, and Brock, 2001; Longnecker, Rogan, and Lucier, 1997). There is also laboratory evidence of carcinogenicity, leading the National Toxicology Program (2005) to classify DDT as reasonably anticipated to be a human carcinogen, and the International Agency for Research on Cancer (1991) to classify it as possibly carcinogenic to humans. A precautionary approach would dictate avoiding the use of such a chemical.
- Continued use of DDT will result in increasing insect resistance, so in the long run this will not be a useful strategy.
- Alternatives to DDT, including nonchemical approaches and synthetic pyrethroids, are readily available.

Arguments in Favor of Continued DDT Use

- DDT has very low acute toxicity for humans (Smith, 2000), and the evidence for human carcinogenicity and other adverse effects is weak (Smith, 2000; Curtis and Lines, 2000). In contrast, the burden of mortality and morbidity from malaria is enormous. Therefore a cost-benefit analysis clearly favors the use of DDT.
- DDT is relatively inexpensive compared to alternatives and therefore more accessible for many poor countries. The cost of alternatives such as malathion and pyrethroid insecticides can be two times to twenty times that of DDT, and bed nets (at several dollars each) are also prohibitively expensive (Tren, 1999).
- DDT is easy to mix and apply, thereby eliminating the need for training and supervision (Tren, 1999). This makes it practical for widespread use in developing nations.
- Malaria (and other arthropod-borne diseases such as dengue fever and urban yellow fever) have surged in many areas following the phaseout of DDT, underlining the importance of DDT in malaria control (Roberts, Loughlin, Hshieh, and Legters, 1997; Roberts, Manguin, and Mouchet, 2000).
- DDT is now used for house spraying, a selective approach that requires much less volume than the previous agricultural and area spraying. This results in a much lower environmental load than resulted from applications in the past.

What do you think? Should the continued use of DDT be permitted for malaria control? (For further information see Kapp, 2004a; Roberts and others, 2004; Stolberg, 1999; Rogan and Chen, 2005.)

available to control specific pests and under what circumstances they may be used. Chemicals that are comparatively less harmful to the environment or the user should be used whenever possible. The pesticide chosen should be effective, so that repeated applications and the use of more chemicals are not necessary. Finally, all labeling directions should be followed, and quantities applied should never exceed the amount prescribed by the label.

Consumer Education

Education of potential users of IPM is also very important. The general public and potential users of IPM must not only be made aware of what IPM is but must also understand its different components and how these components fit into a complete management program, one that reduces hazards to themselves and the environment.

SUMMARY

Pests are plants, animals, or microorganisms that threaten human health or well-being. They include insect pests such as cockroaches, fleas, lice, mosquitoes, and ticks, and vertebrate pests such as rats, mice, and birds. Humans have contended with pests since ancient times; however, most pests also serve valuable ecological and other functions. Each pest has specific biological and ecological characteristics.

Modern pest control has come to rely heavily on chemical agents that act as pesticides. The majority of these fall into four categories: organophosphates, carbamates, organochlorines, and pyrethroids. Pesticides have varying levels of toxicity, both in acute intoxication and in chronic effects such as cancer and neurological disease. People can sustain pesticide exposures in a wide range of settings (home, workplace, and so forth), and through a wide range of pathways (ingestion, inhalation, and skin absorption).

Pesticide regulation is complex, relying on several federal laws. However, the control of pesticide exposure relies not only on laws but also on techniques such as integrated pest management. This is a strategy that combines chemical and nonchemical approaches to pest control, reducing the need to use pesticides.

KEY TERMS

bedbugs

biochemical pesticides

biopesticides

botanical pesticides

carbamates

cockroaches

Federal Food, Drug, and
    Cosmetic Act (FFDCA)

Federal Insecticide,
    Fungicide, and
    Rodenticide Act (FIFRA)

fleas

Food Quality Protection
   Act (FQPA)

general use

integrated pest
   management

lice

mice

microbial pesticides

mosquitoes

organochlorine

organophosphates

organophosphate-induced
   delayed neuropathy

persistent organic
   pollutants (POPs)

pest

pesticides

plant-incorporated
protectants

pyrethroid

restricted use rats

sand flies

termites

ticks

tolerances

Worker Protection
   Standard

DISCUSSION QUESTIONS

1. Pesticides are economic poisons; unlike other toxins or contaminants with which people come into contact, pesticides are intentionally applied to food, living spaces, and people. What are some of the risk-benefit issues in the application of pesticides? Is it worth the risk to apply pesticides?

2. Integrated pest management is a logical approach for many pest problems, but it is not widely used. What are some of the societal trade-offs when using IPM?

3. Pesticide use continues to be a major part of agricultural production; nevertheless, after fifty years of intense chemical use, a quarter to a third of the global harvest is lost to pests. Is this progress? What else can we do to improve the world food supply?

4. Are current pesticide regulations protective of public health, especially for susceptible populations?

5. WHO and other agencies still apply DDT and similar compounds to control many vector-borne diseases, such as malaria. The risks associated with DDT have been known for many decades. Is it appropriate that these compounds are still used for vector control?

REFERENCES

Abdel-Rahman, A. A., and others. "Neurological Deficits Induced by Malathion, DEET, and Permethrin, Alone or in Combination in Adult Rats." *Journal of Toxicology and Environmental Health, Part A*, 2004, *67*(4), 331–356.

Alavanja, M.C.R., Hoppin, J. A., and Kamel, F. "Health Effects of Chronic Pesticide Exposure: Cancer and Neurotoxicity." *Annual Review of Public Health*, 2004, *24*, 155–197.

American Lyme Disease Foundation. "Deer Tick Ecology." http://www.aldf.com/DeerTickEcology.asp, 2005.

Bell, J. W., Veltri, J. C., and Page, B. C. "Human Exposure to N,N-Diethyl-m-Toluamide Insect Repellant Reported to the American Association of Poison Control Centers, 1993–1997." *International Journal of Toxicology*, 2002, *21*, 341–352.

Blondell, J. "Epidemiology of Pesticide Poisonings in the United States, with Special Reference to Occupational Cases." *Occupational Medicine*, 1997, *12*, 209–220.

Blondell, J. M. "Decline in Pesticide Poisonings in the United States from 1995 to 2004." *Clinical Toxicology*, 2007, *45*(5), 589–592.

Buescher, M. D., Rutledge, L. C., Wirtz, R. A., and Nelson, J. H. "The Dose-Persistence Relationship of DEET Against *Aedes Aegypti*." *Mosquito News*, 1983, *43*, 364–366.

Cantor, N. *In the Wake of the Plague: The Black Death and the World It Made*. New York: Free Press, 2001.

Carson, R. *Silent Spring*. Boston: Houghton Mifflin, 1962.

Centers for Disease Control and Prevention. "Hantavirus Pulmonary Syndrome (HPS)." http://www.cdc.gov/ncidod/diseases/hanta/hps, 2005.

Curtis, C. F., and Lines, J. D. "Should DDT Be Banned by International Treaty?" *Parasitology Today*, 2000, *16*(3), 119–121.

Dalaker, J., and Naifeh, M. *Poverty in the United States*. U.S. Bureau of the Census, Current Population Reports, Series P60–201. Washington, D.C.: U.S. Government Printing Office, 1997.

Davis, J. R., Brownson, R. C., and Garcia, R. "Family Pesticide Use in the Home, Garden, Orchard, and Yard." *Archives of Environmental Contamination and Toxicology*, 1992, *22*, 260–266.

"DEET Is Hard to Beat." *Harvard Health Letter*, 2003, *28*, 1–3.

Ecobichon, D. J. "Pesticide Use in Developing Countries." *Toxicology*, 2001, *160*(1–3), 27–33.

Fradin, M. S. "Mosquitoes and Mosquito Repellents: A Clinician's Guide." *Annals of Internal Medicine*, 1998, *128*, 931–940.

Fradin, M. S., and Day, J. F. "Comparative Efficacy of Insect Repellants Against Mosquito Bites." *New England Journal of Medicine*, 2002, *347*, 13–18.

Freeman, N. C., Ettinger, A., Barry, M., and Rhoads, G. "Hygiene- and Food-Related Behaviors Associated with Blood Lead Levels of Young Children from Lead-Contaminated Homes." *Journal of Exposure Analysis and Environmental Epidemiology*, 1997, *7*, 1–15.

Gahan, J. B., Travis, B. V., Morton, F. A., and Lindquist, A. W. "DDT as a Residual-Type Treatment to Control *Anopheles Quadrimaculatus*: Practical Tests." *Journal of Economic Entomology*, 1945, *38*, 223–235.

Gratz, N. G. "Critical Review of the Vector Status of *Aedes Albopictus*." *Medical and Veterinary Entomology*, 2004, *18*, 215–227.

Guillette, L. J., and others. "Reduction in Penis Size and Plasma Testosterone Concentrations in Juvenile Alligators Living in a Contaminated Environment." *General and Comparative Endocrinology*, 1996, *101*, 32–42.

Gurunathan, S., and others. "Accumulation of Chlorpyrifos on Residential Surfaces and Toys Accessible to Children." *Environmental Health Perspectives*, 1998, *106*, 9–16.

Hamilton, G. C., and Racz, A. (eds.). *Pesticide Applicator Training Manual: Mosquito Pest Control, Category 8B*. New Brunswick, N.J.: Rutgers Cooperative Extension, 1998.

Hayes, T. B., and others. "Hermaphroditic, Demasculinized Frogs After Exposure to the Herbicide Atrazine at Low Ecologically Relevant Doses." *Proceedings of the National Academy of Sciences of the United States of America*, 2002, *99*(8), 5476–5480.

Hore, P., and others. "Chlorpyrifos Accumulation Patterns for Child-Accessible Surfaces and Objects and Urinary Metabolite Excretion by Children for Two Weeks After Crack-and-Crevice Application." *Environmental Health Perspectives*, 2005, *113*, 211–219.

International Agency for Research on Cancer. *Occupational Exposures in Insecticide Application, and Some Pesticides.* IARC Monographs on the Evaluation of Carcinogenic Risks to Humans, vol. *53*. Lyon: IARC, 1991.

Kapp, C. "Help or Hazard?" *Lancet*, 2004a, *364*, 1113–1114.

Kapp, C. "New International Convention Allows Use of DDT for Malaria Control." *Bulletin of the World Health Organization*, 2004b, *82*, 472–473.

Keifer, M. C., Wesseling, C., and McConnell, R. "Pesticides and Related Compounds." In L. Rosenstock, M. R. Cullen, C. A. Brodkin, and C. A. Redlich (eds.), *Textbook of Clinical Occupational and Environmental Medicine.* (2nd ed.) Philadelphia: Elsevier Saunders, 2005.

Keithmaleesatti, S., and others. "Concentration of Organochlorine in Egg Yolk and Reproductive Success of *Egretta Garzetta* (Linnaeus, 1758) at Wat Tan-En Non-Hunting Area, Phra Nakhorn Si Ayuthaya Province, Thailand." *Ecotoxicology and Environmental Safety*, 2007, *68*(1), 79–83.

Lewis, R. G., Fortune, C. R., Blanchard, F. T., and Camann, D. E. "Movement and Deposition of Two Organophosphorus Pesticides Within a Residence After Interior and Exterior Applications." *Journal of the Air & Waste Management Association*, 2001, *51*, 339–351.

Longnecker, M. P., Klebanoff, M. A., Zhou, H., and Brock, J. W. "Association Between Maternal Serum Concentration of the DDT Metabolite DDE and Preterm and Small-for-Gestational-Age Babies at Birth." *Lancet*, 2001, *358*, 110–114.

Longnecker, M. P., Rogan, W. J., and Lucier, G. "The Human Health Effects of DDT (Dichlor odiphenyltrichloroethane) and PCBs (Polychlorinated Biphenyls) and an Overview of Organochlorines in Public Health." *Annual Review of Public Health*, 1997, *18*, 211–244.

Lord, C. C. "Featured Creatures." [Brown dog tick.] University of Florida Institute of Food and Agricultural Science; Florida Department of Agriculture and Consumer Services. http://creatures.ifas.ufl.edu/urban/medical/brown_dog_tick.htm#medical, 2001.

Mabaso, M. L., Sharp, B., and Lengeler, C. "Historical Review of Malarial Control in Southern Africa with Emphasis on the Use of Indoor Residual House-Spraying." *Tropical Medicine and International Health*, 2004, *9*, 846–856.

McNeill, W. *Plagues and Peoples.* New York: Anchor Books, 1976.

Nadakavukaren, A. *Our Global Environment: A Health Perspective.* (4th ed.) Prospect Heights, Ill.: Waveland Press, 1995.

Najera, J. A. "Malaria Control: Achievements, Problems and Strategies." *Parassitologia*, 2001, *43*, 1–89.

National Toxicology Program. *Report on Carcinogens.* (11th ed.) Washington, D.C.: Public Health Service, National Toxicology Program, 2005.

New Jersey Department of Environmental Protection, Pesticide Control Program. "Integrated Pest Management." http://www.nj.gov/dep/enforcement/pcp/pcp-pubs.htm, 2005.

North Carolina Agricultural Extension Service. "Ticks." http://ipm.ncsu.edu/AG369/notes/ticks.html, 2005.

Ohbu S., and others. "Sarin Poisoning on Tokyo Subway." *Southern Medical Journal*, 1997, *90*(6), 587–593.

Paramasivan, R., and others. "Serological and Entomological Investigations of an Outbreak of Dengue Fever in Certain Rural Areas of Kanyakumari District, Tamil Nadu." *Indian Journal of Medical Research*, 2006, *123*, 697–701.

Pedigo, L. P. *Agricultural Entomology and Pest Management*. (4th ed.) Upper Saddle River, N. J.: Prentice Hall, 2002.

"Pesticide Control Regulations." *New Jersey Administrative Code*, 7:30–1.2, Definitions. http://michie.lexisnexis.com/newjersey/lpext.dll?f=templates&fn=main-h.htm&cp=uanjadmin, 2009.

Pollack, R. J., Kiszewski, A. E., and Spielman, A. "Repelling Mosquitoes." *New England Journal of Medicine*, 2002, *347*, 2–3.

Priyadarshi, A., Khuder, S. A., Schaub, E. A., and Priyadarshi, S. S. "Environmental Risk Factors and Parkinson's Disease: A Meta-Analysis." *Environmental Research*, 2001, *86*, 122–127.

Punareewattana, K., and others. "Topical Permethrin Exposure Causes Thymic Atrophy and Persistent Inhibition of the Contact Hypersensitivity Response in C57BI/Mice." *International Journal of Toxicology*, 2000, *19*, 383–389.

Rhind, S. M. "Endocrine Disrupting Compounds and Farm Animals: Their Properties, Actions and Routes of Exposure." *Domestic Animal Endocrinology*, 2002, *23*(1–2), 179–187.

Ritter, L., and others. "A Review of Selected Persistent Organic Pollutants." International Program on Chemical Safety (IPCS), WHO. http://www.who.int/ipcs/assessment/en/pcs_95_39_2004_05_13.pdf, 1995.

Roberts, D. R., Loughlin, L. L., Hshieh, P., and Legters, L. J. "DDT, Global Strategies, and a Malaria Control Crisis in South America." *Emerging Infectious Diseases*, 1997, *3*, 295–302.

Roberts, D. R., Manguin, S., and Mouchet, J. "DDT House Spraying and Re-Emerging Malaria." *Lancet*, 2000, *356*, 330–332.

Roberts, D., and others. "Malaria Control and Public Health." *Emerging Infectious Diseases*, 2004, *10*, 1170–1171.

Roberts, J. R., and Reigart, J. R. "Does Anything Beat DEET?" *Pediatric Annals*, 2004, *33*(7), 443–453.

Rogan, W. J., and Chen, A. "Health Risks and Benefits of Bis(4-Chlorophenyl)-1,1,1-Trichloroethane (DDT)." *Lancet*, 2005, *366*, 763–773.

Savage, E. P., and others. "Household Pesticide Usage in the United States." *Archives of Environmental Health*, 1981, *36*, 304–309.

Semenza, J. C., and others. "Reproductive Toxins and Alligator Abnormalities at Lake Apopka, Florida." *Environmental Health Perspectives*, 1997, *105*, 1030–1032.

Siriwong, W. "Organochlorine Pesticide Residues in Aquatic Ecosystem and Health Risk Assessment of Local Agricultural Community." Doctoral dissertation, Graduate School, Chulalongkorn University. 2006.

Smith, A. G. "How Toxic Is DDT?" *Lancet*, 2000, *356*, 267–268.

Stockholm Convention on Persistent Organic Pollutants. [Convention text.] http://www.pops.int/documents/convtext/convtext_en.pdf, 2001.

Stolberg, S. G. "DDT, Target of Global Ban, Finds Defenders in Experts on Malaria." *New York Times*, July 29, 1999, p. 1A.

Sudakin, D. L., and Trevathan, W. R. "DEET: Review and Update of Safety and Risk in the General Population." *Journal of Toxicology: Clinical Toxicology*, 2003, *41*(6), 831–839.

Sullivan, R. *Rats: Observations on the History and Habitat of the City's Most Unwanted Inhabitants.* New York: Bloomsbury, 2004.

Tren, R. *The Economic Cost of Malaria in South Africa: Malaria Control and the DDT Issue.* Johannesburg: Africa Fighting Malaria, 1999.

Triplehorn, C. A., and Johnson, N. F. *Borror and DeLong's Introduction to the Study of Insects.* (7th ed.) Pacific Grove, Calif.: Brooks/Cole, 2005.

Truman, L. C., Bennet, G. W., and Butts, W. L. *Scientific Guide to Pest Control Operations.* Orlando: Harcourt Brace, 1982.

Turusov, V., Rakitsky, V., and Tomatis, L. "Dichlorodiphenyltrichloroethane (DDT): Ubiquity, Persistence, and Risks." *Environmental Health Perspectives,* 2002, *110,* 125–128.

U.S. Environmental Protection Agency. "About Pesticides: Annual Reports." http://www.epa.gov/opp-fead1/annual, 2005a.

U.S. Environmental Protection Agency. "Pesticides: Health and Safety: Toxicity Categories and Pesticide Label Statements." http://www.epa.gov/pesticides/health/tox_categories.htm, 2005b.

U.S. Environmental Protection Agency. "Pesticides: Regulating Pesticides: Laws." http://www.epa.gov/pesticides/regulating/laws.htm, 2005c.

U.S. Environmental Protection Agency. "2000–2001 Pesticide Market Estimates: Usage." http://www.epa.gov/oppbead1/pestsales/01pestsales/usage2001.htm, 2009.

Ware, G. W., and Whitacre, D. M. *The Pesticide Book.* (6th ed.) Willoughby, Ohio: MeisterPro, 2004.

Whitmore, R. W., and others. "Non-Occupational Exposures to Pesticides for Residents of Two U.S. Cities." *Archives of Environmental Contamination and Toxicology,* 1994, *26,* 47–59.

World Health Organization. *DDT and Its Derivatives: Environmental Aspects.* Environmental Health Criteria 83. Albany, N.Y.: WHO. 1989.

Zinsser, H. *Rats, Lice, and History: Being a Study in Biography, Which, After Twelve Preliminary Chapters Indispensable for the Preparation of the Lay Reader, Deals with the Life History of Typhus Fever.* Boston: Little, Brown, 1963.

FOR FURTHER INFORMATION

Book

Reigart, R., and Roberts, J. (eds.). *Recognition and Management of Pesticide Poisonings.* (5th ed.) U.S. Environmental Protection Agency [EPA], Office of Pesticide Programs, 1999. The EPA's Office of Pesticide Programs publishes this work in both English and Spanish. It covers about 1,500 pesticide products, in an easy-to-use format. Toxicology, signs and symptoms of poisoning, and treatment are covered in nineteen chapters on major types of pesticides. The fifth edition adds pesticide products that have come on the market since 1989, includes a new chapter on disinfectants, reviews clinical experiences with pesticide poisonings, and contains detailed references.

U.S. Environmental Protection Agency Web Sites

U.S. Environmental Protection Agency. "About Pesticides." http://www.epa.gov/pesticides/about/types.htm, 2005.

U.S. Environmental Protection Agency. "Pesticides." http://www.epa.gov/pesticides, 2005.

U.S. Environmental Protection Agency. "Pesticides: Health & Safety." http://www.epa.gov/pesticides/safety/healthcare/handbook/handbook.htm, 2005.

Poison Control Centers

The United States has a national network of poison control centers. The national hotline number for the American Association of Poison Control Centers is 1-800-222-1222.

CHAPTER EIGHTEEN

FOOD SAFETY

DAVID MCSWANE

KEY CONCEPTS

- Foodborne illness can threaten public health, incur large costs, and diminish society's well-being in other ways.

- Three classes of hazards—biological, chemical, and physical—can cause foodborne illness.

- Certain groups of people are especially susceptible to foodborne illness and experience more severe symptoms when they contract one.

- Potentially hazardous foods—those that escape time-temperature safety control—are more frequently associated with foodborne illness than properly handled foods.

- Interventions throughout the flow of food, from farm to table, can prevent or control the risk factors that contribute to foodborne illness.

- The "food environment" refers to the availability in schools, communities, and other settings, of both nutritious foods and unhealthy foods. This concept complements traditional food safety approaches.

THE United States has one of the safest food supplies in the world. Yet each year millions of Americans become ill, some with potentially fatal diseases, from eating contaminated food. Foodborne illness poses a significant public health challenge, and prevention of foodborne disease is an essential function of public health, environmental health, and agricultural agencies throughout the nation.

Food safety is the component of environmental health that protects our food supply from farm to table. Food safety programs typically involve a cooperative effort between the food industry and regulatory agencies at the federal, state, and local levels. The collective goal of these programs is to enhance the safety of the food supply and reduce the incidence of foodborne illness.

THE EXTENT OF FOODBORNE ILLNESS

Foodborne illness is the sickness people experience after consuming food and beverages contaminated with pathogenic (disease-causing) microorganisms, chemicals, or physical agents. Victims of foodborne illness commonly experience one or more symptoms such as nausea, vomiting, diarrhea, abdominal pain, headache, fever, and dehydration. The type and the severity of a person's symptoms are influenced by the type of pathogen in the food, the amount of contaminated food consumed, and the individual's health status at the time the contaminated food was eaten.

Foodborne illnesses often occur in *outbreaks*, with two or more people experiencing the same illness as a result of eating contaminated food. The victims of a foodborne disease outbreak may have eaten contaminated food together during a meal or they may have eaten tainted food separately but from a common source, such as a restaurant, supermarket, or manufacturer.

Cases of foodborne illness are the individuals who become ill as a result of eating contaminated food. Cases that occur in outbreaks, together with sporadic cases, make up the *incidence* of foodborne illness—the number of cases per population per unit of time. Foodborne illness is substantially underreported for several reasons: victims frequently experience mild symptoms and do not seek medical care; those who do seek medical care frequently have nonspecific symptoms that are not recognized as foodborne; definitive laboratory diagnoses of vomit, feces, or blood are often not carried out; and even when a diagnosis is made, physicians may not report cases to public health agencies.

David McSwane declares no competing financial interests.

Estimates of the burden of foodborne illness vary greatly, from less than 10 million to over 80 million cases per year, not only because of underreporting but also because many pathogens that cause foodborne illness can also be spread from person to person or through water, thus obscuring the role of foodborne transmission. According to the Centers for Disease Control and Prevention (CDC), the exact cause of a foodborne illness is known in less than 20 percent of cases. In 1996, the CDC implemented the Foodborne Disease Active Surveillance Network (FoodNet), as part of its Emerging Infections Programs network, to monitor and quantify the incidence of foodborne illness. FoodNet conducts active surveillance in ten states for laboratory-confirmed cases of infection caused by nine pathogens. From the data collected through FoodNet and other sources, the CDC estimated in 1999 that there are 76 million cases of foodborne illness in the United States annually, resulting in approximately 325,000 hospitalizations and 5,000 deaths (Mead and others, 1999).

Regional and year-to-year variation in the incidence of foodborne illness has occurred since active surveillance began in 1996. The incidence of certain foodborne illnesses declined over the first decade of FoodNet's data collection but may have stabilized by the mid-2000s. In 2008, the CDC reported that compared with the period from 2004 to 2006, the estimated incidence of infections caused by *Campylobacter, Listeria, Salmonella, Shigella, Vibrio*, and *Yersinia* species and Shiga toxin–producing *Escherichia coli* O157 (STEC O157) had not changed significantly in 2007 and that *Cryptosporidium* species infections had increased (Vugia and others, 2008). Despite the annual and regional fluctuations, reductions in the overall incidence of foodborne illness indicate progress is being made toward preventing foodborne illness and protecting public health. Although less well documented, the burden of foodborne illness in developing countries, where levels of hygiene and sanitation are often substandard, is likely far greater than it is in the United States and other developed nations.

Behind all these statistics are real people who have suffered debilitating, even fatal, diseases from what most of us consider one of life's less risky activities— eating. In addition to pain and suffering, foodborne illness costs society billions of dollars each year in the form of medical expenses, lost productivity, punitive damages and lost business for food companies, and increased surveillance by regulatory agencies.

Foodborne illness remains a significant public health problem for the United States and the rest of the world for at least three major reasons. First, known pathogens are being found in a growing number of foods. *Salmonella* bacteria are commonly found in raw poultry and eggs and have caused foodborne illness for many years. Recently, however, these organisms have also been linked to large foodborne illness outbreaks and product recalls of peanut butter and raw produce. The U.S. Food and Drug Administration (FDA) and CDC recently investigated a foodborne outbreak involving more than 1,440 cases of *Salmonella* Saintpaul infection associated with consumption of raw produce (Jungk and others, 2008). Certain types of raw, red tomatoes were believed to be a vehicle for infection, particularly early in the outbreak. However, information collected late in the investigation points toward jalapeño and serrano peppers grown, harvested, or packed in Mexico as likely food vehicles for the outbreak. *E. coli* O157:H7 bacteria have long been associated with raw or improperly cooked ground beef and pork, but these organisms have also recently been linked to foodborne outbreaks associated with packaged spinach, shredded lettuce, and frozen pizza that contained pepperoni as a topping.

Second, new pathogens are being discovered. *Listeria monocytogenes* and *Cyclospora cayetanensis* are two examples of *emerging* pathogens that have been recently identified as causes of foodborne illness. *Listeria* bacteria have been identified as the cause of recent foodborne outbreaks linked to soft cheeses made with improperly pasteurized milk and to contaminated hot dogs and ready-to-eat luncheon meats. *Cyclospora* is a parasite that has been associated with fresh fruits and vegetables contaminated on the farm.

Third, the number of people who are immunocompromised or otherwise at risk of foodborne illness is growing. Anyone can become ill from eating contaminated food. However, most healthy adults remain asymptomatic or have very mild flu-like symptoms that resolve in a few days. The same is not true for: infants and young children; the elderly; pregnant women and nursing mothers; and people with impaired immune function due to HIV infection, cancer, diabetes, and certain medications that suppress response to infection. The risks associated with foodborne illness are much more serious for immunocompromised individuals than they are for healthy adults. Susceptible individuals typically become ill from smaller doses of pathogens, and the symptoms and durations of their illnesses can be much more severe, even life threatening.

SOURCES OF FOOD CONTAMINATION

Whether food is prepared "from scratch" or arrives ready to eat, it can become contaminated at many points as it flows from harvest through processing and distribution to the consumer. Some common sources of food contamination are presented in Figure 18.1.

Raw foods can become contaminated at the farm, at the ranch, or on board a ship, among other places. Pathogens are present in the intestines of healthy

FIGURE 18.1 Common Sources of Food Contamination

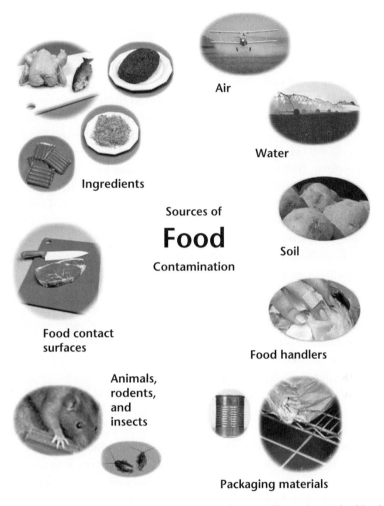

Air

Water

Ingredients

Sources of

Food

Contamination

Soil

Food contact
surfaces

Food handlers

Animals,
rodents,
and
insects

Packaging materials

Source: David McSwane, Nancy Rue, Richard Linton, and Anna Williams, *Essentials of Food Safety and Sanitation*, 4th edition. © 2004. Electronically reproduced by permission of Food Management Institute.

animals raised for food. Similarly, fresh fruits and vegetables can be contaminated if they are washed or irrigated with water that is contaminated with animal manure or human sewage or if pesticides are applied close to the time they are harvested. Contamination can also occur as foods are handled during processing and distribution. Meat and poultry carcasses can become contaminated during slaughter by contact with small amounts of fecal material from the intestines of the animal. Biological hazards can also be introduced by infected food handlers or by cross-contamination, where pathogens from raw animal foods (beef, poultry, fish, and so forth) are transferred to ready-to-eat foods by contaminated hands, equipment, and utensils. Chemical contaminants, such as metals and organic chemicals, may be introduced accidentally during processing, causing outbreaks of toxic foodborne illness.

Foods used every day in the United States come from remote locations around the world. Eating food grown elsewhere in the world means depending on the soil, water, and sanitation conditions in those places and on the way workers in the various parts of the world produce, harvest, process, and transport the products. Because of the globalization of our food supply, the health hazards of one nation easily become those of another. Therefore measures to prevent and control contamination must begin when food is harvested and continue until the food is consumed.

Foodborne illness may be caused by biological, chemical, or physical hazards in food. **Biological hazards** are microscopic organisms, such as bacteria, viruses, and parasites, that pose an invisible challenge to food safety. Bacteria and viruses are the most common causes of foodborne illness, and controlling these biological hazards is a primary goal of every food safety program. **Chemical hazards** are harmful substances that can cause illness if ingested with food. These may be naturally occurring, such as food allergens and the toxins associated with molds, plants (for example, mushrooms), and certain species of fish (for example, puffer fish) and shellfish, or of human origin, such as pesticides, cleaning agents, metals, and polychlorinated biphenyls (PCBs). **Physical hazards** are foreign objects, such as stones, bone fragments from animals, pieces of glass, staples, and jewelry, which can get into food as a result of poor food-handling practices on the farm or ranch, in food-processing plants, and in retail food establishments.

In light of these three causes, acute foodborne illness may be classified as infection, intoxication, or toxin-mediated infection. Foodborne **infections** are caused when biological hazards are consumed along with food. After ingestion the pathogenic organisms multiply in the victim's stomach or intestines and produce such common symptoms of infection as nausea, abdominal pain, fever, and diarrhea. **Intoxications** are poisonings caused by eating food that contains a toxic chemical. Some bacteria produce wastes that are toxic to humans. These toxins can produce illness when ingested with food even when the microbes that produced them are no longer present. Foodborne intoxication may also follow the consumption of poisonous plants or fish or the consumption of food that contains chemicals such as cleaning agents or pesticides. A **toxin-mediated infection** is caused by eating food that contains harmful microorganisms that produce a toxin once inside the human body. A toxin-mediated infection differs from an intoxication because the toxin is produced inside the human body.

Each foodborne illness has a characteristic **onset time**, the amount of time between the consumption of a contaminated food and the appearance of the first symptoms of illness. The onset time varies depending on such factors as the victim's age, health status, body weight, and the amount of contaminant ingested with the food, but usually ranges from a few hours to a few days. However, the onset time for hepatitis A and trichinosis can be several weeks.

It is not possible to cover all the foodborne illnesses of public health significance in this chapter; instead, a few examples are provided in each category. Readers wanting more detailed information or information about other foodborne illnesses are encouraged to consult the *Bad Bug Book* (FDA, 2003) or the CDC's Web page for food-related diseases (CDC, 2005).

Foodborne Illness Caused by Bacteria

Pathogenic bacteria can cause illness when they or their toxins are consumed with food. Unlike spoilage organisms, pathogenic bacteria do not typically change how a food looks, tastes, or smells. Therefore people eat the tainted food not suspecting they are exposing themselves to agents that can make them sick.

Bacterial contamination may occur in raw food, in cooked food that has not been properly handled, and on the surfaces of equipment and utensils that have been contaminated by raw animal foods, humans, or pests such as insects and rodents. In addition, certain food products require time and temperature control to limit the growth of pathogenic microorganisms and toxin formation. These items are called **potentially hazardous foods (time/temperature control for safety foods)**, or PHF/TCS foods. The 2007 Supplement to the 2005 FDA Food Code identifies the following groups of products as potentially hazardous foods (time/temperature control for safety foods) (FDA, 2009c):

- Foods of animal origin that are raw or heat-treated (that is, meat, poultry, eggs, fish, shellfish, and dairy products)
- Foods of plant origin that are heat-treated or consist of raw seed sprouts (for example, cooked rice, steamed or baked potatoes, refried beans, cooked vegetables, and sprouts)
- Cut melons (for example, cantaloupe)
- Garlic and oil mixtures that are not modified in a way to inhibit the growth of pathogenic microorganisms
- Cut tomatoes (including sliced, diced, chopped, and pureed tomatoes) and mixtures of cut tomatoes.

Because PHF/TCS foods have been frequently associated with foodborne disease outbreaks, they are a focal point of most food safety programs. These foods must be handled and stored properly to prevent and control bacterial growth and toxin production that can result in foodborne illness.

Bacterial causes of foodborne illness can be divided into two categories, the spore formers and the non-spore formers. This distinction is important because it has implications for prevention.

Foodborne Illness Caused by Spore-Forming Bacteria   All bacteria exist as vegetative cells that grow, reproduce, and produce wastes. However, some rod-shaped bacteria have the ability to form structures called spores. **Spores** are inactive or dormant forms of bacterial cells that enable the organism to survive when its environment is too hot, cold, dry, or acidic or when there is not enough food. Bacterial spores are commonly found in soil and in the general environment of farms, ranches, and other places where foods are produced. Bacteria can survive for many months as spores. When conditions become more favorable, the spores germinate, much like seeds, and the bacteria start to grow.

Spores are a common contaminant of foods grown in soil, such as vegetables and spices. They may also be found in raw animal foods if the animals have consumed grass and other foodstuffs contaminated with spores. Spores pose a special challenge for food safety because they are much harder to destroy than are vegetative forms of bacteria.

Clostridium perfringens is a species of anaerobic (unable to grow in the presence of oxygen) bacterium that is widely distributed in the environment and is found in the intestines of humans and many domestic and wild animals. Spores of this organism persist in soil, sediments, and areas subject to pollution by human or animal feces. Perfringens food poisoning is a toxin-mediated infection caused by *C. perfringens*. When *C. perfringens* bacteria cells are ingested with food, they colonize in the human intestinal tract and produce an enterotoxin that causes intense abdominal cramps and diarrhea. Symptoms usually begin between eight and twenty-two hours after consumption of foods containing *C. perfringens* bacteria, and the illness usually lasts a day or less. Perfringens is most often associated with PHF/TCS foods such as meat and poultry that have been subjected to temperature abuse. **Temperature abuse** refers to situations in which foods are held in the temperature danger zone (between 41° and 135°F [5° and 57°C]) for enough time to allow growth of harmful organisms and also situations in which foods are not cooked or reheated sufficiently to destroy pathogens. In the case of *C. perfringens*, the bacterial spores can survive high temperatures during the initial cooking process. The spores that survive can germinate into the vegetative forms of the bacteria and then multiply in food that is not properly cooled. If served without adequate reheating, live vegetative forms of *C. perfringens* may be ingested with the food. The bacteria then produce the enterotoxin once they are inside the victim's body.

Clostridium botulinum bacteria are anaerobic organisms that have caused botulism outbreaks associated with improperly home-canned green beans, meats, and fish and with garlic stored in oil. In many of the outbreaks these low-acid foods (pH above 4.6) were inadequately heat processed and then were placed in reduced-oxygen food containers, such as cans, jars, and pouches. When held at room temperature the spores convert to vegetative cells and start to grow. The botulism bacteria then produce a neurotoxin that affects the victim's central nervous system. This toxin is one of the most deadly substances known. Symptoms of botulism usually start within eighteen to thirty-six hours of ingesting contaminated food, and include fatigue, headache, dizziness, double vision, and difficulty breathing and swallowing. If untreated, these symptoms may progress to paralysis of the arms, legs, trunk, and respiratory muscles, which may require ventilator support. After several weeks the paralysis slowly improves. If diagnosed early, foodborne botulism can be treated with an antitoxin that blocks the action of the toxin circulating in the blood.

Botulism toxin is not heat stable and can be destroyed if food is boiled for about twenty minutes. However, botulism cases occur because people do not make a practice of boiling their food, especially home-canned food, for this length of time before eating it.

Foodborne Illness Caused by Non-Spore-Forming Bacteria   Many types of bacteria exist only as vegetative cells and do not form spores. Vegetative bacterial cells are easily destroyed by heat and can be effectively controlled by such processes as cooking and pasteurization. Examples of bacteria in this category that are significant causes of foodborne illness are *E. coli*, *Listeria*, *Salmonella*, and *Staphylococcus*.

Shiga Toxin–Producing E. Coli   The *Escherichia coli* group includes *E. coli* O157:H7 and other *E. coli* bacteria that produce Shiga toxins. These are facultative anaerobic bacteria (that is, they can live with or without oxygen) that can cause an infection or a toxin-mediated infection. Shiga toxin–producing *E. coli* are commonly found in the intestines of warm-blooded animals, especially cows. These bacteria are frequently transferred to foods, such as beef, through contact with feces from the animal's intestines during slaughter. Shiga toxin–producing *E. coli* bacteria have also been found in juice and cider made from apples that have dropped to the ground in the orchard and have been contaminated with fecal waste from grazing animals, These organisms can also be spread by food handlers who are carriers of the bacteria and do not wash their hands properly after going to the toilet and by contaminated equipment and utensils.

The illness begins with flu-like symptoms including severe abdominal pain, nausea, vomiting, and watery or bloody diarrhea. The onset time for the Shiga toxin–producing *E. coli* group is twelve to seventy-two hours, and the illness usually lasts from one to three days. In some people, particularly children under five years of age and the elderly, the infection can also cause a complication called hemolytic uremic syndrome (HUS), in which the red blood cells are destroyed and the kidneys fail. In the United States, HUS is a leading cause of acute kidney failure in children, and most cases of HUS are caused by *E. coli* O157:H7.

Listeria Monocytogenes Listeriosis is an infection caused by eating food contaminated with the bacterium *Listeria monocytogenes*. This disease affects primarily

PERSPECTIVE
Outbreak of *Escherichia Coli* O157:H7 Infections Associated with Fresh Spinach

Widespread concern about *Escherichia coli* O157:H7 began in January 1993, during a multistate outbreak traced to eating undercooked ground beef from a Jack in the Box quick-service restaurant. Once a disease largely associated with contaminated raw or undercooked ground beef, this foodborne illness has since been linked with roast beef, dry salami, raw milk, lettuce, fresh spinach, and unpasteurized apple juice.

In September 2006, the CDC and FDA began investigating an outbreak of *E. coli* O157:H7 epidemiologically linked with Dole brand baby spinach (Centers for Disease Control and Prevention, 2006). The bagged fresh spinach was being sold by grocery stores and other retail outlets. The outbreak caused 205 confirmed illnesses and 3 deaths. The 3 deaths occurred as a result of hemolytic uremic syndrome caused by the *E. coli* infection.

Because *E. coli* bacteria can be spread in many ways, the precise means by which the bacteria were spread to the spinach remain unknown. However, the most plausible theories are that the spinach was contaminated by feces from wild hogs or by surface water runoff from surrounding fields that contained cattle feces.

All of the spinach had come from the Natural Selection Foods processing center in San Juan Batista, California. Accordingly, Natural Selection voluntarily recalled all its spinach products with use-by dates from August 17 to October 1, 2006. The recall included packages of spinach sold under Dole and other private label brands. Further data and study ultimately narrowed the possible sources of the outbreak down to only the Dole brand of packaged greens. It is likely that growers, manufacturers, and distributors lost millions of dollars through lost sales and discarded products as a result of this outbreak and the accompanying recall.

pregnant women, newborns, and adults with weakened immune systems. A person with listeriosis has fever, muscle aches, and sometimes gastrointestinal symptoms such as nausea or diarrhea. If the infection spreads to the nervous system, symptoms such as headache, stiff neck, confusion, loss of balance, or convulsions can occur. Pregnant women who contract listeriosis may experience only a mild, flu-like illness. However, infections during pregnancy may also lead to miscarriage or stillbirth, premature delivery, or infection of the newborn. Onset time is one day to three weeks, and the illness can be of indefinite duration, depending on when treatment is administered.

Listeria monocytogenes is found in soil and water. Vegetables can become contaminated from the soil or from manure used as fertilizer. Animals can carry this bacterium without appearing ill, and thus it can contaminate foods of animal origin such as meats and dairy products. The bacterium has been found in a variety of raw foods, such as uncooked meats and vegetables, as well as in processed foods that become contaminated after processing, such as soft cheeses and cold cuts at the deli counter. Unpasteurized (raw) milk or foods made from unpasteurized milk may contain the bacterium. It is killed by pasteurization and cooking; however, in certain ready-to-eat foods such as hot dogs and deli luncheon meats, contamination may occur after cooking but before packaging, as illustrated in the Perspective discussing deli meats. *Listeria monocytogenes* is an especially important concern in food safety because, unlike most other foodborne pathogens, this organism can grow at refrigeration temperatures, below 41°F (5°C).

Salmonella   *Salmonella* bacteria live in the intestinal tracts of humans and animals, especially birds. *Salmonella* is usually transmitted to humans through consumption of contaminated foods of animal origin, such as beef, poultry, milk, or eggs. However, other foods, including fresh and fresh-cut produce and peanut butter, may become contaminated with fecal material from animals and the unwashed hands of infected food handlers. Most persons infected with *Salmonella* develop diarrhea, fever, and abdominal cramps within twelve to seventy-two hours after infection. The illness usually lasts four to seven days, and most persons recover without treatment. However, elderly people, infants, and individuals with impaired immune systems are more likely to experience severe illness and may need to be hospitalized.

Staphylococcus Aureus   Some strains of *Staphylococcus aureus* produce enterotoxins that cause a condition called staphylococcal food poisoning. The most common symptoms of staphylococcal food poisoning are nausea, vomiting, abdominal cramping, and prostration. The onset of symptoms is usually within two to six hours of exposure, and a person can experience symptoms after consuming only

PERSPECTIVE

Listeria in Ready-to-Eat Deli Meats Causes Foodborne Disease Outbreaks

Officials at the Centers for Disease Control and Prevention reported 120 cases of listeriosis during the summer and early fall of 2002. Cases appeared in eight states: Connecticut, Delaware, Maryland, Massachusetts, Michigan, New Jersey, New York, and Pennsylvania. Most of the victims were hospitalized, seven died, and three pregnant women had miscarriages or stillbirths (Gottlieb and others, 2006).

The Food Safety Inspection Service of the U.S. Department of Agriculture conducted an inspection and found *Listeria* in turkey deli meats from two plants that manufacture fresh and frozen ready-to-eat turkey and chicken products. As a result of the outbreak the plants voluntarily recalled more than 27 million pounds of fresh and frozen poultry products (Food Safety and Inspection Service, 2002).

This outbreak reaffirmed that people who are immunocompromised (very young children, pregnant women, the elderly, and people taking medicines that suppress their response to infection) are especially vulnerable to illness caused by foodborne bacteria such as *Listeria*. Immunocompromised individuals should avoid eating

- Hot dogs and luncheon meats, unless they are reheated until steaming hot
- Soft cheeses and foods made with raw (unpasteurized) milk
- Refrigerated pâtés or meat spreads
- Smoked seafood, unless it is contained in a cooked dish

An outbreak of listeriosis involving processed meats occurred in Canada during the summer and early autumn of 2008. Representatives of the Public Health Agency of Canada identified several dozen confirmed cases and a smaller number of suspected cases, most in Ontario but in other provinces as well. At least twenty deaths were attributed to the outbreak, based on evidence that the victims' *Listeria monocytogenes* infections shared the same genetic fingerprint (Public Health Agency of Canada, 2008b).

Maple Leaf Consumer Foods began a recall of deli meat products after *Listeria* was found in its Toronto plant (Public Health Agency of Canada, 2008a). Subsequently, more than 200 products were recalled after being linked to the outbreak. Dozens of other brands were also pulled off store shelves and from fast-food outlets across the country.

a small amount of toxin in food. Victims experience acute symptoms in many cases, but recovery generally occurs in a few days.

Humans and animals are the primary reservoirs of *Staphylococcus aureus*. Staphylococci are found in the nasal passages and throats and on the hair and skin of 30 to 50 percent of the population, including those who are otherwise healthy. These organisms are also found in infected burns, cuts, pimples, and boils. They can be spread by droplets of saliva when people talk, cough, or sneeze. However, contamination from a worker's hands is the most common way the organism is introduced into foods. Some of the foods that have been incriminated in staphylococcal food-poisoning outbreaks are meat and meat products; poultry and egg products; salads made from eggs, tuna, chicken, potatoes, and macaroni; and cream-filled bakery products. In most outbreaks these foods had been improperly handled by employees during preparation and were temperature abused during preparation, storage, and display.

Foodborne Illness Caused by Viruses

Viruses are currently assuming much greater importance as agents of foodborne illness. Food safety experts now believe the number of cases of foodborne illness caused by viruses is equal to or greater than the number of cases caused by bacteria. The viruses that cause foodborne disease differ from pathogenic bacteria in several ways. Viruses are much smaller in size and cannot grow outside a living host (human or animal). In addition, viruses are not affected by treatment with antibiotics, and a susceptible person needs to consume only a few viral particles in order to develop a foodborne infection. The two viruses of primary importance as food hazards are hepatitis A virus and noroviruses.

Hepatitis A Virus   Hepatitis A virus causes a liver disease called infectious hepatitis. The hepatitis virus is a particular challenge for food establishments because employees can harbor the virus for up to six weeks and not show symptoms of illness. Food workers are generally contagious for one week before onset of symptoms and for two weeks after the symptoms of the disease appear. During that time infected workers may contaminate foods and expose other workers to the virus. The hepatitis A virus is very hardy and can live for several hours in a suitable environment. Infectious hepatitis is usually mild and characterized by jaundice (yellow discoloration of the skin), fatigue, abdominal pain, loss of appetite, nausea, diarrhea, and fever. It can occasionally be severe, especially in people with liver disease.

The virus is most commonly transmitted by the fecal-oral route, when infected workers spread fecal material from unwashed hands and fingernails. Infectious hepatitis can also be spread by the ingestion of food and water that contain the hepatitis A virus. Raw and lightly cooked shellfish harvested from polluted waters, vegetables exposed to polluted water during irrigation, and ready-to-eat foods handled by infected humans offer the largest threats of transmission and disease from hepatitis A.

A large outbreak of infectious hepatitis occurred at a Pennsylvania restaurant in 2003 (Dato and others, 2003). The source was determined to be contaminated green onions. Investigators believe the green onions may have been contaminated with the hepatitis A virus by infected farmworkers during harvesting and preparation and/or by contaminated water used during the irrigation, rinsing, processing, cooling, and icing of the onions.

Noroviruses   Noroviruses are a group of viruses that cause the "stomach flu," or gastroenteritis, in people. Several other names have been used for noroviruses, including Norwalk-like viruses, caliciviruses, and small round structured viruses. The symptoms of Norovirus illness usually include nausea, vomiting, diarrhea, and stomach cramping. Sometimes people additionally have a low-grade fever, chills, a headache, muscle aches, and a general sense of tiredness. The illness often begins suddenly, and the infected person may feel very sick. The illness is usually brief, with symptoms lasting only about one or two days. Sometimes people are unable to drink enough liquids to replace the fluids they have lost through vomiting and diarrhea. This problem with dehydration is usually seen only among the very young, the elderly, and persons with weakened immune systems.

People can become infected by eating food or drinking liquids that are contaminated with a norovirus, by touching surfaces or objects contaminated with a norovirus and then placing their hands in their mouth, and by having direct contact with another person who is infected and showing symptoms. Norovirus outbreaks have been reported in schools and health care facilities, and a norovirus outbreak affected evacuees and relief workers in three temporary shelters the week after Hurricane Katrina in 2005.

Noroviruses are very contagious and can spread easily from person to person. People infected with a norovirus are contagious from the moment they begin feeling ill to at least three days after recovery. Some people may be contagious for as long as two weeks after recovery.

Foodborne Illness Caused by Parasites

Parasites are small creatures that live in or on a living host. Parasitic infections are far less common than either bacterial or viral foodborne illness. Nonetheless,

PERSPECTIVE
Noroviruses Wreak Havoc on Cruise Ships

During 2002, the CDC's Vessel Sanitation Program received reports of twenty-one outbreaks of acute gastroenteritis (AGE) on seventeen cruise ships sailing into U.S. ports (Cramer and others, 2002). Of the twenty-one outbreaks, nine were confirmed by laboratory analysis of stool specimens from ill passengers and crew members to be caused by noroviruses (for example, Norwalk-like viruses). Noroviruses are among the most common causes of viral gastrointestinal outbreaks on cruise vessels. The symptoms of illness caused by Norovirus infection include nausea, vomiting, watery diarrhea, and abdominal pain. The illness usually develops within twelve to forty-eight hours of exposure and lasts from one to three days. Common modes of transmission for these viruses include person-to-person contact and consuming contaminated food or water.

Cruise ships dock in countries where levels of sanitation might be inadequate, thus increasing the risk of contamination in the water and food taken aboard and of having a passenger board with an active infection. After a passenger or crew member brings the virus on board, the close living quarters on ships amplify opportunities for person-to-person transmission. Furthermore, the arrival of new and susceptible passengers every one or two weeks on affected cruise ships provides an opportunity for sustained transmission during successive cruises. The continuation of these outbreaks on consecutive cruises with new passengers and the resurgence of outbreaks caused by the same virus strains that had appeared during previous cruises on the same ship, or even on different ships belonging to the same company, suggest that environmental contamination and infected crew members can serve as reservoirs of infection for passengers.

Because of noroviruses' high infectivity and persistence in the environment, transmission is difficult to control through routine sanitary measures. In addition to emphasizing basic food and water sanitation measures, control efforts should include thorough and prompt disinfection of ships during cruises and isolation of ill crew members and, if possible, passengers for seventy-two hours after clinical recovery. Cruise ships should promote frequent, vigorous hand washing with soap and water by passengers and crew. In addition, passengers and crew should avoid contact with other people on the ship when they are ill.

The increase in reported Norovirus outbreaks on cruise ships in 2002 might reflect an actual increase in these outbreaks or it might be attributable to improved surveillance, with an electronic reporting format implemented in January 2001 and increased application of sensitive molecular assays. The surveillance system captures cases of illness reported to the ship's infirmary or to designated staff on board the ship.

parasites can become biological hazards if they are not properly controlled in retail food establishments. Two examples of foodborne parasites are *Anisakis* spp. and *Cyclospora cayetanensis*.

Anisakis spp. are roundworms found in some species of fish. The worms are about one inch long and the diameter of a human hair. They are beige, ivory, white, gray, brown, or pink. Humans are exposed to this parasite when they eat parasite-infested fish. Symptoms include coughing if worms attach in the throat, vomiting and abdominal pain if worms attach in the stomach, or sharp pain and fever if worms attach in the large intestine. Onset can occur anytime from one hour to two weeks after exposure.

EXHIBIT 18.1
Investigating Foodborne Disease Outbreaks

Protecting the public from foodborne illness depends on rapid detection of outbreaks and a thorough knowledge of the agents and factors responsible for foodborne illness. Various state and local health departments and federal agencies are involved in disease surveillance to detect foodborne disease outbreaks. Surveillance attempts to link individual cases of illness to clusters of illness or outbreaks. The purposes of a foodborne illness investigation are to

- Determine the cause of the outbreak, including the etiologic agent, and verify that the agent is foodborne.
- Detect all cases, the food(s) or beverage(s) involved in the transmission, and the environmental conditions and food-handling practices that may have contributed to the transmission of the agent.
- Control the outbreak, and prevent additional cases from occurring.
- Document foodborne disease occurrence to improve the knowledge of foodborne disease causation.
- Correct poor food-handling practices, and provide training to prevent similar occurrences.
- Revise the HACCP plan (see Exhibit 18.4 later in this chapter) to prevent similar incidents in the future.
- Foster public confidence in the safety of the food supply and the integrity of the industry.

Local health departments play a key role in foodborne illness surveillance, as these agencies are often the first ones notified of cases of illness by family physicians, emergency department doctors, or complaints filed by victims or their families.

Cyclospora cayetanensis is a parasite that has been associated with fresh fruits and vegetables contaminated at the farm. The parasite is passed from person to person by fecal-oral transmission. *C. cayetanensis* frequently finds its way into water and can then be transferred to foods or foods can be contaminated during handling. Symptoms of cyclosporiasis include watery and explosive diarrhea, loss of appetite, and bloating. The illness usually lasts one week or less. (Exhibit 18.1 reviews the process of investigating the kinds of diseases discussed in these sections.)

During the complaint investigation, a health department representative will gather information about the victims and the circumstances surrounding their illness. Individuals filing complaints will be asked to fully describe the situation in their own words and provide basic information such as their name, address, and home and work telephone numbers.

Many complainants attribute their illness to the last place at which they ate and may have already decided what food made them ill. The investigator must consider all possibilities, as the illness may not be food related but may derive from another source or from person-to-person contact.

Although every outbreak is unique, the investigative process generally follows these nine steps (International Association for Food Protection [IAFP], 2007):

1. *Obtain a description of food items and secure any leftover food items.* If the outbreak is associated with a particular event, acquire a list of all food and beverages consumed at the event. If the outbreak is linked with a particular food establishment, obtain a copy of the menu or product list. Determine if leftovers are available from the event. If so, make sure they are collected, labeled, and stored at the proper temperature and where they will not be discarded.

2. *Gather basic data.* Obtain clinical and three-day food histories for the ill people through personal interviews or from medical personnel. This involves collecting information about the food consumed by the victim within the seventy-two hours prior to the onset of symptoms. This time frame is used because the onset time for many foodborne agents is seventy-two hours or less and because recall becomes unreliable for foods consumed earlier than three days prior to onset. The seventy-two-hour food history should include all meals, snacks, and beverages, including water and ice, eaten either at home or commercial establishments. Determine where the foods were prepared—on site, at a caterer's kitchen, or elsewhere. If the foods were prepared at home, find out what ingredients were used, including herbs and spices, and where they were

purchased. Ask if anything unusual was noticed about the foods, such as an off taste, odor, color, or texture. Find out if the foods appeared to be fully cooked and if they were served hot or cold prior to being eaten. The earlier this food history is obtained, the more reliable it is. Clinical information should include signs and symptoms, dates of onset, and common exposures categorized by person, place, and time.

3. *Formulate an initial hypothesis and case definition.* The initial case definition is based on facts about time, place, person, clinical signs, and mode of transmission. This tentative hypothesis is used to direct the investigation; however, it should not be too restrictive. Focusing too closely on one hypothesis can exclude potentially important cases or events. Case definitions can change as the investigation progresses.

4. *Collect clinical specimens for testing.* Determine if any clinical specimens have been collected by health care providers and obtain the results of any tests. If specimens were collected, contact the reference laboratories and have them save the specimens, if possible, for further testing. When specimens have not yet been collected, investigators should attempt to collect clinical specimens, first, from the people who are currently ill and, second, from those who were recently ill. Specimens should also be collected from food handlers who were ill before the outbreak as well as from those who were asymptomatic.

5. *Develop a questionnaire.* A standardized questionnaire is developed, using the initial case definition, food item description, and clinical data. This tool is used to collect

- Exposure data (time and place of exposure, approximate number exposed)
- Patient information (name, address, telephone number)
- Patient demographics (age, gender, and so forth)
- Illness history (whether subject is ill or well, any underlying conditions, medications)
- Clinical data (signs and symptoms, onset date and time, recovery date and time)
- Medical attention sought (provider, sample collection, test results, treatment)
- Contact with other ill individuals
- Menu from suspect meal(s)

Foodborne Illness Caused by Chemicals

Chemicals may occur naturally in food or may be added intentionally or unintentionally during food production, processing, and preparation. Naturally occurring chemicals include food allergens and toxins produced by biological organisms. Chemical contaminants of human origin include agricultural chemicals (for example, pesticides, fertilizers, and antibiotics), food additives (for example,

It is extremely important to interview people who are well in addition to those who are ill. The cause of illness can be identified only by comparing the exposures (foods eaten) of those who are ill (cases) and of those who are not (controls).

6. *Analyze the questionnaires.* This is generally accomplished using a cohort or case-control study format. Analyze the data to identify differences in exposure frequencies between cases and controls to confirm or refute the hypothesis. As data from questionnaires are analyzed, it may be necessary to modify the course of the investigation by formulating a new hypothesis or case definition.

7. *Conduct an environmental investigation.* A health agency representative will audit HACCP processes (make observations and interview employees) and evaluate HACCP records.

8. *Implement control measures.* Control measures may include
    - Providing postexposure prophylaxis to control the spread of the disease
    - Recalling or destroying food
    - Making a public announcement of the outbreak
    - Providing educational information
    - Closing a food establishment to stop the ongoing spread of disease
    - Recommending antibiotic treatment or exclusion from work or child care or other measures

9. *Summarize the investigation.* It is important to prepare a document that summarizes the conditions and causes of the outbreak in order to prevent future occurrences. This summary also serves as the public record of the outbreak.

The revised 5th edition of *Procedures to Investigate Foodborne Illness* is available from the International Association for Food Protection (2007). The information in this manual is based on epidemiological principles and investigative techniques that have been found effective in determining causal factors of disease incidence. The 2007 revision also offers information on intentional contamination. This publication can be a valuable reference for public health personnel or teams who are investigating reports of alleged foodborne illnesses.

preservatives and coloring agents), metals, and industrial by-products. Sometimes such chemicals are added intentionally but have unexpected adverse effects; for example, flavor enhancers such as monosodium glutamate (MSG) can cause headaches in some people. At other times chemicals are added improperly or unintentionally, and the results can be tragic. For example, during the winter of 1971–1972, Iraqi authorities distributed free wheat seeds to people in rural areas. These seeds had been treated with methylmercury as a fungicide and were intended for planting. However, some recipients ground the seeds into flour and made bread with it. An estimated 50,000 people were exposed to the contaminated bread, over 6,000 were hospitalized with acute mercury poisoning, and 459 died (Bakir and others, 1973; Al-Mufti and others, 1976). Ten years later, in 1981, malefactors in Spain denatured large amounts of rapeseed oil with aniline and illicitly sold it as pure olive oil. The contaminant triggered a previously unknown illness that included lung infiltrates, muscle pain, and a high blood count of eosinophils. Nearly 20,000 people became ill, and more than 300 died (Posada de la Paz, Philen, and Borda, 2001). Other chemical contaminants, such as lead and PCBs, have been introduced unintentionally into foods and linked to chronic conditions that developed over years.

Biomagnification occurs when the toxic burden of a large number of organisms at a lower trophic level is accumulated and concentrated by predators at a higher trophic level. For example, phytoplankton and bacteria in aquatic ecosystems take up heavy metals or toxic organic molecules from water or sediments. Their predators—zooplankton and small fish—collect and retain the toxins from many prey organisms, building up higher toxin concentrations. The top carnivores in the food chain—game fish and humans—can accumulate such high toxin levels that they suffer adverse health effects.

Vomiting is the most common symptom of acute chemical intoxication. It usually occurs within fifteen to thirty minutes after ingestion of the chemical, and in most instances victims feel better after expelling the chemical. In other cases more serious results can occur. Examples of chemicals that may cause health problems include food allergens; naturally occurring toxins, such as ciguatoxin and scombrotoxin; and mercury, PCBs, bisphenol A, and pesticides.

Food Allergens   Food allergens can pose a serious health risk to children and adults who are sensitive to these substances. Five to 8 percent of children and 1 to 2 percent of adults are allergic to certain chemicals found in foods and food ingredients. Food allergens cause a person's immune system to overreact and may result in such symptoms as hives, swelling of the lips and tongue, difficulty breathing, vomiting, cramps, and diarrhea. These symptoms can occur within minutes of consuming the allergen. In severe situations a life-threatening allergic reaction called anaphylaxis can occur. Symptoms of anaphylaxis include itching and hives, swelling of the throat and difficulty breathing, dropping blood pressure, and unconsciousness.

The FDA estimates that approximately 90 percent of all allergic reactions are caused by eight types of food: milk, eggs, wheat proteins, peanuts, soy, tree nuts, fish, and shellfish (U.S. Food and Drug Administration, 2007c. These foods have been designated **major food allergens** in the Food Allergen Labeling and

Consumer Protection Act of 2004. In many instances a person who is allergic to a food does not have to eat much of that food in order to experience a severe reaction. As little as half a peanut can cause a severe reaction in a highly sensitive person. The only way people with food allergies can avoid allergic reactions is to avoid eating foods that contain allergens. Proper ingredient labeling and prevention of cross-contamination are important food safety measures for protecting people from food allergens. (Cross-contamination is discussed later in this chapter and summarized in Exhibit 18.3.)

Ciguatoxin   Ciguatoxin is produced by marine algae that live among certain coral reefs. When the algae are eaten by small reef fish, the toxin is stored in their flesh, skin, and organs. When the small reef fish are eaten by larger fish, such as barracuda, mackerel, and snapper, the toxin accumulates in the larger fish. Humans who eat these fish can then suffer ciguatoxin poisoning. Symptoms include vertigo, joint and muscle pain, numbness and tingling in the lips and mouth, temperature reversal sensations (hot things feel cold and vice versa), diarrhea, and vomiting. The onset time ranges from fifteen minutes to twenty-four hours. The toxin is not destroyed by cooking, and there is no commercially known method to determine whether ciguatoxin is present in fish. Purchasing seafood from a reputable supplier is considered the best preventive measure.

Scombrotoxin   The presence of large amounts of scombrotoxin in food can result in scombroid poisoning, also known as histamine poisoning. Histamine is produced by certain bacteria when they decompose foods containing the protein histidine. Tuna, mahi-mahi, sardines, mackerel, anchovies, and amberjack are examples of fish that have high levels of histidine that can be converted to histamine. Cooking does not inactivate the chemical once it has been formed. Symptoms of scombroid poisoning include dizziness, a burning feeling in the mouth, facial rash or hives, a peppery taste in the mouth, headache, itching, teary eyes, and runny nose. The onset time is thirty minutes or less.

Mercury   Mercury contamination of fish has attracted considerable public health attention in recent years. Mercury occurs naturally in the environment. Metallic and inorganic mercury can also be released into the air as industrial emissions, especially from coal-burning power plants (because coal often contains mercury) and from incinerators that burn mercury-containing refuse such as medical waste. Mercury then falls from the air and can enter surface water, accumulating in streams, rivers, and oceans. Mercury may also be a contaminant in wastes that drain directly into waterways from facilities such as paper and chloralkali chemical plants. Bacteria in the water convert the inorganic mercury to an organic form, methylmercury, which then enters the food chain. Fish absorb methylmercury from water as they feed on aquatic organisms. Long-lived, large predator fish such as sharks, swordfish, tilefish, and tuna may accumulate high levels of methylmercury and pose a risk to people who eat them regularly. Methylmercury is a nervous system toxin, and the developing fetus is especially susceptible to its effects. Women of childbearing age have long been warned to limit their fish intake to reduce the risk of exposing their unborn babies to mercury (see Exhibit 18.2).

Polychlorinated Biphenyls   Polychlorinated biphenyls (PCBs) are persistent chlorinated compounds that were manufactured from the 1920s to the 1970s for use in capacitors, transformers, and other applications. These compounds have entered the global ecosystem and have become widely distributed. They are fat soluble, so they concentrate in fatty tissues and are found at high levels in fish that are high on the marine food chain. Results of a recent study (Hites and others, 2004) showed that farmed salmon contain higher levels of PCBs and other persistent organic compounds than wild salmon. Part of the explanation for this is that farmed fish are fed fish meal, a concentrated preparation of smaller fish that represents a source of concentrated fat-soluble chemicals. The extent of the risk

---

EXHIBIT 18.2
FDA Recommendations for Avoiding Mercury in Fish

1. Do not eat shark, swordfish, king mackerel, or tilefish because they contain high levels of mercury.
2. Eat up to 12 ounces (two average meals) a week of a variety of fish and shellfish that are lower in mercury.
   - Five of the most commonly eaten fish that are low in mercury are shrimp, canned light tuna, salmon, pollock, and catfish.
   - Another commonly eaten fish, albacore ("white") tuna has more mercury than canned light tuna. So, when choosing your two meals of fish and shellfish, you may eat up to six ounces (one average meal) of albacore tuna per week.
3. Check local advisories about the safety of fish caught by family and friends in your local lakes, rivers, and coastal areas. If no advice is available, eat up to six ounces (one average meal) per week of fish you catch from local waters, but don't consume any other fish during that week.

Source: FDA, 2004.

to humans is unclear, but based on evidence linking PCBs with cancer, nervous system toxicity, immune dysfunction, and other adverse outcomes, recommendations have also been issued to limit consumption of the most contaminated fish.

Chemical contaminants in fish pose an interesting example of the trade-offs inherent in food safety. Although fish may pose a risk if it is contaminated by mercury or PCBs, fish is an excellent dietary source of protein and omega-3 fatty acids (especially eicosapentaenoic acid, or EPA, and docosahexaenoic acid, or DHA), which are thought to promote cardiovascular health. Food safety involves a careful balance, minimizing the risks of contaminated fish and maximizing benefits by choosing the safest fish.

Bisphenol A   Bisphenol A (BPA) is a chemical found in polycarbonate plastic commonly used in food containers such as baby bottles and water bottles and in the epoxy resins that line some metal food cans. Polycarbonate plastic is sturdy and impact resistant, which makes it an ideal material for food and beverage containers.

The use of bisphenol A in consumer products grabbed headlines in 2008. Longstanding evidence (vom Saal and Hughes 2005; vom Saal and others, 2007) had suggested that BPA could cause toxic effects, especially endocrine disruption, and new epidemiological evidence suggested a link with cardiovascular disease, type 2 diabetes, and liver enzyme abnormalities (Lang and others, 2008). However, competing interpretations of the data abounded. On the one hand, European regulatory authorities concluded that BPA exposures were safe and declined to regulate BPA (European Food Safety Authority, 2006), and the U.S. Food and Drug Administration (FDA) advised the public that "FDA-regulated products containing BPA currently on the market are safe and that exposure levels to BPA from food contact materials, including for infants and children, are below those that may cause health effects" (FDA, 2009a). On the other hand, some scientists called for caution (vom Saal and Myers, 2008), Environment Canada classified BPA as a "toxic" chemical (Environment Canada, 2008) and proposed a ban, and the National Toxicology Program (NTP) released a detailed report that expressed "some concern" (the intermediate level of concern in NTP parlance) for effects on the brain, behavior, and prostate gland in fetuses, infants, and children at current human exposure levels (but "minimal concern" for mammary gland effects and premature puberty, "minimal concern" for reproductive effects among exposed workers, and "negligible concern" for other outcomes such as neonatal mortality and birth defects) (National Toxicology Program, Center for the Evaluation of Risks to Human Reproduction, 2008).

Mindful of public concern, manufacturers such as Nalgene moved to phase out BPA from their products, and retail chains such as Wal-Mart, Toys "R" Us, and Babies "R" Us announced plans to discontinue selling baby bottles containing BPA. Debate focused on a number of issues, including which scientific studies were suitable for consideration, the pharmacokinetics of BPA, and the appropriate policy response to uncertainty about effects at low levels of exposure.

Consumers who are concerned about potential health risks associated with BPA can reduce their exposure by following these tips issued by the National Institute of Environmental Health Sciences (2008):

- Don't microwave polycarbonate plastic food containers as the polycarbonate may break down from overuse at high temperatures.
- Reduce use of canned foods.
- When possible, opt for glass, porcelain, or stainless steel containers, particularly for hot foods and liquids.
- Use baby bottles that are BPA-free.

PERSPECTIVE
Pros and Cons of Natural and Organic Foods

More and more consumers are buying natural and organic foods as they become aware of the connections among the foods they eat and their health and the health of their environment. Natural and organic foods have become a multibillion-dollar industry, and sales of organic foods are likely to increase now that U.S. Department of Agriculture (USDA) national organic standards are in place to further boost consumer confidence.

The terms *natural* and *organic* are not synonymous when applied to foods. Natural foods are generally minimally processed and free of artificial ingredients but not necessarily organically grown. Natural foods may be organic, but it is not required that they be organic. In fact there is no legal definition or system in place that governs what constitutes a natural food.

In contrast, a food that is sold as organic must meet certain standards. When food or feed is produced organically, it means that the crop is grown according to guidelines that prohibit the use of synthetic pesticides, synthetic growth regulators, and conventional, soluble fertilizers. Organic meat, poultry, eggs, and dairy products come from animals that are given no antibiotics or growth hormones. Organic produce is grown without using most conventional synthetic insecticides and herbicides, fertilizers made with synthetic ingredients or sewage sludge, bioengineering, or ionizing radiation. Before a product can be labeled organic, a government-approved certifier must inspect the farm where the food is grown to make sure the farmer is following all the rules necessary to meet the USDA's national organic standards.

The Food Quality Protection Act (FQPA) directed the U.S. Environmental Protection Agency to conduct a reassessment of all food uses of pesticides, taking into account

Pesticides   Pesticides are used widely in agriculture in the United States and worldwide, and many agricultural products such as fruits and vegetables contain trace quantities of pesticides, called *residues*. Foods are not systematically monitored for their pesticide content, but available data suggest that some foods, in at least some instances, can carry nontrivial levels of pesticides. This has encouraged an interest in organic and so-called natural foods. It is also a special issue for children, because their diets include large proportions of fruits and vegetables (or products derived from these foods, such as baby food and juices), resulting in large relative exposures to dietary pesticides. Children may also be more susceptible than adults to these contaminants (for reasons discussed in Chapter Twenty-Five). This issue was studied by the National Academy of Sciences in 1993, and a groundbreaking report, *Pesticides in the Diets of Infants and Children*, recommended renewed attention to the dietary exposures that children sustain (National Research Council, 1993).

the heightened susceptibility of infants and children, the elderly, and other highly susceptible population groups. To improve the accuracy of FQPA pesticide dietary risk assessments, Congress funded the Pesticide Data Program (PDP), which focuses on the foods consumed most heavily by children, and food is tested, to the extent possible, as eaten.

Several years of PDP testing have greatly enhanced our understanding of pesticide residues in the U.S. food supply. The pattern of residues found in organic foods tested by the PDP differs markedly from the pattern in conventional samples in two important ways. First, produce grown organically is less likely to contain detectable levels of pesticide residues than is produce grown using conventional techniques. Second, produce grown using conventional techniques tends to contain multiple pesticide residues more often. Imported foods have consistently contained more residues than domestic samples.

Organic food differs from conventionally produced food in the way it is grown, handled, and processed. Yet the USDA makes no claims that organically produced food is safer or more nutritious than conventionally produced food. One must not lose sight of the fact that bacteria and other pathogens are commonly found in the soil, barns, and general environment on all kinds of farms, including those where organic foods are grown. In addition, foods grown organically can still contain allergens that can trigger an adverse response if eaten by people who have sensitivities to these substances. Finally, organically grown foods are handled by people at various steps from harvest to retail, just as foods grown using conventional methods are. Organic foods are equally vulnerable to contamination from infected workers who do not practice good personal hygiene. For all these reasons, consumers should handle organic foods carefully to protect themselves and their families.

PREVENTION OF FOODBORNE ILLNESS

The CDC has identified several risk factors as primary contributors to foodborne disease outbreaks; these factors are therefore important focus areas for food safety programs. They include (Olsen and others, 2000)

- Improper holding temperatures
- Poor personal hygiene
- Improper cooking temperatures
- Foods from unsafe sources
- Contaminated equipment and cross-contamination

Improper Holding Temperatures

Keeping foods at improper holding temperatures permits the rapid growth of infectious and toxin-producing microorganisms. This rapid growth typically occurs when food is held at temperatures between 41°F and 135°F (5°C and 57°C). This temperature range is referred to as the food **temperature danger zone**. The relationship between temperature and microbial growth is illustrated in Figure 18.2. An important rule in food safety is, "Keep it hot, keep it cold, or don't keep it." This requires keeping hot foods above 135°F (57°C) and cold foods below 41°F (5°C) whenever possible.

There are times during the cooking, cooling, reheating, and food preparation processes when a food must pass through the temperature danger zone. In order to control the growth of pathogens, it is necessary to minimize the amount of time the food remains in that zone during these processes. The objective should be to pass food through the temperature danger zone as quickly as possible (through proper heating and cooling) and as infrequently as possible (by limiting the number of times a food is cooked, cooled, and reheated).

Poor Personal Hygiene

Even healthy people can be a source of the harmful microbes that cause food-borne illness. Therefore good personal hygiene is extremely important when handling foods. Soiled hands and clothing, infected food workers, and workers who do not practice good personal hygiene are major threats to food safety.

Workers in retail food establishments must report to the person in charge when they have been diagnosed with or exposed to Norovirus, hepatitis A virus, *Shigella* spp., enterohemorrhagic or Shiga toxin–producing *E. coli*, and *Salmonella typhi*. All of these diseases can potentially be transmitted by food and are considered severe health hazards. Food handlers who have been exposed to any of these

FIGURE 18.2   Food Temperature Danger Zone

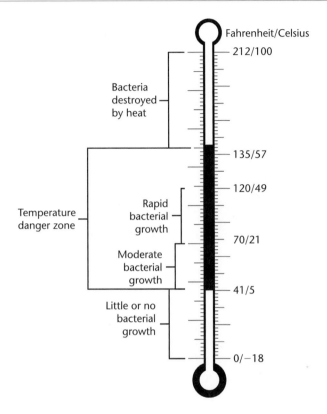

Source: David McSwane, Nancy Rue, Richard Linton, and Anna Williams, *Essentials of Food Safety and Sanitation*, 4th edition. © 2004. Electronically reproduced by permission of Food Management Institute.

pathogens must be excluded from work or assigned to restricted activities where they will have no contact with food.

A food handler's hands and fingers can become contaminated when he or she eats, smokes, uses the toilet, handles raw foods, touches soiled items, or wipes up spills. Saliva, perspiration, feces, juices from raw animal food products, and various types of soil can be significant sources of contamination if they are allowed to get into food. Therefore food workers must wash their hands whenever they have been exposed to these contaminants. Workers should vigorously rub all surfaces of their fingers, fingertips, hands, wrists, and forearms for at least ten to fifteen seconds, using soap or another approved cleaning compound. After washing, the hands and forearms must be rinsed under clean, warm running water and dried with a disposable paper towel or mechanical dryer, as illustrated in Figure 18.3.

FIGURE 18.3   Proper Hand-Washing Procedure

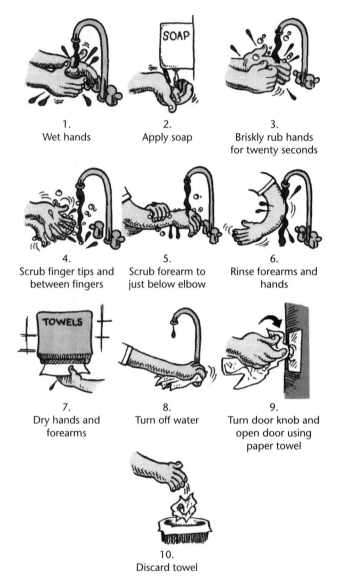

1.
Wet hands

2.
Apply soap

3.
Briskly rub hands
for twenty seconds

4.
Scrub finger tips and
between fingers

5.
Scrub forearm to
just below elbow

6.
Rinse forearms and
hands

7.
Dry hands and
forearms

8.
Turn off water

9.
Turn door knob and
open door using
paper towel

10.
Discard towel

Source: David McSwane, Nancy Rue, Richard Linton, and Anna Williams, *Essentials of Food Safety and Sanitation*, 4th edition. © 2004. Electronically reproduced by permission of Food Management Institute.

Hand-sanitizing lotions may be used by food handlers to reduce the microbial load on clean hands. However, hand sanitizers should never be used as a substitute for proper hand washing.

Food workers may also use disposable gloves to help prevent contamination when handling foods. Gloves are especially useful when working with deli sandwiches, tacos, and other foods that require extensive manual contact during preparation. Workers must treat disposable gloves as a second skin. Whatever can contaminate human hands can also contaminate gloves. Therefore, whenever gloves become soiled, they should be discarded, the worker's hands should be washed thoroughly, and a new pair of disposable gloves put on.

Improper Cooking Temperatures

Raw foods of animal origin, such as red meats, poultry, eggs, fish, and shellfish, are frequently contaminated with microbial pathogens. Practices such as using raw eggs to make a Caesar salad, lightly cooking ground beef and ground pork, and consuming raw oysters on the half shell greatly increase a person's risk of contracting a foodborne illness.

Proper cooking makes food more palatable and safe to eat. When potentially hazardous foods such as meat, poultry, and fish are cooked to proper temperatures, pathogenic bacteria and other harmful organisms found in and on the products are destroyed. Destruction of pathogens depends on the internal temperature of the food product and the amount of time the food is held at that temperature. For instance, to ensure a safe Thanksgiving turkey, it should be cooked to an internal temperature of 165°F (74°C) and held at that temperature for at least fifteen seconds. The internal temperature of foods must be measured periodically throughout the cooking process. For most foods, the internal temperature is measured by inserting the sensing portion of a properly calibrated thermometer or thermocouple into the center or thickest part of the food. This will give an accurate measure of the internal temperature and ensure the food is heated sufficiently to destroy harmful organisms.

Foods from Unsafe Sources

Food from unsafe sources may be contaminated with biological, chemical, and physical hazards. This is the primary reason why foods prepared in a private home may not be used or sold in retail food establishments. These homemade foods are prohibited because of the increased risk of contamination from biological hazards such as *Clostridium botulinum* and *Staphylococcus aureus*. Shellfish harvested from polluted waters can be contaminated with hepatitis A virus. Consumer demand for raw milk and cheese made from raw milk is increasing. However, milk and milk products that are not pasteurized properly can be contaminated with a number of pathogens, including *Listeria monocytogenes*, *E. coli*, and *Salmonella*. The safety and wholesomeness of foods can be enhanced by purchasing foods from sources that are routinely inspected by regulatory agencies and that are in compliance with applicable food safety laws.

Contamination and Cross-Contamination

Pathogens can be transferred to food by contaminated food-contact surfaces. Food-contact surfaces are the parts of equipment, utensils, and work surfaces that normally come into contact with food during storage, preparation, and service. Proper cleaning and sanitizing of these surfaces enhances food safety and quality and increases the life expectancy of equipment and facilities.

Cross-contamination is the transfer of pathogens from one food to another via contaminated hands, equipment, or utensils. Cross-contamination commonly occurs when ready-to-eat foods come into contact with raw animal foods or with surfaces that have had contact with these types of foods. For instance, if the knife and cutting board used when cutting raw chicken into pieces are then used when cutting up lettuce and tomatoes for a salad, the bacteria from the chicken can be transferred to the salad ingredients by the contaminated knife blade and cutting board. Cross-contamination can also occur when raw foods are stored above ready-to-eat foods, and juices from the raw product spill or splash onto the ready-to-eat food. Some measures that can be used to prevent cross-contamination between products are shown in Exhibit 18.3.

EXHIBIT 18.3
Preventing Cross-Contamination Between Products

- Use separate equipment, such as cutting boards, when preparing raw foods and ready-to-eat foods (color coding may be helpful for this task).
- Clean and sanitize food-contact surfaces of equipment and utensils in between working with raw animal foods and ready-to-eat foods.
- Avoid touching ready-to-eat foods with bare hands.
- Prepare ready-to-eat foods first, then the raw foods.
- Keep raw and ready-to-eat foods separate during storage or store ready-to-eat foods above raw products.

Controlling the risk factors that contribute to foodborne illness is not rocket science. However, it does require a concerted effort by both the food industry and consumers to ensure that foods are not temperature abused, proper personal hygiene is practiced, and necessary steps are taken to control contamination and cross-contamination.

HACCP FOOD SAFETY SYSTEM

The **Hazard Analysis and Critical Control Point (HACCP)** approach is a central paradigm of food safety. It is designed to identify and control problems that may cause foodborne illness before they happen. The HACCP concept was developed in 1971 by the Pillsbury Company, in cooperation with the National Aeronautics and Space Administration (NASA) and the U.S. Army, when preparing to produce safe foods for the astronauts in the U.S. space program. By employing the HACCP food safety system, suppliers were able to produce food products for America's space travelers that were nearly 100 percent free of microbial hazards.

HACCP systems are currently used by food processors and retail food establishments to identify food safety hazards and prevent them from contaminating food. HACCP is not a stand-alone program. Rather it is part of a larger system of control procedures that must be in place to ensure food safety. The HACCP system must be supported by standard operating procedures (SOPs) such as good personal hygiene, pest control, and proper cleaning and sanitizing to prevent food from becoming contaminated at points throughout the production process. When SOPs are in place, the HACCP system enables managers to concentrate on food and how it is handled during storage, preparation, display, and service. A brief summary of the HACCP system is presented in Exhibit 18.4.

FOOD SAFETY AGENCIES AND INITIATIVES

There are many opportunities for food products to become contaminated as they flow from the point of production to the point of consumption. Contamination can occur at the farm or ranch, in processing plants, at retail food establishments, and in a consumer's own kitchen. Making food safe is a responsibility that must be shared by producers, processors, transporters, retailers, governmental agencies, and consumers.

EXHIBIT 18.4
HACCP Food Safety System

The HACCP food safety system employs seven steps to identify, evaluate, and control food safety hazards (U.S. Department of Agriculture, 2008).

Step 1: Conduct a Hazard Analysis

Hazard analysis is the process used to identify biological, chemical, or physical hazards of public health significance. The hazards may be found in food due to natural contamination (for example, from raw meat, poultry, or fish), or they may be introduced into the food by workers who practice poor personal hygiene, by improper food-handling practices, or by contaminated equipment. By conducting a hazard analysis, the HACCP team can decide which hazards and conditions are significant for food safety and therefore should be addressed by the HACCP system.

Step 2: Determine Critical Control Points

A **critical control point** (CCP) is a stage in the flow of food where control is essential if one is to prevent or eliminate a hazard or reduce it to an acceptable level. Receiving, storage, cooking, and chilling are a few examples of process stages where CCPs can be employed to control hazards. Loss of control at a CCP can result in an unacceptable health risk and can jeopardize the safety of the finished product and of the consumers who eat it.

Step 3: Establish Critical Limit(s)

Critical limits are the upper and lower boundaries of food safety. When these boundaries are exceeded, a hazard may exist or could develop. A critical limit must be set for each CCP to ensure that the CCP remains under control. When a critical limit is not met, it could mean that the food is not safe.

Protecting food safety is a function of regulatory agencies at all levels of government. Federal agencies are primarily responsible for regulating foods sold through interstate commerce, and state and local agencies enforce food safety rules and regulations in restaurants, supermarkets, institutional feeding operations, and other types of retail food establishments in their jurisdictions. State and local

Step 4: Establish a System to Monitor the CCPs

Once CCPs have been identified and critical limits set, someone must monitor food and food processes to ensure that critical limits are being met. Monitoring involves making observations and measurements of critical limits to determine if a CCP is under control. By routinely monitoring critical control points it is possible to determine when a critical limit has been exceeded before a food safety problem occurs.

Step 5: Establish the Corrective Action to Be Taken When a CCP Is Not Under Control

Corrective action must be taken immediately when monitoring reveals that a critical limit has not been met and it is suspected that a CCP is not under control. For example, if monitoring reveals that a food has not reached the required final cooking temperature, the cooking process must be continued until the required internal product temperature is reached.

Step 6: Verify That the HACCP System Is Working Effectively

The two components of the verification process are (a) verifying that the critical limits established for CCPs will effectively prevent, eliminate, or reduce hazards to acceptable levels, and (b) verifying that the overall HACCP plan is working properly. Verification involves making observations, reviewing monitoring records, and discussing corrective action procedures with employees.

Step 7: Establish Effective Record Keeping

Proper documentation is needed to verify that the HACCP system is working properly. Record keeping will normally involve written records produced during the monitoring and the corrective action steps in the program. Record-keeping requirements must be as simple as possible, and employees must be trained to measure and record data accurately.

regulatory agencies provide a variety of essential services including facility and HACCP plan review, issuance of permits to operate, and routine inspections to assess compliance with food safety regulations. During food establishment inspections, inspectors examine food production, preparation, and service operations to look for evidence of time and temperature abuse, cross-contamination, and poor personal hygiene. In food establishments employing a HACCP system a major part of the inspection involves reviewing records kept as part of that system.

The federal agencies primarily responsible for food safety in the United States are the U.S. Department of Agriculture (USDA), the Food and Drug Administration (FDA), the Centers for Disease Control and Prevention (CDC), and the Environmental Protection Agency (EPA). The following sections present a brief overview of each agency's role in food safety.

U.S. Department of Agriculture

The USDA regulates the production, processing, and interstate sale of domestic and imported meat (for example, cattle, sheep, and swine), poultry (for example, chickens, turkeys, and ducks), and egg products.

The Food Safety and Inspection Service (FSIS) is the agency within USDA that is responsible for ensuring the safety, wholesomeness, and correct labeling and packaging of meat, poultry, and egg products sold in interstate commerce, including imported products. In 2000, FSIS completed implementation of the Pathogen Reduction/Hazard Analysis and Critical Control Point (HACCP) rule. This rule addresses foodborne illness associated with meat and poultry products by focusing more attention on the prevention and reduction of illness-causing microbial pathogens on raw products. It also clarifies the respective roles of government and industry in food safety. Industry is accountable for producing safe food. Government is responsible for setting appropriate food safety standards, maintaining vigorous oversight to ensure that standards are met, and operating a strong enforcement program to deal with plants that do not comply with regulatory standards.

Meat and poultry slaughterhouses and processing plants must implement HACCP programs to control factors affecting the ingredients, products, and processes in their manufacturing plants. The HACCP teams in the meat and poultry plants identify the processing steps they use to produce food commodities and determine what hazards, if any, are likely to occur at each step. After the hazards have been identified, the manufacturers identify critical control points (CCPs) that can be used to prevent, eliminate, or reduce hazards to acceptable levels. Critical limits are then set for each CCP and workers monitor the processes to ensure that CCPs are kept under control and within critical limits. The objective of HACCP programs is to make products safe to consume and to make it possible to prove to agencies and consumers that products are safe.

FSIS inspectors examine animals before and after slaughter at slaughterhouses and processing plants. Inspections are performed on live animals to identify diseased animals and prevent them from entering the food supply. Carcasses are examined after slaughter to identify visible defects that can affect safety and quality. Products are also tested for the presence of harmful pathogens and drug and chemical residues. The traditional organoleptic method, in which inspectors used their senses (principally vision, smell, and touch) to identify high-risk animals, is limited in its ability to identify contaminated foods except in the most severe cases. This limitation was the driving force that prompted USDA officials to make a significant shift toward using HACCP for primary prevention of microbial hazards.

Progress is being made toward reducing pathogenic bacteria in meat, poultry, and eggs as the meat and poultry industries comply with the pathogen reduction and HACCP requirements. This success has prompted the FSIS to strengthen HACCP systems.

Food and Drug Administration

The FDA regulates the production, processing, manufacturing, and interstate sale of all food items except red meats, poultry, and eggs. The FDA's responsibility is to ensure that food is safe, wholesome, sanitary, and honestly packaged and labeled. Specialists at the FDA conduct inspections of food-processing plants, food storage facilities, and imported foods to ensure safety standards are maintained. The agency also promotes public health by protecting food from adulteration and misbranding. Food is considered **adulterated** when it contains filth or harmful substances, is decomposed, or is produced in unsanitary conditions. Food is **misbranded** when it is packaged or labeled in a false or misleading manner.

The FDA has created a variety of programs to protect food safety as products flow from farm to table. In 2007, the FDA published the *Food Protection Plan*, which provides a proactive approach to preventing food safety problems in domestic and imported food (FDA, 2007a). The plan uses a three-pronged approach of prevention, intervention, and response to ensure the safety of our food supply. During the *prevention* phase, the FDA will work with other regulatory agencies and the food industry to identify vulnerabilities and determine the most effective ways to prevent foods from being contaminated. Prevention focuses on reducing risks over the entire life cycle of a product from production to consumption. The *intervention* phase is designed to ensure that preventive measures are properly implemented and that contaminated food is identified when preventive measures are not taken or fail. During the intervention phase, the FDA and other qualified third parties in the public and private sectors will employ risk-based inspections, food sampling, and surveillance activities at critical points in the food supply chain. In addition, FDA will promote the development of tools and procedures that permit more rapid and improved detection of contaminants in foods. Prevention, combined with intervention, will reduce the likelihood of contaminated food products reaching consumers. The goal of the *response* phase is to improve the FDA's ability to respond quickly to food safety problems and communicate more effectively with consumers and other partner organizations. During this phase, FDA will augment the existing emergency response system to shorten the period between detection and containment of a foodborne illness. By doing so, the agency will better protect public health, reduce the adverse economic impact of foodborne illness, and bolster consumer confidence in the U.S. food supply following an incident.

Because fruits and vegetables have become leading vehicles of illnesses associated with foodborne disease outbreaks, the FDA has developed **good agricultural practices** (GAPs) to help farmers protect fruits and vegetables from contamination at the source. Contamination of produce can be reduced by employing GAPs that ensure proper manure management, water use, farmworker health and hygiene, sanitation of food production facilities, and transport of commodities to market. The FDA (2007b) has also published a draft guidance document titled *Guide to Minimize Microbial Food Safety Hazards of Fresh-Cut Fruits and Vegetables*. The purpose of this publication is to advise processors, both domestic companies and those that import fresh-cut produce into the United States, on how to minimize microbial food safety hazards common to the processing of fresh-cut fruits and vegetables. This guidance document targets fresh-cut fruits and vegetables that have been minimally processed (that is, with no lethal kill step) and altered in form by peeling slicing, chopping, shredding, and the like, with or without washing or other treatment prior to being packaged for use by consumers.

Harmful substances can be a part of the food when it arrives at a food processing plant and they can be introduced during processing, handling and transportation. In order to have safe and high-quality food, food processors must reduce these hazards as much as possible. The FDA has created **good manufacturing practices** (GMPs), which are the minimum sanitary and processing requirements employed in food-processing plants. When implemented properly, GMPs help processing plants control the possibility of contamination from poor personal hygiene, pests, and contaminated facilities and equipment to ensure the production of safe and wholesome food. GMPs are an integral part of the nation's control over food safety problems.

When GMPs are not properly implemented by processors, foods can become contaminated and pose a health risk to consumers. When it is known or suspected that a hazard exists in a food product, processors can initiate a food recall to voluntarily remove products from the marketplace to keep consumers safe. A large number of food recalls occur each year due to the presence of pathogens or undeclared allergens in the foods and misbranding of the product containers.

In September 2007, the Topps Meat Company, LLC, announced a recall of frozen ground beef products that had been distributed to retail grocery stores and food service institutions throughout the United States. The recall of more than 25 million pounds of frozen ground beef products was prompted by concern that the ground beef products had been contaminated with *E. coli* O157:H7. *E. coli* bacteria can be found on a small number of cattle farms and can live in the intestines of healthy cattle. Meat can become contaminated during slaughter, and organisms can be thoroughly mixed into beef when it is ground. Improper butchering and processing can also allow *E. coli* to get onto meat. The USDA suspended the grinding of raw products at the Topps plant in Elizabeth, New Jersey, after inspectors found inadequate safety measures. The Topps Meat Company announced that as a result of the economic impact of the second largest beef recall in U.S. history, it was closing its Elizabeth, New Jersey, plant and going out of business immediately (Belson and Fahim, 2007).

In 2007, the Castleberry Food Company recalled more than eighty types of canned chili, beef stew, corned beef hash, and other meat products due to possible botulism contamination. The Department of Agriculture's Food Safety and Inspection Service reported that an equipment malfunction at an Augusta, Georgia, plant may have been responsible for the contamination. Company officials speculate that the meat product was undercooked and therefore not commercially sterilized to ensure proper destruction of the botulism organisms and their spores. As a result, the FDA and USDA asked retailers and food service operations to immediately remove and secure recalled products, making sure that all recalled products were not inadvertently made available for purchase, salvage, or donation and therefore preventing any possibility of human or animal consumption. In addition, consumers who had purchased the suspect products were warned not to open or eat canned products identified as part of the recall or to feed any of the canned products to their pets. Consumers were instructed to throw these products away immediately (Centers for Disease Control and Prevention, 2007).

Health officials in multiple states, with assistance from the CDC and FDA, investigated an outbreak of salmonellosis caused by peanut butter in late 2006 and early 2007. Peanut butter was a new food source for salmonellosis in the United States. Peanuts can become contaminated with salmonellae during growth, harvest, or storage, and the organisms are able to survive high temperatures in a high-fat, low moisture environment such as peanut butter. Because the peanut butter is heated to high temperatures that would normally be expected to kill any germs, investigators suspect the peanut butter may have been contaminated by *Salmonella* bacteria after the heat-treatment step. Possible sources of these bacteria are the raw peanuts and animals (specifically birds) inside the production plant, containers or humans inadvertently carrying the infection into the plant from the outside environment, or the other ingredients used to make peanut butter. This outbreak demonstrates that processed food can become contaminated even when the production process includes a heat-treatment step, underscoring the need for effective preventive controls in food-processing plants to prevent contamination.

Food recalls adversely affect food processors in many ways. They hurt a brand's reputation and can cause consumers to lose confidence in a company's entire line of products. The financial impact of a food recall can be immense. The direct costs of the recall and destruction of the product can cost processors millions of dollars. Besides the direct impact on the affected company, recalls affect other companies. One recall of peanut butter or tomatoes can have a negative effect on all manufacturers of peanut butter and growers of tomatoes. In addition, retailers may be adversely affected by recalls. Consumers often return products similar to but not exactly like the one being recalled, and they stop buying any brand of the product that is the target of the recall. The best way processors can ensure consumer confidence and avoid liability is to follow industry best practices, including the good manufacturing practices created by FDA.

In 1997, the FDA initiated a landmark seafood HACCP program to increase the safety of fish and shellfish and reduce seafood-related illnesses to the lowest possible levels. The seafood HACCP program requires seafood processors, repackers, and warehouses, both domestic firms and foreign exporters to this country, to follow HACCP principles and practices. Under the provisions of the seafood HACCP program, companies are required to identify hazards that in the absence of preventive controls are reasonably likely to affect the safety of seafood products. If even one hazard is identified, the seafood firm is required to adopt and implement an appropriate HACCP plan.

Outbreaks of foodborne illness have been traced to fresh juices that were not pasteurized or otherwise processed to eliminate harmful bacteria such as *E. coli* O157:H7 and *Salmonella*. This led FDA to implement a new safety rule for juices in 2001. Under the rule, juice processors must implement a HACCP plan that addresses all points of production to prevent, reduce, or eliminate hazards in juices. Processors are required to evaluate their manufacturing process to determine whether there are any microbiological, chemical, or physical hazards that could contaminate their products. If a potential hazard is identified, processors are required to implement control measures to prevent, reduce, or eliminate those hazards. Processors are also required to use processes such as pasteurization or UV irradiation or a combination of techniques to achieve a 5-log (99.999 percent) reduction in the numbers of the most resistant pathogens in their finished products, compared to the numbers present in the untreated juice.

Thus HACCP systems are federally required for seafood, juice, meat, and poultry processors. These systems enable food processors to determine where hazards can occur in processing and implement control measures to prevent problems before foodborne illness can occur. The HACCP approach offers a much more comprehensive and effective alternative to spot checks of manufacturing establishments and random sampling of final products to ensure safe foods.

The FDA promotes food safety in retail food establishments by publishing the Food Code, which serves as a model for retail food safety programs (Figure 18.4).

FIGURE 18.4   2005 FDA Food Code

Food Code

U.S. Public Health Service

2005

U. S. DEPARTMENT OF HEALTH AND HUMAN SERVICES

Public Health Service • Food and Drug Administration

College Park, MD 20740

The Food Code is not a federal law or regulation. Rather it is a set of recommendations put forth to promote food safety and sanitation nationwide.

Another function of the FDA is product recalls. The FDA can request a recall of a food product if it believes a potential hazard exists. Food recalls are typically voluntary, except when infant formula is involved. In the vast majority of cases, food processors willingly remove suspect products from the marketplace to keep consumers safe and avoid liability. However, if a company does not agree to a voluntary product recall, the FDA can issue public press releases and proceed to seize or embargo the product to remove it from commerce.

Centers for Disease Control and Prevention (CDC)

The CDC contributes to food safety by helping state and local agencies conduct foodborne disease investigations and compiling statistics on foodborne and waterborne disease outbreaks. These activities support the CDC's goals of preventing and controlling diseases and supporting public health decision making by providing credible information on foodborne diseases.

Environmental Protection Agency (EPA)

The EPA contributes to food safety by regulating the use of toxic substances such as pesticides, sanitizers, and other chemicals. As described in Chapter Seventeen, the EPA regulates pesticides under the authority of the Federal Insecticide, Fungicide, and Rodenticide Act (FIFRA) and the Food Quality Protection Act (FQPA). Under FIFRA the EPA registers pesticides for use in the United States and prescribes labeling and other regulatory requirements to prevent unreasonable adverse effects on health or the environment. The Food Quality Protection Act mandates a single, health-based standard for all pesticides in all foods. It provides special protection for infants and children and expedites approval of safer pesticides. The FQPA requires periodic reevaluation of pesticide registrations and tolerances to ensure that the scientific data supporting pesticide registrations remain up to date.

RECENT INITIATIVES IN FOOD SAFETY

Governmental agencies and the food industry have joined forces to implement other food safety initiatives to lower the incidence of foodborne illness. A brief overview of selected programs is presented here.

PulseNet

PulseNet is a national network of public health laboratories, created by the CDC, that performs DNA "fingerprinting" of bacteria that cause foodborne illness. When cases of disease show similar DNA patterns, this finding suggests a common source, such as a contaminated food product. The fingerprints of strains of bacteria isolated from food products by regulatory agencies can also be compared with those isolated from ill persons. Identifying these connections can help investigators to detect outbreaks and can expedite the recall of foods suspected of being contaminated, removing them from the marketplace.

Fight BAC! Campaign

Consumers are the last line of defense in food safety. The Fight BAC! campaign is an educational program designed to teach consumers about safe food handling. The focal point of the campaign is BAC (short for bacteria), a character used to make consumers aware of the microbes that cause foodborne illness (Figure 18.5).

FIGURE 18.5   Fight BAC! Campaign Logo

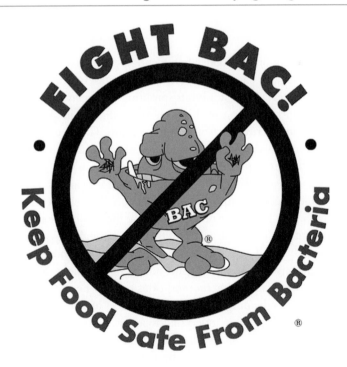

More specifically, consumers are taught that even though they cannot see, smell, or taste BAC, it and millions more germs like it may be in and on food and food-contact surfaces. The Fight BAC! campaign uses a variety of media and community outreach programs to teach consumers how to keep food safe from pathogenic bacteria by washing their hands, cleaning and sanitizing surfaces that touch food, preventing cross-contamination, cooking foods to the proper temperature, and cooling foods quickly.

Consumer Advisories

Food establishments are required to provide **consumer advisories** that inform their customers about the dangers of eating raw or undercooked animal foods or ingredients. The advisories must be provided at the point where customers order or purchase food to inform them of the fact that eating foods such as rare hamburgers, raw oysters, or Caesar salads made with raw eggs may increase their risk of foodborne illness, especially if they have certain medical conditions. Food establishments may use a variety of written communications (for example, brochures, deli case or menu advisories, or statements on labels or table tents) to comply with this the consumer advisory requirement.

Food Irradiation

Food irradiation is a food safety technology that can be used to reduce or eliminate pathogenic bacteria, insects, and parasites. It reduces spoilage, and in certain fruits and vegetables, it inhibits sprouting and delays the ripening process.

Food irradiation uses high-energy radiation in any one of three approved forms: gamma ray, electron beam, or X-ray. Gamma rays may be generated by two approved sources, either cobalt-60 or cesium-137. These substances give off high-energy photons, called gamma rays, which can penetrate foods to a depth of several feet. An electron beam, or e-beam, is a stream of high-energy electrons propelled out of an electron gun. The electrons can penetrate food to a depth of a little over one inch, so the food to be treated must not be thicker than that if it is to be treated all the way through. X-ray irradiation is the newest technology. The X-ray machine employed is a more powerful version of the machines used in many hospitals and dental offices. X-rays can pass through thick foods. Use of this method does require heavy shielding for safety; however, as with e-beams, no radioactive sources are involved.

The FDA has concluded that food irradiation is safe and effective for many foods, a conclusion shared by the World Health Organization (WHO) and the USDA. To date, irradiation has been approved for red meat, poultry, spices, fruits, vegetables, fresh shell eggs, juices, and shellfish. The FDA recently approved the use of irradiation on fresh iceberg lettuce and spinach to protect consumers from *Salmonella* and *E. coli* and to make these products longer lasting.

The FDA requires that irradiated foods be labeled with one of these two statements, "treated with radiation" or "treated by irradiation," and with the *radura*, the international symbol for irradiation. Irradiation labeling requirements apply only to foods sold in stores. For example, containers of irradiated spices must be labeled. However, the same spices do not need to be labeled when used as an ingredient in other foods. Irradiation labeling rules also do not apply to restaurant foods.

Irradiation is not a shortcut that means food hygiene efforts can be relaxed. Irradiated foods need to be stored, handled, and cooked in the same ways as unirradiated foods. They can still become contaminated with germs during processing after irradiation if the rules of basic hygiene are not followed.

Many consumers still question whether irradiation is safe. They wonder if the process transfers radiation to the product or if it causes chemical changes in the food that might be hazardous. Greater public acceptance of food irradiation awaits more understanding that irradiation does not make food radioactive, compromise nutritional quality, or noticeably change food taste, texture, or appearance when it is applied properly to a suitable product.

SAFE FOOD AS HEALTHY FOOD

Other recent initiatives address the public health aspects of food from a somewhat different perspective, focusing on food's nutritional value and the choices that shape what people in different environments eat. The Perspective titled "The Healthy Food Environment" offers three examples of this emerging concern.

EMERGING THREATS TO FOOD SAFETY

Over time new threats to food safety can emerge. Three issues with which regulatory agencies, food producers, and the public are currently concerned are mad cow disease, bioterrorism, and the industrialization of food production.

Mad Cow Disease

Bovine spongiform encephalopathy (BSE), widely referred to as mad cow disease, is a chronic degenerative disease affecting the central nervous system in cattle. Affected

PERSPECTIVE
The Healthy Food Environment

Food safety, as a component of environmental public health, has traditionally focused on keeping hazardous microbes and chemical contaminants out of food. But in recent years a new environmental approach to food has emerged: an emphasis on the environmental context of nutrition and food choices (Story, Kaphingst, Robinson-O'Brien, and Glanz, 2008). Three examples are illustrative: the availability of fresh food in poor neighborhoods, the density of liquor stores in poor neighborhoods, and the availability of "junk food" in and near schools.

Poor neighborhoods, such as those in central cities, have a relative scarcity of supermarkets and other sources of fresh fruits and vegetables. When these products are available, they are often sold in independent grocery stores rather than in national chain supermarkets, at prices out of reach for most neighborhood residents. At the same time, these poor neighborhoods typically have a high density of fast-food stores (Zenk and others, 2005; Moore and Diez-Roux, 2006; Powell and others, 2007). For example, a study in Kansas City showed seventeen fast-food restaurants per 1,000 population in low-income neighborhoods, and only one per 1,000 in high-income neighborhoods (Poston and others, 2002). Evidence suggests that these environmental patterns—and the constrained nutritional choices they imply—predict lower than desirable fruit and vegetable consumption, at least in some ethnic and racial groups (Morland, Wing, and Diez Roux, 2002; Timperio and others, 2008), although social and behavioral factors play an important role as well (Cummins, 2007).

Similarly, poor neighborhoods feature a high density of liquor stores (LaVeist and Wallace, 2000; Romley and others, 2007), posing a different sort of environmental cue. Although this density has not been linked directly to drinking in poor neighborhoods,

animals may display agitated or aggressive behavior, abnormal posture, and lack of coordination. There is neither any treatment nor a vaccine to prevent the disease.

BSE was first diagnosed in 1986 in Great Britain. The first case discovered in the United States was diagnosed in Washington State in December of 2003. Even though the heifer affected with the disease appears to have been an anomaly, the episode created great concern in the United States and abroad. BSE belongs to the family of diseases known as the transmissible spongiform encephalopathies (TSEs). These diseases include scrapie, which affects sheep and goats, chronic wasting disease in deer and elk, and Creutzfeldt-Jakob disease in humans. TSEs create holes in the brain. As the disease progresses, more and more brain and central nervous system tissue is affected. Initial symptoms involve tremors and twitching. Later symptoms include blindness and loss of memory. Death follows.

a study of college students showed that the density of liquor stores predicted the students' drinking habits (Weitzman, Folkman, Folkman, and Wechsler, 2002).

Finally, a lively debate has arisen about the *school nutrition environment*, which concerns such features as the placement of soft drink and junk food vending machines in schools. Two leading sources of information are the School Health Policies and Programs Study, administered by the CDC, and the School Nutrition and Dietary Assessment Study, administered by the USDA. Data from these studies (O'Toole, Anderson, Miller, and Guthrie, 2007; Finkelstein, Hill, and Whitaker, 2008) show that vending machines are common in schools. They are found in about one in five elementary schools, rising to 85 to 97 percent of high schools. In the CDC data, 77 percent of the schools surveyed sold soft drinks, sports drinks, and fruit drinks, and 62 percent sold salty snacks and baked goods not low in fat. In contrast, only 12 percent sold low-fat or nonfat yogurt, only 18 percent sold fruits or vegetables, and only 20 percent sold low-fat or skim milk (O'Toole and others, 2007). And these conditions are not limited to the schools themselves; in neighborhoods surrounding schools, especially those that serve poor (and possibly minority) students, there is a disproportionate concentration of convenience and fast-food stores (Zenk and Powell, 2008; Sturm 2008). Although available data do not conclusively link the school nutrition environment with students' eating habits, studies suggest that healthier food selections are associated with healthier food choices (Timperio and others, 2008) and that environmental interventions can successfully increase fruit consumption in schools (French and Stables, 2003). Critics charge that selling nonnutritious foods may discourage and even preclude healthy nutritional choices.

A broad view of food safety might well include attention to the nutritional opportunities and choices that play a role in shaping what people in different environments eat.

The USDA's BSE surveillance program has historically focused on the cattle populations in which BSE is most likely to be found. These include cattle condemned at slaughter because of signs of central nervous system disorders, nonambulatory cattle, and cattle that die on farms.

In March 2004, Secretary of Agriculture Ann M. Veneman announced an expanded surveillance effort for BSE in the United States. The primary focus of USDA's enhanced surveillance effort will continue to be on the highest-risk populations for the disease, but the USDA will greatly increase the number of target animals surveyed and will include a random sampling of apparently normal, aged animals. According to statements released by the USDA, the enhanced program, when fully implemented, will be able to detect BSE at the rate of 1 positive in 10 million adult cattle with a 99 percent confidence level.

Bioterrorism

Since September 11, 2001, terrorism in the United States has become a national concern. Security experts believe the food supply is vulnerable to attacks by international terrorist groups, and this has prompted governmental agencies and the food industry to join forces to develop food defense plans and guidelines for responding to threats to food security. Food security is different from food safety. **Food security** involves protecting food against deliberate contamination, whereas food safety is protecting food against accidental or unplanned contamination.

The CDC has identified and ranked several foodborne pathogens as agents for possible terrorist attacks (Sobel, Khan, and Swerdlow, 2002). *Bacillus anthracis* (anthrax) and *Clostridium botulinum* (botulism) have been rated by the CDC as high-priority biological agents (Category A) because they are easy to disseminate and cause severe morbidity and moderate to high mortality. Most of the foodborne biological agents identified by CDC have been classified as Category B agents because they are moderately easy to disseminate and cause moderate morbidity and low mortality. The Category B biological agents include *Salmonella* spp., *Shigella dysenteriae*, *E. coli* O157:H7, and ricin, a toxin. Several of the pathogens identified by CDC as critical biological agents are also known to pose a significant threat as unintentional food contaminants, as discussed earlier in this chapter. In addition, the CDC has identified certain chemicals as possible agents for a terrorist attack. These include heavy metals, such as arsenic, lead, and mercury, and pesticides, dioxins, furans, and PCBs, all of which can be used to contaminate food. These toxins too have been introduced inadvertently into foods at times and linked to human health effects.

Terrorists frequently rely on readily available, low-technology approaches to induce fear and produce death and mass destruction. The ideal agent for a terrorist is one that is easily spread, produces high morbidity and mortality, and can be spread from person to person after the initial exposure. Security experts believe terrorists might use a combination of the biological and chemical agents noted here, attack in more than one location simultaneously, use new agents, or use organisms that are not on the critical list (for example, common, drug-resistant, or genetically engineered pathogens).

These actions have been recommended to producers, processors, and retailers for responding to the threat of sabotage in a rational manner (U.S. Food and Drug Administration, 2009b):

- Allow only employees who have proper identification into production areas.
- Use sign-in and sign-out records to track visitors and keep areas secure.
- Prohibit personal items, such as lunch containers, briefcases, purses, and similar items, from processing areas.

- Report any unusual or suspicious activity to supervisors or managers, and contact the Federal Bureau of Investigation (FBI) and the FDA's Office of Crime Investigation when a problem is identified.
- Designate a spokesperson to deal with media or other inquiries.
- Advise managers and employees to be alert and to report any unusual activity promptly.

The Industrial Production of Food

Modern agriculture has become increasingly consolidated, with large farms producing crops and livestock on an industrial scale. Although large-scale food production has made more food available to more people, at more affordable prices, than ever before, critics have raised several concerns. Modern agriculture is heavily dependent on fossil fuels, and the energy invested in producing and transporting food often far exceeds the energy consumers derive from eating it. As petroleum becomes increasingly scarce and expensive, this approach to agriculture may not be sustainable over the long term (Pfeiffer, 2006; see also Chapter Thirteen). Moreover, agriculture is a substantial contributor to climate change (Food and Agriculture Organization, 2006; McMichael, Powles, Butler, and Uauy, 2007; also see Chapter Ten), in part due to industrial practices. A second concern relates to the wholesomeness of the food supply. Author Michael Pollan has argued that extensive reliance on corn and corn products, such as high fructose corn syrup, has diminished the nutritional value (and taste!) of many foods (Pollan, 2006). A third concern relates to the environmental impact of what has been called *factory farming*; large-scale farm facilities may be significant sources of pollutants such as nitrates, phosphates, microbes, and chemicals, including antibiotics (Silbergeld, Graham, and Price, 2008; see also Chapter Sixteen). In coming years, an important challenge will be to produce enough food to feed everybody in ways that are sustainable, efficient, economically viable, environmentally friendly, and healthy.

FOOD SAFETY CAREERS

Preventing foodborne illness and deaths from such illness remains a major public health challenge, and there are as many varieties of food safety careers as there are challenges to solve. There has never been a case of foodborne illness that could not have been prevented, and prevention is a theme that is common to all food safety careers.

Food safety professionals protect and promote public health by investigating foodborne disease outbreaks to learn about their causes and by implementing food safety strategies to prevent future outbreaks from occurring. They also inspect production facilities, food-processing plants, and retail food establishments to ensure that products are safe, wholesome, and suitable for human consumption. Food safety professionals work in a variety of settings including private industries, governmental agencies, health care facilities, and academic institutions.

College and graduate areas of study for those who work in the food safety field range from veterinary medicine and microbiology to food science and environmental health. Those who choose a career in food safety use the principles of biology, chemistry, physics, and other sciences to solve problems. Food safety professionals routinely prepare reports, so good written and oral communication skills are essential.

SUMMARY

Even though the United States has one of the safest food supplies in the world, foodborne illness poses a significant challenge to public health. Foodborne illness threatens the health and well-being of millions of Americans each year and costs billions of dollars in lost productivity, medical expenses, legal fees, lost business, and increased surveillance by regulatory agencies. Outbreaks of foodborne illness receive widespread media attention, and consumer confidence falls whenever a foodborne disease outbreak is reported. The bad publicity associated with such outbreaks can cause financial problems for the company whose product caused the outbreak and for the food industry. The entire food industry is affected when consumers begin to doubt the safety of food products.

Foodborne illness can be prevented, and the responsibility for making food safe must be shared by producers, processors, retailers, governmental officials, and consumers. A comprehensive and coordinated effort by all these entities is required to ensure the safety of our food supply from the farm to the table.

Data recently released by the CDC indicate measurable reductions in the incidence of some foodborne diseases. These data, although inconclusive for all foods, show that current approaches to combating pathogens in meat, poultry, and egg products; seafood, and juices have been effective (Shallow and others, 2004). However, the days when these foods were the primary sources of foodborne illnesses are gone—now fresh produce is the chief villain. The CDC reported 190 outbreaks of foodborne illness associated with fresh produce between 1972 and 1997. During the five years that followed, the number of outbreaks jumped to 249 and included outbreaks linked to lettuce, melons, and tomatoes (Institute of Food Technologists, 2007). Progress is being made toward the goal of preventing foodborne illness and protecting public health, but efforts to control foodborne pathogens are far from complete. The food industry, governmental agencies, and consumers must continue their vigilance over the nation's food supply to achieve even higher levels of safety and confidence.

KEY TERMS

adulterated

biological hazards

biomagnification

chemical hazards

consumer advisories

critical limits

critical control point

cross-contamination

food security

foodborne illness

good agricultural practices

good manufacturing
  practices

hazard analysis

Hazard Analysis Critical
  Control Point (HACCP)

infections

intoxications

major food allergens

misbranded

onset time

physical hazards

potentially hazardous foods
  (time/temperature
  control for safety foods)

spores

temperature abuse

temperature danger zone

toxin-mediated infections

DISCUSSION QUESTIONS

1. How do infections, intoxications, and toxin-mediated infections cause food-borne illness?
2. What four groups of people tend to be most susceptible to foodborne illness?
3. What are the three classes of foodborne hazards? Give an example of each class.
4. What are potentially hazardous foods (time-temperature control for safety foods)? What characteristics cause these foods to be frequently associated with foodborne disease outbreaks? And what is the temperature danger zone, and why is it important to food safety?
5. What is meant by poor personal hygiene, and how can it lead to foodborne illness?
6. What is cross-contamination, and what are some ways to prevent it?
7. What are the advantages of using HACCP rather than traditional food safety programs in retail food establishments? What are critical control points and critical limits as they are used in HACCP programs? Why is monitoring an important step in an HACCP system?
8. How do food recalls contribute to the safety of our nation's food supply?
9. Please discuss this statement: *Access to healthy food is an environmental justice issue.*

REFERENCES

Al-Mufti, A. W., and others. "Epidemiology of Organomercury Poisoning in Iraq, I: Incidence in a Defined Area and Relationship to the Eating of Contaminated Bread." *Bulletin of the World Health Organization*, 1976, *53*(suppl.), 23–36.

Bakir, F., and others. "Methylmercury Poisoning in Iraq." *Science*, 1973, *181*(96), 230–241.

Belson, K., and Fahim, K. "After Extensive Beef Recall, Topps Goes Out of Business." *New York Times*, October 6, 2007, 1.

Centers for Disease Control and Prevention, National Center for Infectious Diseases. *Foodborne Illness*. http://www.cdc.gov/ncidod/dbmd/diseaseinfo/foodborneinfections_g.htm, 2005.

Centers for Disease Control and Prevention. "Multi-State Outbreak of *E. coli* O157:H7 Infections From Spinach." http://www.cdc.gov/ecoli/2006/september/. 2006.

Centers for Disease Control and Prevention. "Botulism Associated with Canned Chili Sauce, July-August 2007." http://www.cdc.gov/botulism/botulism.htm. 2007.

Cramer, E.H., and others. "Outbreaks of Gastroenteritis Associated with Noroviruses on Cruise Ships—United States, 2002." *Morbidity and Mortality Weekly Report*, 2002, *51*(49);1112–1115.

Cummins, S. "Neighbourhood Food Environment and Diet: Time for Improved Conceptual Models?" *Preventive Medicine*, 2007, *44*, 196–197.

Dato, V., and others. "Hepatitis A Outbreak Associated with Green Onions at a Restaurant—Monaca, Pennsylvania, 2003." *Morbidity and Mortality Weekly Report*, 2003, *52*(47), 1155–1157.

Environment Canada. "Draft Screening Assessment for The Challenge: Phenol, 4,4'-(1-methylethylidene) bis- (Bisphenol A)." Chemical Abstracts Service Registry No. 80-05-7. http://www.ec.gc.ca/substances/ese/eng/challenge/batch2/batch2_80–05–7.cfm, 2008.

European Food Safety Authority. "Opinion of the Scientific Panel on Food Additives, Flavourings, Processing Aids and Materials in Contact with Food (AFC) Related to 2,2-Bis(4-Hydroxyphenyl) Propane." Question number: EFSA-Q-2005-100. *EFSA Journal*. http://www.efsa.europa.eu/EFSA/efsa_locale-1178620753812_1178620772817.htm., 2006.

Food and Agriculture Organization of the United Nations. *Livestock's Long Shadow. Environmental Issues and Options*. ftp://ftp.fao.org/docrep/fao/010/a0701e/a0701e.pdf, 2006.

Finkelstein, D. M., Hill, E. L., and Whitaker, R. C. "School Food Environments and Policies in US Public Schools." *Pediatrics*, 2008, *122*(1), e251–259.

Food Safety and Inspection Service, U.S. Department of Agriculture. "Pennsylvania Firm Expands Recall of Turkey and Chicken Products for Possible *Listeria* Contamination." 2002. http://www.fsis.usda.gov/OA/recalls/prelease/pr090-2002.htm.

French, S. A., and Stables, G. "Environmental Interventions to Promote Vegetable and Fruit Consumption Among Youth in School Settings." *Preventive Medicine*, 2003, *37*, 593–610.

Gottlieb, S.L. and others. "Multistate Outbreak Of Listeriosis Linked to Turkey Deli Meat and Subsequent Changes in U.S. Regulatory Policy." *Clinical Infectious Diseases*, 2006, *42*(1), 29–36.

Hites, R. A., and others. "Global Assessment of Organic Contaminants in Farmed Salmon." *Science*, 2004, *303*, 226–229.

Institute of Food Technologists. "Foodborne Illness: Increased Scrutiny on Fresh Produce." http://www.ift.org/cms/?pid51001625. 2007.

International Association for Food Protection. *Procedures to Investigate Foodborne Illness.* (5th ed.) Des Moines, Iowa: International Association for Food Protection, 1999.

International Association for Food Protection. *Procedures to Investigate Foodborne Illness.* (5th ed., revised.) Des Moines, Iowa: International Association for Food Protection, 2007.

Jungk, J., and others. "Outbreak of *Salmonella* Serotype Saintpaul Infections Associated with Multiple Raw Produce Items—United States, 2008." *Morbidity and Mortality Weekly Report*, 2008, *57*, 929–934.

Lang I. A., and others. "Association of Urinary Bisphenol A Concentration with Medical Disorders and Laboratory Abnormalities in Adults." *JAMA*, 2008, *300*(11), 1303–1310.

LaVeist, T. A., and Wallace, J. M., Jr. "Health Risk and Inequitable Distribution of Liquor Stores in African American Neighborhoods." *Social Science & Medicine*, 2000, *51*(4), 613–617.

McMichael, A. J., Powles, J. W., Butler, C. D., and Uauy, R. "Food, Livestock Production, Energy, Climate Change, and Health." *Lancet* 2007, *370*:1253–1263.

McSwane, D., Rue, N., Linton, R., and Williams, A. *Essentials of Food Safety and Sanitation.* (4th ed.) Upper Saddle River. N.J.: Pearson Education, 2004.

Mead, P. S., and others. "Food-Related Illness and Death in the United States." *Emerging Infectious Diseases*, 1999, *5*(5), 607–625.

Moore, L. V., and Diez Roux, A. V. "Associations of Neighborhood Characteristics with the Location and Type of Food Stores." *American Journal of Public Health*, 2006, *96*, 325–331.

Morland, K., Wing, S., and Diez Roux, A. "The Contextual Effect of the Local Food Environment on Residents' Diets: The Atherosclerosis Risk in Communities Study." *American Journal of Public Health*, 2002, *92*, 1761–1767.

National Institute of Environmental Health Sciences. "Since You Asked—Bisphenol A: Questions and Answers about the National Toxicology Program's Role in Evaluating Bisphenol A." http://www.niehs.nih.gov/news/media/questions/sya-bpa.cfm#17, 2008.

National Research Council, Committee on Pesticides in the Diets of Infants and Children. *Pesticides in the Diets of Infants and Children.* Washington, D.C.: National Academies Press, 1993.

National Toxicology Program, Center for the Evaluation of Risks to Human Reproduction. *NTP-CERHR Monograph on the Potential Human Reproductive and Developmental Effects of Bisphenol A.* NIH Publication No. 08-5994. http://cerhr.niehs.nih.gov/chemicals/bisphenol/bisphenol.pdf, 2008.

Olsen, S. J., and others. "Surveillance for Foodborne Disease Outbreaks—United States, 1993–1997." *Morbidity and Mortality Weekly Report*, 2000, *49*(SS01), 1–51.

O'Toole, T. P., Anderson, S., Miller, C., and Guthrie, J. "Nutrition Services and Foods and Beverages Available at School: Results from the School Health Policies and Programs Study 2006." *Journal of School Health*, 2007, *77*, 500–521.

Pfeiffer, D. A. *Eating Fossil Fuels: Oil, Food and the Coming Crisis in Agriculture.* Gabriola Island, B.C.: New Society Publishers, 2006.

Pollan, M. *The Omnivore's Dilemma: A Natural History of Four Meals.* New York: Penguin Press, 2006.

Posada de la Paz, M., Philen, R. M., and Borda, A. I. "Toxic Oil Syndrome: The Perspective After 20 Years." *Epidemiologic Reviews*, 2001, *23*(2), 231–247.

Poston, W.S.C., and others. "Obesity and the Environment: A Tale of Two Kansas Cities." Poster presented at the 23rd annual Scientific Sessions of the Society of Behavioral Medicine, San Diego, Apr. 2002.

Powell, L. M., and others. "Food Store Availability and Neighborhood Characteristics in the United States." *Preventive Medicine*, 2007, *44*, 189–195.

Public Health Agency of Canada. "Listeria Investigation and Recall—2008." http://www.inspection .gc.ca/english/fssa/concen/2008listeriae.shtml, 2008a.

Public Health Agency of Canada. "Listeria Monocytogenes Outbreak." http://www.phac-aspc.gc.ca/ alert-alerte/listeria/listeria_2008-eng.php, 2008b.

Romley, J. A., Cohen, D., Ringel, J., and Sturm, R. "Alcohol and Environmental Justice: The Density of Liquor Stores and Bars in Urban Neighborhoods in the United States." *Journal of Studies on Alcohol*, 2007, *68*(1), 48–55.

Shallow, S., and others. "Preliminary FoodNet Data on the Incidence of Foodborne Illnesses? Selected Sites, United States, 2002." *Morbidity and Mortality Weekly Report*, 2004, *53*(16), 338–343.

Silbergeld, E. K., Graham, J., and Price, L. B. "Industrial Food Animal Production, Antimicrobial Resistance, and Human Health." *Annual Review of Public Health* 2008, *29*, 151–169.

Sobel J., Khan A. S., and Swerdlow D. L. "Threat of a Biological Terrorist Attack on the U.S. Food Supply: The CDC Perspective." *Lancet*, 2002, *359*(9309), 874–880.

Story, M., Kaphingst, K.M., Robinson-O'Brien, R., and Glanz, K. "Creating Healthy Food and Eating Environments: Policy and Environmental Approaches." *Annual Review of Public Health*, 2008, *29*, 253–272.

Sturm, R. "Disparities in the Food Environment Surrounding US Middle and High Schools." *Public Health*, 2008, *122*(7), 681–690.

Timperio, A., and others. "Children's Fruit and Vegetable Intake: Associations with the Neighbourhood Food Environment." *Preventive Medicine*, 2008, *46*(4), 331–335.

U.S. Department of Agriculture, Food Safety Research Information Office. "A Focus on Hazard Analysis and Critical Control Points." http://fsrio.nal.usda.gov/document_fsheet. php?product_id5155. 2008.

U.S. Food and Drug Administration. *Foodborne Pathogenic Microorganisms and Natural Toxins Handbook: The "Bad Bug Book."* http://vm.cfsan.fda.gov/~mow/intro.html, 2003.

U.S. Food and Drug Administration. "What You Need to Know About Mercury in Fish and Shellfish." http://www.cfsan.fda.gov/~dms/admehg3.html, 2004.

U.S. Food and Drug Administration. *Food Protection Plan.* http://www.fda.gov/oc/initiatives/advance/ food/plan.html, 2007a.

U.S. Food and Drug Administration. *Guide to Minimize Microbial Food Safety Hazards of Fresh-Cut Fruits and Vegetables.* http://www.cfsan.fda.gov/~dms/prodgui3.html, 2007b.

U.S. Food and Drug Administration. "Food Allergies: What You Need to Know." http://www.fda.gov/ Food/ResourcesForYou/Consumers/ucm079311.htm. 2007c.

U.S. Food and Drug Administration. Bisphenol A. http://www.fda.gov/NewsEvents/ PublicHealthFocus/ucm064437.htm. 2009a.

U.S. Food and Drug Administration. Food Security Preventative Measures Guidance. http://www.fda. gov/Food/FoodDefense/FoodSecurity/default.htm. 2009b.

U.S. Food and Drug Administration. *2005 Food Code.* http://www.fda.gov/Food/FoodSafety/ RetailFoodProtection/FoodCode/FoodCode2005/default.htm, 2009c.

Vom Saal, F. S., and Hughes, C. "An Extensive New Literature Concerning Low-Dose Effects of Bisphenol A Shows the Need for a New Risk Assessment." *Environmental Health Perspectives*, 2005, *113*(8), 926–933.

Vom Saal, F. S., and Myers, J. P. "Bisphenol A and Risk of Metabolic Disorders." *JAMA*, 2008, *300*, 1353–1355.

Vom Saal, F. S., and others. "Chapel Hill Bisphenol A Expert Panel Consensus Statement: Integration of Mechanisms, Effects in Animals and Potential to Impact Human Health at Current Levels of Exposure." *Reproductive Toxicology*, 2007, *24*(2), 131–138.

Vugia, D., and others. "Preliminary FoodNet Data on the Incidence of Infection with Pathogens Transmitted Commonly Through Food—10 States, 2007." *Morbidity and Mortality Weekly Report*, 2008, *57*, 366–370.

Weitzman, E. R., Folkman, A., Folkman, K. L., and Wechsler, H. "The Relationship of Alcohol Outlet Density to Heavy and Frequent Drinking and Drinking-Related Problems Among College Students at Eight Universities." *Health & Place*, 2002, *9*(1), 1–6.

Zenk, S. N., and Powell, L. M. "US Secondary Schools and Food Outlets." *Health & Place*, 2008, *14*, 336–346.

Zenk, S., and others. "Neighborhood Racial Composition, Neighborhood Poverty, and the Spatial Accessibility of Supermarkets in Metropolitan Detroit." *American Journal of Public Health*, 2005, *95*(4), 660–667.

FOR FURTHER INFORMATION

Books and Guides

Bryan, F. L., and others. *Procedures to Implement the Hazard Analysis Critical Control Point System*. Ames, Iowa: International Association for Food Protection, 1991.

Heymann, D. (ed.). *Control of Communicable Diseases in Man*. (18th ed.) Washington, D.C.: American Public Health Association Press, 2005.

Jay, J. M. *Modern Food Microbiology*. (6th ed.) Gaithersburg, Md.: Aspen, 2000.

McSwane, D., Linton, R., and Rue, N. *SuperSafeMark Guide to Food Safety*. Arlington, Va.: Food Marketing Institute, 2007.

Potter, N., and Hotchkiss, J. *Food Science*. (5th ed.) Gaithersburg, Md.: Aspen, 1998.

Agencies and Organizations

Centers for Disease Control and Prevention, http://www.cdc.gov.

Food Allergy Network, http://www.foodallergy.org.

Food and Agriculture Organization of the United Nations, http://www.fao.org.

Food Marketing Institute, http://www.fmi.org.

Gateway to Government Food Safety Information, http://www.foodsafety.gov.

International Association for Food Protection, http://www.foodprotection.org. Use this site to order copies of *Procedures to Investigate Foodborne Illness*.

International Food Information Council, http://www.ific.org.

National Restaurant Association, http://www.restaurant.org.

Partnerships for Food Safety Education, http://www.fightbac.org.

U.S. Department of Agriculture, http://www.usda.gov.

U.S. Environmental Protection Agency http://www.epa.gov.

U.S. Food and Drug Administration, http://www.fda.gov.

CHAPTER NINETEEN

HEALTHY BUILDINGS

HOWARD FRUMKIN

KEY CONCEPTS

- People spend more than 90 percent of their time in buildings, so building conditions may have an important impact on health.

- Principal building types include homes, schools, workplaces, and health care facilities.

- Important health-related aspects of buildings include injury risks, exposure to pests, exposure to mold and moisture, indoor air quality, toxic exposures, and mental health effects.

- Some populations are disproportionately exposed to building-related hazards and merit special public health attention.

- Some people are especially vulnerable to building-related hazards; among these people are the elderly and people with disabilities.

- Many techniques are available to achieve safe, healthy buildings.

- *Green buildings*—buildings designed for environmental performance—offer a complementary approach to safe, healthy buildings.

"WE give shape to our buildings, and they in turn shape us," said Winston Churchill in a 1943 speech to the House of Commons. Indeed, we spend most of our time in buildings—more than 90 percent by some estimates (Leech and others, 2002). Homes top the list; studies in North America (Leech and others, 2002) and Europe (Brasche and Bischot, 2005) show that people average between fifteen and sixteen hours per day at home. Employed people typically spend about eight hours per day at their workplaces, and students spend almost as much time in their schools. In specialized buildings, such as hospitals and prisons, people (sometimes especially vulnerable people) may spend prolonged periods of time. Buildings are a typical human environment, and they matter greatly for our health and well-being.

This chapter explores environmental health on the scale of buildings. We focus on homes, schools, and health care facilities because workplaces are discussed in Chapter Twenty. We mention safety only briefly because injury risks are discussed in Chapter Twenty-Two, and we focus on health instead. We focus on buildings in developed nations because health issues in buildings in poor countries—especially indoor air problems related to burning biofuels (Zhang and Smith, 2003)—are discussed in Chapter Eleven. Finally, we take a broad view of health, extending beyond physical ailments to mental health and well-being. Buildings that are well built and maintained, welcoming, easily navigated, clean, safe, and comfortable can promote mental health (Evans, Wells, Chan, and Saltzman, 2000) and enhance comfort and well-being (Alexander and others, 1977; de Botton, 2006)—important parts of health in the broadest sense.

THE RANGE OF BUILDINGS

Homes are where people spend more time than they do in any other building, and homes have long been recognized as a critical influence on health. In the words of Florence Nightingale, "The connection between the health and the dwelling of the population is one of the most important that exists" (quoted in Lowry, 1991).

The American Housing Survey, conducted about every six years by the U.S. Census Bureau for the Department of Housing and Urban Development, is a rich source of information. According to the 2005 survey (U.S. Census Bureau, 2006), there are approximately 124 million homes in the United States, and 109 million of them are occupied year-round. Of these 124 million, approximately

Howard Frumkin declares no competing financial interests.

75 million are owner-occupied and the remainder rented. About 70 million homes are detached, single-family houses, and about 26 million are parts of multiple-unit structures such as apartment houses. (The remainder belong to other categories, such as trailers.) The median year of construction is 1973, and more than 20 million homes are more than fifty years old (Figure 19.1).

Some homes are substandard, posing obvious dangers to their inhabitants. In the 2005 American Housing Survey, safety hazards were common and included missing roofing material (5.1 million homes), broken windows (5.0 million), loose stairway railings (3.7 million), sagging roofs (3.2 million), cracked or crumbling foundations (3.2 million), loose steps (3.0 million), deficient plumbing (2.5 million), and room heaters without flues (1.8 million). Substandard housing threatens well-being in a global sense by undermining residents' dignity and security (Dunn, 2002; Dupuis and Thorns, 1998). In addition, substandard housing can directly cause injury and death. According to the Home Safety Council (Runyan and Casteel, 2004), about 18,000 deaths occur in homes each year in the United States, of which about 33 percent are due to falls, 26 percent to poisonings, 19 percent to burns, and the remainder to other causes. In addition to safety hazards, substandard housing may pose exposures to lead paint, cockroaches and dust mites, rats and mice, carbon monoxide, and other hazards (Matte and Jacobs, 2000; Krieger and Higgins, 2002; Howden-Chapman, 2004). Some of these hazards especially target people with particular susceptibilities, such as the very young, the very old, and people with respiratory diseases such as asthma.

Low-income families and members of ethnic minorities disproportionately live in substandard housing. But some housing hazards affect people across the population. For example, about one in seventeen U.S. homes has a radon level above 4 pCi/L, the Environmental Protection Agency action level (National Research Council, Committee on Health Risks of Exposure to Radon, 1998). As described in Chapter Twenty-One, this exposure contributes substantially to lung cancer risk, especially among smokers.

Schools are a second important category of building (Figure 19.3). There are 94,000 public schools in the United States, and more than 48 million students attend them. An additional 5.3 million students attend 30,000 private schools. Children spend more time in their schools than in any other environment except home. And it is not only children who spend time in schools. They are joined by more than 4.7 million teachers, and hundreds of thousands of administrators, custodians, food service workers, security guards, and other personnel (Frumkin, Geller, Rubin, and Nodvin, 2006).

Like homes, schools may confront their occupants with a range of environmental hazards (Frumkin, Geller, Rubin, and Nodvin, 2006). In the mid-1990s, the U.S. General Accounting Office (GAO) issued detailed reports on conditions

FIGURE 19.1   Housing Can Take Many Forms and Vary Greatly in Desirability and Safety

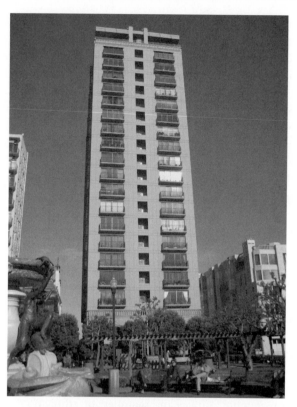

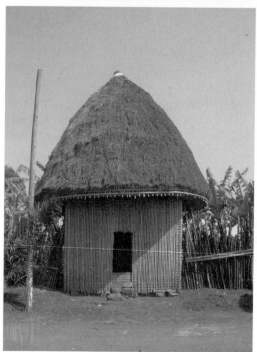

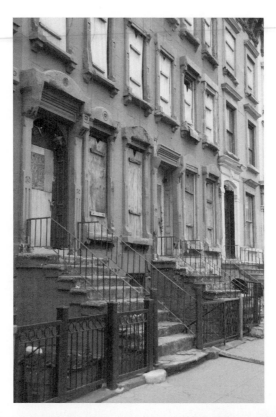

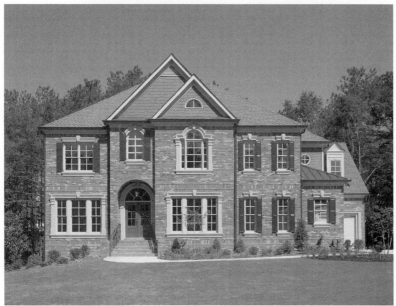

PERSPECTIVE
Manufactured Structures

In the aftermath of Hurricanes Katrina and Rita in 2005, more than 120,000 manufactured housing units (Figure 19.2) were deployed in the Gulf of Mexico region to shelter people who had been displaced from their homes. Within the first year, concerns
arose about possible health problems among these residents. Many of these concerns
focused on formaldehyde, but other concerns—such as moisture and mold—were
raised as well.

What were these units? Sometimes lumped together under the term *trailers*, **manufactured structures** in fact come in a variety of designs. Most common among the
units used after Hurricanes Katrina and Rita were **travel trailers**—small (generally under
320 square feet), wheel-mounted trailers, originally designed to provide temporary living

FIGURE 19.2   Katrina Trailer

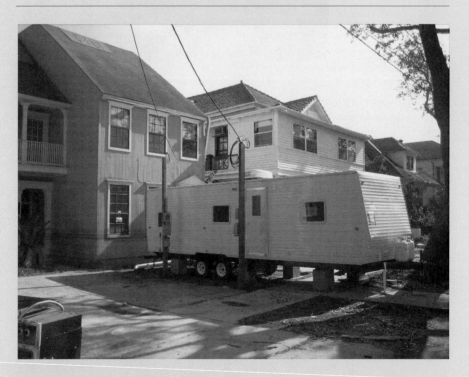

Source: Infrogmation, http://commons.wikimedia.org/wiki/File:FEMAtrailerNapoleonFreret.jpg,
2006. Permission granted under the terms of the GNU Free Documentation License, Version
1.2 or any later version published by the Free Software Foundation.

quarters during recreation, camping, or travel and regulated as vehicles rather than as buildings. There were also **manufactured homes** (formerly known as mobile homes)—larger (generally more than 320 square feet) structures built on a permanent chassis; containing plumbing, heating, air-conditioning, and electrical systems; and designed to be used as dwellings (with or without a permanent foundation) when connected to the required utilities. Still another design used was the **park model**, a larger version of a travel trailer, used as temporary living quarters.

These housing units deployed after the 2005 hurricanes were only a small part of a much larger universe. Millions of Americans live, go to school, and work in manufactured structures every day. With regard to housing, some units are used on a long-term basis, others for short-term recreational and travel use, and still others as temporary housing following disasters. In the 2005 American Housing Survey, of 124.4 million housing units in the United States, 8.7 million (7 percent) were manufactured homes, housing 17.2 million Americans. With regard to schools, a 2005 U.S. Department of Education survey of public school principals showed that 37 percent of all public schools use portable buildings (sometimes called **modular classrooms**) (Chaney and Lewis, 2007). In California, one in three students learns in a portable building (Shendell, Winer, Weker, and Colome, 2004; Shendell and others, 2004). Of note, urban schools are more likely to have portable buildings than are suburban or large-town schools and rural or small-town schools (52 percent versus 27 percent and 36 percent, respectively), and the prevalence of portable buildings rises with minority enrollment, from a low of 19 percent in schools with less than 6 percent minority enrollment to a high of 53 percent in schools with 50 percent or more minority enrollment (Chaney and Lewis, 2007). No data are available on how many people work each day in manufactured structures, but construction trailers, sales offices, and other such uses are common.

Could manufactured structures raise health concerns? Indoor air quality is one such issue. Manufactured structures are built with particleboard, oriented strand board, fiberboard, and similar materials, and these can release volatile compounds, especially formaldehyde, over time. A study of 519 temporary housing units in the Gulf Region showed elevated formaldehyde levels. The geometric mean was 77 parts per billion (ppb), two or three times the typical level in U.S. houses, and measurements ranged as high as several hundred ppb. Certain factors, such as small size (travel trailers as opposed to manufactured homes), high temperatures, and closed windows, predicted higher levels of formaldehyde. Because formaldehyde levels tend to be higher in newly constructed manufactured structures and during warmer weather, the Centers for Disease Control and Prevention (CDC) cautioned that observed levels likely underrepresented long-term exposures; many of the units studied were approximately two years old, and the study was conducted during the winter (CDC, 2008). Formaldehyde is irritating and may contribute to the development of respiratory and allergic symptoms in children (Mendell, 2007). In addition it is considered a probable human carcinogen by several agencies, although there are uncertainties in estimating formaldehyde's cancer risks.

Formaldehyde is not the only indoor air concern in manufactured structures; among the others are pesticides, environmental tobacco smoke, other volatile organic compounds, and carbon monoxide, as in any building. And indoor air is not the only potential health issue in manufactured structures. Others exist, as is the case for any building: moisture and mold, fire safety issues, injury risks, and pests such as rats and mice, cockroaches, and dust mites. In addition, manufactured structures pose some unique challenges related to utility hookups (including water, sewage, and electricity), structural integrity, and proper tethering. The combination of light weight and lack of tethering helps to explain the devastation that tornadoes and other severe storms can wreak in trailer communities. Some of these problems may be widespread. For example, the 2005 American Housing Survey (U.S. Census Bureau, 2006) reported that of 8.7 million manufactured homes, 401,000 had a sagging roof, 329,000 had a

of U.S. schools (GAO, 1995, 1996a, 1996b). According to the GAO, one in three schools had buildings in need of extensive repair or replacement, and almost 60 percent reported a major building feature that needed extensive repairs, an overhaul, or replacement. In addition, about half the schools reported one or more unsatisfactory environmental conditions such as poor ventilation, heating or lighting problems, or poor physical security. There were schools in warm climates without functioning air-conditioning, schools in cold climates without adequate heating systems, and schools across the country without good lighting. The report described overcrowded schools, noisy schools, and schools with blatant safety hazards. In one example, a school ceiling that had been weakened by leaking water collapsed just forty minutes after students had left the building. Such incidents regularly appear in media reports: an elementary school in Cleveland whose staff discovered hidden structural problems in the roof after a ceiling leak was noted (Okoben, 2006); a high school on Long Island, New York, in which a ceiling collapsed onto a chemistry class, injuring nine students (Keane, 2003); an elementary school in Austin that evacuated all 777 pupils and closed for gutting and renovation when large amounts of Stachybotrys and *Penicillium* molds resulted from roof leaks (Mann, 2000). In the GAO reports, most problems were not isolated; a school with one problem often had multiple problems.

Later research by the National Center for Education Statistics (2000) found similar results. Nearly half the schools in this study reported at least one environmental factor in unsatisfactory condition: ventilation in 26 percent of the schools, visible hole in the roof and 188,000 a visible hole in the floor, 308,000 had sloping outside walls, 668,000 had broken windows, and 183,000 had a foundation with either visible crumbling or open cracks or holes.

Manufactured structures offer important advantages. They are affordable, flexible, and rapidly installed. At a time when affordable housing is an ever more important national goal, and when school districts need affordable, convenient options, manufactured structures will continue to play an important role. Standard public health principles apply in keeping people safe and healthy as they live, study, and work in these structures. Good design involves such features as adequate ventilation. Good construction involves using materials that do not emit dangerous levels of formaldehyde. Good installation involves secure placement and tethering. Good maintenance involves caring for the entire structure, avoiding leaks, maintaining good hygiene, and avoiding the introduction of hazards. Through these measures, the health and safety of the millions of people who use manufactured structures can be protected.

acoustics or noise control in 18 percent, indoor air quality in 18 percent, heating in 17 percent, and lighting in 12 percent. Ongoing research has continued to corroborate these findings. For example, a recent review of air quality in schools revealed that inadequate ventilation, excessive levels of carbon dioxide, volatile organic compounds, **bioaerosols**, bacteria, dust mites, and animal allergens are common (Daisey, Angell, and Apte, 2003). In a Michigan study of sixty-four elementary and middle school classrooms, only one in four classrooms had recommended levels of ventilation, and one in six had levels of carbon dioxide above 1,000 ppm (Godwin and Batterman, 2007)—a marker of low air circulation. Conditions such as these pose both short-term and long-term threats to children's health and academic performance (Mendell and Heath, 2005) and may translate into higher health care costs as well.

Health care facilities are a special category of buildings. Patients with various ailments may be especially susceptible to environmental hazards and may stand to benefit greatly from healthy, restorative buildings. In addition, health care workers spend long hours in these facilities, often in high-stress jobs, so careful design offers promise for them as well.

Health care facilities use a wide range of potentially toxic chemicals, such as mercury (in thermometers and other instruments), plastics (containing such components as phthalates), sterilizing agents (such as ethylene oxide), and cleaning materials (which are heavily used because sanitation is so important in health care facilities). Some medications, such as chemotherapeutic agents and radionuclides, can be toxic.

FIGURE 19.3   School Design

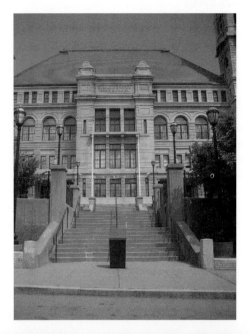

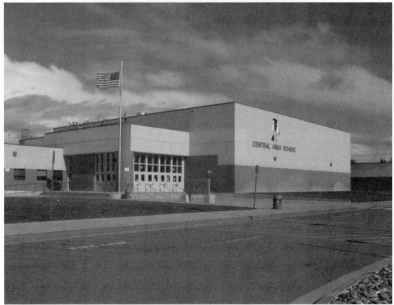

Sources: Neighborhood school: Infrogmation, http://commons.wikimedia.org/wiki/File:FallRiverMADurfe eShcoolEntrance.jpg, 2007; community school: Tewy, http://commons.wikimedia.org/wiki/File:Central_ High_School_(Grand_Junction,_Colorado).jpg, 2006. Permission granted under the terms of the GNU Free Documentation License, Version 1.2 or any later version published by the Free Software Foundation.

School design has changed dramatically over recent decades, from small, multistory schools embedded in neighborhoods to low-rise, rambling structures on large suburban or exurban parcels of land.

However, safe and healthy clinical facilities do more than prevent exposure to dangerous chemicals. Growing evidence suggests that well-designed facilities can help prevent medical errors, reduce stress in both patients and staff, improve sleep, and improve clinical outcomes (as measured by reduced pain, reduced need for some medications, and speedier recovery). The features that promote health and well-being include single rooms (as opposed to multibed rooms), reduced noise, improved lighting (including natural daylight), better ventilation, and better ergonomic designs (Ulrich and others, 2004; Marberry, 2006; Rashid and Zimring, 2008).

Design features that promote health can also advance environmental goals. For example, avoiding the use of volatile organic chemicals protects both health and the environment. The use of natural daylight for lighting not only improves well-being and performance but also reduces energy demand. An exciting development in recent years has been the alignment of *healthy health care design*, with its primary focus on the health of patients and staff, and *green health care*, with its primary focus on environmental performance (Guenther and Vittori, 2007).

LIGHTING

Good **lighting** is an important part of a healthy building. Whereas our ancestors used a variety of light sources—candles, fires, lanterns, and so forth—(or simply went to sleep when it got dark), modern buildings use two general sources of light: natural light and electric light. *Sunlight* refers to the direct, parallel rays of the sun; it is very bright, casts strong shadows, and may cause glare at close range. **Daylight** (or diffuse sunlight) is sunlight diffused by clouds, the earth's atmosphere, reflection off a surface, or passage through translucent material. It is a soft, even source of light. Electric light comes from a variety of bulb types, including incandescent, fluorescent, and high-intensity discharge bulbs, and light-emitting diodes (LEDs).

Good lighting promotes health, well-being, and performance. In a school-based study, investigators found that more daylight in classrooms was associated with 20 percent faster progress in acquiring math and reading skills (Heschong Mahone Group, 1999). In a hospital study, patients in intensive care units recovered faster if they were in rooms with windows (Guzowski, 2000). Office workers with windows report better health and job satisfaction (California Energy Commission, 2003). Conversely, poor lighting has negative consequences. Excessively bright lighting can cause squinting and headaches, dim lighting can cause eye strain, and flickering can cause headaches and discomfort. Adequate lighting in buildings is needed not only for comfort and performance but for safety; people need to be able to see potential trip and fall hazards and to find their way to exits in case of emergency.

Many guidelines for good lighting are available (Ander, 2003; Boubekri, 2008). Daylighting should be prioritized, not only because it is beneficial for people, but because it reduces energy demand. Daylight may come from windows, skylights, louvers, and clerestories. But because daylight is variable, it should be integrated with electric lighting. Areas where people need good illumination, such as at desks in schools and offices and at workstations in workplaces, should be well provided with soft, even light. Glare—as comes from direct views of a direct light source—should be minimized.

INJURY RISKS

Many types of injuries can occur in buildings. Some are work related, and are discussed in Chapter Twenty. Others are common in homes, schools, and other buildings. Of these, the two most common are falls and burns.

Falls are a common cause of injuries in buildings, especially in homes. Several risk factors are well recognized. These include stairs without banisters or handrails (a danger for both small children and the elderly), windows on upper floors without window locks or safety guards (a danger for small children), bathtubs without mats or nonskid strips, poor lighting, slippery floors, uneven surfaces, and tripping hazards such as electrical cords (Tinetti, Speechley, and Ginter, 1988; American Academy of Pediatrics, 2001). Personal risk factors combine with environmental risk factors to play a role; among the elderly, for example, risks include having medical conditions such as orthostatic hypotension, visual or cognitive impairment, and balance and gait abnormalities, and taking certain medications (Todd and Skelton, 2004; Chang and others, 2004). Although falls have been recognized as a major problem for the elderly (Rubenstein and Josephson, 2006), children are also at risk, both in the United States (Nagaraja and others, 2005; Phalen, Khoury, Kalkwarf, and Lanphear, 2005) and in developing nations (Hyder, Sugerman, Ameratunga, and Callaghan, 2007). Many preventive strategies have been proposed, including banisters, railings, and stairway gates; locks and safety guards on windows; padded or carpeted floor surfaces; correction of hazards such as loose electrical cords; and attention to personal risk factors. Sometimes these approaches are combined in multifactorial risk reduction programs, in both home and institutional settings, although the evidence to support such interventions is not always convincing (Coussement and others, 2008; Gates and others, 2008).

Burns are another common cause of injuries in buildings, and fire safety has long been recognized as a priority for safe buildings. In 2006, there were 524,000 structural fires in the United States, causing 2,705 deaths and 14,350 injuries (excluding those suffered by firefighters) and $9.6 billion in property damage

(National Fire Protection Association, 2006). Fire extinguishers, fire escapes (especially on multistory buildings), sprinkler systems (Hall, 2007), design features such as stairways that are separated from floor spaces, nonflammable structural elements such as steel beams, and the use of fireproofing are all important safety measures (Buchanan, 2001; Purkiss, 2006). Many of these measures have been incorporated into the Fire Code and the related standards issued by the National Fire Protection Association (www.nfpa.org) and implemented at the state and local levels.

Smoke alarms are a key means of preventing injury or death due to home fires. They are associated with reduction in injuries and deaths due to residential fires in the range of 50% (Warda and Ballesteros, 2007) and possibly as much as 80% (Mallonee and others, 1996).

However, as is the case for falls, environmental measures need to be supplemented by behavioral interventions. One promising residential fire prevention program, for example, included smoke alarms, educational activities, and cooperation among local health departments, fire departments, community organizations, and the media (Ballesteros, Jackson, and Martin, 2005). In commercial buildings, schools, and other institutional settings, fire drills are an important adjunct to environmental approaches. Extensive recommendations are available at a Web site hosted jointly by the Centers for Disease Control and Prevention, the Consumer Product Safety Commission, and the U.S. Fire Administration (www.firesafety.gov).

PESTS

For as long as people have built and used buildings, they have shared them with pests. Chief among these pests are insects such as mites, termites, and cockroaches, and rodents such as mice and rats. These unwelcome visitors can have important consequences for health. Cockroach allergy, for instance, is a major contributor to asthma among inner-city children whose homes are infested (Rosenstreich and others, 1997). Flies can spread foodborne pathogens such as salmonella. Rats can spread diseases such as rat-bite fever and plague and can infect people with hantavirus, aggravate allergies, and cause electrical damage by chewing wires. Termites can cause structural damage by destroying wooden beams. Strategies for controlling pests are described in Chapter Seventeen.

MOISTURE AND MOLD

Molds are those fungi that grow in the form of multicellular filaments, called *hyphae*. Many thousands of species of mold are recognized, but only a small subset of them are described as occurring in buildings, with names such as *Alternaria, Aspergillus, Cladosporium, Fusarium, Penicillium, Rhizopus, Stachybotrys,* and *Trichoderma.* Molds share several features. First, they reproduce through spores, which can often survive for prolonged periods in inhospitable conditions. Second, they require moisture to reproduce and grow. Third, they derive their energy not through photosynthesis but from organic matter such as starch and cellulose. Molds are ubiquitous in nature, where they play essential roles in breaking down organic waste such as dead leaves. Molds have many useful applications; some are used to make cheese, soy sauce, and other foods, and others have given rise to medications such as penicillin (from *Penicillium chrysogenum*) and lovastatin (from *Aspergillus terreus*).

Mold spores are common throughout the environment, including building interiors, where they generally cause no problems. For mold to grow, three conditions are required: warmth, moisture, and nutrients. Most buildings contain plenty of nutrients, in walls, carpets, insulation, and other materials. Hence warm, moist conditions—say, in basements or showers—complete the requirements and may trigger excessive mold growth. Some buildings or parts of buildings routinely have conditions that encourage mold growth; think of a greenhouse, an indoor pool, or a laundry room. If a portion of a building becomes moist—say, if water infiltrates a roof or wall or accumulates under a carpet—then mold growth may result. Following a flood, when parts of a building have been immersed in water, mold growth is common (see Figure 19.4). Mold is not the only exposure that may occur in damp indoor spaces; others include bacteria such as *Legionella*, bacterial endotoxins, and dust mites.

Mold can threaten health in several ways (Institute of Medicine, Committee on Damp Indoor Spaces and Health, 2004; Bush and others, 2006; Seltzer and Fedoruk, 2007). First, some molds produce chemicals. These may be volatile organic compounds (VOCs), such as alcohols, ketones, and esters. These VOCs can cause the musty odors sometimes associated with mold growth, and they can cause symptoms in some people, such as irritation of the mucous membranes and headaches. Molds may also produce metabolic by-products called *mycotoxins,* which are toxic to humans (and other animals). The best known example, aflatoxin (from *Aspergillus flavus*), is not building related; it is encountered as a food contaminant. But some building-related molds, such as *Stachybotrys*, can also produce mycotoxins. Mycotoxins are not usually volatile; instead they settle on spores, on hyphal fragments, and on dust, become airborne, and are inhaled (Institute of Medicine, Committee on Damp Indoor Spaces and Health, 2004). Mycotoxins have been suspected of causing human disease after building exposures, especially in an outbreak of acute pulmonary hemorrhage in children in Cleveland in the early 1990s, but there remains scientific uncertainty about the nature and extent

FIGURE 19.4   Mold-Damaged Building in New Orleans Following
Hurricane Katrina

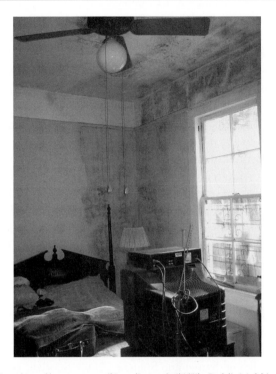

Source: Infrogmation, http://commons.wikimedia.org/wiki/File:DublinMold.jpg, 2005.
Permission granted under the terms of the GNU Free Documentation License, Version 1.2 or
any later version published by the Free Software Foundation.

of such mycotoxin-related disease (Institute of Medicine, Committee on Damp
Indoor Spaces and Health, 2004; Bennett and Klich, 2003).

A second way in which mold can affect health is by eliciting immune responses.
Some immune responses, such as allergies, are familiar; symptoms include sneezing, coughing, and having a runny nose, red eyes, or a skin rash. Asthma commonly has an immune component, and exposure to damp indoor spaces and
mold can aggravate this condition (Institute of Medicine, Committee on the
Assessment of Asthma and Indoor Air, 2000; Institute of Medicine, Committee
on Damp Indoor Spaces and Health, 2004). More severe immune responses, such
as a lung disease called hypersensitivity pneumonitis, are far less common. Third,
people can suffer infections from some molds. The victims of these infections are
typically people with compromised immune systems, such as transplant patients,

people on chemotherapy, or people with infections such as HIV. Aspergillosis, caused by *Aspergillus*, is the best known example of such an infection.

A mold problem is usually initially recognized by visual inspection—discolored patches on walls or other surfaces, sometimes with a fuzzy texture—or by the musty smell that often accompanies mold. It is possible to measure mold growth in buildings and to identify the species that are growing, but the value of this measurement is unclear (Horner, Barnes, Codina, and Levetin, 2008), as any significant infestation needs to be cleaned up, irrespective of species.

There are two key actions for remediating a mold problem: cleaning up the mold that has accumulated and correcting the moisture problem that allowed the mold to grow in the first place. Limited patches of mold are cleaned up with materials such as detergent or bleach, but if mold has infiltrated more broadly—say, after a major flood—then entire sections of wall or other building components may need to be replaced. Preventing the formation of mold is key, and several guidelines exist: keeping the relative humidity between 40 and 60 percent; promptly correcting moisture sources such as leaky roofs, windows, and pipes; promptly cleaning up after flooding; and ventilating shower, laundry, and cooking areas (Warsco and Lindsey, 2003).

INDOOR AIR QUALITY

The quality of the air in a building can have a substantial impact on the people in that building (Samet and Spengler, 2003; Sundell, 2004). In schools, for example, there is evidence that indoor air contaminants can affect student health and performance both directly and indirectly (Daisey and others, 2003; Mendell and Heath, 2005). Many contaminants can undermine **indoor air quality**, including radon, tobacco smoke, carbon monoxide, and asbestos.

Radon is a colorless, odorless, radioactive gas that occurs naturally in the rock and soil of many parts of the world. When building foundations are sunk into the ground in such areas, radon can off-gas from the soil, enter the basement air, and go on to permeate the building air. In the 1980s, radon gained notoriety when media reports described a Pennsylvania home with such high radon levels that the resident, a nuclear power plant worker, set off alarms when he arrived at work. Data from underground miners and from case-control studies of lung cancer patients have established that radon exposure is a risk factor for lung cancer. Radon in buildings is readily managed; it can be measured inexpensively and relatively accurately, and ventilation can generally bring levels down to a range associated with very low risk (National Research Council, Committee on Health Risks of Exposure to Radon, 1998).

PERSPECTIVE
Indoor Air Pollution from Biomass Burning in Poor Countries

Buildings in developing nations and in wealthy nations pose very different sets of health challenges in several areas, including indoor air quality (Zhang and Smith, 2003). About half the world's population relies on **biomass fuel** for cooking and heating at home. Biomass, as explained in Chapter Thirteen, includes such materials as crop residues, animal dung, wood, and peat. In some parts of the world, such as China, coal is burned in homes. Often the stoves used are inefficient, burning at low temperatures; producing relatively large quantities of hydrocarbons, carbon monoxide, particulate matter, and other pollutants; and not venting these emissions to the outside. Studies from Africa (Rumchev, Spickett, Brown, and Mkhweli, 2007), China (Mestl and others, 2007), India (Sinha and others, 2006), and other parts of the world have documented extremely high levels of these contaminants in the indoor air of homes. In fact, the exposure to air pollutants at home can eclipse the exposure people sustain outside, even in polluted urban areas.

These exposures cause considerable morbidity. Indoor air pollution in developing nations has been implicated as a major cause of respiratory disease, especially in women and children whose home exposure is greatest (Smith, Samet, Romieu, and Bruce, 2000; Shrestha and Shrestha, 2005; Mishra, 2003; Peabody and others, 2005; Rumchev and others, 2007).

Many solutions have been proposed. Some are technological, such as using more efficient stoves and better stovepipes for improved ventilation; these are often out of reach economically. Other solutions focus on using cleaner fuel; as described in Chapter Thirteen, a shift to cleaner fuel often accompanies increasing prosperity. In the long run, an important challenge for environmental health in developing nations will be the provision of ample, clean fuel for cooking and heating.

Tobacco smoke is also a well recognized contaminant of indoor air in buildings in which people smoke—offices, homes, restaurants, and others. By the 1980s, epidemiologic research had established that this exposure increases the risk of cancer, cardiovascular disease, asthma and respiratory disease in children, and other adverse outcomes (U.S. Public Health Service, Office of the Surgeon General, 1986; National Research Council, Committee on Passive Smoking, 1986; Institute of Medicine, Committee on the Assessment of Asthma and Indoor Air, 2000; Nazaroff, 2004). Based on this evidence, a broad movement to limit or ban smoking in public places, including workplaces, restaurants, airports, and other buildings, has spread rapidly, representing a major public health success. Evidence suggests that such limits result in substantial reductions in exposure to tobacco smoke, and in corresponding health benefits (Fichtenberg and Glantz, 2002; Fong and others, 2006; Eisner, 2006; Koh and others, 2007).

Carbon monoxide is a unique indoor air contaminant. It can accumulate in buildings when combustion sources are present and the air is not adequately ventilated. One source, for example, is generators that burn diesel or other fuel in or near buildings, a common practice after disasters and when electric power is otherwise interrupted. Another, less common source of carbon monoxide exposure is the ice maintenance machines (called Zambonis) found at ice skating rinks. When inhaled, carbon monoxide bonds with hemoglobin in red blood cells, preventing these cells from transporting oxygen properly. Low levels of exposure can cause headaches, fatigue, and aggravation of ischemic heart disease, and high levels of exposure can be fatal. The best approach is prevention—preventing combustion from occurring in indoor spaces and ensuring plenty of ventilation when it does occur, so that dangerous levels of carbon monoxide cannot accumulate.

Asbestos has been recognized as a hazard for many decades (Figure 19.5). Until the 1970s it was widely used to insulate commercial buildings, schools, and homes and to manufacture building materials such as floor tiles. As a result, asbestos has emerged as an important indoor air contaminant. The initial approach to remediation, in the 1980s, was to remove the asbestos, a costly and sometimes dangerous job. More recently, in-place management through containment and encapsulation has gained more acceptance. A more recently recognized dimension of the asbestos problem relates to vermiculite, a fibrous insulating material contaminated by tremolite asbestos and other asbestos-like minerals. This material, marketed as Zonolite and also under other trade names, was used in millions of homes and commercial buildings. The associated risk has not yet been fully quantified.

TOXIC EXPOSURES

Lead is a well-recognized hazard. When ingested or inhaled, it can cause toxicity to the nervous and gastrointestinal systems and to the kidneys. Children are especially vulnerable, and even low levels of exposure can cause cognitive and behavioral abnormalities. Lead exposure has historically occurred in many ways—through inhalation of lead when it was used as a gasoline additive; ingestion of lead when it was used in tin cans, consumer goods, and medications; contamination of stills used to make moonshine; and workplace exposure in facilities such as battery factories. One of the major uses of lead in past years was as a component of paint, because it made the paint more durable. Although lead is

FIGURE 19.5   Deteriorating Asbestos Insulation Can Pose a Serious Health Hazard

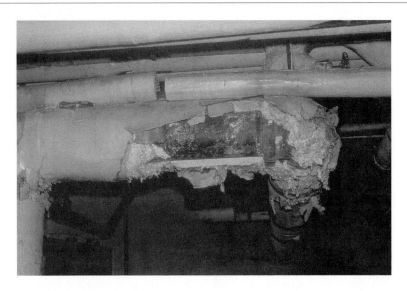

Source: © www.earldotter.com.

no longer used in paint, tens of millions of homes still contain lead-based paint; fortunately, this number is declining steadily (Jacobs and others, 2002). As lead-based paint breaks down over time, lead can be found in paint chips on window sills or other woodwork, in household dust, and in soil near the house. When older homes are renovated, large amounts of lead can be released.

In many ways the story of lead-based paint embodies of a public health success (Jacobs, Kelly, and Sobolewski, 2007). First, the science base was built. This included developing and validating methods for measuring lead in dust (Lanphear and others, 1995), and showing that lead-based paint and contaminated dust and soil were major pathways of childhood lead exposure (Lanphear and Roghmann, 1997; Lanphear and others, 1998). Remediation approaches were studied, and the most and least effective ones identified (Amitai, Graef, Brown, and Gerstle, 1987; Aschengrau and others, 1997; Charney, Kessler, Farfel, and Jackson, 1983). In addition, scientists and economists showed that the benefits of lead hazard control far outweighed the costs. Studies have estimated the benefits of eliminating lead-based paint hazards in housing to be as high as 221 times the cost, a highly favorable return on investment (U.S. Department of Housing and Urban Development, 1999; Gould, 2009).

All of this information was a powerful spur to a health-protective public policy involving standardized procedures for removing lead safely (U.S. Department of Housing and Urban Development, 1995); health-based exposure standards for paint, dust, and soil in housing undergoing remediation, renovation, or repainting (EPA, 2001); and a multiagency, ten-year plan that charted a course to eliminating lead-based paint hazards in houses (President's Task Force, 2000). Although this plan has not yet been fully implemented, and more remains to be done, the proportion of children with elevated levels of lead in their blood has continued to decline (Schwemberger and others, 2005).

Pesticides are commonly applied in buildings and can be a source of toxic exposures. Some classes of pesticides, such as organophosphates, are especially toxic, and others, such as pyrethroids, are less toxic. Solutions include choosing less toxic pesticides, applying them as sparingly as possible, and using other forms of pest control such as physical barriers and careful food storage techniques (often as part of an integrated pest management approach). (The health consequences of pesticide exposure and preventive approaches are discussed in Chapter Seventeen.)

Cleaning materials are commonly used in buildings. Three basic processes are used in cleaning: *mechanical* processes, such as sweeping and vacuuming; *chemical* processes, which employ substances such as detergents or ammonia to dissolve dirt or to create barriers (as stripping and waxing floors does); and *surface-abrasion* processes, such as burnishing. A study of janitorial practices in Santa Clara County, California, estimated that the average janitor uses twenty-eight gallons of chemicals per year, weighing 234 pounds; hazardous ingredients constituted about 25 percent of this total (Barron, Berg, and Bookman, 1999). The extent to which such materials are used in homes is not known. Examples of dangerous ingredients in cleaners are shown in Table 19.1.

There are many ways to reduce the risk associated with such chemicals. Dangerous chemicals can be replaced with safer ones. Cleaning procedures can be altered. For example, instead of cleaning on a rigid schedule, cleaning can be done only when conditions warrant. Similarly, cleaning can be scheduled during hours when other people are least likely to be present. Those who do the cleaning, such as janitors, can be trained in the careful use of chemicals. And steps can be taken to reduce the soiling of buildings, through such measures as wiping feet when entering, to reduce the frequency of needed cleaning. *Sick building syndrome* is a term applied to buildings in which symptoms seem to cluster—often in connection with suspected chemical exposures. This situation is described in the accompanying Perspective.

MENTAL HEALTH

Buildings may play an important role in mental health. Housing is at the center of this relationship. Although a *house* is simply a structure, the term *home* carries much more meaning. It suggests a source of permanence and continuity in a changing

TABLE 19.1   Hazardous Ingredients of Cleaners (Partial Listing)

Product Category	Hazardous Ingredients	Health Effects
Glass cleaners, general purpose cleaners, carpet spot removers	2-Butoxyethanol (ethylene glycol monobutyl ether)	Blood and liver toxicity; possible carcinogenicity.
Toilet cleaners	Acids (hydrochloric, phosphoric)	Acid burns.
Oven cleaners, heavy-duty degreasers	Lye (sodium hydroxide)	Lye burns.
Floor strippers	Ammonium hydroxide.	Skin, eye, and respiratory irritation and burns.
	Ethanolamine	Skin, eye, and respiratory irritation and burns; central nervous system toxicity.
	2-Butoxyethanol	Blood and liver toxicity; possible carcinogenicity.
Sanitizers, laundry whiteners	Bleach (sodium hypochlorite)	Skin and eye irritation. Mixing bleach with ammonia or acids can release highly toxic gases.
Metal polishes	Tetrachloroethylene, other volatile organic compounds	Central nervous system, liver, and kidney toxicity; carcinogenicity (some compounds).

Sources: Western Sustainability and Pollution Prevention Network, 2002; Ashkin and Ellis, 2006.

world; a setting for the establishment of predictable, comforting routines; a source of intergenerational support and help; and a place where people can feel in control and construct their identities—functions that together have been called *ontological security* (Dupuis and Thorns, 1998).

Specific features of buildings may also promote (or threaten) mental health. Crowding offers one example (Gove and Hughes, 1983). Crowding is not easy to define. As an objective measurement, crowding is the number of people per unit of area or the number of people per room, but there is no widely accepted density that defines crowding. As a subjective experience, crowding is marked by a feeling of inability to control interactions with other people or by interference with activities such as reading, conversing, or studying. Two hallmarks of crowding are loss of privacy and overstimulation.

Crowding is associated with psychological distress and dysfunction. In more crowded homes, parents are more critical of and less responsive to their children

PERSPECTIVE
Sick Building Syndrome

From time to time, people who share space in a building develop shared health complaints. Workers in an office building might develop irritation of the eyes, nose, and throat. Students in a school might develop headaches. Or guests in a hotel might develop respiratory disease. These and other illnesses are often called *building-related illnesses*. Health care providers and public health officials often need to evaluate such situations, to search for and control possible causes, and to treat the affected individuals.

In some cases, outbreaks of illness in a building can be traced to a specific cause. One example is legionellosis, an infectious disease caused by the gram-negative bacterium *Legionella pneumophila*. This organism was famously identified after a disease outbreak in a Philadelphia hotel during the 1976 American Legion convention. Legionella can colonize cooling towers, air-conditioning systems, hot water systems, and fountains, which explains why legionellosis can be a building-associated disease. Another cause of building-related illness is toxic exposures to such things as organic chemicals from roofing, cleaning, or other building activities.

But often no specific cause can be identified when illness clusters in a building. This situation is termed **sick building syndrome**. The hallmark of sick building syndrome is the presence of acute symptoms such as headache; eye, nose, or throat irritation; cough; dry or itchy skin; dizziness and nausea; difficulty in concentrating; fatigue; and sensitivity to odors. In general it is difficult to document the medical dysfunction with clinical testing or to identify a specific cause of the symptoms. Symptoms usually resolve promptly when people leave the building.

Although standard diagnosis may be difficult, investigation of sick buildings may reveal remediable problems. These may include air contaminants; malfunction of the heating, ventilating, and air-conditioning system; and problems in the social environment such as low job satisfaction, stress, and interpersonal conflict. Air sampling may seem an appealing approach, but it is costly and often uninformative.

Solutions generally include controlling any identified sources of air contaminants and making general improvements in building systems, including providing increased ventilation and perhaps air filtration. Education and communication are key, because sick building syndrome is typically accompanied by a high level of concern and even panic among those affected.

Sources: U.S. Environmental Protection Agency, Office of Air and Radiation . . . , 2008; Marmot and others, 2006; Brauer, Kolstad, Orbaek, and Mikkelsen, 2006a, 2006b.

(Bradley and Caldwell, 1984; Evans, Maxwell, and Hart, 1999), and children show more psychological distress (Evans, Saegert, and Harris, 2001). People who live in crowded conditions may show more aggressive behavior and social withdrawal (Regoeczi, 2003) or experience more interpersonal conflict within families (Evans, Lepore, Shejwal, and Palsane,1998; Saegert, 1982). Nor are such problems confined to the home. At school, children from crowded homes show more behavioral problems (Evans and others, 1998, 2001; Saegert, 1982), less motivation and less persistence with problem solving (Evans and others, 1998, 2001), and lower reading scores and more restricted vocabularies (Saegert, 1982). College students who feel crowded in their living situations perform less well in the classroom (Stokols, Ohlig, and Resnick, 1978). Crowding in schools can also contribute to dysfunction. Elementary students in more crowded classrooms have lower academic achievement (Weldon, Loewy, Winer, and Elkin, 1981), and less crowded schools enjoy improved attitudes about the school environment among both teachers and students and also show less faculty absenteeism (McCain and others, 2006).

Other features of buildings have been shown to affect mental health, some intuitive, such as being noisy (Lercher, Evans, Meis, and Kofler, 2002); and some less clear, such as being a high-rise building (Gifford, 2007) or having a relatively high level of moisture (Hopton and Hunt, 1996). (These factors may be proxies for other building conditions.) Overall, buildings that are in poor condition—especially housing units—seem to threaten mental health (Gifford and Lacombe, 2006). In one study (Evans and others, 2000), investigators identified and measured these aspects of housing quality:

- Cleanliness/clutter
- Privacy
- Presence or absence of hazards
- Structural quality
- Child resources, such as play areas and child care

They found that better housing quality predicted less psychological distress (as measured with the Demoralization Index of the Psychiatric Epidemiology Research Instrument).

UNIVERSAL DESIGN

Certain features of building design can pose barriers to some people. For example, people with poor vision have difficulty with dim lighting, elderly people have difficulty with stairs, and people who use wheelchairs have difficulty with narrow doorways. As described in Chapter Twenty-Five, children are especially vulnerable to some exposures, and this is true in homes, schools, and other buildings (Breysse and others, 2004). Observations such as these gave rise to the concept of **universal design**, which the Center for Universal Design (1997) defines as the "design of products and environments to be usable by all people, to the greatest extent possible, without the need for adaptation or specialized design." The principles of universal design are listed in Exhibit 14.2 in Chapter Fourteen. The accompanying Perspective, "Building Design for the Elderly," describes a particular instance of good design.

PERSPECTIVE
Building Design for the Elderly

As the population ages, more and more elderly people need buildings designed to protect them against risk factors and to help them thrive and function optimally. One challenge is mobility limitations. Design principles include having an outside entrance that requires neither steps nor a ramp, placing all the basics (kitchen, bathroom, bedroom) on the first floor to obviate the need to climb stairs, and widening hallways and doorways to allow easy passage of wheelchairs. Good lighting is important because many elderly people experience decreased visual acuity. Light switches should be positioned so as to avoid the need to walk through darkened areas, and fixtures should be installed within easy reach (say, mounted on walls instead of on ceilings) for changing light bulbs. Fall prevention is also important, given the high risk of falls in the elderly. Additional design principles include

- Minimizing changes in walking surfaces
- Using slip-resistant surfaces, such as rough tile and carpet with short, dense pile
- Installing handrails on both sides of stairs
- Installing secure grab bars in tubs and showers and near toilets
- Minimizing the use of extension cords and other trip hazards

These principles can be applied not only in private homes and apartments but also in nursing homes and other facilities where the elderly reside and in hotels, libraries, and other facilities that serve elderly visitors. Many of these principles are part of universal design, so other groups of people may benefit from these design principles as well.

Sources: Bakker, 1997; Mitka, 2001; Rollins, 2000.

TOWARD SAFE, HEALTHY BUILDINGS

As in much of the environmental health field, many strategies exist for promoting health in buildings. Some are policies that may be implemented, others are technical or environmental solutions, and still others are behavioral.

Public policies that ensure safe, healthy buildings are elusive. For some environmental health challenges—say, outdoor air pollution (as described in Chapter Twelve)—there are specific laws, dedicated agencies, and clear strategies to protect health. But for buildings this is not the case. No agencies at the federal, state, or local levels have overall responsibility for conditions in homes, schools, or health care facilities. (Certain specific issues, such as elevator safety, are assigned to agencies.) Jacobs and others (2007) note the lack of concerted public action for indoor air quality in homes and suggest that this has come about because "there is not a perceived Shared Common for which the public feels a communal benefit and responsibility"—in contrast to, say, public concern over outdoor air pollution. In some cases nongovernmental organizations offer guidance. For example, the American National Standards Institute (ANSI) and the American Society of Heating, Refrigerating, and Air-Conditioning Engineers (ASHRAE) publish standards for ventilation to achieve acceptable indoor air quality (American Society of Heating, Refrigerating, and Air-Conditioning Engineers, 2007), and many in government and industry use these standards as a benchmark. (The For Further Information section at the end of this chapter identifies other organizations that promote healthy homes, schools, and health care facilities.)

Many local public health departments have initiated *healthy homes* programs to promote interventions that protect health and safety in residences. These are collaborative efforts because the public health agencies must work in concert with housing authorities, homeowners and landlords, environmental agencies, and others. A cardinal feature of these programs is their cross-cutting agendas. Community health workers who visit homes are typically equipped to assess a wide range of housing conditions, including asthma triggers, moisture and mold, lead and other chemical exposures, safety measures such as smoke detectors, and more (Krieger and Higgins, 2002; Krieger and others, 2002). Popular sources of information, such as handbooks, assist families wishing to make their homes healthy (Bower, 2000; CDC and HUD, 2006).

In recent years the science base that guides public health protection in buildings has expanded considerably (Matte and Jacobs, 2000; Thomson, Pettigrew, and Morison, 2001; Krieger and Higgins, 2002; Saegert and others, 2003; Sandel and others, 2004; Wu and others, 2007; Zimring and Bosch, 2008; Rashid and Zimring, 2008; Ulrich and others, 2008). Several conclusions emerge from this work. First, many solutions are well understood and empirically supported. Second, few solutions are as simple as they seem; even the most straightforward approach can have hidden costs and risks. Third, many approaches can be bundled to achieve greater public health impact more efficiently. Fourth, environmental interventions are often combined with other approaches, such as education, policy change, and so on. Fifth, many interventions do more than protect health and safety; they can be economical, environmentally friendly, and aesthetically pleasing. Examples of these features are shown in Table 19.2.

ARCHITECTURE, ENVIRONMENT, AND HUMAN HEALTH

Neighborhood Context

This chapter discusses buildings, rather than the larger scale of neighborhoods, communities, and cities. However, there is no sharp line separating the two. Buildings exist in a context, and the impacts of buildings on health may stem both from features of the buildings themselves and from what surrounds the buildings. One example of applying this idea is the *broken windows* theory, which holds that signs of disorder in a community—broken windows, graffiti, untended yards, and so on, some evident in buildings and others on the neighborhood scale—predict uncivil behavior and poor health (Wilson and Kelling, 1982; Cohen and others, 2000). Another example comes from studies of people who have moved from poor housing in poor neighborhoods to better housing in neighborhoods with higher incomes (Orr and others, 2003; Acevedo-Garcia and others, 2004). Although the evidence base is limited, it appears that such moves improve health. The features of a healthy home can be reinforced when the surrounding community provides opportunities for routine physical activity, nearby destinations such as shopping and schools, clean air, nearby parks and green space, and similar assets. (These topics are discussed in Chapter Fourteen.)

Green Building

Green building (also known as sustainable or high-performance building), according to the EPA (2009), is "the practice of creating structures and using processes that are environmentally responsible and resource-efficient throughout a building's life-cycle from siting to design, construction, operation, maintenance, renovation and deconstruction." As this definition suggests, green building arose from the intersection of building science and environmental concerns. The principal components of green building are

TABLE 19.2 Approaches to Protecting Health and Safety in Buildings

Goal	Strategies	Comments
Reducing asthma triggers in homes	Placing impermeable covers on mattresses and pillows Treating carpets and bedding with acaricides (to eliminate dust mites) Using air filtration Removing old carpets and bedding Intensive cleaning and extermination (to eliminate cockroaches) Installing central ventilation and humidity control	Many trials show little or no success. Success tends to depend on using multiple strategies. Additional benefit of education on home maintenance and asthma care.
Reducing lead exposure in homes	Removing (abatement) or encapsulating of lead-containing paint Replacing windows and door frames Repainting deteriorated paint Using professional dust control	Strong evidence for reducing dust lead levels, but less evidence for reducing blood lead. Incorrect abatement techniques can increase exposure. Additional benefit of education regarding hygiene.
Controlling injuries in homes, day-care facilities, and nursing homes	Installing smoke alarms Installing window guards (to prevent falls, especially among children) Reducing hot water temperature (to prevent scalds) Using radiator covers (to prevent burns) Improving lighting (to prevent falls, especially among the elderly) Putting visual cues on floors, such as tile patterns (to prevent falls, especially among the elderly)	Demonstrated benefit of home visits with counseling. Benefit of addressing multiple injury risks. Different risks for children and the elderly.
Reducing mold and moisture	Repairing leaks Replacing water-damaged materials (walls, carpets, and so forth) Maintaining optimal humidity	

(continued)

TABLE 19.2   (Continued)

Goal	Strategies	Comments
Reducing stress, infection, and medical errors in health care facilities	Installing effective air quality control Having hand-washing stations at key locations Using easy-to-clean floor, wall, and furniture coverings Having single-bed, acuity-adaptable rooms Using natural lighting, with views of nature Putting noise-absorbing materials on ceilings and walls Planting hospital gardens	Measures are designed to benefit both patients and health care workers.
Reducing pesticide exposure	Applying integrated pest management (see Chapter Seventeen)	

- Appropriate site selection
- Energy efficiency and renewable energy
- Water efficiency
- Environmentally preferable building materials and specifications
- Waste reduction
- Toxics reduction
- Good indoor air quality

The design and architecture fields are displaying a growing interest in green building. A prime example is **LEED (Leadership in Energy and Environmental Design)**, an initiative of the U.S. Green Building Council. To encourage the adoption of sustainable green building practices, LEED provides specific performance criteria for such issues as site selection, water management, and energy systems. It also offers a certification process that measures building sustainability. LEED criteria are available for many categories of buildings, such as homes, commercial buildings, schools, and retail stores.

Increasingly, there is also recognition that aspects of green building offer public health benefits. Some of these are direct; for example, reducing pesticide use in favor of integrated pest management reduces exposure to potentially toxic chemicals. Other benefits are indirect; for example, a more energy efficient building draws less electricity from power plants, helping to reduce air pollution and making fewer contributions to climate change (and thus reducing health threats). A growing literature offers advice on green design and construction for homes (Yudelson, 2008; Baker-Laporte, Elliott, and Banta, 2008), schools (Karliner, 2005; National Research Council, 2007; U.S. Green Building Council, 2008), and health care facilities (Purves, 2002; Frumkin and Coussens, 2007; Guenther and Vittori, 2007).

Biophilic Design

Biophilic design is another way in which architecture intersects with human health and well-being. Biophilic design is based on the theory of *biophilia*—the notion that humans have an affinity with nature, as described in Chapter Twenty-Four. This leads to the concept of *restorative design*—the idea that if buildings embody natural design elements, they can offer people the same kind of restorative experience that occurs with nature contact. Biophilic design includes an organic (or naturalistic) dimension—shapes and forms that reflect the human affinity for nature—and a place-based (or vernacular) dimension—design that connects to the culture and ecology of a locale. Examples of such design elements include natural materials such as wood, stone and clay; water features; natural daylight; botanical and animal motifs; and building shapes that fit into the landscape. Increasing evidence suggests that buildings with such features offer health benefits to the people who live, work, and study in them (Knowles, 2006; Kellert, Heerwagen, and Madoe, 2008).

SUMMARY

Much of modern life is lived indoors—in homes, schools, workplaces, and other specialized settings, such as health care facilities. The conditions in buildings therefore have great potential to affect health, well-being, and comfort. Ambient conditions such as lighting, crowding, and air quality; injury risks such as fall and burn hazards; exposure to such hazards as toxins and mold; and even the less tangible aesthetic qualities of buildings, may all play an important role.

Not everybody is equally affected by buildings. People with disabilities, the elderly, and people living in substandard housing are examples of populations with specific vulnerabilities and needs. Efforts to provide safe, healthy, and accessible buildings need to take these needs into account.

Many techniques are available to achieve safe, healthy buildings, building on many of the core tools of public health. These range from design decisions, such as installing wide doorways to permit mobility, to primary preventive strategies, such as lead paint removal, to maintenance and to such devices as carbon monoxide detectors and smoke alarms. In some cases these strategies dovetail with green strategies designed for environmental performance. Such co-benefits are welcome, as they help us to achieve health and environmental goals simultaneously.

KEY TERMS

asbestos

bioaerosols

biomass fuel

biophilic design

carbon monoxide

cleaning materials

daylight

green building

indoor air quality

lead

LEED (Leadership in Energy and Environmental Design)

lighting

manufactured homes

manufactured structures

modular classrooms

moisture and mold

pesticides

park models

radon

sick building syndrome

stachybotrys

tobacco smoke

travel trailers

universal design

DISCUSSION QUESTIONS

1. Why is outdoor air quality regulated more effectively than indoor air quality?
2. Examine your own home taking a public health perspective. Can you identify at least three hazards? How would you correct them?
3. Why might children and the elderly face different injury risks in buildings?
4. People with disabilities face special challenges in buildings and may need various accommodations to ensure access, health, and safety. What is the concept of universal design, and how does it address these challenges? Also discuss three accommodations that may be needed.
5. Promoting health, protecting the environment, and saving money can be highly compatible goals when designing and operating buildings, but sometimes these goals are in opposition. Describe a situation in which trade-offs among these goals are necessary, and explain how you would handle the situation.

REFERENCES

Acevedo-Garcia, D., and others. "Does Housing Mobility Policy Improve Health?" *Housing Policy Debate*. http://www.fanniemaefoundation.org/programs/hpd/pdf/hpd_1501_Acevedo .pdf, 2004.

Alexander, C., and others. *A Pattern Language*. New York: Oxford University Press, 1977.

American Academy of Pediatrics. "Falls from Heights: Windows, Roofs, and Balconies." *Pediatrics*, 2001, *107*, 1188–1191.

American Society of Heating, Refrigerating, and Air-Conditioning Engineers. *Ventilation for Acceptable Indoor Air Quality*. ANSI/ASHRAE 62.1–2007. Washington, D.C.: American National Standards Institute and American Society of Heating, Refrigerating, and Air-Conditioning Engineers, 2007.

Amitai, Y., Graef, J. W., Brown, M. J., and Gerstle, R. S. "Hazards of Deleading Homes of Children with Lead Poisoning." *American Journal of Diseases of Children*, 1987, *141*, 758–760.

Ander, G. D. *Daylighting Performance and Design*. Hoboken, N.J.: Wiley, 2003.

Aschengrau, A., and others. "Residential Lead Paint Hazard Remediation and Soil Lead Abatement: Their Impact Among Children with Mildly Elevated Blood Lead Levels." *American Journal of Public Health*, 1997, *87*, 1698–1702.

Ashkin, S., and Ellis, R. "Cleaning Materials and Methods." In H. Frumkin, R. J. Geller, I. L., Rubin, and J. Nodvin (eds.), *Safe and Healthy School Environments* (pp. 169–188), New York: Oxford University Press, 2006.

Baker-Laporte, P., Elliott, E., and Banta, J. *Prescriptions for a Healthy House: A Practical Guide for Architects, Builders & Homeowners*. (3rd ed.) Gabriola Island, B.C.: New Society, 2008.

Bakker, R. *Elder Design: Designing and Furnishing a Home for Your Later Years*. New York: Penguin, 1997.

Ballesteros, M. F., Jackson, M. L., and Martin, M. W. "Working Toward the Elimination of Residential Fire Deaths: The Centers for Disease Control and Prevention's Smoke Alarm Installation and Fire Safety Education (SAIFE) Program." *Journal of Burn Care and Rehabilitation* 2005; *26*(5):434–439.

Barron, T., Berg, C., and Bookman, L. *How to Select and Use Safe Janitorial Chemicals*. Janitorial Products Pollution Prevention Project. http://www.wrppn.org/Janitorial/05%20Report.pdf, Dec. 1999.

Bennett, J. W., and Klich, M. "Mycotoxins." *Clinical Microbiology Reviews*, 2003, *16*, 497–516.

Boubekri, M. *Daylighting, Architecture and Health: Building Design Strategies*. Burlington, Mass.: Elsevier, Architectural Press, 2008.

Bower, L. M. *Creating a Healthy Household*. Bloomington, Ind.: Healthy House Institute, 2000.

Bradley, R. H., and Caldwell, M. "The HOME Inventory and Family Demographics." *Developmental Psychology*, 1984, *20*, 315–320.

Brasche, S., and Bischof, W. "Daily Time Spent Indoors in German Homes—Baseline Data for the Assessment of Indoor Exposure of German Occupants." *International Journal of Hygiene and Environmental Health*, 2005, *208*(4), 247–253.

Brauer, C., Kolstad, H., Orbaek, P., and Mikkelsen, S. "No Consistent Risk Factor Pattern for Symptoms Related to the Sick Building Syndrome: A Prospective Population Based Study." *International Archives of Occupational and Environmental Health*, 2006a, *79*(6), 453–464.

Brauer, C., Kolstad, H., Orbaek, P., and Mikkelsen, S. "The Sick Building Syndrome: A Chicken and Egg Situation?" *International Archives of Occupational and Environmental Health*, 2006b, *79*(6), 465–471.

Breysse, P., and others. "The Relationship Between Housing and Health: Children at Risk." *Environmental Health Perspectives*, 2004, *112*, 1583–1588.

Buchanan, A. H. *Structural Design for Fire Safety*. Hoboken, N.J.: Wiley, 2001.

Bush, R. K., and others. "The Medical Effects of Mold Exposure." *Journal of Allergy and Clinical Immunology*, 2006, *117*, 326–333.

California Energy Commission. *Windows and Offices: A Study of Worker Performance and the Indoor Environment*. Technical Report P500–03–082-A-9. White Salmon, Wash.: New Buildings Institute, 2003.

Center for Universal Design. *The Principles of Universal Design, Version 2.0*. North Carolina State University. http://design.ncsu.edu/cud/about_ud/udprinciplestext.htm, 1997.

Centers for Disease Control and Prevention. "Carbon monoxide exposures—United States, 1999–2004." *Morbidity and Mortality Weekly Report*, 2007, *56*(50), 1309–1312.

Centers for Disease Control and Prevention. *Final Report on Formaldehyde Levels in FEMA-Supplied Travel Trailers, Park Models, and Mobile Homes*. http://www.cdc.gov/nceh/ehhe/trailerstudy/pdfs/FEMAFinalReport.pdfs, 2008.

Centers for Disease Control and Prevention and U.S. Department of Housing and Urban Development. *Healthy Housing Reference Manual*. Atlanta: U.S. Department of Health and Human Services, 2006.

Chang, J. T., and others. "Interventions for the Prevention of Falls in Older Adults: Systematic Review and Meta-Analysis of Randomised Clinical Trials." *British Medical Journal*, 2004, *328*(7441), 680.

Chaney, B., Lewis, L. *Public School Principals Report on Their School Facilities: Fall 2005* (NCES 2007–007). Washington: U.S. Department of Education, National Center for Education Statistics, 2007.

Charney, E., Kessler, B., Farfel, M., and Jackson, D. "A Controlled Trial of the Effect of Dust-Control Measures on Blood Lead Levels." *New England Journal of Medicine*, 1983, *309*, 1089–1093.

Cohen, D., and others. "'Broken Windows' and the Risk of Gonorrhea." *American Journal of Public Health*, 2000, *90*, 230–236.

Coussement, J., and others. "Interventions for Preventing Falls in Acute- and Chronic-Care Hospitals: A Systematic Review and Meta-Analysis." *Journal of the American Geriatrics Society*, 2008, *56*(1), 29–36.

Daisey, J. M., Angell, W. J., and Apte, M. G. "Indoor Air Quality, Ventilation, and Health Symptoms in Schools: An Analysis of Existing Information." *Indoor Air*, 2003, *13*, 53–64.

de Botton, A. *The Architecture of Happiness*. New York: Pantheon, 2006.

Dunn, J. R. "Housing and Inequalities in Health: A Study of Socioeconomic Dimensions of Housing and Self-Reported Health from a Survey of Vancouver Residents." *Journal of Epidemiology and Community Health*, 2002, *56*, 671–682.

Dupuis, A., and Thorns, D. C. "Home, Home Ownership and the Search for Ontological Security." *The Sociological Review*, 1998, *46*, 24–47.

Eisner, M. D. "Banning Smoking in Public Places: Time to Clear the Air." *JAMA*, 2006, *296*, 1778–1779.

Evans, G. W., Lepore, S. J., Shejwal, B. R., and Palsane, M. N. "Chronic Residential Crowding and Children's Well-Being: An Ecological Perspective." *Child Development*, 1998, *69*, 1514–1523.

Evans, G. W., Maxwell, L. M., and Hart, B. "Parental Language and Verbal Responsiveness to Children in Crowded Homes." *Developmental Psychology*, 1999, *35*, 1020–1023.

Evans, G. W., Saegert, S., and Harris, R. "Residential Density and Psychological Health Among Children in Low-Income Families." *Environment and Behavior*, 2001, *33*, 165–180.

Evans, G. W., Wells, N. M., Chan, H.-Y. E., and Saltzman, H. "Housing Quality and Mental Health." *Journal of Consulting and Clinical Psychology*, 2000, *68*, 526–530.

Fichtenberg, C. M., and Glantz, S. A. "Effect of Smoke-Free Workplaces on Smoking Behaviour: Systematic Review." *British Medical Journal*. 2002, *325*, 188–191.

Fong, G. T., and others. "Reductions in Tobacco Smoke Pollution and Increases in Support for Smoke-Free Public Places Following the Implementation of Comprehensive Smoke-Free Workplace Legislation in the Republic of Ireland: Findings from the ITC Ireland/UK Survey." *Tobacco Control*, 2006, *15*(suppl. 3), iii51–iii58.

Frumkin, H., and Coussens, C. *Green Healthcare Institutions: Health, Environment and Economics*. Washington, D.C.: National Academies Press, 2007.

Frumkin, H., Geller, R. J., Rubin, I. L., and Nodvin, J. (eds.). *Safe and Healthy School Environments*. New York: Oxford University Press, 2006.

Gates, S., and others. "Multifactorial Assessment and Targeted Intervention for Preventing Falls and Injuries Among Older People in Community and Emergency Care Settings: Systematic Review and Meta-Analysis." *British Medical Journal*, 2008, *336*, 130–133.

Gifford, R. "The Consequences of Living in High-Rise Buildings." *Architectural Science Review* 2007, *50*, 2–17.

Gifford, R., and Lacombe, C. "Housing Quality and Children's Socioemotional Health." *Journal of Housing and the Built Environment*, 2006, *21*, 177–189.

Godwin, C., and Batterman, S. "Indoor Air Quality in Michigan Schools." *Indoor Air*, 2007, *17*, 109–121.

Gould, E. Childhood Lead Poisoning: Conservative Estimates of the Social and Economic Benefits of Lead Hazard Control. *Environmental Health Perspectives* 2009, *117*, 1162–67.

Gove, W. R., and Hughes, M. *Overcrowding in the Household: An Analysis of Determinants and Effects*. San Diego: Academic Press, 1983.

Guenther, R., and Vittori, G. *Sustainable Healthcare Architecture*. Hoboken, N.J.: Wiley, 2007.

Guzowski, M. *Daylighting for Sustainable Design*. New York: McGraw-Hill, 2000.

Hall, J. R., Jr. *U.S. Experience with Sprinklers and Other Fire Extinguishing Equipment*. National Fire Protection Association. http://www.nfpa.org/assets/files/PDF/OSsprinklers.pdf, June 2007.

Heschong Mahone Group. *Daylighting in Schools: An Investigation into the Relationship Between Daylighting and Human Performance*. HMG Project No. 9803. San Francisco: Pacific Gas and Electric, 1999.

Hopton, J. L., and Hunt, S. M. "Housing Conditions and Mental Health in a Disadvantaged Area in Scotland." *Journal of Epidemiology and Community Health*, 1996, *50*, 56–61.

Horner, W. E., Barnes, C., Codina, R., and Levetin, E. "Guide for Interpreting Reports from Inspections/Investigations of Indoor Mold." *Journal of Allergy and Clinical Immunology*, 2008, *121*(3), 592–597.

Howden-Chapman, P. "Housing Standards: A Glossary of Housing and Health." *Journal of Epidemiology and Community Health*, 2004, *58*, 162–168.

Hyder, A. A., Sugerman, D., Ameratunga, S., and Callaghan, J. A. "Falls Among Children in the Developing World: A Gap in Child Health Burden Estimations?" *Acta Paediatrica*, 2007, *96*(10), 1394–1398.

Institute of Medicine, Committee on Damp Indoor Spaces and Health, Board on Health Promotion and Disease Prevention. *Damp Indoor Spaces and Health.* Washington, D.C.: National Academies Press, 2004.

Institute of Medicine, Committee on the Assessment of Asthma and Indoor Air. *Clearing the Air: Asthma and Indoor Air Exposures.* Washington, D.C.: National Academies Press, 2000.

Jacobs, D. E., Kelly, T., and Sobolewski, J. "Linking Public Health, Housing, and Indoor Environmental Policy: Successes and Challenges at Local and Federal Agencies in the United States." *Environmental Health Perspectives*, 2007, *115*, 976–982.

Jacobs, D. E., and others. "The Prevalence of Lead-Based Paint Hazards in U.S. Housing." *Environmental Health Perspectives*, 2002, *110*, A599–A606.

Karliner, J. *The Little Green Schoolhouse: Thinking Big About Ecological Sustainability, Children's Environmental Health and K-12 Education in the USA.* http://www.greenschools.net/greenschools.pdf, 2005.

Keane, C. "Ceiling Collapses in Third Floor Science Wing. Sewanhaka High School Students, Staff Evacuated." *Floral Park Dispatch.* http://www.antonnews.com/floralparkdispatch/2003/03/07/news, Mar. 7, 2003.

Kellert, S.R., Heerwagen, J., and Mador, M. *Biophilic Design: The Theory, Science and Practice of Bringing Buildings to Life.* New York: Wiley, 2008.

Knowles, R. L. *Ritual House: Drawing on Nature's Rhythms for Architecture and Urban Design.* Washington, D.C.: Island Press, 2006.

Koh, H. K., Joossens, L. X., and Connolly, G. N. "Making Smoking History Worldwide." *New England Journal of Medicine*, 2007, *356*(15), 1496–1498.

Krieger, J., and Higgins, D. L. "Housing and Health: Time Again for Public Health Action." *American Journal of Public Health*, 2002, *92*, 758–768.

Krieger, J., and others. "The Seattle-King County Healthy Homes Project: Implementation of a Comprehensive Approach to Improving Indoor Environmental Quality for Low-Income Children with Asthma." *Environmental Health Perspectives*, 2002, *110*(suppl. 2), 311–322.

Lanphear, B. P., and Roghmann, K. J. "Pathways of Lead Exposure in Urban Children." *Environmental Research*, 1997, *74*, 67–73.

Lanphear, B. P., and others. "A Side-By-Side Comparison of Dust Collection Methods for Sampling Lead-Contaminated House Dust." *Environmental Research*, 1995, *68*, 114–123.

Lanphear, B. P., and others. "The Contribution of Lead-Contaminated House Dust and Residential Soil to Children's Blood Lead Levels: A Pooled Analysis of 12 Epidemiological Studies." *Environmental Research*, 1998, *79*, 51–68.

Leech, J. A., and others. "It's About Time: A Comparison of Canadian and American Time-Activity Patterns." *Journal of Exposure Analysis and Environmental Epidemiology*, 2002, *12*, 427–432.

Lercher, P., Evans, G. W., Meis, M., and Kofler, W. W. "Ambient Neighbourhood Noise and Children's Mental Health." *Occupational and Environmental Medicine*, 2002, *59*(6), 380–386.

Lowry, S. "Housing." *British Medical Journal*, 1991, *303*(6806), 838–840.

Mallonee, S., and others. "Surveillance and Prevention of Residential-Fire Injuries." *New England Journal of Medicine*, 1996, *335*, 27–31.

Mann, A. "Mold in Schools: A Health Alert." *USA Weekend.* http://www.usaweekend.com/00_issues/000820/000820mold.html, Aug. 20, 2000.

Marberry, S. O. (ed.). *Improving Healthcare with Better Building Design.* Chicago: Health Administration Press, 2006.

Marmot, A. F., and others. "Building Health: An Epidemiological Study of 'Sick Building Syndrome' in the Whitehall II Study." *Occupational and Environmental Medicine*, 2006, *63*(4), 283–289.

Matte, T. D., and Jacobs, D. E. "Housing and Health—Current Issues and Implications for Research and Programs." *Journal of Urban Health*, 2000, *77*, 7–25.

McCain, G., and others. "Some Effects of Reduction of Extra-Classroom Crowding in a School Environment." *Journal of Applied Social Psychology*, 2006, *15*(6), 503–515.

Mendell, M. J. "Indoor Residential Chemical Emissions as Risk Factors for Respiratory and Allergic Effects in Children: A Review." *Indoor Air*, 2007, *17*, 259–277.

Mendell, M. J., and Heath, G. A. "Do Indoor Pollutants and Thermal Conditions in Schools Influence Student Performance? A Critical Review of the Literature." *Indoor Air*, 2005, *15*, 27–52.

Mestl, H. E., and others. "Urban and Rural Exposure to Indoor Air Pollution from Domestic Biomass and Coal Burning Across China." *Science of the Total Environment*, 2007, *377*(1), 12–26.

Mishra, V. "Indoor Air Pollution from Biomass Combustion and Acute Respiratory Illness in Preschool Age Children in Zimbabwe." *International Journal of Epidemiology*, 2003, *32*(5), 847–853.

Mitka, M. "Home Modifications to Make Older Lives Easier." *JAMA*, 2001, *286*, 1699–1700.

Nagaraja, J., and others. "Deaths from Residential Injuries in U.S. Children and Adolescents, 1985–1997." *Pediatrics*, 2005, *116*, 454–461.

National Fire Protection Association. *The U.S. Fire Problem.* http://www.nfpa.org, 2006.

National Center for Education Statistics. *Condition of America's Public School Facilities: 1999.* http://nces.ed.gov/surveys/frss/publications/2000032, 2000.

National Research Council. *Green Schools: Attributes for Health and Learning.* Washington: National Academies Press, 2007.

National Research Council, Committee on Health Risks of Exposure to Radon, *Health Effects of Exposure to Radon (BEIR VI).* http://books.nap.edu/html/beir6, 1998.

National Research Council, Committee on Passive Smoking. *Environmental Tobacco Smoke: Measuring Exposures and Assessing Health Risks.* Washington: National Academies Press, 1986.

Nazaroff, W. W. "Inhalation of Hazardous Air Pollutants from Environmental Tobacco Smoke in US Residences." *Journal of Exposure Analysis and Environmental Epidemiology*, 2004, *14*(suppl. 1), S71–S77.

Okoben, J. "Roof Collapse Danger Closes Cleveland School." *Cleveland Plain Dealer*, Jan. 6, 2006, p. B1.

Orr, L., and others. *Moving to Opportunity for Fair Housing Demonstration: Interim Impacts Evaluation.* U.S. Department of Housing and Urban Development, Office of Policy Development and Research. http://www.huduser.org/publications/fairhsg/mtoFinal.html, 2003.

Peabody, J. W., and others. "Indoor Air Pollution in Rural China: Cooking Fuels, Stoves, and Health Status." *Archives of Environmental & Occupational Health*, 2005, *60*(2), 86–95.

Phalen, K. J., Khoury, J., Kalkwarf, H., and Lanphear, B. P. "Residential Injuries in U.S. Children and Adolescents." *Public Health Reports*, 2005, *120*, 63–70.

President's Task Force on Environmental Health Risks and Safety Risks to Children. *Eliminating Childhood Lead Poisoning: A Federal Strategy Targeting Lead Paint Hazards.* http://www.cdc.gov/nceh/lead/about/fedstrategy2000.pdf, 2000.

Purkiss, J. A. *Fire Safety Engineering: Design of Structures.* (2nd ed.) Boston: Butterworth-Heinemann, 2006.

Purves, G. *Healthy Living Centres: A Guide to Primary Health Care Design.* Oxford, U.K.: Architectural Press, 2002.

Rashid, M., and Zimring, C. "A Review of the Empirical Literature on the Relationships Between Indoor Environment and Stress in Health Care and Office Settings: Problems and Prospects of Sharing Evidence." *Environment and Behavior,* 2008, *40,* 151–190.

Regoeczi, W. C. "When Context Matters: A Multilevel Analysis of Household and Neighborhood Crowding on Aggression and Withdrawal." *Journal of Environmental Psychology,* 2003, *23,* 457–470.

Rollins, G. *Designs on Building Safe Homes for the Elderly.* National Safety Council. http://www.nsc.org/resources/issues/articles/fallfalls.aspx, 2000.

Rosenstreich, D. L., and others. "The Role of Cockroach Allergy and Exposure to Cockroach Allergen in Causing Morbidity Among Inner-City Children with Asthma." *New England Journal of Medicine,* 1997, *336,* 1356–1363.

Rubenstein, L. Z., and Josephson, K. R. "Falls and Their Prevention in Elderly People: What Does the Evidence Show?" *Medical Clinics of North America,* 2006, *90*(5), 807–824.

Rumchev, K., Spickett, J. T., Brown, H. L., and Mkhweli, B. "Indoor Air Pollution from Biomass Combustion and Respiratory Symptoms of Women and Children in a Zimbabwean Village." *Indoor Air,* 2007, *17*(6), 468–474.

Runyan, C. W., and Casteel, C. (eds.). *The State of Home Safety in America: Facts About Unintentional Injuries in the Home.* (2nd ed.) Home Safety Council. http://homesafetycouncil.org/state_of_home_safety/sohs_2004_p017.pdf, 2004.

Saegert, S. "Environment and Children's Mental Health: Residential Density and Low Income Children." In A. Baum and J. E. Singer (eds.), *Handbook of Psychology and Health.* Vol. 2 (pp. 247–281). Mahwah, N.J.: Erlbaum, 1982.

Saegert, S. C., and others. "Healthy Housing: A Structured Review of Published Evaluations of US Interventions to Improve Health by Modifying Housing in the United States, 1990–2001." *American Journal of Public Health,* 2003, *93,* 1471–1477.

Samet, J. M., and Spengler, J. D. "Indoor Environments and Health: Moving into the 21st Century." *American Journal of Public Health,* 2003, *93,* 1489–1493.

Sandel, M., and others. "The Effects of Housing Interventions on Child Health." *Pediatric Annals,* 2004, *33,* 474–481.

Schwemberger, J. G., and others. "Blood Lead Levels—United States, 1999–2002." *Morbidity and Mortality Weekly Report,* 2005, *54*(20), 513–516.

Seltzer, J. M., and Fedoruk, M. J. "Health Effects of Mold in Children." *Pediatric Clinics of North America,* 2007, *54*(2), 309–333.

Shendell, D. G., Winer, A. M., Weker, R., Colome, S. D. "Evidence of Inadequate Ventilation in Portable Classrooms: Results of a Pilot Study in Los Angeles County." *Indoor Air* 2004, *14,* 154–158.

Shendell, D. G., and others. "Air Concentrations of VOCs in Portable and Traditional Classrooms: Results of a Pilot Study in Los Angeles County." *Journal of Exposure Analysis and Environmental Epidemiology* 2004, *14,* 44–59.

Shrestha, I. L., and Shrestha, S. L. "Indoor Air Pollution from Biomass Fuels and Respiratory Health of the Exposed Population in Nepalese Households." *International Journal of Occupational and Environmental Health*, 2005, *11*(2), 150–160.

Sinha, S. N., and others. "Environmental Monitoring of Benzene and Toluene Produced in Indoor Air Due to Combustion of Solid Biomass Fuels." *Science of the Total Environment*, 2006, *357*(1–3), 280–287.

Smith, K. R., Samet, J. M., Romieu, I., and Bruce, N. "Indoor Air Pollution in Developing Countries and Acute Lower Respiratory Infections in Children." *Thorax*, 2000, *55*(6), 518–532.

Stokols, D., Ohlig, W., and Resnick, S. M. "Perception of Residential Crowding, Classroom Experiences, and Student Health." *Human Ecology*, 1978, *6*, 233–252.

Sundell, J. "On the History of Indoor Air Quality and Health." *Indoor Air*, 2004, *14*, 51–58.

Thomson, H., Pettigrew, M., and Morrison, D. "Health Effects of Housing Improvement: Systematic Review of Intervention Studies." *British Medical Journal*, 2001, *323*, 187–190.

Tinetti, M. E., Speechley, M., and Ginter, S. F. "Risk Factors for Falls Among Elderly Persons Living in the Community." *New England Journal of Medicine*, 1988, *319*, 1701–1707.

Todd, C., and Skelton, D. *What Are the Main Risk Factors for Falls Amongst Older People and What Are the Most Effective Interventions to Prevent These Falls?* WHO Regional Office for Europe, Health Evidence Network. http://www.euro.who.int/document/E82552.pdf, 2004.

Ulrich, R., and others. *The Role of the Physical Environment in the Hospital of the 21st Century: A Once-in-a-Lifetime Opportunity.* Center for Health Design. http://www.healthdesign.org/research/reports/physical_environ.php, Sept. 2004.

Ulrich, R. S., and others. "A Review of the Research Literature on Evidence-Based Healthcare Design (Part I)." *Health Environments Research & Design Journal*, 2008, *1*, 16–125.

U.S. Census Bureau. *American Housing Survey for the United States: 2005.* Current Housing Report, Series H150/05.http://www.census.gov/hhes/www/housing/ahs/ahs.html, Aug. 2006.

U.S. Department of Housing and Urban Development. *Guidelines for the Evaluation and Control of Lead Paint Hazards in Housing.* HUD-1547-LBP. http://www.hud.gov/offices/lead/lbp/hudguidelines/index.cfm, 1995.

U.S. Department of Housing and Urban Development. *Economic Analysis of the Final Rule on Lead-Based Paint.* http://www.nhl.gov/offices/lead/library/enforcement/completeRIA1012.pdf, 1999.

U.S. Environmental Protection Agency. "Lead; Identification of Dangerous Levels of Lead." Final Rule. *Federal Register*, *66*, 1206 (2001). http://www.epa.gov/fedrgstr/EPA-TOX/2001/January/Day-05/t84.pdf.

U.S. Environmental Protection Agency. *Green Building: Basic Information.* http://www.epa.gov/greenbuilding/pubs/about.htm, 2009.

U.S. Environmental Protection Agency, Office of Air and Radiation, Office of Research and Development, Office of Radiation and Indoor Air. *Indoor Air Facts No. 4 (revised): Sick Building Syndrome.* http://www.epa.gov/iaq/pubs/sbs.html, 2008.

U.S. General Accounting Office. *School Facilities: Condition of America's Schools.* GAO/HEHS-95–61. http://www.gao.gov/archive/1995/he95061.pdf, 1995.

U.S. General Accounting Office. *School Facilities: America's Schools Report Differing Conditions.* GAO/HEHS-96–103. http://www.gao.gov/archive/1996/he96103.pdf, 1996a.

U.S. General Accounting Office. *School Facilities: Profiles of School Conditions by State.* GAO/HEHS-96–148. http://www.gao.gov/archive/1996/he96148.pdf, 1996b.

U.S. Green Building Council. *Build Green Schools.* http://www.buildgreenschools.org, 2008.

U.S. Public Health Service, Office of the Surgeon General. *The Health Consequences of Involuntary Smoking: A Report of the Surgeon General.* DHHS Publication CDC 87–8398. Rockville, Md.: U.S. Department of Health and Human Services, 1986.

Warda, L. J. and Ballesteros, M. F. "Interventions to Prevent Residential Fire Injury." In Doll, L. S. and others, Eds. *Handbook of Injuyry and Violence Prevention.* New York: Springer, 2007, pp. 97–116.

Warsco, K., and Lindsey, P. F. "Proactive Approaches for Mold-Free Interior Environments." *Archives of Environmental Health*, 2003, *58*(8), 512–522.

Weldon, D. E., Loewy, J. H., Winer, J. I., and Elkin, D. J. "Crowding and Classroom Learning." *Journal of Experimental Education*, 1981, *49*, 160–176.

Western Sustainability and Pollution Prevention Network. "Janitorial Products Pollution Prevention Project." http://www.westp2net.org/Janitorial/jp4.cfm, 2002.

Wilson, J. Q., and Kelling, G. L. "Broken Windows: The Police and Neighborhood Safety." *Atlantic Monthly.* http://www.theatlantic.com/doc/198203/broken-windows, Mar. 1982.

Wu, F., and others. "Improving Indoor Environmental Quality for Public Health: Impediments and Policy Recommendations." *Environmental Health Perspectives*, 2007, *115*, 953–957.

Yudelson, J. *Choosing Green: The Homeowner's Guide to Good Green Homes.* Gabriola Island, B.C.: New Society, 2008.

Zhang, J., and Smith, K. R. "Indoor Air Pollution: A Global Health Concern." *British Medical Bulletin*, 2003, *68*, 209–225.

Zimring, C., and Bosch, S. "Building the Evidence Base for Evidence-Based Design: Editors' Introduction." *Environment and Behavior*, 2008, *40*, 147–150.

FOR FURTHER INFORMATION

Organizations for Healthy Buildings

Healthy Building Network, http://www.healthybuilding.net. A national network of green building professionals, environmental and health activists, and others who promote healthier building materials as a means of improving public health and preserving the global environment.

Organizations for Healthy Health Care Design

Academy of Architecture for Health (AAH), http://www.aia.org/aah_default. This component of the American Institute of Architects specializes in health care architecture.

Center for Health Design, http://www.healthdesign.org. Through research, education, advocacy, and technical assistance, this organization supports health care and design professionals all over the world in their quest to improve the quality of health care through evidence-based building design.

Health Care Without Harm, http://www.noharm.org/us. A coalition of organizations working to protect health by reducing pollution in the health care sector.

Hospitals for a Healthy Environment (H2E), http://www.h2e-online.org. A national movement for environmental sustainability in health care, jointly founded by the American Hospital

Association, the U.S. Environmental Protection Agency, Health Care Without Harm, and the American Nurses Association. H2E educates health care professionals about pollution prevention opportunities and provides tools and resources to facilitate the industry's movement toward environmental sustainability.

Green Guide for Health Care, http://www.gghc.org. Green Guide for Health Care compiles a best practices guide for healthy and sustainable building design, construction, and operations for the health care industry.

Practice Greenhealth, http://www.practicegreenhealth.org. A nonprofit membership organization formed through a merger of Hospitals for a Healthy Environment, Green Guide for Health Care, and Healthcare Clean Energy Exchange. It offers environmental solutions for the health care sector to use to achieve better, safer, and greener workplaces and communities.

Organizations for Healthy Homes

U.S. Department of Housing and Urban Development, Healthy Homes Initiative, http://www.hud.gov/offices/lead/hhi/index.cfm. A federal program that holistically addresses a variety of environmental health and safety concerns including mold, lead, allergens, asthma, carbon monoxide, home safety, pesticides, and radon.

National Center for Healthy Housing, http://www.centerforhealthyhousing.org. Founded as the National Center for Lead-Safe Housing to bring the public health, housing, and environmental communities together to combat childhood lead poisoning, and renamed National Center for Healthy Housing to reflect an expanded mission to help to decrease children's exposure to additional biological, physical, and chemical hazards in the home.

Alliance for Healthy Homes, http://www.afhh.org. A national, nonprofit, public interest organization working to prevent and eliminate hazards in homes such as lead, mold, carbon monoxide, radon, pests, and pesticides.

Organizations for Healthy Schools

Healthy Schools Network, http://www.healthyschools.org. A national nonprofit organization that does research and education, coalition building, and advocacy to ensure that every child has a healthy learning environment that is clean and in good repair.

U.S. Environmental Protection Agency, Healthy Schools Web site, http://www.epa.gov/schools. A federal agency Web site designed to provide one-stop access to the many programs and resources available to prevent and resolve environmental issues in schools. It includes the EPA's Healthy School Environments Assessment Tool (HealthySEATv2), a customizable, user-friendly software program that helps school districts evaluate and manage environmental, safety, and health issues.

Organizations for Green Building

U.S. Green Building Council, http://www.usgbc.org. A nonprofit organization that promotes environmentally friendly buildings and is well known for its Leadership in Energy and Environmental Design (LEED) Green Building Rating System™, which provides tools and performance criteria for those designing, building, and operating buildings. LEED standards are available for new construction, existing buildings, specific building types such as schools and retail stores, and neighborhoods.

U.S. Environmental Protection Agency, Green Building Web site, http://www.epa.gov/greenbuilding. A federal agency Web site that provides information on various aspects of green building, including energy efficiency, water efficiency, and waste reduction.

Southface Energy Institute, http://www.southface.org. A nonprofit organization that promotes sustainable homes, workplaces, and communities through the use of environmentally friendly technologies and techniques. Provides information on residential and commercial buildings.

Organizations for Building Design for the Elderly

Environmental Geriatrics, Cornell Medical School, http://www.environmentalgeriatrics.org. Defining *environmental geriatrics* as the study and application of design principles to interiors and products to optimize the health, function, and well-being of older adults, this Web site offers information and links on elder-friendly building design.

CHAPTER TWENTY

WORKPLACE HEALTH AND SAFETY

MELISSA PERRY

HOWARD HU

KEY CONCEPTS

- The workplace is a unique environmental setting because it is the setting in which adults spend most of their time outside the home, it may entail long-term, high-level, and diverse exposures, it carries specific social and legal connotations, and for other reasons.

- Industries that pose high risk for injury and disease include mining, construction, agriculture, and manufacturing.

- On a global scale, the risks of occupational injury and disease are especially high in poor countries.

- A range of strategies exist for preventing workplace injuries and disease, including process re-engineering, work environment controls, administrative controls, and behavioral controls.

THE workplace can be thought of as a localized subset of the larger environment, a place where people confront environmental exposures each day as they earn their living. But occupational health is more than small-scale environmental health; it is a complex and fascinating topic that deserves special consideration. Why? First, work remains the central activity for adults, the one in which they spend most of their time outside of the home. In their work environments, people have enormous potential for exposures (both healthy and hazardous) over many years. Second, many hazardous exposures are experienced at their highest level in the workplace. In fact, this is reflected in long-standing policy; regulations typically allow higher exposures in the workplace than in the general environment. Third, the workplace presents an extraordinarily broad range of exposures, from acute chemical poisoning to catastrophic injuries, from long-term chemical effects to psychological stress. This variety is only partially captured in the term *occupational safety and health*, in which the concept of **occupational safety** refers to protection from injuries and the concept of **occupational health** refers to protection from illnesses. These long-term, high-level, and diverse exposures account for a fourth special feature of the workplace: it has been a "laboratory" for many exposures, with workers the inadvertent guinea pigs. Many environmental hazards were first recognized in the workplace through observations of highly exposed workers. Fifth, occupational health is not only a subset of public health; it is also a subset of labor relations, a sociopolitical context that embodies unique issues of power, history, justice, and law. Sixth, the workplace as a social construct offers many opportunities for health interventions, from health education to medical screening to drug screening. Finally, employment—and lack of employment, for those needing but unable to find jobs—has health ramifications, particularly in countries like the United States, where health insurance and other benefits are often tied to employment. Occupational health is a unique and important part of environmental health.

HISTORY OF OCCUPATIONAL HEALTH

Since antiquity scholars have written about the specific exposures and diseases associated with occupations. Hippocrates recognized and recorded lead toxicity in the mining industry in the fourth century BCE. Pliny the Elder, a Roman scholar of the first century BCE, described hazards associated with handling zinc and sulfur as well as perhaps the first recorded industrial hygiene protective device, a

Melissa Perry and Howard Hu declare no competing financial interests.

mask constructed from an animal bladder that was used by miners and smelter workers exposed to dust or fumes. Working conditions remained abysmal in the Middle Ages, but feudal guilds were established that assisted ill workers and their families. Formal study of occupational disease was undertaken by Ulrich Ellenbog in 1473, when he published a pamphlet on occupational diseases and injuries among gold miners, wrote about the toxic effects of carbon monoxide, mercury, lead, and nitric acid, and offered specific recommendations on hygiene and other preventive measures. In *De Re Metallica*, a book published in 1556, the Saxon physician and geologist **Georgius Agricola** described injuries and illnesses among miners, including silicosis—a deadly lung disease brought on by inhaling granite dust—and proposed methods for mine ventilation and other forms of worker protection.

In Italy in 1700, **Bernardino Ramazzini** (1633–1714), widely regarded as the "father of industrial medicine," published the first comprehensive book on industrial medicine, *De Morbis Artificum Diatriba* ("The Diseases of Workmen"). The book contained accurate descriptions of the occupational diseases of many of the trades of his time as well as his famous admonition that "when a doctor visits a working-class home he should be content to sit on a three-legged stool, if there isn't a gilded chair, and he should take time for examination; and to the questions recommended by Hippocrates, he should add one more: What is your occupation?" Ramazzini's writing also influenced the development of the field of industrial hygiene through his assertion that occupational diseases should be studied in the work environment rather than in hospital wards.

Later, in eighteenth-century England, **Percival Pott** (1715–1788) recognized soot as one of the causes of scrotal cancer among chimney sweeps, one of the first recorded connections between occupational exposures and cancer. Moreover, he used his reputation as a prominent London surgeon to advocate for passage of the Chimney-Sweepers Act of 1788, which formally recognized the disease connection and offered protections.

During the industrial revolution of the late eighteenth and nineteenth centuries, technology advanced rapidly, new and often dangerous machines were deployed in industry after industry, and mass production became common. Textile mills and factories sprung up, employing workers who no longer owned the means of production, worked for hourly wages, and had to depend on employers for their working conditions. These mills and factories also generated a huge increase in the use of chemicals, such as the acids, alkalis, soaps, and mordants needed for processing textiles. The conditions in the mills and factories, including worker exposure to chemicals, were often abominable.

Charles Turner Thackrah (1795–1833), a Yorkshire physician, developed an interest in the diseases he observed among the poorer classes of people living in the city of Leeds. He became a major figure in occupational health with the publication of his 200-page book felicitously titled *The Effects of the Principal Arts, Trades and Professions, and of Civic States and Habits of Living, on Health and Longevity, with Suggestions for the Removal of Many of the Agents which Produce Disease and Shorten the Duration of Life.* In it he proposed guidelines for the prevention of certain diseases, recommending the elimination of lead as a glaze in the pottery industry and the use of ventilation and respiratory protection among knife grinders, for example. Public outcry and the efforts of early Victorian reformers such as Thackrah led to passage of the Factory Act in 1833 and the Mines Act in 1842.

The first article on occupational disease in the United States appeared in 1837 and relied on Thackrah as an authority. But it was not until the turn of the twentieth century that the first major champion of occupational health in the United States emerged, the remarkable **Alice Hamilton** (1869–1970; Figure 20.1). A social reformer and keen firsthand observer of industrial conditions, she startled

FIGURE 20.1　Alice Hamilton, Pioneer in Occupational Health in the United States

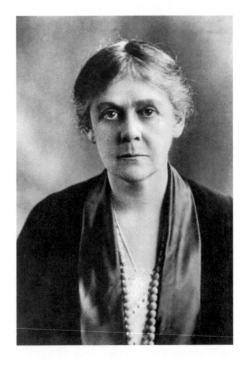

Source: AP/Wide World Photos.

mine owners, factory managers, and state officials in Chicago with evidence of links between illness and exposure to toxins. Hamilton was appointed by the governor of Illinois to direct that state's Occupational Disease Commission from 1910 to 1919, and she became a key proponent of legislation establishing early forms of occupational health regulation and workers' compensation. In 1919, she moved to Boston and became the first female professor at Harvard Medical School, and later, in 1925, the Harvard School of Public Health. At Harvard, Hamilton conducted industrial research and, between 1924 and 1930, served on the Health Committee of the League of Nations, which allowed her to investigate industrial health conditions in other countries as well. She published *Industrial Poisons in the United States* in 1925, *Industrial Toxicology* in 1934, and perhaps the most inspiring of her works, her autobiography, *Exploring the Dangerous Trades*, in 1943. In 1947, she became the first woman to receive the Albert Lasker Public Service Award.

The efforts of Hamilton and others to increase awareness of occupational health issues in the 1920s and 1930s were reinforced by a series of occupational health disasters. A prime example was the Gauley Bridge disaster (also known as the Hawk's Nest incident), in which several thousand workers, mostly African Americans, were employed to drill tunnels through rock during the construction of a new hydroelectric plant in West Virginia. There were no controls to reduce ex vposure to rock dust containing silica, and an estimated 700 workers died of acute silicosis—a catastrophic lung disease brought on by silica fibers. By 1935, the West Virginia House of Delegates had promulgated a compensation program for silicosis victims.

The latter half of the twentieth century saw the development of modern academic departments of occupational health. One of the most prominent was led by **Irving Selikoff** (1915–1992) at the Mount Sinai School of Medicine. Selikoff was a physician who conducted some of the first studies linking asbestos exposure to the development of cancer and went on to lead the international effort to control asbestos exposure. Another winner of the Lasker Public Service Award (1952) and a tireless advocate who later lobbied for better recognition and control of other occupational carcinogens, Selikoff wrote: "By the time an agent is discovered and under control, millions of workers may have been exposed. Stopping cancer by stopping exposure may be too late. Tens of thousands will die of cancer because of seeds planted decades ago, unless those seeds can be destroyed. Their families may share the same risk because of contamination brought home, because of reproductive changes made by the same agents, and because of hazardous wastes in the air, water and on the land of their communities" (Ramazzini Institute for Occupational and Environmental Health Research, 2004).

VARIETIES OF WORKPLACE ENVIRONMENTS

The nature of work has changed and continues to change for millions of workers, in parallel with profound changes in the world's economies. These changes include a rapid rise in the size of the service and information technology sectors, a relative contraction of manufacturing employment, and a marked transfer of some industries, particularly labor-intensive manufacturing and service work, from developed to developing countries. Such changes have radically changed the profile of workplace risks. Nevertheless, hazards remain, even in the advanced economies of the most developed countries.

The International Labour Organization (ILO) estimates that nearly half the world's population, about 2.84 billion people worldwide, are engaged in some form of economic activity. The amount of time workers spend at work varies, from 1,421 hours per year in Germany to 2,316 in Korea according to 2007 data (Organization for Economic Cooperation and Development, 2009a); the levels may be even higher in some poor countries such as Peru (Lee, McCann, and Messenger, 2007). The U.S. figure is intermediate, at 1,792 hours per year.

Employment patterns vary in part by the level of a country's economic development. In most developed nations the largest share of employment is in the services sector, followed by industry, with a small proportion, usually less than 10 percent, in agriculture. In other nations, predominantly transitional economies, agriculture accounts for the largest proportion of employment, followed by services and then industry (ILO, 2007). China has a unique pattern: the largest share of employment remains in agriculture, followed by industry and then the services sector. In recent years agriculture has lost its place as the main sector of employment globally and has been replaced by the services sector, which in 2006 constituted 42.0 percent of world employment compared to 36.1 percent for agriculture. After showing steady declines in the early 1990s, the proportion of world employment in manufacturing had leveled off in 2006, at 21 percent (ILO, 2007).

Given the hazards often associated with both agriculture and manufacturing, these trends signal some progress toward safer and healthier workplaces, a trend reflected in occupational safety and health data in some places and in some industries. However, the reality is that all work—including work that at first glance would seem to be benign—may carry risks of injury or illness. Whereas industries such as mining and construction present obvious dangers to life and limb, others pose more subtle threats—infectious diseases for health care workers, stress for office workers, chemical exposures for dry cleaners.

In many countries a secondary, or informal, economy accounts for a substantial proportion of employment. Window washers and vendors on the streets of Mexico

City or Bangkok, undocumented farmworkers in the fields of California or North Carolina, Turkish construction workers in Germany, and African dishwashers in Spain, all labor in this setting. Such workers usually enjoy few labor rights and tend to be excluded from official statistics and workplace protection programs. Little is known about their health and safety status. However, it is likely that they work longer hours, face more uncontrolled hazards, suffer higher rates of injury and illness, and have fewer protections than workers in more mainstream employment do.

WORKPLACE HEALTH AND SAFETY PROBLEMS

The health and safety problems that arise in the workplace cover a wide range and include

- Occupational lung diseases
- Musculoskeletal disorders
- Occupational cancer
- Acute injuries
- Cardiovascular disease
- Disorders of reproduction
- Neurotoxic disorders
- Psychological disorders, including stress
- Noise-induced hearing loss
- Dermatologic conditions
- Infectious diseases
- Symptom-defined disorders, such as multiple chemical sensitivity

Some specific instances of these problems, such as the lung disease silicosis, have been recognized since ancient times, and others, such as reproductive toxicity from solvent exposure, have been more recently characterized. Some, such as asbestosis, are unique to the workplace (or nearly so), and others, such as lung cancer, may arise both from occupational and from nonoccupational exposures. Some are minor nuisances, and others are fatal. Each category is briefly described in the following sections.

Occupational Lung Diseases

Lung diseases among workers who breathe high concentrations of contaminated air have been recognized for centuries. One group of occupational lung diseases, the *pneumoconioses*, results when workers breathe dust that penetrates into the lungs, accumulates in the lung parenchyma (the lung tissue), and causes pathological reactions. These diseases include **asbestosis** from breathing asbestos (for example, asbestos miners, insulators and other construction workers, and manufacturers of asbestos products such as brake linings and textiles are at risk), **silicosis** from breathing silica (miners, quarry workers, and sandblasters are at risk), **coal workers' pneumoconiosis** (or black lung) from breathing coal dust (miners are at risk), and **berylliosis** from breathing beryllium (hard metal workers are at risk). Victims of these diseases typically suffer from shortness of breath, cough, and weakness and have characteristic findings on chest X-ray. These diseases are largely irreversible and often progress even after exposure has ended.

A second group of occupational lung diseases affects the airways more than the lung parenchyma. **Occupational asthma** is one example. Hundreds of exposures have been reported to cause occupational asthma, including exposures to chemicals such as toluene diisocyanate (for example, workers who make polyurethane foam products are at risk), trimellitic anhydride (workers exposed to epoxy resins are at risk), and polyvinyl chloride (meat wrappers are at risk). Other causes are naturally occurring molecules found in biological matter, such as wheat and other grains (for example, bakers and millers are at risk), certain wood dusts (timber cutters, carpenters, and cabinetmakers are at risk), colophony (solderers are at risk), and latex (health care workers are at risk). Occupational asthma was traditionally thought to result from long-term exposures, but in recent years immediate onset of asthma following acute, high-dose exposure to irritants such as may occur during chemical spills has been recognized. This unfortunate turn of events has been termed **reactive airways dysfunction syndrome**.

Some diseases affect both the lung parenchyma and the airways. An example is **byssinosis** (also called brown lung, or Monday morning asthma). This disease, caused by inhaling the dust of cotton or other vegetable fibers (such as hemp, flax, or sisal), causes an asthmalike syndrome that improves after a few days away from work and flares upon the worker's return.

A final category of occupational lung disease is lung cancer. Many workplace exposures have been linked to lung cancer, including asbestos, diesel exhaust, chromium, nickel, and arsenic. A classic example of an occupational lung carcinogen is a chemical called bis-chloromethyl ether (BCME), which caused an outbreak of lung cancer affecting dozens of workers in a chemical factory manufacturing Plexiglas in Philadelphia in the 1960s.

Musculoskeletal Disorders

Work-related musculoskeletal disorders (MSDs) affect primarily the tendons, muscles, and ligaments of the upper extremities and back. Physical factors, especially repetition, force, awkward positioning, and vibration, play an important role in the onset of upper-extremity disorders, whereas heavy lifting, frequent bending and twisting, and whole body vibration are risk factors for low-back disorders (Bernard, 1997). Musculoskeletal disorders associated with office work have increased since the early 1990s and can range in severity from mild symptoms to functional impairment. These problems are quite prevalent in keyboard operators who type for prolonged periods, with more than 50 percent of newly hired computer users experiencing MSDs within the first year on a job (Gerr and others, 2002). **Carpal tunnel syndrome** is a common example of peripheral nerve entrapment syndrome; it can occur in both wrists and be completely disabling. Tendonitis and nerve entrapments, as well as many back injuries, often result from cumulative trauma over time, rather than a single acute injury, accounting for terms such as **repetitive strain injuries** or **cumulative trauma disorders**. Although it is usually easy to identify the cause of such acute work injuries such as fractures and lacerations, MSDs, by their nature, usually have a slow and insidious onset, which makes identifying causal factors especially difficult. Problems with recognition are complicated further by the facts that non-work-related activities can cause MSDs too and that stress and other psychosocial factors may increase susceptibility to MSDs.

Occupational Cancer

Workplace exposures can contribute to the causation of cancers. Cancers associated with workplace exposures typically occur following a **latency period** of at least ten years and at body sites that have had extensive contact with the agents involved—the lungs and skin when they are directly exposed or the liver and urinary tract when they are pathways for the metabolism and excretion of carcinogens—or at sites with unusually susceptible cells, such as bone marrow. In addition to the lung cancers noted previously, examples include cancers of the skin (from sun exposure in outdoor workers and from arsenic, coal tar, and soot); the pleura and peritoneum, the linings of the lung and abdomen, respectively (almost exclusively from asbestos); the nasal cavity and sinuses (from chromium, nickel, wood, and leather dusts); the liver (from arsenic and vinyl chloride); the bone marrow (from benzene and ionizing radiation); and the bladder (from aromatic amines). In assessing individual cases of cancer, it is often difficult to quantify the relative roles of workplace carcinogens and of other potential contributors such as cigarette smoking or genetic susceptibility (as reflected by, for example, familial predisposition).

Acute Injuries

According to the **National Institute for Occupational Safety and Health** (NIOSH) and the **Bureau of Labor Statistics** (BLS), about 4 million traumatic injuries occur in U.S. workplaces each year, of which between 5,000 and 6,000 are fatal. The full range of traumatic injuries occurs at work, including amputations, fractures, eye loss, and lacerations.

Injury rates are highest in transportation, construction, and manufacturing (see Figure 20.2 and also the case example in the accompanying Perspective). Fatality rates, however, demonstrate a different pattern. Between 5,000 and 6,000 workers are killed on the job each year, or about 100 every week. Fatality rates are highest in agriculture, mining, and transportation (BLS 2008a) resulting from

PERSPECTIVE
Occupational Fatalities Resulting from Falls

Falls have surpassed workplace homicides to become the second leading cause (after motor vehicle crashes) of work-related death across all industries. Between 1980 and 1994, for example, deaths due to falls accounted for 10 percent of all occupational fatalities, with an average of 540 deaths per year—10 each week, 2 each working day. The Census of Fatal Occupational Injuries (Bureau of Labor Statistics [BLS], 2008a) reported that the number of fatal falls in 2007 rose to a high of 835—a 39 percent increase since 1992 when the CFOI was first conducted. In many of these fatalities, investigation revealed that noncompliance with regulations contributed to the falls and that the deaths were potentially preventable. Injury and fatality rates are high in the construction industry, and falls are the leading cause of workplace fatalities among construction workers.

Case Example

On August 29, 2002, a twenty-three-year-old Hispanic roofer died from injuries he sustained when he fell over the unprotected edge of an elementary school gymnasium roof to an asphalt walkway approximately fifteen feet below. The victim was part of a seven-man roofing crew. He was last seen standing near the edge of the roof pulling on a power cord. No fall protection system was in place. A coworker standing nearby saw the victim fall over the edge. The foreman was working at ground level at the time of the incident and heard coworkers' calls for help. He called 911 from his cell phone while coworkers and school personnel ran to help the victim. Emergency responders arrived within a few minutes and, on observing the severity of the victim's head injury, called for a medical helicopter for transport. The medical helicopter was delayed by weather problems. A military helicopter responded approximately thirty minutes after the incident and transported the victim to a regional trauma center, where he was pronounced dead on arrival. The roofing company had operated for thirty-eight years and had thirty employees.

such incidents as mine collapses and tractor rollovers. The transportation sector deserves special mention, since about half of work-related fatalities are motor vehicle related. Falls play an important role, as does workplace violence, which accounts for the largest share of workplace deaths among women. The highest numbers of occupational homicides occur in retail stores (including liquor stores, gas stations, grocery stores, and jewelry stores), restaurants, hotels, and justice and public order facilities such as courts and prisons. Taxi drivers have the highest rate of occupational fatalities (BLS, 2008a).

Employees were trained and required to use fall protection, but none was used on the day of the incident (NIOSH, 2003).

Recommendations and Requirements

NIOSH recommends that employers should, at a minimum, (1) incorporate safety in work plans, (2) identify all fall hazards at a worksite, (3) conduct safety inspections regularly, (4) train employees in recognizing and avoiding unsafe conditions, and (5) provide employees with appropriate protective equipment and train them in its use. Passive fall prevention systems, such as guardrails and safety nets, are preferred over active systems, such as personal fall arrest systems (PFASs), because passive systems do not require workers to actively patrol their own safety. A PFAS involves a full-body harness that distributes the fall arrest forces over the body upon impact, self-retracting lifelines that limit the distance a worker can fall, and possibly also rope grabs, lanyards, and anchorage points. The Occupational Safety and Health Administration (OSHA) defines low-slope roofing as roofing with a slope less than or equal to a four-foot rise over twelve feet. For low-slope roofs six feet or more aboveground (as in this case), a warning line system is required; this involves a barrier erected on the roof to warn employees that they are approaching an unprotected roof edge. Within the warning line, employees are not required to use a guardrail, body belt, or safety net system. Employees working beyond the warning line require at least a safety monitor, a person responsible for recognizing fall hazards and warning employees about them. Safety monitors are the least protective of all fall protection systems permitted by OSHA, however, and combining the warning line system with other acceptable methods of fall protection is recommended. In this case no warning line system was in place nor was anyone assigned to be the safety monitor, despite the fact that both were required by the company's fall protection plan. In addition, instead of using battery-powered tools, the construction workers had plugged their tools into outlets at ground level. The worker is believed to have fallen while tugging on the entangled power cord of the electric screw gun he was using. Power cords should not be used in areas where they can become entangled (fall risk), near roof edges (fall risk), or where they could be damaged (electrocution risk).

FIGURE 20.2   Incidence Rate* of Nonfatal Occupational Injury Cases by Sector, 2007 (Private Employers Only)

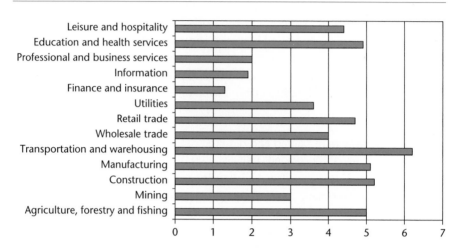

*Injuries/100 full-time workers.
Source: Bureau of Labor Statistics, 2008c.

Cardiovascular Disease

Several occupational exposures can contribute to cardiovascular disease. Some are chemicals, such as carbon monoxide, found in motor vehicle exhaust; methylene chloride, a solvent used by furniture refinishers and others in paint stripping; and carbon disulfide, a chemical that is used in the manufacture of rayon and that accelerates atherosclerotic plaque formation. An interesting example of work-related cardiovascular disease occurs among workers involved in nitroglycerin manufacturing; in drug form this chemical is used medically to dilate the coronary arteries, but when workers who have become habituated to it through workplace exposure leave the workplace for a few days, they may experience coronary vaso-constriction. Chronic lead exposure among, for example, workers who manufacture lead batteries or who remove lead paint, increases the risk of hypertension and its subsequent outcomes (such as stroke and heart attack), as well as abnormalities of cardiac conduction. Psychosocial stress and physical exposures, such as to noise, may also contribute to cardiovascular disease.

Disorders of Reproduction

A number of workplace exposures can threaten reproductive health. Examples include exposures to insecticides and herbicides, PCBs and polybrominated biphenyls (PBBs), ethylene oxide (a gas used in hospitals to sterilize equipment), metals (lead, arsenic, cadmium, mercury), and solvents. Dibromochloropropane, a nematicide, caused a well-known epidemic of sterility among production workers and farmers using the product. There is concern that exposures to some pesticides and other chlorinated organic chemicals may disrupt the function of the endocrine system, leading to disorders of development in children of exposed workers and contributing to the risk of such diseases as testicular cancer and breast cancer.

Neurotoxic Disorders

The central nervous system is a complex and delicate system that is a common target of toxic exposures. Most people are familiar with the neurotoxic effects of ethanol, a common chemical that is the active ingredient in alcoholic beverages. Many chemicals encountered in the workplace have similar effects. Painters, metal degreasers, plastics workers, cleaners, and other workers who are exposed to solvents such as toluene and perchloroethylene are at risk of central nervous system symptoms such as fatigue, memory loss, difficulty concentrating, and emotional lability. These effects may occur acutely and typically improve after hours or a day away from work. However, long-term exposures may lead to chronic effects and even to a syndrome termed *chronic solvent encephalopathy*. Abnormalities can often be detected on neurobehavioral testing. Some workers improve after discontinuation of exposure, but in other cases the effects appear to be irreversible. Other substances associated with neurobehavioral dysfunction include metals, particularly lead, mercury, arsenic, and manganese; pesticides, such as organophosphates and organochlorines; polychlorinated biphenyls (PCBs); and gases such as carbon monoxide. There is growing evidence that some nervous system toxicants may interact with genetic susceptibility factors to contribute to neurodegenerative diseases such as Alzheimer's, Parkinson's, and amyotrophic lateral sclerosis (Lou Gehrig's disease).

The peripheral nervous system may also be a target of workplace exposures. Organic solvents such as n-hexane, heavy metals such as lead and arsenic, and some organophosphate compounds can damage peripheral nerves, leading to weakness or even paralysis of the hands and feet. Some neurotoxins have unique and specific effects. For example, dimethylaminopropionitrile (DMAPN), an industrial catalyst, can cause paralysis of the bladder.

Psychological Disorders, Including Stress

Stress has emerged as a major occupational health concern. Not only does stress undermine quality of life, but it is a risk factor for hypertension, cardiovascular disease, immune dysfunction, asthma, and possibly other conditions (Lovallo, 2004; McEwen, 2007). The leading model for understanding workplace stress was laid out by Karasek (1979) and Karasek and Theorell (1990) (Figure 20.3). This **demand-control model** emphasizes two dimensions of the workplace experience: job demand and decision control. People with high job demands perceive excessive task requirements or workload, time pressure, and conflicting demands. They describe themselves as "working very hard," "working very fast," and "not having enough time to get the job done." People with low workplace control say that they lack influence at work and are unable or unauthorized to make decisions or influence their jobs. Jobs with high demands and low control are those that are most stressful, as indicated by the downward arrow in Figure 20.3. However, high job demands are not necessarily bad; when combined with high control, demanding jobs can be highly stimulating and motivating. A third dimension of the workplace, social support, can mitigate some of the effects of stress.

FIGURE 20.3   Karasek Job Strain Model

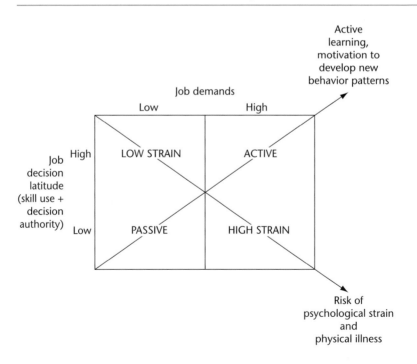

Source: Schnall, Landsbergis, and Baker, 1994.

The demand-control model is not the only theoretical construct for understanding workplace stress (Siegrist, 2002). According to the **person-environment fit model**, stress arises from mismatches between what work provides and what the worker needs, and between work demands and the worker's abilities. And the **effort-reward imbalance model** focuses on the mismatch between efforts made at work and the rewards, such as earnings, self-esteem, and job security, that result (Tsutsumi and Kawakami, 2004).

Unemployment deserves specific attention because unemployed workers experience increased psychological and emotional distress and are at higher risk for suicide. Unemployment may refer to either a community's aggregate unemployment rate or an individual's personal unemployment experience (Dooley, Fielding, and Levi, 1996). As of early 2009, according to Organization for Economic Co-operation and Development (OECD) standardized unemployment rates for twenty-nine OECD member countries, unemployment rates ranged from 16.6 percent in Spain to 3.7 percent in Switzerland (OECD, 2009b). The United States had an unemployment rate of 8.1 percent, which was projected to increase with the continued economic crisis. Unemployment disproportionately affects young people and ethnic minorities. However, a downturn in the economy can have further-reaching effects. Moreover, people may be forced to remain in or accept employment at low wages, with too few hours, with low job security, or with intense work demands. Being out of work or underemployed takes a toll on both physical and psychological well-being, as reflected in rates of physical illness, admission to mental hospitals, and psychiatric diagnoses. Although sound economic policies need to lower unemployment rates and ensure optimal employment for all workers, it is also important that occupational health practitioners recognize that individuals need social and psychological support following job loss.

Noise-Induced Hearing Loss

Loud noises are a feature of many workplaces. Exposure to noise can be acute, as with the sudden burst of an explosion or metal-on-metal impact noise, or chronic, as with the routine daily use of tools in the construction trades, machines in manufacturing, or equipment in numerous other jobs. **Noise-induced hearing loss** occurs when loud sounds damage the delicate hair cells critical to hearing in the inner ear. According to NIOSH, 30 million Americans are exposed to hazardous noise at work, and 10 million have suffered permanent hearing loss as a result. Sound is measured in decibels. The decibel scale is logarithmic, so a noise at 110 decibels is ten times louder than a noise at 100 decibels. A humming refrigerator reaches about 40 decibels, a normal conversation takes place at about 60 decibels, and traffic noise in a city may reach 80 decibels. In a woodshop the noise level is about 100 decibels, chainsaw noise measures about 110 decibels, and the loud noises produced by motorcycles, firecrackers, and firearms can reach 120 to 140 decibels. Prolonged exposure to noise above 85 decibels can cause hearing loss.

Like many occupational exposures, noise can be addressed through primary prevention—reducing the noise at the source if possible, or enclosing the noise source so noise exposure is reduced in the work zone. If these measures are impossible, then personal protective equipment such as noise-reducing earmuffs or earplugs may be used. However, earplugs exemplify some of the limits of personal protective equipment. Many workers do not like them, they offer inadequate protection if selected or used improperly, and they may introduce problems of their own, such as inhibiting social interaction and blocking workers' ability to hear shouted warnings or alarms.

Dermatologic Conditions

Skin disorders account for about one in eight reported occupational diseases. Although several patterns may occur, such as burns, abrasions, and lacerations, the most common workplace skin disease is **contact dermatitis**. This condition is a reaction to substances that come into contact with the skin. It may represent an allergic reaction, or it may result simply from irritation. Not surprisingly, the most common sites of contact dermatitis are the hands and arms. Rates of contact dermatitis are highest in agriculture, forestry, and fishing, followed by manufacturing. A wide range of chemicals and other materials can cause contact dermatitis, including cutting oils in the machine tool trades, grease and lubricating oils among mechanics, formaldehyde and dyes among textile workers, and latex (in gloves) among health care workers. With chronic contact dermatitis, a worker's skin may become thickened, hyperpigmented, dry, fissured, and itchy. Skin in this condition not only causes troubling symptoms for the worker but may also function poorly as a barrier, permitting chemicals to cross the skin and enter the person's general circulation. At times even intact skin may be a pathway by which chemicals enter the body, as described in Chapter Two. Examples of chemicals that undergo percutaneous absorption include organophosphates, carbon disulfide, and methyl butyl ketone and other organic solvents.

Infectious Diseases

Many categories of workers are at risk of occupational infections. Health care workers confront blood-borne pathogens such as hepatitis B virus and HIV/AIDS; prevention requires scrupulous attention to avoiding contact with body fluids, handling needles and other sharps properly, and using protective equipment.

Health care workers are also at risk of airborne infections, with tuberculosis being the most feared because the mycobacterium involved can be transported over relatively long distances in infectious droplets. Other workers at risk for infectious disease include farmworkers, slaughterhouse workers, and other workers who come into contact with animals and may contract illnesses (the zoonoses) usually affecting animals. Outdoor workers may be bitten and infected by insects, and teachers and child-care workers are exposed to diseases of children. Infections in workers may be a problem in broader public health terms as well. For example, a restaurant worker with active hepatitis A may transmit the disease to large numbers of customers.

Symptom-Defined Disorders

The range of occupational illnesses also includes syndromes for which the pathophysiology remains obscure. One example is **sick building syndrome** (SBS), a constellation of symptoms including headache, fatigue, nasal irritation, and confusion. As explained in Chapter Nineteen, SBS typically presents as a cluster of symptoms among occupants of an office building with limited fresh air intake and with point sources of indoor air pollution (such as copy machine emissions). Another symptom-based syndrome is **multiple chemical sensitivity** (MCS), which is characterized by symptoms similar to those of sick building syndrome (headache, fatigue, respiratory irritation, confusion, muscle aches, and abdominal distress). MCS sufferers, after an initial workplace (or nonoccupational) exposure event, begin to report exacerbations when exposed to relatively low levels of irritants such as fragrances, motor vehicle exhaust, and marker pen odors. Some cases of MCS begin as SBS.

EPIDEMIOLOGY OF OCCUPATIONAL INJURIES AND ILLNESSES

Are workplace injuries and illnesses a large public health problem? To answer this question we need to assess data on the magnitude of the problem. And to do this we need to understand the data and where they come from.

There are two main sources of primary occupational injury and illness data: employer reports and insurance system reports. In the United States, employers are required to maintain records of injuries and illnesses in their workplaces. Each year the Department of Labor's Bureau of Labor Statistics collects these reports from a national sample of employers in its Survey of Occupational Injuries and Illnesses, compiles the data, extrapolates them to the entire workforce, and issues annual reports. Insurance data in the United States come primarily from workers' compensation systems, but useful information may also come from private health insurance systems such as health maintenance organizations (HMOs). Both employer reports and workers' compensation data are likely to underreport; those who collect data have incentives not to report, and although most occupational injuries are readily recognized and attributed to work, many cases of illness go unrecognized or unacknowledged and they may also manifest years after the original causative exposure.

A third source of data is the health care system. For example, the Census of Fatal Occupational Injuries (CFOI) compiles multiple data sources on workplace deaths, the National Electronic Injury Surveillance System uses hospital emergency department information, and the National Health Interview Survey annually surveys U.S. household members on health issues, including injuries. These sources are informative only when information on occupation is collected at the time health care services are delivered. For example, emergency departments must seek and record information on whether or not injuries are work related if this source is to yield useful occupational data.

Finally, a variety of secondary data sources—sources not specifically intended to collect occupation-related health data—can yield statistics on specific populations or types of illness or injury. These sources may offer indirect access to statistics that are normally hard to collect. Examples of secondary data sources on work-related injury and illness include vital records (death certificates), labor union pension records, police and justice system reports (data on transportation crashes and interpersonal violence events), regulatory agency records (for example, national transportation agency records), emergency medical service (EMS) records, coroners' reports, employment records, and trauma registries (if they collect work-related injury information).

With this general understanding of the sources of occupational health statistics, we can consider the data available on occupational mortality and morbidity. As discussed previously, between 5,000 and 6,000 workers are killed on the job each year in the United States. However, this fatality picture changes considerably once fatal illnesses are taken into account. In the United States, estimates of the annual number of fatalities from work-related disease range from 49,000 to 65,000 (Leigh and others, 1997; Steenland and others, 2003; Schulte, 2005), approximately ten times higher than the acute fatality count. The causes of these deaths include occupational cancer, respiratory and cardiovascular disease, chronic renal failure, and hepatitis. Many of these work-related deaths are not individually attributed to occupational exposures and go uncounted in official data.

Globally, workplace injuries and illnesses are an even larger problem, due to the transfer of hazards from developed to developing nations and inadequate safeguards in many poor nations (see Chapter Eleven). The World Health Organization and the International Labour Organization have recently estimated that about 2 million workers lose their lives each year to occupational injuries and illnesses (Nelson and others, 2005; Driscoll and others, 2005; ILO, 2005); this burden exceeds the toll from traffic crashes and war combined. The occupational fatality rate varies greatly, from 5.3 per 100,000 workers per year in established market economies such as the United States, Europe, and Japan, to 21.0 in sub-Saharan Africa, 22.5 in the Middle East, and 23.1 in parts of Asia (Takala, 1999, 2000). Again, official statistics probably underestimate the true burden of occupational fatalities, due to underreporting, misdiagnosis, and in many poor countries, the existence of a substantial informal economy in which no reporting occurs at all.

When we turn from fatalities to nonfatal injuries and illnesses, the workplace is also an important contributor. According to the BLS, a total of 4 million injuries and illnesses were reported in private industry workplaces in the United States during 2007, an annual incidence of 4.2 cases per 100 full-time worker equivalents. The highest incidence was in the manufacturing sector (with 5.4 cases per 100 workers per year) and the lowest was in the financial services sector (BLS, 2008e). Although the most recent BLS data do not report the types of cases, data from the late 1990s suggest that nearly two-thirds of cases were accounted for by musculoskeletal diseases, such as carpal tunnel syndrome and tendonitis, and noise-induced hearing loss. Skin diseases such as dermatitis accounted for about one case in eight. Other diseases, such as asbestosis, cancers, and lead-induced hypertension, account for a small proportion of cases. However, diseases that develop over a long period (such as asbestosis) or that have workplace associations that are not immediately obvious (such as cancers or lead-induced hypertension) are known to be greatly underrecorded in databases such as the BLS survey.

Not only do these injuries and illnesses cause suffering for workers and inconvenience for both workers and employers, they are also costly. The Liberty Mutual 2007 Workplace Safety Index estimated that direct costs for occupational injuries in 2007 rose to $48.3 billion (Liberty Mutual, 2008).

The risks of occupational injury and disease vary by age, occupation, industry, geographic location, and even the size of the workplace. A foundry worker clearly faces a higher risk than an insurance underwriter (Figure 20.5). Similarly, two occupations accounted for more than 63 percent of work-related anxiety, stress, and neurotic disorder cases in the United States in 2001: technical, sales, and administrative support workers (2,250 cases) and managerial and professional specialty occupations (1,331 cases) (NIOSH, 2004). Workplace size is also an important variable; smaller workplaces generally experience higher rates of injury and illness, partly because fewer resources are available to control health and safety risks. In mining, for example, the highest fatal injury rates occur

PERSPECTIVE
Occupational Health in India

India is the world's second most populous nation, encompassing a diverse range of cultures and languages and spanning a broad range of climates and ecologies. It is also arguably the world's largest democracy, one that is undergoing vast and rapid changes related to rural-urban demographic shifts, industrialization and development, a globalizing economy, and associated alterations in people's lifestyles. India has grown a huge middle class, fueled by a productive education system and growth in the manufacturing, information technology, and biotechnology sectors—all while substantial segments of the population remain afflicted by poverty, unemployment, malnutrition, infectious diseases (such as malaria and tuberculosis), and disability.

One of the most prominent and universal symbols of the hazards of industrialization and globalization remains the 1984 disaster in Bhopal, India, in which a pesticide plant owned by the U.S.-based Union Carbide Corporation experienced a chemical leak resulting in the release of massive clouds of methyl isocyanate over the city of Bhopal. By 1994, the death toll was estimated at 6,000. Independent agencies now estimate that the number of deaths related to this disaster has reached between 15,000 and 20,000, and several hundred thousand residents have experienced subsequent chronic health effects such as respiratory impairments, adverse reproductive outcomes, and cognitive deficits (Dhara and Dhara, 2002). Efforts to provide support for victims and settle claims resulting from the disaster became enmeshed in politics and a tug-of-war between the government's interests in justice and in continued foreign investment. Nevertheless Bhopal—and the rest of the country—has continued to develop, with the city now a thriving industrial hub of textile manufacturing, food processing, and electrical manufacturing.

Occupational health in India currently poses the same huge challenges that confront many rapidly developing countries. These challenges include enforcing lax health and safety standards, training a workforce with uneven levels of education, promoting health and safety concerns to the many thousands of small businesses and families engaged in home-based industries, and dealing with foreign industries that offer the promise of jobs but also carry substantial occupational health risks. At the same time, some of India's occupational health issues are somewhat specific to India. For example, many of the estimated 100 million women in India who work outside the home are employed by industries engaged in such hazardous activities as the manufacturing of fireworks and matches (high exposures to potassium chloride, tetraphosphorus trisulfide, and lead tetroxide and high risks of fire and explosions), the manufacturing of *bidi*, or cigarettes (nicotine exposures several times higher than those of smokers), agriculture (exposures to pesticides), and electronics manufacturing (exposures to solvents, arsine, phosphine, lead, and cadmium). **Child labor** is also a major problem in India (Venkateswarlu and others, 2003), with an estimated 70 to 115 million children between the ages of five and fourteen in the workforce, primarily in the agricultural sector (Figure 20.4). Many work twelve hours a day, are frequently exposed to pesticides, and are not provided with safety equipment or even shoes to protect their feet or water to wash their hands and clothes. Some materials banned for industrial use in other countries, such as asbestos, continue to be used in India, with an estimated 10 million industrial and mine workers in India exposed to asbestos or other dusts at concentrations of health concern.

FIGURE 20.4   Occupational Health in India: A Child Worker in a Marketplace

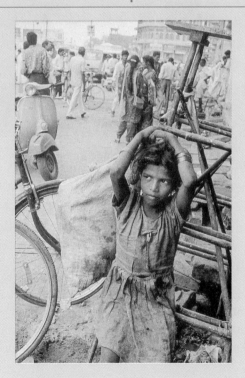

FIGURE 20.5   Foundry Worker Pours Molten Metal

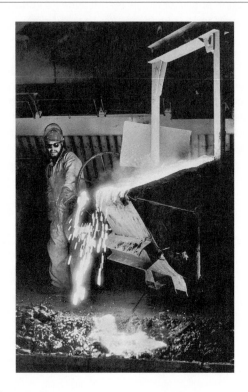

Source: © www.earldotter.com.

Among the risks of foundry work are heat effects, burns, and silicosis (from shaking out the molds).

in mines employing fewer than ten workers. Internationally, the availability and adequacy of health and safety protections vary greatly, with workers in some countries facing a substantially higher risk than workers in other countries (even after accounting for differences in reporting).

Three industries deserve special mention, because they have unusually high work-related morbidity and mortality: mining, agriculture, and construction.

Mining

There are 500,000 miners in the United States and at least 13 million miners working worldwide. Miners face risks of injuries from mine collapses, explosions, and power equipment and risks of illnesses from inhaling dusts and diesel fumes and from chemical exposures. In the United States, fatalities in mining have decreased over time due to the passage of mine health and safety legislation and due to improvements in mining technology, such as the use of roof bolting to prevent roof cave-ins, of dust suppression and ventilation techniques, and of noncombustible materials to prevent fires and explosions. Despite these improvements, mining remains one of the most hazardous U.S. occupations.

Agriculture

Farming is also one of the most hazardous occupations. In the United States the leading agents of fatal and nonfatal injuries to farmers and other farmworkers are tractors, other farm machinery, livestock, building structures, falls, and bodies of water. Environmental exposures include pesticides, volatile organic compounds (fuel and solvents), noxious gases, airborne irritants, noise, vibration, zoonotic infectious diseases, and stress. Farm family members may also be exposed to these hazards, making agriculture a unique example of the intersection of occupational and environmental exposures. On the approximately 2.08 million farms in the United States in 2007 (USDA, 2008), there were 1.8 million farmworkers (BLS, 2008b). Farming is also unique in that child labor is common. The Childhood Agricultural Injury Surveillance Project found that in 2006 an estimated 1,120,000 youths less than twenty years of age lived on farms in the United States (NIOSH, 2008). An estimated 23,100 children under the age of twenty years who lived on, worked on, or visited farms and ranches were injured in 2006, and approximately 100 unintentional injury deaths occur annually among children and adolescents on U.S. farms (NIOSH, 2008). Although the exact number of youths exposed to farm hazards annually is unknown, it has been estimated at more than 2 million.

Construction

The construction trades also rank high on the list of most hazardous occupations, in terms of both fatal and nonfatal occupational injuries. In 2005, construction ranked second after the transportation industry in the rate of nonfatal injuries and illnesses (239.5 per 10,000 full-time workers) and fourth in the rate of fatal injuries (11.1 per 100,000 full-time workers) (Center for Construction Research and Training, 2007). In 2007, falls to a lower level accounted for the highest number of fatal injuries among construction workers (448 deaths), and highway crashes accounted for the next highest number (141 deaths) (BLS, 2008a).

SPECIAL WORKING POPULATIONS

Occupational health professionals are concerned with the safety of all workers, but certain populations of workers are especially vulnerable to workplace risks. This may occur for one or more of several reasons: they may confront excessive risks on the job, they may be susceptible to certain risks due to social or biological factors, or they may enjoy fewer protections than other workers. Four categories of workers deserve mention here: women, socially and economically disadvantaged groups, children, and elders.

Women Workers

Women in the United States and internationally are more likely than men to work in low-skilled, low-paying jobs. These jobs may feature exposures to chemicals that can threaten reproductive health, repetitive movements that can lead to musculoskeletal injuries, and other hazards. The reasons women are at higher risk than men are for work-related health problems have more to do with the social and economic influences affecting women's work than with biological sex differences. Less attention is paid to health risks specific to female-dominated occupations such as health care worker, cleaner, or keyboard operator; there is a (mis)perception that women's work is harmless and does not require major occupational health consideration; and the dual roles that women usually face as wage earners and family caregivers are not typically accommodated in the workplace.

Although over 49 million women worked full time at wage and salary jobs in the United States in 2005 (BLS, 2006), women remain at a salary disadvantage when compared to men. Full-time working women as a group earned only about 80 percent of what men earned in 2007 (BLS, 2008c). A 2007 Department of Labor report on women's employment and wage patterns attributed this disparity, in part, to the overrepresentation of women in traditionally lower-paying jobs. Although women are more likely than men to work in professional and related occupations, they are not well represented in the higher paying job groups within this broad sector. In 2007, 9 percent of female professionals were employed in the high-paying computer and engineering fields, compared with 43 percent of their male counterparts. Professional women are more likely to work in the education and health care occupations, in which pay has been generally lower. Sixty-seven percent of female professionals worked in these fields in 2007, compared with 30 percent of male professionals (BLS, 2008d).

Lower-paying positions can mean more mentally and physically demanding work. Many female-dominated jobs, such as cleaning and child care, are also socially isolating. Women's work is erroneously perceived as not being overtly dangerous compared to male-dominated work, such as mining or construction. However, injury statistics demonstrate that injury rates in some female-dominated industries are excessive. Health care workers experience high rates of overexertion from physically handling patients and are at risk of blood-borne pathogen exposures due to needlestick injuries, and precision industry assemblers and food service workers experience high rates of repetitive strain and cumulative trauma injuries due to repetitive manual work and static postures. Underestimating the health risks in such gender-segregated jobs results in insufficient health and safety protections for women.

Socially and Economically Disadvantaged Workers

In the United States and internationally, ethnic minorities who are socially marginalized are also more likely than other groups to be employed in physically demanding jobs with inherent hazards, such as construction, farmwork, mining, or meat packing (Murray, 2003). In the United States, problems related to this marginalization are compounded for undocumented immigrant workers, who are frequently employed in farm or service work but who are hidden from occupational safety regulatory authority. Undocumented immigrants often have no alternative to enduring unsafe working conditions and have no recourse if they are injured or become ill as a result of their work. The vulnerability of undocumented immigrant workers in the United States is now starting to receive increased attention among workplace safety advocates, and addressing their circumstances is becoming a major thrust of occupational health advocacy campaigns (American Public Health Association, 2005). This issue, like many other social and economic injustice problems, will likely be solved only when the requisite political will is in place to realize broad-reaching legislative protections for immigrant workers. The next decade will undoubtedly witness active debate around this issue, and occupational health professionals from clinicians to safety professionals to labor union representatives will contribute to that debate, with their ultimate goal being the protection of immigrant workers.

Child Workers

Another example of an especially vulnerable group in terms of workplace health and safety protections is young workers. In the United States, child labor laws are in place that are intended to recognize the inherent vulnerabilities that youths face, including an increased risk that they will be exploited in the workplace. However, the lack of comprehensive regulatory enforcement and the wide-scale lack of information among child workers, parents, and employers about child worker rights and protections contribute to the thousands of preventable work-related injuries and illnesses among youths each year. The conditions of child farmworkers are illustrative. U.S. child labor laws include exceptions for youths working in agriculture, and enforcement programs are weak. These two realities result in excessively hazardous conditions for teenage and younger farmworkers. Globally, estimates are that 150 million children are trapped in child labor, with approximately 70 percent working in agriculture. The International Labor Organization has declared the abolition of child labor a global cause for the new millennium and is reporting major declines in the number of children affected, especially among children involved in hazardous work (ILO, 2006).

PERSPECTIVE
Recollections of a Child Farmworker

When I was fourteen I worked in the fields for two weeks, chopping the weeds around the cotton plants. . . . I woke up one night, I couldn't breathe; I was allergic to something they were spraying in the fields. I stopped breathing . . . I tried to drink water but I couldn't so I ran into my mom's room 'cause I didn't have no air in me and I was like [wheezing gasps] trying to get air in there but I couldn't . . .

At the hospital they said I was allergic to something out there . . . something they were spraying. . . . They sprayed the fields in the morning. We'd be out there when they were doing it, or when they were leaving, or we could see them doing other fields. They'd spray by plane.

Source: Richard M., seventeen years old, in an interview conducted in Casa Grande, Arizona, October 27, 1998; quoted in Human Rights Watch, 2000.

Older Workers

Another special workplace population consists of older workers. With average life expectancy now over seventy-five years in developed countries and sixty-four years in developing countries, people are staying in the workplace at older ages than was typical in the twentieth century. Recent downturns in the global economy that have reduced retirement savings have reinforced this trend. Productivity might be expected to decline with age, but occupational capacity studies to date do not consistently support this relationship (Silverstein, 2008). In many contexts both life experience and years of experience on the job better predict job performance. It is perhaps most useful to think about age and work performance in terms of specific tasks. Performance in jobs requiring knowledge-based judgments without time pressure is enhanced by age; skilled manual work is not necessarily affected by age if it requires average exertion; however, fast-paced data-processing performance can be impaired by age.

Special health concerns of older workers pertain most to injury. In general the frequency of injury decreases with age, although injury severity, including the likelihood of death, increases with age. However, as with the relationship between age and job performance, the relationship between injury severity and age varies by job type. Older construction workers are at higher risk than younger workers for nonfatal falls from ladders, whereas younger farmers are at higher risk for fatal machinery accidents. Older workers are at risk for unfair treatment when they are selectively used as part-time or occasional workers without the same pay and benefits as full-time coworkers. Hiring and employment practices must be equitable regardless of age to ensure that older workers are not forced into marginalized positions.

OCCUPATIONAL INJURY AND ILLNESS PREVENTION

Prevention is central to the approach to any occupational health problem. It is critical to appreciate that prevention is most effective when it is considered and practiced on multiple levels.

Approaches to Prevention

In a workplace with an assortment of hazards, what is the best approach to preventing injury and disease? A useful way of thinking about prevention is to adopt an integrated strategy that draws on key aspects from public health, industrial hygiene, and environmental stewardship models. Occupational disease and injury are caused by exposure to hazards on the job, and prevention requires controlling exposures. Anticipation of hazardous exposures, surveillance of hazards and health effects, analysis of health effects, and ultimately hazard control are all critical parts of an integrated approach to prevention. (Prevention strategies are discussed further in Chapter Twenty-Six.)

A wide variety of tactics and technologies is available for controlling hazards. Four basic choices are **process reengineering**, **environment controls**, **administrative controls**, and worker **behavioral controls** including **personal protective equipment**. As explained in more detail in Chapter Twenty-Six, a hierarchy of strategies exists, with a clear preference for workplace design that eliminates or minimizes exposures.

An example of healthy workplace design, and one of the best strategies, is **product substitution** or **process substitution**, that is, replacing a toxic hazard or a risky process with a safer alternative. For example, polyvinyl chloride (PVC) manufacturing might be replaced by production of another, less hazardous material. This would definitely eliminate hazardous workplace exposures to vinyl chloride monomer, and it would also offer upstream and downstream benefits: a reduced need for chlorine production (which often occurs at hazardous chloralkali plants), a reduced need for phthalate plasticizers (which can enter the human food chain), and a reduced need for incineration of chlorine-containing plastic products (which form dioxins when burned). Such changes require consideration of occupational hygiene at the earliest stage of planning a new industry or industrial plant. Such consideration remains underemphasized in the training of most engineering and business executives, but it constitutes a strategic goal that should be a part of the movement to make industry green (protective of the environment) in the twenty-first century.

Examples of possible work environment controls, continuing with the case of PVC manufacturing, are setting up automatic unloading of vinyl chloride monomer (instead of having workers manually open and pour from the bags), installing ventilation to reduce dust exposure, and enclosing the polymerization process to reduce worker exposures. **Industrial hygienists** are specialists in documenting the need for such controls and in designing and implementing them. Least preferable are protocols that call for workers to wear personal protective equipment,

PERSPECTIVE
Occupational Lead Exposure and Reproductive Health

General population exposures to lead in the United States have declined over 70 percent in the past twenty years, largely due to the phaseout of leaded gasoline and the elimination of lead solder in food cans. However high exposures to lead can still occur in many different ways, including occupational exposure.

Case Presentation

A twenty-eight-year-old woman works as a torch burner, cutting steel coated with lead paint. She is now considering having a child. During the past eight years, her blood lead level has twice exceeded 40 μg/dL, the OSHA occupational standard, but currently it is 22 μg/dL. She is concerned that if she has a child it may face risks stemming from her current and past lead exposures.

such as protective clothing and respirators, because this equipment relies for its effectiveness on human behavior and compliance (never infallible), is often uncomfortable to wear (especially for an eight-hour work shift), and sometimes poses safety hazards of its own (for example, a respirator reduces the worker's ability to communicate during an emergency). Occupational health specialists prefer using worker-focused interventions only when no other control alternatives exist.

Finally, administrative controls involve changes in how tasks are organized and performed. For example, in a workplace with a record of back injuries from lifting, the employer might provide training in proper lifting techniques and require that all lifts above a certain weight be performed by teams of two workers rather than by single individuals. Another administrative control strategy is to restrict hazardous jobs to workers considered less susceptible to their effects, but such an approach can discriminate against certain classes of workers. For example, one firm that used lead in its production process restricted women of childbearing age from lead-exposed jobs (unless they could show that they were unable to bear children). This practice was challenged as discriminatory, and a landmark Supreme Court decision, *United Auto Workers* v. *Johnson Controls*, found for the plaintiff, limiting the scope of administrative controls (as discussed in the Perspective on occupational lead exposure).

Toxicity of Lead

High exposure to lead can occur through multiple sources, such as eating food contaminated by lead (from cooking in ceramic ware with a lead-based glaze, for example), drinking water contaminated by lead-soldered plumbing, taking part in hobbies that use lead (such as making stained glass), using personal products that contain lead (such as kohl, an eyeliner cosmetic sometimes contaminated with lead), living in a home where lead paint was used and is now peeling, and working in an environment where lead is used or handled (such as automobile battery plants [see Figure 20.6], smelters, or construction projects that involve disturbing existing lead paint). NIOSH recently estimated that occupational exposures alone mean that every year more than 25,000 workers experience blood lead levels exceeding 40 μg/dL, the maximum allowable level under current regulations.

The routes of lead absorption are inhalation and ingestion. After lead is absorbed it reaches the blood and is rapidly distributed across membranes into organs such as the brain, testes, and bone. High exposures in both children and

FIGURE 20.6   Workers in an Automobile Battery Plant, a Source of
Occupational Lead Exposure

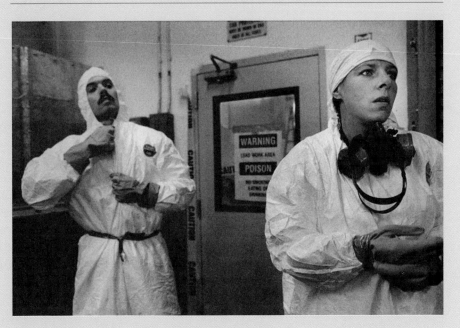

Source: © www.earldotter.com.

adults (producing blood lead levels greater than 40 to 80 μg/dL) can result in a
wide spectrum of nonspecific symptoms of poisoning, including abdominal pain,
lethargy and confusion, and joint pain. In children, recent studies indicate that
even relatively low blood lead levels (in the single digits of μg/dL) can be enough
to impair mental development (Lanphear and others, 2005). Screening for blood
lead levels in children six months to five years of age is mandatory in many states,
with current federal guidelines recommending interventions when blood lead levels exceed 10 μg/dL. Excretion occurs primarily through the kidneys into urine;
treatment with chelating agents (drugs that bind with metal and hasten their
excretion) is sometimes warranted.

   In addition to creating a threat of acute toxicity, chronic lead exposure contributes to the risk of later chronic disease. Recent epidemiological studies have

outlined this risk by using noninvasive techniques to measure lead in bone, where, by virtue of being the site of deposition for more than 95 percent of the adult lead body burden, lead levels serve as a biomarker for cumulative exposure as well as a potential internal source of lead reentering the blood, operating over long periods of time, and increasing the risk of central nervous system toxicity, kidney damage, hypertension, and reproductive effects. The rate of reentry is greatly accelerated during times of high bone resorption, such as pregnancy. Recent studies suggest that during pregnancy maternal bone lead stores are transferred into blood, cross the placenta, and affect fetal development, resulting in reduced birthweight, reduced skeletal growth, and lower performance on cognitive testing at two years of age (Hu and Hernández-Avila, 2002). Calcium supplementation in pregnant mothers has been recently shown to reduce fetal lead exposure by up to 30 percent by reducing bone resorption and the intestinal absorption of lead (Ettinger and others, 2008).

Legal Issues

A famous class action lawsuit occurred in 1984 after Johnson Controls, a large manufacturing company, excluded women of childbearing age from lead-exposed jobs in that company (unless they could provide medical evidence that they were unable to bear a child). After a long court battle that saw the policy upheld in federal district and appeals courts, the U.S. Supreme Court overturned the lower court decisions, saying that "the bias in the policy was obvious and that fertile men but not fertile women are given a choice as to whether they wish to risk their reproductive health for a particular job" (Annas, 1991). This case set a landmark precedent that has essentially restricted OSHA from promulgating regulations that protect female workers in ways different from protections for male workers.

OSHA's lead standard sets forth lengthy and detailed regulations for different kinds of potential occupational lead exposures. These regulations specify under what conditions an employee may be exposed to lead, what levels of exposure are permissible, and in what ways an employer is responsible for monitoring these exposures. The regulations also outline the steps that must be taken for an employee who has had an unacceptable exposure (over the limits), including access to medical care and wage protection during time off from work. However, pursuant to the Johnson Controls decision, there is no provision for gender differences in exposure, and should a woman become pregnant the fetus is not protected from lead exposure. The regulations do state that an employee can seek out medical advice "with respect to reproductive health . . . and may request pregnancy testing or lab evaluation of male fertility" (OSHA, 2005).

Occupational Safety and Health Regulation

Regulatory approaches are central to any discussion of occupational hazard prevention. Workplace regulations—what they are, which governmental agency creates and enforces them, their effectiveness, and so on—vary widely from country to country. In most countries, government has intervened in the private market, with standard setting, enforcement, and health and safety training, in response to a range of factors: the inability of voluntary efforts in the free market to protect workers adequately, the regular occurrence of widely publicized occupational health disasters, pressure from labor unions, and the existence of international guidelines from the International Labour Organization. Some countries subscribe to regional policies (such as those set by the European Union), but most have developed their own approaches to safety and health regulation.

In the United States (the focus of most of the ensuing discussion), the primary law regulating health in the workplace is the Occupational Safety and Health Act (OSH Act) of 1970. This legislation established the federal Occupational Safety and Health Administration (OSHA) to set and enforce standards and the National Institute for Occupational Safety and Health to conduct research and carry out site-specific health hazard evaluations. Among other important laws are the Mine Safety and Health Act (MSHA) of 1969 and the Toxic Substances Control Act (TSCA) of 1976.

There are limits to OSHA's regulatory authority. In 1979, Congress exempted businesses with ten or fewer employees from routine OSHA inspections (although specific complaints can still trigger inspections). States may opt to maintain their own occupational safety and health regulatory programs; in theory these must be at least as protective as OSHA regulations, although some states have been notably lax in their enforcement. OSHA's jurisdiction also does not extend to federal or state workers; such workers must be covered by safety and health programs maintained by their own agencies.

What is OSHA's obligation in terms of setting standards? Section 6(b)(5) of the OSH Act requires the U.S. Secretary of Labor to set a standard that "most adequately assures, to the extent feasible, on the basis of the best available evidence, that no employee will suffer material impairment of health or functional capacity, even if such employee has a regular exposure to the hazard dealt with by such standard for the period of his working life." With regard to toxics, the burden of proving that a substance is hazardous is placed on OSHA. OSHA is also required to prove that any controls it proposes are technically feasible.

Not surprisingly, many of the regulations proposed by OSHA are heavily contested, usually by the affected industries or labor unions, or by both, and several challenges have had to be addressed in federal court. Among precedents that have been set in such rulings and are now codified in the *Code of Federal Regulations (CFR)* are that OSHA must conduct quantitative risk assessment as part of the standard-setting process (Occupational Safety and Health Standard for Benzene, 29 *CFR* 1910.1028), that OSHA may require medical monitoring and, based on that monitoring, may require removal of an employee from work while he or she maintains full pay and benefits (Occupational Safety and Health Standard for Lead, 29 *CFR* 1910.1025), and that an OSHA standard is legally acceptable even if some employers are forced out of business, as long as the entire affected industry is not disrupted (Occupational Safety and Health Standard for Asbestos, 29 *CFR* 1910.1011).

Perhaps the most far-reaching of all OSHA standards was established under the Hazard Communication Act (Occupational Safety and Health Standard, 29 *CFR* 1910.1200; also known as the right-to-know standard), which requires manufacturers and employers to disclose information regarding chemical exposures to their employees (and to select others, such as employees' health providers). Under this Act, employers need to make available material safety data sheets (MSDSs) that list chemical ingredients and basic information on associated health risks for all potentially toxic substances used in the workplace. The Act also gives employees legal access to their workplace medical and exposure records.

Of course the effectiveness of regulations is dependent on enforcement. Occupational safety and health enforcement is carried out in large part by a national network of regional and area offices that perform workplace inspections to check for violations of health and safety standards. OSHA makes random inspections of workplaces (sometimes without advance notice), with an emphasis on workplaces entailing a higher than average level of risks. In addition, certain events, such as workplace fatalities, trigger automatic inspections, and any employee can request an OSHA inspection while also requesting that his or her name be kept confidential. Violations of standards that are uncovered in such inspections are punishable by fines. However, OSHA's capacity to perform inspections is limited by the small number of OSHA inspectors (around 1,000) relative to the millions of U.S. workplaces and by antiregulatory political pressure. Instead of conducting inspections, OSHA often simply relays a complaint to an employer by mail, requiring as a response only a reply that discusses how the complaint will be addressed. Industries with high risks of toxic chemical exposures—as opposed to high risks of injuries—are often given less attention. Finally, OSHA's ability to conduct its work is heavily dependent on a budget that has historically been vulnerable to political interventions.

SUMMARY

The workplace is a keenly important environment in terms of human health and safety. For many people, it rivals the home as the environment in which the most time is passed. It is also the environment in which the risks of hazardous exposures are often highest. In fact much of what we know about the toxic effects of environmental chemicals derives from workplace studies, underlining the role of the workplace as an unintentional laboratory for human exposures. Workplace exposures also occur in settings that are socially complex, politically complex, and shaped by labor-management relations. Efforts to control workplace hazards have been highly contested, with labor unions claiming safe, healthy work as a human right, and employers insisting on their right to control workplace conditions and their need to control production costs.

In the United States, workplace injuries and illnesses have declined in recent years, as a result of numerous factors. One factor may be progressive underreporting. Other factors reflect real improvements: technical improvements in many industrial processes and the shift in the economy from manufacturing to services and information have brought about a reduction in risk for the most dangerous exposures. Another factor is the export of hazards to poorer countries as part of the globalization of production. In the twenty-first century, occupational health and safety will increasingly need to focus on vulnerable working populations—those in the United States that are marginalized, such as migrant and undocumented workers, and those in poor nations that lack effective regulatory protection. For all these working populations, public health protection will grow out of traditional workplace protection strategies: workplace redesign, workplace exposure controls, personal protection, and administrative controls.

KEY TERMS

administrative controls

Agricola, Georgius

asbestosis

behavioral controls

berylliosis

Bureau of Labor Statistics

byssinosis

carpal tunnel syndrome

child labor

coal workers' pneumoconiosis (black lung)

contact dermatitis

cumulative trauma disorders

demand-control model

effort-reward imbalance model

Hamilton, Alice

industrial hygienists

latency period

multiple chemical sensitivity

National Institute for Occupational Safety and Health

noise-induced hearing loss

occupational asthma

occupational health

occupational safety

personal protective
    equipment

person-environment fit
    model

pneumoconiosis

Pott, Percival

process reengineering

process substitution

product substitution

Ramazzini, Bernardino

reactive airways
    dysfunction syndrome

repetitive strain injuries

Selikoff, Irving

sick building syndrome

silicosis

Thackrah, Charles Turner

work environment controls

work-related musculoskel-
    etal disorders

DISCUSSION QUESTIONS

1. Other than the fact that the workplace is where many people spend much of their lives, what environmental health characteristics distinguish the workplace from other settings?

2. What role did the textile industry play in the history of occupational health?

3. What health effects can be caused by lead exposure? What workplace exposures (name at least two) can increase the risk of heart disease?

4. Why are earplugs a less than ideal solution for protecting workers from noise-induced hearing loss?

5. What factors play a role in the underreporting of workplace illnesses and deaths?

6. Why are children particularly vulnerable to occupational health risks, and in what industries do children make up a major segment of the workforce?

7. What are administrative controls in the context of occupational health prevention strategies?

8. In the United States, occupational health regulations are set by the Occupational Safety and Health Administration (OSHA). What are some of the major factors that limit the effectiveness of these regulations?

REFERENCES

American Public Health Association. *Policy Statement on Occupational Health and Safety Protections for Immigrant Workers*. http://www.apha.org/advocacy/policy/policysearch/default.htm?id=1318, 2005.

Annas, G. J. "Fetal Protection and Employment Discrimination: The Johnson Controls Case." *New England Journal of Medicine*, 1991, *325*, 740–743.

Bernard, B. P. *Musculoskeletal Disorders (MSDs) and Workplace Factors*. National Institute for Occupational Safety and Health. http://www.cdc.gov/niosh/ergosci1.html, 1997.

Bureau of Labor Statistics. "Table 20: Employed Persons by Full- and Part-Time Status and Sex, 1970–2005 Annual Averages." In *Current Population Survey 2005*: http://www.bls.gov/cps/wlf-table20–2006.pdf, 2006.

Bureau of Labor Statistics. *Census of Fatal Occupational Injuries Summary 2007*. http://www.bls.gov/news.release/cfoi.nr0.htm, 2008a.

Bureau of Labor Statistics. "Table 18: Employed Persons by Detailed Industry, Sex, Race, and Hispanic or Latino Ethnicity." In *Current Population Survey 2007*. http://www.bls.gov/cps/cpsaat18.pdf, 2008b.

Bureau of Labor Statistics. Incidence rate and number of nonfatal occupational injuries by selected industries, 2007. http://data.bls.gov/cgi-bin/print.pl/news.release/osh.t05.htm. 2008c.

Bureau of Labor Statistics. *Highlights of Women's Earnings in 2007*. Report 1008. http://www.bls.gov/cps/cpswom2007.pdf, 2008d.

Bureau of Labor Statistics. *Workplace Injuries and Illnesses in 2007*. http://www.bls.gov/iif/oshsum.htm, 2008e.

Center for Construction Research and Training. *Construction Chartbook*. http://www.cpwr.com/rp-chart-book31–50.html, 2007.

Dhara, V. R., and Dhara, R. "The Union Carbide Disaster in Bhopal: A Review of Health Effects." *Archives of Environmental Health*, 2002, *57*, 391–404.

Dooley, D., Fielding, J., and Levi, L. "Health and Unemployment." *Annual Review of Public Health*, 1996, *17*, 449–465.

Driscoll, T., and others. "Review of Estimates of the Global Burden of Injury and Illness Due to Occupational Exposures." *American Journal of Industrial Medicine*, 2005, *48*, 491–502.

Ettinger A. S., and others. "Effect of Calcium Supplementation on Blood Lead Levels in Pregnancy: A Randomized Control Trial." *Environmental Health Perspectives*, 2008, *117*, 26–31.

Gerr, F., and others. "A Prospective Study of Computer Users, I: Study Design and Incidence of Musculoskeletal Symptoms and Disorders." *American Journal of Industrial Medicine*, 2002, *41*, 221–235.

Hu, H., and Hernández-Avila, M. "Lead, Bones, Women, and Pregnancy: The Poison Within?" *American Journal of Epidemiology*, 2002, *156*, 1088–1091.

Human Rights Watch. "Fingers to the Bone: United States Failure to Protect Child Farmworkers." http://www.hrw.org/reports/2000/frmwrkr, 2000.

International Labour Organization. *Global Estimates of Fatal Work-Related Diseases and Occupational Accidents, World Bank Regions 2005*. http://www.ilo.org/public/english/protection/safework/accidis/globest_2005/world.pdf, 2005.

International Labour Organization. *The End of Child Labour: Within Reach*. http://www.ilo.org/ipec/lang—en/index.htm, 2006.

International Labour Organization. *Key Indicators of the Labor Market*. http://www.ilo.org/public/english/employment/strat/kilm/download/kilm04.pdf, 2007.

Karasek, R. "Job Demands, Job Decision Latitude, and Mental Strain: Implications for Job Redesign." *Administrative Science Quarterly*, 1979, *24*, 285–308.

Karasek, R., and Theorell, T. *Healthy Work: Stress, Productivity, and the Reconstruction of Working Life*. New York: Basic Books, 1990.

Lanphear, B. P., and others. "Low-Level Environmental Lead Exposure and Children's Intellectual Function: An International Pooled Analysis." *Environmental Health Perspectives*, 2005, *113*, 894–899.

Lee, S., McCann, D., and Messenger, J. C. *Working Time Around the World: Trends in Working Hours, Laws and Policies in a Global Comparative Perspective*. Geneva: International Labour Organization, 2007.

Leigh, J. P., and others. "Occupational Injury and Illness in the United States: Estimates of Costs, Morbidity, and Mortality." *Archives of Internal Medicine*, 1997, *157*, 1557–1568.

Liberty Mutual. *2007 Workplace Safety Index*. http://www.libertymutualgroup.com/omapps/ ContentServer?cid=1138365240689&pagename=LMGResearchInstitute%2Fcms_ document%2FShowDoc&c=cms_document, 2008.

Lovallo, W. R. *Stress and Health: Biological and Psychological Interactions*. (2nd ed.) Thousand Oaks, Calif.: Sage, 2004.

McEwen, B. S. "Physiology and Neurobiology of Stress and Adaptation: Central Role of the Brain." *Physiological Reviews*, 2007, *87*(3), 873–904.

Murray, L. R. "Sick and Tired of Being Sick and Tired: Scientific Evidence, Methods, and Research Implications for Racial and Ethnic Disparities in Occupational Health." *American Journal of Public Health*, 2003, *93*(2), 221–226.

National Institute for Occupational Safety and Health. "Hispanic Roofer Dies After 15-Foot Fall from a Roof—North Carolina." *Fatality Assessment Control Evaluation Program*. http://www.cdc.gov/ niosh/face/In-house/full200303.html, 2003.

National Institute for Occupational Safety and Health. "Fatal and Nonfatal Injuries, and Selected Illnesses and Conditions." In *Worker Health Chartbook 2004*. NIOSH Publication No. 2004– 146. http://www2a.cdc.gov/niosh-chartbook/ch2/ch2–1.asp, 2004.

National Institute for Occupational Safety and Health. *The NIOSH Childhood Agricultural Injury Surveillance Project*. http://www.cdc.gov/niosh/childag/childagsurvproj.html, 2008.

Nelson, D. I., and others. "The Global Burden of Selected Occupational Diseases and Injury Risks: Methodology and Summary." *American Journal of Industrial Medicine*, 2005, *48*, 400–418.

Occupational Safety and Health Administration. *Regulations (Preambles to Final Rules), Section 4-IV: Summary and Explanation of the Standard: Occupational Exposure to Lead*. http://www.osha.gov/pls/ oshaweb/owadisp.show_document?p_table=PREAMBLES&p_id=950, 2005.

Organization for Economic Cooperation and Development. Average Annual Hours Actually Worked per Worker. OECD StatExtracts. http://stats.oecd.org/Index.aspx?DatasetCode=ANHRS. 2009a.

Organization for Economic Cooperation and Development. Labour Force Statistics (MEI): Survey based unemployment rates and levels. http://stats.oecd.org/Index.aspx?QueryName=253& QueryType=View. 2009b.

Ramazzini Institute for Occupational and Environmental Health Research. *The Selikoff Fund for Environmental and Occupational Cancer Research*. http://www.ramazziniusa.org/oct00/selikoff_ fund.htm, 2004.

Schnall, P. L., Landsbergis, P. A., and Baker, D. "Job Strain and Cardiovascular Disease." *Annual Review of Public Health*, 1994, *15*, 381–411.

Schulte, P. "Characterizing the Burden of Occupational Injury and Disease." *Journal of Occupational and Environmental Medicine*, 2005, *47*, 607–622.

Siegrist, J. "Effort–Reward Imbalance at Work and Health." In P. L. Perrowe and D. C. Ganster, Editors, *Historical and Current Perspectives on Stress and Health*. Amsterdam: JAI Elsevier, 2002, pp. 261–291.

Silverstein, M. "Meeting the Challenges of an Aging Workforce." *American Journal of Industrial Medicine*, 2008, *51*(4), 269–280.

Steenland, K., and others. "Dying for Work: The Magnitude of U.S. Mortality from Selected Causes of Death Associated with Occupation." *American Journal of Industrial Medicine*, 2003, *43*(5), 461–482.

Takala, J. "Global Estimates of Fatal Occupational Accidents." *Epidemiology*, 1999, *10*, 640–646.

Takala, J. "Indicators of Death, Disability and Disease at Work." *Asian-Pacific Newsletter on Occupational Health and Safety*, 2000, *7*(1), 4–8.

Tsutsumi, A., and Kawakami, N. "A Review of Empirical Studies on the Model of Effort-Reward Imbalance at Work: Reducing Occupational Stress by Implementing a New Theory. *Social Science & Medicine*, 2004, *59*, 2335–2359.

U.S. Department of Agriculture, National Agricultural Statistics Service. *Farms, Land in Farms and Livestock Operations—2007 Summary*. http://usda.mannlib.cornell.edu/usda/current/ FarmLandIn/FarmLandIn-02–01–2008_revision.pdf, Feb. 2008.

Venkateswarlu, D., and others. "Child Labour in India: A Health and Human Rights Perspective." *Lancet*, 2003, *362*(suppl.), S32–S33.

FOR FURTHER INFORMATION

Books and Encyclopedia

International Labour Organization. *Encyclopedia of Occupational Safety and Health*. (4th ed.) http://www. ilocis.org/mainpage.html, n.d.

LaDou, J. (ed.). *Current Occupational and Environmental Medicine*. (4th ed.) New York: Lange Medical Books/McGraw–Hill, 2006.

Levy, B. S., Wegman, D. H., Baron, S. L., and Sokas, R. K. (eds.). *Occupational and Environmental Health: Recognizing and Preventing Disease and Injury*. (5th ed.) Philadelphia: Lippincott, 2005.

Rosenstock, L., Cullen, M. R., Brodkin, C. A., and Redlich, C. A. (eds.). *Textbook of Clinical Occupational and Environmental Medicine*. (2nd ed.) Philadelphia: Saunders, 2005.

Journals and Magazines

American Journal of Industrial Medicine, http://www3.interscience.wiley.com/journal/34471/home.
International Journal of Occupational and Environmental Health, http://www.ijoeh.com/index. php/ijoeh/index.

Journal of Occupational and Environmental Medicine, http://www.joem.org.
Occupational and Environmental Medicine, http://oem.bmj.com.
Occupational Health & Safety magazine, http://ohsonline.com/home.aspx.

Agencies and Professional Organizations

Bureau of Labor Statistics, http://www.bls.gov.
Center for Construction Research and Training, http://www.cpwr.com.
International Labour Organization, http://www.ilo.org/global/lang-en/index.htm.
National Council of Occupational Safety and Health, http://www.coshnetwork.org.
National Institute of Occupational Safety and Health, http://www.cdc.gov/NIOSH.
National Labor Relations Board, http://www.nlrb.gov.
Occupational Safety and Health Administration, http://www.osha.gov/index.html.
World Health Organization, "Occupational Health" Web page, http://www.who.
        int/topics/occupational_health/en.

CHAPTER TWENTY-ONE

RADIATION

ARTHUR C. UPTON

KEY CONCEPTS

- There are several forms of radiation, and each may interact with living cells, although their molecular mechanisms vary.

- Each form of radiation has associated injuries of public health concern.

- The risk of each type of radiation-induced injury varies with the dose of radiation.

- Exposure to each form of radiation occurs from specific sources and via specific pathways, and there are public health policies intended to limit such exposures.

RADIANT **energy** exists in two forms: (1) **electromagnetic waves** of widely differing energies and wavelengths and (2) **accelerated atomic particles** varying in energy, mass, and charge. The diverse forms of radiation are shown in Figure 21.1. They differ in their physical characteristics and, accordingly, in the ways in which they transfer energy. Some types of radiation can deposit enough sharply localized energy to disrupt atoms and molecules in their paths, whereas others can deposit only enough energy to excite atoms and molecules. Radiations of different types thus vary markedly in their biological effects. For this reason the health effects of each form of radiation are considered separately in this chapter. Also discussed are the health effects of **ultrasound**, a form of energy often classified with radiation for public health purposes but that actually consists of high-frequency mechanical vibrations and is not a component of the **electromagnetic spectrum**.

FIGURE 21.1   The Electromagnetic Spectrum

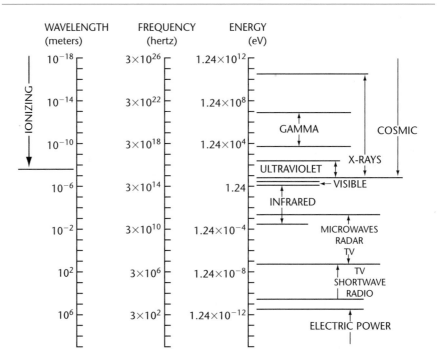

Source: Mettler and Upton, 2008, reprinted with permission from Elsevier.

Arthur C. Upton declares no competing financial interests.

HISTORICAL BACKGROUND

Since time immemorial, the sun and fire flames have both been known to be sources of light and heat to which overexposure could be injurious. Other sources of potentially hazardous radiation were not generally recognized, however, until after Roentgen's discovery of the **X-ray**, in 1895. The X-ray was then introduced into medical practice so rapidly that within barely a year ninety-six cases of radiation injury were reported (Stone-Scott, 1897). Initially, most of the injuries were acute skin reactions on the hands of those working with the early radiation equipment (see, for example, Figure 21.2), but in a short time many other types of injury also had been reported, including the first cancers attributed to **ionizing radiation** (Table 21.1).

In the years since Roentgen's discovery, knowledge of radiation injury has been greatly advanced by extensive studies of the effects of radiation in humans, laboratory animals, and other model systems (Upton, 1986, 1987; National Research Council [NRC], 2006). Historical findings of particular public health significance include (1) the occurrence of rapidly fatal reactions to irradiation in heavily exposed

FIGURE 21.2   A Pioneer Radiologist Testing His Fluoroscope by Examining His Own Hand, Fully Exposing Himself and His Patient in the Process

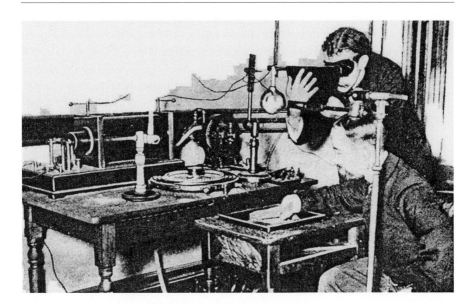

Source: Percy Brown, *American Martyrs to Science Though the Roentgen Rays,* 1936. Courtesy of Charles C. Thomas Publisher Ltd., Springfield, Illinois.

TABLE 21.1 Radiation Injuries During the First Decades Following Roentgen's 1895 Discovery of the X-Ray

Date	Type of Injury	Reported By
1896	Dermatitis of hands	Grubbe
1896	Smarting of eyes	Edison
1897	Epilation	Daniel
1897	Constitutional symptoms	Walsh
1899	Degeneration of blood vessels	Gassman
1902	Cancer in X-ray ulcer	Frieben
1903	Inhibition of bone growth	Perthes
1903	Sterilization	Albers-Schonberg
1904	Blood changes	Milchner and Mosse
1906	Bone marrow changes	Warthin
1911	Leukemia in five radiation workers	Jagic
1912	Anemia in X-ray workers	Belere

Source: Stone, 1959.

radiation accident victims and atomic bomb victims; (2) the delayed occurrence of dose-dependent increases in the frequency of lung cancers in underground hard rock miners, skeletal cancers in radium dial painters, skin cancers and leukemias in early radiologists, and cancers of the many types found in atomic bomb survivors and other irradiated populations; and (3) the occurrence of dose-dependent increases in the frequency of severe mental retardation, and other developmental disturbances in children irradiated prenatally (Upton, 1986, 1987; Mettler and Upton, 2008). Over the years, research into the health effects of various forms of radiation has received continuing impetus from radiation's expanding uses in medicine, science, and industry. The resulting knowledge of radiation effects has contributed importantly to the development of measures for protecting human health against radiation and other environmental hazards as well.

IONIZING RADIATION

Ionizing radiations are those forms of radiation that can deposit enough localized energy in living cells to break chemical bonds and give rise to ions and free radicals. Such radiations include electromagnetic waves of extremely short wavelength

(Figure 21.1) and accelerated atomic particles (for example, **electrons**, **protons**, **neutrons**, and **alpha particles**). Doses of ionizing radiation are customarily measured in terms of the corresponding amounts of energy that are deposited in the absorbing tissues (Table 21.2).

Natural sources of ionizing radiation include (1) **cosmic rays**; (2) **radium** and other radioactive elements in the earth's crust; (3) internally deposited **potassium-40**, **carbon-14**, and other radionuclides normally present in living cells; and (4) inhaled **radon** and its daughter elements (Table 21.3). The dose received from cosmic rays varies with one's elevation, being twice as high in mountainous regions as at sea level, and up to two orders of magnitude higher at jet aircraft altitudes (National Council on Radiation Protection and Measurements [NCRP], 1987; United Nations Scientific Committee on the Effects of Atomic Radiation [UNSCEAR], 2000). Likewise, the dose received from radium may be increased by a factor of two or more in regions where the earth is rich in this element (NCRP, 1987). The largest dose from natural sources is typically the dose to the bronchial epithelium from inhaled radon (Table 21.3), which can vary by an order of magnitude or more, depending on the concentration of radon in indoor

TABLE 21.2 Quantities and Dose Units of Ionizing Radiation

Quantity Being Measured	Dose Unit*	Definition
Absorbed dose	Gray (Gy)	Energy deposited in tissue (1 joule/kg)
Equivalent dose	Sievert (Sv)	Absorbed dose weighted for the ion density (potency) of the radiation
Effective dose	Sievert (Sv)	Equivalent dose weighted for the sensitivity of the exposed organ(s)
Collective effective dose	Person-Sv	Effective dose applied to a population
Committed effective dose	Sievert (Sv)	Cumulative effective dose to be received from a given intake of radioactivity
Radioactivity	Becquerel (Bq)	One disintegration per second

Note: The units of measure listed are those of the International System, introduced in the 1970s to standardize usage throughout the world (International Commission on Radiological Protection [ICRP], 1991; Mettler and Upton, 2008). They have largely supplanted the earlier units; namely, the rad (1 rad = 100 ergs per gm = 0.01 Gy), the rem (1 rem = 0.01 Sv), and the curie (1 Ci = 3.7×10^{10} disintegrations per second).

TABLE 21.3 Average Amounts of Ionizing Radiation Received Annually by a Resident of the United States

Source	Dose (mSv)[a]	% of Total
Natural		
Radon[b]	1.9	31
Cosmic	0.27	4
Terrestrial	0.28	4
Internal	0.39	7
Total natural	2.84	46
Artificial		
X-ray diagnosis	2.4	39
Nuclear medicine	0.8	13
Consumer products	0.10	2
Occupational	<0.01	<0.03
Nuclear fuel cycle	<0.01	<0.03
Nuclear fallout	<0.01	<0.03
Miscellaneous[c]	<0.03	<0.03
Total artificial	3.35	54
Total natural and artificial	6.2	100

Note: The values tabulated represent average values for the entire population; doses to specific individuals and subgroups may be substantially lower or higher.

[a] Average effective dose to soft tissues.

[b] Average effective dose to respiratory epithelium.

[c] Department of Energy facilities, smelters, transportation, and so forth.

Sources: Adapted from NRC, 1990; UNSCEAR, 2006; Mettler and Upton, 2008.

air (NCRP, 1984; UNSCEAR, 2000). Cigarette smokers may sustain even larger doses (up to 0.2 Sv [20 rem] per year) to the bronchial epithelium from polonium, another alpha-emitter that is normally present in tobacco smoke (NCRP, 1984).

In addition to the radiation received from natural sources, people are also exposed to radiation from artificial sources, the largest being the use of X-rays in medical diagnosis (Table 21.3). The effective doses received in various types of diagnostic examinations vary widely, ranging from less than 0.01 millisievert (mSv) for examination of an arm or leg to more than 4 mSv for a barium enema. Lesser sources of exposure to man-made radiation include radioactive minerals (for example, uranium-238, thorium-232, potassium-40, and radium-226) in building materials, phosphate fertilizers, crushed rock, and combustible fuels; radiation-emitting components of TV sets, video display terminals, smoke detectors, and other consumer products; radioactive fallout from atomic weapons (for example, cesium-137, strontium-90, strontium-89, carbon-14, hydrogen-3, zirconium-95); nuclear power (for example, hydrogen-3, carbon-14, krypton-85, iodine-129, and cesium-137); and nuclear waste (Table 21.3). Contrary to popular conception, the irradiation of food to rid it of microbial contaminants does not render the food radioactive or cause subsequent consumers of the food to be exposed to radiation.

Workers in certain occupations receive additional doses, depending on their job assignments and working conditions. Such occupations include, among others, medical and industrial radiography, nuclear reactor construction and operation, well logging, uranium mining and enrichment, and serving on airline crews. The average dose received occupationally by monitored radiation workers in the United States each year is less than that received from natural sources, and less than 1 percent of such workers receive a dose approaching the maximum permissible limit (50 mSv [5 rem]) in any given year (NCRP, 1989). (The cancer risk of workers in nuclear facilities is discussed in Chapter Thirteen.) In less developed countries, however, where adequate facilities, equipment, and safety measures are often lacking, occupational doses tend to be larger (UNSCEAR, 1988, 2006).

Types and Mechanisms of Injury

Ionizing radiation, impinging on living cells, collides randomly with atoms and molecules in its path, giving rise to ions and free radicals, which break chemical bonds and cause other molecular alterations that may injure the cells. The spatial distribution of such events along the path of the radiation, known as the **linear energy transfer** (**LET**) of the radiation, depends on the energy, mass, and charge of the radiation. X-rays and **gamma rays** are sparsely ionizing in comparison with charged particles; for example, an alpha particle typically gives up all of its energy in traversing only a few cells (Goodhead, 1988; Mettler and Upton, 2008). The initial physicochemical alterations occur almost instantaneously, but the evolution and expression of any resulting biological effects may take minutes, days, or years, depending on the types of effects.

Any molecule in the cell may be altered by radiation, but DNA is the most critical biological target because of the limited redundancy of the genetic information it contains. A dose of radiation large enough to kill the average dividing cell (2 Sv [200 rem]) suffices to cause hundreds of lesions in its DNA (Ward, 1988). Most such lesions are reparable, but those produced by a densely ionizing radiation (such as a proton or an alpha particle) are generally less reparable than those produced by a sparsely ionizing radiation (such as an X-ray or a gamma ray)

(Goodhead, 1988; Ward, 1988; Mettler and Upton, 2008). For this reason, the **relative biological effectiveness** (**RBE**) of densely ionizing radiations exceeds that of sparsely ionizing radiations for most forms of injury (NCRP, 2001a; Mettler and Upton, 2008).

Genetic Effects   Damage to DNA that remains unrepaired or that is misrepaired may be expressed in the form of mutation rate, with a frequency of approximately 10^{-5} to 10^{-6} per locus per Sv (NRC, 2006). The mutation rate appears to increase as a linear nonthreshold function of the dose, implying that a single ionizing particle traversing the DNA may suffice to cause a mutation (NCRP, 2001a; NRC, 2006). With low-LET (sparsely ionizing) radiation, however, the yield of mutations per unit dose typically decreases with decreasing dose rate, passing through a minimum in the range of 0.1 to 1.0 cGy (centigray) per minute, below which it rises again with further reduction of the dose rate (Vilenchik and Knudson, 2000). This variation in the mutagenic effectiveness of low-LET radiation is interpreted to signify that dose rates in the range of 0.1 to 1.0 cGy per minute are optimal for the error-free repair of DNA damage, and that repair is progressively less effective as the dose rate decreases below about 0.1 cGy per minute (Vilenchik and Knudson, 2000). Of note, a similar, DNA repair-enhancing adaptive response can be elicited by prior exposure to an appropriate "conditioning" dose of radiation in some cells; however, it is not clear whether all types of DNA repair are enhanced by the response or whether all types of cells share this response (Wojcik, 2000; NRC, 2006). Furthermore, the mechanisms that normally facilitate DNA repair or eliminate cells with unrepaired damage may not operate effectively in cells in which one or more of the responsible homeostatic genes has been mutated or lost (Mettler and Upton, 2008).

In addition to its mutagenic effects, radiation may also cause changes in chromosome number and chromosome structure. The type and frequency of this damage vary with the stage of the cell cycle in which it occurs. The dose-response relationships for such chromosome aberrations are typically linear-quadratic at high doses and dose rates, and more nearly linear, with shallower slopes, at lower doses and dose rates of low-LET radiation (NCRP, 2001a). Such aberrations in blood lymphocytes are elevated to a similar extent in radiation workers and in human populations residing in areas of high natural background radiation levels; they serve as a useful biological dosimeter in radiation workers, radiation accident victims, and other exposed persons (Bender and others,, 1988; Mettler and Upton, 2008). Irradiation can also cause chromosome aberrations to arise in the progeny of exposed cells, many cell generations later, owing to the induction of a transmissible genomic instability in the exposed cells (Morgan and others, 1996). In some types of cells irradiated in vitro, moreover, preexposure to a conditioning dose can reduce the frequency of chromosome aberrations produced by a subsequent "test" dose (UNSCEAR, 1994). However, it is questionable whether such an adaptive response affords significant protection against the effects of chronic low-level irradiation, because a dose of at least 5 mGy (milligrays) delivered at a rate of at least 50 mGy per minute appears to be required to elicit the response, the protective effect of the response lasts but a few hours, and the response varies markedly from person to person, some individuals appearing to be entirely nonresponsive (Wojcik, 2000; NRC, 2006).

Heritable genetic effects of irradiation have been well documented in other organisms but have yet to be demonstrated conclusively in humans. Extensive studies in the more than 76,000 children of Japanese atomic bomb survivors have not detected any elevations in untoward pregnancy outcomes, neonatal deaths, malignancies, balanced chromosomal rearrangements, sex-chromosome aneuploids, alterations of serum or erythrocyte protein phenotypes, changes in sex ratio, or disturbances in growth and development (NRC, 1990, 2006; Mettler and Upton, 2008). Likewise, although a case-control study has suggested an excess of leukemia and non-Hodgkin's lymphoma in young people in the village of Seascale, England, related to the occupational irradiation of their fathers (Gardner and others, 1990), there are strong reasons for rejecting this hypothesis (Doll, Evans, and Darby, 1994; Wakeford and others, 1994a, 1994b).

In the absence of definitive evidence of heritable effects of radiation in humans, estimates of the risks of such effects must rely heavily on extrapolation from findings in laboratory animals. From the available data, it is inferred that human germ cells are probably no more radiosensitive than those of the mouse and that a dose of at least 1.0 Sv would be required to double the rate of heritable mutations in humans (NRC, 2006). On this basis, it is estimated that less than 1 percent of inherited disease in the human population is attributable to natural background irradiation (NRC, 2006; Mettler and Upton, 2008).

Somatic Effects This section considers the early, acute effects of radiation on body tissues. Radiation damage to genes, chromosomes, and other vital organelles can be lethal to affected cells, especially dividing cells, which are highly radiosensitive as a class (Hall and Giaccia, 2006; Mettler and Upton, 2008). Measured in terms of their proliferative capacity, the survival of dividing cells tends to decrease exponentially with increasing dose, 1 to 2 Sv (100 to 200 rem) generally sufficing to reduce the surviving population by about 50 percent (Hall and Giaccia, 2006). Although a dose below 0.5 Sv (50 rem) kills too few cells to cause clinically detectable injury in most organs other than those of the embryo, a larger dose may kill enough of the progenitor cells in a tissue to interfere with the orderly replacement of its senescent cells, thereby causing tissue atrophy. The rapidity of the atrophy depends in part on cell population dynamics within the affected tissue; atrophy is slower in organs characterized by slow cell turnover, such as liver and vascular endothelium, and faster in organs characterized by rapid cell turnover, such as bone marrow, epidermis, and intestinal mucosa (Mettler and Upton, 2008). Also, if only a small volume of tissue is irradiated, or if the dose is accumulated gradually over an extended period of time, the severity of the injury tends to be reduced by the compensatory proliferation of surviving cells.

The acute effects of radiation are diverse and vary markedly in their dose-response relationships, clinical manifestations, timing, and prognosis (Mettler and Upton, 2008). Such reactions generally result from the severe depletion of progenitor cells in the exposed tissues and can be elicited only by doses above the thresholds high enough to kill many such cells. These reactions are therefore classified as **nonstochastic** (or **deterministic**) effects, in contrast to the mutagenic and carcinogenic effects of radiation, which are classified as **stochastic** effects, because they are thought to result from random molecular alterations in individual cells that increase in frequency as linear nonthreshold functions of the dose (ICRP, 1991; NCRP, 2001a; Mettler and Upton, 2008).

Although some degree of radiation injury is inevitable in radiotherapy patients, few treated with modern methods experience severe or disabling radiation injuries. By the same token, modern safety practices have all but eliminated injuries from excessive occupational exposure as were prevalent among pioneer radiation workers. Radiation accidents, however, remain a significant cause of injury. Some 285 nuclear reactor accidents (excluding the Chernobyl accident) were reported in various countries between 1945 and 1987, resulting in the irradiation of more than 1,350 persons, 33 of whom were injured fatally (Lushbaugh, Fry, and Ricks, 1987). The most serious such accident to date was the Chernobyl accident, in 1986, which released enough radiation and radioactive materials to cause radiation sickness and burns in more than 200 emergency personnel and firefighters, injuring 31 of them fatally. The heaviest contamination occurred near the reactor, necessitating evacuation of tens of thousands of inhabitants from the area, but doses to the thyroid gland averaging more than 20 mSv (2 rem) were received by infants in some areas of neighboring countries, largely through the ingestion of radioiodine via cow's milk, and the incidence of thyroid cancer in such children rose dramatically (Mettler and Upton, 2008). Organs other than the thyroid typically received such a small fraction of the dose normally accumulated each year from natural background radiation that the long-term health effects of such exposure cannot be predicted with certainty. The collective dose commitment to the population of the Northern Hemisphere as a whole, however, is estimated to approximate 600,000 person-Sv (60 million person-rem) (UNSCEAR, 1988), which could be predicted (on the basis of the nonthreshold risk models discussed later) to cause up to 30,000 extra cancer deaths within the next seventy years (U.S. Department of Energy [DOE], 1987).

PERSPECTIVE
Chernobyl

On April 26, 1986, an accident occurred at the Chernobyl nuclear power station, owing to serious operator errors in the testing of a turbine generator during a normal, scheduled shutdown. The accident resulted in a meltdown of the reactor core, a fire, a series of explosions, and the release of large amounts of radioactive materials from the plant over the ensuing ten days.

After the accident, hundreds of the firefighters and other emergency workers who had been employed at the site were hospitalized for burns and radiation injuries; thousands of people and domestic animals were evacuated from the surrounding areas in order to limit their exposure to radioactive fallout; and millions of people living elsewhere in the USSR were given prophylactic doses of potassium iodide to prevent their uptake of toxic quantities of radioiodine.

In spite of efforts to limit exposure to the radioactive materials released by the accident, the incidence of thyroid cancer in children living in contaminated areas has risen significantly, in parallel with their uptake of radioiodine in cow's milk.

Radiation accidents have become less frequent, but they continue to occur from time to time (Gusev, Guskova, and Mettler, 2001). Also, accidents involving medical and industrial gamma ray sources, although less catastrophic than reactor accidents, have been far more numerous and have sometimes caused severe injury and loss of life. The improper disposal of a cesium-137 source in Goiania, Brazil, in 1987, for example, resulted in the irradiation of dozens of unsuspecting victims, four of whom were injured fatally (UNSCEAR, 1993).

Prominent features of the acute effects of ionizing radiation on the more radiosensitive tissues of the body are described briefly in the following list (also see Table 21.4).

Skin. Brief exposure of the skin to a dose of 6 Sv or more suffices to produce a sunburn-like rash and loss of hair in the exposed area. If the dose exceeds 10 to 20 Sv, blistering and ulceration may ensue, followed by scarring of the underlying tissue, and a second wave of atrophy and ulceration months or years later (Mettler and Upton, 2008).

Bone marrow and lymphoid tissue. A dose of 2 to 3 Sv delivered rapidly to the whole body leads to a marked depression of the lymphocyte count and immune response within hours and a comparable depression of the leukocyte and platelet counts within three to five weeks. After a larger dose, the latter

TABLE 21.4 Major Forms and Features of Acute Radiation Syndrome

Time After Irradiation	Cerebral Form (>50 Sv)	Gastrointestinal Form (10–20 Sv)	Hemopoietic Form (2–10 Sv)	Pulmonary Form (>6 Sv to lungs)
First day	Nausea Vomiting Diarrhea Headache Disorientation Ataxia Coma Convulsions Death	Nausea Vomiting Diarrhea	Nausea Vomiting Diarrhea	Nausea Vomiting
Second week		Nausea Vomiting Diarrhea Fever Erythema Prostration Death		
Third to sixth weeks			Weakness Fatigue Anorexia Fever Hemorrhage Epilation Recovery (?) Death (?)	
Second to eighth months				Cough Dyspnea Fever Chest pain Respiratory failure (?)

Sources: Adapted from UNSCEAR, 1988; Mettler and Upton, 2008.

changes may be severe enough to result in fatal infection or hemorrhage, or both (Table 21.4). In Hiroshima and Nagasaki, for example, the majority of the many thousands of fatally injured victims who were exposed to atomic bomb radiation within 1 km of ground zero and did not die from blast injuries or burns succumbed from damage to the bone marrow (Ohkita, 1975).

Intestine. An acute dose of 10 Sv causes the lining of the small intestine to become denuded within days (Mettler and Upton, 2008), and if a large enough area of the lining is affected, a fulminating, rapidly fatal dysentery-like syndrome results (Table 21.4).

Gonads. A dose of 0.15 Sv delivered rapidly to both testes can kill enough immature sperm-forming cells to lower the sperm count, and a dose of 2 to 4 Sv is likely to cause permanent sterility. Likewise, a dose of 1.5 to 2.0 Sv delivered rapidly to both ovaries kills enough oocytes to cause temporary sterility, and a larger dose permanent sterility, depending on the age of the woman at the time of exposure (ICRP, 1984; Mettler and Upton, 2008).

Respiratory tract. The lung is not highly radiosensitive, but a dose of 6 to 10 Sv can cause the exposed area to become severely inflamed within one to three months. If a large enough volume of the lung is affected, respiratory failure may follow within weeks, or other complications may occur months or years later (ICRP, 1984; UNSCEAR, 1988; Mettler and Upton, 2008).

Lens of the eye. Acute exposure of the lens to more than 1 Sv may be followed within months by the formation of a microscopic lens opacity; and 2 to 3 Sv received in a single brief exposure (or 5.5 to 14 Sv accumulated over a period of months) may cause a vision-impairing cataract (ICRP, 1984; Mettler and Upton, 2008).

Other tissues. The other tissues of the body have thresholds for acute injury that are substantially higher than those for the reactions described above (Mettler and Upton, 2008). All tissues, however, tend to be more radiosensitive when in a rapidly growing state (ICRP, 1984; Mettler and Upton, 2008).

Whole-body radiation injury. Rapid exposure of a major part of the body to more than 1 Sv may cause the *acute radiation syndrome* ("radiation sickness"). This syndrome is characterized by (1) an initial prodromal stage with malaise, anorexia, nausea, and vomiting; (2) an ensuing asymptomatic, latent period; (3) a second (main) phase of illness; and (4) finally, either recovery or death (Table 21.4). The main phase of illness typically takes one of the following four forms, depending on the predominant locus of radiation injury: hematological, gastrointestinal, cerebral, or pulmonary. Another syndrome, termed **chronic radiation sickness**, has been reported in chronically exposed workers of the Mayak Nuclear facility and in people residing downriver from the facility who were exposed to radioactive effluents from the plant. The clinical findings in these groups, yet to be reported in other irradiated populations, include varying and persistent leukopenia, thrombocytopenia, arthralgia, asthenia, and various other ill-defined neurological complaints (Kossenko and others, 1994).

Localized radiation injury. In contrast to the clinical manifestations of acute whole-body radiation injury, which are often dramatic and prompt, the reaction to sharply localized irradiation, whether from an external radiation source or from an internally deposited radionuclide, tends to evolve more slowly and to produce few symptoms unless the volume of tissue irradiated or the dose is relatively large. Of note, some radionuclides (such as, tritium, carbon-14, and cesium -137) tend to be distributed systemically and to irradiate the whole body to varying degrees, whereas others are characteristically concentrated in specific organs. Radium and strontium-90, for example, are deposited predominantly in bone, causing skeletal injuries primarily, whereas radioactive iodine concentrates in the thyroid gland, which is the chief site of any resulting injury (Stannard, 1988; Mettler and Upton, 2008).

Carcinogenic Effects   The carcinogenic effects of ionizing radiation, first manifested early in this century by skin cancers and leukemia in pioneer radiation workers, have since been documented extensively by the occurrence of dose-dependent excesses of osteosarcomas and cranial sinus carcinomas in radium dial painters, carcinomas of the respiratory tract in underground hard-rock miners, and cancers of many organs in atomic bomb survivors, radiotherapy patients, and experimentally irradiated laboratory animals (Upton, 1986; Mettler and Upton, 2008). The tumors caused by irradiation characteristically take years or decades to appear and exhibit no features distinguishing them from other tumors. With few exceptions, moreover, they have been detectable only after relatively large doses (0.5 Sv [50 rem]) and have varied in frequency with the type of neoplasm as well as the age and sex of the exposed individuals. The neoplasms typically evolve through a succession of stages, and in experimental animals the carcinogenic effects of radiation have included initiating effects, promoting effects, and effects on the progression of neoplasia, depending on the experimental conditions (NRC, 2006). The molecular mechanisms of these effects remain to be fully elucidated, but the activation of oncogenes or the inactivation or loss of tumor-suppressor genes, or both, appear to be involved in many if not all instances (NRC, 2006). Furthermore, the carcinogenic effects of radiation resemble those of chemical carcinogens in being modifiable by hormones, nutritional variables, and other modifying factors; and in combination with chemical carcinogens, the effects of radiation may be additive, synergistic, or mutually antagonistic, depending on the specific chemicals and exposure conditions (UNSCEAR, 2000; Mettler and Upton, 2008).

Effects on the Developing Embryo Radiosensitivity is relatively high throughout prenatal life. The effects of a given dose can vary markedly, however, depending on the developmental stage of the embryo or fetus at the time of exposure (Mettler and Upton, 2008). During the preimplantation period, the embryo is maximally susceptible to killing by irradiation. Subsequently, during critical stages in organogenesis, it is susceptible to the induction of malformations and other disturbances of development. The latter are dramatically exemplified in the dose-dependent increase in the frequency of mental retardation and the dose-dependent decrease in IQ test scores observed in atomic bomb survivors who were irradiated between the eighth and fifteenth weeks (and, to a lesser extent, between the sixteenth and twenty-fifth weeks) after conception (UNSCEAR, 1986; NRC, 1990; Mettler and Upton, 2008). Susceptibility to the carcinogenic effects of radiation also appears to be comparatively high throughout the prenatal period; that is, the available data suggest that irradiation in utero may increase a child's risk of leukemia and other cancers by as much as 40 percent per Sv (Doll and Wakeford, 1997; Mettler and Upton, 2008).

Risk Assessment

Although nonstochastic effects of radiation are produced only by relatively large doses, genetic and carcinogenic effects appear to increase in frequency as non-threshold functions of the dose (NCRP, 2001a; Mettler and Upton, 2008). The existing data, however, do not suffice to describe the dose-incidence relationship unambiguously for any type of neoplasm in the low-dose domain or to define how long after irradiation the risk of the growth may remain elevated in an exposed population. Therefore, any risks attributable to low-level irradiation can be estimated only by extrapolation, based on models (NCRP, 2001a), a process described in detail in Chapter Thirty. Various dose-effect models have been used to estimate the risks of low-level irradiation, and most of these models involve the assumption that the overall risk of cancer increases in proportion with the dose at low-dose levels; however, because the carcinogenic potency of X-rays and gamma rays in laboratory animals has been found to be reduced by as much as an order of magnitude when the exposure is prolonged, the risk to humans is generally estimated to increase less steeply with the dose at low doses and dose rates than at high doses and dose rates. Furthermore, as has been emphasized elsewhere (NCRP, 2001a; NRC, 2006), the available data do not exclude the possibility of a threshold in the mSv dose range below which the carcinogenicity of radiation is lacking altogether. For this reason the existing estimates must be used with caution in attempting to predict the risks of cancer from small doses or doses accumulated over weeks, months, or years (NRC, 2006; Mettler and Upton, 2008).

These uncertainties notwithstanding, models have been applied to epidemiological data from the atomic bomb survivors and other irradiated populations and have yielded estimates of the lifetime risks of different forms of cancer that may be attributable to ionizing irradiation (see the examples in Table 21.5). In interpreting the estimates, however, it must be recognized that they are based on population averages and hence cannot be assumed to apply equally to all individuals. Susceptibility to certain types of cancer (notably cancers of the thyroid and breast) is substantially higher in children than in adults, and susceptibility is also increased in association with certain hereditary disorders, such as retinoblastoma and nevoid basal cell carcinoma syndrome (Sankaranarayanan and Chakraborty,

TABLE 21.5   Estimated Lifetime Risks of Fatal Cancer Attributable to 0.1 Sv (10 Rem) Low-Dose-Rate, Whole-Body Irradiation

	Excess Cancer Deaths Per 100,000	
Type or Site of Cancer	**(No.)**	**(% excess above baseline)[a]**
Colon	61	3
Lung	200	7
Bone marrow (leukemia)	65	13
Stomach	22	4
Breast	40	2
Urinary bladder	25	4
Esophagus	20	6
Liver	16	9
Gonads	24	5
Thyroid	8	8
Bone	5	5
Skin	2	2
Remainder	87	2
Total	575	2

[a] Percentage increase in the baseline risk expected for a nonirradiated population.

Source: Adapted from NRC, 2006.

1995; ICRP, 1998; Little, 2000; Mettler and Upton, 2008). Although quantitative estimates are therefore limited by various sources of uncertainty, some view them as the only rational basis for attributing cancer in a previously irradiated person to the dose of radiation in question (Land and others, 2003; Kocher and others, 2008).

Studies to ascertain whether the rates of cancer and other diseases vary detectably with natural background radiation levels have been inconclusive thus far. A few studies have even suggested an inverse relationship, which some observers have interpreted as evidence of beneficial (or *hormetic*) effects of low-level irradiation (Luckey, 1991; Calabrese and Baldwin, 2000; Tubiana, Arengo, Averbeck, and Masse, 2007). However, such a relationship has not usually persisted after controlling for the effects of confounders (UNSCEAR, 2000; NCRP, 2001a; Upton, 2001; NRC, 2006). The fact that populations residing in areas of elevated natural background radiation have not exhibited significant increases in cancer rates (UNSCEAR, 2000) is not unexpected in view of the low exposure levels; the estimates tabulated in Table 21.5 imply that no more than 2 percent of all cancer deaths in the general population are attributable to natural background radiation (NRC, 1990). At the same time, however, it is noteworthy that indoor exposure to radon is estimated to account for up to 9 to 10 percent of the lung cancers in the United States (Krewski and others, 2005) and Europe (Darby and others, 2005), amply justifying efforts to assess and control indoor levels of this naturally occurring radionuclide (U.S. Environmental Protection Agency [EPA], 2007).

When we turn to occupational risks, although some cohorts of underground hard rock miners continue to exhibit elevated mortality from lung cancer (NRC, 1998), carcinogenic effects of occupational irradiation are no longer readily demonstrable in most U.S. radiation workers, thanks to modern radiation protection practices. The data for several large cohorts of nuclear workers, however, suggest a dose-dependent excess of leukemia and other cancers in this population (Cardis and others, 2007) that is comparable in magnitude with the estimate displayed in Table 21.5. Excesses of multiple myeloma and other forms of cancer have also been reported in some cohorts of occupationally exposed workers, but such excesses have been observed only inconsistently and are of equivocal significance (UNSCEAR, 2000; Mettler and Upton, 2008).

Among populations exposed to radioactive fallout, carcinogenic effects on the thyroid gland have been well documented. One example is Marshall Islanders who received large doses to the thyroid in childhood and infancy (possibly up to 20 Gy [2,000 rad]) from radioactive iodine, tellurium, and external gamma ray emitters in fallout released by a thermonuclear weapons test at Bikini atoll in 1954 (Robbins and Adams, 1989). Other examples are children who lived downwind of the Nevada nuclear weapons test site (Kerber and others,, 1993; Simon, Bouville, and Land, 2006) and children in Belarus and the Ukraine following the Chernobyl accident (Heidenreich and others, 1999; Mettler and Upton, 2008).

Although nuclear accidents can be catastrophic, as demonstrated by the Chernobyl accident, the public health impacts of nuclear power compare favorably overall with those of most other electricity-generating systems. Under normal operating conditions, and allowing for accidents, the lives lost per terawatt-hour (TWh) of electricity generated have been estimated to approximate 25.2 for nuclear power, versus 138 for coal, 359 for oil, 43 for natural gas, and 1 for wind (Krewitt, Hurley, Trukenmuller, and Friedrich, 1998). The safe disposal of nuclear wastes poses special challenges, because long half-lives make some of them hazardous for many thousands of years. In part for this reason, considerable public fear and political opposition to nuclear power persist (Crowley and Ahearne, 2002). However, rising energy costs and the need to respond to global climate change may herald renewed interest in this source of energy (see Chapters Ten, on climate change, and Thirteen, on energy).

Radiation Protection and Prevention

To minimize any associated risks of radiation injury, it is recommended that (1) no activity involving ionizing radiation should be considered justifiable unless it produces a sufficient benefit to those who are exposed, or to society at large, to offset any harm it may cause; (2) in any such activity the dose or likelihood of exposure should be kept **as low as reasonably achievable (ALARA)**, taking all relevant economic and social factors into account; and (3) the radiation exposure of individuals resulting from any combination of such activities should be subject to dose limits low enough to prevent nonstochastic effects altogether and also low enough to prevent the risks of any stochastic effects (which may have no thresholds) from exceeding socially acceptable levels. For members of the public, therefore, it is generally recommended that the effective dose not exceed 5 mSv in any given year or 1 mSv per year on average over any three years (NCRP, 1993; International Atomic Energy Agency [IAEA], 1996; Mettler and Upton, 2008).

To comply with these precautionary guidelines, any facility dealing with ionizing radiation must (1) be properly designed, (2) carefully plan and oversee its operating procedures, (3) maintain a meticulous radiation protection program, (4) ensure that its workers are adequately trained and supervised, and (5) maintain a well-developed and well-rehearsed emergency preparedness plan, in order to be able to respond promptly and effectively in the event of a malfunction, spill, or other type of radiation accident (Shapiro, 1990; IAEA, 1996; NCRP, 1998; Gusev and others, 2001). These guidelines apply both to developed countries and to developing countries (UNSCEAR, 1988; IAEA, 1996).

Because medical radiographic examinations and indoor radon constitute the most important controllable sources of exposure to ionizing radiation for the general public (Table 21.3), prudent measures to limit irradiation from these sources are clearly warranted (NCRP, 1993; IAEA, 1996; EPA, 2007). Other potential risks to human health and the environment that call for increased attention are the millions of cubic feet of radioactive and mixed wastes (mine and mill tailings, spent nuclear fuel, waste from the decommissioning of nuclear power plants, dismantled industrial and medical radiation sources, radioactive pharmaceuticals and reagents, heavy metals, polycyclic aromatic hydrocarbons, and other contaminants) that are present in ever-growing quantities and severely tax existing storage capacities at numerous sites (see, for example, NRC, 1989; DOE, 1993; Crowley and Ahearne, 2002). Furthermore, whereas the atomic bombs detonated over Hiroshima and Nagasaki were of 12.5 kiloton and 22 kiloton magnitudes, respectively, it is estimated that a nuclear detonation of only 0.01 kiloton magnitude could deliver whole-body doses of 4 Gy or more to persons within 250 meters of ground zero, fatally injuring 50 percent of them instantaneously, and that its residual radioactive fallout could deliver comparable doses to persons remaining within 1.3 kilometers of the detonation (NCRP, 2001a). The need to keep nuclear and other radioactive materials out of the hands of terrorists and to prepare for the threat to public health that their involvement in a terrorist event could pose is thus particularly urgent and calls for special precautions at local as well as national and global levels (NCRP, 2001b).

ULTRAVIOLET RADIATION

Ultraviolet radiation (UVR) consists of electromagnetic waves, subdivided for convenience into three bands of the spectrum (Figure 21.1): UVA, 315 to 440 nm (or black light); UVB, 280 to 315 nm; and UVC, 100 to 280 nm (which is germicidal). The chief source of UVR for members of the public is sunlight, which varies in intensity with latitude, elevation, and season (Driscoll and Cridland, 2000). Important man-made sources of high-intensity exposure include sunlamps and tanning lamps, welding arcs, plasma torches, germicidal and black-light lamps, electric arc furnaces, hot-metal operations, mercury-vapor lamps, and lasers. Common low-intensity sources include fluorescent lamps and certain laboratory equipment (Driscoll and Cridland, 2000).

Types and Mechanisms of Injury

Because UVR does not penetrate deeply into human tissues, the injuries it causes are confined chiefly to the skin and eyes. Dermal reactions to UVR, common among fair-skinned people, include sunburn; pigmentation; skin cancers (basal cell and squamous cell carcinomas, and possibly, to a lesser extent, melanomas); aging of the skin; telangiectasia; solar elastoses; and solar keratoses (Figure 21.3) (Driscoll and Cridland, 2000; Yashar and Lim, 2003; Berwick, Lachiewicz, Pestak, and Thomas, 2008). Injuries of the eye include photokeratitis and photoconjunctivitis, which may result from brief exposure to a high-intensity UVR source (*welder's flash*) or from more prolonged exposure to intense sunlight (*snow blindness*); prolonged exposure may also cause pterygium, climatic droplet keratopathy, cortical lens cataract, solar retinitis, and macular degeneration (Driscoll and Cridland, 2000; McCarty and Taylor, 2002; Sliney, 2002).

The effects of UVR result chiefly from its absorption in DNA, leading to the production of pyrimidine dimers and mutational changes in exposed cells (Ehrhart, Gosselet, Culerrier, and Sarasin, 2003). Sensitivity to UVR may therefore be

FIGURE 21.3   A Basal Cell Carcinoma of the Skin of Twenty Years Duration in a Fifty-Eight-Year-Old Man

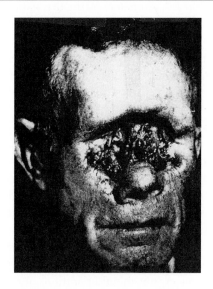

Source: Warren, 1953. Reprinted with permission from Elsevier.

Such tumors are the commonest of cancers and occur primarily in sun-exposed areas of the skin.

increased by DNA repair defects (for example, xeroderma pigmentosum), by agents (such as caffeine) that inhibit the repair enzymes, and by photosensitizing agents (such as psoralens, sulfonamides, tetracyclines, nalidixic acid, sulfonylureas, thiazides, phenothiazines, furocumarins, and coal tar), that produce UVR-absorbing DNA photoproducts (Harper and Bickers, 1989; Yashar and Lim, 2003). The carcinogenic action of UVR is mediated primarily through direct effects on the exposed cells but may involve depression of local immunity as well (Ichihashi and others, 2003; Rana and others, 2008). UVB, although far less intense than UVA in sunlight, plays a more important role in sunburn and skin carcinogenesis (English, Armstrong, Kricker, and Fleming, 1997), but UVA contributes to the latter also, as well as to tanning, some photosensitivity reactions, aging of the skin, photokeratitis, and cortical lens opacities (Driscoll and Cridland, 2000).

Radiation Protection and Prevention

Excessive exposure to sunlight or other sources of UVR should be avoided, especially by fair-skinned individuals. In addition to engineering and administrative controls for limiting exposure (enclosures, interlocks, restriction of access, training, supervision, and so forth), protective clothing, UVR-screening lotions or creams, and UVR-blocking sunglasses should be used for this purpose when necessary. To protect occupationally exposed workers under conditions where the duration of exposure is not less than 0.1 μs, it is recommended that exposures of the skin and eye to UVR be kept below 30 J/m^2 effective irradiance and that exposure of the eye to UVA be kept below 10^4 J/m^2 (Driscoll and Cridland, 2000).

From a global perspective it is significant that the protective layer of ozone in the stratosphere has been gradually depleted by chlorofluorocarbons and other air pollutants (Rex and others, 1997; McKenzie, Bjorn, Bais, and Ilyasd, 2003; Diffey, 2004), and that every 1 percent decrease in ozone is estimated to increase the UVR reaching the earth by 1 to 2 percent, raising the risk of nonmelanotic skin cancer by 2 to 6 percent (Henriksen, Dahlback, Larsen, and Moan, 1990). The rise in cancer rates is only one of the adverse outcomes expected from increased levels of UVR; perhaps the most serious is the far-reaching impacts on vegetation and crop production (Worrest and Grant, 1989; Caldwell and others, 2003).

VISIBLE LIGHT

Visible light consists of electromagnetic waves ranging in wavelength from 380 nm (violet) to 760 nm (red) (Figure 21.1). Sources of visible light in the environment vary widely in the intensity of their emissions. Common high-intensity sources other than the sun include lasers, electric welding or carbon arcs, and tungsten filament lamps.

Types and Mechanisms of Injury

A light that is too bright can injure the eye through photochemical reactions in the retina. Sustained exposure to intensities exceeding 0.1 mW/cm^2, such as can result from gazing at a bright source of light, may produce photochemical blue-light injury, and brief exposure of the retina to intensities exceeding 10 mW/cm^2, depending on image size, may cause a retinal burn, resulting in a scotoma (blind spot), which may be permanent (Sliney and Wolbarsht, 1980; Frank and Slesin, 1998). The lens, iris, cornea, and skin also are vulnerable to injury from the thermal effects of laser radiation (Sliney and Wolbarsht, 1980). Too little illumination, conversely, can also be harmful, causing eyestrain (Huer, 1983) and aggravating seasonal affective disorder (SAD) (Rosenthal and others, 1988).

Radiation Protection and Prevention

Bright, continuously visible light normally elicits an aversion response that acts to protect the eye against injury, so few sources of light are sufficiently large and bright to cause a retinal burn under normal viewing conditions. A solar eclipse must never be viewed directly, however, and in situations involving potential exposure to carbon arcs, lasers, or other high-intensity sources appropriate training, equipment, and protective eye shields are indicated (American National Standards Institute [ANSI], 1986; American Conference of Governmental Industrial Hygienists [ACGIH], 2005).

INFRARED RADIATION

Infrared radiation (IR) consists of electromagnetic waves ranging in wavelength from 7×10^{-5} m to 3×10^{-2} m (Figure 21.1). Such radiation is emitted by all objects with temperatures above absolute zero, but potentially hazardous sources of IR include furnaces, ovens, welding arcs, molten glass, molten metal, and heating lamps.

Types and Mechanisms of Injury

The injuries caused by IR are mainly burns of the skin and cataracts of the lens of the eye. The warning sensation of heat usually prompts aversion in time to prevent the skin from being burned by IR, but the lens of the eye lacks heat-sensing and heat-dissipating ability and is therefore vulnerable. Consequently, glassblowers, blacksmiths, oven operators, and those working around heating and drying lamps are at risk of IR-induced cataracts (Lydahl, 1984).

Radiation Protection and Prevention

Control of IR hazards requires appropriate shielding of sources, proper training and supervision of potentially exposed persons, and use of protective clothing and goggles. As a further precaution, it is recommended that exposures to IR not exceed 10 mW/cm^2 (ACGIH, 2005).

MICROWAVE RADIATION

Microwave and radiofrequency radiation (**MW/RFR**) consists of electromagnetic waves ranging in frequency from about 3 kHz to 300 GHz (Figure 21.1). Sources of MW/RFR occur in radar, television, radio, cellular phones, cell phone towers, and other telecommunications systems and in various industrial operations (such as heating, welding, and melting of metals; processing of wood and plastic; and using high-temperature plasma), household appliances (such as microwave ovens), and medical applications (such as diathermy and hyperthermia) (Sliney and Colville, 2000).

Types and Mechanisms of Injury

The biological effects of MW/RFR appear to be primarily thermal. MW/RFR can penetrate deeply enough, however, to burn dermal and subcutaneous tissues, burns that heal slowly. Cataracts of the lens of the eye also can result from high-intensity exposures (1.5 kW/m^2 (Lipman, Tripathi, and Tripathi, 1988), and death from hyperthermia has occurred in the industrial use of MW/RFR sources (Roberts and Michaelson, 1985). MW/RFR can also interfere with cardiac pacemakers and other medical devices. Although the biological effects of MW/RFR are attributed primarily to thermal mechanisms, there is growing evidence suggesting that MW/RFR may elicit some effects through nonthermal mechanisms as well. Such effects, yet to be demonstrated conclusively, have been suggested to include damage to DNA (Mazor and others, 2008; Blank, 2008), impairment of fertility, developmental disturbances, neurobehavioral abnormalities, depression of immunity, stimulation of cell proliferation, and carcinogenic effects (Tenforde, 1998; International Commission on Non-Ionizing Radiation Protection [ICNIRP], 2004: Hardell and others, 2007; Sadetski and others, 2008). The question of cancer risk has gained much attention thanks to the widespread use of cell phones (Figure 21.4).

PERSPECTIVE
Cell Phones and Cancer

Suggestions that the radiofrequency radiation from cellular phones may increase the risk of cancer have caused growing concern in recent years, prompting public objections to the siting of TV, radio, and cell phone transmission towers. To date, epidemiological and experimental data provide no conclusive evidence that low-level MW/RFR radiation is carcinogenic or genotoxic (ICNIRP, 2004; Hardell and others, 2007; Sadetski and others, 2008). However, there is some evidence that the risks of ipsilateral parotid gland tumors, acoustic neuromas, and gliomas may be increased in long-term (>10 years) users of cell phones (Hardell and others, 2007; Sadetski and others, 2008). As cell phone use grows, it will become a leading source of RFR exposure, and ongoing epidemiological studies will be critical in helping to clarify the nature and magnitude of any risks that cell phones may pose.

FIGURE 21.4   Cell Phones, Now Virtually Ubiquitous, Increase the Level of Radiofrequency Radiation Throughout the Environment

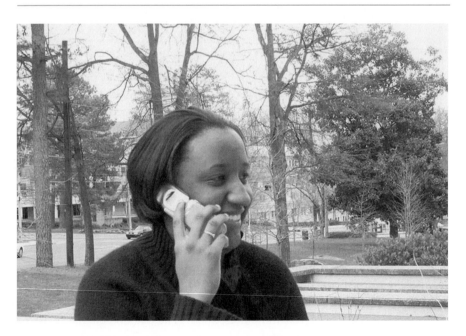

Radiation Protection and Prevention

Prevention of injury from MW/RFR requires proper design and shielding of MW/RFR sources, along with appropriate training and supervision of potentially exposed persons (especially those wearing cardiac pacemakers or other sensitive devices). To prevent detectable heating of tissue, exposures to MW/RFR of different frequencies should be kept below the relevant threshold limit values, which are based on the amount of radiofrequency energy absorbed in tissue, or the **specific absorption rate** (**SAR**) (ICNIRP, 1998; Sliney and Colville, 2000; ACGIH, 2005). The current SAR limit for cell phones, as set by the Federal Communications Commission, is 1.6 watts per kilogram (National Institute of Environmental Health Sciences, 2002). Also, in the face of uncertainty about the risks that may be involved, some observers recommend limiting the time spent on the phone or employing a headset or earpiece to increase the distance between the phone's microwave antenna and the user's head. As a further precaution, the governments of Germany, France, and the United Kingdom have all recommended severely restricting the use of cell phones by children.

EXTREMELY LOW-FREQUENCY ELECTROMAGNETIC FIELDS

Extremely low-frequency (ELF) electromagnetic fields (EMFs) consist of time-varying magnetic fields with frequencies below 300 Hz (Sliney and Colville, 2000). They are widely present throughout the environment, the largest arising intermittently from solar activity and thunderstorms and reaching intensities on the order of 0.5 T (teslas) (Grandolfo and Vecchia, 1985). Stronger EMFs, however, are the localized 50 to 60 Hz fields generated by electric power lines, transformers, motors, household appliances, video display tubes (VDTs), and various medical devices, notably magnetic resonance imaging (MRI) systems (Office of Technology Assessment [OTA], 1989; Tenforde, 1992). For example, the field strength on the ground beneath a 765 kV, 60 Hz power line carrying 1 kA (kiloampere) per phase is on the order of 15 T; and the field strength in close proximity to common household appliances may range up to 2.5 mT (milliteslas) (Tenforde, 1992). The strength of such fields decreases rapidly with distance, however, so that the average ambient value in the home environment is less than 0.3 T (3 mG [milligauss] (Silva, Hummon, Rutter, and Hooper, 1989). Similarly, although field strengths at VDTs typically range up to 5 T, those at the location of the operator are generally less than 1 T (Tenforde, 1992).

Types and Mechanisms of Injury

Extremely-low-frequency EMFs may have biological effects. The electrical currents they induce can alter electrical activity in the body—in cell membranes; in electrically active tissues such as nerves, muscles, and the retina; and in cardiac pacemakers. Low exposures (current density under 10 mA/m^2) produce few, if any, effects, because this level of electrical activity occurs naturally in many tissues. However, higher exposures (current densities above 10 mA/m^2) can change the biochemistry and physiology of some cells. These changes may include alterations in growth rate, melatonin secretion, endocrine activity, and immune response, although probably not genotoxicity. And even higher exposures (current densities above 1 A) can excite nerves and cause potentially irreversible effects, such as cardiac fibrillation (Tenforde, 1992, 1998).

The possibility that long-term exposure to weaker EMFs may cause other, severe effects has been suggested by epidemiological observations that the risks of leukemia in children may be increased by residential exposure to household EMFs, the risks of brain cancer and leukemia may be increased by occupational exposure to EMFs in utility workers, and the risks of reproductive disorders may be increased in pregnant women by chronic exposure to EMFs through the operation of VDTs (Tenforde, 1992, 1996; NRC, 1996). Although the weight of the evidence argues against the latter possibility, the relevant epidemiological data are inconclusive as yet, and their interpretation is complicated by uncertainties in exposure assessment and by the lack of established biological mechanisms for the effects in question (NRC, 1996; Tenforde, 1998). Nevertheless, the fact that such fields have been reported to influence ion transport, melatonin secretion, and tumor promotion in some model systems (Tenforde, 1992, 1998) has reinforced public health concern (OTA, 1989; NRC, 1996).

Radiation Protection and Prevention

Areas containing EMFs stronger than 0.5 mT (such as exist around transformers, accelerators, MRI systems, and other electric devices) should be posted with warning signs and should be avoided by persons wearing pacemakers. In addition, it is recommended that the strength of any 60 Hz time-varying magnetic field, such as typically exists around an MRI system, should be limited to 1 mT for occupational exposures, and to 0.1 mT for exposure of those wearing cardiac pacemakers or for continuous exposures involving members of the general public (ACGIH, 2005). Also, as a precautionary measure to minimize any risks that might be associated with the use of electric blankets or VDTs, most manufacturers have introduced design changes to eliminate or reduce the EMFs to which the users of such devices could otherwise be exposed (Tenforde, 1992, 1996; Sliney and Colville, 2000).

ULTRASOUND

Ultrasound is often classified for public health purposes with nonionizing radiation, but it is not a component of the electromagnetic spectrum and actually consists of mechanical vibrations at frequencies above the audible range (that is, 16 kHz). High-power, low-frequency ultrasound is used widely in science and industry for cleaning, degreasing, plastic welding, liquid extracting, atomizing, homogenizing, and emulsifying operations, as well as in medicine for lithotripsy and other applications. Low-power, high-frequency ultrasound is used widely in analytical work and in medical diagnosis, such as in ultrasonography (NCRP, 1983, 1992, 2002).

Types and Mechanisms of Injury

The biological effects of ultrasound occur through mechanisms similar in many respects to those of mechanical vibration, involving thermal (NCRP, 1992) as well as nonthermal (NCRP, 2002) changes. High-power, low-frequency ultrasound, transmitted through the air or through bodily contact with the generating source, has been observed to cause a variety of effects in occupationally exposed workers, including headache, earache, tinnitus, vertigo, malaise, photophobia, hyperacusia, peripheral neuritis, and autonomic polyneuritis. The possibility that it may harm the embryo also has been suggested (NCRP, 1983; 2002).

Excessive exposure to high-frequency ultrasound may be expected, in principle, to cause complaints similar to those just noted; however, no adverse effects have been shown to result from exposure to high-frequency ultrasound at the low power levels used in medical ultrasonography (NCRP, 2002). Nevertheless, the existing epidemiological data do not suffice to exclude the possibility that ultrasonography as it is currently employed in clinical practice may carry a small risk of adverse effects (NCRP, 2002).

Radiation Protection and Prevention

Protection against potential injury by ultrasound requires appropriate isolation and insulation of generating sources, proper training and use of ear protective devices by those working around such sources, and care to ensure that sound levels do not exceed relevant exposure limits (ACGIH, 2005). In addition, yearly audiometric and neurological examinations of occupationally exposed workers are recommended (World Health Organization, 1982).

SUMMARY

The adverse health effects of different forms of radiant energy are highly diverse, ranging from rapidly fatal reactions to cancers, birth defects, and hereditary disorders that do not appear until months, years, or decades later. The nature, frequency, and severity of the effects depend on the type of radiant energy and the particular conditions of exposure. Most such effects are produced only by moderate to high levels of exposure and can therefore be prevented by keeping any exposures below the relevant thresholds. On the other hand the genotoxic and carcinogenic effects of ionizing and ultraviolet radiations appear to increase in frequency as nonthreshold functions of the dose; therefore prevention may require avoiding exposure to these forms of radiation altogether. Given that complete avoidance is not feasible, exposure should be limited sufficiently to prevent any resulting risks of mutagenic and carcinogenic effects from exceeding acceptable levels.

To achieve the desired level of protection against each of the different forms of radiation requires appropriate design, control, and operation of all radiation sources; proper training and supervision of operating and potentially exposed personnel; and education of the public in prudent protective health measures. These requirements can be met satisfactorily in most situations involving radiation hazards if the necessary effort is made and resources are provided. Public health problems that remain to be adequately addressed at this time include the risks associated with residential exposure to indoor radon, the hazards posed by the large and growing quantities of radioactive and mixed wastes, the need to assess the potential risks of radio-frequency radiation and 60 Hz electromagnetic fields; and the ultraviolet radiation–induced impacts on human health and the environment that can be expected to result from further depletion of stratospheric ozone levels.

KEY TERMS

accelerated atomic particles

alpha particles

as low as is reasonably achievable (ALARA)

carbon-14

chronic radiation sickness

cosmic rays

deterministic

electromagnetic spectrum

electromagnetic waves

electrons

extremely low-frequency (ELF) electromagnetic fields (EMFs)

gamma rays

infrared radiation (IR)

ionizing radiation

linear energy transfer (LET)

microwave and radiofrequency radiation (MW/RFR)

neutrons

nonstochastic

potassium-40

protons

radiant energy

radium

radon

relative biological
  effectiveness (RBE)

specific absorption rate
  (SAR)

stochastic

ultrasound

ultraviolet radiation
  (UVR)

visible light

X-ray

DISCUSSION QUESTIONS

1. What are the mechanisms through which the different forms of radiation interact with living cells at the molecular level, and how may they lead to adverse effects on human health?
2. What types of injury of public health concern are associated with exposure to each of the different forms of radiation, and how does the risk of each such injury vary with the dose of the radiation in question?
3. Dental X-rays are performed routinely in many dental offices and clinics. How would you evaluate the risks and benefits of routine dental X-rays?
4. A cell phone company proposes to erect a cell phone tower on the roof of your university building. Would you approve of this installation? If not, why not?

REFERENCES

American Conference of Governmental Industrial Hygienists. *Threshold Limit Values and Biological Exposure Indices for 2005*. Cincinnati, Ohio: American Conference of Governmental Industrial Hygienists, 2005.

American National Standards Institute. *Safe Use of Lasers*. New York: American National Standards Institute, 1986.

Bender, M. A., and others. "Current Status of Cytogenetic Procedures to Detect and Quantify Previous Exposures to Radiation." *Mutation Research*, 1988, *196*, 103–159.

Berwick, M., Lachiewicz, A., Pestak, C., and Thomas, N., "Solar UV Exposure and Mortality from Skin Tumors." *Advances in Experimental Medicine and Biology*, 2008, *624*, 117–124.

Blank, M. "Protein and DNA Reactions Stimulated by Electromagnetic Fields." *Electromagnetic Biology and Medicine*, 2008, *27*, 3–23.

Brown, P. *American Martyrs to Science Though the Roentgen Rays*. Springfield, Ill.: Thomas, 1936.

Calabrese, E. J., and Baldwin, L. A. "Radiation Hormesis: The Demise of a Legitimate Hypothesis." *Human and Experimental Toxicology*, 2000, *19*, 76–84.

Caldwell, M. M., and others. "Terrestrial Ecosystems, Increased Solar Ultraviolet Radiation and Interactions with Other Climatic Change Factors." *Photochemical & Photobiological Sciences*, 2003, *2*, 29–38.

Cardis, E., and others. "The 15-Country Collaborative Study of Cancer Risk Among Radiation Workers in the Nuclear Industry: Estimates of Radiation-Related Cancer Risks." *Journal of Radiation Research*, 2007, *167*, 396–416.

Crowley, K. D., and Ahearne, J. F. "Managing the Environmental Legacy of U.S. Nuclear-Weapons Production." *American Scientist*, 2002, *90*, 514–523.

Darby, S., and others. "Radon in Homes and Risk of Lung Cancer: Collaborative Analysis of Individual Data from 13 European Case-Control Studies." *British Medical Journal*, 2005, *330*, 223–225.

Diffey, B. "Climate Change, Ozone Depletion and the Impact on Ultraviolet Exposure of Human Skin." *Physics in Medicine & Biology*, 2004, *49*(1), R1–R11.

Doll, R., Evans, N. J., and Darby, S. C. "Paternal Exposure Not to Blame." *Nature*, 1994, *367*, 678–680.

Doll, R., and Wakeford, R. "Risk of Childhood Cancer from Fetal Irradiation." *British Journal of Radiology*, 1997, *70*, 130–139.

Driscoll, C.M.H., and Cridland, N. A. "Ultraviolet Radiation." In M. Lippmann (ed.), *Environmental Toxicants* (pp. 851–887). (2nd ed.) Hoboken, N.J.: Wiley-Interscience, 2000.

Ehrhart, J. C., Gosselet, F. P., Culerrier, R. M., and Sarasin, A. "UVB-Induced Mutations in Human Key Gatekeeper Genes Governing Signaling Pathways and Consequences for Skin Tumourigenesis." *Photochemical & Photobiological Sciences*, 2003, *2*, 825–834.

English, D. R., Armstrong, B. K., Kricker, A., and Fleming, C. "Sunlight and Cancer." *Cancer Causes and Control*, 1997, *8*, 271–283.

Frank, A. L., and Slesin, L. "Nonionizing Radiation." In R. B. Wallace (ed.), *Maxcy-Rosenau-Last Public Health and Preventive Medicine* (pp. 627–635). (14th ed.) Stamford, Conn.: Appleton & Lange, 1998.

Gardner, M. J., and others. "Results of Case-Control Study of Leukaemia and Lymphoma Among Young People Near Sellafield Nuclear Plant in West Cumbria." *British Medical Journal*, 1990, *300*, 423–429.

Goodhead, D. J. "Spatial and Temporal Distribution of Energy." *Health Physics*, 1988, *55*, 231–240.

Grandolfo, M., and Vecchia, P. "Natural and Man-Made Exposures to Static and ELF Magnetic Fields." In M. Grandolfo, S. M. Michaelson, and A. Rindi (eds.), *Biological Effects and Dosimetry of Static and ELF Electromagnetic Fields* (pp. 49–70). New York: Plenum, 1985.

Gusev, I. A., Guskova, A. K., and Mettler, F. A. (eds.). *Medical Management of Radiation Accidents*. (2nd ed.) Boca Raton, Fla.: CRC Press, 2001.

Hall, E., and Giaccia, A. *Radiobiology for the Radiologist*. Philadelphia: Lippincott Williams & Wilkins, 2006.

Hardell, L., and others. "Long-Term Use of Cellular Phones and Brain Tumours: Increased Risk Associated with Use for ≥10 Years." *Journal of Occupational and Environmental Medicine*, 2007, *64*, 626–632.

Harper, L. C., and Bickers, D. R. *Photosensitivity Diseases: Principles of Diagnosis and Treatment*. (2nd ed.) Toronto: Decker, 1989.

Heidenreich, W. F., and others. "Time Trends of Thyroid Cancer Incidence in Belarus After the Chernobyl Accident." *Radiation Research*, 1999, *181*, 617–625.

Henriksen, T., Dahlback, A., Larsen, S., and Moan, J. "Ultraviolet Radiation and Skin Cancer: Effect of an Ozone Layer Depletion." *Photochemical & Photobiological Sciences*, 1990, *51*, 579–582.

Huer, H. H. "Lighting." In L. Parmeggiana (ed.), *Encyclopedia of Occupational Health and Safety* (pp. 1225–1231). Geneva: International Labour Organization, 1983.

Ichihashi, M., and others. "UV-Induced Skin Damage." *Toxicology*, 2003, *189*, 21–39.

International Atomic Energy Agency. *International Basic Safety Standards for Protection Against Ionizing Radiation and for the Safety of Radiation Sources*. Vienna: International Atomic Energy Agency, 1996.

International Commission on Non-Ionizing Radiation Protection. "Guidelines for Limiting Exposure to Time-Varying Electric, Magnetic, and Electromagnetic Fields (up to 300 GHz)." *Health Physics*, 1998, *74*, 494–522.

International Commission on Non-Ionizing Radiation Protection. "Epidemiology of Health Effects of Radiofrequency Exposure." *Environmental Health Perspectives*, 2004, *112*, 1741–1754.

International Commission on Radiological Protection. "Nonstochastic Effects of Ionizing Radiation." *Annals of the ICRP*, 1984, *14*(3), 1–33.

International Commission on Radiological Protection. "1990 Recommendations of the International Commission on Radiological Protection." *Annals of the ICRP*, 1991, *21*(entire issue 1–3).

International Commission on Radiological Protection. "Genetic Susceptibility to Cancer." *Annals of the ICRP*, 1998, *28*(1–2), 1–157.

Kerber, R. A., and others. "A Cohort Study of Thyroid Disease in Relation to Fallout from Nuclear Weapons Testing." *JAMA*, 1993, *270*, 2076–2082.

Kocher, D., and others. "Interactive Radioepidemiological Program (IREP): A Web-Based Tool for Estimating Probability of Causation/Assigned Share of Radiogenic Cancers." *Health Physics*, 2008, *95*, 119–147.

Kossenko, M. M., and others. Analysis of Chronic Radiation Sickness in the Population of the Southern Urals. AFFRI Contract Report 94–1. Springfield, Va.: Armed Forces Radiobiological Research Institute, 1994.

Krewitt, W., Hurley, F., Trukenmuller, A., and Friedrich, R. "Health Risks of Energy Systems." *Risk Analysis*, 1998, *18*, 377–383.

Krewski, D., and others. "Residential Radon and Risk of Lung Cancer: A Combined Analysis of 7 North American Case-Control Studies." *Epidemiology*, 2005, *16*, 137–145.

Land, C. E., and others. Report of the NCI-CDC Working Group to Revise the 1985 NIH Radioepidemiological Tables. NIH Publication No. 035387. Bethesda, Md.: National Institutes of Health, 2003.

Lipman, R. M., Tripathi, B. J., and Tripathi, R. C. "Cataracts Induced by Microwave and Ionizing Radiation." *Survey of Ophthalmology*, 1988, *33*, 200–210.

Little, J. B. "Radiation Carcinogenesis." *Carcinogenesis*, 2000, *21*, 397–404.

Luckey, T. D. *Radiation Hormesis*. Boca Raton, Fla.: CRC Press, 1991.

Lushbaugh, C. C., Fry, S. A., and Ricks, R. C. "Nuclear Reactor Accidents: Preparedness and Consequences." *British Journal of Radiology*, 1987, *60*, 1159–1183.

Lydahl, E. "Infrared Radiation and Cataract." *Acta Ophthalmologica*, 1984, *166* (suppl.), 1–63.

Mazor, R., and others. "Increased Levels of Numerical Aberrations After in Vivo Exposure of Human Lymphocytes to Radiofrequency Electromagnetic Fields for 72 Hours." *Radiation Research*, 2008, *169*, 28–37.

McCarty, C. A., and Taylor, H. R. "A Review of the Epidemiological Evidence Linking Ultraviolet Radiation and Cataracts." *Developments in Ophthalmology*, 2002, *35*, 21–31.

McKenzie, R. L., Bjorn, L. O., Bais, A., and Ilyasd, M. "Changes in Biologically Active Ultraviolet Radiation Reaching the Earth's Surface." *Photochemistry and Photobiology*, 2003, *2*, 5–15.

Mettler, F. A., and Upton, A. C. *Medical Effects of Ionizing Radiation*. (3rd ed.) Philadelphia: Saunders, 2008.

Michaelson, S. M. "Effects of Exposure to Microwaves: Problems and Perspectives." *Environmental Health Perspectives*, 1974, *8*, 133–156.

Morgan, W. F., and others. "Genomic Instability Induced by Ionizing Radiation." *Radiation Research*, 1996, *146*, 247–258.

National Council on Radiation Protection and Measurements. Biological Effects of Ultrasound: Mechanisms and Clinical Implications. NCRP Report No. 74. Bethesda, Md.: National Council on Radiation Protection and Measurements, 1983.

National Council on Radiation Protection and Measurements. Evaluation of Occupational and Environmental Exposures to Radon and Radon Daughters in the United States. NCRP Report No. 78. Bethesda, Md.: National Council on Radiation Protection and Measurements, 1984.

National Council on Radiation Protection and Measurements. Ionizing Radiation Exposure of the Population of the United States. NCRP Report No. 93. Bethesda, Md.: National Council on Radiation Protection and Measurements, 1987.

National Council on Radiation Protection and Measurements. Exposure of the U.S. Population from Occupational Radiation. NCRP Report No. 101. Bethesda, Md.: National Council on Radiation Protection and Measurements, 1989.

National Council on Radiation Protection and Measurements. Exposure Criteria for Medical Diagnostic Ultrasound, I: Criteria Based on Thermal Mechanisms. NCRP Report No. 113. Bethesda, Md.: National Council on Radiation Protection and Measurements, 1992.

National Council on Radiation Protection and Measurements. Limitation of Exposure to Ionizing Radiation. NCRP Report No. 116. Bethesda, Md.: National Council on Radiation Protection and Measurements, 1993.

National Council on Radiation Protection and Measurements. Operational Radiation Safety Program. NCRP Report No. 127. Bethesda, Md.: National Council on Radiation Protection and Measurements, 1998.

National Council on Radiation Protection and Measurements. Evaluation of the Linear-Nonthreshold Dose-Response Model For Ionizing Radiation. NCRP Report No. 136. Bethesda, Md.: National Council on Radiation Protection and Measurements, 2001a.

National Council on Radiation Protection and Measurements. Management of Terrorist Events Involving Radioactive Materials. NCRP Report No. 138. Bethesda, Md.: National Council on Radiation Protection and Measurements, 2001b.

National Council on Radiation Protection and Measurements. Exposure Criteria for Medical Diagnostic Ultrasound, II: Criteria Based on All Known Mechanisms. NCRP Report No. 140. Bethesda, Md.: National Council on Radiation Protection and Measurements, 2002.

National Institute of Environmental Health Sciences. *EMF: Questions and Answers*. Research Triangle Park, N.C.: National Institute of Environmental Health Sciences, 2002.

National Research Council. *The Nuclear Weapons Complex*. Washington, D.C.: National Academies Press, 1989.

National Research Council. *Health Effects of Exposure to Low Levels of Ionizing Radiation: BEIR V*. Washington, D.C.: National Academies Press, 1990.

National Research Council. *Possible Health Effects of Exposure to Residential Electric and Magnetic Fields.* Washington, D.C.: National Academies Press, 1996.

National Research Council. *Health Effects of Exposure to Radon.* Washington, D.C.: National Academies Press, 1998.

National Research Council. *Health Risks from Exposure to Low Levels of Ionizing Radiation: BEIR VII Phase 2.* Washington, D.C.: National Academies Press, 2006.

Office of Technology Assessment. *Biological Effects of Power Frequency Electric & Magnetic Fields. Background Paper: OTA-BP-E-53.* Washington, D.C.: U.S. Government. Printing Office, 1989.

Ohkita, T. "Acute Effects." In S. Okada and others (eds.), "A Review of Thirty Years Study of Hiroshima and Nagasaki Atomic Bomb Survivors, II: Biological Effects." *Radiation Research*, 1975, *16*(suppl.), pp. 49–66.

Rana, S., and others. "Ultraviolet B Suppresses Immunity by Inhibiting Effector and Memory T Cells." *American Journal of Pathology*, 2008, *172*, 993–1004.

Rex, M., and others. "Prolonged Stratospheric Ozone Loss in the 1995–96 Arctic Winter." *Nature*, 1997, *389*, 835–838.

Robbins, J., and Adams, W. "Radiation Effects in the Marshall Islands." In S. Nagataki (ed.), *Radiation and the Thyroid* (pp. 11–24). Amsterdam: Excerpta Medica, 1989.

Roberts, N. J., Jr., and Michaelson, S. M. "Epidemiological Studies of Human Exposures to Microwave Radiation: A Critical Review." *International Archives of Occupational and Environmental Health*, 1985, *56*, 169–178.

Rosenthal, N. E., and others. "Phototherapy for Seasonal Affective Disorder." *Journal of Biological Rhythms*, 1988, *3*, 101–120.

Sadetski, S., and others. "Cellular Phone Use and Risk of Benign and Malignant Parotid Gland Tumors—A Nationwide Case-Control Study." *American Journal of Epidemiology*, 2008, *167*, 457–467.

Sankaranarayanan, K. and Chakraborty, R., "Cancer Predisposition, Radiosensitivity and the Risk of Radiation-Induced Cancers, I: Background." *Radiation Research*, 1995, *143*, 121–143.

Shapiro, J. *Radiation Protection: A Guide for Scientists and Physicians.* (3rd ed.) Cambridge, Mass.: Harvard University Press, 1990.

Silva, M., Hummon, N., Rutter, D., and Hooper, C. "Power Frequency Magnetic Fields in the Home." *IEEE Transactions on Power Delivery*, 1989, *4*, 465–477.

Simon, S. L., Bouville, A., and Land, C. E. "Fallout from Nuclear Weapons Tests and Cancer Risks." *American Scientist*, 2006, *94*, 48–57.

Sliney, D. H. "How Light Reaches the Eye and Its Components." *International Journal of Toxicology*, 2002, *21*, 501–509.

Sliney, D. H., and Colville, F. "Microwaves and Electromagnetic Fields." In M. Lippmann (ed.), *Environmental Toxicants* (pp. 577–593). (2nd ed.) Hoboken, N.J.: Wiley-Interscience, 2000.

Sliney, D. H., and Wolbarsht, M. *Safety with Lasers.* New York: Plenum, 1980.

Stannard, J. N. *Radioactivity and Health: A History.* DOE/RL/01830-T5. Washington, D.C.: National Technical Information Services, 1988.

Stone, R. S. "Maximum Permissible Standards." In P. B. Sonnenblick (ed.), *Protection in Diagnostic Radiology*. New Brunswick, N.J.: Rutgers University Press, 1959.

Stone-Scott, N. "X-Ray Injuries." *American X-Ray Journal*, 1897, *1*, 57–67.

Tenforde, T. S. "Biological Interactions and Potential Health Effects of Extremely-Low-Frequency Magnetic Fields from Power Lines and Other Common Sources." *Annual Review of Public Health*, 1992, *13*, 173–196.

Tenforde, T. S. "Interaction of ELF Magnetic Fields with Living Systems." In C. Polk and E. Postow (eds.), *Handbook of Biological Effects of Electromagnetic Fields* (pp. 185–230). (2nd ed.) Boca Raton, Fla.: CRC Press, 1996.

Tenforde, T. S. "Electromagnetic Fields and Carcinogenesis—An Analysis of Biological Mechanisms." In G. L. Carlo (ed.), *Wireless Phones and Health: Scientific Progress* (pp. 183–196). Boston: Kluwer Academic, 1998.

Tubiana, M., Arengo, A., Averbeck, D., and Masse, R., "Low-Dose Risk Assessment." *Radiation Research*, 2007, *167*, 742–744.

United Nations Scientific Committee on the Effects of Atomic Radiation. *Genetic and Somatic Effects of Ionizing Radiation. 1986 Report to the General Assembly, with Annexes.* New York: United Nations, 1986.

United Nations Scientific Committee on the Effects of Atomic Radiation. *Sources, Effects, and Risks of Ionizing Radiation. 1988 Report to the General Assembly, with Annexes.* New York: United Nations, 1988.

United Nations Scientific Committee on the Effects of Atomic Radiation. Sources and Effects of Ionizing Radiation. *UNSCEAR 1993 Report to the General Assembly, with Scientific Annexes.* New York: United Nations, 1993.

United Nations Scientific Committee on the Effects of Atomic Radiation. *Sources and Effects of Ionizing Radiation. UNSCEAR 1994 Report to the General Assembly, with Scientific Annexes.* New York: United Nations, 1994.

United Nations Scientific Committee on the Effects of Atomic Radiation. *Sources and Effects of Ionizing Radiation. UNSCEAR 2000 Report to the General Assembly, with Scientific Annexes.* New York: United Nations, 2000.

United Nations Scientific Committee on the Effects of Atomic Radiation. *Sources and Effects of Ionizing Radiation. UNSCEAR 2006 Report to the General Assembly, with Scientific Annexes.* New York: United Nations, 2006.

U.S. Department of Energy. *Health and Environmental Consequences of the Chernobyl Nuclear Power Plant Accident.* DOE/ER-0332. Washington, D.C.: U.S. Department of Energy, 1987.

U.S. Department of Energy. *Interim Mixed Waste Inventory Report: Waste Streams, Treatment Capacities and Technologies.* DOE/NBM-1100. Springfield, Va.: National Technical Information Services, 1993.

U.S. Environmental Protection Agency. *A Citizen's Guide to Radon: The Guide to Protecting Yourself and Your Family from Radon.* EPA-402-K-07–009. Washington, D.C.: U.S. Environmental Protection Agency, 2007.

Upton, A. C., "Historical Perspectives on Radiation Carcinogenesis." In A. C. Upton, R. E. Albert, F. J. Burns, and R. E. Shore (eds.), *Radiation Carcinogenesis* (pp. 1–10). New York: Elsevier, 1986.

Upton, A. C. "Prevention of Work-Related Injuries and Diseases: Lessons from Our Experience with Ionizing Radiation." *American Journal of Industrial Medicine*, 1987, *12*, 291–309.

Upton, A. C. "Radiation Hormesis: Data and Interpretations." *Critical Reviews in Toxicology*, 2001, *31*, 681–695.

Vilenchik, M. M., and Knudson, A. G., Jr. "Inverse Radiation Dose-Rate Effects on Somatic and Germ-Line Mutations and DNA Damage Rates." *Proceedings of the National Academy of Sciences of the United States of America*, 2000, *97*, 5381–5386.

Wakeford, R., and others. "The Descriptive Statistics and Health Implications of Occupational Radiation Doses Received by Men at the Sellafield Nuclear Installation Before the Conception of Their Children." *Journal of Radiology Protection*, 1994a, *14*, 3–16.

Wakeford, R. and others. "The Seascale Childhood Leukaemia Cases—The Mutation Rates Implied by Paternal Preconceptional Radiation Doses." *Journal of Radiology Protection*, 1994b, *14*, 17–24.

Ward, J. F. "DNA Damage Produced by Ionizing Radiation in Mammalian Cells: Identities, Mechanisms of Formation, and Repairability." *Progress in Nucleic Acid Research and Molecular Biology*, 1988, *35*, 96–128.

Warren, S. "Neoplasms." In W.A.D. Anderson (ed.), *Anderson's Pathology*. St. Louis: Mosby, 1953.

Wojcik, A. "The Current Status of the Adaptive Response to Ionizing Radiation in Mammalian Cells." *Human and Ecological Risk Assessment*, 2000, *6*, 281–300.

World Health Organization. *Ultrasound. Environmental Health Criteria 22*. Geneva: World Health Organization, 1982.

Worrest, R. C., and Grant, L. D. "Effects of Ultraviolet-B Radiation on Terrestrial Plants and Marine Organisms." In R. R. Jones and T. Wigley (eds.), *Ozone Depletion: Health and Environmental Consequences* (pp. 197–206). Hoboken, N.J.: Wiley, 1989.

Yashar, S. S., and Lim, H. W. "Classification and Evaluation of Photodermatoses." *Dermatologic Therapy*, 2003, *16*, 1–7.

FOR FURTHER INFORMATION

Organizations

Many organizations address various aspects of radiation health and safety.

International Atomic Energy Agency, Vienna, Austria (www.iaea.org) The IAEA, an independent international organization related to the United Nations, was established in 1957 as the world's "Atoms for Peace" organization. It works with Member States and multiple partners worldwide to promote safe, secure and peaceful nuclear technologies.

International Commission on Radiological Protection, Ottawa, Ontario, Canada (www.icrp.org) The ICRP is a non-governmental organization established in 1928. Its parent organization is the International Society of Radiology, but its scope is broader than the medical field; it addresses all aspects of protection against ionizing radiation. The Commission is supported by a number of international organizations and by many governments. It issues recommendations on the principles of radiation protection.

International Commission on Non-Ionizing Radiation Protection, Oberschleissheim, Germany (http://www.icnirp.de/) The ICNIRP is a non-governmental organization of experts that disseminates information on the potential health hazards of exposure to non-ionizing radiation.

National Council on Radiation Protection and Measurements, Bethesda, MD (http://www.ncrponline.org/) The NCRP is a congressionally chartered U.S. organization that develops and disseminates information, guidance and recommendations on radiation protection and measurements.

U.S. Nuclear Regulatory Commission, Washington, D.C. (www.nrc.gov) The NRC is a government
agency that formulates policies, develops regulations governing nuclear reactor and nuclear
material safety, issues orders to licensees, and adjudicates legal matters.

Other agencies and organizations that address various aspects of radiation health and safety include
the U.S. Centers for Disease Control and Prevention (CDC), the U.S. Environmental
Protection Agency, the American Conference of Governmental Industrial Hygienists, and
the U.S. Department of Labor Occupational Safety and Health Administration.

Publications

The BEIR (Biologic Effects of Ionizing Radiation) Reports, from the National Academy of Sciences,
are authoritative compilations of information on various aspects of radiation and health.
While somewhat dated, they provide a useful framework.

Other important texts are included in the chapter references.

Kusunoki, Y. and Hayashi, T.: "Long-lasting alterations of the immune system by ionizing radiation
exposure: implications for disease development among atomic bomb survivors." *International
Journal of Radiation Biology*, 2008, *84*, 1–14.

National Council on Radiation Protection and Measurements (NCRP): *Ionizing Radiation Exposure
of the Population of the United States*. NCRP Report No. 160. Bethesda: National Council on
Radiation Protection and Measurements, 2009.

CHAPTER TWENTY-TWO

INJURIES

Jeremy J. Hess

Junaid A. Razzak

KEY CONCEPTS

- Injuries result when the human body is briefly exposed to intolerable levels of energy or is deprived of elements essential to life and function.

- Injuries, both intentional and unintentional, are preventable.

- Injuries constitute a major public health burden, particularly in the developing world, and are the tenth leading cause of mortality worldwide.

- Injuries affect the poor, the marginalized, and women and children disproportionately.

- The injury pyramid illustrates that for every injury resulting in death, there are often thousands of injuries resulting in short- or long-term disability.

- The Haddon Matrix is a staple of injury prevention and control; it guides conceptualization of the factors facilitating injury and the management of these factors.

- Injury control includes education of people at risk, enforcement of relevant laws and regulations, and engineering of passive controls.

- Injury prevention and control is context specific, and abundant examples exist of successful injury control measures in specific contexts.

THE word **injury** originates from the Latin *in jur* (from *jus*), which literally means "not right." In cellular terms, injury is physical damage caused by the excessive transfer of energy (whether mechanical, electrical, chemical, thermal, or radiant) or by the lack of essential factors for energy production (such as a lack of oxygen, resulting in suffocation or drowning, for example), or for maintenance of homeostasis (resulting in frostbite, for example).

Traditionally, public health officials ignored injuries because they were assumed to be random, unavoidable "accidents," without a clear causal pathway. We now know, however, that many injuries, like diseases, affect identifiable high-risk groups and follow a predictable chain of events and are therefore preventable. When prevention fails, the severity of an injury may still be reducible. The likelihood of death or long-term disability can be reduced by prompt provision of acute care and, subsequently, of rehabilitation. The combination of these three strategies—prevention, acute care, and rehabilitation—is termed **injury control**.

This chapter provides a general outline of injuries, following a public health approach and focusing on environmental factors. It begins with definitions, provides some epidemiological data to frame the scope of the injury problem, and proceeds to a general analysis of injury outcomes as well as risk and preventive factors. It then discusses general principles of **injury prevention** and control and examines certain injuries and environments in greater detail to illustrate key points about injury causes and prevention. This last section illustrates ways to conceptualize injuries and creative strategies to reduce the significant burdens that injuries impose.

INJURY PREVENTION AND CONTROL

Injury control draws on the expertise of many disciplines, including epidemiology, disease prevention, health promotion, biomechanics, acute care, rehabilitation, law, and public administration. It follows the traditional public health approach, which involves four generic steps (Centers for Disease Control and Prevention [CDC], 2002):

1. Define the health problem;
2. Identify causes, risk factors, and protective factors associated with the problem;
3. Develop and test interventions to reduce the problem's impact; and

Jeremy J. Hess and Junaid A. Razzak declare no competing financial interests.

4. Implement successful interventions, evaluate their impact, and ensure widespread acceptance and implementation of prevention principles and strategies of control.

Defining the Problem

The World Health Organization (WHO) defines injury as "the physical damage when a human body is suddenly or briefly subjected to intolerable levels of energy. It can be a bodily lesion resulting from acute exposure to energy in amounts that exceed the threshold of physiological tolerance, or it can be an impairment of function resulting from the lack of one or more vital elements (i.e., oxygen, water, warmth), as in drowning, strangulation, or freezing. The time between exposure to the energy and the appearance of an injury is short" (Holder and others, 2001, p. 5).

Injury control involves characterizing the distribution of injuries in given populations, quantifying the scope of an injury problem, monitoring patterns and trends, and evaluating the impact of countermeasures. Several information sources may be used for this purpose. Vital records or death certificates can be used to document overall rates of mortality, but they do not provide information about nonfatal injuries. Hospital records as well as trauma registries, emergency department (ED) data, emergency medical services (EMS) reports, and police reports, or a combination of these sources, may be used to provide essential information about cases of major trauma, depending on local resources and the nature of the information being sought. In the United States the National Hospital Discharge Survey and the National Hospital Ambulatory Medical Care Survey: Emergency Department Summary, are important sources of injury data. Other high-income countries (HICs) have similar systems for monitoring morbidity and mortality data associated with injuries. Although middle-income and low-income countries (MICs and LICs, respectively) often do not have similar extensive surveillance systems in place, data on injuries can be gathered from death certificates, hospital discharge summaries, emergency department records, and other sources (Razzak and Luby, 1998; Razzak, Marsh, and Stansfield, 2002).

Types of Injuries   Relying on these sources of data, investigators have identified a wide range of injuries and classified them according to several schemes. The most widely used approach divides injuries by intent. Purposefully inflicted injuries, or **intentional injuries,** are subdivided into those caused by self-directed harm, such as suicide, attempted suicide, or a suicidal gesture (sometimes called *parasuicide*), and those due to interpersonal violence. Violence-related injuries are further subdivided into individual violence (for example, assault or homicide), group violence (for example, gang violence), and collective violence (for example, religious or ethnic violence or state-sanctioned warfare). **Unintentional injuries** are often subdivided by mechanism—road traffic injuries, falls, burns, poisonings, drownings, and so on. Injuries may also be classified in other ways: according to the environment or circumstances in which they occur (for example, home, workplace, or roadways), by the body parts or systems most affected (for example, spinal cord injury), or by a particular pattern or context that results in injuries (for example, intimate partner violence).

Global Burden of Injury   Injuries are a significant cause of both morbidity and mortality throughout the world, ranking among the ten leading causes of death worldwide (Krug, 1999) and killing over 16,000 people a day (Krug and others, 2000). According to WHO, injury ranks as a leading cause of death and disability among all age groups up to the age of sixty (Peden, McGee, and Krug, 2002). An estimated 5 million people worldwide died from injuries in 2000, accounting for 9 percent of global deaths and 12 percent of the global burden of disease. As injuries commonly target young men during their most productive years, the burden of injuries is often distributed far beyond the injured individual.

Injuries place a disproportionate burden on the world's poor; more than 90 percent of injuries in 2000 occurred in LICs and MICs (Peden and others, 2002). The LICs and MICs of Europe have the highest injury mortality rates, but the Southeast Asia and Western Pacific regions account for the highest number of injury deaths worldwide. Even in HICs such as the United States, injuries account for just over 35 percent of ED visits (Pitts, Niska, Xu, and Burt, 2008). In the United States, injuries are the number one cause of death between the ages of one and forty-four and account for more years of potential life lost before age sixty-five than all causes of cancer and all causes of heart disease combined.

Injury mortality has a multimodal age distribution, most heavily affecting children, adolescents, young adults, and parents of young children. Young people between the ages of fifteen and forty-four years account for nearly half of the world's fatal injuries. Because of their vulnerability and often close proximity to water and fire, children under five years of age account for approximately 25 percent of drowning deaths and just over 15 percent of fire-related deaths worldwide.

Injury rates are higher in males than in females. For example, global injury mortality is twice as high among males as among females, and for some types of injuries—road traffic injuries and interpersonal violence—the disparity approaches threefold. However, this pattern varies by injury type; in some regions female mortality rates from suicide and burns are as high as or even higher than male rates.

In contrast to the progress that has been made in the control of many infectious diseases, little has been done to stem the tide of injuries around the world. In fact the World Bank predicts that the global burden of injuries, especially road traffic injuries, self-inflicted injuries, and injuries from interpersonal violence, will increase dramatically by the year 2020 (Murray and Lopez, 1996). Road traffic injuries alone are expected to rise from the ninth leading cause of death worldwide to fifth by 2030 (Table 22.1) (WHO, 2008).

The Injury Pyramid   Injury mortality data represent only a small fraction of the total injury burden. For every injured victim who dies, there are typically many more who sustain serious but nonfatal injuries. Many of these victims suffer long-lasting or even permanent disabilities. Because, in general, nonfatal events greatly outnumber fatalities, the relationship among injury deaths, hospitalizations, and ED or office visits can be viewed as an **injury pyramid** (Figure 22.1). For example, a study of injuries in Missouri and Nebraska from 1996 through 1998 identified 13,052 fatal injuries, 131,210 hospital admissions for injuries, and 1.9 million injury visits to emergency departments. For each fatal injury there were approximately 10 hospitalizations and more than 100 injury visits, a difference of one order of magnitude between the different levels of injury. Road traffic injuries and firearm-related injuries were the leading causes of fatal injury in both states, but falls were a far more common cause of hospital admissions and ED visits than firearms were, ranking second only to road traffic injuries (Wadman, Muelleman, Coto, and Kellermann, 2003).

It is likely that similar ratios of fatal to nonfatal injuries by cause prevail in LICs and MICs. However, many countries lack the data systems necessary to tabulate these counts routinely and reliably. As a result, mortality data are often the only information available to quantify the public health impact of injuries. This means that conclusions are based on only the tip of a very large pyramid.

TABLE 22.1   Global Ranking of Injury-Related Mortality, 2004 and 2030

	Rank (according to number of deaths)	
	2004	**2030 (projected)**
Road traffic injuries	9	5
Self-inflicted injuries	16	12
Interpersonal violence	22	16

Source: Data from WHO, 2008.

FIGURE 22.1   The Injury Pyramid

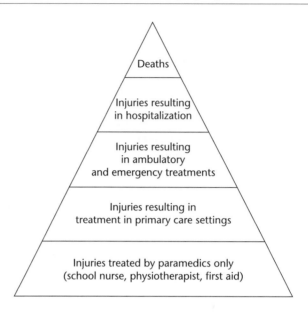

Identifying Risk and Protective Factors

The second step of the public health approach calls for characterizing risk and protective factors associated with injuries. In practice this is done through descriptive epidemiological studies. These studies characterize who is injured, what injuries are involved, and where, when, and, why particular injuries occur. These data can also generate hypotheses for further investigation with analytical studies. In some cases the link between a risk factor and injury is so strong that no additional research is needed. For example, early studies of road traffic injuries in the United States revealed that half of all fatal crashes and 60 percent of fatal single-vehicle crashes involved alcohol (Polen and Friedman, 1988). In other cases, in order to quantify the impact of particular risk factors, it is necessary to compare the rate of injury among those with the risk factors of interest to the rate among similar individuals without these risk factors. Conversely, protective factors, essentially negative risk factors, can diminish the effect of an injury or prevent it from occurring at all. The protective effect of bicycle helmets against closed head injuries is an excellent example of a strong protective factor that mitigates the effect of a potentially devastating injury.

Developing and Testing Interventions

Once risk and protective factors have been investigated, interventions can be conceived, developed, and tested. Careful attention must be given to the characteristics of the target population, the feasibility of the candidate countermeasure(s), the acceptability of the countermeasure(s) among the target population, and the countermeasure cost. Pilot programs are often helpful to test various strategies. The most promising can then be selected for widespread implementation. The **Haddon matrix** is particularly useful for managing this process of injury prevention and control.

William Haddon, a physician, established the field of injury control by applying the core principles of public health to the prevention and mitigation of injuries. Using the time-tested concept of the epidemiological triangle—the idea that many diseases result from harmful interactions among the host, the disease vector, and the environment—Haddon showed how these same three factors interact to cause many injuries. To facilitate the identification of opportunities for prevention and control, Haddon divided injury-causing events into three temporal phases: the pre-event phase, the event itself, and the post-event phase. This yielded a phase-factor matrix of nine cells, as shown in Table 22.2 (Haddon, 1972). Examining each cell can suggest various strategies to prevent or control injuries. Since its introduction in 1972, the Haddon matrix has proven to be an invaluable tool for injury prevention and control.

Haddon (1973) later outlined ten generic injury-control strategies that can be used to break the chain of injury causation (Table 22.3). Examining this list to identify the most promising approaches is known as *options analysis*. The best strategy is not always the most obvious one or the one most proximate to the injury itself. Often a combination of strategies is superior to any single one.

Haddon's ideas were first applied to the prevention and control of motor vehicle crashes, an application that is illustrated in the accompanying Perspective. They yielded dramatic results. According to the Centers for Disease Control and Prevention (CDC), between 1925 and 1999 the number of drivers increased six-fold, the number of motor vehicles increased elevenfold, and the number of vehicle miles traveled (VMT) increased tenfold. Despite this dramatic increase in automobile use, the death rate per 100 million VMT plummeted from 18 in 1925

TABLE 22.2   The Haddon Matrix Applied to Motor Vehicle Crashes

Phases	Host	Agent	Environment
Pre-event	Alcohol; speed	Tires, brakes	Signs; signals; road surface
Event	Belt use; helmet use	Seat belt; air bags	Side slope; guardrails
Post-event	Health, age	Fuel system; materials	EMS response; road shoulders

Source: Haddon, 1972.

TABLE 22.3   Options Analysis in Injury Control

Options	Examples
1. Prevent creation of hazard.	Ban production and civilian sale of assault weapons.
2. Reduce the amount of hazard.	Limit water heater temperature to 125°F (47.25°C).
3. Prevent the release of a hazard that already exists.	Put dangerous medications in childproof containers.
4. Modify the rate of distribution of release of the hazard from its source.	Require fire-safe cigarettes that cannot easily ignite furniture or bedding.
5. Separate, by time or space, the hazard from the host.	Construct overpasses or underpasses to eliminate crossing streams of traffic.
6. Physically separate, by barriers, the hazard from the host.	Equip taxicabs with bulletproof and knifeproof partitions.
7. Modify surfaces and basic structures to minimize injury.	Equip all new cars with driver-side and passenger-side air bags.
8. Make that which is to be protected more resistant to damage.	Issue bulletproof vests to law enforcement officers and security guards.
9. Mitigate damage already done.	Promote citizen training in first aid and cardiopulmonary resuscitation (CPR).
10. Stabilize, repair, and rehabilitate the injured person.	Implement trauma care.

Source: Haddon, 1973.

to only 1.7 in 1997, a 90 percent decrease (CDC, 1999). On the strength of this accomplishment the CDC acclaimed the reduction in road and traffic fatalities as one of the top ten public health achievements of the twentieth century. Other developed countries, such as Sweden and United Kingdom, have achieved equal if not more impressive improvements in road traffic safety (Evans, 2004). Assuredly, this reduction in mortality began before Haddon applied his theories to injury control, and there were significant advances in road safety and automobile engineering that resulted in substantial safety gains. Nevertheless, Haddon's approach to traffic safety was revolutionary and facilitated a great public health accomplishment.

Implementing Interventions and Ensuring Acceptance of Control Strategies

The fourth component of the public health approach, implementing interventions and pursuing widespread adoption of the most effective strategies, is best considered jointly with the third component, developing and testing interventions. So in this section we outline some of the basic concepts of injury prevention

PERSPECTIVE
The Car Crash in Which Princess Diana Died

On August 31, 1997, Diana Princess of Wales and her companion, Dodi al-Fayed, were involved in a high-speed car crash in a roadway underpass in Paris, France. The princess, her companion, and the car's chauffeur, Henri Paul, were all killed; Trevor Rees-Jones, a restrained front-seat passenger, survived with facial trauma. The crash—the details of which are well known and have been broadcast around the world—the emergency medical response, and the ultimately fatal outcomes lend themselves to Haddon Matrix analysis. This analysis illustrates several principles of injury prevention and control.

Using the terms of Haddon's matrix, the hosts of the injury were the princess, al-Fayed, Rees-Jones, and Paul; only Rees-Jones was restrained. The princess and al-Fayed were in the backseat. The vector was deceleration precipitated by the impact of the car against a supporting column in the underpass, and in turn the deceleration injuries sustained by the vehicle's passengers. The hosts' environment included the interior of the car and the backseat in particular; the car's environment included an underpass with central support columns, rather than a smooth wall or a guardrail to separate the columns from the road way.

Dividing the event further, important pre-event phase factors included the chauffeur's intoxication and the car's high speed. Important factors affecting the event itself included the lack of restraints (seat belts) in use and the lack of supplemental passive measures (airbags) that could deploy during a fatal impact. A key post-event factor affecting the outcome was the emergency medical service (EMS) response, which was focused on on-scene extraction and treatment rather than expedited transport to a trauma care facility. Rees-Jones was extricated and treated for facial injuries; the chauffeur and al-Fayed were pronounced dead on EMS arrival; the princess was still alive when EMS arrived. The delay in transporting the extricated princess to a hospital was approximately forty-five minutes to an hour. Despite her significant injuries, had the post-event phase of her injury been managed more expeditiously, the ultimate outcome might have been less tragic, illustrating another key component of injury control: mitigation of an injury's effect.

This brief analysis illustrates a host of injury prevention and control principles and suggests multiple ways in which injuries can be prevented and their effects mitigated and controlled.

strategies and illustrate that developing such strategies and ensuring their widespread adoption form something of a continuum. (Another part of the fourth component is evaluation, and we discuss that separately later.)

Active Versus Passive Interventions Most injury prevention strategies can be classified as either active or passive. Active countermeasures require the conscious cooperation of the individual to be effective. Examples include the use of manual safety belts, motorcycle helmets, child safety seats, and protective eyewear in the workplace. Passive countermeasures require little or no cooperation by the person being protected. Examples include air bags in cars, sprinkler systems in public buildings, flotation hulls on watercraft, and shields that prevent workers from becoming ensnared in hazardous equipment.

The Three E's of Injury Control Most injury control countermeasures, whether active or passive, employ one of three generic strategies: *education, enforcement of regulations*, or *engineering of physical structures* (including environmental changes). Each approach offers advantages and disadvantages.

  Education is often the first approach taken to promote safe behavior. Educational interventions encourage the public to adopt safe behaviors and practices voluntarily. Implicit in this approach is the belief that once people know what to do to reduce their risk of injury, they will change their behavior. Examples of such interventions are driver's education, child pedestrian training (Burke and others, 1996), education of parents and caregivers to reduce playground injuries among children (Withaneachi and Meehan, 1998), education through posters and videos that promote safe behavior in the workplace (Smith, 2001), and various training materials that promote burn prevention (Herd, Widdowson, and Tanner, 1986; Keswani, 1986). Recent innovations include training to prevent dog bites and educating all-terrain-vehicle consumers at vehicle dealerships (Mello and others, 2007).

  Public education campaigns are popular because they are voluntary. Although educational programs do lead to an increase in knowledge, they may have little impact on behavior and on injury rates, especially if they are carried out in isolation. For example, a systematic review of randomized, controlled trials on improving pedestrian safety showed improvements in some road safety behaviors among trained pedestrians but no consistent, overall behavioral change (Duperrex, Bunn, and Roberts, 2002). The impact of public education is often blunted by attenuation of effect. No matter how powerful, pervasive, and repetitive a safety message may be, some people never encounter it. Among those who do, some will actively reject the message. Some who accept the message will be insufficiently motivated to change their behavior. Among those who change their behavior, some will relapse overtime, and some will fail to follow the message consistently. Finally, not everyone who adopts a protective strategy escapes injury.

  Enforcement of laws and regulations may increase compliance when voluntary acceptance of an effective countermeasure is poor. Motorcycle helmets provide a telling example. Wearing a motorcycle helmet reduces the risk of death or severe traumatic brain injury in a crash by approximately 55 percent. In states where helmet use is voluntary, only about half of motorcyclists wear one, whereas in states where helmet use is mandated and the law is aggressively enforced, helmet usage exceeds 98 percent (National Highway Traffic Safety Administration, 2003). Evaluations have conclusively shown that states with mandatory helmet laws have lower motorcycle crash fatality rates than do states that lack these laws (Ulmer and Preusser, 2003). A recent review of the effect of helmet laws in the fifty U.S. states from 1975 to 2004 supports these findings: after controlling for other factors, states with universal helmet laws have motorcyclist mortality rates 22 to 33 percent lower than the rates in states without such laws (Houston and Richardson, 2008). It follows that states that repeal mandatory motorcycle helmet laws see a rise in injury rates and deaths: in Pennsylvania after that state's 2003 repeal of a mandatory helmet law, helmet use among riders involved in crashes decreased from 82 percent to 58 percent, and head-injury deaths increased by 66 percent (Mertz and Weiss, 2008).

Bicycle helmet use can be increased with legislation as well (Graitcer, Kellermann, and Christoffel, 1995). In Montgomery County, Maryland, educational efforts to encourage bicycle helmet use increased self-reported use from 8 to 13 percent. In nearby Howard County, where educational efforts were supplemented by a mandatory bicycle helmet law, helmet use increased from 11 to 37 percent (Dannenberg and others, 1993). A recent study evaluated the effect of a 1995 law mandating helmet use for riders under eighteen in Montreal and found a drop of 55 percent in the mortality rate for riders aged fifteen and under but little change in the rate for adults, supporting the efficacy of the law and suggesting that it should be extended to adults as well (Wesson and others, 2008).

Combining education and enforcement usually works better than relying on either strategy alone. In Elmira, New York, a publicity campaign combined with high-visibility enforcement of the state's seat belt law boosted rates of use from 49 to 77 percent. Four months after the effort ceased, seat belt use declined to 66 percent, but it rebounded to 80 percent during a reminder campaign (Williams, Preusser, Blomberg, and Lund, 1987). In Houston, Texas, the use of seat belts increased from 39 to 54 percent after a multifaceted program that included education, a media campaign, and high-profile law enforcement (Hanfling, Mangus, Gill, and Bailey, 2000). In Brazil a 20 percent reduction in traffic fatalities followed the implementation of speed limits (Poli de Figueiredo and others, 2001). In the cities of Bogotá and Cali, Colombia, a widely publicized and visibly enforced ban on the carrying of firearms during elections and high-risk holidays was associated with a significant decrease in the rate of homicides compared to the rate when the ban was not in effect (Villaveces and others, 2000).

Although mandatory use laws are often effective, they may be difficult to enact. Opponents of such laws argue that they infringe on personal freedom and that individuals have the right to choose hazardous behavior if the risk is acceptable to them. Moreover, enforcement of regulations can be difficult in many LICs due to limited resources. In Ghana, for example, a nation of 18 million, the entire 16,000-member police force has only 145 vehicles available for enforcement and other purposes (Forjuoh, 2003). Laws may be of little benefit without enforcement, however; a recent observational study of helmet use among motorcyclists in an area of southern China with mandatory helmet laws that are not routinely enforced showed high awareness of the benefits of helmet use, but little adoption (Li, Li, and Cai, 2008).

In workplace settings, rules to promote safe behavior by employees may be easily introduced, but they are unlikely to be effective unless they are visibly and consistently enforced. Examples include requiring the use of hard hats in construction zones, safety goggles near ocular hazards, and safety straps when working in high places, and enforcing a strict no-smoking policy around flammable materials.

Engineering solutions are the injury control strategy that draws most directly on the preventive paradigm of environmental health (see Chapter Twenty-Six). Many injuries can be prevented by designing and building safety into products or environments. The up-front cost of engineering may exceed the cost of education or enforcement campaigns, but the downstream benefits are often greater as well. Engineering is usually more effective than behavioral change because it does not require the cooperation of users to exert its protective effects.

Consider the following examples. In contrast to unsuccessful efforts to "fix the nut behind the wheel," adoption of federal standards for passenger restraint systems (seat belts), safety glass, fuel system integrity, and nonflammable interior fabric saved an estimated 37,000 lives between 1975 and 1978 alone. The subsequent introduction of air bags cut the annual toll of crash-related deaths and injuries still further (Kahane, 1998).

Seat belts in cars are a good example of successful engineering for injury prevention. When properly used, they reduce motor vehicle fatalities by about 50 percent and serious injuries by about 55 percent. They are affordable and feasible in countries where automobile use is prevalent or rapidly increasing, but it is difficult to encourage widespread use of seat belts without high-visibility enforcement (Forjuoh, 2003).

LICs differ from HICs in their patterns of road traffic deaths. Whereas in HICs motor vehicle occupants make up the majority of fatal road traffic injury victims, in LICs the majority of victims are vulnerable road users—pedestrians, passengers riding in large vehicles such as trucks and buses, and riders of two-wheelers (bicycles and motorcycles) (Razzak, Laflamme, Luby, and Chotani, 2004; Peden and others, 2004). Because it is difficult if not impossible to get pedestrians to change their behavior consistently, engineering interventions are often the most effective strategy for protecting them. Some options include installation of sidewalks, imposition of roadway barriers between pedestrians and traffic, placement of flexible "pedestrian crossing" signs in the center of a roadway, creation of one-way-street networks in urban areas, school zone signage and other measures, and installation of adequate lighting so that pedestrians crossing roadways are visible at night (Retting, Ferguson, and McCartt, 2003). Other effective strategies include red-light cameras, traffic-calming measures, and provision of bicycling and pedestrian facilities (Mohan, 2004). Many of these interventions can be adopted by LICs, particularly in locations where pedestrian injuries occur with great frequency (Forjuoh, 2003).

In South Asia, high death rates from burns among females result from using portable stoves on uneven surfaces (where they can overturn and explode) or on the floor (where long skirts can catch fire and where refueling and maintenance are difficult) (Fauveau and Blancet, 1989; Marsh and others, 1996). Simple changes in stove design to keep heat and flames away from clothing and out of reach of children could prevent many burns. Loose, flammable clothing is another important risk factor for burns among children and women in some LICs. Proven interventions from HICs (Baker, O'Neill, Ginsburg, and Li, 1992), such as use of fabrics that are less flammable, fire-resistance standards for children's sleepwear, and a change from loose, frilly dresses to more close-fitting clothes, can be applied in LIC settings with significant advantage. A recent review applies the Haddon Matrix to the issue and identifies a host of potential strategies, including alternative energy sources, better kerosene containment, modifications to appliance engineering, improved ventilation in cooking areas, consumer education, and training for caregivers and emergency responders (Peck and others, 2008).

Engineering strategies can be applied to equipment and devices, or they can be applied on a larger scale, to environments. Seat belts are an example of an engineering change within an automobile; banked curves, guardrails, and separation of opposing lanes of traffic are examples of larger-scale environmental changes. Both of these types of change are usually considered engineering strategies, but in the examples later in this chapter, we distinguish engineering and environmental change, in part to emphasize the role of environmental health approaches in injury control. Certain interventions, including early warning systems for severe weather events such as floods, storms, and heat waves, apply engineering methods to larger-scale environmental concerns. They employ solutions such as remote-sensing technology and computer modeling to project hazards and provide targeted prevention messaging before the hazardous exposure arrives.

PERSPECTIVE
Early Warning Systems for Severe Weather: Tropical Storm Nargis

With global climate change, changes in ambient and sea-surface temperatures have resulted in increasingly severe weather throughout the globe, including more severe heat waves, storms, and floods, as discussed in Chapter Ten. Population pressures and other trends, such as the retirement of baby boomers in the United States, are resulting in increased settlement of coastal areas particularly vulnerable to these hazards, compounding the effect. From a public health perspective, morbidity and mortality from injuries are the primary health outcomes of extreme weather events. Injuries continue to be an issue in the clean-up phase, and significant outcomes also arise from population displacement, including infectious disease outbreaks, mental health effects such as depression and suicide, and exacerbations of chronic disease resulting from interruptions in medical care. Infrastructure damage is often extensive, hindering recovery and ongoing development efforts.

The impacts are particular severe in the developing world, where populations often settle ecologically vulnerable marginal areas, early warning communications are limited, and evacuations must often be done on foot due to lack of transportation infrastructure. Tropical cyclone Nargis, a storm roughly equal in intensity to Hurricane Katrina, which struck Myanmar (formerly Burma) in May 2008, provides a good example of the effects of such a storm. Nargis killed over 130,000 people and severely affected 1.5 million people; it was the worst natural disaster in Myanmar's recorded history. The storm was focused on a very populous area and the inhabitants received little to no warning from Myanmar's government, despite adequate tracking and forecasting done by other governments and communicated to Myanmar's Department of Meteorology and Hydrology.

Nargis's devastation could have been significantly minimized had early warnings been communicated effectively. There is clearly a political component to injury prevention in this context, as Myanmar is a military dictatorship that maintains a closed society with little information exchange. Nevertheless, the case highlights several important concerns regarding effective preparation for severe weather events in the developing world. Peter Webster (2008), a climatologist, has outlined three primary improvements that would be beneficial:

1. Extending the time horizon of severe weather forecasts
2. Adding storm surge forecasts to the mandate of Regional Specialized Meteorological Centers
3. Developing resilient national disaster plans

Webster points to Bangladesh's experience with developing national disaster and flood response plans that make effective use of meteorological and climatological forecasts. When that country used forecasts for river flow and storm surge in its planning, mortality from tropical storm Sidr in 2007 was dramatically lower than the mortality rate for similar storms in both 1991 and 1970, each of which killed approximately 200,000 people. Sidr, in contrast, killed approximately 6,000, and much more infrastructure was preserved as well (Webster, 2008). Webster has also done work generating flood forecasts for Bangladesh; these ten-day probabilistic forecasts are used to inform authorities in a timely manner of the need to evacuate people and critical infrastructure, enhancing recovery and community resilience.

Such forecasting and early warning systems are an increasingly important component of large-scale injury prevention efforts. Similar strategies have been employed with great effect in response to heat waves and other increasingly prevalent and severe natural hazards. Engineering solutions that allow anticipation of hazardous environmental exposures facilitate primary prevention and will be an increasingly important tool in a warming world.

FIGURE 22.2   Startled Man Ready to Run After Hurricane Driven
Wave Smashes into Seawall

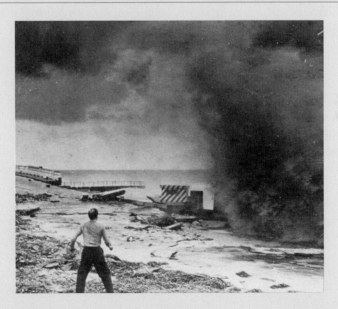

Source: National Oceanic and Atmospheric Administration, http://www.photolib.noaa.gov/htmls/wea00411.htm.

Because engineering solutions can increase the cost of a product, they are often unpopular with manufacturers. For this reason many advocates of injury prevention support consumer product safety laws to compel manufacturers to act. Manufacturers often oppose product safety legislation because they fear it will raise the prices of their products, discourage sales, and reduce their ability to compete with less regulated manufacturers in other countries. When efforts to regulate a hazardous product fail, product liability lawsuits may be the only way to force a needed change in product design. That can elicit another form of legislative backlash, as manufacturers seek protection from product liability lawsuits under the guise of "tort reform" (Vernick, Mair, Teret, and Sapsin, 2003).

Evaluating and Refining Interventions

Program evaluation is an important part of the public health approach. Without continuing surveillance and other well-designed modes of program evaluation, it is difficult to assess which interventions have the greatest impact and likely should be reinforced and which have the least impact and likely should be changed or curtailed. Program evaluation uses established methods to reach valid conclusions about the effects of a given intervention. This large field is beyond the scope of this chapter, but in general, many prevention programs are evaluated by determining their impact on morbidity or mortality in the target population. When good surveillance systems are in place, this approach is worthwhile and can produce valid results. However, large-scale surveillance is not always possible or might fail to detect the effects of small-scale demonstration projects. In some instances surrogate measures may be used to assess program impact. For example, rates of smoke detector use in a target neighborhood before and after a promotional program might be used in evaluating that program because quantifying fire-related injuries—which are rare events— might take too long. Also, as surveillance is time consuming and expensive, sampling techniques can establish patterns in subsets of a given population; these patterns can then be extrapolated to the population as a whole. This technique can be useful for MICs and LICs, where resource constraints can limit sample size. Regardless of the form the evaluation takes, it must be tailored to the intervention and the outcome of interest, and the methodology should yield valid results. Once a good program evaluation has been performed, intervention priorities can be reorganized, the Haddon matrix can be revisited, and new prevention goals can be pursued.

INJURY PREVENTION IN PRACTICE

Now that we have outlined the public health approach and explored several of its key components with regard to injury control, we turn to several specific types of injuries to illustrate how that approach is applied.

Intentional Injuries (Violence)

In the *World Report on Violence and Health*, published by the World Health Organization in 2002, Krug and others (2002) defined violence as "the intentional use of physical force or power, threatened or actual, against oneself, another person, or against a group or community that either results in or has a high likelihood of resulting in injury, death, psychological harm, mal-development or deprivation" (p. 5). This report divides violence into three broad categories: *self-directed violence*, *interpersonal violence*, and *collective violence*. These terms describe, respectively, attempted and completed suicides (as well as parasuicides); violence inflicted by another individual or by small groups of individuals; and violence inflicted by larger groups such as states, organized political groups, militia groups, and terrorist organizations. These three broad categories may each be divided further to reflect specific subsets of violence, including physical, sexual, and psychological violence and violence involving deprivation or neglect. This typology is graphically presented in Figure 22.3.

Epidemiology and Risk Factors   Violence caused 51,175 deaths and 2,102,099 nonfatal injuries in 2005 in the United States (National Center for Injury Prevention and Control [NCIPC], 2008). The economic impact of gunshot wounds in the United States alone is estimated at $126 billion each year, and cutting or stab wounds cost an additional $51 billion annually (Miller and Cohen, 1997). In 2002, an estimated 1.6 million people worldwide died as a result of violence and intentional injuries (WHO, 2004). Violence is a leading cause of death for people aged fifteen to forty-four worldwide, accounting for about 14 percent of deaths among males and 7 percent of deaths among females in this age group. Most of these deaths occur in low- and middle-income countries. Nearly half of violence-related deaths in any given year are suicides, almost one-third are homicides, and about one-fifth are war related. Mortality figures represent the tip of the iceberg. For every person who dies as a result of violence, many more sustain nonfatal injuries. Many survivors of violence suffer a range of physical, sexual, reproductive, and mental health problems.

Countermeasures   Countermeasures for intentional injuries include a range of strategies. Many countries attempt to reduce the degree of harm caused by

FIGURE 22.3 Typology of Violence

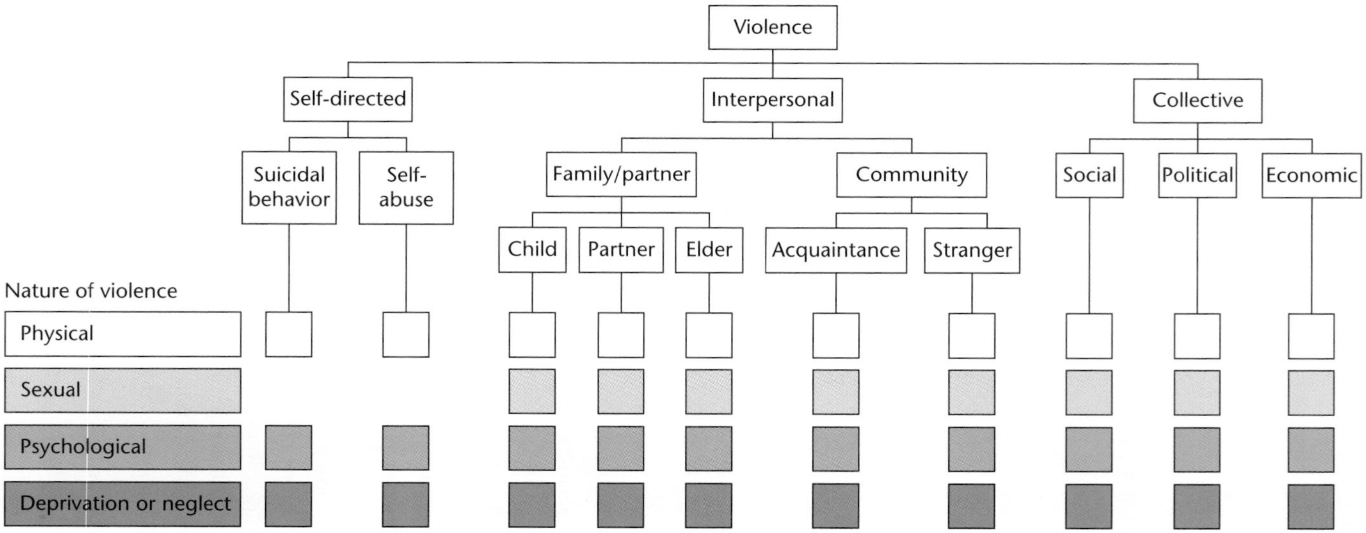

violence by controlling access to or use of firearms, the most common means of interpersonal violence (Krug and others, 2002; Kellermann, Lee, Mercy, and Banton, 1991). Using local agencies to perform background checks was found to reduce gun-related suicide by 27 percent and homicide by 22 percent (Sumner, Layde, and Guse, 2008). Although some of the best-known violence countermeasures rely on education and enforcement, a surprising number relate to environmental change. These measures are sometimes known as *crime prevention through environmental design*, or CPTED (Sherman and others, 1998). The measures are broadly applicable and have been shown to reduce robberies and violent crime (Carter, Carter, and Dannenberg, 2003; Casteel, Peek-Asa, Howard, and Kraus, 2004). Some examples are shown in Table 22.4.

Burns

A burn occurs when some or all of the layers of the skin are destroyed by a hot liquid (*scald*), a hot solid (*contact burn*), or a flame (*flame burn*). Burns can also be produced by exposure to ultraviolet radiation, radioactivity, electricity, and certain chemicals.

Epidemiology and Risk Factors   In the United States in 2007 there were 1,557,500 fire responses, 3,430 fire fatalities, and 17,675 fire injuries among civilians. Total property loss was estimated at $14.6 billion. Home fires account for 84 percent of the civilian fire deaths (Karter, 2008). Globally, fire-related burns accounted for 311,535 deaths in 2002 (WHO, 2004). At least 80 percent of these deaths occurred in homes. More than 95 percent of fatal fire-related burns worldwide

TABLE 22.4   Countermeasures for Intentional Injuries

Education	Anger management interventions
Enforcement	Community policing
	Targeted patrols, to discourage the carrying of concealed weapons
	Earlier closing hours for bars
Engineering	Safety locks on guns
Environmental change	Improved street lighting
	Safe pedestrian routes
	Bulletproof booths at all-night gas stations and selected retail outlets
	Drop safes, to limit cash on hand
	Protective shields between the front and back seats in taxicabs

occur in LICs and MICs. Two thirds of fire-related mortality is in Southeast Asia, where females have the highest fire-related burn mortality rates in the world, followed by males in Africa and females in the Eastern Mediterranean. Children under five years of age and the elderly (those over seventy years old) have the highest burn mortality rates. In India alone there are approximately 100,000 deaths due to burns each year; 600,000 burn victims require hospital admission and treatment in a burn unit.

Countermeasures   Countermeasures for burns include a wide range of strategies, as shown in Table 22.5.

Poisoning

A poison exposure is the ingestion of or contact with a substance that can produce toxic effects. Poisonings can be acute or chronic, as discussed in Chapter Two. Acute poisonings are classified as injuries.

Epidemiology and Risk Factors   In 2005, there were 32,691 poisoning deaths in the United States, and U.S. poison centers reported approximately 2.4 million human poison exposure calls (Bronstein and others, 2007). More than 90 percent of poison exposures occur at home, and just over half of these exposures involve children younger than age six. The most common poison exposures for children are ingestion of household products, such as cosmetics and personal care products, cleaning substances, pain relievers, foreign bodies, and plants. For adults, the

TABLE 22.5   Countermeasures for Burns

Education	Burn prevention campaigns
Enforcement	Building codes
	Smoking rules around flammable material
Engineering	Tap water temperature reduction
	Temperature regulating valves
	Modified tap handles
	Smoke detectors
	Automatic sprinklers
	Control of ignition sources (cigarettes, matches, and lighters)
	Reduction of clothing flammability
Environmental	Elevated hearths for cooking and heating fires

most common poison exposures are pain relievers, sedatives, cleaning substances, antidepressants, and bites or stings. Carbon monoxide (CO) results in more fatal unintentional poisonings in the United States than any other agent, with the highest number occurring during the winter months.

Medical spending for poisoning totaled $26 billion in 2000 (Finkelstein, Corso, and Miller, 2006). Spending would be considerably higher in the United States without the established network of poison control centers that aid in the triage and treatment of acute poisonings (Darwin, 2003; Miller and Lestina, 1997).

Worldwide, poisonings rank sixth as a cause of injury, and in 2002, there were 350,365 poisoning deaths (WHO, 2004). Data on poisonings in developing countries are scarce (though in recent years there has been increasing discussion on the role of poison centers in the developing world; Laborde, 2004) but suggest that pesticides, kerosene, and other chemicals are most often implicated; pesticides have the largest role in fatal exposures (Konradsen and others, 2003). This has led to calls for regulation of the most harmful pesticides and removal of certain pesticides from distribution entirely (Konradsen and others, 2003).

Countermeasures   Countermeasures for poisoning rely more heavily on education, enforcement, and engineering than on environmental changes, as shown in Table 22.6.

Falls

A fall is an event that results in a person coming inadvertently to rest on the ground or floor or other lower level.

TABLE 22.6   Countermeasures for Poisoning

Education	Warning labels
	Physician-based education programs
	Community-based education programs
	Poison control centers
Enforcement	Carbon monoxide alarms
Engineering	Child-resistant packaging
	Carbon monoxide alarms
	Distinctive shapes and sizes for tablets of medicine
Environmental	Locked storage for pesticide stocks on farms

Epidemiology and Risk Factors   More than one in three U.S. adults aged sixty-five and older falls each year, making falls a leading cause of fatal injuries and the most common cause of nonfatal injuries and hospital admissions for trauma among that age group in the United States. Globally, an estimated 391,764 people died due to falls in 2002 (WHO, 2004). A quarter of all fatal falls occurred in the HICs. Europe and the Western Pacific region combined account for nearly 60 percent of the total number of fall-related deaths worldwide. Males in the LICs and MICs of Europe have by far the highest fall-related mortality rates worldwide.

There are two distinct at-risk populations for falls, children and the elderly. In all regions of the world, adults over the age of seventy years, particularly females, have significantly higher fall-related mortality rates than younger people do. However, children account for the most morbidity, with almost 50 percent of the total number of fall-related **disability-adjusted life years (DALYs)**, a standardized measure that accounts for both premature death and disability. In lowland areas of tropical countries where tree agriculture is widespread, occupational falls from trees and other tree-related injuries are a leading cause of death, hospitalization, or permanent disability from spinal cord injury. In some countries, building-related falls from unprotected rooftops, windows, and stairs are a common source of injury for children. The home environment has been identified as a potential contributor to as many as 50 percent of falls occurring among the elderly. Falls among children, in contrast, are related to their age. Young children most frequently fall in and around the home, for example, from chairs, from beds, and down stairs. Older children fall from playground equipment, during play and recreational activities, and during sports.

Countermeasures   Countermeasures for falls rely heavily on environmental interventions, as shown in Table 22.7.

Drowning

Drowning is fatal respiratory impairment from submersion or immersion in liquid.

Epidemiology and Risk Factors   In the United States more than 3,000 people die in unintentional drownings each year, averaging 9 people per day. About three times that number receive care in emergency departments for near drownings. In 2002, 382,312 people drowned worldwide, making drowning the third leading cause of unintentional injury death after road traffic injuries and falls (WHO, 2004). These global burden of disease figures underestimate drowning deaths, because they exclude drowning due to floods, boating, and water transport. Ninety-seven percent of all drowning deaths occur in LICs and MICs. The Western Pacific and Southeast Asia regions account for 60 percent of the mortality and DALYs. Males in Africa and in the Western Pacific have the highest drowning mortality rates worldwide. Among the various age groups, children under five years of age have the highest drowning mortality rates. Over half the global mortality due to drowning and 60 percent of the total number of DALYs due to drowning occur among children younger than fifteen years old.

Countermeasures   Drowning countermeasures are summarized in Table 22.8.

TABLE 22.7   Countermeasures for Falls

Education	Physical activity and balancing exercises
Enforcement	Legislation for roof, window, and stairway barriers in high-rise buildings
Engineering	Barriers in high-rise buildings
Environmental	Removal of obstructed pathways and loose throw rugs
	Well-maintained stairways
	Improved lighting and visibility
	Modification of hard surfaces on which people might fall
	Safety devices, such as grab bars
	Barriers in high-rise buildings

TABLE 22.8   Countermeasures for Drowning

Education	Swimming instruction
	Training in resuscitation techniques
Enforcement	Supervision; lifeguards
Engineering	Pool alarms; pool covers
	Personal flotation devices
Environmental	Fencing that completely encloses pools

INJURY CONTROL IN SPECIAL SETTINGS

Certain settings have special importance for injury control, either because they pose a particular risk or because specific control strategies are available. This section discusses four such settings: the workplace, playgrounds, roadways, and the home.

The Workplace

Occupational injuries represent a considerable part of the injury burden on society, affecting people in the most productive years of their lives.

Epidemiology   Globally, almost 1,000 workers are killed by injuries every day, and about 6 of every 1,000 workers will be fatally injured at work during a forty-year worklife. Nonfatal injuries are an even more pervasive problem, though in the United States they have been on the decline from a 1990 high of 6.4 million annually to 4.1 million in 2001. Nonfatal workplace injury incidence from 1976 to 2001 declined 39 percent overall. This parallels the historical trend for fatal injuries as well: the annual rate for workplace deaths from injury has declined from 37 per 100,000 full-time workers in 1933 to 4 per 100,000 in 2002 (Sestito, Lunsford, Hamilton, and Rosa, 2004).

Occupational injuries cover a wide spectrum. They range from skin cuts to piercing wounds, burns, amputations, crush injuries, eye injuries, and chemical exposures. In certain occupational groups, such as law enforcement personnel and commercial truck drivers, violent acts or road traffic injuries are leading causes of occupational injuries and deaths.

Countermeasures   Countermeasures for workplace injuries are shown in Table 22.9 (and are discussed in more detail in Chapter Twenty).

TABLE 22.9   Countermeasures for Workplace Injuries

Education	Job safety training
Enforcement	Occupational safety and health standards that require use of protective gear, such as eyewear, hard hats, and safety belts
Engineering	Machine guards
	Automated sensors to interrupt hazardous equipment
Environmental	Conversion to automated production lines
	Barriers that divide workers from vehicles

Playgrounds

In terms of Haddon's approach, children are the host of playground injuries; the vector is often potential energy, in the form of gravity, as many playground injuries result from falls (from swings, slides, or other equipment, for example). As children may not be supervised and cannot be relied on to generate active injury control themselves, the playground environment must be engineered with passive injury control in mind.

Epidemiology   More than 200,000 children are treated for playground equipment–related injuries in U.S. hospital emergency rooms each year. Two-thirds of these injuries occur on public playgrounds. Four out of five injuries involve falls, primarily to the surface below playground equipment (Tinsworth and McDonald, 2001).

Countermeasures   Countermeasures for playground injuries rely heavily on engineering and environmental changes, as shown in Table 22.10.

Roadways

Transportation injuries, especially those that occur on and near roadways, represent one of the leading categories of injuries worldwide. A road traffic injury is defined as any injury due to a crash involving one or more vehicles and originating or terminating on a public roadway.

Epidemiology   The worldwide epidemic of road traffic injuries is only just beginning. At present over a million people die each year and some 10 million people

TABLE 22.10   Countermeasures for Playground Injuries

Education	Education of children, parents, and teachers
Enforcement	Adult playground supervision to prevent bullying and hazardous behavior
Engineering	Average inclines of no more 30 degrees on slides
	Handrails on stairways and stepladders
	Playground surfaces that are covered with wood chips, double-shredded bark mulch, or pea gravel.
Environmental	Organization of equipment to prevent injuries from conflicting activities and from children running between activities
	Separation of equipment by user age

sustain permanent disabilities in road traffic crashes. For people under forty-four years of age, road traffic crashes are a leading cause of death and disability, second only to HIV/AIDS. Many developing countries are still at comparatively low levels of motorization, and the incidence of road traffic injuries in these countries is likely to increase as motor vehicle use proliferates. It is estimated that by 2020, road traffic crashes will have moved from ninth to third in the world disease burden ranking, as measured in DALYs.

Several categories of risk factors for road injuries can be identified. These relate to road users, the road itself, and vehicles. These factors, in turn, suggest a variety of injury control strategies (Peden and others, 2004). All road users are at risk of being injured or killed in a road traffic crash, although especially vulnerable road users, such as pedestrians and people using two-wheelers, usually bear the greatest burden. In a review of road traffic collisions in thirty-eight developing countries, it was found that pedestrian fatalities outnumbered other road-user deaths in 75 percent of the studies (Odero, Garner, and Zwi, 1997). Young male drivers and their passengers were at higher risk. Multicountry studies have shown that individuals from less privileged socioeconomic groups or living in poorer areas are at greatest risk of being killed or injured. Seat belt use among drivers and vehicle occupants has been found to decrease death and nonfatal injuries by 50 percent. Similarly, a child who is properly restrained in a safety seat is 71 percent less likely to die in a crash than is a child who is not properly restrained. Another major risk factor for road traffic injuries is use of alcohol. Alcohol consumption increases the probability both that a crash will occur and that death or serious injury will follow. A survey of studies in LICs and MICs found that a positive blood alcohol level was noted in 8 to 29 percent of drivers involved in crashes who were not fatally injured and in 33 to 69 percent of fatally injured drivers.

Roadway factors are also extremely important. Roads built to facilitate transport without consideration of safety can dramatically increase the incidence of serious and fatal traffic injuries. In many countries roads have multiple users, ranging from pedestrians to two-wheelers to automobiles and large vehicles. From the perspective of pedestrians and cyclists, proximity to motor vehicles capable of traveling at high speeds is the most important road safety problem. A road network planned for safety includes a hierarchy of roads, each intended to serve a certain function. It should also include infrastructure that protects pedestrians and bicyclists from automobiles and large transport vehicles. Each road should be designed according to its particular function in the network. A key characteristic of a well-designed road is that it protects vulnerable road users from large vehicles and makes compliance with the intended speed limit a natural choice for drivers. Such design can not only prevent injuries but also achieve other public health goals, such as promoting walking and bicycling (see Chapter Fourteen).

Vehicle design can have considerable influence on crash injuries. The risk of injury can be increased by many factors, such as poor design of the crush zone so it fails to absorb energy, failure of the structural cage around the passenger compartment to provide a protective shell, absence of features that protect occupants from side impacts or stop them from being ejected from the vehicle, and lack of high-mounted brake lights in the rear. Similarly, vehicles that are not clearly visible are at high risk of involvement in crashes, especially at night, and slow-moving vehicles on fast-moving roadways are at risk for rear-end crashes. Daytime running lights for cars, though not required in many countries, reduce the incidence of daytime crashes by 10 to 15 percent (Elvik, 1996). Bus and truck fronts designed to reduce injuries to pedestrians and cyclists could also lower the injury burden, as could minimizing differences in vehicle design in ways that would reduce injuries when a higher-riding vehicle and a lower-riding vehicle collide.

Countermeasures Countermeasures to reduce road injuries draw on a broad spectrum of strategies, from driver and pedestrian education to environmental modifications. Examples appear in Table 22.11 and the Perspective on highway and railroad crossings.

TABLE 22.11 Countermeasures for Road Injuries

Education	Pedestrian safety education
	Bicyclist training schemes
	Motorist education
	Helmet and seat belt promotion
Enforcement	Speed limits
	Graduated driver's licenses
	Strategies for reducing alcohol-impaired driving
	Helmet and seat belt use laws
Engineering	Puncture-resistant gas tanks
	Energy-absorbing interiors
	Crush zones and reinforced cages around occupants
	Air bags
Environmental	Areawide traffic calming
	Bicycle paths and lanes
	Energy-absorbing materials in front of bridge columns and other fixed objects
	Breakaway light poles
	Roadway lighting at high-frequency pedestrian crossings

PERSPECTIVE
Highway-Railroad Crossings

The United States has over 200,000 miles of railroad tracks, and railroads carry approximately 40 percent of the country's freight traffic. In 2003, according to the Federal Railroad Administration (FRA), there were over 750 million train miles traveled, and there were 368 fatalities involving highway-rail crossings. According to FRA surveillance data, the rate of fatalities at highway-rail crossings has steadily declined since the 1990s while total rail traffic has significantly increased. Safety officials attribute the drop in fatality rates to several factors. These measures include education, engineering, and enforcement activities and provide an interesting example of injury prevention and control.

Railroad crossings are engineered environments. Crash injuries at crossings involve kinetic energy transferred from a moving train, with limited capacity to brake, to a moving or stationary highway vehicle and its passengers. Engineering solutions to crossing injuries have been aimed at limiting the ability of motor vehicles to enter the crossing—and thus the zone where injury is likely to occur—at the same time a train enters the crossing. Passive measures are the most reliable, as they do not require active motorist compliance. Crossing arms are a longstanding example of a passive measure, though motorists may circumvent simple arms and enter the crossing. Innovations have included medians that tightly direct traffic flow at crossings, cable netting at crossing sites, and automated regional traffic redirection systems to redirect automobile traffic based on rail traffic flow. Driver education about crossings and safety measures, as well as increased enforcement of laws such as whistle laws and moving violations specific to highway-rail crossings have also contributed to mortality reduction in recent years.

Although no studies have been done to show a clear causal relationship between any particular interventions and changes in mortality rates, highway-rail intersections offer an excellent model of a unique environment in which engineering, education, and enforcement have all been profitably used to control injury. (See Federal Railroad Administration, Office of Safety Analysis, 2005, for surveillance data and additional information.)

Home Injuries

Injuries that occur in the home are conceptually grouped according to the environment in which they occur, rather than by the particular mechanism of injury or by intent. The most common home injuries are falls, being struck or hit by an object (including intentional acts of violence), being cut, and overexertion injuries (such as back strain). Other home injuries include burns and scalds (Figure 22.5), poisoning, animal bites, and a host of less common types (Home Safety Council, 2004).

Epidemiology Given the wide range of injuries in the home environment, it is difficult to present a unifying epidemiological picture, but recent studies have

FIGURE 22.4   Railroad Crossings Are the Site of Many Accidents Each Year

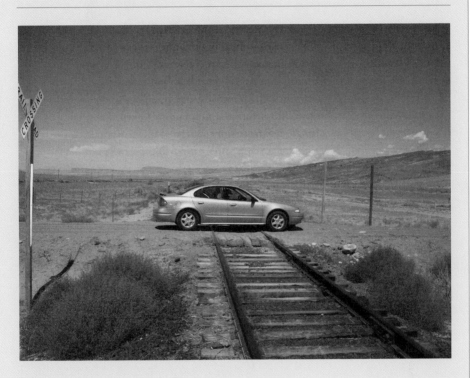

Source: ©iStockphoto.com/Jim Lopes.

provided significant insight into this constellation of injuries. In total, there are more than 18,000 fatalities from unintentional home injuries annually in the United States (Runyan and others, 2005a), and nonfatal home injuries requiring medical attention numbered more than 12 million each year from 1992 to 1999 (Runyan and others, 2005b). Generally, home injuries are responsible for more than 10 million ED visits annually in the United States, and account for approximately 20 percent of ED visits for injuries as a whole (NCIPC, 2002). Epidemiological data on some of the most common home injuries—notably falls, a particularly important home injury—have been presented in other sections of

FIGURE 22.5   Kitchens Often Contain Many Dangers

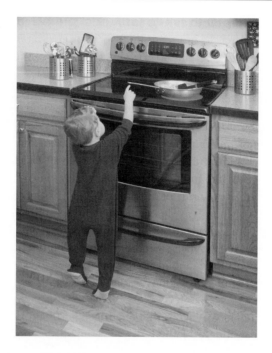

Source: ©iStockphoto.com/ Robert Dant.

this chapter. Unintentional injuries in the home are quite costly: $217 billion in 1998, by one estimate (Zaloshnja, Miller, Lawrence, and. Romano, 2005).

Countermeasures   A wide range of interventions have been shown to be effective at reducing home injuries. Some of the more notable interventions that have not been presented in other parts of this chapter are displayed in Table 22.12.

SUMMARY

Injury, whether caused by unintentional or intentional events, is a significant public health problem. The burden of injury is greatest in LICs and MICs and among individuals of low socioeconomic status in HICs. Most of these injuries are preventable.

Public health professionals can play an important role in reducing the global burden of injuries by identifying, implementing, and evaluating population-based countermeasures to prevent and control injuries. Which strategy is employed in a particular country

TABLE 22.12   Countermeasures for Home Injuries

Education	Fire hazard and escape route education for children and families
	Poison control education for children
	Babysitter training
	Choking response training
	Gun safety education (store guns safely or do not keep them at home)
Enforcement	Building code enforcement
	Sprinkler and fire alarm system code enforcement
Engineering	Hot water heater temperature controls
	Gun trigger locks; trigger fingerprint recognition
	Childproof cigarette lighters
	Fire-resistant fabrics for sleepwear and furnishings
	Fire escapes and escape routes
	Child safety caps on medications
Environmental	Cupboard locks
	Electrical outlet covers
	Fire hazard reduction
	Fire alarms
	Stair gates

will depend in large part on the nature of the local problem, the concerns of the population, the availability of resources, and competing demands. Nonetheless, there is ample reason to believe that even simple countermeasures may make a big impact on reducing the global burden of death and disability due to injury.

KEY TERMS

disability adjusted life   injury control   intentional injuries
years (DALYs)   injury prevention   transportation injuries
Haddon matrix   injury pyramid   unintentional injuries
injury

DISCUSSION QUESTIONS

1. What is the difference between an injury and an accident? Why is it important to make the distinction? Discuss some strategies for highlighting the difference between accidents and injuries.

2. How do injury control and environmental health overlap?

3. Describe an injury sustained by you or a member of your family. How well does it meet the injury definition laid out in this chapter? Create a Haddon matrix for the injury. What are several solutions that could minimize the incidence or impact of the injury among others? Make sure you have at least one educational, one environmental, and one engineering solution.

4. Scan the headlines of the last week, and identify a type of injury mentioned there. What would a public health approach for reducing morbidity and mortality from that injury look like? Your response should (a) create a precise definition of the injury; (b) outline strategies for clarifying its distribution, risk factors, and protective factors; (c) suggest intervention strategies for reducing the injury's morbidity and mortality; and (d) describe how you would evaluate the effectiveness of your proposed interventions.

5. Gun violence poses a significant burden on citizens of the United States. Create a Haddon matrix for interpersonal violence involving firearms in the United States (identify a subset of gun violence, such as shootings in the home or hunting injuries, if you wish). What are at least three interventions that are not listed in this chapter and that could be used for reducing morbidity and mortality from gun-related injuries? Conduct an options analysis of these interventions, and identify those that you believe would have the highest yield.

6. For one hour of your day, catalogue all the injury prevention mechanisms that you encounter (directly or indirectly). For instance, when you get in your car, list the major injury prevention and control measures there, including seat belts, air bags, and supplemental restraint systems, and so forth. Attempt to include educational, environmental, and engineering solutions in your list.

7. Sometimes, a measure to control injuries may collide with another public health priority. For example, playground safety may collide with "natural playground" design that encourages children to be imaginative and take risks, fireproofing clothing may expose consumers to toxic chemicals, or controlling pedestrian injuries may reduce physical activity. Pick one of these instances, or another example, and discuss the issues involved.

REFERENCES

Baker, S. P., O'Neill, B., Ginsburg, M. J., and Li, G. *The Injury Fact Book.* (2nd ed.) New York: Oxford University Press, 1992.

Bronstein, A. C., and others. "2006 Annual Report of the American Association of Poison Control Centers' National Poison Data System (NPDS)." *Clinical Toxicology,* 2007, *45,* 815–917.

Burke, G., and others. "Evaluation of the Effectiveness of a Pavement Stencil in Promoting Safe Behavior Among Elementary School Children at School Bus Stops." *Pediatrics*, 1996, *97*, 520–530.

Carter, S. P., Carter, S. L., and Dannenberg, A. L. "Zoning Out Crime and Improving Community Health in Sarasota, Florida: Crime Prevention Through Environmental Design." *American Journal of Public Health*, 2003, *93*, 1442–1445.

Casteel, C., Peek-Asa, C., Howard, J., and Kraus, J. F. "Effectiveness of Crime Prevention Through Environmental Design in Reducing Criminal Activity in Liquor Stores: A Pilot Study." *Journal of Occupational Environmental Medicine*, 2004, *46*, 450–458.

Centers for Disease Control and Prevention. "Achievements in Public Health, 1900–1999 Motor-Vehicle Safety: A 20th Century Public Health Achievement." *Morbidity and Mortality Weekly Report*, 1999, *48*(18), 369–374.

Centers for Disease Control and Prevention. *Injury Fact Book 2001–2002.* Atlanta, Ga.: Centers for Disease Control and Prevention, National Center for Injury Prevention and Control, 2002.

Dannenberg, A. L., and others. "Bicycle Helmet Laws and Educational Campaigns: An Evaluation of Strategies to Increase Children's Helmet Use." *American Journal of Public Health*, 1993, *83*, 667–674.

Darwin, J. "Reaffirmed Cost-Effectiveness of Poison Centers." *Annals of Emergency Medicine*, 2003, *41*, 159–160.

Duperrex, O., Bunn, F., and Roberts, I. "Safety Education of Pedestrians for Injury Prevention: A Systematic Review of Randomised Controlled Trials." *British Medical Journal*, 2002, *324*, 1129.

Elvik, R. "A Meta-Analysis of Studies Concerning the Safety Effects of Daytime Running Lights on Cars." *Accident Analysis and Prevention*, 1996, *28*, 685–694.

Evans, L. "Evans Responds to Letters on 'Roles of Litigation and Safety Belts.'" *American Journal of Public Health*, 2004, *94*, 171–172.

Fauveau, U., and Blancet, T. "Deaths from Injuries and Induced Abortion Among Rural Bangladesh Women." *Social Science & Medicine*, 1989, *29*, 1121–1127.

Federal Railroad Administration, Office of Safety Analysis. http://safetydata.fra.dot.gov/OfficeofSafety/publicsite/query/query.aspx, 2005.

Finkelstein, E., Corso, P., and Miller, T. *The Incidence and Economic Costs of Injury in the United States.* New York: Oxford University Press, 2006.

Forjuoh, S. N. "Traffic-Related Injury Prevention Interventions for Low-Income Countries." *Injury Control and Safety Promotion*, 2003, *10*, 109–118.

Graitcer, P. L., Kellermann, A. L., and Christoffel, T. A. "Review of Educational and Legislative Strategies to Promote Bicycle Helmets." *Injury Prevention*, 1995, *1*, 122–129.

Haddon, W. A. "Logical Framework for Categorizing Highway Safety Phenomena and Activity." *Journal of Trauma*, 1972, *12*, 193–207.

Haddon, W. "Energy Damage and the Ten Countermeasure Strategies." *Journal of Trauma*, 1973, *13*, 321–331.

Hanfling, M. J., Mangus, L. G., Gill, A. C., and Bailey, R. "A Multifaceted Approach to Improving Motor Vehicle Restraint Compliance." *Injury Prevention*, 2000, *6*, 125–129.

Herd, A. N., Widdowson, P., and Tanner, N.S.B. "Scalds in the Very Young: Prevention or Cure." *Burns*, 1986, *12*, 246–249.

Holder, Y., and others (eds.). *Injury Surveillance Guidelines.* Geneva: World Health Organization, in Conjunction with the Centers for Disease Control, 2001.

Home Safety Council. *State of Home Safety in America.* Washington: Home Safety Council. http://homesafety-council.org/AboutUs/Research/re_sohs_w001.asp, 2004.

Houston, D. J., and Richardson, L. E. "Motorcyclist Fatality Rates and Mandatory Helmet-Use Laws." *Accident Analysis & Prevention,* 2008, *40*: 200–208.

Kahane, C. J. *Fatality Reduction by Air Bags: Analysis of Accident Data Through Early 1996.* National Highway Traffic Safety Administration (NHTSA) Report No. DOT-HS-808–470. Washington, D.C.: National Highway Traffic Safety Administration, 1998.

Karter, M. J. *Fire Loss in the United States 2007.* National Fire Protection Association, Fire Analysis and Research Division. http://www.nfpa.org/assets/files/PDF/OS.fireloss.pdf, 2008.

Kellermann, A. L., Lee, R. K., Mercy, J. A., and Banton, J. "The Epidemiological Basis for the Prevention of Firearm Injuries." *Annual Review of Public Health,* 1991, *12*, 17–40.

Keswani, M. H. "The Prevention of Burning Injury." *Burns,* 1986, *12*, 533–539.

Konradsen, F., and others. "Reducing Acute Poisoning in Developing Countries—Options for Restricting the Availability of Pesticides." *Toxicology,* 2003, *192*, 249–261.

Krug, E. G. (ed.). *Injury: A Leading Cause of the Global Burden of Disease.* Geneva: World Health Organization, 1999.

Krug, E. G., and others. "The Global Burden of Injuries." *American Journal of Public Health,* 2000, *90*, 523–526.

Krug, E. G., and others (eds.). *World Report on Violence and Health.* Geneva: World Health Organization, 2002.

Laborde, A. "New Roles for Poison Control Centres in the Developing Countries." *Toxicology,* 2004, *198*, 273–277.

Li, G. L., Li, L. P., and Cai, Q. E. "Motorcycle Helmet Use in Southern China: An Observational Study." *Traffic Injury Prevention,* 2008, *9*, 125–128.

Marsh, D., and others. "Epidemiology of Adults Hospitalized with Burns in Karachi, Pakistan." *Burns,* 1996, *22*, 225–229.

Mello, M. J., and others. "Innovations in Injury Prevention Education." *Journal of Trauma,* 2007, *63* (3 suppl.), S7–S9.

Mertz, K. J., and Weiss, H. B. "Changes in Motorcycle-Related Head Injury Deaths, Hospitalizations, and Hospital Charges Following Repeal of Pennsylvania's Mandatory Motorcycle Helmet Law." *American Journal of Public Health,* 2008, *98*(8), 1464–1467.

Miller, T. R., and Cohen, M. A. "Costs of Gunshot and Cut/Stab Wounds in the United States, with Some Canadian Comparisons." *Accident Analysis and Prevention,* 1997, *29*, 329–341.

Miller, T. R., and Lestina, D. C. "Costs of Poisoning in the United States and Savings from Poison Control Centers: A Benefit-Cost Analysis." *Annals of Emergency Medicine,* 1997, *49*(2), 239–245.

Mohan, D. "Evidence-Based Interventions for Road Traffic Injuries in South Asia." *Journal of the College of Physicians & Surgeons—Pakistan,* 2004, *14*, 746–747.

Murray, C. J., and Lopez, A. D. *The Global Burden of Disease: A Comprehensive Assessment of Mortality and Disability from Diseases, Injuries and Risk Factors in 1990 and Projected to 2020.* Global Burden of Disease and Injury Series, Vol. I. Cambridge, Mass.: Harvard School of Public Health on behalf of the World Health Organization and the World Bank, 1996.

National Center for Injury Prevention and Control. *Injury Research Agenda*. Atlanta, Ga.: National Center for Injury Prevention and Control, 2002.

National Center for Injury Prevention and Control. *Web-Based Injury Statistics Query and Reporting System (WISQARS)*. http://www.cdc.gov/ncipc/wisqars, 2008.

National Highway Traffic Safety Administration. *Motorcycle Safety Program*. Washington, D.C.: U.S. Department of Transportation, 2003.

Odero, W., Garner, P., and Zwi, A. "Road Traffic Injuries in Developing Countries: A Comprehensive Review of Epidemiological Studies." *Tropical Medicine and International Health*, 1997, *2*, 445–460.

Peck, M. D., and others. "Burns and Injuries from Non-Electric-Appliance Fires in Low- and Middle-Income Countries, Part II: A Strategy for Intervention Using the Haddon Matrix." *Burns*, 2008, *34*, 312–319.

Peden, M., McGee, K., and Krug, E. (eds.). *Injury: A Leading Cause of the Global Burden of Disease, 2000*. Geneva: World Health Organization, 2002.

Peden, M., and others (eds.). *World Report on Road Traffic Injury Prevention*. Geneva: World Health Organization, 2004.

Pitts, S.R., Niska, R.W., Xu, J., and Burt, C.W. *National Hospital Ambulatory Medical Care Survey: 2006 Emergency Department Summary*. National Health Statistics Report Number 7. Hyattsville, MD: National Center for Health Statistics. August, 2008. http://www.cdc.gov/nchs/data/nhsr/nhsr007.pdf.

Polen, M. R., and Friedman, G. D. (U.S. Preventive Services Task Force). "Automobile Injury: Selected Risk Factors and Prevention in the Health Care Setting." *JAMA*, 1988, *259*, 76–80.

Poli de Figueiredo, L. F., and others. "Increases in Fines and Driver License Withdrawal Have Effectively Reduced Immediate Deaths from Trauma on Brazilian Roads: First-Year Report on the New Traffic Code." *Injury*, 2001, *32*(2), 91–94.

Razzak, J. A., Laflamme, L., Luby, S. P., and Chotani, H. "Childhood Injuries in Pakistan: When, Where and How?" *Public Health*, 2004, *118*(2), 114–120.

Razzak, J. A., and Luby, S. P. "Estimating Deaths and Injuries Due to Road Traffic Accidents in Karachi, Pakistan, Through the Capture-Recapture Method." *International Journal of Epidemiology*, 1998, *27*, 866–870.

Razzak, J. A., Marsh, D. M., and Stansfield, S. "District Hospital-Based Injury Data: Is It an Option in a Developing Country?" *Injury Prevention*, 2002, *8*, 345–346.

Retting, R. A., Ferguson, S. A., and McCartt, A. T. "A Review of Evidence-Based Traffic Engineering Measures Designed to Reduce Pedestrian-Motor Vehicle Crashes." *American Journal of Public Health*, 2003, *93*, 1456–1462.

Runyan, C. W., and others. "Unintentional Injuries in the Home Environment in the United States, Part I: Mortality." *American Journal of Preventive Medicine*, 2005a, *28*, 73–79.

Runyan, C. W., and others. "Unintentional Injuries in the Home Environment in the United States, Part II: Morbidity." *American Journal of Preventive Medicine*, 2005b, *28*, 80–87.

Sestito, J. P., Lunsford, R. A., Hamilton, A. C., and Rosa, R. R. (eds.). *Worker Health Chartbook 2004*. National Institute of Occupational Safety and Health. http://www.cdc.gov/niosh/docs/2004–146/pdfs/2004–146.pdf, 2004.

Sherman, L. W., and others. *Preventing Crime: What Works, What Doesn't, What's Promising*. Washington, D.C.: National Institute of Justice, 1998.

Smith, G. S. "Public Health Approaches to Occupational Injury Prevention: Do They Work?" *Injury Prevention*, 2001, *7*, 3–10.

Sumner, S. A., Layde, P. M., and Guse, C. E. "Firearm Death Rates and Association with Level of Firearm Purchase Background Check." *American Journal of Preventive Medicine*, 2008, *35*, 1–6.

Tinsworth, D. K., and McDonald, J. E. *Special Study: Injuries and Deaths Associated with Children's Playground Equipment.* Washington D.C.: U.S. Consumer Product Safety Commission, Apr. 2001.

Ulmer, R. G., and Preusser, D. F. *Evaluation of the Repeal of Motorcycle Helmet Laws in Kentucky and Louisiana.* NHTSA Report No. DOT-HS-809–530. Washington D.C.: National Highway Traffic Safety Administration, 2003.

Vernick, J. S., Mair, J. S., Teret, S. P., and Sapsin, J. W. "Role of Litigation in Preventing Product-Related Injuries." *Epidemiologic Reviews*, 2003, *25*, 90–98.

Villaveces, A., and others. "Effect of a Ban on Carrying Firearms on Homicide Rates in Two Colombian Cities." *JAMA*, 2000, *283*, 1205–1209.

Wadman, M. C., Muelleman, R. L., Coto, J. A., and Kellermann, A. L. "The Pyramid of Injury: Using E-Codes to Accurately Describe the Burden of Injury." *Annals of Emergency Medicine*, 2003, *42*, 468–478.

Webster, P. J. "Myanmar's Deadly Daffodil." *Nature Geoscience*, 2008, *1*, 488–490.

Wesson, D. E., and others. "Trends in Pediatric and Adult Bicycling Deaths Before and After Passage of a Bicycle Helmet Law." *Pediatrics*, 2008, *122*, 605–610.

Williams, A. F., Preusser, D. F., Blomberg, R. D., and Lund, A. D. "Seat Belt Use Law Enforcement and Publicity in Elmira, New York: A Reminder Campaign." *American Journal of Public Health*, 1987, *77*, 1450–1451.

Withaneachi, D., and Meehan, T. "Promoting Safer Play Equipment in Primary Schools: Evaluation of an Educational Campaign." *Health Promotion Journal of Australia*, 1998, *8*, 125–129.

World Health Organization. *Revised Global Burden of Disease (GBD) 2002 Estimates.* http://www.who.int/healthinfo/bodgbd2002revised/en/index.html, 2004.

World Health Organization. *World Health Statistics 2008.* http://www.who.int/whosis/whostat/EN_WHS08_Full.pdf, 2008.

Zaloshnja, E., Miller, T. R., Lawrence, B. A., and Romano, E. "The Costs of Unintentional Home Injuries." *American Journal of Preventive Medicine*, 2005, *28*, 88–94.

FOR FURTHER INFORMATION

Books

Barss, P., Smith, G. S., Baker, S. P., and Mohan, D. *Injury Prevention: An International Perspective: Epidemiology, Surveillance and Policy.* New York: Oxford University Press, 1998.

Christoffel, T., and Gallagher, S. S. *Injury Prevention and Public Health Practical Knowledge, Skills, and Strategies.* Gaithersburg, Md.: Aspen, 1999.

Mohan, D., and Tiwari, G. (eds.). *Injury Prevention and Control.* Boca Raton, Fla.: CRC Press, 2000.

Rivara, F. P., and others. *Injury Control: Research and Program Evaluation.* New York: Cambridge University Press, 2000.

Robertson, L. S. *Injury Epidemiology*. New York: Oxford University Press, 1999.

Smith, G., and others. *Injury Prevention: An International Perspective: Epidemiology, Surveillance, and Policy*. New York: Oxford University Press, 1998.

Journals

Accident Analysis and Prevention, http://www.elsevier.com/wps/find/journaldescription.cws_home/336/ description#description. Published by Elsevier and affiliated with the Association for the Advancement of Automotive Medicine (AAAM).

Injury Control and Safety Promotion, http://www.tandf.co.uk/journals/titles/17457300.asp. Published by Taylor & Francis and associated with EuroSafe (European Association for Injury Prevention and Safety Promotion.

Injury Prevention, http://ip.bmjjournals.com. Published by BMJ Publishing Group, this is the official journal of the International Society for Child and Adolescent Injury Prevention (ISCAIP) and the Society for Advancement of Violence and Injury Research (SAVIR).

Journal of Safety Research. http://www.nsc.org/lrs/res/jsr.aspx and http://www.elsevier.com/wps/find/ journaldescription.cws_home/679/description#description. A joint publication of Elsevier and the National Safety Council (NSC).

Traffic Injury Prevention, http://www.tandf.co.uk/journals/titles/15389588.asp. Published by Taylor & Francis, this is the official journal of the Association for the Advancement of Automotive Medicine (AAAM), International Traffic Medicine Association (ITMA), International Council on Alcohol, Drugs and Traffic Safety (ICADTS), and International Research Council on the Biomechanics of Impact (IRCOBI).

Agencies and Organizations

American College of Emergency Physicians (ACEP). [Homepage.] http://www.acep.org This professional organization of emergency physicians addresses a number of injury control issues in its policies and resources.

Centers for Disease Control and Prevention (CDC), National Center for Injury Control and Prevention (NCICP). [Homepage.] http://www.cdc.gov/ncipc, 2005. The NCICP maintains information on injury control, including surveillance data and statistics, for the United States. The NCICP's Web site also offers program information and funding sources.

Injury Prevention Web. [Homepage.] http://www.injuryprevention.org, 2005. The Injury Prevention Web is a meta-site that hosts the Web pages of several injury prevention organizations and serves as an excellent source for injury prevention resources.

SafetyLit. [Homepage.] http://www.safetylit.org, 2005. SafetyLit is an online resource for recent injury prevention research.

World Health Organization. "Injuries and Violence Prevention." http://www.who.int/violence_ injury_prevention/en, 2005. WHO's Department of Violence and Injury Prevention and Disability maintains a clearinghouse for information about injury control, including epidemiology and prevention, the world over, with a regularly updated list of campaigns, conferences, and other injury control activities.

CHAPTER TWENTY-THREE

ENVIRONMENTAL DISASTERS

MARK E. KEIM

KEY CONCEPTS

- Environmental disasters occur when three things come together: population exposure to an environmental hazard, conditions of vulnerability in that population and its environment, and insufficient capacity or strategies to reduce or cope with negative consequences.

- Environmental hazards that lead to disasters may be natural or technological.

- The hazards that cause disasters may vary greatly but the public health consequences and the public health and medical needs of affected populations do not.

- Disaster risk is the product of the probability of disaster occurrence and the probability of a vulnerable population becoming affected minus the absorptive capacity of that population.

- Disaster risk management is a comprehensive, all-hazard approach that entails developing and implementing strategies for all phases of the disaster life cycle—prevention, mitigation, preparedness, response, and recovery—in the context of sustainable development.

DEFINING DISASTER

A **disaster** is "a serious disruption of the functioning of a community or a society causing widespread human, material, economic or environmental losses that exceed the ability of the affected community or society to cope using its own resources" (United Nations/International Strategy for Disaster Reduction [UN/ISDR], 2009). If a disruptive event does not exceed a community's or society's capacity to cope, it is classified as an *emergency* (World Health Organization [WHO], 1998, p. 16). Emergencies and disasters are thus part of a continuum of events that differ only in their degree of severity.

EXHIBIT 23.1
Definitions of Key Terms

Absorptive capacity. A limit to the rate or quantity of impact that can be absorbed (or adapted to) without exceeding the threshold of disaster declaration.

All-hazard approach. Developing and implementing emergency management strategies for the full range of likely emergencies or disasters, both natural and technological (the latter category includes hazards arising from terrorism and warfare).

Building code. A set of ordinances or regulations and associated standards intended to control aspects of the design, construction, materials, alteration, and occupancy of structures in order to ensure human safety and welfare and to make the structures resistant to collapse and damage.

Capability. The ability to achieve a desired operational effect under specified standards and conditions through combinations of means and ways to perform a set of tasks.

Capacity. The combination of all the strengths, attributes and resources available within a community, society or organization that can be used to achieve agreed goals.

Critical facilities. The primary physical structures, technical facilities, and systems that are socially, economically, or operationally essential to the functioning of a society or community, both in routine circumstances and in the extreme circumstances of an emergency.

Disaster risk. The potential disaster losses, in lives, health status, livelihoods, assets, and services, that could occur to a particular community or a society over some specified future time period.

Mark E. Keim declares no competing financial interests.

Disaster *consequences* may include "loss of life, injury, disease, and other negative effects on human physical, mental and social well-being, together with damage to property, destruction of assets, loss of services, social and economic disruption, and environmental degradation" (UN/ISDR, 2009). The severity of the consequences is referred to as *disaster impact*. Exhibit 23.1 defines additional key terms in disaster risk reduction.

Environmental disasters occur when three things come together: (1) population exposure to an environmental **hazard**, (2) conditions of **vulnerability**, and (3) insufficient **capacity** or measures to reduce or cope with the potential negative consequences.

Disaster risk management. The systematic process of using administrative directives, organizations, and operational skills and capacities to implement strategies, policies, and improved coping capacities in order to lessen the adverse impacts of hazards and the possibility of disaster.

Disaster risk reduction. The concept and practice of reducing disaster risks through systematic efforts to analyze and manage the causal factors of disasters, by, for example, reducing exposure to hazards, lessening the vulnerability of people and property, managing land and the environment wisely, and improving preparedness for adverse events.

Early warning system. The set of capacities needed to generate and disseminate timely and meaningful warning information that enables individuals, communities, and organizations threatened by a hazard to prepare and to act appropriately and in sufficient time to reduce the possibility of harm or loss.

Emergency services. The set of specialized agencies that have specific responsibilities and objectives in serving and protecting people and property in emergency situations.

Exposure. People, property, systems, or other elements present in hazard zones that are thereby collectively subject to potential losses.

Forecast. A definite statement or statistical estimate of the likely occurrence of a future event or conditions for a specific area.

Hazard. A dangerous phenomenon, substance, human activity, or condition that may cause loss of life, injury, or other health impacts, property damage, loss of livelihoods and services, social and economic disruption, or environmental damage.

Land-use planning. The process undertaken by public authorities to identify, evaluate, and decide among the different options for the use of land, including consideration of long-term economic, social, and environmental objectives and the implications for different communities and interest groups, and the subsequent formulation and promulgation of plans that describe the permitted or acceptable uses.

Mitigation. The lessening or limiting of the adverse impacts of hazards and related disasters.

Natural hazard. A natural process or phenomenon that may cause loss of life, injury, or other health impacts, property damage, loss of livelihoods and services, social and economic disruption, or environmental damage.

Nonstructural measure. Any measure not involving physical construction that uses knowledge, practice, or agreement to reduce risks and impacts, in particular through promoting policies and laws, raising public awareness, training, and education.

Preparedness. The knowledge and capacities developed by governments, professional response and recovery organizations, communities, and individuals to effectively anticipate, respond to, and recover from the impacts of likely, imminent, or current hazard events or conditions.

Prevention. The outright avoidance of adverse impacts of hazards and related disasters.

Public awareness. The extent of common knowledge about disaster risks, the factors that lead to disasters, and the actions that can be taken individually and collectively to reduce exposure and vulnerability to hazards.

Recovery. The restoration, and improvement where appropriate, of facilities, livelihoods, and living conditions of disaster-affected communities, including efforts to reduce disaster risk factors.

Residual risk. The risk that remains unmanaged even when effective disaster risk reduction measures are in place and for which emergency response and recovery capacities must be maintained.

Resilience. The ability of a system, community, or society exposed to hazards to resist, absorb, accommodate to, and recover from the effects of a hazard in a timely and efficient manner, including its ability to preserve and restore its essential basic structures and functions.

Response. The provision of emergency services and public assistance during or immediately after a disaster in order to save lives, reduce health impacts, ensure public safety, and meet the basic subsistence needs of the people affected.

Environmental disasters may be classified in terms of the hazards that cause them and whether these hazards are natural or technological in origin (see Table 23.1). **Natural hazards** may be further classified as meteorological or geophysical. **Technological hazards** include those that are toxic, thermal, or mechanical.

Risk. The probability of harmful consequences, that is, the expected losses (deaths, injuries, property damaged, livelihoods harmed, economic activity disrupted, or environment damaged), resulting from interactions between natural or human-induced hazards and vulnerable conditions.

Risk assessment. The determination of the nature and the extent of risk by analyzing potential hazards and evaluating existing conditions of vulnerability that might act together to harm exposed people, property, services, livelihoods, and the environment on which they depend.

Risk management. The systematic approach and practice of managing uncertainty to minimize potential harm and loss.

Risk retention. A set of procedures for responding and recovering, once a loss has occurred; applied to risks that cannot be avoided or transferred.

Risk transfer. The process of formally or informally shifting the financial consequences of particular risks from one party to another, whereby a household, community, enterprise, or state authority will obtain resources from the other party after a disaster occurs in exchange for ongoing or compensatory social or financial benefits provided to that other party.

Structural measures. Any physical construction to reduce or avoid possible impacts of hazards or any application of engineering techniques to achieve hazard resistance and resilience in structures or systems.

Susceptibility. The state of being at risk, if exposed to a hazard.

Sustainable development. Development that meets the needs of the present without compromising the ability of future generations to meet their own needs.

Technological hazard. A hazard originating from technological or industrial conditions, such as an accident, dangerous procedure, infrastructure failure, or specific human activity, that may cause loss of life, injury, illness or other health impacts, property damage, loss of livelihoods and services, social and economic disruption, or environmental damage.

Vulnerability. The characteristics and circumstances of a community, system or asset that make it susceptible to the damaging effects of a hazard.

Source: Slightly adapted from UN/ISDR, 2009; Henry, 2005–2006.

Industrial chemical disasters may be unintentional (due to equipment failure or worker error or fatigue) (Lillibridge, 1997), or they may be intentional. In fact, industrial disasters may differ from acts of sabotage, warfare, and terrorism only in malicious intent (Keim, 2002).

TABLE 23.1   A Typology of Environmental Disasters

Natural		Technological	
Hydrometeorological	Drought	Toxic	Chemical
	Wildfires		Radiological
	Heat waves		
	Storms[a]		
	Floods		
Geophysical	Earthquakes	Thermal	Fires
	Landslides[b]		Explosions
	Volcanic eruptions		Nuclear
	Tsunamis		
		Mechanical	Transport accidents

[a] Storms include cyclones, tornadoes, windstorms, snow or ice storms, and dust storms.

[b] Landslides include debris flows, mud flows, volcanic lahars, and snow avalanches.

Disaster risk is the product of the probability of disaster occurrence and the probability of a vulnerable population becoming affected minus the **absorptive capacity** of the society. Thus a disaster is defined by the vulnerability of the population to a hazard event and not by the mere fact that the event has occurred (de Ville de Goyet and Lechat, 1976). Absorptive capacity and resilience are not synonymous. **Resilience** is "the ability of a system, community or society exposed to hazards to resist, absorb, accommodate to and recover from the effects of a hazard in a timely and efficient manner, including through the preservation and restoration of its essential basic structures and functions" (UN/ISDR, 2009). It is made up of (1) the absorbing capacity, (2) the buffering capacity, and (3) the response to the event and the recovery from the damage sustained. Absorptive capacity is the *rate or limit* of this ability.

For any hazard the risk varies with the vulnerability of the population (that is, the degree of population **susceptibility**, **exposure**, and resilience to the hazard). **Risk reduction** actions reduce the number of events that exceed the community's or society's ability to respond, thereby preventing some emergencies from ever becoming disasters (UN ISDR, 2004).

Risk assessment is widely used to quantify environmental health risk. The risk equation has also been applied to estimate disaster risk, according to the following relationship:

$$p(D) = k[p(H) \times p(V)] - AC$$

where $p(D)$ = risk of disaster occurrence, k is a constant, $p(H)$ = the probability of hazard occurrence, $p(V)$ = the probability of population vulnerability, and AC = absorptive capacity (also known as adaptive capacity). According to this equation, disaster risk may be reduced among populations at risk by reducing the hazard itself; by decreasing the vulnerability; and by increasing the absorptive capacity (Keim, 2002).

SCOPE OF THE PROBLEM

The incidence of environmental disasters, both natural and technological, is increasing worldwide (Centre for Research on the Epidemiology of Disasters [CRED], 2005; Noji, 1997). During the decade 1997 to 2006, 6,806 environmental disasters (not including wars, conflict-related famines, and epidemics) were reported to have killed 1.2 million people worldwide, affected 2.7 billion lives, and resulted in property damage exceeding $800 billion (International Federation of Red Cross and Red Crescent Societies [IFRC], 2007).

Natural disasters constituted 54 percent of these events. The most frequent types of disasters reported, whether natural or technological, were floods (32 percent), transport accidents (28 percent), and windstorms (10 percent). Meteorological hazards (perhaps related to climate change; see Chapter Ten) are affecting increasing numbers of people and causing increasingly large economic losses (Thomalla, 2006). Between 1970 and 1999, victims of meteorological hazards made up 90 percent of the world's disaster-related fatalities (CRED, 2005).

The terminology of storms is complex. A *storm* is any disturbed state of an astronomical body's atmosphere, especially affecting its surface, and strongly implying severe weather. It may be marked by strong wind, thunder and lightning (a thunderstorm), by heavy precipitation (such as ice [ice storm]), or by wind transporting some substance through the atmosphere (as in a dust storm, snowstorm, hailstorm, and so forth). A *cyclone* is a weather phenomenon featuring a central region of low pressure surrounded by air flowing in an inward spiral and generating maximum sustained winds speeds of seventy-four miles per hour or more. Cyclones that form over warm water are known as *tropical cyclones*. A tropical cyclone is referred to as a *hurricane* in the Atlantic basin and the western Coast of Mexico, as *typhoon* in the western Pacific, and as a *cyclone* in the Indian Ocean and Australasia (Malilay, 1997). *Tornadoes* are different from cyclones in that they generally form over land in areas of large vertical temperature gradients, and they are smaller and briefer in duration. When tropical cyclones make landfall, they sometimes give rise to tornadoes.

The world's poor nations are disproportionately affected by disasters, and the most vulnerable and marginalized people in these nations bear the brunt (Munich

Re Group, 2002; Burkle, 2006; Clack, Keim, MacIntyre, and Yeskey, 2002; IFRC, 2007; Brouewer and others, 2007; National Science and Technology Council [NSTC] . . . , 1996; Nelson, 1990). Table 23.2 shows the major environmental disasters that occurred from 1997 to 2006 and the number of fatalities associated with each event.

Two separate environmental disasters in May 2008 resulted in a death toll equivalent to 21 percent of the total for the entire previous decade. Cyclone Nargis struck Myanmar on May 2, 2008, causing catastrophic destruction and at least 146,000 fatalities (BBC News, 2008). Ten days later, an earthquake with a magnitude of 7.9 on the Richter scale struck Sichuan province in central China, killing an estimated 86,000 people and leaving about 4.8 million homeless (Relief Web, 2008).

PUBLIC HEALTH IMPACT

Populations at risk for disasters face a vast range of hazards within a nearly infinite set of scenarios. This unpredictability is poorly suited to scenario-based approaches to risk management (Henry, 2005). However, even though the hazards that cause disasters may vary greatly, the potential public health consequences and subsequent public health and medical needs of the population do not (Keim, 2006a; Federal Emergency Management Agency [FEMA], 1996). For example, warfare, chemical releases, floods, hurricanes, and earthquakes all displace people from their homes. These hazards all require the same sheltering capability with only minor adjustments based on the rapidity of onset, scale, duration, location, and intensity. Regardless of the hazard, disasters can be seen as causing fifteen public

TABLE 23.2   Environmental Disasters Ranked by Number of Lives Lost, Worldwide, 1997–2006

Disaster Type	Year	Location	Estimated Fatalities
Tsunami	2004	Indian Ocean	226,408
Earthquake	2005	Pakistan	74,647
Heat wave	2003	Europe	70,000
Flood or landslide	1999	Venezuela	30,000
Earthquake	2003	Iran	26,796
Earthquake	2001	India	20,005
Tropical cyclone	1998	Central America	18,791
Earthquake	1999	Turkey	17,791

Source: IFRC, 2007.

health consequences that are addressed by thirty-two categories of public health and medical capabilities (Keim, 2006a). By using an all-hazard, capability-based approach, communities can prepare for and respond to disasters by applying their own capabilities to any hazard. Table 23.3 lists the consequences and public health capabilities that are most commonly addressed in a disaster response. The range of public health consequences actually varies little among disaster hazards. The application of public health capabilities may vary more, according to the severity of disaster consequences (impact of the disaster) rather than the hazard type.

Natural Disasters

Table 23.4 summarizes the relative public health impacts of various types of **natural disasters**. This table illustrates that very similar public health capabilities are applied across many disaster types, regardless of the specific hazard or scenario.

Compared to meteorological disasters, geophysical disasters tend to create higher rates of injuries. Geophysical disasters also tend to occur with less opportunity for advance warning (Krug and others, 1998; Lutgendorf, 1995). Injuries are the leading cause of death in all natural disasters. For geophysical disasters, burns, asphyxia, and forms of blunt and penetrating trauma are the main causes of death.

For cyclones and floods, the main cause of death is drowning. (Malilay, 1997; Centers for Disease Control and Prevention [CDC], 2002). In the case of tropical cyclones, most of the mortality occurs during the storm surge, especially in low-income nations (Chowdhury and others, 1992; Diacon, 1992). Most injuries (such as nail puncture wounds, lacerations, falls, burns, electrocutions, and carbon monoxide [CO] poisonings), are sustained during the disaster recovery and cleanup phase. The main cause of death in tornadoes and landslides is traumatic injury sustained during the disaster impact. The main causes of death in heat waves are heat illness and exacerbations of chronic respiratory and cardiovascular disease (Wilhite, 1993). Drought-related deaths are generally mediated by agricultural, economic, and medical effects such as malnutrition, poverty, poor sanitation and hygiene, unsafe water, infectious diseases, and conflict (Bailey and Walker, 2007; Wilhite, 1993). The main causes of death during wildfires are burn and smoke inhalation injuries. The public health impact of wildfires may include burn injuries, exacerbations of chronic obstructive pulmonary disease and asthma, and temporary population displacement that results in a need for humanitarian assistance (Sanderson, 1997).

Infectious disease epidemics following natural disasters are rare and differ according to the affected nation's level of economic development (CDC, 1998,

TABLE 23.3   Public Health Consequences and Capabilities Associated with all Disasters

Public Health Consequences	Public Health Capabilities
All consequences	Resource management
	Mental health services
	Reproductive health services
	Social services
	Occupational health and safety
	Business continuity
Deaths	Mortuary services
	Social services
	Mental health services
Illness and injuries	Health services
	Injury prevention and control
	Epidemiology
	Disease prevention and control
Loss of clean water	Access to safe water
Loss of shelter	Shelter and settlement
	Social services
	Security
Loss of personal and household goods	Replacement of personal and household goods
Loss of sanitation and routine hygiene	Sanitation, excreta disposal, and hygiene promotion
Disruption of solid waste management	Solid waste management
Public concern for safety	Risk communication
	Public information
	Security
Increased pests and vectors	Pest and vector control
Loss or damage of health care system	Health system and infrastructure support
Worsening of chronic illnesses	Health services
Food scarcity	Food safety, security, and nutrition
Standing surface water	Public works and engineering
Toxic exposures	Risk assessment
	Population protection
	Health services
	Hazmat emergency response
	Occupational health and safety

Source: Adapted from Keim, 2006a.

TABLE 23.4 The Relative Public Health Impact of Natural Environmental Disasters

| Public Health Impact | Geophysical | | | Meteorological | | | | |
| | Seismic | | Volcanic | High Precipitation | | | Low Precipitation | |
	Earthquake	Tsunami	Volcanic Eruption	Landslide	Tropical Cyclone	Flood	Drought	Wildfire
Deaths	Many	Many	Few to moderate	Few to moderate	Few, but many in poor nations	Few, but many in poor nations	Few, but many in poor nations	Few
Injuries	Many	Many	Few to moderate	Few to moderate	Few	Few	Unlikely	Few
Loss of clean water	Focal to widespread	Focal to widespread	Focal to widespread	Focal	Focal to widespread	Focal to widespread	Widespread	Focal
Loss of shelter	Focal to widespread	Focal to widespread	Focal to widespread	Focal	Focal to widespread	Focal to widespread	Focal to widespread	Focal
Loss of personal and household goods	Focal to widespread	Focal to widespread	Focal to widespread	Focal	Focal to widespread	Focal to widespread	Focal to widespread	Focal
Major population movements	Focal to widespread	Focal to widespread	Focal to widespread	Focal	Focal to widespread	Focal to widespread	Focal to widespread	Focal
Loss of routine hygiene	Focal to widespread	Focal to widespread	Focal to widespread	Focal	Focal to widespread	Focal to widespread	Widespread	Focal
Loss of sanitation	Focal to widespread	Focal to widespread	Focal to widespread	Focal	Focal to widespread	Focal to widespread	Focal	Focal
Disruption of solid waste management	Focal to widespread	Focal to widespread	Focal to widespread	Focal	Focal to widespread	Focal to widespread	Focal	Focal

(continued)

TABLE 23.4 Continued

Public Health Impact	Geophysical				Meteorological			
	Seismic		Volcanic		High Precipitation		Low Precipitation	
	Earthquake	Tsunami	Volcanic Eruption	Landslide	Tropical Cyclone	Flood	Drought	Wildfire
Public concern for safety	High	High	High	Moderate to high	High	Moderate to high	Low to moderate	Moderate to high
Increased pests	Focal to widespread	Focal to widespread	Unlikely	Unlikely	Focal to widespread	Focal to widespread	Focal to widespread	Unlikely
Loss or damage of health care system	Focal to widespread	Focal to widespread	Focal to widespread	Focal	Focal to widespread	Focal to widespread	Focal	Focal to widespread
Worsening of chronic illnesses	Focal to widespread	Focal to widespread	Focal to widespread	Focal	Focal to widespread	Focal to widespread	Widespread	Focal to widespread
Loss of electrical power	Focal to widespread	Focal to widespread	Focal to widespread	Focal	Focal to widespread	Focal to widespread	Focal	Unlikely
Toxic exposures	Widespread for CO poisoning	Widespread for CO poisoning	Widespread for air, soil, and surface water	Focal	Widespread for CO poisoning	Widespread for CO poisoning	Focal	Widespread for air
Food scarcity	Focal	Focal	Focal	Focal	Common in low-lying coastal areas	Focal to widespread	Widespread in poor nations	Focal

Note: Darker shading denotes a more severe impact.

2002; Guill and Shandera, 2001; WHO, 1979; Toole, 1997). Geophysical disasters are almost never associated with epidemics of communicable disease (Floret and others, 2006; Guha-Sapir and van Panhuis, 2005). Meteorological disasters are only rarely associated with epidemics of communicable disease, mostly in low-income nations (Keim, 2008; WHO, 1979). Behavioral health effects are among the most debilitating long-term outcomes of environmental disasters (WHO, 1992; Ursano, Fullerton, and McCaughey,1994; Krug and others, 1998; Keenan and others, 2004; Sattler and others, 2002; Caldera and others, 2001; Goenjian and others, 2001).

All natural disaster hazards can markedly affect the ability of the population to maintain and access adequate shelter, water, sanitation, hygiene, health care, nutrition, security, and public services or utilities in order to maintain their health during a disaster event. These factors have a significant influence on morbidity following a disaster.

Technological Disasters

Technological disasters may occur as the result of fires, explosions (Hull, Grindlinger, and Hirsch, 1985), and releases or spills (Duclos and others, 1987; Binder, 1989). The event itself may be overt or insidious in its onset, and acute or chronic in duration (Lillibridge, 1997). The main cause of death is injury in the form of poisonings, burns, and blunt and penetrating trauma. Table 23.5 summarizes the relative public health impacts of various types of technological disasters.

Incidents involving either slow or explosive releases of chemicals are common and on the increase (Quarantelli and Gray, 1986; Bertazzi, 1989). Growing population densities in areas where chemicals are manufactured and transported have increased the numbers of persons potentially exposed (Sanderson, 1992). In many rapidly industrializing countries, less elaborate measures than developed countries use for the protection of the environment, human health, and safety have often led to disproportionate risk of technological disasters (Lillibridge, 1997; de Souza Porto and de Freitas, 1996; Brown, Himelberger, and White, 1993; Glickman, Golding, and Terry, 1993; Mehta and others, 1990). This phenomenon has been described as "sociopolitical amplification" and "exportation of risk" (de Souza Porto and de Freitas, 1996; also see Chapter Eleven).

Terrorism Disasters

U.S. policy on combating terrorism has been evolving over the past thirty years. During this time, at least six terror-related disasters have occurred in the United

TABLE 23.5 The Relative Public Health Impact of Technological Environmental Disasters (Related to Industry, Terrorism, or Conflict)

Public Health Impact	Toxicological		Thermal	Mechanical	
	Hazardous Material Release	Urban Fire	Explosions or bombings	Transport Crash	Structural Failure
Deaths	Moderate to many	Few to moderate	Moderate to many	Few to moderate	Moderate to many
Severe injuries	Moderate to many	Moderate to many	Moderate to many	Moderate to many	Moderate to many
Loss of clean water	Focal to widespread	Focal	Focal	Focal	Focal
Loss of shelter	Focal to widespread	Focal	Focal	Focal	Focal
Loss of personal and household goods	Focal to widespread	Focal	Focal	Focal	Focal
Major population movements	Focal to widespread	Focal	Focal	Focal	Focal
Loss of routine hygiene	Focal to widespread	Focal	Focal	Focal	Focal
Loss of sanitation	Focal to widespread	Focal	Focal	Focal	Focal
Disruption of solid waste management	Unlikely	Unlikely	Unlikely	Unlikely	Unlikely
Public concern for safety	High	High	High	High	High
Increased pests and vectors	Unlikely	Unlikely	Unlikely	Unlikely	Unlikely
Loss or damage of health care system	Focal	Focal	Focal	Focal	Focal
Worsening of existing chronic illnesses	Focal to widespread	Focal to widespread	Focal	Focal	Focal
Loss of electricity	Focal	Focal	Focal	Focal	Focal
Toxic exposures	Focal to widespread	Focal to widespread	Focal	Focal	Focal
Food scarcity	Focal	Unlikely	Unlikely	Unlikely	Unlikely

Note: Darker shading denotes a more severe impact.

States. These six disasters are estimated to have killed 3,179 and injured 8,163 (Keim, 2006b). Of the six, four involved conventional weapons (improvised explosive devices), and two involved unconventional weapons (biological warfare agents). Table 23.6 lists recent domestic U.S. terrorist events that have influenced U.S. policy (Keim, 2006b).

TABLE 23.6   Recent Terrorist Events that have Influenced U.S. Policy

Date	Event	Description
1984	Bhagwan Rajneesh salmonella release	Salmonella bacteria released in ten The Dalles, Oregon, restaurants. Outbreak linked to Bhagwan Rajneesh religious cult years later. None killed; over 800 infected.
1993	World Trade Center (WTC) bombing	Truck bomb detonated in the WTC parking garage. Linked to Middle East, including multiple Arab nationalities. Killed 6; wounded 1,042.
1995	Bombing of the Murrah Federal Building in Oklahoma City	Truck bomb detonated near the Alfred P. Murrah Federal Building in Oklahoma City, Oklahoma. Linked to U.S. right-wing extremists. Killed 169; injured more than 500.
1996	Bombing at Atlanta Olympic Games	Pipe bomb exploded in Centennial Olympic Park, Atlanta, Georgia, on the ninth day of the 1996 Summer Olympics. Killed 1; injured 112.
2001	World Trade Center and Pentagon attacks	Hijacked airliners deliberately flown into WTC towers and Pentagon. Linked to Middle East, Al Qaeda terrorist network. Killed over 2,998; injured 6,291.
2001	Anthrax letter attacks	Letters containing anthrax spores mailed to news media personnel and Congress. Caused first cases of intentional anthrax infection in the United States. Followed a 3-year history of over 1,500 anthrax letter hoaxes. Perpetrators remain at large. Killed 5; infected 18.

Source: Keim, 2006b.

Of the terrorism deaths in the United States during these three decades, 94 percent occurred in one day as a result of the 2001 attack on the World Trade Center in New York City. This event also had the single largest impact on U.S. policy (Keim, 2006b). These domestic events, together with other acts of terrorism overseas (for example, the 1995 sarin attacks carried out by Aum Shinrikyo members in Japan; the 1998 U.S. embassy bombings in Kenya and Tanzania; the 2000 attack on the U.S.S. *Cole* in Yemen; and the bombings in Bali in 2002, Madrid in 2004, and London in 2005) helped drive a significant change in U.S. policy. Exhibit 23.2 lists some of the major "lessons learned" that have influenced U.S. policy toward disaster risk management in recent times.

PRINCIPLES OF DISASTER RISK MANAGEMENT

Risk management is activity directed toward assessing, controlling and monitoring risks. Strategies for risk management include risk assessment and control measures; these in turn include transferring the risk to another party, avoiding

---

EXHIBIT 23.2
Lessons Learned from Terrorist Attacks That Have Influenced U.S. Policy

- Need for a comprehensive and coordinated disaster risk reduction strategy
- Need for comprehensive analytical risk assessment
- Need for improved coordination and information-sharing among
  - U.S. federal agencies
  - Civilian and military assets
  - Regional assets
- Need for improved occupational health and safety
- Importance of interoperability of communications
- Importance of mutual aid and assistance
- Importance of risk communication
- Importance of incident management systems
- Importance of a capabilities-based approach
- Need for awareness that public health and hospital preparedness remains variable throughout the United States

---

Source: Keim, 2006b.

the risk, reducing the negative effect of the risk, and accepting some or all of the consequences of a particular risk.

Disaster risk management

Disaster risk management applies the general principles of risk management to disasters. Figure 23.1 and Table 23.7 describe the components of disaster risk management, including both assessment and control. Disaster risk management is a comprehensive, **all-hazard approach** that entails developing and implementing strategies for each phase of the disaster. All disasters are said to follow a cyclical pattern, which is known as the *disaster life cycle* (Hogan and Burstein, 2007) and that has five stages: **prevention**, **mitigation**, **preparedness**, **response**, and **recovery** (Ciottone, 2006), phases that often overlap each other in time and in scope. Thus, the life cycle approach to risk management (King, 1988) must also be emphasized when it comes to management of disaster risk.

Figure 23.2 depicts the process of risk management as applied to the disaster cycle. It compares **risk avoidance** and reduction measures (on the upper left) to **risk retention** measures (on the lower right) (Keim, 2008). This depiction of disasters as cyclical may seem to imply that disasters are inevitable. This is not the case. The goals of risk avoidance and risk reduction are to avert disasters and to reduce the retained risk, thus breaking the disaster cycle. *The ultimate goal of disaster risk management is to break the disaster life cycle.*

Ideally, disaster risk management is based on a prioritization process. Once risks have been identified, they are assessed in terms of the potential severity of loss and the probability of occurrence. The risks with the greatest loss and the greatest probability of occurrence are handled first, and risks with lower losses and lower probabilities of occurrence are handled in descending order. In practice this process can be very difficult. One fundamental difficulty in disaster risk assessment is determining the probability of occurrence, because the needed statistical information is not available on many kinds of incidents. Furthermore, evaluating the severity of the consequences (impact) is often difficult; outcomes such as mental illness can defy quantification. Thus expert opinion and available statistics are the primary sources of information. Nevertheless, risk assessment can produce useful information that clarifies risks and supports decisions.

The criteria for measuring disaster consequence severity (impact) vary but usually address issues related to the following (British Columbia Ministry of Public Safety and Solicitor General, 2003):

- Number of fatalities and injuries
- Critical facilities and community lifelines

FIGURE 23.1 Schematic Overview of the Components and the
Process of Risk Management

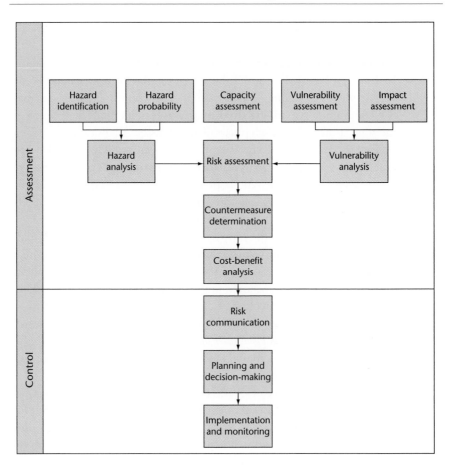

- Property and environmental damage
- Economic, social, and political disruption
- Size of the area or number of people affected

Once risks have been identified and assessed, techniques to manage the risk fall into one or more of these four major categories (Dorfman and others, 2007):

- Avoidance (eliminate)
- Reduction (mitigate)

TABLE 23.7　Key Components and Activities of Disaster Risk Management

Component	Activities
Hazard analysis 　Hazard identification 　Hazard probability	Identifying hazards with the potential to cause loss or damage of an asset Determining frequency of past hazard events
Impact assessment 　Asset assessment 　Loss assessment	Determining critical assets (that is, population, medical facilities, and so forth) Identifying expected loss or damage of each asset for each hazard Prioritizing assets based on consequence of loss
Capacity assessment	Identifying strengths, attributes, and resources available for responding to and recovering from a disaster
Vulnerability assessment 　Exposure 　Susceptibility	Estimating degree of vulnerability of each asset for each hazard Identifying preexisting countermeasures and their level of effectiveness
Countermeasure determination 　Avoidance or reduction 　Transfer or retention	Identifying new countermeasures that may be taken to eliminate or lessen hazards and vulnerabilities
Cost-benefit analysis	Identifying countermeasure costs and benefits Prioritizing options
Risk communication	Preparing a range of recommendations for decision makers and the public
Risk management plan	Developing a plan for disaster risk treatment for each phase of the emergency cycle
Implementation and monitoring	Implementing the risk management program and monitoring it, according to the plan

Source: Slightly modified from Keim, 2002.

- Transfer (outsource or insure)
- Retention (accept and add to budget)

Table 23.8 compares the four major categories of risk management techniques to the three stages of prevention, the five stages of the disaster life cycle, and the three major components of disaster risk management. It can be seen that these various stages are complementary and can be combined to create a unified

FIGURE 23.2   The Disaster Cycle and Corresponding Risk
Management Measures

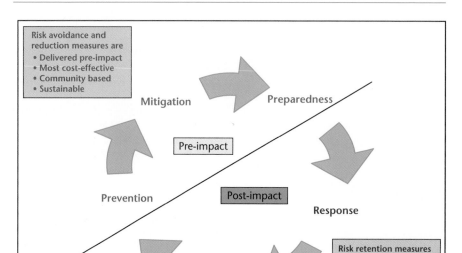

approach to the management of environmental health disaster risk (Dorfman and others, 2007; Lind, 1988).

Disaster Risk Avoidance

Even though people may not always have the ability to prevent disasters from occurring, the health sector can play an important role in preventing the public health impact. The risk of a public health disaster occurs when vulnerable populations are both exposed and susceptible to environmental hazards (Keim, 2008). Primary prevention seeks to prevent the disaster hazard exposure from ever occurring (see Chapter 26). This function is consistent with the category of risk treatment known as risk avoidance; examples include land use zoning and regulations that prevent settlement in disaster-prone areas (such as floodplains).

Disaster Risk Reduction

Risk reduction involves methods that reduce the severity of the loss or the likelihood of the loss. Risk reduction activities seek to prepare for and mitigate the

TABLE 23.8 Comparison of Various Techniques for Disaster Prevention, Emergency Management, and Risk Management

Stages of Prevention	Stages of Disaster Life Cycle Management	Categories of Risk Management Techniques	Components of Disaster Risk Management
Primary prevention	Prevention	Risk avoidance	Hazard avoidance
Secondary prevention	Mitigation		Vulnerability reduction
	Structural (exposure)	Risk reduction	
	Financial (susceptibility or resilience)	Risk transfer	
	Preparedness (susceptibility or resilience)	Risk reduction	
Tertiary prevention	Response		
	Recovery	Risk retention	Residual risk

health effects of disasters that cannot be prevented. Secondary prevention aims to detect the disaster hazard event early to control its advance and reduce the resulting health burden (see Chapter 26). **Disaster risk reduction** has emerged as a core element of **sustainable development** in the United States and abroad (NSTC, 1996).

Disaster Risk Transfer

Insurance contracts and *risk retention* pools are mechanisms for **risk transfer** (Dorfman and others, 2007). By purchasing an insurance contract, people are able to transfer and share risk across a large population. Risk retention pools are also used to share risk among a group. They are different from traditional insurance in that no premium is assessed in advance; instead, losses are assessed among all members of the group once they occur.

Disaster Risk Retention

Risk retention involves accepting the loss when it occurs and then attempting to respond and recover, if possible. All **residual risks** that are not avoided or transferred are retained by default. Tertiary prevention seeks to prevent additional risk once the adverse event has occurred. This stage of prevention aims to reduce morbidity, avoid complications, and restore function (see Chapter 26). Examples of risk retention activities are the provision of medical care and supplying of temporary shelter to disaster-affected populations, Risk retention thus corresponds well to the disaster cycle phases of response and recovery (Keim, 2008).

Disaster Risk Management Plan

A disaster risk management plan selects appropriate controls or countermeasures to manage each risk. An effective risk management plan should include a schedule for control implementation and should designate responsible persons for those actions. **Public awareness** of disaster risk and risk treatment options is necessary. **Risk communication** is therefore a key part of the disaster risk management plan.

PUBLIC HEALTH TOOLS FOR DISASTERS

Applying the principles of disaster risk management, public health takes steps across the spectrum of prevention, preparedness, response, and recovery.

Preventing the Public Health Impact of Disasters

Primary prevention seeks to prevent adverse events from occurring. Effective management of natural hazards has prevented the risk of numerous disasters caused by floods, cyclones, droughts, and wildfires. For example, floodplain management in areas of frequent flooding may actually prevent flood disasters altogether.

The primary prevention of environmental disaster risk relies heavily on hazard avoidance through **structural measures**. These measures include modification of the physical environment through architectural design, engineering controls, and construction methods and materials in order to prevent hazard exposure (Malilay, 1997; Floodplain Management Association, 2007). Structural measures for primary prevention are better developed for meteorological disasters than that for geophysical disasters. **Nonstructural measures** (for example, land use strategies, policies, and laws and public awareness raising, training, and education) may be the most effective means of preventing many geophysical disaster impacts.

Much of the approach to primary prevention of technological disasters is based on regulation of industrial and commercial practices, including the manufacture, storage, transport, and use of hazardous materials, as well as promotion of safe practices in the construction and transportation industries.

Mitigating the Public Health Impact of Disasters

Secondary prevention of environmental disaster risk includes mitigation measures. Mitigation serves to reduce population vulnerability by reducing population exposure, as well as susceptibility, to disaster hazards (Keim, 2008). Mitigation may include both structural measures and nonstructural measures (United Nations Disaster Relief Office, 1991). Disaster-related mitigation activities reduce deaths and injuries by ensuring structural safety through enforcing adequate building codes, promulgating legislation to relocate structures away from disaster-prone areas, engaging in **land use planning** and regulation, and managing high-hazard zones (Malilay, 1997). **Critical facilities** can be identified before disaster occurrence, and engineering measures may be taken to mitigate loss of critical health infrastructure and assets during extreme weather events.

Although disasters involve the destruction of lives and property, they also create something important: opportunities to improve safety, enhance equity, and rebuild in new or different ways through promotion of "healthy people, healthy homes and healthy communities" (Srinivasan, O'Fallon, and Dearry, 2003). Ideally, those opportunities will be used to produce safer communities with more equitable and sustainable livelihoods for people (Bolin and Stanford, 1998). Healthy homes are disaster resilient and are designed and built to stay safe during extreme weather events. Healthy communities minimize exposure of people and property to natural disasters; sustainable communities are disaster-resilient communities (Beatley, 1998).

Preparing for Disasters

The secondary prevention of environmental disaster risk includes preparedness measures. Preparedness implies a behavioral approach focused on actions taken in advance of a disaster in order to reduce its impact. This reduces population vulnerability. Public health preparedness activities should be based on developing and maintaining a core readiness among the thirty-two public health response capabilities identified by Keim (2006a) as needed to address the fifteen most common public health impacts of disasters (also see Table 23.3). The eleven E's of public health preparedness (Exhibit 23.3) offer an easy way to recall those capabilities commonly involved in public health preparedness.

According to FEMA (1996), "The centerpiece of comprehensive emergency management is the emergency operations plan." Emergency operations plans describe "who will do what, as well as when, and with what resources, and by what authority—before, during and immediately after an emergency" (FEMA 1996). FEMA's National Response Framework (NRF) presents the guiding principles

EXHIBIT 23.3

The 11 E's of Public Health Preparedness

- Evaluation and monitoring of hazard
- Early warning
- Evacuation
- Emergency operations planning
- Education and training
- Exercises and drills
- Engagement of the public
- Electronic media and communication
- Epidemiology
- Equipment and supplies
- Economic and political incentive

designed to enable all levels of domestic response partners to prepare for and provide a unified national response to disasters and emergencies (FEMA, 2008b). Public health has a well-defined role under Emergency Support Function #8 (ESF-8) of the NRF, which addresses all public health and medical issues (FEMA, 2003).

Responding to the Public Health Impact of Disasters

Tertiary prevention of environmental disaster risk involves measures taken during the response and recovery phase as a component of risk retention. Disaster response is predominantly focused on immediate and short-term needs and is sometimes called *disaster relief*. Response usually includes those actions immediately necessary to remove the affected population from ongoing exposure or risk of harm. Public health disaster response capabilities are applied during the disaster response (see Table 23.3).

The Incident Command System (ICS) is a standardized, on-scene, all-hazard incident management concept in the United States. It is a management protocol based upon a flexible, scalable response organization providing a common framework within which people can work together effectively. The National Incident Management System (NIMS) is a form of incident command system used in the United States in order to provide a systematic proactive approach to guide departments and agencies at all levels of government, nongovernmental organizations, and the private sector to work seamlessly work together before, during and after emergencies (FEMA, 2008a). Building on the existing National Incident Management

System (NIMS) the NRF's coordinating structures are always in effect for implementation at any level and at any time for local, state, and national emergency or disaster response (FEMA, 2008a, 2008b).

Immediately after the disaster impact, rapid needs assessments are first conducted in order to determine any gap between the health and medical needs of an affected community and the resources that are available. Although communicable disease outbreaks are rare after natural disasters in the United States, some potential does exist for disease transmission; therefore affected communities are placed under an active disease surveillance system (CDC, 1983).

Public health is often involved in temporary sheltering and settlement decisions that concern the rapid reinstatement of healthy homes and healthy communities and that have a direct impact on the public health of disaster-affected populations. Public health assists in delivery of health care, inspection of food safety and water quality, and assessment of sanitation and hygiene in mass care shelters. The demands for environmental health services and consultation are high during natural disasters (CDC, 1993). Public health also becomes involved in health risk assessments and technical assistance related to any suspected hazardous material exposures after an environmental disaster (Euripidou and Murray, 2004).

Health communication is a valuable tool in educating the public before and after disaster impact (conveying protective behaviors to prevent drowning or heat illness, for example). Injuries such as electrocutions, burns, and carbon monoxide poisonings are examples of disaster-related morbidity that can be prevented through public awareness and health education.

Recovering from the Public Health Impact of Disasters

Rehabilitation and reconstruction begin soon after the emergency phase has ended and should be based on preexisting strategies and policies that facilitate clear institutional responsibilities for recovery actions and enable public participation. The division between the response stage and the subsequent recovery stage is not clear-cut. Some response actions, such as the supply of temporary housing and water supplies, may extend well into the recovery stage.

Recovery programs, coupled with the heightened public awareness after a disaster, also afford a valuable opportunity to develop and implement disaster risk reduction measures and to apply the "build back better" principle (UN/ISDR, 2009).

Full recovery from the public health impact of environmental disasters may take years to achieve. Additional financial, health, and emotional costs may continue long after basic utilities and shelters have been reinstated (Cohen, 1991).

The disaster recovery phase may also offer a window of opportunity for improving risk reduction strategies, such as preparedness and mitigation efforts.

SUMMARY

The frequency of environmental disasters is increasing worldwide. The public health impacts of environmental disasters include death, injuries, and diminished ability to maintain adequate shelter, water, sanitation, hygiene, public services, and utilities. A primary focus on response and recovery is an impractical and inefficient strategy for dealing with disaster threats. Disaster risk management is a comprehensive, all-hazard approach that entails developing and implementing strategies for all the phases of the disaster life cycle—prevention, mitigation, preparedness, response, and recovery—in the context of sustainable development. Disaster risk management begins with a risk assessment that evaluates hazard frequency and impact as well as the vulnerability of the population and its absorptive capacity to respond to the disaster. This risk assessment is then communicated to stakeholders and a plan is developed for hazard avoidance (prevention); risk reduction (mitigation and preparedness), and risk retention (response and recovery). Disaster risk management then applies a capability-based approach to treat residual risk not otherwise avoided or transferred.

KEY TERMS

absorptive capacity

all-hazard approach

capability-based approach

capacity

critical facilities

disaster

disaster risk

disaster risk management

disaster risk reduction

early warning system

emergency preparedness

emergency services

environmental disasters

exposure

forecast

hazard

land-use planning

mitigation

natural disasters

natural hazard

nonstructural measures

preparedness

prevention

public awareness

recovery

residual risk

resilience

response

risk assessment

risk avoidance

risk communication

risk management

risk reduction

risk retention

risk transfer

susceptibility

structural measures

sustainable development

technological disasters

technological hazard

vulnerability

DISCUSSION QUESTIONS

1. What are three major natural and technological hazards that currently place your community at risk for disaster?
2. Who are the people and facilities in your community most vulnerable to these disasters?
3. What risk reduction measures would you recommend in order to reduce the risk of the top three disasters in your community? (Include at least one measure each for prevention, mitigation, and preparedness.) Discuss the reasons for your recommendations.
4. Please discuss this statement: *An all-hazards approach is preferable to hazard-by-hazard preparedness.*
5. Please discuss this statement: *A disaster life cycle analysis is essential to effective management of public health consequences of disasters.*

REFERENCES

Bailey, G., and Walker, J. "Heat Related Disasters." In D. E. Hogan and J. L. Burstein (eds.), *Disaster Medicine.* (2nd ed.) Philadelphia: Lippincott Williams & Wilkins, 2007.

BBC News. "Burma Death Toll Jumps to 78,000." http://news.bbc.co.uk/2/hi/asia-pacific/7405260.stm, 2008.

Beatley, T. "The Vision of Sustainable Communities." In R. Burby (ed.), *Cooperating with Nature* (pp. 233–262). Washington, D.C.: National Academies Press, 1998.

Bertazzi, P. "Industrial Disasters and Epidemiology." *Scandinavian Journal of Work, Environment & Health,* 1989, *15*, 85–100.

Binder, S. "Deaths, Injuries and Evacuations from Acute Hazardous Materials Releases." *American Journal of Public Health,* 1989, *79*, 1042–1044.

Bolin, R. and Stanford, L. *The Northridge Earthquake: Vulnerability and Disaster.* London: Routledge, 1998.

British Columbia Ministry of Public Safety and Solicitor General. *Hazard, Risk and Vulnerability Analysis Toolkit.* Victoria, B.C.: National Library of Canada, 2003.

Brouewer, R., and others. "Socioeconomic Vulnerability and Adaptation to Environmental Risk: A Case Study of Climate Change and Flooding in Bangladesh." *Risk Analysis,* 2007, *27*(2), 313–326.

Brown, H., Himelberger, J., and White, A. "Development of Environment Interactions in the Export of Hazardous Technologies." *Technological, Forecasting and Social Change,* 1993, *43*, 125–155.

Burkle, F. M. "Globalization and Disasters: Issues of Public Health, State Capacity and Political Action." *Journal of International Affairs,* 2006, *59*(2), 241–265.

Caldera, T., and others. "Psychological Impact of the Hurricane Mitch in Nicaragua in a One-Year Perspective." *Social Psychiatry and Psychiatric Epidemiology,* 2001, *36*, 108–114.

Centers for Disease Control and Prevention. "Outbreak of Diarrheal Illness Associated with a Natural Disaster—Utah." *Morbidity and Mortality Weekly Report,* 1983, *32*, 662–664.

Centers for Disease Control and Prevention. "Morbidity Surveillance Following the Midwest Flood—Missouri, 1993."*Morbidity and Mortality Weekly Report*, 1993, *42*, 797–798.

Centers for Disease Control and Prevention. "Needs Assessment Following Hurricane Georges—Dominican Republic."*Morbidity and Mortality Weekly Report*, 1998, *48*, 93–95.

Centers for Disease Control and Prevention. "Tropical Storm Allison Rapid Needs Assessment: Houston, Texas, June 2001."*Morbidity and Mortality Weekly Report*, 2002, *51*, 365–369.

Centre for Research on the Epidemiology of Disasters. *EM-DAT: The International Disaster Database.* Université Catholique de Louvain, Ecole de Santé Publique. http://www.emdat.be, 2005.

Chowdhury, M., and others. "Cyclone Aftermath: Research and Directions for the Future." In H.Hossain, C. P. Dodge, and F. H. Abed (eds.), *From Crisis to Development: Coping with Disasters in Bangladesh* (pp. 101–133). Dhaka: University Press, 1992.

Ciottone, G. "Introduction to Disaster Medicine." In G. Ciottone (ed.), *Disaster Medicine*. Philadelphia: Mosby-Elsevier, 2006.

Clack, Z., Keim, M., MacIntyre, A., and Yeskey, K. "Emergency Health and Risk Management in Sub-Saharan Africa: A Lesson from the Embassy Bombings in Tanzania and Kenya."*Prehospital and Disaster Medicine*, 2002, *17*(2), 59–66.

Cohen, D. *Aftershock: The Psychological and Political Consequences of Disaster.* London: Paladin, 1991.

de Souza Porto, M. F., and de Freitas, C. M. "Major Chemical Accidents and Industrializing Countries: The Socio-Political Amplification of Risk."*Risk Analysis*, 1996, *16*(1), 19–29.

de Ville de Goyet, C., and Lechat, M. "Health Aspects in Natural Disasters."*Tropical Doctor*, 1976, *6*, 152–157.

Diacon, D. "Typhoon Resistant Housing in the Philippines: The Core Shelter Project."*Disasters*, 1992, *16*, 266–271.

Dorfman, M. S. *Introduction to Risk Management and Insurance.* (9th ed.) Englewood Cliffs, N.J.: Prentice Hall, 2007.

Duclos, P., and others. "Community Evacuation Following a Chlorine Release, Mississippi."*Disasters*, 1987, *11*(4), 286–289.

Euripidou, E., and Murray, V. "Public Health Impacts of Floods and Chemical Contamination." *Journal of Public Health*, 2004, *26*(4), 376–383.

Federal Emergency Management Agency. *SLG 101: Guide for All-Hazard Emergency Operations Planning.* http://www.fema.gov/plan/gaheop.shtm, 1996.

Federal Emergency Management Agency. *Emergency Support Function #8: Health and Medical Services Annex.* http://www.au.af.mil/au/awc/awcgate/frp/frpesf8.htm, Jan. 2003.

Federal Emergency Management Agency. *National Incident Management System.* http://www.fema.gov/pdf/emergency/nims/NIMS_core.pdf, 2008a.

Federal Emergency Management Agency. *National Response Framework.* http://www.fema.gov/pdf/emergency/nrf/nrf-core.pdf, 2008b.

Floodplain Management Association. *Overview of Floodplain Management.* http://www.floodplain.org/overview_of_floods.htm, 2007.

Floret, N., and others. "Negligible Risk for Epidemics After Geophysical Disasters."*Emerging Infectious Diseases*, 2006, *12*(4), 543–548.

Frumkin, H., and others. "Climate Change: The Public Health Response."*American Journal of Public Health*, 2008, *98*, 435–445.

Glickman, T., Golding, D., and Terry, K. *Fatal Hazardous Materials Accidents in Industry: Domestic and Foreign Experience from 1945 to 1991*. Washington, D.C.: Center for Risk Management, 1993.

Goenjian, A. K., and others. "Posttraumatic Stress and Depressive Reactions Among Nicaraguan Adolescents After Hurricane Mitch."*American Journal of Psychiatry*, 2001, *158*, 788–794.

Guha-Sapir, D., and van Panhuis, W. *The Andaman Nicobar Earthquake and Tsunami 2004: Impact on Diseases in Indonesia*. Brussels: Centre for Research on the Epidemiology of Disasters, 2005.

Guill, C. K., and Shandera, W. X. "The Effects of Hurricane Mitch on a Community in Northern Honduras."*Prehospital and Disaster Medicine*, 2001, *16*, 124–129.

Henry, R. "Defense Transformation and the 2005 Quadrennial Defense Review."*Parameters*, Winter 2005–2006, pp. 5–15.

Hogan, D., and Burstein, J. "Basic Physics of Disasters." In D. Hogan and J. Burstein (eds.), *Disaster Medicine*. Philadelphia: Lippincott Williams & Wilkins, 2007.

Hull, D., Grindlinger, G., and Hirsch, E. "The Clinical Consequences of an Industrial Plant Explosion." *Journal of Trauma*, 1985, *25*(4),303–307.

International Federation of Red Cross and Red Crescent Societies. "Disaster Data." In *World Disaster Report 2007* (pp. 172–181). http://www.ifrc.org/Docs/pubs/disasters/wdr2007/WDR2007-English.pdf, 2007.

Keenan, H. T., and others. "Increased Incidence of Inflicted Traumatic Brain Injury in Children After a Natural Disaster."*American Journal of Preventive Medicine*, 2004, *26*, 189–193.

Keim, M. "Intentional Chemical Disasters." In D. Hogan and J. Burstein (eds.), *Disaster Medicine* (pp. 340–348). Philadelphia: Lippincott Williams & Wilkins, 2002.

Keim, M. "Disaster Preparedness." In G. Ciottone (ed.), *Disaster Medicine*. Philadelphia: Mosby-Elsevier, 2006a.

Keim, M. "Lessons Learned as a Result of Terrorist Attacks." In G. Ciottone (ed.), *Disaster Medicine*. Philadelphia: Mosby-Elsevier, 2006b.

Keim, M. "Building Human Resilience: The Role of Public Health Preparedness and Response as an Adaptation to Climate Change."*American Journal of Preventive Medicine*, 2008, *35*(5), 508–516.

King, F. "The Role of Risk Assessment in Life-Cycle Risk Management." In G. Lafond (ed.), *Risk Assessment and Management: Emergency Planning Perspective*. Waterloo, Canada: University of Waterloo Press, 1988.

Krug, E. G., and others. "Suicide After Natural Disasters."*New England Journal of Medicine*, 1998, *338*, 373–378.

Lillibridge, S. "Industrial Disasters." In E. K. Noji (ed.), *The Public Health Consequences of Disasters* (pp. 354–372). New York: Oxford University Press, 1997.

Lind, N. "Risk Analysis for Risk Management." In G. Lafond (ed.), *Risk Assessment and Management: Emergency Planning Perspectives*. Waterloo, Canada: University of Waterloo Press, 1988.

Lutgendorf, S., and others. "Physical Symptoms of Chronic Fatigue Syndrome Are Exacerbated by the Stress of Hurricane Andrew."*Psychosomatic Medicine*, 1995, *57*, 310–323.

Malilay, J. "Floods." In E. K. Noji (ed.), *The Public Health Consequences of Disasters* (pp. 287–300). New York: Oxford University Press, 1997.

Mehta, P. S., and others. "Bhopal Tragedy's Health Effects." *JAMA*, 1990, *264*, 2781–2787.

Munich Re Group. *Annual Review: Natural Catastrophes 2002*. http://www.munichre.com/publications/302–03631_en.pdf, 2002.

National Science and Technology Council, Committee on the Environment and Natural Resources, Subcommittee on Natural Disaster Reduction. *Natural Disaster Reduction: A Plan for the Nation.* Washington, D.C.: U.S. Government Printing Office, 1996.

Nelson, D. "Mitigating Disasters: Power to the Community."*International Nursing Review*, 1990, *37*(6), 371.

Noji, E. K. "The Nature of isaster: General Characteristics and Public Health Effects." In E. K.Noji (ed.), *The Public Health Consequences of Disasters* (pp. 3–20). New York: Oxford University Press, 1997.

Quarantelli, E., and Gray, J. "Research Findings on Community and Organizational Preparations for and Responses to Acute Chemical Emergencies."*Public Management*, 1986, *68*, 11–13.

Relief Web. "More Than 4.8 Million Homeless in Sichuan Quake." Agence France-Presse. http://www.reliefweb.int/rw/RWB.NSF/db900SID/PANA-7EPG6V?OpenDocument, 2008.

Sanderson, L. "Toxicologic Disasters: Natural and Technologic." In J. Sullivan and G. Krieger (eds.), *Hazardous Materials Toxicology: Clinical Principles of Environmental Health.* Philadelphia: Lippincott Williams & Wilkins, 1992.

Sanderson, L. "Fires." In E. K. Noji (ed.), *The Public Health Consequences of Disasters* (pp. 373–396). New York: Oxford University Press, 1997.

Sattler, D. N., and others. "Hurricane Georges: A Cross-National Study Examining Preparedness, Resource Loss, and Psychological Distress in the U.S. Virgin Islands, Puerto Rico, Dominican Republic, and the United States." *Journal of Traumatic Stress*, 2002, *15*, 339–350.

Srinivasan, S., O'Fallon, L. R., and Dearry, A. "Creating Healthy Communities, Healthy Homes, Healthy People: Initiating a Research Agenda on the Built Environment and Public Health."*American Journal of Public Health*, 2003, *93*(9), 1446–50.

Thomalla, F. "Reducing Hazard Vulnerability: Towards a Common Approach Between Disaster Risk Reduction and Climate Adaptation," *Disasters*, 2006, *30*(1), 39–48.

Toole, M. J. "Communicable Disease and Disease Control." In E. K. Noji (ed.), *The Public Health Consequences of Disasters* (pp. 79–100). New York: Oxford University Press, 1997.

United Nations Disaster Relief Office. *Mitigating Natural Disasters: Phenomena, Effects and Options.* New York: United Nations, 1991.

United Nations International Strategy for Disaster Reduction. *Terminology: Basic Terms of Disaster Risk Reduction.*http://www.unisdr.org/eng/library/lib-terminology-eng-p.htm, 2004.

United Nations International Strategy for Disaster Reduction. *Terminology on Disaster Risk Reduction.* http://www.unisdr.org/eng/terminology/UNISDR-terminology-2009-eng.pdf, 2009.

Ursano, R. J., Fullerton, C. S., and McCaughey, B. G. "Trauma and Disaster." In R. J.Ursano, B. G.McCaughey, and C. S.Fullerton (eds.), *Individual and Community Responses to Trauma and Disaster: The Structure of Human Chaos* (pp. 3–27). New York: Cambridge University Press, 1994.

Wilhite, D. A. *Drought Mitigation Technologies in the United States: With Future Policy Recommendations.* Technical Report Series 93–1. Lincoln, Neb.: International Drought Information Center, 1993.

World Health Organization. "The Risk of Disease Outbreaks After Natural Disasters."*WHO Chronicle*, 1979, *33*, 214–216.

World Health Organization. *Psychosocial Consequences of Disasters:* Prevention and Management. Report No. WHO/MNH/PSF/91.3. Geneva: World Health Organization, 1992.

World Health Organization. *Health Sector Emergency Preparedness Guide.* Geneva: World Health Organization, 1998.

FOR FURTHER INFORMATION

Books, Reports, and Other Documents

Ciottone, G. R., (ed.). *Disaster Medicine.* Philadelphia, Mosby-Elsevier, 2006. This book is both a comprehensive text and a quick resource. Part 1 introduces the many topics of disaster medicine and management with an emphasis on the multiple disciplines. Part 2 introduces the reader to every conceivable disaster scenario and its management issues.

Hyogo Framework for Action 2005–2015: Building the Resilience of Nations and Communities to Disasters. http://www.unisdr.org/eng/hfa/docs/Hyogo-framework-for-action-english.pdf, n.d. The Hyogo Framework for Action (HFA), the product of the United Nations World Conference on Disaster Reduction, held in 2005, is a key instrument for implementing disaster reduction and has been adopted by the member states of the United Nations. Its overarching goal is to build the resilience of nations and communities to disasters by achieving substantial reduction of disaster losses by 2015.

Landesman, L. *Public Health Management of Disasters: The Practice Guide.* Washington, D.C.: American Public Health Association, 2005. Among the useful features of this book is the recognition of the public health component of disasters—a neglected area. Frequently, emergency response focuses on environmental degradation or terrorism concerns but not on the basic health concerns of each disaster, which are at least as likely to pose challenges. In support of this idea, the author delineates various types of disasters and the public health implications of each.

National Science and Technology Council. *Grand Challenges for Disaster Reduction.* http://www.nehrp.gov/pdf/grandchallenges.pdf, 2005. In this document, the Subcommittee on Disaster Reduction, an element of the President's National Science and Technology Council, describes a ten-year strategy for meeting six grand challenges of disaster reduction and provides a framework for prioritizing the federal investments in science and technology.

Noji, E. K. (ed.). *The Public Health Consequences of Disasters.* New York, Oxford University Press, 1997. Illustrated with examples from recent research in the field, this collection of chapters summarizing the most pertinent and useful information about the public health impact of disasters is divided into four sections dealing with general issues, geophysical events, weather-related problems, and human generated disasters.

United Nations Development Programme. *Reducing Disaster Risk: A Challenge for Development.* http://www.undp.org/cpr/disred/documents/publications/rdr/english/rdr_english.pdf, 2004. Mapping out an agenda for change in the way disaster risk is perceived within the development community, this report presents a range of opportunities for moving development pathways toward meeting the UN Millennium Development Goals by integrating disaster risk reduction into development planning.

Yokohama Strategy and Plan of Action for a Safer World: Guidelines for Natural Disaster Prevention, Preparedness and Mitigation. http://www.unisdr.org/eng/about_isdr/bd-yokohama-strat-eng.htm, n.d. A product of the United Nations 1994 World Conference on Natural Disaster Reduction, this document provides guidelines for natural disaster prevention, preparedness, and mitigation. It describes the principles on which a disaster reduction strategy should be based, outlines the plan of action agreed upon by member states of the United Nations, and gives some guidelines on action follow-up.

Guidebooks

Following is a listing of guidebooks commonly used for response to environmental disasters. Also see the discussion in this chapter of FEMA's National Incident Management System (http://www.fema.gov/pdf/emergency/nims/NIMS_core.pdf) and National Response Framework (http://www.fema.gov/pdf/emergency/nrf/nrf-core.pdf), two national management and response systems intended to coordinate all levels of disaster response and recovery.

Centers for Disease Control and Prevention. *Public Health Emergency Response Guide for State, Local, and Tribal Public Health Directors.* http://www.bt.cdc.gov/planning/responseguide.asp, 2004.

Pan American Health Organization. *WHO/PAHO Guidelines for the Use of Foreign Field Hospitals in the Aftermath of Sudden-Impact Disasters.* San Salvador: Pan American Health Organization, 2003.

Protein-Calorie Advisory Group of the United Nations System. *A Guide to Food and Health Relief Operations for Disasters.* New York: United Nations, 1977.

The Sphere Project. *Humanitarian Charter and Minimum Standards in Disaster Response.* http://www.sphere-project.org, 2004.

United Nations High Commissioner for Refugees. *Handbook for Emergencies.* (2nd ed.) Geneva: United Nations High Commissioner for Refugees, June, 2000. United Nations Children's Fund. *Emergency Field Handbook: A Guide for UNICEF Staff.* New York: United Nations Children's Fund, 2005.

U.S. Agency for International Development. *Field Operations Guide for Disaster Assessment and Response, Version 3.0.* http://www.usaid.gov/our_work/humanitarian_assistance/disaster_assistance/resources/pdf/fog_v3.pdf, n.d.

World Health Organization. *Emergency Response Manual: Guidelines for WHO Representatives in Country Offices in the Western Pacific Region.* Manila: World Health Organization, 2003.

World Health Organization. *Handbook For Emergency Field Operations.* EHA/Field/99.1. n.p.: World Health Organization.

Agencies and Organizations

American Medical Association (AMA), Center for Public Health Preparedness and Disaster Response (CPHPDR), http://www.ama-assn.org/ama/pub/physician-resources/public-health/center-public-health-preparedness-disaster-response.shtml. CPHPDR is a national educational resource for enhancing the disaster preparedness and response capabilities of both civilian and military providers.

Centers for Disease Control and Prevention (CDC), Centers for Public Health Preparedness (CPHP), http://www.bt.cdc.gov/cotper/cphp/background.asp. Initiated in 2000 to strengthen terrorism and emergency preparedness by linking academic expertise to state and local health agency needs, the CPHP program brings together community colleges, colleges, and universities with a common focus on public health preparedness to establish a national network of education and training resources.

National Voluntary Organizations Active in Disaster (National VOAD), http://www.nvoad.org/ Default.aspx. As coalition of coalition of nonprofit organizations that respond to disasters as part of their overall mission, National VOAD) is also a forum where organizations can share knowledge and resources throughout the disaster cycle—preparation, response, and recovery—to help disaster survivors and their communities.

United Nations: International Strategy for Disaster Reduction (UN/ISDR), http://www.unisdr. org/eng/about_isdr/isdr-mission-objectives-eng.htm. UN/ISDR aims at building disaster-resilient communities by promoting increased awareness of the importance of disaster reduction as an integral component of sustainable development, with the goal of reducing human, social, economic, and environmental losses due to natural hazards and related technological and environmental disasters.

CHAPTER TWENTY-FOUR

NATURE CONTACT

HOWARD FRUMKIN

KEY CONCEPTS

- The theory of biophilia suggests that people may have an innate affinity for living things. This theory has been expanded to suggest that people have a broad affinity to nature.

- Contact with nature may offer a range of health benefits. Several mechanisms have been suggested that may explain these benefits.

- Evidence is available for the health benefits of nature contact in at least four domains: animal contact, plant contact, viewing nature, and entering wilderness.

- There are many potential opportunities to advance public health through nature contact.

MUCH of this book is about hazards. We learn that contaminated food can cause diarrheal diseases (Chapter Eighteen), that air pollution can cause respiratory disease (Chapter Twelve), that poorly designed road-ways can result in injuries (Chapters Fourteen and Twenty-Two), that degraded urban environments may encourage violence (Chapter Fourteen). Clearly, environmental exposures can threaten health—and this is a central focus of the environmental health field.

But the environment, broadly conceived, may also enhance health. One example is the many pharmaceuticals that derive from plants and animals, a compelling argument for preserving biodiversity (Wilson, 1992; Daily, 1997; Cassis, 1998; Chivian and Bernstein, 2008). Another example is even more intuitive: contact with the natural world may directly benefit health. If so, then the field of environmental health needs to extend beyond controlling toxicity in order to consider health-promoting environments. This chapter reviews the evidence for health benefits linked with the natural environment.

THE LINKS BETWEEN HEALTH AND ENVIRONMENT

Many people appreciate a walk in the park or the sound of a bird's song or the sight of ocean waves lapping at the seashore. Even if these were only aesthetic preferences they would deserve attention because they are so common as to seem nearly universal. In the words of University of Michigan psychologist Rachel Kaplan (1983): "Nature matters to people. Big trees and small trees, glistening water, chirping birds, budding bushes, colorful flowers—these are important ingredients in a good life" (p. 155). But perhaps these are more than aesthetic preferences. Perhaps we as a species find tranquility in certain natural environments—a sense of comfort, restoration, even healing. If so, contact with nature might be an important component of our well-being.

From an evolutionary perspective, a deep-seated connection with the natural world would be no surprise. Primate evolution began at least 65 million years ago, and the first hominids appeared as much as 5 million years ago. Two million years ago australopithecines were fashioning primitive stone tools and hunting in bands on the grassy savannas of Africa. *Homo habilis* probably appeared 2 or 3 million years ago, and our immediate predecessor, *Homo erectus*, appeared about 1.5 million years ago. Human history as we now know it began during the Neolithic period, just 10,000 or 15,000 years ago, when the last great ice age

Howard Frumkin declares no competing financial interests.

ended and climate and ecology came to resemble those of our current world. Our ancestors—true *Homo sapiens*—began to form settlements, cultivate crops, domesticate animals, dig mines, and even make art. If the last 2 million years of our species' history were scaled to a single human lifetime of seventy years, then the first humans would not have begun settling into villages until eight months after their sixty-ninth birthday. Some people—aboriginal groups in Australia, South America, the Pacific Islands, and elsewhere—would remain hunter-gatherers until a day or two before their seventieth birthday. We have broken with long-established patterns of living rather late in our life as a species.

For the great majority of human existence, human lives have been embedded in the natural environment. Those who could navigate it well—who could smell the water, find the plants, follow the animals, recognize the safe haven—must have enjoyed survival advantages. According to biologist E. O. Wilson (1993), "It would . . . be quite extraordinary to find that all learning rules related to that world have been erased in a few thousand years, even in the tiny minority of peoples who have existed for more than one or two generations in wholly urban environments" (p. 32). In a 1984 book, Wilson hypothesized the existence of **biophilia**, "the innately emotional affiliation of human beings to other living organisms" (Wilson, 1984, p. 31). Building on this theory, others have postulated an affinity for nature that goes beyond living things to include streams, ocean waves, and wind (Heerwagen and Orians, 1993).

The human connection to nature and the idea that this connection might be a component of good health have a long history in philosophy, art, and popular culture (see, for example, Nash, 1982; McLuhan, 1994). The New England transcendentalists, almost two centuries ago, argued that the human spirit was rooted in nature, and a leading exponent, Henry David Thoreau, wrote of the "tonic of wildness." A century later the conservationist John Muir (Figure 24.1) observed, "Thousands of tired, nerve-shaken, over-civilized people are beginning to find out that going to the mountains is going home; that wilderness is a necessity; and that mountain parks and reservations are useful not only as fountains of timber and irrigating rivers, but as fountains of life" (Fox, 1981, p. 116).

But the history of human culture has also in many ways been the history of separation from nature. David Abram (1996) argues that this separation began with the very development of language, which replaced nature images with abstract symbols as central elements of human cognition and communication. Although our ancestors lived in close proximity to nature, their struggle to survive was in many ways a struggle to vanquish nature, or at least to shape it to their ends and to control its most drastic exigencies. The book of Genesis, which dates from about 3,000 years ago, included the often-repeated divine mandate, "Be fertile and multiply. Fill the land and conquer it. Dominate the fish of the sea, the

FIGURE 24.1   John Muir

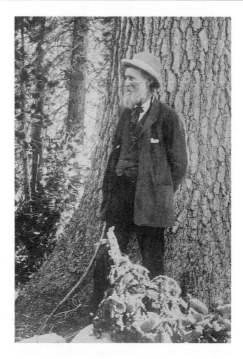

Source: Undated, unattributed, public domain photo, http://commons.wikimedia.org/wiki/
Image:John_Muir.jpg.

John Muir (1838–1914) was a naturalist and conservationist whose writings had a profound
influence on American attitudes toward nature.

birds of the sky, and every beast that walks the land." (Contemporary thinkers
have imputed a gentler meaning to this passage, emphasizing stewardship rather
than conquest.) The ancient Greeks abstracted human learning from nature. In
the Platonic dialogue *Phaedrus*, Socrates finds himself outside the city walls, and
grumbles to his companion, "I'm a lover of learning, and trees and open country
won't teach me anything, whereas men in town do" (Hamilton and Cairns, 1961,
p. 479). For Socrates, wisdom and comfort were to be found in human society,
apart from, and above, the world of nature. And subsequent developments have
led most people, at least in developed nations, to live lives that are effectively
insulated from the natural world. In the words of historian Roderick Nash (1982),
"For thousands of years after our race opted for a civilized existence, we dreamed
of and labored toward an escape from the anxieties of a wilderness condition only

to find, when we reached the promised land of supermarkets and air conditioners, that we had forfeited something of great value" (p. 267).

Through what mechanisms might nature contact benefit health? Environmental psychology offers some possible answers to this question. Kaplan and Kaplan (1982) emphasized the importance of *directed attention*, the ability to focus and block competing stimuli during purposeful activity. They proposed that people can develop *attentional fatigue* from excessive concentration, resulting in memory loss, diminished ability to focus, and greater impatience and frustration in interpersonal interactions. Moreover, they suggested that contact with nature could be restorative by renewing attention and improving cognitive abilities—a construct known as **attention restoration** (Kaplan, 1995). They noted four aspects of restorative environments: *fascination* (effortless interest or curiosity), a sense of *being away* from one's usual setting, *extent or scope* (being part of a larger whole), and *compatibility* with one's preferences (Kaplan and Kaplan, 1989).

Research has supported the link between nature contact and attention restoration. For example, one study (Tennessen and Cimprich, 1995) showed that college students with more natural views from their dormitory windows had higher levels of attention and cognitive function than those without. A study of apartment dwellers (Kaplan, 2001) showed that those with nature views from their windows scored higher on measures of effective functioning (including "focused," "effective," and "attentive") and lower on measures of distraction (including "forgetful," "disorganized," and "difficult to finish things you have started"). Among the components of nature views, landscaping and gardens were most important in predicting effective functioning, and trees, farms, and fields were most important in predicting less distraction. Studies of people taking different types of vacations (wilderness backpacking or urban) or no vacation and studies of people taking different walks (in a natural setting or in a city) or no walk found that proofreading performance, a measure of attention, was highest in the groups with nature contact (Hartig, Mang, and Evans, 1991). A study of children who had moved from substandard housing found that those who moved to "greener" homes (with more views of nearby nature) had higher levels of cognitive functioning (Wells, 2000), and a study of girls in a low-income housing project found that those with nature views had greater self-discipline (Faber Taylor, Kuo, and Sullivan, 2002). A study of children with attention deficit/hyperactivity disorder (Kuo and Taylor, 2004), using parents' ratings of their children's symptoms, found that playing in relatively green, or natural, settings reduced ADHD symptoms substantially more than playing in built outdoor and indoor settings. Nature contact may help, at least in part, through attention restoration.

Nature contact may also help by stress reduction. This is an intuitive notion; many people choose vacations in beautiful natural locations, probably expecting their stress to diminish. Again, research supports this notion. For example, Ulrich and others (1991) exposed undergraduate students to a stressful film, followed by a variety of videotapes of natural and urban settings. The students' stress recovery, as measured by self-report and measures of cardiovascular variables, was significantly faster when they viewed the nature scenes. In another study (Parsons and others, 1998), students viewed a stressful film (showing workplace injuries), followed by a video of a roadside scene (a forest, a golf course, a mixed development, or a commercial urban setting), followed by a second stressor (solving mathematical problems under time pressure). As measured by several (but not all) stress-related outcomes, such as blood pressure and skin conductance, students experienced higher levels of stress and recovered more slowly after viewing the artifact-dominated scenes relative to the nature-dominated scenes. And in a third study (Wells and Evans, 2003), 337 children in rural towns in upstate New York were classified according to the naturalness of their homes, including the views from the windows, the number of plants inside the home, and the composition of the yard. Children in the high-nature homes reacted to stressful life events with significantly less psychological distress than children in the low-nature homes did. Results such as these suggest that nature contact may function, at least acutely, to mitigate stress.

Nature contact might be healthy in a third way, by playing a role in wholesome child development. Psychologists and others (Nabhan and Trimble, 1994; Kahn, 1999; Kahn and Kellert, 2002; Louv, 2005) have argued that children's ability to develop perceptual and expressive skills, imagination, moral judgments, and other attributes is greatly enhanced by contact with nature. Chapter Twenty-Five introduces the concept that children have windows of vulnerability to toxic exposures; children may also have developmental windows during which nature contact fills important needs.

In considering the benefits of animal contact, Beck and Katcher (2003) suggest a fourth mechanism—social support. They point out that social contact is a strong predictor of good health and that pets provide companionship and intimacy for many people. This may be a beneficial aspect of nature contact more generally. For example, a study in Zurich found that children who regularly played outside in natural areas had more than twice as many playmates as children restricted to indoor play because of heavy nearby traffic (Hüttenmoser, 1995). Interestingly, the same disparity in the quantity of friends was found among the corresponding groups of parents as well. And a study in England found that the well-established relationship between income-related deprivation and mortality was reduced among people who lived near green space (Mitchell and Popham, 2008). Perhaps both biophilia-related mechanisms and social mechanisms function to yield health benefits.

Suppose, then, that humans have an affiliation with nature, an affiliation that conferred a survival advantage over evolutionary time, and that is now part of our genetic heritage. Suppose further that in modern life we contain and suppress this affiliation—not only with technology and lifestyle choices but even with such basic means as the structure of our language. Is there any evidence that we can promote health by promoting this affiliation?

DOMAINS OF NATURE CONTACT

Evidence that our contacts with nature can be beneficial to health is available from at least four aspects of the natural world—animals, plants, landscapes, and wilderness experiences.

Animals

Animals have always played a prominent part in human life (Clutton-Brock, 1981). More people go to zoos each year than to all professional sporting events (Wilson, 1993, p. 32). Almost two-thirds of U.S. households have a pet, including about 39 percent with a dog and about 34 percent with a cat (corresponding to national populations of about 75 million dogs and 88 million cats) (American Pet Products Association, 2007; Fleishman-Hillard International Communications, 2007) (Figure 24.2). More than 90 percent of the characters used in preschool books to teach children language and counting are animals (Kellert, 1993, p. 52). Numerous studies have established that household animals are considered family members; people talk to their pets as if they were human, carry their photographs, buy them birthday presents, and share their bedrooms with them (Beck and Katcher, 1983). Large numbers of pet owners report that, if faced with financial hardship, they would cut back on groceries, entertainment, and household goods before they would cut back on pet care (Fleishman-Hillard International Communications, 2007). During disasters such as Hurricane Katrina, many pet owners refuse to evacuate without their pets, and those who lose their pets suffer considerable psychopathology (Hunt, Hind, and Johnson, 2008). Fifty percent of adults and 70 percent of adolescents confide in their animals (Beck and Meyers, 1996).

A wide body of evidence links animals with human health (Headey, 2003). In a study in a Melbourne cardiovascular disease risk clinic, nearly 6,000 patients were divided into those who owned pets and those who did not. The pet owners had lower systolic blood pressure, cholesterol, and triglycerides than the non-pet owners, an effect that reached statistical significance among men but not women.

FIGURE 24.2   The Human-Animal Bond

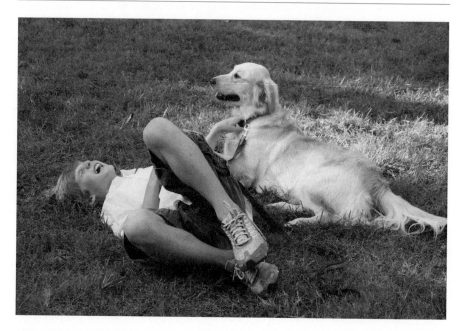

Source: Photo © 2008 Trisha Addicks, http://www.trishaaddicksphotography.com. Used with permission.

These findings could not be explained by differences in exercise levels (say, from dog walking), in diet, in social class, or in other confounders (Anderson, Reid, and Jennings, 1992). In a 1995 study, 369 survivors of myocardial infarction were followed for one year. Of these, 112 owned pets and 257 did not. The dog owners had a one-year survival rate six times higher than that of the non-dog owners, and this benefit was not due to physiological differences (cat owners showed no such advantage) (Friedmann and Thomas, 1995). In a study of 240 married couples, half with pets and half without, participants were exposed to two stressors (a mathematical task and immersing the hand in cold water) under one of four conditions: alone, with a companion (the pet for pet owners, and a friend for non-pet owners), with the spouse, or with both companion and spouse. Pet owners had lower baseline heart rate and blood pressure, lower cardiovascular reactivity to the stressors, and faster recovery, and the advantage was most marked when the pet was present during the testing (Allen, Blascovich, Wendy, and Mendes, 2002).

Investigators in Cambridge, England, followed 71 adults who had just acquired pets and compared them with 26 petless controls over a ten-month period. Within a month of acquiring the pet the pet owners showed a statistically significant decrease in minor health problems. In the dog owners (but not the cat owners) this improvement was sustained for the entire ten months of observation (Serpell, 1991). In another study, this one in the United States, 938 Medicare enrollees were divided into pet owners and non-pet owners. The pet owners, especially the dog owners, had fewer physician visits than non-pet owners. Moreover, stressful life events triggered more doctor visits among those without pets but not among pet owners, suggesting that owning a pet helped mediate stress (Siegel, 1990). (Not all studies have found decreased use of medical services among elderly pet owners; for negative findings see Jorm and others, 1997; Parslow and other, 2005.)

Animal-assisted therapy has been evaluated in the treatment of mental illness. For example, in a Virginia psychiatric hospital, 230 patients with mood disorders, schizophrenia, substance abuse disorders, and other diagnoses were treated with both a session of animal-assisted therapy (featuring interaction with a dog) and a session of conventional recreational therapy, using a crossover design. Both therapies reduced the patients' anxiety levels as measured by the State-Trait Anxiety Inventory, but in all diagnostic groups except the group with mood disorders, the animal-assisted therapy achieved substantially greater reductions (Barker and Dawson, 1998).

The role of animals in helping people handle stress has been tested specifically. In one study patients about to undergo oral surgery were randomly assigned to one of five conditions: a half-hour of looking at an aquarium, with or without hypnosis, a half-hour of looking at a picture of a waterfall, with or without hypnosis, and a half-hour of sitting quietly (the control group). The patients' comfort and relaxation during surgery were graded independently by the oral surgeon, the investigator, and the patients themselves. The most relaxed patients were those who looked at the aquarium, irrespective of whether they had been hypnotized. The patients who looked at the waterfall picture and were also hypnotized were almost as relaxed. Those who looked at the waterfall picture without being hypnotized, however, had low relaxation scores, as low as those of the control patients (Katcher, Segal, and Beck, 1984). In another study, forty-five women were exposed to a stressful stimulus alone, in the presence of a human friend, and in the presence of their dog. Their autonomic nervous system responses to stress, such as heart rate, were measured. The stress response was marked when subjects were alone and even more marked when a friend was present. But having a dog present significantly reduced the stress response (Allen, 1997). *Animal-facilitated therapy* in the treatment of psychiatric conditions is widely used (Draper, Gerber, and Layng, 1990; Beck and Katcher, 2003).

The mechanisms of benefit from animal contact are unclear. They may relate to the link to nature, to companionship, or to other factors (Beck and Katcher,

1983). Some benefit may grow from the social interactions, favor exchanges, and sense of community that follow animal companionship (Wood, Giles-Corti, and Bulsara, 2005; Wood, Giles-Corti, Bulsara, and Bosch, 2007). Whatever the mechanism, the bulk of the evidence supports the conclusion of animal researchers Alan Beck and N. Marshall Meyers (1996): "Preserving the bond between people and their animals, like encouraging good nutrition and exercise, appears to be in the best interests of those concerned with public health" (p. 249).

Plants

People feel good around plants. In the 1989 National Gardening Survey of more than 2,000 randomly selected households, 50.1 percent of respondents agreed with the statement, "The flowers and plants at theme parks, historic sites, golf courses, and restaurants are important to my enjoyment of visiting there," and 40 percent agreed with the statement, "Being around plants makes me feel calmer and more relaxed" (Butterfield and Relf, 1992). Among residents of retirement communities, 99 percent indicate that "living within pleasant landscaped grounds" is either essential or important, and 95 percent indicate that windows facing green, landscaped grounds are either essential or important (Browne, 1992). Office employees report that plants make them feel calmer and more relaxed, and that an office with plants is a more desirable place to work (Randall, Shoemaker, Relf, and Geller, 1992; Larsen and others, 1998), although work performance does not necessarily improve (Larsen and others, 1998). In a nationwide poll conducted by the National Gardening Association in 2006, 33 percent of households reported that "I enjoy gardening" and 27 percent reported that "gardening makes me happy" (Butterfield, 2006). In urban settings, gardens and gardening have been linked to a range of social benefits, ranging from improved property values to greater conviviality (for example, Patel, 1992). Psychologist Michael Perlman (1994) has written of the psychological power of trees, as evidenced by mythology, dreams, and self-reported emotional responses.

Empirical evidence of mental health benefits is scarce but intriguing. For example, in the Dubbo Study, a longitudinal cohort study of 2,805 elderly people in New South Wales, 56 percent of men and 41 percent of women gardened daily. Compared with those not gardening, daily gardeners enjoyed a 40 percent lower risk of admission for dementia, and those gardening weekly or less often had an 11 percent reduction (Simons, Simons, McCallum, and Friedlander, 2006). Indeed, the concept that plants have a role in mental health has given rise to a treatment approach called *horticultural therapy* (Lewis, 1996; Simson and Straus, 2003; Haller and Kramer, 2006). Horticultural therapy is also used in community-based programs, geriatrics programs, prisons, developmental disabilities programs, and special education (Mattson, 1992). In prisons, observers have noted that gardening has a "strangely soothing effect," making "pacifists of potential battlers" (Neese, 1959) and seemingly decreasing the numbers of assaults among prisoners (Hunter, 1970, reported in Lewis, 1990). Community gardening may offer many health and social benefits to community residents.

Could contact with plants also contribute to healing from physical ailments (Lewis, 1990)? Oliver Sacks raised this possibility in a memorable passage in his 1984 account of recovery from a serious leg injury, *A Leg to Stand On*. After more than two weeks in a small hospital room with no outside view, and a third week on a dreary surgical ward, he was finally taken out to the hospital garden:

> This was a great joy—to be out in the air—for I had not been outside in almost a month. A pure and intense joy, a blessing, to feel the sun on my face and the wind in my hair, to hear birds, to see, touch, and fondle the living plants. Some essential connection and communion with nature was re-established after the horrible isolation and alienation I had known. Some part of me came alive, when I was taken to the garden, which had been starved, and died, perhaps without my knowing it [pp. 133–134].

Sacks credited his garden contact with an important role in his recovery and mused that perhaps more hospitals should have gardens or even be set in the countryside or near woods.

Another anecdotal account comes from Swee-Lian Yi, a twenty-nine-year-old severe stroke victim, who was hospitalized in New York's Rusk Institute of Rehabilitation Medicine. Like Sacks, she found her first visit to the hospital greenhouse a turning point: "It was when I walked through that building, perfectly quiet, filled with green and growing plants and the sweet smell of healthy soil that my anxiety began to ebb away. In its place came a tranquility I had not experienced since the day of my stroke" (Yi, 1985). In fact hospitals have traditionally had gardens as an adjunct to recuperation and healing, and notable examples survive in many parts of the country (Gerlach-Spriggs, Kaufman, and Warner, 1998; Hartig and Marcus, 2006). Empirical evidence of efficacy is scarce (Soderback, Soderstrom, and Schalander, 2004; Frumkin, 2004), but what is available is suggestive. For example, researchers at New York's Rusk Institute of Rehabilitation Medicine compared horticultural therapy with routine patient education in cardiac rehabilitation patients. Horticultural therapy significantly reduced both the heart rate and the total mood disturbance as measured by the Profile of Mood States (POMS) inventory, whereas patient education classes did not (Wichrowski and others, 2005). As further evidence accumulates, it may confirm a longstanding

PERSPECTIVE
Community Gardens

Community gardens are an increasingly common initiative in many communities, especially in urban neighborhoods where people otherwise have little or no access to land for cultivation (Figure 24.3). Community gardens are parcels of land that are typically community managed, and individuals or families are allocated patches within the garden for their own use. Participants grow vegetables, herbs, flowers, and other edible or ornamental plants. Among the benefits claimed for community gardens are that they help to

- Build a sense of community among participants
- Restore blighted neighborhoods
- Provide improved access to fresh, nutritious, affordable food
- Build skills among participants
- Improve mental health and well-being
- Provide physical activity

Few public health interventions offer such a range of benefits at such low cost and with so few downsides.

Sources: Armstrong, 2000; Bartolomei, Corkery, Judd, and Thompson, 2003; Giesecke, and Sherman, 1991; Flanigan and Varma, 2006; Schukoske, 2000.

belief that proximity to plants, like proximity to animals, may in some circumstances enhance health.

Landscapes

Natural landscapes may have a similar effect. Returning to an evolutionary perspective, human history probably began on the African savanna, a region of open grasslands punctuated by scattered copses of trees and denser woods near rivers and lakes. If this sounds like the choicest real estate in most cities and towns, that may not be a coincidence. As E. O. Wilson (1984) points out, "certain key features of the ancient physical habitat match the choices made by modern human beings when they have a say in the matter" (p. 109)—a pattern that repeats in parks, cemeteries, golf courses, and lawns. "It seems that whenever people are given

FIGURE 24.3   A Community Garden

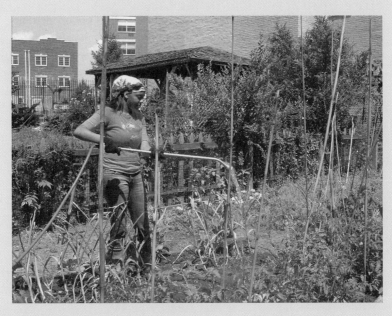

Source: Courtesy of Council on the Environment of New York City.

Community gardens offer participants, including urban residents, the opportunity to connect with nature, learn valuable skills, and raise some of their own food.

a free choice, they move to open tree-studded land on prominences overlooking water" (p. 110).

Could evolution have selected for certain landscape preferences? Perhaps. A crucial step in the lives of most organisms, including humans, is selection of a habitat. If a creature gets into the right place, everything is likely to be easier. "Habitat selection depends on the recognition of objects, sounds, and odors to which the organism responds as if it understood their significance for future behavior and success" (Heerwagen and Orians, 1993, p. 140). For example, many birds use patterns of tree density and vertical arrangement of branches as primary settling cues; presumably these cues correlate with crucial information about such benefits as food availability and concealment from predators. For early humans a place with an open view would have offered better opportunities than a spatially restricted setting to identify food and shelter and to avoid predators. But not too open a view: clumps

PERSPECTIVE
Nature Contact in the Inner City

An important line of research from the University of Illinois Landscape and Human Health Laboratory has focused on nature contact in a rarely studied setting: inner-city housing projects. Investigators took advantage of a natural experiment at Chicago's Robert Taylor Homes. This complex, which no longer stands, consisted of twenty-eight identical high-rise buildings arrayed along a three-mile stretch of land bounded by busy roadways and railway lines. Some of the buildings were surrounded by pleasant stands of trees, whereas others opened onto barren stretches of ground (Figure 24.4). Residents were essentially randomly assigned to a building with one landscape type or the other, because assignment depended on where a vacancy existed when their names came up on the Housing Authority list. The research compared residents of the buildings with and without trees, and was limited to those who lived on the lower floors (to ensure that participants in buildings surrounded by trees did have tree views from their windows).

FIGURE 24.4   Robert Taylor Homes, Chicago (top: aerial view; middle: buildings with nearby trees; bottom: buildings without nearby trees)

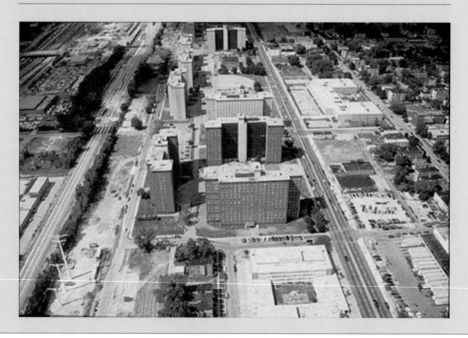

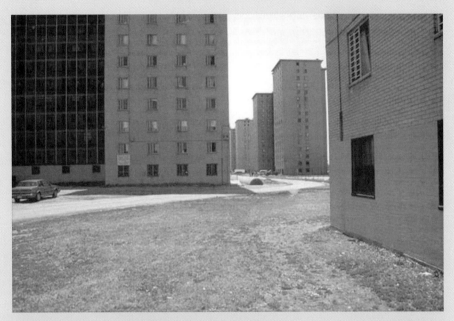

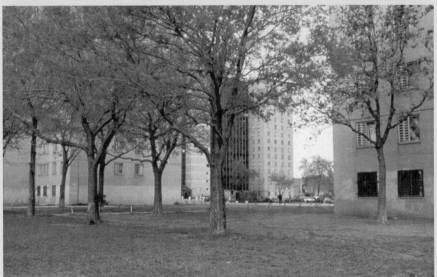

Source: William Sullivan, University of Illinois. Used with permission.

In use from 1962 to 1997, this project was home to as many as 27,000 people. It provided a setting for studying the effects of nearby nature on residents' health and well-being.

This research yielded surprising and important findings. Compared to living in buildings with barren surroundings, living in buildings with trees was associated with

- Higher levels of attention and greater effectiveness in managing major life issues (Kuo, 2001)
- Substantially lower levels of aggression and violence (both as victims and as perpetrators) among women (Kuo and Sullivan, 2001a)
- Lower levels of reported crime (Kuo and Sullivan, 2001b)
- Higher levels of self-discipline (as measured by tests of concentration, impulse inhibition, and delay of gratification) among girls (but not among boys) (Taylor, Kuo, and Sullivan, 2002)

These findings suggest that nature contact in otherwise deprived urban environments—even relatively simple forms of contact such as having trees outside an apartment building—can offer powerful benefits to the people who live there.

of trees would offer hiding places in a pinch and, like streams and lakes, might also signal the presence of prey for the hunter (Ulrich, 1993). Going further, perhaps the ability to identify relaxing, restorative settings and the capacity to recover from fatigue and stress could also have been adaptive (Ulrich, 1993; Kaplan and Kaplan, 1989). If you can run away from a saber-toothed tiger, your survival is enhanced. But if, having run away, you can then get to a peaceful place, relax, and gather your strength, that may further enhance your survival. Perhaps individuals who chose such settings gained a survival advantage (Ulrich, 1993).

There is considerable evidence that people's aesthetic preferences conform to this prediction. When offered a variety of landscapes, people react most positively to savanna-like settings, with moderate to high depth or openness, relatively smooth or uniform-length grassy vegetation or ground surfaces, scattered trees or small groupings of trees, and water (Schroeder and Green, 1985; Kaplan, 1984). Notably, these findings emerge cross-culturally, in studies of North Americans, Europeans, Asians, and Africans (see, for example, Hull and Revell, 1989; Purcell, Lamb, Peron, and Falchero, 1994; Korpela and Hartig, 1996).

The effect of landscapes may extend beyond aesthetics to restoration or stress recovery. Research on recreational activities has shown that savanna-like settings are associated with self-reported feelings of peacefulness, tranquility, or relaxation (Ulrich, 1983). Viewing such settings leads to decreased fear and anger and enhanced positive affect on the Zuckerman Inventory of Personal Reactions (ZIPERS) (Honeyman, 1992). Moreover, viewing nature scenes is associated with enhanced mental alertness, attention, and cognitive performance, as measured by tasks such as proofreading and by formal psychological testing (Cimprich, 2003; Tennessen and Cimprich, 1995).

Interesting evidence comes from the study of urban parks (Nielsen and Hansen, 2007). In Copenhagen, investigators found, not surprisingly, that living near a park predicted more frequent visits to the park. But living near a park also predicted a lower level of self-reported stress and a lower risk of obesity—a relationship not fully explained by more visits to the park. In a two-year longitudinal study in Indianapolis, investigators found that children who lived in "greener" neighborhoods experienced less weight gain than children in neighborhoods with less green space (Bell, Wilson, and Liu, 2008). It seems that proximity to green space confers health benefits through both physical activity and other mechanisms. Parks are increasingly viewed as a health amenity.

The same results emerge from studies that directly consider other health endpoints. In 1981, Ernest Moore, a University of Michigan architect, took advantage of a natural experiment at the State Prison of Southern Michigan, a massive depression-era structure. Half the prisoners occupied cells along the outside wall, with a window view of rolling farmland and trees, and the other half occupied cells that faced the prison courtyard. Assignment to one or the other kind of cell was random. Compared to the prisoners in the exterior cells, the prisoners in the inside cells had a 24 percent higher frequency of sick call visits. Moore could not identify any design feature to explain this difference and concluded that the outside view "may provide some stress reduction" (Moore, 1981–1982). Likewise, employees with views of nature at work report fewer headaches (as well as less job pressure and greater job satisfaction) than do those without such a view (Kaplan, Talbot, and Kaplan, 1988, reported in Kaplan, 1992).

Similar observations have come from health care settings. A short 1984 article in *Science* bore the provocative title "View Through a Window May Influence Recovery from Surgery." Like the Michigan prison study, this study also took advantage of an inadvertent architectural experiment. On the surgical floors of a 200-bed suburban Pennsylvania hospital, some rooms faced a stand of deciduous trees and others faced a brown brick wall. Postoperative patients were assigned essentially randomly to one or the other kind of room. The records of all cholecystectomy patients over a ten-year interval, restricted to the summer months when the trees were in foliage, were reviewed. End points were the length of hospitalization, the need for pain and anxiety medications, the occurrence of minor medical complications, and nurses' notes. Compared to patients with brick views, patients with tree views had statistically significantly shorter hospitalizations (7.96

PERSPECTIVE
Parks and Public Health

Parks have long been prized as features of towns and cities. Pioneering urban planners such as Frederick Law Olmsted, and municipal officials of the nineteenth

FIGURE 24.5   *A Sunday Afternoon on the Island of La Grande Jatte,*
1884–1886, by Georges Seurat

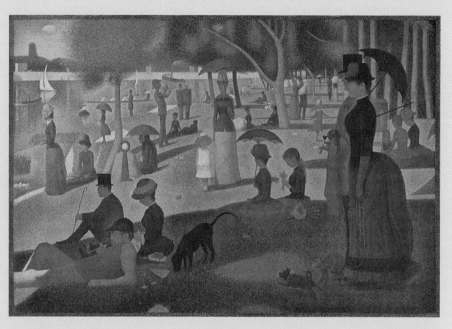

This is not only a famous example of pointillist painting, it also illustrates the long-standing appreciation of parks as venues for nature contact, relaxation, social interaction, and physical activity.

days compared to 8.70 days), less need for pain medications, and fewer negative comments in the nurses' notes (Ulrich, 1984).

Other evidence is available from therapeutic settings. In a study of dental patients, researchers placed a large mural of an open, natural scene on the wall of a dental waiting room on some days and removed it on others. Dental patients and early twentieth centuries considered parks essential oases in cities, allowing urban dwellers to connect with nature, enjoy each other's company, breathe fresh air, and pursue recreational activities (Olmsted, [1870] 1999; Cranz, 1982) (Figure 24.5).

Parks may range from small pockets of green space deep within urban canyons to vast reserves of natural land in rural areas. Parks offer a range of health benefits (Sherer, 2006). One of the best studied is physical activity; living near a park predicts more physical activity, and certain park features, such as greenery, good maintenance, recreational facilities, and amenities such as restrooms, are known to predict greater use (Bedimo-Rung, Mowen, and Cohen, 2007; Cohen and others, 2007). Parks also offer mental health benefits, perhaps through stress reduction (Orsega-Smith, Mowen, Payne, and Godbey, 2004)—benefits that result not only from visiting parks but from living near them. Indirect health benefits arise from the role of parks in protecting watersheds, reducing air pollution, and cooling urban heat islands.

The ways in which these benefits operate may vary across the population. Ethnic and racial groups differ in their preferences and in the ways they use parks (Virden and Walker, 1999; Gobster, 2002; Ho and others, 2005). Children benefit from specific features of parks, as do older adults (Payne, Orsega-Smith, Godbey, and Roy, 1998). Parks and recreation professionals, like public health professionals, need to take these differences into account as they address the needs of a diverse population and assure equitable service delivery.

Many park systems recognize parks' links with public health, and some have even adopted health themes in promoting park use. The slogan of the parks department of the state of Victoria, Australia, for example, is "Healthy Parks, Healthy People" (http://www.parkweb.vic.gov.au). Public health initiatives have been launched by such groups as the National Parks and Recreation Association (http://www.nrpa.org) and the City Parks Alliance (http://www.cityparksalliance.org). These groups emphasize not only the health benefits but also the synergistic environmental and economic benefits of parks.

Parks exemplify the role of nature contact in promoting public health.

with appointments on the days when the mural was visible had lower blood pressure and less self-reported anxiety than the patients with appointments on the days when the mural was taken down (Heerwagen, 1990). In a study of psychiatric inpatients, patients were exposed to two kinds of wall art: nature scenes such as landscapes and abstract or symbolic art. Interviews suggested more positive responses to the nature scenes. And in fifteen years of records on patient attacks on the wall art, every attack was on abstract art, none was on a nature scene (Ulrich, 1986, reported in Ulrich, 1993). (No information was provided on how many of the psychiatric patients were artists or art critics.) And in a randomized clinical trial of patients undergoing bronchoscopy (insertion of a flexible fiber-optic tube through the trachea into the lungs), patients who viewed a nature scene (a mountain stream in a spring meadow) and heard recorded nature sounds (water in a stream or chirping birds) experienced better pain control than did patients who received only conventional sedation (although anxiety levels did not differ between the two groups) (Diette and others, 2003). Viewing landscapes and related nature scenes, whether in actuality or in pictures, seems to have a salutary effect.

Wilderness Experiences

Wilderness experiences—entering the landscape rather than only viewing it— may also be therapeutic. David Cumes (1998a, 1998b) has described "wilderness rapture," involving self-awareness; feelings of awe, wonder, and humility; a sense of comfort in and connection to nature; increased appreciation of others; and a feeling of renewal and vigor. Others have described the spiritual inspiration that comes from wilderness experiences (Fredrickson and Anderson, 1999). These outcomes are often cited in favorable accounts of so-called wilderness therapy for psychiatric patients (Jerstad and Stelzer, 1973; Witman, 1987; Plakun, Tucker, and Harris, 1981; Berman and Anton, 1988), emotionally disturbed children and adolescents (Hobbs and Shelton, 1972; Marx, 1988; Davis-Berman and Berman, 1989), bereaved persons (Moyer, 1988; Birnbaum, 1991), and rape and incest survivors (Levine, 1994) and also for patients with cancer (Pearson, 1989), end-stage renal disease (Warady, 1994), posttraumatic stress disorder (PTSD) (Hyer and others, 1996), addiction disorders (Bennett, Cardone, and Jarczyk, 1998; Kennedy and Minami, 1993), and other ailments (Easley, Passineau, and Driver, 1990). **Green exercise** may represent a less intense version of this same phenomenon.

Most documented examples of beneficial effects from wilderness experiences relate to mental health end points. In one such study, a group of 5.5-to 11.5-year-old, emotionally disturbed boys attending an outdoor day camp was compared to a group of similar boys not attending the camp. The campers' self-ratings of their emotional adjustment and also their teachers' ratings were significantly better than those of the controls, although neither parents' ratings nor scores on formal psychological testing showed an improvement (Shniderman, 1974). In another study, a group of adolescents being treated for

PERSPECTIVE
Green Exercise

Exercise is clearly good for health; the benefits include weight loss, blood pressure and cholesterol reduction, and decreased risk of heart attacks, stroke, diabetes, and some cancers. Exercise is also good for mental health; it improves attention, lifts mood, and relieves depression. Could it matter where you exercise?

Access to nature, it turns out, is a powerful inducement to being physically active. Research on correlates of physical activity has shown that after controlling for such factors as age and socioeconomic status, access to green space is a strong predictor of physical activity, especially walking (Giles-Corti and Donovan, 2003; Bird, 2004; Giles-Corti and others, 2005). This has become an important consideration in "active living by design" trends.

Research has also suggested that exercise in natural settings may be more beneficial than exercise in barren or heavily built settings (Pretty, Griffin, Sellens, and Pretty, 2003). In a Swedish study, twelve people who ran regularly, took two hour-long runs, one through a nature reserve of pine and birch forest, open fields, and a lakeshore and the other through an urban route with mid-rise apartment houses, commercial development, and heavy traffic. The runners preferred the park route and rated it more psychologically restorative than the urban route. In addition, self-rated anxiety or depression and anger decreased more and self-rated revitalization and tranquility improved more with the park than with the urban route (although these differences did not reach statistical significance) (Bodin and Hartig, 2003).

In another study volunteers exercised on a treadmill while viewing different scenes on a screen—some rural and other urban, some pleasant and others unpleasant. Exercising while viewing the pleasant rural scenes led to greater blood pressure reductions and more consistent improvements in psychological measures (self-esteem, anger-hostility, fatigue-inertia, tension-anxiety, and vigor-activity) than occurred in any other study condition (although not always with statistical significance) (Pretty, Peacock, Sellens, and Griffin, 2005).

If these findings can be replicated, they suggest that the well-known health benefits of exercise may be further enhanced by exercising in pleasing natural settings—something that golfers, hikers, and resort owners (among others) may already believe.

depression, substance abuse, or adjustment reactions improved on measures of cooperation and trust following a wilderness experience, whereas controls did not (Witman, 1987). Psychiatric inpatients showed improvements in coping ability and locus of control following a wilderness adventure program (Plakun, Tucker, and Harris, 1981). Inpatients at the Oregon State Mental Hospital showed improved function and greater probability of discharge following wilderness adventure programs (Jerstad and Stelzer, 1973). In a convenience sample of more than 700 people who had participated in wilderness excursions lasting two to four weeks, 90 percent described "an increased sense of aliveness, well-being, and energy," and 90 percent reported that the experience had helped them break an addiction (defined broadly and ranging from nicotine to chocolate) (Greenway, 1995).

This literature is more extensive than the literature on plants and animals (Colan, 1986), but several limitations make it difficult to interpret (McNeil, 1957; Byers, 1979). Much of the published research comes from proponents, such as adventure companies with a personal or commercial interest in wilderness experiences. Much of the research refers to structured trips or summer camp programs rather than to the more general phenomenon of contact with wilderness. Beneficial outcomes may be due to the vacation quality of the experience, to the psychological value of setting and achieving difficult goals, or to the group bonding that occurs on some such trips (or to some combination of these), rather than (or in addition to) the wilderness contact itself. Few studies have been randomized, and selection bias can rarely be excluded. Blinding of subjects is impossible, and blinding of investigators has not been attempted.

Despite these limitations, many published accounts do suggest some benefit from wilderness experiences. Mental health has been more studied than somatic conditions, and short-term benefit has been demonstrated more than long-term benefit.

There is evidence, then, that contact with the natural world—with animals, plants, landscapes, and wilderness—may offer health benefits. Perhaps this reflects ancient learning habits, preferences, and tastes, echoes of human origins as creatures of the wild. Satisfying these preferences by promoting contact with the natural world may be an effective way to enhance health (not to mention cheaper and freer of side effects than medications). If so, this implies a broad vision of environmental health, one that stretches from urban planning to landscape architecture, from interior design to forestry, from botany to veterinary medicine.

THE GREENING OF ENVIRONMENTAL HEALTH

A paradigm of environmental health that considers nature contact as well as toxicity, good places as well as bad ones, health as well as illness, has implications in at least three arenas: research, collaboration, and public health intervention.

Research

Clinical and epidemiological research in environmental health addresses many variants of the same question: Is there an association between exposure and outcome? A focus on nature contact suggests a research agenda directed not only at potentially hazardous exposures but also at potentially healthy ones, and at outcomes that reflect not only impaired health but also enhanced health (Frumkin, 2003). If people have regular contact with flowers or trees, do they report greater well-being, better sleep, fewer headaches, reduced joint pain? Do inner-city children who attend a rural summer camp have better health during the next semester of school than their friends who spent the summer in the city? Do patients with cancer or AIDS survive longer, or have fewer infections or less pain or higher T cell counts, if they have pets? Do gardens in hospitals speed postoperative recovery? Does psychotherapy that employs contact with nature—known as *ecopsychology* (Roszak, Gomes, and Kanner, 1995)—have an empirical basis? If these or related therapeutic approaches show promise, which patients will benefit and what kinds of contact with nature will have the greatest efficacy and cost effectiveness?

Answering these questions requires an orientation toward empirical research among professions, from landscape architecture to horticulture, that have traditionally not emphasized such research. It also requires an ability to define and operationalize variables currently unfamiliar to health researchers. What is exposure to nature, what does the concept of a *dose* mean in this context, and how do we measure it? Similarly, the outcome variables that reflect health instead of disease are less familiar and need to be developed and validated. These challenges offer broad opportunities for methods development and hypothesis testing.

Collaboration

Environmental health specialists, from researchers to clinicians, have long recognized the need to collaborate with other professionals. They work with mechanical engineers to build exposure chambers, with chemists to measure exposures, and with software engineers to apply geographic information systems to health data. A focus on natural environments requires collaborations with other kinds of professionals: landscape architects, who can help with identifying the salient features of outdoor exposures; interior designers, who can do the same for microenvironments; veterinarians, who can help with understanding human relationships with animals; and urban and regional planners, who can help with linking environmental health principles with large-scale environmental design.

Public Health Intervention

Finally, as data accumulate about the health benefits of particular environments, research needs to be translated into action. On the clinical level this may have implications for patient care. Perhaps physicians and nurses will advise patients

---

PERSPECTIVE
Leave No Child Inside

Do children have a special need to connect with nature? Child development theory suggests that this may be the case. As children mature, they have a growing need to explore and manipulate their environments (Heerwagen and Orians, 2002). Children's affinity for "secret spaces"—hidden spots under low tree canopies or within clumps of shrubbery—may exemplify this process (Kirkby, 1989). There is evidence that contact with nature offers children benefits as diverse as stress reduction (Wells and Evans, 2003) and improved cognitive function (Wells, 2000).

In an influential 2005 book, *Last Child in the Woods*, author Richard Louv called attention to a problem he dubbed "nature deficit disorder"—the notion that contemporary children suffer from a lack of unstructured play and exploration in natural settings. This idea resonated widely and has helped spur federal, state, and local initiatives to reconnect children with nature. In Chicago in 2007, a consortium of over 200 community and environmental groups launched Leave No Child Inside, an initiative designed to reconnect children in that city with nature (http://www.kidsoutside.info). State initiatives have proliferated—the 2006 bill in Washington State that mandated a study of the effects of outdoor education, with a priority on underserved children; the Outdoor Bill of Rights in California in 2007; the No Child Left Inside Act in New Mexico in 2008 (funded by a tax on televisions and video games). A 2007 federal bill, the No Child Left Inside Act, proposed to amend the No Child Left Behind law with a provision for training teachers in environmental and outdoor education, funding environmental education programs in schools, and promoting environmental literary.

The rapid spread of these initiatives suggests that nature contact among children may become a mainstream strategy in environmental health.

to take a few days in the country, to spend time gardening, or to adopt a pet if clinical evidence offers support for such measures. Perhaps hospitals will be built in scenic locations, and rehabilitation centers will routinely include gardens. Health promotion professionals may include nature contact among the healthy behaviors they encourage (St. Leger, 2003). Perhaps the employers and managed care organizations that pay for health care will come to fund such interventions, especially if they prove to rival pharmaceuticals in cost and efficacy.

PERSPECTIVE
Green Gym

The Green Gym was developed in 1977 by William Bird, a general practitioner, advocate of the countryside as a health resource, and adviser to Natural England. The Green Gym is a volunteer program consisting of group sessions, typically held weekly, during which participants perform conservation or gardening work such as coppicing, clearing scrubland, path building, and tree planting; they also take time for exercises and for socializing. Dozens of Green Gym projects are active across the United Kingdom, involving thousands of participants. Some are targeted to special groups, such as people with disabilities, caregivers requiring respite, and employees suffering workplace stress.

The Green Gym program stresses the health benefits of working in the outdoors. It grew out of several existing programs, including Conservation Volunteering, in which people perform environmental work as a community service under the auspices of a large charity, the BTCV (formerly the British Trust for Conservation Volunteers), and Health Walks, a public health effort to get sedentary people more active. The Green Gym concept stresses the importance of the relationships among the local community, the local environment, and the health and well-being of residents.

The Green Gym has been systematically evaluated in a series of reports from Oxford Brookes University's Centre for Health Care Research & Development (Reynolds, 1999, 2000, 2002). Evaluation findings include the development of camaraderie and social capital (reflected in very high retention rates), increases in physical activity both during Green Gym sessions and at other times of the week, and self-reported improvement in mental health, well-being, and quality of life. There are also environmental benefits, many of which are enjoyed by the entire community.

PERSPECTIVE
Biophilic Design

If nature contact offers health benefits, then the obvious public health strategy would be to get people into nature. But a complementary strategy is also available: bringing nature to people. Because people spend most of their time indoors, this means designing buildings that build on people's affinity with nature. *Biophilic design* is "an approach that fosters beneficial contact between people and nature in modern buildings and landscapes" (Kellert, 2008, p. 5). Biophilic design is characterized by two basic design elements. One is an organic or naturalistic approach, with shapes and forms that reflect people's affinity for nature; examples include such features as water, sunlight, plants, and natural materials. The second is place-based, or vernacular, design that connects to the culture and ecology of a locality; this might involve geography, history, landscape orientation, and a host of other features. Biophilic design can be seen on the small scale in a window planter or an artfully designed walkway and on the large scale in such iconic buildings as the Sydney Opera House, with its soaring bird- and sail-like forms over the waterfront of Sydney Harbour (also see Figure 24.6).

FIGURE 24.6   Frank Lloyd Wright's Fallingwater

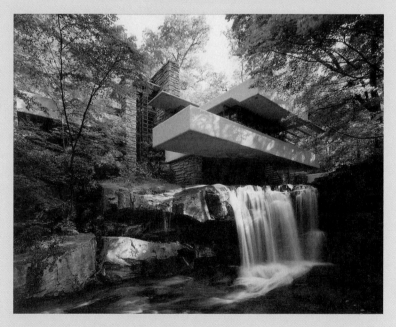

Source: Figura, 2007, http://commons.wikimedia.org/wiki/File:Falling_Water_01.jpg. Permission granted under the terms of the GNU Free Documentation License, Version 1.2 or any later version published by the Free Software Foundation.

This house illustrates some of the principles of biophilia: the use of natural materials and motifs and close contact with nature.

SUMMARY

On the public health level, environmental health has a long history of providing data and advocating action based on these data to achieve control of environmental hazards, seeking more protective air pollution regulations, lower automobile emissions, safer pesticide practices, and cleaner rivers and streams. In the same way, public health will need to act on emerging evidence of environmental health benefits. We take it for granted that health experts play a prominent role at the Food and Drug Administration and the Environmental Protection Agency; how about a role at the National Park Service or the local zoo? Examples of programs that aim to promote public health by promoting nature contact include the Leave No Child Inside movement in the United States and the Green Gym projects in the United Kingdom. Building design that embodies biophilic principles has been promoted and may be an important public health opportunity. As we learn more about the health benefits of contact with the natural world, we need to apply this knowledge in ways that directly enhance the health of the public.

KEY TERMS

Attention restoration

Biophilia

Green exercise

DISCUSSION QUESTIONS

1. Describe your last contact with a natural setting—on a vacation, a weekend outing, or even a recent visit to a park. How did it make you feel? How would you design research to demonstrate these effects across a broad population?
2. Consider the availability of parks and green space in your city or town. Are they available near the places where people live and work? Do some sections have better access to them than others? What about poor and minority communities? Is this an environmental justice issue?
3. Suppose your community is considering a land conservation initiative that would set aside tracts of green space and prohibit future development on them. Environmental advocates are leading this effort, but they ask you to support it based on public health considerations. How would you make the case?

REFERENCES

Abram, D. *The Spell of the Sensuous: Perception and Language in a More-Than-Human World.* New York: Vintage Books, 1996.

Allen, D. T. "Effects of Dogs on Human Health." *Journal of the American Veterinary Medicine Association,* 1997, *210,* 1136–1139.

Allen, K., Blascovich, J., Wendy, B., and Mendes, W. B. "Cardiovascular Reactivity and the Presence of Pets, Friends, and Spouses: The Truth About Cats and Dogs." *Psychosomatic Medicine,* 2002, *64,* 727–739.

American Pet Products Association. *2007–2008 National Pet Owners Survey.* http://www.americanpet-products.org/pubs_survey.asp, 2007.

Anderson, W. P., Reid, C., and Jennings, G. "Pet Ownership and Risk Factors for Cardiovascular Disease." *Medical Journal of Australia,* 1992, *157,* 298–301.

Armstrong, D. A. "Survey of Community Gardens in Upstate New York: Implications for Health Promotion and Community Development." *Health & Place,* 2000, *6,* 319–327.

Barker, S. B., and Dawson, K. S. "The Effects of Animal-Assisted Therapy on Anxiety Ratings of Hospitalized Psychiatric Patients." *Psychiatric Services,* 1998, *49*(6), 797–801.

Bartolomei, L., Corkery, L., Judd, B., and Thompson, S. *A Bountiful Harvest: Community Gardens and Neighbourhood Renewal in Waterloo.* Sydney: University of New South Wales Press, 2003.

Beck, A. M., and Katcher, A. H. *Between Pets and People: The Importance of Animal Companionship.* New York: Perigree Books, 1983.

Beck, A. M., and Katcher, A. H. "Future Directions in Human-Animal Bond Research." *American Behavioral Scientist,* 2003, *47,* 79–93.

Beck, A. M., and Meyers, N. M. "Health Enhancement and Companion Animal Ownership." *Annual Review of Public Health,* 1996, *17,* 247–257.

Bedimo-Rung, A. L., Mowen, A. J., and Cohen, D. A. "The Significance of Parks to Physical Activity and Public Health: A Conceptual Model." *American Journal of Preventive Medicine,* 2005, *28*(suppl. *2*), 159–168.

Bell, J. F., Wilson, J. S., and Liu, G. C. "Neighborhood Greenness and 2-Year Changes in Body Mass Index of Children and Youth." *American Journal of Preventive Medicine,* 2008, *35,* 547–553.

Bennett, L. W., Cardone, S., and Jarczyk, J. "Effects of a Therapeutic Camping Program on Addiction Recovery: The Algonquin Relapse Prevention Program." *Journal of Substance Abuse Treatment,* 1998, *15,* 469–474.

Berman, D. S., and Anton, M. T. "A Wilderness Therapy Program as an Alternative to Adolescent Psychiatric Hospitalization." *Residential Treatment for Children and Youth,* 1988, *5,* 41–53.

Bird, W. *Natural Fit: Can Green Space and Biodiversity Increase Levels of Physical Activity?* Royal Society for the Protection of Birds. : http://www.rspb.org.uk/Images/natural_fit_full_version_tcm9–133055.pdf, 2004.

Birnbaum, A. "Haven Hugs & Bugs." *American Journal of Hospice Palliative Care,* 1991, *8,* 23–29.

Blair, D., Giesecke, C. C., and Sherman, S. A. "Dietary, Social and Economic Evaluation of the Philadelphia Urban Gardening Project." *Journal of Nutrition and Education,* 1991, *23,* 161–167.

Bodin, M., and Hartig, T. "Does the Outdoor Environment Matter for Psychological Restoration Gained Through Running?" *Psychology of Sport and Exercise,* 2003, *4,* 141–153.

Browne, A. "The Role of Nature for the Promotion of Well-Being in the Elderly." In D. Relf (ed.), *The Role of Horticulture in Human Well-Being and Social Development*. Portland, Ore.: Timber Press, 1992.

Butterfield, B. *What Gardeners Think*. National Gardening Association. : http://www.gardenresearch.com, 2006.

Butterfield, B., and Relf, D. "National Survey of Attitudes Toward Plants and Gardening." In D. Relf (ed.), *The Role of Horticulture in Human Well-Being and Social Development*." Portland, Ore.: Timber Press, 1992.

Byers, E. S. "Wilderness Camping as a Therapy for Emotionally Disturbed Children: A Critical Review." *Exceptional Children*, 1979, *45*, 628–635.

Cassis, G. "Biodiversity Loss: A Human Health Issue." *Medical Journal of Australia*, 1998, *169*, 568–569.

Chivian, E., and Bernstein, A. (eds.). *Sustaining Life: How Human Health Depends on Biodiversity*. New York: Oxford University Press, 2008.

Cimprich, B. "An Environmental Intervention to Restore Attention in Women with Newly Diagnosed Breast Cancer." *Cancer Nursing*, 2003, *26*, 284–292.

Clutton-Brock, J. *Domesticated Animals from Early Times*. Austin: University of Texas Press, 1981.

Cohen, D. A., and others. "Contribution of Public Parks to Physical Activity." *American Journal of Public Health*, 2007, *97*, 509–514.

Colan, N. B. *Outward Bound: An Annotated Bibliography 1976–1985*. Greenwich, Conn.: Outward Bound USA, 1986.

Cranz, G. *The Politics of Park Design: A History of Urban Parks in America*. Cambridge, Mass.: MIT Press, 1982.

Cumes, D. *Inner Passages Outer Journeys: Wilderness, Healing, and the Discovery of Self*. Minneapolis: Llewellyn, 1998a.

Cumes, D. "Nature as Medicine: The Healing Power of the Wilderness." *Alternative Therapies*, 1998b, *4*, 79–86.

Daily, G. C. (ed.). *Nature's Services: Societal Dependence on Natural Ecosystems*. Washington D.C.: Island Press, 1997.

Davis-Berman, J., and Berman, D. S. "The Wilderness Therapy Program: An Empirical Study of Its Effects with Adolescents in an Outpatient Setting." *Journal of Contemporary Psychotherapy*, 1989, *19*, 271–281.

Diette, G. B., and others. "Distraction Therapy with Nature Sights and Sounds Reduces Pain During Flexible Bronchoscopy." *Chest*, 2003, *123*, 141–148.

Draper, R. J., Gerber, G. J., and Layng, E. M. "Defining the Role of Pet Animals in Psychotherapy." *Psychiatric Journal of the University of Ottawa*, 1990, *15*(3), 169–172.

Easley, A. T., Passineau, J. F., and Driver, B. L. (comps.). The Use of Wilderness for Personal Growth, Therapy, and Education. Fort Collins, Colo.: U.S. Department of Agriculture, Forest Service, Rocky Mountain Forest and Range Experiment Station, 1990.

Faber Taylor, A., Kuo, F. E., and Sullivan, W. C. "Views of Nature and Self-Discipline: Evidence from Inner City Children." *Journal of Environmental Psychology*, 2002, *22*, 49–63.

Flanigan, S., and Varma, R. "Promoting Community Gardening to Low-Income Urban Participants in the Women, Infants and Children Program (WIC) in New Mexico." *Community Work and Family*, 2006, *9*, 69–74.

Fleishman-Hillard International Communications. *Pet Spending Survey*. http://pov.fleishman.com/wp-content/themes/fhbrand/docs/Fleishman-Hillard%20Pet%20Spending%20Survey.pdf, 2007.

Fox, S. *John Muir and His Legacy*. Boston: Little, Brown, 1981.

Fredrickson, L. M., and Anderson, D. H. "A Qualitative Exploration of the Wilderness Experience as a Source of Spiritual Inspiration." *Journal of Environmental Psychology*, 1999, *19*, 21–39.

Friedmann, E., and Thomas, S. A. "Pet Ownership, Social Support, and One-Year Survival After Acute Myocardial Infarction in the Cardiac Arrhythmia Suppression Trial (CAST)." *American Journal of Cardiology*, 1995, *76*, 1213–1217.

Frumkin, H. "Healthy Places: Exploring the Evidence." *American Journal of Public Health*, 2003, *93*, 1451–1456.

Frumkin, H. "White Coats, Green Plants: Clinical Epidemiology Meets Horticulture." *Acta Horticulturae*, 2004, *639*, 15–26.

Gerlach-Spriggs, N., Kaufman, R. E., and Warner, S. B. *Restorative Gardens: The Healing Landscape*. New Haven, Conn.: Yale University Press, 1998.

Giles-Corti, B., and Donovan, R. "Relative Influences of Individual, Social Environmental, and Physical Environmental Correlates of Walking." *American Journal of Public Health*, 2003, *93*, 1583–1589.

Giles-Corti, B., and others. "Increasing Walking: How Important Is Distance to, Attractiveness, and Size of Public Open Space?" *American Journal of Preventive Medicine*, 2005, *28*(suppl. 2), 169–176.

Gobster, P. "Managing Urban Parks for a Racially and Ethnically Diverse Clientele." *Leisure Sciences*, 2002, *24*, 143–159.

Greenway, R. "The Wilderness Effect and Ecopsychology." In T. Roszak, M. E. Gomes, and A. D. Kanner (eds.), *Ecopsychology: Restoring the Earth, Healing the Mind*. San Francisco: Sierra Club Books, 1995.

Haller, R. L., and Kramer, C. L. *Horticultural Therapy Methods: Making Connections in Health Care, Human Service, and Community Programs*. Philadelphia: Haworth Press, 2006.

Hamilton, E., and Cairns, H. (eds.). *Plato: The Collected Dialogues*. Princeton, N.J.: Princeton University Press, 1961.

Hartig, T., Mang, M., and Evans, G. "Restorative Effects of Natural Environmental Experiences." *Environment and Behavior*, 1991, *23*, 3–26.

Hartig, T., and Marcus, C. C. "Healing Gardens—Places for Nature in Health Care." *Lancet*, 2006, *368*, S36–S37.

Headey, B. "Pet Ownership: Good for Health?" *Medical Journal of Australia*, 2003, *179*, 460–461.

Heerwagen, J. H. "The Psychological Aspects of Windows and Window Design." In K. H. Anthony, J. Choi, and B. Orland (eds.), *Proceedings of the 21st Annual Conference of the Environmental Design Research Association*. Oklahoma City, Okla.: Environmental Design Research Association, 1990.

Heerwagen, J. H., and Orians, G. H. "Humans, Habitats, and Aesthetics." In S. R. Kellert and E. O. Wilson (eds.), *The Biophilia Hypothesis*. Washington, D.C.: Island Press, 1993.

Heerwagen, J. H., and Orians, G. H. "The Ecological World of Children." In P. H. J. Kahn and S. R. Kellert (eds.), *Children and Nature: Psychological, Sociocultural, and Evolutionary Investigations* (pp. 29–63). Cambridge, Mass.: MIT Press, 2002.

Ho, C., and others. "Ethnic Variations in Urban Park Preferences, Visitation, and Perceived Benefits." *Journal of Leisure Research*, 2005, *37*, 281–306.

Hobbs, T. R., and Shelton, G. C. "Therapeutic Camping for Emotionally Disturbed Adolescents." *Hospital & Community Psychiatry*, 1972, *23*, 298–301.

Honeyman, M. K. "Vegetation and Stress: A Comparison Study of Varying Amounts of Vegetation in Countryside and Urban Scenes." In D. Relf (ed.), *The Role of Horticulture in Human Well-Being and Social Development*. Portland, Ore.: Timber Press, 1992.

Hull, R. B., and Revell, G.R.B. "Cross-Cultural Comparison on Landscape Scenic Beauty Evaluations: A Case Study in Bali." *Journal of Environmental Psychology*, 1989, *9*, 177–191.

Hunt, M., Hind, A.-A., and Johnson, M. "Psychological Sequelae of Pet Loss Following Hurricane Katrina." *Anthrozoös*, 2008, *21*, 109–121.

Hunter, N. L. *Horticulture Programs in Prisons*. San Luis Obispo: California State Polytechnic College, Horticulture Department, 1970.

Hüttenmoser, M. "Children and Their Living Surroundings: Empirical Investigations into the Significance of Living Surroundings for the Everyday Life and Development of Children." *Children's Environments*, 1995, *12*, 403–413.

Hyer, L., and others. "Effects of Outward Bound Experience as an Adjunct to Inpatient PTSD Treatment of War Veterans." *Journal of Clinical Psychology*, 1996, *52*, 263–278.

Jerstad, L., and Stelzer, J. "Adventure Experiences as Treatment for Residential Mental Patients." *Therapeutic Recreation*, 1973, *7*, 8–11.

Jorm, A. F., and others. "Impact of Pet Ownership on Elderly Australians' Use of Medical Services: An Analysis Using Medicare Data." *Medical Journal of Australia*, 1997, *166*, 376–377.

Kahn, P. H., Jr. *The Human Relationship with Nature: Development and Culture*. Cambridge, Mass.: MIT Press, 1999.

Kahn, P. H. Jr., and Kellert, S. R. (eds.). *Children and Nature: Psychological, Sociocultural, and Evolutionary Investigations*. Cambridge, Mass.: MIT Press, 2002.

Kaplan, R. "The Role of Nature in the Urban Context." In I. Altman and J. F. Wohlwill (eds.), *Human Behavior and Environment*, Vol. *6*: *Behavior and the Natural Environment*. New York: Plenum, 1983.

Kaplan, R. "Dominant and Variable Values in Environmental Preference." In A. S. Devlin and S. L. Taylor (eds.), *Environmental Preference and Landscape Preference*. New London: Connecticut College, 1984.

Kaplan, R. "The Psychological Benefits of Nearby Nature." In D. Relf (ed.), *The Role of Horticulture in Human Well-Being and Social Development*. Portland, Ore.: Timber Press, 1992.

Kaplan, R. "The Nature of the View from Home: Psychological Benefits." *Environment and Behavior*, 2001, *33*, 507–542.

Kaplan, R., and Kaplan, S. *The Experience of Nature: A Psychological Perspective*. New York: Cambridge University Press, 1989.

Kaplan, S. "The Restorative Benefits of Nature: Toward an Integrative Framework." *Journal of Environmental Psychology*, 1995, *15*, 169–182.

Kaplan, S., and Kaplan, R. *Cognition and Environment*. New York: Praeger, 1982.

Kaplan, S., Talbot, J. F., and Kaplan, R. *Coping with Daily Hassles: The Impact of Nearby Nature on the Work Environment*. Washington, D.C.: USDA Forest Service, North Central Forest Experiment Station, 1988.

Katcher, A., Segal, H., and Beck, A. "Comparison of Contemplation and Hypnosis for the Reduction of Anxiety and Discomfort During Dental Surgery." *American Journal of Clinical Hypnosis*, 1984, *27*, 14–21.

Kellert, S. R. "*The Biological Basis for Human Values of Nature*." In S. R. Kellert and E. O. Wilson (eds.), *The Biophilia Hypothesis*. Washington, D.C.: Island Press, 1993.

Kellert, S. R. "Dimensions, Elements, and Attributes of Biophilic Design." In S. R. Kellert, J.
    Heerwagen, and M. Mador (eds.), *Biophilic Design: The Theory, Science and Practice of Bringing
    Buildings to Life* (pp. 3–19). Hoboken, N.J.: Wiley, 2008.

Kellert, S. R., Heerwagen J., and Mador M. (eds.). *Biophilic Design: The Theory, Science and Practice of
    Bringing Buildings to Life.* Hoboken, N.J.: Wiley, 2008.

Kennedy, B. P., and Minami, M. "The Beech Hill Hospital/Outward Bound Adolescent Chemical
    Dependency Treatment Program." *Journal of Substance Abuse Treatment*, 1993, *10*, 395–406.

Kirkby, M. "Nature as Refuge in Children's Environments." *Children's Environments Quarterly*, 1989, *6*,
    7–12.

Korpela, K., and Hartig, T. "Restorative Qualities of Favorite Places." *Journal of Environmental
    Psychology*, 1996, *16*, 221–233.

Kuo, F. E. "Coping with Poverty: Impacts of Environment and Attention in the Inner City." *Environment
    and Behavior*, 2001, *33*(1), 5–34.

Kuo, F. E., and Sullivan, W. C. "Aggression and Violence in the Inner City: Effects of Environment via
    Mental Fatigue." *Environment and Behavior*, 2001a, *33*(4), 543–571.

Kuo, F. E., and Sullivan, W. C. "Environment and Crime in the Inner City: Does Vegetation Reduce
    Crime?" *Environment and Behavior*, 2001b, *33*(3), 343–367.

Kuo, F. E., and Taylor, A. F. "A Potential Natural Treatment for Attention-Deficit/Hyperactivity
    Disorder: Evidence from a National Study." *American Journal of Public Health*, 2004, *94*,
    1580–1586.

Larsen, L., and others. "Plants in the Workplace: The Effects of Plant Density on Productivity,
    Attitudes, and Perceptions." *Environment and Behavior*, 1998, *30*, 261–282.

Levine, D. "Breaking Through Barriers: Wilderness Therapy for Sexual Assault Survivors." *Women and
    Therapy*, 1994, *15*(3–4), 175–184.

Lewis, C. A. "Gardening as Healing Process." In M. Francis and R. T. Hester (eds.), *The Meaning of
    Gardens.* Cambridge, Mass.: MIT Press, 1990.

Lewis, C. A. *Green Nature/Human Nature: The Meaning of Plants in Our Lives.* Urbana: University of Illinois
    Press, 1996.

Louv, R. *Last Child in the Woods: Saving our Children from Nature-Deficit Disorder.* Chapel Hill, N.C.:
    Algonquin Press, 2005.

Marx, J. D. "An Outdoor Adventure Counseling Program for Adolescents." *Social Work*, 1988, *33*,
    517–520.

Mattson, R. H. "Prescribing Health Benefits Through Horticultural Activities." In D. Relf (ed.), *The Role
    of Horticulture in Human Well-Being and Social Development.* Portland, Ore.: Timber Press, 1992.

McLuhan, T. C. *The Way of the Earth: Encounters with Nature in Ancient and Contemporary Thought.* New York:
    Simon & Schuster, 1994.

McNeil, E. B. "The Background of Therapeutic Camping." *Journal of Social Issues*, 1957, *13*, 3–14.

Mitchell, R., and Popham, F. "Effect of Exposure to Natural Environment on Health Inequalities: An
    Observational Population Study." *Lancet*, 2008, *372*, 1655–1660.

Moore, E. O. "A Prison Environment's Effect on Health Care Service Demands." *Journal of
    Environmental Systems*, 1981–1982, *11*, 17–34.

Moyer, J. A. "Bannock Bereavement Retreat: A Camping Experience for Surviving Children." *American
    Journal of Hospice Care*, 1988, *5*, 26–30.

Nabhan, G. P., and Trimble, S. *The Geography of Childhood: Why Children Need Wild Places*. Boston: Beacon Press, 1994.

Nash, R. *Wilderness and the American Mind*. (3rd ed.) New Haven, Conn.: Yale University Press, 1982.

Neese, R. "Prisoner's Escape." *Flower Grower*, 1959, *46*, 39–40.

Nielsen, T. S., and Hansen, K. B. "Do Green Areas Affect Health? Results from a Danish Survey on the Use of Green Areas and Health Indicators." *Health & Place*, 2007, *13*, 839–850.

Olmsted, F. L. "Public Parks and the Enlargement of Towns." In R. T. LeGates and F. Stout (eds.), *The City Reader* (pp. 314–320). (2nd ed.) London: Routledge, 1999. (Olmsted's essay originally published 1870.)

Orsega-Smith, E., Mowen, A., Payne, L., and Godbey, G. "The Interaction of Stress and Park Use on Psycho-Physiological Health in Older Adults." *Journal of Leisure Research*, 2004, *36*, 232–257.

Parslow, R. A., and others. "Pet Ownership and Health in Older Adults: Findings from a Survey of 2,551 Community-Based Australians Aged 60–64." *Gerontology*, 2005, *51*, 40–47.

Parsons, R., and others. "The View from the Road: Implications for Stress Recovery and Immunization." *Journal of Environmental Psychology*, 1998, *18*, 113–140.

Patel, I. C. "Socio-Economic Impact of Community Gardening in an Urban Setting." In D. Relf (ed.), *The Role of Horticulture in Human Well-Being and Social Development*. Portland, Ore.: Timber Press, 1992.

Payne, L., Orsega-Smith, E., Godbey, G., and Roy, M. "Local Parks and the Health of Older Adults: Results from an Exploratory Study." *Parks Recreation*, 1998, *33*(10), 64–70.

Pearson, J. "A Wilderness Program for Adolescents with Cancer." *Journal of the Association of Pediatric Oncology Nurses*, 1989, *6*, 24–25.

Perlman, M. *The Power of Trees: The Reforesting of the Soul*. Woodstock, Conn.: Spring, 1994.

Plakun, E., Tucker, G. J., and Harris, P. Q. "Outward Bound: An Adjunctive Psychiatric Therapy." *Journal of Psychiatric Treatment and Evaluation*, 1981, *3*, 33–37.

Pretty, J., Griffin, M., Sellens, M., and Pretty, C. Green Exercise: Complementary Roles of Nature, Exercise and Diet in Physical and Emotional Well-Being and Implications for Public Policy. CES Occasional Paper 2003–1. Centre for Environment and Society, University of Essex. http://www2.essex.ac.uk/ces/ResearchProgrammes/CESOccasionalPapers/GreenExercise.pdf, Mar. 2003.

Pretty, J., Peacock, J., Sellens, M., and Griffin, M. "The Mental and Physical Health Outcomes of Green Exercise." *International Journal of Environmental Health Research*, 2005, *15*, 319–337.

Purcell, A. T., Lamb, R. J., Peron, E. M., and Falchero, S. "Preference or Preferences for Landscape?" *Journal of Environmental Psychology*, 1994, *14*, 195–209.

Randall, K., Shoemaker, C. A., Relf, D., and Geller, E. S. "Effects of Plantscapes in an Office Environment on Worker Satisfaction." In D. Relf (ed.), *The Role of Horticulture in Human Well-Being and Social Development*. Portland, Ore.: Timber Press, 1992.

Reynolds, V. The Green Gym: An Evaluation of a Pilot Project in Sonning Common, Oxfordshire. Research Report #8. Oxford Brookes University, School of Health and Social Care, Oxford Centre for Health Care Research & Development.. : http://shsc.brookes.ac.uk/research/reports, 1999.

Reynolds, V. "The Green Gym." *Voluntary Action*. 2, 15–25. http://voluntaryaction.ivr.org.uk, 2000.

Reynolds, V. Well-Being Comes Naturally: An Evaluation of the BTCV Green Gym at Portslade, East Sussex. Research Report #17. Oxford Brookes University, School of Health and Social

Care, Oxford Centre for Health Care Research & Development. http://shsc.brookes.ac.uk/research/reports, 2002.

Roszak, T., Gomes, M. E., and Kanner, A. D. (eds.). *Ecopsychology: Restoring the Earth, Healing the Mind.* San Francisco: Sierra Club Books, 1995.

Sacks, O. *A Leg to Stand On.* New York: HarperCollins, 1984.

Schroeder, H. W., and Green, T. L. "Public Preferences for Tree Density in Municipal Parks." *Journal of Arboriculture,* 1985, *11,* 272–277.

Schukoske, J. E. "Community Development Through Gardening: State and Local Policies Transforming Urban Open Space." *Legislation and Public Policy,* 2000, *3,* 351–393.

Serpell, J. "Beneficial Effects of Pet Ownership on Some Aspects of Human Health and Behaviour." *Journal of the Royal Society of Medicine,* 1991, *84,* 717–720.

Sherer, P. M. The Benefits of Parks: Why America Needs More City Parks and Open Space. Trust for Public Land. http://www.tpl.org/content_documents/parks_for_people_Jul2005.pdf, 2006.

Shniderman, C. M. "Impact of Therapeutic Camping." *Social Work,* 1974, *19,* 354–357.

Siegel, J. "Stressful Life Events and Use of Physician Services Among the Elderly: The Moderating Role of Pet Ownership." *Journal of Personality and Social Psychology,* 1990, *58,* 1081–1086.

Simons, L. A., Simons, J., McCallum, J., Friedlander, Y. "Lifestyle Factors and Risk of Dementia: Dubbo Study of the Elderly." *Medical Journal of Australia,* 2006, *184,* 68–70.

Simson, S., and Straus M. C. *Horticulture as Therapy: Principles and Practice.* Philadelphia: Haworth Press, 2003.

Soderback, I., Soderstrom, M., and Schalander, E. "Horticultural Therapy: The 'Healing Garden' and Gardening in Rehabilitation Measures at Danderyd Hospital Rehabilitation Clinic, Sweden." *Pediatric Rehabilitation,* 2004, *7,* 245–260.

St. Leger, L. "Health and Nature–New Challenges for Health Promotion." [Editorial.] *Health Promotion International,* 2003, *18,* 173–175.

Taylor, A. F., Kuo, F. E., and Sullivan, W. C. "Views of Nature and Self-Discipline: Evidence from Inner City Children." *Journal of Environmental Psychology,* 2002, *22*(1–2), 49–63.

Tennessen, C. M., and Cimprich, B. "Views to Nature: Effects on Attention." *Journal of Environmental Psychology,* 1995, *15,* 77–85.

Ulrich, R. S. "Aesthetic and Affective Response to Natural Environment." In I. Altman and J. F. Wohlwill (eds.), *Human Behavior and Environment, Vol. 6: Behavior and the Natural Environment.* New York: Plenum, 1983.

Ulrich, R. S. "View Through a Window May Influence Recovery from Surgery." *Science,* 1984, *224,* 420–421.

Ulrich, R. S. Effects of Hospital Environments on Patient Well-Being. Research Report 9(55). Trondheim, Norway: University of Trondheim, Department of Psychiatry and Behavioral Medicine, 1986.

Ulrich, R. S. "Biophilia, Biophobia, and Natural Landscapes." In S. R. Kellert and E. O. Wilson (eds.), *The Biophilia Hypothesis.* Washington, D.C.: Island Press, 1993.

Ulrich, R. S., and others. "Stress Recovery During Exposure to Natural and Urban Environments." *Journal of Environmental Psychology,* 1991, *11,* 201–230.

Virden, R. J., and Walker, G. J. "Ethnic/Racial and Gender Variations Among Meanings Given to, and Preferences for, the Natural Environment." *Leisure Sciences,* 1999, *21,* 219–239.

Warady, B. A. "Therapeutic Camping for Children with End-Stage Renal Disease." *Pediatric Nephrology*, 1994, *8*, 387–390.

Wells, N. M. "At Home with Nature: Effects of "Greenness" on Children's Cognitive Functioning." *Environment and Behavior*, 2000, *32*, 775–795.

Wells, N. M., and Evans, G. W. "Nearby Nature: A Buffer of Life Stress Among Rural Children." *Environment and Behavior*, 2003, *35*, 311–330.

Wichrowski, M., and others. "Effects of Horticultural Therapy on Mood and Heart Rate in Patients Participating in an Inpatient Cardiopulmonary Rehabilitation Program." *Journal of Cardiopulmonary Rehabilitation*, 2005, *25*, 270–274.

Wilson, E. O. *Biophilia: The Human Bond with Other Species.* Cambridge, Mass.: Harvard University Press, 1984.

Wilson, E. O. *The Diversity of Life.* Cambridge, Mass.: Harvard University Press, 1992.

Wilson, E. O. "Biophilia and the Conservation Ethic." In S. R. Kellert and E. O. Wilson (eds.), *The Biophilia Hypothesis.* Washington, D.C.: Island Press, 1993.

Witman, J. P. "The Efficacy of Adventure Programming in the Development of Cooperation and Trust with Adolescents in Treatment." *Therapeutic Recreation Journal*, 1987, *21*, 22–29.

Wood, L., Giles-Corti, B., and Bulsara, M. "The Pet Connection: Pets as a Conduit for Social Capital." *Social Science & Medicine*, 2005, *61*, 1159–1173.

Wood, L. J., Giles-Corti, B, Bulsara, M. K. and Bosch, D. A. "More Than a Furry Companion: The Ripple Effect of Companion Animals on Neighborhood Interactions and Sense of Community." *Society and Animals*, 2007, *15*, 43–56.

Yi, S.-L. "A Life Renewed." *National Gardening*, 1985, *8*, 19–21.

FOR FURTHER INFORMATION

Books

Altman, I., and Wohlwill, J. F. (eds.). *Human Behavior and Environment*, Vol. 6: *Behavior and the Natural Environment.* New York: Plenum, 1983.

Caras, R. A. *A Perfect Harmony: The Intertwining Lives of Animals and Humans Throughout History.* New York: Fireside, 1996.

Fine, A. (ed.) *Handbook on Animal-Assisted Therapy: Theoretical Foundations and Guidelines for Practice.* San Diego: Academic Press, 2000.

Flagler, J., and Poincelot, R. P. *People-Plant Relationships: Setting Research Priorities.* Binghamton, N.Y.: Food Products Press, 1994.

Francis, M., Lindsey, P., and Rice, J. S. (eds.). *The Healing Dimensions of People-Plant Relations: Proceedings of a Research Symposium.* Davis: University of California Davis, Center for Design Research, 1994.

Kellert, S. R., and Wilson, E. O. (eds.). *The Biophilia Hypothesis.* Washington, D.C.: Island Press, 1993.

Maller, C., and others. *Healthy Parks, Healthy People: The Health Benefits of Contact with Nature in a Park Context: A Review of Relevant Literature.* (2nd ed.) Deakin University and Parks Victoria. http://www.parkweb.vic.gov.au/resources/mhphp/pv1.pdf, 2008.

Marcus, C. C., and Barnes, M. *Healing Gardens: Therapeutic Benefits and Design Recommendations*. Hoboken, N.J.: Wiley, 1999.

Relf, D. (ed.). *The Role of Horticulture in Human Well-Being and Social Development: A National Symposium, 19–21 April 1990, Arlington, Virginia*. Portland, Ore.: Timber Press, 1992.

Tyson, M. M. *The Healing Landscape: Therapeutic Outdoor Environments*. New York: McGraw-Hill, 1998.

Three books already listed in the chapter References are also especially useful; they are Gerlach-Spriggs, Kaufman, and Warner, 1998; Lewis, 1996; and Louv, 2005.

University-Based Web Sites

Edinburgh College of Art, OPENspace, http://openspace.eca.ac.uk. OPENspace is a research center for inclusive access to outdoor environments. Its Web site includes reviews on the health benefits of access to open space and nature (with titles such as Health, Well-Being, and Open Space focusing on such groups as ethnic minorities and teenagers).

Purdue University, Center for the Human-Animal Bond, http://www.vet.purdue.edu/chab. This research and education center investigates the health effects of animal contact. Its Web site provides research results and links to a number of related sites.

University of Illinois, Landscape and Human Health Laboratory, http://www.lhhl.uiuc.edu. This laboratory is a leader in research on benefits of nature contact. Its Web site contains information in a variety of interesting categories, such as "Canopy & Crime," "Girls & Greenery," "Kids & Concentration," "Neighbors & Nature," "Plants & Poverty," and "Vegetation & Violence."

University of Essex, Centre for Environment and Society, http://www2.essex.ac.uk/ces/ResearchProgrammes/NewPageCollaborative ResProg.htm‥ This university center has a research focus on human health, including the benefits of nature contact. Its Web site offers research papers on topics such as green exercise and links to other useful sites.

Professional Organizations

People-Plant Council, http://www.hort.vt.edu/HUMAN/PPC.html.
American Horticultural Therapy Association, http://www.ahta.org.
Delta Society (the human-animal health connection), http://www.deltasociety.org.

Nongovernmental Organizations

Children & Nature Network (C&NN), http://www.childrenandnature.org. CN&N is dedicated to reconnecting children with nature. Its Web site includes news, reviews of current research, and links to key resources.

Government Project

European Cooperation in Science and Technology (COST), http://www.cost.esf.org. Among COST's wide range of projects is one, COST 39, that focuses on forests, trees, and human health and well-being. Its five working groups, with experts from across Europe, address physical and mental health and well-being, forest products, forest environment and health, therapeutic aspects including rehabilitation and outdoor education, evaluation in terms of best practice and economic contribution, and physical activity, well-being and prevention of illness. COST 39 can be visited at several web sites:

http://www.e39.ee
http://www.cost.esf.org/index.php?id=143&action_number=e39
http://www.forestresearch.gov.uk/fr/INFD-66LJNL

CHAPTER TWENTY-FIVE

CHILDREN

Maida P. Galvez

Joel Forman

Philip J. Landrigan

KEY CONCEPTS

- As medicine has advanced, the pattern of illness in children has changed, from episodic outbreaks of infectious diseases to chronic illnesses such as asthma, developmental disorders, cancer, and obesity, which have been termed the *new pediatric morbidity*. The environmentally attributable contribution to pediatric chronic diseases is substantial.

- The chemical revolution that began in the 1950s has led to widespread exposure of children to thousands of synthetic chemicals. The majority of these chemicals have not been tested for toxicity to children.

- A fundamental concept in pediatric environmental health is that children are uniquely vulnerable to toxic environmental exposures. A careful environmental history is critical to the evaluation of possible toxic exposures in children.

- Many gaps remain in our knowledge about environmental hazards to children. Traditional risk assessment approaches have not adequately protected children. New approaches are needed that place children and not chemicals at the center of the paradigm.

- Public health policies that reduce the use of toxins can successfully reduce children's exposure. This has been dramatically demonstrated with the reduction in childhood lead poisoning after the removal of lead from gasoline.

THE environment in which children live today is very different from that of fifty years ago. The chemical revolution has been one major engine of environmental change. As a result of advances in chemistry, there now exist more than 80,000 synthetic chemicals, nearly all of them invented since the 1950s (U.S. Environmental Protection Agency [EPA], 1998). They include plastics, pesticides, motor fuels, building materials, antibiotics, chemotherapeutic agents, flame retardants, and synthetic hormones. Children are especially at risk of exposure to the more than 3,000 synthetic chemicals that are produced in quantities of 1 million pounds or more per year (EPA, 2007b). These high production volume (HPV) chemicals are distributed widely in the environment—in air, food, water, and consumer products. In recent national surveys conducted by the Centers for Disease Control and Protection (CDC), measurable quantities of more than 100 HPV synthetic chemicals were detected in the bodies of American children (CDC, 2005). Only 43 percent of HPV chemicals have been tested for their potential to cause toxicity (EPA, 2007b). This lack of toxicological data creates a setting in which new chemicals can cause and have caused adverse effects in children (and in adults) without warning.

Population growth, rapid urbanization, and development of the macroenvironment represent a second dimension of environmental change in the past fifty years. Especially rapid evolution has occurred in the **built environment**—housing, roads and walkways, transportation networks, shops and markets, and parks and public spaces (Weich and others, 2001). Urban, rural, suburban, agricultural, and developing areas each have unique environmental features, and the impacts of chemical exposures on children's health are mediated by the contextual settings of these built environments.

It is now understood that the environment, on both the micro (chemical) and the macro (structural) level, has a profound ability to affect children's growth and development, exerting positive as well as negative influences (Briggs, 2003). Health and disease are the products of complex interactions among multiple genetic, behavioral, cultural, familial, socioeconomic, and environmental factors. The study of environmental factors and their effects on children's health is critical to understanding the etiology of a vast array of common childhood conditions from, asthma to obesity, and to developing evidence-based strategies for disease prevention and health promotion.

Children's environmental health issues are important not only to parents and pediatricians but to society at large. Children's unknowing exposure to hundreds

Maida P. Galvez, Joel Forman, and Philip J. Landrigan declare no competing financial interests.

of new chemicals makes them the experimental subjects in a lifelong uncontrolled experiment. Children unduly bear the burden of such permanent and irreversible effects of toxic environmental exposures as decreased intelligence, birth defects, and developmental delays. This chapter introduces the field of children's environmental health with a historical account of the recognition that children are a special population, discusses general considerations in examining environmental etiologies for children's health problems, and presents case studies of specific environmental exposures, including pesticides, lead, solvents, mold, and neighborhood design. It concludes with a discussion of risk assessment and risk communication as they apply to children.

CHILDREN AS A SPECIAL POPULATION

Our understanding that children require special attention with respect to environmental exposures involves the changing patterns of disease among children, the economic burden of children's diseases, and children's particular sensitivity to environmental exposures.

Changing Patterns of Disease

Patterns of illness among children in the United States and other industrially developed nations have changed substantially in the past century (Haggerty and Rothmann, 1975). The major diseases confronting children in developed nations today are chronic illnesses, such as asthma, which doubled in prevalence from 1980 to the 1990s and remains at historically high levels (Akinbami, 2006); congenital malformations, deformations, and chromosomal abnormalities, which, combined, remain the leading cause of infant death (Matthews and MacDorman, 2008); developmental disorders, such as attention deficit/hyperactivity disorder (Pastor and Reuben, 2008); and childhood cancer, which has increased in incidence since the 1970s (Ries and others, 2004). Collectively, these diseases are termed the **new pediatric morbidity**. The traditionally critical infectious diseases are much reduced in incidence, and in developed nations (in contrast to the situation in developing nations) they are no longer the leading causes of illness and death (DiLiberti and Jackson, 1999). Infant mortality has been lowered, although not equally across U.S. society, and life expectancy increased.

Evidence is increasing that toxic chemicals in the environment are important causes of disease in children. It is now hypothesized that the majority of disease in childhood is the consequence of interactions between the environment— defined broadly to include diet and lifestyle factors as well as toxic chemical exposures—and individual, genetically determined susceptibility (Olden and Wilson, 2000).

Economic Burden of Pediatric Environmental Disease

The contribution of environmental pollutants to the incidence, prevalence, mortality, and costs of disease in U.S. children is substantial. Landrigan and others (2002b) examined this burden for four categories of illness—lead poisoning, asthma, cancer, and neurobehavioral disorders. They found that the costs of these environmentally related diseases in children amount to $54.9 billion annually, approximately 2.8 percent of the total annual cost of illness in the United States. These costs may be compared to the annual health care costs attributable to motor vehicle crashes ($80.6 billion) and those due to stroke ($51.5 billion) (Conover, n.d.). The projected costs of military weapons research in 2003 totaled $53.9 billion (Center for Defense Information, 2002). The costs of pediatric disease of environmental origin are large compared with the relatively meager amount of money spent on research related to children (Office of Science and Technology Policy, National Science and Technology Council, 1997). Landrigan and others concluded that diseases of toxic environmental origin among children make an important and insufficiently recognized contribution to total health care costs in the United States.

The costs of pediatric disease of environmental origin will likely become yet greater in the years ahead if children's exposures to inadequately tested chemicals are permitted to continue. Increased investment is required in tracking and surveillance (Pew Environmental Health Commission, 2000), in basic studies of disease mechanisms, and in prevention-oriented epidemiological research, such as the National Children's Study (Berkowitz and others, 2001; Landrigan and others, 2006). Most important, increased investment in pollution prevention is needed.

Children's Sensitivity to Environmental Exposures: A Historical Perspective

Environmental pediatrics originated in early studies of major outbreaks of acute disease of toxic origin in children. These analyses formed the basis for the current understanding that children are uniquely vulnerable to many toxins in the environment. The following are some of the more notable of these early analyses:

- A 1904 report from Queensland, Australia, describing an epidemic of lead poisoning in young children (Gibson, 1904). Clinical and epidemiological investigation traced the source of the outbreak to the ingestion of lead-based paint by children playing on verandas. This study was the first report of lead poisoning from paint in children, and it led to the banning of lead-based paint in many nations.

- A study of an epidemic of leukemia in the 1940s and 1950s among young children in Hiroshima and Nagasaki who were exposed to ionizing radiation in the 1945 atomic bombings (Miller, 1956). This study and subsequent studies of fetuses exposed in utero (see, for example, Gurney and others, 1996) established that infants and fetuses are more susceptible than adults to leukemia after radiation exposure. In addition, an increased risk of microcephaly was observed among infants who were exposed to radiation in the first trimester of pregnancy during the bombings (Miller and Blot, 1972).

- A report from Minamata, Japan, in the 1960s of an epidemic of cerebral palsy, mental retardation, and convulsions among children living in a fishing village on the Inland Sea (Harada, 1978). This epidemic was traced to ingestion of fish and shellfish contaminated with methylmercury. The source of the mercury was found to be a plastics factory that had discharged metallic mercury into the sediments on the floor of Minamata Bay. The mercury was transformed by microorganisms into methylmercury, and it then bioaccumulated as it moved up the marine food chain, eventually reaching people who ate fish and shellfish. The most devastating effects were seen among children exposed in utero. Similar epidemics of **Minamata disease** occurred subsequently in Guatemala (Ordonez, Carrillo, Miranda, and Gale, 1966), Iraq (Bakir and others, 1973), and New Mexico (Pierce and others, 1972).

- Studies of the epidemic of phocomelia (congenital limb malformations) that followed the ingestion of **thalidomide** as an antiemetic agent in early pregnancy (McBride, 1961; Taussig, 1962). More than 15,000 cases were reported worldwide.

- A report on cases of adenocarcinoma of the vagina among young women who had been exposed in utero to the synthetic estrogen diethylstilbestrol, taken in pregnancy by their mothers to prevent premature labor (Herbst, Hubby, Azizi, and Makii, 1981).

Robert W. Miller, a pediatrician who served for many years as an epidemiologist with the U.S. National Cancer Institute, deserves great recognition as the first scientist to move beyond the study of specific outbreaks of acute environmental disease in children to the realization that children are unusually sensitive to a broad range of environmental toxins. Miller stressed the key role of the alert clinician in identifying associations between environmental exposures and pediatric disease. Early in his career Miller was assigned by the U.S. Public Health Service to the Atomic Bomb Casualty Commission (now the Radiation Effects

Research Foundation) in Hiroshima, Japan. His research there elucidated the epidemiology of leukemia in children exposed to the atomic bombings (Miller, 1956). He returned to the United States, and in the late 1960s he established the Committee on Environmental Hazards (now the Committee on Environmental Health) of the **American Academy of Pediatrics**, a scholarly body that has been of seminal importance for development of the discipline of environmental pediatrics.

Herbert L. Needleman is a second pediatrician who contributed enormously to the development of environmental pediatrics. Needleman's research centered on the study of lead neurotoxicity in children (Needleman and others, 1979, 1990). His seminal contribution was the recognition that lead can cause toxic effects at levels of exposure too low to produce clinically overt symptoms. This recognition gave rise to the now widely applied concept of *subclinical toxicity*, the idea that toxic agents such as lead produce a spectrum of effects ranging from coma, convulsions, and death at high-end exposures to silent brain injury with loss of intelligence and disruption of behavior at low-end exposures. Needleman's other great contribution was in the realm of evidence-based advocacy. When he was charged falsely by the lead industry with having fabricated his results, he demonstrated great courage in standing his ground and in allowing his data to be examined objectively by the National Institutes of Health. For his scientific contributions to the health of children as well as for his courage, Needleman was subsequently awarded the Heinz Award in the Environment.

Four key historical milestones that further advanced the development of environmental pediatrics were the publication by the National Research Council in 1993 of *Pesticides in the Diets of Infants and Children*, passage of the Food Quality Protection Act in 1996, promulgation of a presidential Executive Order on children's health and the environment in 1997, and passage of the Consumer Product Safety Improvement Act in 2008.

Report on Pesticides in the Diets of Infants and Children, 1993   An event of catalytic importance in bringing environmental threats to children's health to the attention of policymakers was the formation in 1988 of the National Research Council (NRC) Committee on Pesticides in the Diets of Infants and Children. This committee, chaired by physician Philip Landrigan, was convened at the request of the Senate Committee on Agriculture. The congressional charge to the committee was threefold:

1. To explore differences in exposure to pesticides between children and adults and the implications of those differences for risk assessment
2. To explore differences in susceptibility to pesticides between children and adults and their implications for risk assessment

3. To analyze federal laws and regulations regarding food use pesticides to determine whether those rules adequately protected the health of infants and children

The committee issued its final report in 1993 (NRC, 1993). The major conclusion was that "children are not little adults." By that phrase the committee meant that children are qualitatively different from adults both in their patterns of exposure and in their vulnerability to pesticides and other toxic chemicals. Specifically, the committee noted four fundamental differences between children and adults:

1. Children have disproportionately heavy exposures to environmental toxicants.
2. Children's metabolic pathways, especially in the first months after birth, are immature. In many instances children are less able than adults are to deal with toxic compounds.
3. Children are undergoing rapid growth and development. These developmental processes create windows of unique vulnerability in which the course of development can be disrupted permanently by environmental toxins.
4. Because children have more future years of life than do adults, they have more time to develop chronic diseases that may be triggered by early exposures with long latency periods.

The NRC committee also concluded that the federal laws and regulations governing the use of agricultural pesticides were not sufficiently strict to protect the health of children. The committee found that these laws and regulations were targeted toward protecting the health of healthy adults and accounted for neither the unique exposures nor the special susceptibilities of children. The committee recommended that federal policies for regulating agricultural pesticides be revamped fundamentally. Specific recommendations included the following:

- Collect better data on children's exposure to pesticides.
- Improve toxicological testing of pesticides to include assessments of developmental toxicity.
- Perform toxicological studies that examine the long-term and delayed effects of early exposures to pesticides.
- Examine the possible interactive effects among multiple pesticides, especially those that act through similar mechanisms of action.
- Protect the health of children by imposing an extra margin of safety in setting standards for pesticides when data on children's unique exposures or special susceptibilities to a particular pesticide are lacking or when the data show that children are uniquely susceptible to that pesticide.

PERSPECTIVE
The Unique Susceptibility of Children

Children are highly vulnerable to environmental toxins. **Children's unique susceptibility** stems from several sources. Children have greater exposures to environmental toxins than do adults (NRC, 1993). Children drink more water, eat more food, and breathe more air per kilogram of body weight than do adults. For example, in the first six months of life infants consume seven times as much water (in total) per kilogram as do average adults. Children aged one through five years eat three to four times more food per kilogram than do adults. Furthermore, children have unique food preferences. For example, the average one-year-old drinks twenty-one times more apple juice and eleven times more grape juice and eats two to seven times more grapes, bananas, pears, carrots, and broccoli than does the average adult (Wiles and Campbell, 1993). The air intake of a resting infant, per unit of body weight, is twice that of an adult. These patterns of increased consumption reflect the rapid metabolism of children as well as their need to fuel growth and development.

The implication for health is that children may have substantially greater exposure per kilogram to toxic materials that are present in water, food, or air. Two additional characteristics of children further magnify their exposures to toxins in the environment: they frequently put their hands in their mouths, which increases their ingestion of any toxins in dust or soil, and they play close to the ground, which increases their exposure to toxins in dust, soil, and carpets as well as to toxins that form low-lying layers in the air, as certain pesticide vapors do.

The metabolic pathways of children, especially in the first months after birth, are immature compared with those of adults (Spielberg, 1992). As a consequence of this biochemical immaturity, the ability of a child to detoxify and excrete certain toxins is different from that of an adult. In some instances children are actually better able than adults to deal with environmental toxins. More commonly, however, they are less able than adults to deal with toxic chemicals and thus are more vulnerable to them (NRC, 1993).

Children undergo rapid growth and development, and their delicate developmental processes are easily disrupted (NRC, 1993). Many organ systems in young children, such as the nervous, reproductive, and immune systems, undergo very rapid growth, development, and differentiation during the first months and years of life. During this period, structures are developed and vital connections are established. These developmental processes create windows of great vulnerability to environmental toxicants, in which even minute exposures can produce devastating results. The nervous system, for example, is not well able to repair any structural damage that is caused by environmental toxins. If cells in the developing brain are destroyed by chemicals such as lead, mercury, or solvents or if formation of vital connections between nerve cells is blocked, then there is a high risk that the resulting neurobehavioral dysfunction will be permanent and irreversible. The consequences can be loss of intelligence and alteration of normal behavior (Eriksson and others, 2001). Similar considerations pertain in the reproductive, immune, endocrine, and cardiovascular systems.

Food Quality Protection Act, 1996   In 1996, three years after release of the NRC report *Pesticides in the Diets of Infants and Children*, the U.S. Congress, by unanimous vote of both Houses, passed the **Food Quality Protection Act** (FQPA), the major federal legislation governing the use of pesticides in agriculture. The FQPA incorporates all the major recommendations of the NRC committee. It requires that pesticide standards be based primarily on health considerations and that standards be set at levels that protect the health of infants and children. It requires that an extra margin of safety be incorporated into pesticide risk assessment when data show that a particular pesticide is especially toxic to infants and children or when data on the toxicity to infants and children are lacking. It requires that interactive effects among pesticides be considered. Finally, the FQPA requires that pesticides be assessed systematically for possible endocrine-disrupting effects.

Passage of the FQPA was a watershed event for children's environmental health. As the first federal environmental statute to call explicitly for protecting children's health against environmental hazards, it marked a paradigm shift in federal policy. The consequences of the FQPA have extended far beyond the regulation of agricultural pesticides.

Executive Order on Children's Health and the Environment, 1997   In April 1997, President Clinton and Vice President Gore signed an Executive Order titled **Protection of Children from Environmental Health Risks and Safety Risks**. This order declared that protection of children's environmental health would be a high priority of that administration. It established a cabinet-level oversight committee on children's environmental health, cochaired by the administrator of the U.S. Environmental Protection Agency and the secretary of the U.S. Department of Health and Human Services. This committee was given broad responsibility to review the programs of all cabinet agencies to ensure that they were protective of children's health. Never previously had children's environmental health enjoyed such a high profile within the federal government. Consequences of the work of this cabinet-level committee include the establishment of a national network of children's environmental health and disease prevention research centers and the launching of the National Children's Study; both of these developments are discussed later in this chapter.

The Consumer Product Safety Improvement Act of 2008   In 2007, millions of toys found to be contaminated with lead were recalled from store shelves, including lead-contaminated toy trains, dolls, vinyl lunch boxes, and toy jewelry. Lead is a highly toxic chemical and brain injury is the most serious consequence of pediatric lead poisoning. Young children are especially vulnerable to lead because their brains are rapidly developing and because their normal hand-to-mouth behavior increases the risk that they will take lead into their bodies from the environment.

This situation highlighted the lack of federal controls on imported toys. To address these issues, the **Consumer Product Safety Improvement Act** of 2008 was passed by the House and Senate by overwhelming margins and subsequently signed into law by President Bush. Of particular significance, the Act now requires mandatory third-party safety testing and certification of all toys and products marketed to children twelve years of age and younger. It also bans all but trace amounts of lead and the plasticizers called **phthalates** in children's toys and products (discussed later in this chapter). This groundbreaking legislation thus addresses the previous lack of required premarket testing of children's toys and products.

However, even though the Consumer Product Safety Improvement Act of 2008 makes major strides with respect to protecting children from environmental toxins in children's toys and products, the lack of premarket testing of synthetic chemicals in widespread use in everyday items remains a concern. The U.S. government's failure to require premarket testing of synthetic chemicals leaves pediatricians and the American public to learn about toxicities through recognition of the unanticipated consequences of human exposure, thus in effect making all inhabitants of the Earth canaries in a coal mine.

FIGURE 25.1   A Children's Playground Located Near a Source of Toxic Emissions

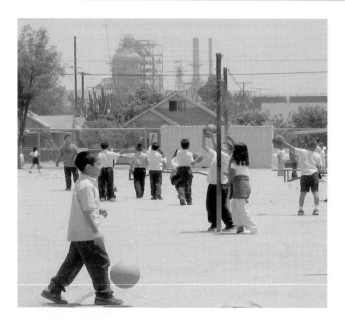

Source: Photo by Andrea Hricko; used with permission.

FIGURE 25.2   Children Bathing in a Drum That
Once Held a Toxic Chemical

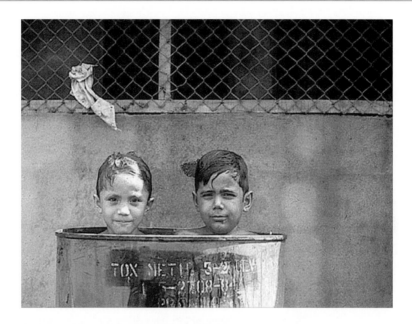

Source: Photo by Don Cole; used with permission.

As a consequence of these advances, environmental pediatrics has emerged as a new field of research and practice and has systematically begun to address questions about the role of environmental factors in the etiology of a diverse range of childhood illnesses. Since the late 1990s, children's environmental health has become an increasingly important and visible component of pediatric practice. The American Academy of Pediatrics (AAP) published the *Handbook of Pediatric Environmental Health* in 1999 (and a second edition five years later), a resource commonly referred to as the Green Book. National conferences have been held on the impact of environmental toxins on the health of children, and journals have devoted entire issues to topics in children's environmental health (Weiss and Landrigan, 2000; Paulson and Gitterman, 2007a, 2007b; Alimonti, Böse-O'Reilly, Moshammer, and van den Hazel, 2008). The national network of research-oriented **Centers for Children's Environmental Health and Disease Prevention** and a parallel network of clinically oriented **Pediatric Environmental Health Specialty Units** have been established in the United States and abroad. As the field of environmental pediatrics grows as a specialty so does the body of research by leading scientists and clinicians who seek to further our understanding of the impact of environmental exposures on the growth and development of children.

CASE STUDIES IN ENVIRONMENTAL PEDIATRICS

Clinicians who evaluate patients need to consider the possibility of environmental contributions to symptoms and disease (as described in Chapter Twenty-Seven). This is as true for children as it is for adults. A high index of suspicion is critical to making a correct diagnosis. This suspicion will guide environmental screening questions when taking a history. Integral to an environmental history is obtaining information about current and past exposures, potential sources of toxic exposures, exposure settings, and potential routes of exposures (Figures 25.1 and 25.2). Particular attention must be paid to those factors unique to the age and

PERSPECTIVE
The Dilemma of Breast Feeding

Human milk is without question the best source of nutrition for human infants. Breast milk contains the optimal balance of fats, carbohydrates, and proteins for developing babies, and it provides a range of benefits for growth, immunity, and development (Institute of Medicine, Food and Nutrition Board, 1991). Breast milk contains immune factors that help infants fight infections (Oddy, 2001), and it contains growth factors that appear to influence brain development and increase resistance to chronic diseases such as asthma, allergies, and diabetes. Breast feeding builds a bond between a mother and her child, and this bond enhances health and well-being across the generations. For these reasons, the American Academy of Pediatrics recommends exclusive breast feeding for a minimum of six months.

Unfortunately, breast milk is not pristine. Contamination of human milk is widespread, the result of decades of inadequately controlled pollution of the environment by toxic chemicals. Polychlorinated biphenyls (PCBs), dichlorodiphenyltrichloroethane (DDT) and its metabolites, dioxins, dibenzofurans, polybrominated diphenyl ethers (**PBDEs**), and heavy metals are among the toxic chemicals most often found as **breast milk contaminants** (Hooper and McDonald, 2000; Solomon and Weiss, 2002). These compounds are encountered to varying extents among women in developed as well as developing nations. Some of the highest levels of contamination are seen among women in agricultural areas of the developing world that are extensively treated with pesticides (Hooper and others, 1999) and among women in remote areas. An example of the latter are the Canadian Inuit, who eat a diet rich in seal, whale, and other species high on the marine food chain developmental stage of the child. These principles are illustrated in the case studies that follow and that examine typical routes of exposure and exposure settings.

Routes of Exposure

When the possibility of environmental etiology is under diagnostic consideration, it is important to determine whether a plausible pathway of exposure exists. Exposure pathways vary by chemical and by stage of life. As described in Chapter Two, the major routes for adults are inhalation, ingestion, and skin absorption, with parenteral (intravenous and intramuscular) routes sometimes being important. For children, it is important also to consider transplacental transfer and breast milk. At times multiple pathways may be involved—for example, both skin absorption and inhalation, as in the case of metallic mercury, to which children may be exposed both by skin contact and by inhalation of vapors.

that accumulate heavy burdens of persistent organic pollutants (**POPs**) (Dewailly and others, 1993).

The finding of toxic chemicals in breast milk raises a series of important issues for pediatric practice, for the practice of public health, and for the environmental health research community (Landrigan and others, 2002a; Solomon, Weiss, Owen, and Citron, 2005). It also illuminates gaps in current knowledge, including insufficient information on the nature and levels of contaminants in breast milk, lack of consistent protocols for collecting and analyzing breast milk samples, lack of toxicokinetic data, and lack of data on children's health outcomes following exposure to chemicals in breast milk. These gaps impede risk assessment and make it difficult to formulate evidence-based health guidance.

In the clinical setting mothers often pose the question of potential harms from breast feeding. Yet the longitudinal studies of babies who consumed breast milk that are needed to answer this question are lacking. Though there are tests available to measure the levels of chemical contaminants such as dioxins in breast milk, there are no standard reference values that define a "safe" level of exposure. In the absence of such standards the information that results from breast milk testing is, except in extreme cases, difficult to interpret and of little use clinically.

The American Academy of Pediatrics (2005) does not recommend that mothers routinely have their breast milk tested for environmental contaminants. The benefits of human milk far outweigh the risks, so women should not stop breast feeding because of concerns about environmental contamination, unless specifically advised to do so by a pediatrician or pediatric environmental specialist. The take-home message is that "breast is best" in terms of infant feedings, but large-scale, prospective studies are still needed to clarify the health effects of environmental contaminants commonly found in breast milk.

In keeping with the principles of developmental toxicology, the diagnostic evaluation should identify specific behaviors unique to a child's age that may place him or her at increased risk. The following cases illustrate routes of exposure and highlight the unique susceptibility of children to environmental exposures in the context of everyday experiences.

Exposure Through Inhalation: Case Study on Air Pollutants   In a New York inner-city neighborhood, community-based organizations, **environmental justice** coalitions, parents' associations, community board members, and schools came together to oppose the reopening of a depot for diesel-powered buses across the street from a public elementary school and adjacent to low-income housing projects (Northridge and others, 1999; West Harlem Environmental Action, 2005). The primary concern was the potential health effects, particularly asthma, related to diesel exhaust. This neighborhood has the highest rates of asthma citywide.

Diesel exhaust is recognized to be a serious health hazard (as discussed in Chapter Twelve). It is a known respiratory irritant and has been shown to exacerbate asthma in susceptible individuals. It contains many toxic chemicals, and two pose especially critical risks to human health. The first, oxides of nitrogen (NO_x), is a major contributor to ground-level ozone. These oxides are corrosive to lung tissue and act as powerful respiratory irritants, worsening asthma and causing bronchitis. The second, particulate matter, can also be inhaled and can lodge deep in the lungs. The particulates contain abundant polycyclic aromatic hydrocarbons (**PAHs**), a class of chemicals recognized by the Environmental Protection Agency as human carcinogens.

Children are particularly sensitive to NO_x and airborne particulate matter in diesel exhaust for several reasons. First, children breathe more rapidly than adults, allowing for the inhalation of more pollutants per kilogram of body weight. Children also spend more time playing outdoors and close to the ground, increasing their likelihood of being exposed to outdoor air pollutants. Also, children have an entire lifetime over which to develop chronic illnesses related to environmental exposures incurred early on.

Grassroots activism has raised awareness of the disproportionate siting of bus depots in predominantly low-income, minority communities as an environmental justice issue (see Chapter Eight). Despite these efforts the groups were unable to defeat the opening of the bus depot in 2003. Still, concessions were made, including the addition of a roof on the depot building. Activists have not backed down, however, and continue to press for conversion of the city's bus fleet to ultra low sulfur diesel fuel or compressed natural gas. They are also advocating for enforcement of anti-idling laws, which prohibit buses from running their engines while standing in the city streets.

Exposure Through Ingestion: Case Study on Pesticides in Food and Water   A program in the Yakima and Columbia River valleys in Washington State is reaching out to adolescent and adult female migrant and seasonal farmworkers at risk for health effects from pesticide exposure. By definition, migrant workers are those who move from one agricultural community to another, as dictated by the crops that are in season. For these workers and their children the risk of pesticide exposure is heightened by the indoor and outdoor contamination of their homes through spraying, take-home exposures, and soil and water contamination. This combination of exposures from many routes may result in widespread contamination of areas where children eat, sleep, and play. Both the water supply and food products, including locally grown produce, may also be affected.

Ingestion of contaminated food products is the predominant source of exposure to pesticides for the general population. In one study (Curl, Fenske, and Elgethun, 2003), parents kept records of what foods their children ate, and investigators found that children whose diets were predominantly organic had significantly lower levels of pesticides in their urine than children who ate a conventional diet. In another study (Lu and others, 2006), parents agreed to replace their children's conventional diets with organic diets for five days, and collected urine samples before, during, and after this period. As shown in Figure 25.3, urinary detection of pesticide residues (in this case, malathion) declined dramatically while the children ate organic diets. As expressed by the investigators of the first study, "consumption of organic fruits, vegetables and juices can reduce children's exposure levels from above to below the U.S. Environmental Protection Agency's current guidelines, thereby shifting exposures from a range of uncertain risk to a range of negligible risk. Consumption of organic produce appears to provide a relatively simple way for parents to reduce their children's exposure to organophosphate pesticides" (p. 382).

Even though there are known benefits to pesticide use, such as increased crop yield and prevention of insect- and rodent-borne diseases, the benefits must be tempered by consideration of potential risks (see Chapter Seventeen). Depending on the pesticide of concern, a variety of health effects have been detected. Multiple organ systems may be affected, including the lungs, kidneys, digestive tract, immune system, and central nervous system. In addition, the EPA considers several organophosphate pesticides to be probable carcinogens. Epidemiological studies support a relationship between pesticide exposure and subsequent development of brain cancer, non-Hodgkin's lymphoma, and leukemia (Zahm and Ward 1998; Sanborn and others, 2004). In examining the effects of exposures to pesticides during pregnancy, studies have suggested an association with limb reduction defects (Engel, O'Meara, and Schwartz, 2000); cryptorchidism, or undescended testes (Weidner, Moller, Jensen, and Skakkebaek, 1998;

FIGURE 25.3   Daily Average Excretion of Malathion Dicarboxylic
Acid (MDA), a Metabolite of Malathion, in Children Aged 3-11
Before, During, and After a Diet of Organic Food

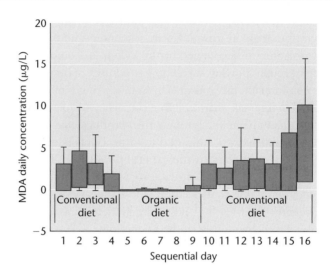

Source: Lu and others, 2006; reproduced with permission from *Environmental Health Perspectives.*

Damgaard and others, 2006; Andersen, 2008); neural tube defects (Shaw and others, 1999; Brender, 2002; Rull, 2006); heart problems (Loffredo, Silbergeld, Ferencz, and Zhang, 2001); and impaired fetal growth (Longnecker, Klebanoff, Zhou, and Brock, 2001; Whyatt and others, 2005).

To remove pesticide residues from produce, parents are advised to rinse fresh produce thoroughly with water before it is cooked or eaten. Peeling reduces the levels of pesticides that may be on the surface, though some residues remain because they have been absorbed into the food. Eating a diet with many different fruits, vegetables, and grains is a healthy practice that may also prevent overexposure to a single pesticide residue found in a particular crop. The most effective method to reduce intake is consumption of certified organic produce grown with minimal or no synthetic chemicals.

For seasonal and migrant workers, pesticide exposures from the food supply are compounded by occupational exposures. Many farm workers are not aware of the risks associated with pesticide exposure or have not been educated about preventive measures that can reduce negative health impacts of such exposure. Some workers choose not to practice behaviors that could minimize negative health effects. A cooperative effort of the National Catholic Rural Life Conference (NCRLC), organizations engaged in pesticide education or providing services to migrants, Radio Cadena and other Hispanic media, the Diocese of Yakima, and four Catholic parishes is helping adolescent and adult, female migrant and seasonal farmworkers to reduce the negative health impacts of agricultural pesticides. As part of this project the parishes involved have developed and implemented educational sessions on the reduction of health impacts from agricultural pesticides and have evaluated the effects of these sessions. They have also created an educational series of radio minidramas, news pieces, and public service announcements. This is one example of how a religious group has identified a need in the community and mobilized resources to provide pesticide safety and sanitation education. Church-based initiatives such as this one provide a unique opportunity to reach many members of a community.

Exposure Through the Skin: Case Study on DEET   The members of a family living in the United States are returning to their native country in sub-Saharan Africa for a four-week vacation and are discussing concerns about malaria with their family pediatrician. The parents are bringing along on the trip their three children: a fifteen-month-old infant son, a four-year-old son, and a nine-year-old daughter. They plan to use malaria prophylaxis in addition to insecticide-treated mosquito netting at night. However, they have also seen a number of insect repellants available in the local pharmacy. Today they are bringing in a specific repellant for the pediatrician's review; they want to know if it is approved for use in children. The active ingredient is **DEET** (N,N-diethyl-m-toluamide, also known as N,N-diethyl-3-methylbenzamide), at a concentration of 10 percent.

The pediatrician advises the family that DEET is a widely used product that repels a variety of insects including mosquitoes and ticks. Concentrations range from 10 to 100 percent, but only concentrations below 30 percent are recommended for children. A common misperception among families is that "more is better," particularly when they see that DEET in concentrations greater than 90 percent is widely available in retail stores. The main route of DEET exposure is dermal, and very high exposures may occur with frequent reapplication, as has been reported with combination sunscreens and insect repellants. For this reason combination sunscreens and repellants are not recommended. The pediatrician also recommends that the children wear long-sleeved clothing that covers their extremities as a protective measure. DEET may then be applied to their clothing rather than directly on the skin. Otherwise, DEET should be applied only once daily, in sparse amounts, to exposed areas of the skin. Strict avoidance of the child's face and hands is necessary to prevent accidental ingestion through hand-to-mouth behaviors.

Acute DEET toxicity is rare but may include skin or eye irritation and, following high-dose exposures, central nervous system disorders such as seizures (Lipscomb, Kramer, and Leikin, 1992; Menon, 2004) and encephalopathy (Briassoulis, Narlioglou, and Hatzis, 2001; Sudakin, 2003). Animal studies of acute and chronic high-dose exposure suggest potential effects on the liver, kidney, and brain.

Exposure in Utero: Case Study on Polychlorinated Biphenyls   Polychlorinated biphenyls (**PCBs**) are a family of synthetic chlorinated hydrocarbon compounds that were used widely from the 1930s until the 1970s as coolants and lubricants and as insulators in transformers, electrical equipment, capacitors, insulation, the fluorescent lighting of the time, and air conditioners. They were also used as solvents in carbonless carbon paper, plastics, and paints. They resist burning and are difficult to break down, traits that made them ideal for these uses. In 1977, use of PCBs was banned because of concerns about their persistence in the environment and their effects on human health.

Much was learned about the devastating effects of high-dose PCB **exposure in utero** from a large-scale community outbreak that occurred in Kyushu province, Japan, in 1968 (Masuda, 1985). The source of the contamination was PCBs that had leaked from heat exchangers to contaminate rice oil. Rice oil is widely used for cooking in that area, and women who consumed food cooked with the contaminated oil accumulated PCBs in their fatty tissue. When these women subsequently became pregnant, the lipophilic PCBs were able to cross the placenta, thus exposing babies in utero. PCBs also concentrated in breast milk. Approximately 1,000 babies were affected. Infants born to the PCB-poisoned mothers had a constellation of symptoms, including mental retardation, developmental delays, eye and skin defects, darkening of the skin, and liver disease. These health effects came to be known as **Yusho disease** (Taylor, Lawrence, Hwang, and Paulson, 1984).

Lower-dose exposure to PCBs in the prenatal period, at levels too low to produce obvious symptoms, has also been shown to have adverse effects on central nervous function, including decreased intelligence, memory, and attention span (Grandjean and others, 2001; Tilson, Jacobson, and Rogan, 1990; Yu, Hsu, Gladen, and Rogan, 1991). These effects appear permanent and irreversible. Quite strikingly, similar effects have not been seen following exposure to PCBs during infancy and childhood. This difference in susceptibility suggests a special **window of vulnerability** for the developing brain in utero.

Though levels of PCBs can be measured accurately in blood and in breast milk, there are no standard clinical reference values that define a "normal" level of exposure. All Americans have some level of PCBs in their bodies as a result of environmental contamination decades ago, and the CDC provides information on population norms, but the link between low-level adult exposure to PCBs and health effects is not clear (CDC, 2005). For that reason, results of PCB testing are difficult to interpret and of little use clinically.

There is no known treatment to reduce the levels of PCBs in the body. The mainstay of therapy is to minimize exposure to PCBs; the most important action is to avoid eating fish caught from PCB-contaminated waters. Adherence to fish consumption advisories is particularly critical for pregnant women and women who hope to become pregnant in the future. State health departments issue advisories that list local areas considered unsafe for fishing due to PCB contamination.

Exposure Settings

Routes of exposure are often very much tied to a particular exposure setting. Exposure settings for children include the home, day-care centers, schools, public areas, and neighborhoods. The nature of the exposure setting may either enhance or mitigate the impact of the exposure, depending on the amount of time the child spends there, the condition of the area, and the degree of social control. Often all areas in which a child spends time must be explored in determining the exact source of an exposure. The following cases highlight the interactions between an exposure setting and a specific contaminant.

Home Exposure: Case Study on Lead   On routine blood testing a two-year-old girl was found to have a blood lead level of 22 micrograms per deciliter (µg/dL). A prior lead level obtained one year earlier had been 8 µg/dL. She is currently healthy though she has also been diagnosed with a mild iron deficiency anemia. According to her parents she has never been diagnosed with developmental delays, and her behavior is typical for a two-year-old. The child's seven-year-old sister was also tested and found to have a lead level of 2 µg/dL. The CDC's current level of concern is 10 µg/dL. Blood lead levels of 10 µg/dL, and even levels lower than 5 µg/dL, have been associated with behavioral problems and decreased intelligence (Lanphear, 2005). Children with blood lead levels above 20 µg/dL may exhibit gastrointestinal symptoms such as poor appetite, nausea, vomiting, abdominal pain, and constipation. These children may have difficulty with learning and school performance and also behavioral problems such as hyperactivity. Severe **lead poisoning**, with blood lead levels above 60 µg/dL, may be associated with neurological symptoms such as changes in mental status, difficulty walking, seizures, and coma, though even at high levels, overt clinical symptoms are not apparent.

The two-year-old girl's pediatrician elicited an environmental history, adapted from the AAP Green Book, to determine whether there were any potential sources of exposure in the home (Etzel and Balk, 2003). Here are the key questions asked in that history; each question is followed by the parents' answer in italics:

- What is the age and condition of the home? U.S. homes built pre-1978 may contain leaded paint. *We live in a two-bedroom apartment in a building that was built in the early 1900s. We have lived there for about ten years.*
- Are the windowsills peeling? Do the window wells contain solid material? Friction areas such as windows and door jambs can produce lead-containing dust and paint chips, which young children may then ingest through hand-to-mouth behaviors. *The window wells are solid but the windowsills have been peeling for many years now. We have complained to our landlord, but he has never addressed the problem.*
- Are you renovating a room or planning to? Renovations in older homes, without proper precautions for lead-based paint hazards, can be a potential source of exposure to pregnant women and children. *There have been no major renovations while we have been living here, though we did sand and paint the family room about 8 months ago. We did all the work ourselves and stayed in the home while the work was going on.*
- Have there been any recent renovations in common areas of your building or in your neighborhood? Renovations in close proximity to the home, such as a neighbor's home, or in common areas of a building, such as the fire escape or basement, may also generate leaded dust and paint chips. *There are no renovations that we are aware of.*
- Does your neighborhood have any local industries that may be potential sources of lead exposure? *Our neighborhood is predominantly residential and always has been as far as we know.*
- Do you use tap water? Some older homes have leaded pipes, which may then contaminate the water supply. *We drink city tap water, which is safe to drink according to the local department of health.*
- Do you use imported herbal remedies? Some traditional and herbal remedies contain lead; this is especially important in communities with new immigrants. *We don't use any herbal remedies.*
- What do you and your spouse do for a living? Are there any potential occupational take-home exposures? *My husband works in a restaurant as a manager, and I am a full-time mom.*
- Do you work at home with substances that may be hazardous? *No hobbies or projects at home.*
- Do you use any imported spices or products that may contain lead? *None.*
- Do you use any traditional ceramic pottery or other imported dishware where lead may be found in the glaze? *No.*

- Have you recently traveled outside the country, as there are a variety of lead exposures to consider in foreign settings and in fact leaded gasoline is still used in many parts of the world? *We haven't traveled outside of the U.S.*
- Does your child exhibit frequent hand-to-mouth behaviors? Has she been observed directly ingesting paint chips? *She constantly has her hands in her mouth though we have never witnessed her ingesting paint chips.*
- Have you checked her toys for the possible toy recalls related to lead including toy charms and jewelry? *We did check the Consumer Product Safety Commission Web site but her toys seemed to be OK. She also doesn't have any toy jewelry, though her older sister does. We'll be sure to remove those from the house.*

As part of the investigation, the local department of health (DOH) conducted an evaluation to identify any lead hazards in the home. This evaluation included an inventory of the child's daily activities, including time spent outside the home. **X-ray fluorescence** (**XRF**) identified the presence of leaded paint throughout the apartment and multiple areas of chipped peeling paint, particularly around the door frames and windows. This was a clear violation of the city's lead laws. No other sources of lead were found. Local lead laws require landlords in this city to conduct annual visits to homes with children aged six years and under. Lead hazards must be identified and appropriately abated by a certified lead abatement contractor within a specified time period. In this case the family was relocated while abatement was conducted. Lead dust swipe sampling was conducted after the renovations had been completed and prior to the family's return to the apartment. Blood lead levels were followed every three months for the two-year-old girl and her lead levels subsequently declined to below 10 µg/dL without the need for chelation therapy. The child was placed on supplemental iron for iron deficiency anemia, and her parents were advised to ensure that her diet was rich in iron and calcium.

Day-Care Exposure: Case Study on Solvents   Several families raised concerns to the Environmental Protection Agency and the local health department about work going on in close proximity to a suburban day-care center, sited in a former industrial area. A hazardous material team had been seen conducting testing of outdoor areas within fifty yards of the center. The day-care center had been in operation for five years and served about 150 children aged six weeks to five years. The building had fourteen rooms and there was an outside play area.

Investigation by the EPA and health department revealed that a steel company had been in operation for thirty years on a site adjacent to the site where the day-care center was now located. The steel company site had been designated an **EPA Superfund site** owing to hazardous waste. Degreasers had been used, including tetrachloroethylene (PERC), trichloroethylene, and trichloroethane. Sludge from the degreasing equipment was stored in drums. The steel company had been cited in the past for improper spill control, and ensuing investigations revealed elevated levels of the degreasers at depths down to forty feet below the ground surface. Levels of these chemicals were also found in groundwater samples collected from monitoring wells.

Due to concerns that exposures from the Superfund site might pose a problem to nearby facilities, including the day-care center, environmental testing was conducted for PERC, the chemical being found at the highest levels. Other volatile organic compounds (VOCs) were also measured. Air samples were collected by means of passive organic vapor sampling devices for twenty-four-hour periods on three separate occasions. The results for PERC in the day-care center ranged from 46 to 260 micrograms per cubic meter ($\mu g/m^3$). The New York State Department of Health recommends that the air level of PERC in a residential community not exceed 100 $\mu g/m^3$. These levels are set to protect the health of healthy adults and do not take into consideration vulnerable populations such as young children. Repeat testing conducted after improvements to the day-care center's ventilation system revealed levels of 7.0 to 20.7 $\mu g/m^3$. Families with children attending the day-care center were notified about the elevated levels of PERC found there. A series of community forums was convened, and representatives from the EPA, the local DOH, the regional Pediatric Environmental Health Specialty Unit, and the department of pediatrics at a nearby community hospital were present in order to help explain the potential health impacts from these exposures.

According to the Agency for Toxic Substances and Disease Registry (ATSDR) (2007b), tetrachloroethylene (also known as perchloroethylene [**PCE**, or **PERC**] and tetrachloroethene) is a synthetic chemical widely used for fabric dry cleaning and metal degreasing. At room temperature it is nonflammable and liquid in form. It evaporates easily into the air and has a sharp, sweet odor. Most people can smell tetrachloroethylene when it is present in air at a level of 30,000 $\mu g/m^3$ or more, although some people can detect it at even lower levels. High concentrations of tetrachloroethylene can cause dizziness, headache, sleepiness, confusion, nausea, difficulty in speaking and walking, unconsciousness, and death. Skin irritation may result from repeated or extended skin contact. These symptoms occur almost entirely in work environments when people have been accidentally exposed to high concentrations. Results of animal studies, conducted with amounts much higher than those that most people are exposed to, show that tetrachloroethylene can cause liver and kidney damage. The health effects of breathing air or drinking water with low levels of tetrachloroethylene are not known.

Given the levels found at the day-care center and information from prior studies assessing levels of exposure in children living adjacent to dry-cleaning stores, the consensus was that the children who had been at the center were not at significant risk for long-term health effects related to their exposures. However, given the fact that the levels were elevated above background levels and that children may in fact be particularly vulnerable to exposures incurred early in life due to their rapid growth and ongoing development, in general it was felt to be prudent to minimize these exposures. The day-care center voluntarily closed upon receiving the results of the elevated PERC levels. The children remained asymptomatic. Although blood or urine testing is available for some of these exposures, it was not recommended for these families as there are no standardized reference values for "normal" levels of exposure, particularly for children. Further studies are needed to assess the health effects of chronic, low-level PERC exposures for children.

School Exposure: Case Study on Mold   One October a school nurse at a public elementary school noted an increased frequency of asthma exacerbations in fourth-grade students from one particular homeroom. In an effort to identify potential triggers the nurse surveyed the room. There were no carpets or pets present in the classroom, and it had not undergone any recent renovations. The classroom was used for history and English classes, and no arts and crafts or scientific experiments were conducted there. Upon entering the room the nurse noted a musty odor. The ceiling was found to have an area of water damage, with a small area of mold visible on the ceiling. The principal of the school was notified. In order to obtain further information about potential health effects related to mold, the local department of health was consulted, in addition to the regional Pediatric Environmental Health Specialty Unit (PEHSU). The school also elected to have an industrial hygienist survey the school to make recommendations for mold abatement.

Health effects from **mold** range from irritant effects such as eye, ear, nose, and throat irritations to allergy or asthma symptoms such as sneezing, coughing, and wheezing. (See Chapter Nineteen for further information.) It is not known whether mold exposure causes asthma. For susceptible individuals it may exacerbate asthmatic conditions. The relationship between mold exposure and chronic symptoms such as fatigue is unclear. Some molds, such as *Stachybotrys*, produce toxins, but it is not known whether exposure to these toxins causes chronic health effects. If a family has a strong family history of *atopy* (allergy symptoms), it is possible that the children are predisposed to allergies and that the subsequent exposure to mold is exacerbating their symptoms. In general the best test to determine sensitivity is to observe whether the symptoms improve when the exposure is removed. Do the child's symptoms improve when the child is out of the school for a significant period of time, such as during vacations? If so, this is the best evidence that symptoms are being aggravated by mold exposure. Usually, mold-related symptoms resolve once exposure has been removed.

Determining the source of the moisture is of utmost importance in preventing any further mold growth. Ideally, humidity in schools should be kept between 30 and 50 percent, adequate ventilation with indoor-outdoor air exchange should be ensured, and any water leaks should be addressed immediately. It is recommended that a certified industrial hygienist evaluate the area of concern to make recommendations about further cleanup. Extensive areas of mold (more than ten square feet) should be addressed by certified contractors, as outlined in the Environmental Protection Agency's "Mold in Schools" fact sheet (EPA, Indoor Environments Division, 2004).

In this case the hygienist, after surveying the affected classroom and other classrooms, determined the etiology to be an isolated pipe leak affecting this classroom alone. Children were removed from the classroom for the duration of the abatement. Parents were informed of the proceedings from the start of the investigation, were provided with information about the health effects of mold, and were given the opportunity to discuss their concerns with health professionals through the local DOH and the regional PEHSU. Parents were also referred to the Healthy Schools Network (HSN) for further information. Founded in 1995, HSN is a national not-for-profit organization centered on children's environmental health and dedicated to assuring every child and school employee an environmentally safe and healthy school through research, information, referral, and advocacy.

For further assistance, the IAQ (Indoor Air Quality) Design Tools for Schools Web site (EPA, 2009) provides guidance and links to other information resources for those involved in the design of new schools and the repair, renovation, and maintenance of existing school facilities. Though the primary focus is on indoor air quality, the IAQ tools Web site also promotes energy efficiency, day lighting, materials efficiency, and safety.

Play Area Exposure: Case Study on Arsenic   A news release alerted the public to the potential hazards of arsenic-treated wood, used commonly since the 1930s in decks, in playground equipment, and for other outdoor uses. Upon hearing the news, families in a suburban California community became concerned about the playground equipment in the nearby state park. The playground, refurbished two years previously, was widely used by the community year round. One family identified the manufacturer of the playground equipment and found that the lumber did in fact consist of wood treated with chromated copper arsenic (CCA). This preservative is used to protect wood against rot and fungus.

A child's hand-to-mouth behavior is the major source of exposure to arsenic from **CCA-treated wood** in playsets. Children aged six and younger frequently exhibit hand-to-mouth behaviors, which allow the direct ingestion of arsenic. The risk of exposure to arsenic is greatest when the wood is in poor condition. As this playground set was only two years old, it was in fairly good condition, though there were a few areas of obvious wear. The playground surface was made from recycled rubber, which diminished potential exposures from arsenic leaching into soil and subsequent hand-to-mouth ingestion through this pathway.

Although the predominant sources of exposure to arsenic are food, soil, and water (especially the groundwater of certain areas, as described in Chapter Fifteen), arsenic exposure via playgrounds may contribute to a child's daily level of exposure. Concerns have been raised about arsenic due to its association with an increased risk of developing lung or bladder cancer over a child's lifetime (ATSDR, 2007a). Epidemiological studies from Taiwan have shown an increased incidence of lung and bladder cancer from elevated levels of arsenic in the drinking water (Chiou and others, 1995, 2001). Due to these potential health effects, the manufacturers of CCA-treated products reached a voluntary agreement with the EPA to end the manufacture of CCA-treated wood for most consumer applications as of December 2003. However, some CCA-treated wood may have remained on store shelves through mid-2004.

To minimize exposure to arsenic-treated wood, diligent maintenance of playground equipment is warranted to prevent wear and tear and the subsequent leaching of arsenic. One method of upkeep is routine annual staining of the wood with a polyurethane stain to prevent deterioration. Another option is to choose wood alternatives such as cedar or redwood, which do not require pretreatment. Frequent hand washing is recommended, particularly after outdoor play, in order to decrease potential for direct ingestion.

In this case, local parents spearheaded an effort to replace the CCA-treated equipment with a cedar playset. In the meantime the local parks department performed regular upkeep and maintenance of the equipment.

Exposure Through Urban and Suburban Neighborhood Design: Childhood Obesity Obesity is a global problem. The World Health Organization (2002) has declared overweight to be one of the top ten health risks in the world and one of the top five in developed nations. Studies designed to assess the impact of environmental determinants of overweight are now exploring how neighborhood design (urban, suburban, or rural) influences diet and physical activity levels and the subsequent prevalence of childhood obesity.

Many of the structural features of the urban built environment—its enormous size, its large and densely clustered population, its social institutions, its psychosocial stressors, its economy, its rapid pace, its violence, its ways of configuring its streets, parks, schools, and playspaces—affect children's health, growth, and development. The adverse effects of the urban environment are especially magnified in low-income, predominantly minority communities where crowded streets, lack of outdoor playspaces, limited access to fresh and healthy food, and substandard housing all contribute to substantial and well-documented disparities in child health (Jackson, 2003; Wendel, Dannenberg, and Frumkin, 2008; also see Chapter Fourteen in this volume).

In suburban and rural communities, environmental factors contribute to childhood overweight and obesity in a unique way. As cities rapidly encroach upon neighboring areas, the phenomenon of urban sprawl is becoming common. Urban sprawl is characterized by low-density land use, separation of homes from other land uses such as stores and schools, and low "connectivity" along surface roads. In the United States and other developed countries, people are relying more and more on cars to get from place to place instead of walking or taking public transportation. Too many suburban towns have no sidewalks and no safe bicycle paths (Frumkin, Frank, and Jackson, 2004). Neighborhood design is one factor promoting this method of transportation, as residential areas are segregated from stores, schools, and other resources.

The impression is widespread that obesity is solely a problem of the individual. Although it is true that individual choice is an important factor in the genesis of obesity, it is also true, especially in the case of childhood obesity, that environmental factors in the home, school, and neighborhood that promote poor dietary habits and sedentary lifestyles are important. Obesity is a problem not only of the individual but also of neighborhoods, schools, modes of transportation, local food availability, food advertising practices, and government policies (Maziak, Ward, and Stockton, 2008). Further exploration of the impact of the environment on everyday behaviors is critical to understanding the current trend of rising obesity.

Environmental risk factors that may influence everyday behaviors and risk of obesity include a *food environment* that poses increased exposure to high-calorie fast foods, junk foods, and refined sugars (Ford and Dzewaltowski, 2008). Low-income families must often depend on smaller stores that have a limited selection of fresh foods, often at relatively high cost. The presence of a supermarket within a census tract is associated with a 32 percent increase in fruit and vegetable intake compared to the average intake in neighborhoods without supermarkets (Morland, Wing, and Diez Roux, 2002). Supermarkets have twice the amount of healthy foods that neighborhood grocery stores do and four times the amount carried by convenience stores (Sallis and others, 1986). Yet there are four times as many supermarkets located in white neighborhoods as there are in black neighborhoods (Morland, Wing, Diez Roux, and Poole, 2002). Public health workers and health care providers need to consider factors in the local food environment level when recommending dietary changes.

Patterns of physical activity may also be influenced by the built environment. Lack of access to playgrounds, a dearth of organized sports activities, and concerns for physical safety that lead parents to keep their children indoors may further increase the risk of childhood obesity. Increased television viewing, which may be a marker of an increasingly sedentary lifestyle, is now widely recognized as a risk factor for childhood obesity, and this is one potential area in which to target interventions (Dietz and Gortmaker, 1985). In fact, reducing television viewing has been shown in several studies to reduce childhood obesity (Robinson, 1999; Dennison, Russo, Burdick, and Jenkins, 2004).

Improved access to recreational facilities is associated with higher levels of participation in vigorous activity, regardless of individuals' socioeconomic status (Sallis and others, 1990). Disadvantaged areas tend to have fewer recreational facilities, raising concerns that lack of access is a barrier to physical activity, putting some communities at higher risk for inactivity and obesity (MacIntyre, MacIver, and Sooman, 1993). This reinforces the role of the built environment as a potentially modifiable risk factor for physical inactivity.

Recognizing the contribution of the environment to this growing epidemic is just the beginning. Further work is needed to develop and implement strategies to prevent and control obesity. Identifying and addressing environmental determinants of obesity through research studies provides a unique opportunity to institute change on a population-wide level through both structural changes in the environment and public policy changes in conjunction with individual behavioral changes (Srinivasan, O'Fallon, and Dearry, 2003).

RISK ASSESSMENT AND COMMUNICATION

Traditional **risk assessment** has generally failed to consider the special exposures and the unique susceptibilities of infants and children (see Chapter Twenty-Nine). Children represent a unique subgroup within the population, one that requires special consideration in risk assessment. In calling for a new paradigm for environmental research and risk assessment, Landrigan and Carlson (1995) wrote: "The essence of this paradigm is to place the child, not the chemical or hazard, at the center of the analysis. The analysis would then begin with the child, his or her biology, exposure patterns, and developmental stage. This paradigm calls for a new way of thinking, and a retooling of the risk assessment process so that it takes into account not only the increased vulnerability of children but also the effects of multiple and cumulative exposures over the course of a lifetime" (p. 50).

Adoption of a new child-centered agenda for research and risk assessment will be necessary if disease of toxic environmental origin in children is to be identified, understood, controlled, and prevented. This agenda needs to be multidisciplinary. It needs to focus specifically on (1) exploration and quantification of unique patterns and pathways of exposure for children; (2) adoption of new, more sensitive approaches to testing chemicals that can recognize the consequences of exposure during early development and throughout the life span; (3) identification, through clinical and epidemiological studies, of etiologic associations between cumulative environmental exposures and pediatric diseases (EPA, 2007a); and (4) elucidation, at the cellular and molecular levels, of the pathogenic mechanisms of pediatric environmental illness.

If high-risk groups such as children do not receive appropriate consideration, then risk assessment and the regulatory decisions that follow from it will in many cases fail to protect these most vulnerable members of society from environmentally induced disease and dysfunction. As outlined for the new agenda, several specific tasks need to be part of developing and implementing this new child-centered paradigm, including improved **exposure assessment**, enhanced **toxicity testing**, new toxicodynamic and toxicokinetic models, a mechanistic approach to hazard assessment, and application of **uncertainty factors** and safety factors that specifically consider children's risks (Landrigan, Kimmel, Correa, and Eskenazi, 2004). In addition, application of the **precautionary principle** can provide an overarching framework for considering children's risks.

Improved Exposure Assessment

Additional data are needed on children's patterns and levels of exposures to chemicals in the environment. Because exposures vary by age, this information will need to be collected for different age groups, from the developing baby in utero through adolescence. Accurate and frequently updated information is needed on children's diets at different ages and on the concentrations of **xenobiotics** (chemicals foreign to the human body) in those diets. Surveys also should be regularly conducted of levels of chemical contaminants in breast milk. Better data are needed on the extent of exposure that results from children's unique mouthing behaviors.

All sources of exposure need to be considered in evaluating the potential risks that environmental chemicals present to infants and children (NRC, 1993). Models need to be developed that can account for children's simultaneous exposures to multiple chemicals of differing potency via multiple routes of exposure that together may contribute to a specific health outcome. These models need to be able to assess the cumulative effects of chemicals that may have either synergistic or antagonistic actions. The EPA's recent work in assessing exposures to multiple organophosphate pesticides is a useful first step in this direction (EPA, 2008).

Exposure estimates for acute effects and exposure estimates for chronic effects need to be constructed differently. The incorporation of biomarkers into data collection may be useful. The essential element is to examine the full distribution of children's exposures to chemicals in the environment. Point estimates of average exposure are no longer sufficient. The actual distribution of the range of children's exposures across the population needs to be determined through field studies. Appropriate mathematical models, such as Monte Carlo models (see Chapter Twenty-Nine), must be constructed in order to permit the combination of various data sets and thus an examination of full exposure distributions (National Academy of Sciences (NAS), 1992). Of special concern are children whose exposures fall into the top 10, 5, or 1 percent of the population.

Enhanced Toxicity Testing

New, more sensitive approaches to chemical toxicity testing are needed that can reliably detect the unanticipated developmental consequences of exposures during critical windows of prenatal and postnatal vulnerability (Selevan, Kimmel, and Mendola, 2000; Buschmann, 2006). These new models of developmental toxicity testing need to generate data on organ systems that have not been adequately addressed in the past, for example, the nervous, immune, respiratory, reproductive, cardiovascular, and endocrine systems.

A shortcoming of much current toxicity testing is that test chemicals are administered to experimental animals in adolescence, and the animals are subsequently sacrificed at a point in life that corresponds roughly to a human age of sixty to sixty-five years. Thus both the unique effects of early exposures and any late effects of early exposures are not captured (EPA, Risk Assessment Forum, 2002); these effects might include cancer, heart disease, neurological disorders, or diabetes. To improve current toxicity testing for certain classes of chemicals, investigators may need to undertake studies in which chemicals and possibly multiple chemicals are administered to experimental animals either in utero or shortly after birth and the subjects then followed over their entire natural life spans. For other classes of compounds, it may be necessary to expose animals throughout the life span. The approach should attempt to replicate the human experience, and this may enhance detection of delayed effects (NAS, 1992).

Excessive reliance on observation of birth anomalies and insufficient testing of organ system function have been features of much traditional toxicity testing. To improve the situation, enhanced functional tests of neurobehavioral, immune, endocrine, and reproductive toxicity will be of great importance (EPA, 1986, 2008; EPA, Risk Assessment Forum, 1991, 2002). One particular area of growing concern is the potential for recently introduced chemicals such as phthalates to act as endocrine disrupters (EDs). Recent national surveys conducted by the Centers for Disease Control and Prevention found that biomarker residues of EDs are present almost universally in Americans but also that significant disparities in body burdens by age, sex, and race and ethnicity exist, with the highest levels found in children and minorities. Animal studies have shown a relationship between phthalates and fetal death, malformation, and reproductive toxicity (Shea, 2003; Foster, 2006). Concerns about the potential for human health effects led to the inclusion of a phthalates ban in the Consumer Product Safety Improvement Act of 2008. Still, an exploration of the potential for endocrine disruption through phthalate exposure from commonplace items such as plastic toys and other plasticizers, including **bisphenol A (BPA)**, which is widely found in food packaging and baby bottles, is urgently needed. Yet very few short- or long-term follow-up studies have evaluated possible phthalate toxicity (Shea, 2003) and even fewer studies have looked at cumulative exposures to endocrine disruptors (Howdeshell and others, 2007; Howdeshell and others, 2008; Rider and others, 2009) and other contributory exposures throughout the life span. These functional assessments need to be applied on a more routine basis, especially when data from other studies, for example, adult target organ toxicity or multigenerational studies, raise concerns about possible developmental effects.

New Toxicodynamic and Toxicokinetic Models

The physiological and biochemical characteristics of children that influence the metabolism and disposition of chemicals at different stages of development need to be considered in risk assessment. Physiological parameters such as tissue growth rates, and biochemical parameters such as enzyme induction, may differentially affect the responses of infants and children at different developmental stages to environmental chemicals (Cresteil, 1998; Ginsberg and others, 2002). Physiologically based pharmacokinetic models (**PBPK models**) can be used to estimate the dose of toxic metabolites reaching target tissues at different developmental stages (O'Flaherty, 1997; Welsch, Blumenthal, and Conolly, 1995; Ginsberg, Hattis, Miller, and Sonawane, 2004; Ginsberg, Slikker, Bruckner, and Sonawane, 2004); Emond, 2005).

A Mechanistic Approach to Hazard Assessment

The pathogenic mechanisms of environmentally induced disease in children need to be elucidated at functional, organ, cellular, and molecular levels (Birnbaum, 1994; Campbell, Seidler, and Slotkin, 1997; Whitney, Seidler, and Slotkin, 1995; Garcia, Seidler, and Slotkin, 2005; Yang and others, 2008). These assessments could be undertaken in conjunction with toxicity testing of chemicals and also in the context of epidemiological studies. Clinical and epidemiological studies are of proven value for studying etiologic associations between environmental exposures and pediatric disease (Bellinger and others, 1987; Jacobson and Jacobson, 1996; Needleman and others, 1990), and the National Children's Study (discussed later) will be invaluable in this regard.

Application of Uncertainty and Safety Factors Specific to Children's Risks

In the absence of data to the contrary, children must be presumed to be more vulnerable than adults to environmental toxic agents, a presumption specifically recommended by the NRC Committee on Pesticides in the Diets of Infants and Children (1993). Traditional approaches to risk assessment are now being modified to account more carefully and explicitly for risks to children (EPA, Risk Assessment Forum, 2002). However, a number of data gaps in exposure assessment and in developmental toxicity must be addressed through the development and implementation of additional testing guideline protocols (EPA, 1999; EPA, Risk Assessment Forum, 2002), the acquisition of better information on children's exposure patterns and sources, and basic research both on mechanisms of underlying development and on chemical interactions of environmental agents with developing organ systems (NRC, 2000).

Application of the Precautionary Principle

The 1998 Wingspread "Statement on the Precautionary Principle" summarizes the precautionary principle as follows: "When an activity raises threats of harm to human health or the environment, precautionary measures should be taken even if some cause and effect relationships are not fully established scientifically." (This principle is described in detail in Chapter Twenty-Six.) It has special relevance to children, because the notion of protecting children from harm is so widely accepted.

Risk Communication

Concern for one's children's health and well-being is a defining aspect of parenting. Indeed, even adults who minimize the risks of their own environmental exposures may have deep concerns about those their children confront. Clear **risk communication** on the part of health care providers and collaborative partnerships with agencies and academic centers can do much to provide parents with useful information and to help them respond appropriately to environmental exposures. Examples of this exchange of information appear in the case studies presented earlier and in the Perspective on risk communication and further information appears in Chapter Thirty-One.

PERSPECTIVE
Risk Communication and the World Trade Center

A difficulty in risk assessment targeted toward children is that we have so little knowledge about normal background levels of exposure for the general population aged zero to eighteen years and babies in utero. Current acceptable thresholds of exposure for many environmental exposures are based on studies of healthy adults in the workplace setting and do not take into account vulnerable populations.

After the fall of the World Trade Center (WTC) towers in New York City, officials and investigators were faced with concerns about pediatric exposures to environmental toxins for which there are no good child health standards. The strategy they employed was to compare the WTC exposures to both the current and the historical background exposure levels. This method is useful for comparison of both dose and duration of exposure. Although this information has a limited ability to answer questions about health effects related to the exposure or about safety, it provides families with a frame of reference. When the magnitude of the exposure is in line with either current or historical background levels and is of brief duration, this sort of comparison can provide some reassurance even when a true risk assessment is not possible in the absence of evidence-based reference values or environmental thresholds specific to children.

This general approach proved very useful when dealing with such WTC exposures as releases of volatile organic compounds, dioxins, polychlorinated biphenyls, and even toxins with reference ranges for sensitive populations, such as particulate matter and lead. For example, the collapse of the World Trade Center led to the release of particulate matter (**PM$_{2.5}$** and **PM$_{10}$**) from the breakdown of the building's structures and contents. This resulted in tons of dust, rubble, and debris at ground zero. The fact that gases, dust, soot, and smoke were also released, as a result of the fires at the site, was clearly evidenced by the smoke plumes seen in varying degrees for the duration of the fires, through December 2001.

THE FUTURE OF CHILDREN'S ENVIRONMENTAL HEALTH: NATIONAL CHILDREN'S STUDY

In December 2000, the U.S. Congress appropriated funds to plan the **National Children's Study**, a national, longitudinal cohort study of children's health (National Children's Study, 2009). An important goal of this study is to examine systematically the impact on children's health and development of early exposure to environmental toxins. In addition, the study will examine interactions among

In the immediate aftermath of the WTC collapse, EPA data indicated large increases in hourly levels of $PM_{2.5}$ at and above the Air Quality Index level of 40 $\mu g/m^3$. In general these short-term elevations of particulate matter followed the path of the smoke plumes, as determined by wind direction. Levels of particulate matter were higher at nighttime and lower on rainy days because moisture decreased the amounts of airborne particulate matter. Though some hourly levels were reported to be as high as 200 $\mu g/m^3$, twenty-four-hour averages for these same areas were significantly lower at 40 to 90 $\mu g/m^3$.

Although these twenty-four-hour levels were elevated, they were similar to background levels of air pollution seen previously in New York City. Routine EPA monitoring of particulate matter provides us with these historical levels. Data prior to September 2001 indicated outdoor particulate matter levels of 18.4 $\mu g/m^3$ for $PM_{2.5}$ (year 2000 average) and levels of 25 $\mu g/m^3$ for PM_{10} (1998 average). Twenty-four-hour levels for New York City as high as 40 to 89 $\mu g/m^3$ for $PM_{2.5}$ and 51 to 121 $\mu g/m^3$ for PM_{10} (1996 to 2001) had been previously reported. This indicated that even pre-9/11 levels of particulate matter exceeded the National Ambient Air Quality Standards (NAAQS), most likely reflecting background levels of air pollution in urban areas. This stresses that much work has yet to be done to improve the overall quality of outdoor air.

Guidance provided to families in the surrounding community explained that long-term health effects were unlikely to result from short-term exposures to particulate matter. However, acute reversible health effects, including asthma exacerbations and eye, ear, nose, and throat irritation, were possible. This was in contrast to the more substantial exposures experienced by the workers and volunteers at ground zero, for whom significant long-term health effects were possible. Studies are now underway to assess whether health effects are seen in the infants of pregnant women present at the WTC site the day of the collapse of the towers. A registry of ground zero workers and volunteers is also under way, enabling long-term follow-up of health conditions with long latency periods.

environmental toxins, socioeconomic factors, behavioral factors, and genetic inheritance and their effects on the health of children. It is anticipated that beginning in 2009, the study will enroll as many as 100,000 children and families and that it will follow the children prospectively to at least age eighteen (Berkowitz and others, 2001)—a pediatric counterpart to the landmark Framingham Heart Study, one of the major sources of insight into adult health over the last half century (Futterman and Lemberg, 2000; Messerli and Mittler, 1998). Although other cohort studies have studied children prospectively (Broman, 1984; Rutter, 1989;

Silva, 1990), no longitudinal study has examined the impact of environmental toxins on children's health or has studied the interactions between environmental toxins and other social, behavioral, and environmental risk factors.

The National Children's Study will have the statistical power to explore the simultaneous impact of many risk factors—environmental toxicants, health behaviors, socioeconomic factors, and genetics—on the long-term health of U.S. children. Prospective epidemiological research can quantify environmental exposures and evaluate factors that are not recorded routinely in medical charts or birth certificates. Such research can also assess the effects of early exposures to environmental toxicants on neurobehavioral development. The longitudinal design will permit direct examination of risk factors from earliest exposure through to the clinical appearance of dysfunction, thus permitting recognition of the sequence of causality. Recent advances in epidemiological technique, in computer technology, in the management of biological specimens, and in the evaluation of genetic markers increase the potential of this study to yield important etiologic insights (Berkowitz and others, 2001; Landrigan and others, 2006).

Establishing this national longitudinal study will be an enormously complex and costly task (Berkowitz and others, 2001). When focusing on relatively rare outcomes, such as some of those that may occur in children, a large sample size is required, and this study will enroll thousands of participants, resulting in enough new cases of disease and death to ensure statistically reliable findings. Retaining and tracking thousands of participants over many years is a challenge. The collection, processing, storage, and maintenance of biological specimens will need to be controlled carefully. Data will be obtained on environmental exposures and psychosocial aspects in the home environment. Standardized, age-appropriate, developmental assessments will be the main outcome measures. The successful establishment and maintenance of such a cohort will require teams drawn from a range of disciplines, including epidemiology, exposure assessment, toxicology, developmental psychology, neurobiology, biostatistics, and pediatrics. In return, however, the National Children's Study promises to yield unprecedented insights into the determinants of health and illness in children.

SUMMARY

Environmental pediatrics is an area of pediatric medicine that has advanced remarkably in the past fifty years. It has risen to importance in parallel with two developments: first, the conquest in the industrialized nations of the major infectious diseases and the corresponding rise in chronic conditions such as asthma, cancer, developmental disabilities, and birth defects as the primary causes of illness and death in children and, second, the growing recognition that environmental factors are responsible, at least in part, for these changes in patterns of disease.

The challenge now for children's environmental health is to understand better the impact of environmental exposures on the patterns of health and disease in children and to design evidence-based approaches to the prevention and treatment of childhood disease of environmental origin. "Children are not merely a special vulnerable group within our population but rather the current inhabitants of a developmental stage through which all future generations must pass. Protection of fetuses, infants and children is essential for the sustainability of the human species" (Landrigan, Kimmel, Correa, and Eskenazi, 2004, p. 263). We have a strong foundation of data, clinicians and researchers, concerned parents, policymakers, and training programs; we must continue the tradition of inquiry into the role of the environment in children's health and into action that can protect children from environmental hazards.

KEY TERMS

American Academy of Pediatrics

bisphenol A (BPA)

breast milk contaminants

built environment

CCA treated wood

Centers for Children's Environmental Health and Disease Prevention

children's unique susceptibility

Consumer Product Safety Improvement Act

DEET

environmental justice

environmental pediatrics

EPA Superfund site

Executive Order on Protection of Children

from Environmental Health Risks and Safety Risks (1997)

exposure assessment

exposure in utero

Food Quality Protection Act

lead poisoning

Minamata Disease

mold

National Children's Study

new pediatric morbidity

NO_x

PAHs

PBDEs

PBPK models

PCBs

PCE

Pediatric Environmental Health Specialty Units

PERC

phthalates

$PM_{2.5}$

PM_{10}

POPs

precautionary principle

risk assessment

risk communication

thalidomide

toxicity testing

trichloroethylene

uncertainty factors

windows of vulnerability

xenobiotics

X-ray fluorescence (XRF)

Yusho disease

DISCUSSION QUESTIONS

1. Examine the statistics on childhood lead poisoning in your area to determine which populations are at risk. In particular, carefully examine demographics and geographic distributions of childhood lead poisoning cases. Explore the local lead laws and compare them to the lead laws of other areas to determine whether they are adequately protective. If necessary, how might you advocate for stricter lead laws in your area?

2. Name potential pathways of exposure for a specific toxin (such as cigarette smoke, carbon monoxide, endocrine disruptors, or dioxins), and name the factors unique to a child's developmental stage that may place him or her at increased risk. Explore the current scientific literature on subsequent health effects related to this exposure at each critical window of vulnerability (pregnancy, infancy, early childhood, and adolescence).

3. What are the current recommendations for fish intake in pregnant women and children? Where can families in your area obtain information on local fish advisories? What are the potential health effects related to in utero or childhood exposures to mercury or PCBs in fish? Use the current scientific literature, including population-based studies of fish intake, to support your response. Explore current regulations on mercury and PCB pollution, and identify areas where your advocacy may be beneficial.

4. Neighborhood factors influence lifestyle habits. What are some of the neighborhood design factors that might improve a child's level of physical activity? Differentiate between urban and suburban design. In particular, address factors in the schools that might be addressed to improve both diet and physical activity. Which groups in your area could you convene to address making positive changes in these various factors?

5. What environmental justice (EJ) issues in your area may disproportionately affect children's health? How might you reach out to communities disproportionately affected by environmental toxins? Explore past EJ issues that have negatively affected children's health, and identify the groups or factors that were largely responsible for implementing change.

6. What can be done on the local, state, national, and international levels to secure the future of children's environmental health research, clinical services, advocacy, and policy? Use a current environmental concern as an example.

REFERENCES

Agency for Toxic Substances and Disease Registry. "ToxFAQs for Arsenic." http://www.atsdr.cdc.gov/tfacts2.html, 2007a.

Agency for Toxic Substances and Disease Registry. "ToxFAQs for Tetrachloroethylene (PERC)." http://www.atsdr.cdc.gov/tfacts18.html, 2007b.

Akinbami, L. J. "The State of Childhood Asthma, United States, 1980–2005." *Advance Data from Vital Health Statistics*, 2006, *381*.

Alimonti, A., Böse-O'Reilly, S., Moshammer, H., and van den Hazel, J. P. (eds.). Special Issue on Children's Health and the Environment. *International Journal of Environment and Health*, 2008, 2(3/4, entire issue).

American Academy of Pediatrics, Section on Breastfeeding. "Breastfeeding and the Use of Human Milk." *Pediatrics*, 2005, *115*, 496–506.

Andersen, H. R. "Impaired Reproductive Development in Sons of Women Occupationally Exposed to Pesticides During Pregnancy." *Environmental Health Perspectives*, 2008, *116*(4), 566–572.

Bakir, F., and others. "Methylmercury Poisoning in Iraq." *Science*, 1973, *181*(4096), 230–241.

Bellinger, D., and others. "Longitudinal Analyses of Prenatal and Postnatal Lead Exposure and Early Cognitive Development." *New England Journal of Medicine*, 1987, *316*(17), 1037–1043.

Berkowitz, G. S., and others. "The Rationale for a National Prospective Cohort Study of Environmental Exposure and Childhood Development." *Environmental Research*, 2001, *85*(2), 59–68.

Birnbaum, L. S. "The Mechanism of Dioxin Toxicity: Relationship to Risk Assessment." *Environmental Health Perspectives*, 1994, *102*(suppl. 9), 157–167.

Brender, J. "Parental Occupation and Neural Tube Defect-Affected Pregnancies Among Mexican Americans." *Journal of Occupational and Environmental Medicine*, 2002, *44*(7), 650–656.

Briassoulis, G., Narlioglou, M., and Hatzis, T. "Toxic Encephalopathy Associated with Use of DEET Insect Repellents: A Case Analysis of Its Toxicity in Children." *Human & Experimental Toxicology*, 2001, *20*(1), 8–14.

Briggs, D. *Making a Difference: Indicators to Improve Children's Environmental Health*. World Health Organization. http://www.who.int/phe/children/en/cehindic.pdf, 2003.

Broman, S. "The Collaborative Perinatal Project: An Overview." In S. A. Mednick, M. Harway, and K. M. Finello (eds.), *Handbook of Longitudinal Research*. New York: Praeger, 1984.

Buschmann, J. "Critical Aspects in Reproductive and Developmental Toxicity Testing of Environmental Chemicals." *Reproductive Toxicology*, 2006, *22*(2), 157–163.

Campbell, C. G., Seidler, F. J., and Slotkin, T. A. "Chlorpyrifos Interferes with Cell Development in Rat Brain Regions." *Brain Research Bulletin*, 1997, *43*(2), 179–189.

Center for Defense Information. *Highlights of the FY'03 Budget Request*. http://www.cdi.org/issues/budget/FY03Highlights-pr.cfm, 2002.

Centers for Disease Control and Prevention. *Third National Report on Human Exposure to Environmental Chemicals*. NCEH Publication No. 05–0725. Atlanta, Ga.: Centers for Disease Control and Prevention, 2005.

Chiou, H. Y., and others. "Incidence of Internal Cancers and Ingested Inorganic Arsenic: A Seven-Year Follow-Up Study in Taiwan." *Cancer Research*, 1995, *55*(6), 1296–1300.

Chiou, H. Y., and others. "Incidence of Transitional Cell Carcinoma and Arsenic in Drinking Water: A Follow-Up Study of 8,102 Residents in an Arseniasis-Endemic Area in Northeastern Taiwan." *American Journal of Epidemiology*, 2001, *153*(5), 411–418.

Conover, C. J. "Annual Cost of Illness and Injury, Most Costly Health Conditions in U.S. (billions of dollars, Year 2000)." Duke University Center for Health Policy, Law & Management. http://wiki.aas.duke.edu/hpolicy/cost-of-illness, n.d.

Cresteil, T. "Onset of Xenobiotic Metabolism in Children: Toxicological Implications." *Food Additives and Contaminants*, 1998, *15*(suppl.), 45–51.

Curl, C. L., Fenske, R. A., and Elgethun, K. "Organophosphorus Pesticide Exposure of Urban and Suburban Preschool Children with Organic and Conventional Diets." *Environmental Health Perspectives*, 2003, *111*(3), 377–382.

Damgaard, I. I. N., and others. "Persistent Pesticides in Human Breast Milk and Cryptorchidism." *Environmental Health Perspectives*, 2006, *114*(7), 1133–1138.

Dennison, B. A., Russo, T. J., Burdick, P. A., and Jenkins, P. L. "An Intervention to Reduce Television Viewing by Preschool Children." *Archives of Pediatrics & Adolescent Medicine*, 2004, *158*(2), 170–176.

Dewailly, E., and others. "Inuit Exposure to Organochlorines Through the Aquatic Food Chain in Arctic Quebec." *Environmental Health Perspectives*, 1993, *101*(7), 618–620.

Dietz, W. H., Jr., and Gortmaker, S. L. "Do We Fatten Our Children at the Television Set? Obesity and Television Viewing in Children and Adolescents." *Pediatrics*, 1985, *75*(5), 807–812.

DiLiberti, J. H., and Jackson, C. R. "Long-Term Trends in Childhood Infectious Disease Mortality Rates." *American Journal of Public Health*, 1999, *89*(12), 1883–1885.

Emond, C. "Comparison of the Use of a Physiologically-Based Pharmacokinetic Model and a Classical Pharmacokinetic Model for Dioxin Exposure Assessments." *Environmental Health Perspectives*, 2005, *113*(12), 1666–1668.

Engel, L. S., O'Meara, E. S., and Schwartz, S. M. "Maternal Occupation in Agriculture and Risk of Limb Defects in Washington State, 1980–1993." *Scandinavian Journal of Work, Environment & Health*, 2000, *26*(3), 193–198.

Eriksson, J. G., and others. "Early Growth and Coronary Heart Disease in Later Life: Longitudinal Study." *British Medical Journal*, 2001, *322*(7292), 949–953.

Etzel, R. A., and Balk, S. J. (eds.). *Handbook of Pediatric Environmental Health*. (2nd ed.) Elk Grove, Ill.: American Academy of Pediatrics, 2003.

Ford, P. B., and Dzewaltowski, D. A. "Disparities in Obesity Prevalence Due to Variation in the Retail Food Environment: Three Testable Hypotheses." *Nutrition Reviews*, 2008, *66*(4), 216–228.

Foster, P. M. D. "Disruption of Reproductive Development in Male Rat Offspring Following in Utero Exposure to Phthalate Esters." *International Journal of Andrology*, 2006, *29*(1), 140–147.

Frumkin, H., Frank, L., and Jackson, R. J. *Urban Sprawl and Public Health*. Washington, D.C.: Island Press, 2004.

Futterman, L. G., and Lemberg, L. "The Framingham Heart Study: A Pivotal Legacy of the Last Millennium." *American Journal of Critical Care*, 2000, *9*(2), 147–151.

Garcia, S. J., Seidler, F. J., and Slotkin, T. A. "Developmental Neurotoxicity of Chlorpyrifos: Targeting Glial Cells." *Environmental Toxicology and Pharmacology*, 2005, *19*(3), 455–461.

Gibson, J. L. "A Plea for Painted Railing and Painted Walls of Rooms as the Source of Lead Poisoning Among Queensland Children." *Australian Medical Gazette*, 1904, *23*, 149–153.

Ginsberg, G., and others. "Evaluation of Child/Adult Pharmacokinetic Differences from a Database Derived from the Therapeutic Drug Literature." *Toxicological Sciences*, 2002, *66*(2), 185–200.

Ginsberg, G., Hattis, D., Miller, R., and Sonawane, B. "Pediatric Pharmacokinetic Data: Implications for Environmental Risk Assessment for Children." *Pediatrics*, 2004, *113*(4), 973–983.

Ginsberg, G., Slikker, W., Jr., Bruckner, J., and Sonawane, B. "Incorporating Children's Toxicokinetics into a Risk Framework." *Environmental Health Perspectives*, 2004, *112*(2), 272–283.

Grandjean, P., and others. "Neurobehavioral Deficits Associated with PCB in 7-Year-Old Children Prenatally Exposed to Seafood Neurotoxicants." *Neurotoxicology and Teratology*, 2001, *23*(4), 305–317.

Gurney, J. G., and others. "Trends in Cancer Incidence Among Children in the U.S." *Cancer*, 1996, *78*(3), 532–541.

Haggerty, R., and Rothmann, J. *Child Health and the Community*. Hoboken, N.J.: Wiley, 1975.

Harada, H. "Congenital Minamata Disease: Intrauterine Methylmercury Poisoning." *Teratology*, 1978, *18*(2), 285–288.

Herbst, A. L., Hubby, M. M., Azizi, F., and Makii, M. M. "Reproductive and Gynecologic Surgical Experience in Diethylstilbestrol-Exposed Daughters." *American Journal of Obstetrics and Gynecology*, 1981, *141*(8), 1019–1028.

Hooper, K., and McDonald, T. A. "The PBDEs: An Emerging Environmental Challenge and Another Reason for Breast-Milk Monitoring Programs." *Environmental Health Perspectives*, 2000, *108*(5), 387–392.

Hooper, K., and others. "Analysis of Breast Milk to Assess Exposure to Chlorinated Contaminants in Kazakhstan: Sources of 2,3,7,8-Tetrachlorodibenzo-p-Dioxin (TCDD) Exposures in an Agricultural Region of Southern Kazakhstan." *Environmental Health Perspectives*, 1999, *107*(6), 447–457.

Howdeshell, K. L. and others. "Cumulative Effects of Dibutyl Phthalate and Diethylhexyl Phthalate on Male Rat Reproductive Tract Development: Altered Fetal Steroid Hormones and Genes." *Toxicological Sciences* 2007, *99*(1), 190–202.

Howdeshell K. L. and others. "A Mixture of Five Phthalate Esters Inhibits Fetal Testicular Testosterone Production in the Sprague-Dawley Rat in a Cumulative, Dose-Additive Manner." *Toxicological Sciences*, 2008, *105*(1), 153–65.

Institute of Medicine, Food and Nutrition Board. *Nutrition During Lactation*. Washington, D.C.: National Academies Press, 1991.

Jackson, R. J. "The Impact of the Built Environment on Health: An Emerging Field." *American Journal of Public Health*, 2003, *93*(9), 1382–1384.

Jacobson, J. L., and Jacobson, S. W. "Intellectual Impairment in Children Exposed to Polychlorinated Biphenyls in Utero." *New England Journal of Medicine*, 1996, *335*(11), 783–789.

Landrigan, P. J., and Carlson, J. E. "Environmental Policy and Children's Health." *Future Child*, 1995, *5*(2), 34–52.

Landrigan, P. J., Kimmel, C. A., Correa, A., and Eskenazi, B. "Children's Health and the Environment: Public Health Issues and Challenges for Risk Assessment." *Environmental Health Perspectives*, 2004, *112*(2), 257–265.

Landrigan, P. J., and others. "Chemical Contaminants in Breast Milk and Their Impacts on Children's Health: An Overview." *Environmental Health Perspectives*, 2002a, *110*(6), A313–A315.

Landrigan, P. J., and others. "Environmental Pollutants and Disease in American Children: Estimates of Morbidity, Mortality, and Costs for Lead Poisoning, Asthma, Cancer, and Developmental Disabilities." *Environmental Health Perspectives*, 2002b, *110*(7), 721–728.

Landrigan, P. J., and others. "The National Children's Study: A 21-Year Prospective Study of 100,000 American Children." *Pediatrics*, 2006, *118*(5), 2173–2186.

Lanphear, B. P. "Low-Level Environmental Lead Exposure and Children's Intellectual Function: An International Pooled Analysis." *Environmental Health Perspectives*, 2005, *113*(7), 894–899.

Lipscomb, J. W., Kramer, J. E., and Leikin, J. B. "Seizure Following Brief Exposure to the Insect Repellent N,N-Diethyl-m-Toluamide." *Annals of Emergency Medicine*, 1992, *21*(3), 315–317.

Loffredo, C. A., Silbergeld, E. K., Ferencz, C., and Zhang, J. "Association of Transposition of the Great Arteries in Infants with Maternal Exposures to Herbicides and Rodenticides." *American Journal of Epidemiology*, 2001, *153*(6), 529–536.

Longnecker, M. P., Klebanoff, M. A., Zhou, H., and Brock, J. W. "Association Between Maternal Serum Concentration of the DDT Metabolite DDE and Preterm and Small-for-Gestational-Age Babies at Birth." *Lancet*, 2001, *358*(9276), 110–114.

Lu, C., and others. "Organic Diets Significantly Lower Children's Dietary Exposure to Organophosphorus Pesticides." *Environmental Health Perspectives*, 2006, *114*(2), 260–263.

MacIntyre, S., MacIver, S., and Sooman, A. "Area, Class and Health: Should We Be Focusing on Places or People?" *Journal of Social Policy*, 1993, *22*(2), 213–243.

Masuda, Y. "Health Status of Japanese and Taiwanese After Exposure to Contaminated Rice Oil." *Environmental Health Perspectives*, 1985, *60*, 321–325.

Matthews, T. J., and MacDorman, M. F. *Infant Mortality Statistics from the 2005 Period Linked Birth/Infant Death Dataset.* National Center for Health Statistics, 2008.

Maziak, W., Ward, K. D., and Stockton, M. B. "Childhood Obesity: Are We Missing the Big Picture?" *Obesity Reviews*, 2008, *9*(1), 35–42.

McBride, W. G. "Thalidomide and Congenital Abnormalities." *Lancet*, 1961, *2*, 1358.

Menon, K. S. "Exposure of Children to DEET and Other Topically Applied Insect Repellents." *American Journal of Industrial Medicine*, 2005, *47*(1), 91–97.

Messerli, F. H., and Mittler B. S. "Framingham at 50." *Lancet*, 1998, *352*(9133), 1006.

Miller, R. W. "Delayed Effects Occurring Within the First Decade After Exposure of Young Individuals to the Hiroshima Atomic Bomb." *Pediatrics*, 1956, *18*(1), 1–18.

Miller, R. W., and Blot, W. J. "Small Head Size After In-Utero Exposure to Atomic Radiation." *Lancet*, 1972, *2*(7781), 784–787.

Morland, K., Wing, S., and Diez Roux, A. "The Contextual Effect of the Local Food Environment on Residents' Diets: The Atherosclerosis Risk in Communities Study." *American Journal of Public Health*, 2002, *92*(11), 1761–1767.

Morland, K., Wing, S., Diez Roux, A., and Poole, C. "Neighborhood Characteristics Associated with the Location of Food Stores and Food Service Places." *American Journal of Preventive Medicine*, 2002, *22*(1), 23–29.

National Academy of Sciences. *Environmental Neurotoxicology.* Washington, D.C.: National Academies Press, 1992.

National Children's Study. [Homepage]. http://www.nationalchildrensstudy.gov, 2009.

National Research Council, Committee on Pesticides in the Diets of Infants and Children. *Pesticides in the Diets of Infants and Children*. Washington, D.C.: National Academies Press, 1993.

National Research Council. *Scientific Frontiers in Developmental Toxicology and Risk Assessment*. Washington, D.C.: National Academies Press, 2000.

Needleman, H. L., and others. "Deficits in Psychologic and Classroom Performance of Children with Elevated Dentine Lead Levels." *New England Journal of Medicine*, 1979, *300*(13), 689–695.

Needleman, H. L., and others. "The Long-Term Effects of Exposure to Low Doses of Lead in Childhood: An 11-Year Follow-Up Report." *New England Journal of Medicine*, 1990, *322*(2), 83–88.

Northridge, M. E., and others. "Diesel Exhaust Exposure Among Adolescents in Harlem: A Community-Driven Study." *American Journal of Public Health*, 1999, *89*(7), 998–1002.

Oddy, W. H. "Breastfeeding Protects Against Illness and Infection in Infants and Children: A Review of the Evidence." *Breastfeeding Review*, 2001, *9*(2), 11–18.

Office of Science and Technology Policy, National Science and Technology Council. *Investing in Our Future: A National Research Initiative for America's Children for the 21st Century*. Washington, D.C.: Executive Office of the President, Office of Science and Technology Policy, 1997.

O'Flaherty, E. J. "Pharmacokinetics, Pharmacodynamics, and Prediction of Developmental Abnormalities." *Reproductive Toxicology*, 1997, *11*(2–3), 413–416.

Olden, K., and Wilson, S. "Environmental Health and Genomics: Visions and Implications." *Nature Reviews: Genetics*, 2000, *1*(2), 149–153.

Ordonez, J. V., Carrillo, J. A., Miranda, M., and Gale, J. L. [Epidemiologic study of a disease believed to be encephalitis in the region of the highlands of Guatemala.] [Article in Spanish.] *Boletin de la Oficina Sanitaria Panamericana*, 1966, *60*(6), 510–519.

Pastor, P. N., and Reuben, C. A. "Diagnosed Attention Deficit Hyperactivity Disorder and Learning Disability—United States, 2004–2006." National Center for Health Statistics. *Vital Health Statistics*, 2008, *10*(237), 1–14.

Paulson, J. A., and Gitterman, B. A. (eds.). "Children's Health and the Environment, Part I." *Pediatric Clinics of North America*, 2007a, *54*(1, entire issue).

Paulson, J. A., and Gitterman, B. A. (eds.). "Children's Health and the Environment, Part II." *Pediatric Clinics of North America*, 2007b, *54*(2, entire issue).

Pew Environmental Health Commission. *Attack Asthma: Why America Needs a Public Health Defense System to Battle Environmental Threats*. http://healthyamericans.org/reports/files/asthma.pdf, Apr. 2000.

Pierce, P. E., and others. "Alkyl Mercury Poisoning in Humans: Report of an Outbreak." *JAMA*, 1972, *220*(11), 1439–1442.

Rider C.V. and others. "Cumulative Effects of In Utero Administration of Mixtures of 'Antiandrogens' on Male Rat Reproductive Development." *Toxicologic Pathology*, 2009, *37*(1), 100–113.

Ries, L. A. G., and others. *SEER Cancer Statistics Review, 1975–2004*. National Cancer Institute. http://seer.cancer.gov/csr/1975_2004, 2004.

Robinson, T. N. "Reducing Children's Television Viewing to Prevent Obesity: A Randomized Controlled Trial." *JAMA*, 1999, *282*(16), 1561–1567.

Rull, R. P. "Neural Tube Defects and Maternal Residential Proximity to Agricultural Pesticide Applications." *American Journal of Epidemiology*, 2006, *163*(8), 743–753.

Rutter, M. "Isle of Wight Revisited: Twenty-Five Years of Child Psychiatric Epidemiology." *Journal of the American Academy of Child and Adolescent Psychiatry*, 1989, *28*(5), 633–653.

Sallis, J. F., and others. "San Diego Surveyed for Heart-Healthy Foods and Exercise Facilities." *Public Health Reports*, 1986, *101*(2), 216–219.

Sallis, J. F., and others. "Distance Between Homes and Exercise Facilities Related to Frequency of Exercise Among San Diego Residents." *Public Health Reports*, 1990, *105*(2), 179–185.

Sanborn, M., and others. *Systematic Review of Pesticide Human Health Effects*. Ontario College of Family Physicians. http://www.ocfp.on.ca/local/files/Communications/Current%20Issues/Pesticides/Final%20Paper%2023APR2004.pdf, 2004.

Selevan, S. G., Kimmel, C. A., and Mendola, P. "Identifying Critical Windows of Exposure for Children's Health." *Environmental Health Perspectives*, 2000, *108*(suppl. 3), 451–455.

Shaw, G. M., and others. "Maternal Pesticide Exposure from Multiple Sources and Selected Congenital Anomalies." *Epidemiology*, 1999, *10*(1), 60–66.

Shea, K. M. (American Academy of Pediatrics Committee on Environmental Health). "Pediatric Exposure and Potential Toxicity of Phthalate Plasticizers." *Pediatrics*, 2003, *111*(6, pt. 1), 1467–1474.

Silva, P. A. "The Dunedin Multidisciplinary Health and Development Study: A 15-Year Longitudinal Study." *Paediatric and Perinatal Epidemiology*, 1990, *4*(1), 76–107.

Solomon, G. M., and Weiss, P. M. "Chemical Contaminants in Breast Milk: Time Trends and Regional Variability." *Environmental Health Perspectives*, 2002, *110*(6), A339–A347.

Solomon, G., Weiss, P., Owen, B., and Citron, A. *Healthy Milk, Healthy Baby: Chemical Pollution and Mother's Milk*. Natural Resources Defense Council. http://www.nrdc.org/breastmilk/default.asp, 2005.

Spielberg, S. P. *"Anticonvulsant Adverse Drug Reactions: Age Dependent and Age Independent."* In P. S. Guzelian, C. J. Henry, and S. S. Olin (eds.), *Similarities and Differences Between Children and Adults: Implications for Risk Assessment*. Washington, D.C.: International Life Sciences Institute Press, 1992.

Srinivasan, S., O'Fallon, L. R., and Dearry, A. "Creating Healthy Communities, Healthy Homes, Healthy People: Initiating a Research Agenda on the Built Environment and Public Health." *American Journal of Public Health*, 2003, *93*(9), 1446–1450.

Sudakin, D. D. L. "DEET: A Review and Update of Safety and Risk in the General Population. *Clinical Toxicology*, 2003, *41*(6), 831–839.

Taussig, H. "A Study of the German Outbreak of Phocomelia." *JAMA*, 1962, *180*, 1106–1114.

Taylor, P. R., Lawrence, C. E., Hwang, H. L., and Paulson, A. S. "Polychlorinated Biphenyls: Influence on Birthweight and Gestation." *American Journal of Public Health*, 1984, *74*(10), 1153–1154.

Tilson, H. A., Jacobson, J. L., and Rogan, W. J. "Polychlorinated Biphenyls and the Developing Nervous System: Cross-Species Comparisons." *Neurotoxicology and Teratology*, 1990, *12*(3), 239–248.

U.S. Environmental Protection Agency. "Guidelines for the Health Assessment of Suspect Developmental Toxicants." *Federal Register*, *51*, 34028–34040 (1986).

U.S. Environmental Protection Agency. *Chemicals in Commerce Information System: Chemical Update System Database*. Washington, D.C.: U.S. Environmental Protection Agency, 1998.

U.S. Environmental Protection Agency. *Toxicology Data Requirements for Assessing Risks of Pesticide Exposure to Children's Health*. Report of the Toxicology Working Group of the 10X Task Force. http://www.epa.gov/scipoly/sap/1999/index.htm#may, 1999.

U.S. Environmental Protection Agency. *Concepts, Methods, and Data Sources for Cumulative Health Risk Assessment of Multiple Chemicals, Exposures and Effects: A Resource Document (Final Report)*. EPA/600/R-06/013F. Washington, D.C.: U.S. Environmental Protection Agency, 2007a.

U.S. Environmental Protection Agency. *HPV Chemical Hazard Data Availability Study*. http://www.epa .gov/HPV/pubs/general/hazchem.htm, 2007b.

U.S. Environmental Protection Agency. *Assessing Pesticide Cumulative Risk*. http://www.epa.gov/ oppsrrd1/cumulative, 2008.

U.S. Environmental Protection Agency. *IAQ Tools for Schools Program*. http://www.epa.gov/iaq/schools, 2009.

U.S. Environmental Protection Agency, Indoor Environments Division. "Fact Sheet: Mold in Schools." EPA-402-F-03-029. http://www.epa.gov/iaq/schools/pdfs/publications/moldfactsheet.pdf, 2004.

U.S. Environmental Protection Agency, Risk Assessment Forum. *Guidelines for Developmental Toxicity Risk Assessment*. EPA/600/FR-91/001. http://cfpub.epa.gov/ncea/cfm/recordisplay. cfm?deid=23162, 1991.

U.S. Environmental Protection Agency, Risk Assessment Forum. *A Review of the Reference Dose and Reference Concentration Processes*. EPA/630/P-02/002F. http://www.epa.gov/raf/publications/ review-reference-dose.htm, 2002.

Weich, S., and others. "Measuring the Built Environment: Validity of a Site Survey Instrument for Use in Urban Settings." *Health & Place*, 2001, *7*(4), 283–292.

Weidner, I. S., Moller, H., Jensen, T. K., and Skakkebaek, N. E. "Cryptorchidism and Hypospadias in Sons of Gardeners and Farmers." *Environmental Health Perspectives*, 1998, *106*(12), 793–796.

Weiss, B., and Landrigan, P. J. "The Developing Brain and the Environment: An Introduction." *Environmental Health Perspectives*, 2000, *108*(suppl. 3), 373–374.

Welsch, F., Blumenthal, G. M., and Conolly, R. B. "Physiologically Based Pharmacokinetic Models Applicable to Organogenesis: Extrapolation Between Species and Potential Use in Prenatal Toxicity Risk Assessments." *Toxicology Letters*, 1995, *82–83*, 539–547.

Wendel, A. M., Dannenberg, A. L., and Frumkin, H. "Designing and Building Healthy Places for Children." *International Journal of Environment and Health*, 2008, *2*(3/4), 338–355.

West Harlem Environmental Action. "We Act." http://www.weact.org, 2008.

Whitney, K. D., Seidler, F. J., and Slotkin, T. A. "Developmental Neurotoxicity of Chlorpyrifos: Cellular Mechanisms." *Toxicology and Applied Pharmacology*, 1995, *134*(1), 53–62.

Whyatt, R.M., and others. "Biomarkers in Assessing Residential Insecticide Exposures During Pregnancy and Effects on Fetal Growth." *Toxicology and Applied Pharmacology*, 2005, *206*(2), 246–254.

Wiles, R., and Campbell, C. *Pesticides in Children's Food*. Washington, D.C.: Environmental Working Group, 1993.

World Health Organization. *The World Health Report 2002: Reducing Risks, Promoting Healthy Life*. Geneva: World Health Organization, 2002.

Yang, D., and others. "Chlorpyrifos and Chlorpyrifos-Oxon Inhibit Axonal Growth by Interfering with the Morphogenic Activity of Acetylcholinesterase." *Toxicology and Applied Pharmacology*, 2008, *228*(1), 32–41.

Yu, M. L., Hsu, C. C., Gladen, B. C., and Rogan, W. J. "In Utero PCB/PCDF Exposure: Relation of Developmental Delay to Dysmorphology and Dose." *Neurotoxicology and Teratology*, 1991, *13*(2), 195–202.

Zahm, S. H., and Ward, M. H. "Pesticides and Childhood Cancer." *Environmental Health Perspectives*, 1998, *106*(suppl. 3), 893–908.

FOR FURTHER INFORMATION

Books

Needleman, H. L., and Landrigan, P. J. *Raising Children Toxic Free: How to Keep Your Child Safe from Lead, Asbestos, Pesticides, and Other Environmental Hazards.* New York: HarperCollins, 1994.

Wigle, D. T. *Child Health and the Environment.* New York: Oxford University Press, 2003.
Another book deserving emphasis is Etzel and Balk, 2003, listed in the chapter References.

Journal

Environmental Health Perspectives. [Homepage.] http://ehp.niehs.nih.gov. This journal produced by the National Institute of Environmental Health Sciences (NIEHS) has a monthly section dedicated to children's environmental health and is a valuable source of emerging research in this area.

Agencies and Organizations

American Academy of Pediatrics (AAP), Committee on Environmental Health. [Homepage.] http://www.aap.org/visit/cmte16.htm, 2005. Active in promoting children's environmental health within the pediatrics profession and more broadly, the AAP Committee on Environmental Health produces the *Handbook of Pediatric Environmental Health*, issues policy statements, and maintains an informative Web site:

U.S. Environmental Protection Agency (EPA), Office of Children's Health Protection. [Homepage.] http://yosemite.epa.gov/ochp/ochpweb.nsf/homepage, 2005. The EPA's Office of Children's Health Protection coordinates children's environmental health activity within EPA and with other partners; its Web site is an excellent source of information and links to other information sources.
The following nongovernmental organizations also offer useful information.

Children's Environmental Health Network (CEHN), http://www.cehn.org.

Children's Health Environment Coalition (CHEC), http://www.checnet.org.

Healthy Schools Network, Inc (HSN), http://www.healthyschools.org.

Learning Disabilities Association of America, http://www.ldanatl.org.

Clinical Services and Training Programs

Association of Occupational and Environmental Clinics (AOEC). "Pediatric Environmental Health
      Specialty Units." http://www.aoec.org/PEHSU.htm, 2005. In 1998, the AOEC, in
      association with the EPA and ATSDR, established a network of clinical centers in children's
      environmental health, the Pediatric Environmental Health Specialty Units (PEHSUs).
      Located throughout the United States and in some foreign countries, PEHSUs provide
      clinical assessments, education, and consultation. Visit the Web site for more information and
      links to each unit.
Ambulatory Pediatric Association (APA). In 2001, the APA established the Pediatric Environmental
      Health Fellowship Program, a national training program in environmental pediatrics. This
      training is available at Boston Children's Hospital of Harvard Medical School, Mount Sinai
      School of Medicine, Cincinnati Children's Hospital, Children's National Medical Center,
      and University of Washington School of Medicine.

Research

National Institute of Environmental Health Sciences (NIEHS). "Centers for Children's Environmental
      Health and Disease Prevention Research." http://www.niehs.nih.gov/translat/children/
      children.htm, 2005. In 1998, the EPA, NIEHS, and CDC jointly established the Centers for
      Children's Environmental Health and Disease Prevention Research, a national network of
      research centers at major medical centers. The creation of these centers marked the largest
      federal research investment to date in children's environmental health.
Centers for Disease Control and Prevention. "National Report on Human Exposure to Environmental
      Chemicals." http://www.cdc.gov/exposurereport, 2008. The CDC periodically publishes
      the National Report on Human Exposure to Environmental Chemicals, an ongoing assess-
      ment, using biomonitoring, of the exposure of the U.S. population, including children, to
      environmental chemicals. Visit the Web site for information on methods and results and to
      view existing reports.

PART FIVE

THE PRACTICE OF ENVIRONMENTAL HEALTH

CHAPTER TWENTY-SIX

PREVENTION IN ENVIRONMENTAL HEALTH

LYNN R. GOLDMAN

KEY CONCEPTS

■ Prevention lies at the core of environmental public health. It includes not only the control of hazards, but also health promotion through environmental strategies.

■ Prevention in environmental health extends upstream to the root causes of environmental change and to the resulting environmental pressures that eventually have an impact on human health and well-being.

■ Prevention efforts can be divided into primary, secondary, and tertiary prevention. All are relevant in environmental health.

■ The prevention hierarchy ranges from definitive approaches, such as completely removing a hazard (more preferable), to administrative, behavioral, and end-of-pipeline approaches (less preferable).

■ The precautionary principle proposes that cost-effective preventive measures should proceed even in the face of scientific uncertainty.

■ In environmental public health practice, all the core functions of public health—in the categories of assessment, policy development, and assurance—are used to pursue prevention.

THE mission of environmental public health extends well beyond remediating, cleaning up, or otherwise making up for past mistakes. It is to assure conditions that enhance the health of humans and other species. This chapter examines the concept of prevention and its application in environmental public health. It explores the principles and frameworks that underlie prevention in environmental public health, and how prevention strategies in environmental public health fit within the general practice of public health.

The environment has a major impact on individuals' risk of chronic diseases and conditions, such as cancers, chronic lung disease, and birth defects, and on the risk of acute illnesses, such as viral gastroenteritis, respiratory infections, and such vector-borne diseases as malaria. Accordingly, environmental public health is concerned with the prevention of these conditions.

But the environment has far broader impacts on health. Some environmental conditions confer resilience to the most harmful impacts of natural disasters, whereas others put people directly in harm's way (through building homes and other structures on flood plains and earthquake faults, for example.) Some environments promote health by providing nutritious food, adequate supplies of drinking water, opportunities for outdoor recreation, and aesthetic and mental health benefits of nature contact. The state of knowledge about causation of communicable diseases is more advanced that that for chronic diseases and natural disasters, which are in turn better understood than environmental aspects of health promotion. However, prevention efforts in environmental health need to address all of these concerns.

From the outset it is important to emphasize that certain environmental health problems are much more serious in developing countries than in wealthy countries. In developing nations, for example, drinking water contaminated by microorganisms and toxic substances causes considerable morbidity and mortality, and burning coal, wood, and other biomass fuel sources for cooking and heating contributes to indoor air and outdoor air pollution (see Chapter Eleven). Chemical releases are more common, and there are fewer means to protect workers, nearby communities, and passersby. Worldwide there are large numbers of preventable deaths and injuries due to earthquakes, storms, and floods; many of these deaths are preventable with appropriate environmental measures, such as construction standards for homes and buildings.

René Dubos noted in 1965 that indices of environmental health are "expressions of the success or failure experienced by the [human] organism in its efforts to respond adaptively to environmental challenges" (Dubos, 1965). Prevention in environmental health is at its core a continuous effort to adapt to environmental challenges, most of which are created by human activities. With rapid population growth, development, and technological change on a global scale, prevention efforts have become more and more complex.

Lynn R. Goldman declares no competing financial interests.

Despite these challenges, there is evidence of remarkable success in environmental health protection over the last two centuries. The sanitary movement of the 1800s resulted in enormous reductions in mortality from infectious diseases. This accounted for remarkable increases in life expectancy in much of the world (in the United States, from forty-seven years in 1900 to seventy-eight in 2007). In the last forty years in the industrialized nations, stronger environmental laws have resulted in cleaner air, safer drinking water, and recovery of some rivers and lakes that in 1970 had unacceptable levels of pollution for fishing and recreation. In many parts of the world the easiest problems have to a great extent been addressed, leaving the environmental threats that are much more difficult to control and require more participation from a broader range of society. Environmental health problems today often involve multiple small sources of pollutants rather than a few large and visible ones. Many of these small sources are from sectors such as agriculture and small business, which are less familiar than other sectors now are with environmental regulations and are often resistant to change. Further, as developed countries confront climate change by reducing carbon emissions, new technologies will emerge, and with them, new challenges for prevention of health threats.

As discussed in Chapter Eleven, global trends in environmental health are more disturbing. In developing countries, economic development and the rapid pace of urbanization have resulted in alarming increases in air and water pollution and in waste generation. Drinking water is under pressure both from pollution and from consumption, and in many parts of the world there are serious shortages of potable water. Weather extremes associated with global warming are associated with increased risk of heat-related mortality, increased intensity of severe weather events and of their resultant impacts on human health and well-being, and changes in ranges of vector-borne diseases, alterations in agricultural productivity, and greater uncertainty in water supplies. Pollution and overfishing are threatening fish harvests. At the same time, efforts to produce more fish via fish farming have too often had other undesirable environmental consequences, such as water pollution. Globally, there is little control of chemicals and pesticides in commerce and disposal. Prevention of noncommunicable diseases is especially challenging for developing countries because these diseases are multifactorial and because the scarcity of local data makes prevention efforts highly dependent on international practices instead of approaches rooted in local culture, lifestyles, and climate (McMichael, Woodruff, and Hales, 2006).

CONCEPTS OF PREVENTION

The **DPSEEA** (driving forces-pressures-state-exposure-effects-actions) model, presented in the Introduction to this book, is useful in understanding environmental health prevention efforts. For environmental health, **driving forces** are factors such as population growth and technology development that motivate environmental processes. These result in the generation of environmental **pressures**, for example, increases in vehicle miles driven or the numbers of coal-fired power plants. The **state** of the environment, such as the concentration of pollutants in the air (and whether such concentrations potentially are hazardous), is modified by such pressures. **Exposure** occurs when people are present both at the place and time that the hazard occurs and when there is an intact pathway for exposure. Depending on the timing and the amount of exposure (dose), along with other factors like life stage and coexposures, exposure may lead to health **effects**. **Actions** to reduce or control the hazards (or to promote environmental health) can be taken at all points in this chain of events. In 1958, Leavell and Clark defined a three-stage model for **prevention** that remains relevant:

- **Primary prevention** involves interventions prior to the development of any signs of ill health. In the case of environmental health, strategies directed toward modifying driving forces, pressures, and the state of the environment are primary prevention efforts. Such efforts are divided into two categories:
  Health promotion: interventions that are not directed toward the prevention of a specific disease but rather to further general health and well-being. Education about safe household pest management strategies and safe use of household pesticides is an example.
  Specific protection: interventions taken to intercept known causes of diseases. The phaseout of lead (a known developmental neurotoxicant) in gasoline is an example.
- **Secondary prevention** is early detection of a health problem, prior to the onset of disease, for the purpose of intervening at an early stage to prevent the development of the disease. In environmental health this is usually a preventive effort targeting the phase when exposure has begun to occur but prior to disease development. An example is occupational or childhood lead screening, where the objective is to identify people at an early stage of exposure and to take steps to prevent further exposure.
- **Tertiary prevention** involves early identification and treatment of people with a disease in order to prevent or forestall disability or death. An example is the effort to diagnose children with asthma promptly and to ensure that physicians and families follow recommended guidelines for medical treatment and environmental remediation in order to reduce the severity of health impacts of this disease on children.

The practice of industrial hygiene, as described in Chapter Four, takes an approach to prevention in occupational health that hews to a **prevention**

PERSPECTIVE
Moving Childhood Lead Poisoning Prevention from Tertiary to Primary Prevention

Childhood lead poisoning prevention is a good example of the change over time from a tertiary prevention to a primary prevention approach to environmental health. As a result of long-standing, widespread misuse of lead, the United States suffered an epidemic of lead poisoning. This was a particular hazard for poor children living in dilapidated housing with deteriorating lead-based paint, but potentially a hazard to all children where such paint had been applied. In 1971, the American Academy of Pediatrics urged clinicians and the federal government to undertake a massive effort to screen children for lead poisoning by assessment of blood lead levels, and in the 1970s the Centers for Disease Control and Prevention (CDC) and state and local public health agencies embarked on lead-screening campaigns in many U.S. urban areas. The aim of such programs was to identify children with clinically elevated blood lead levels (initially 60 μg/dL and above) so that such children could be treated in order to avert the most severe consequences of lead poisoning. In many communities, local environmental and housing agencies abated lead hazards in these homes, but such activities were not funded by the federal government. This approach, in retrospect, basically involved tertiary prevention, early identification and treatment of children who already were lead poisoned to prevent the worst consequences.

As a result of discoveries about lead toxicity the CDC lowered the lead level of concern in several steps from 60 to (by 1993) 10 μg/dL. At the same time, the approach to prevention continued to be clinically based; efforts to remediate household lead contamination continued to start with lead screening and identification of children with elevated blood lead levels. When blood lead levels were lowered, this became secondary prevention; when the standard was lowered to 10 or 15 μg/dL, most children found to be above those levels did not require specific medical therapy, although general nutrition and health supervision were needed. In the United States, overlapping with blood lead screening efforts, primary prevention efforts had also begun, starting with the control of lead in paint, pipe solder and other plumbing materials, and numerous other consumer products in the 1970s, and the phasedown of lead in gasoline in the 1980s. These measures were generally effective in lowering lead exposures across the entire population. Most recently, primary prevention approaches have been developed to mitigate lead exposures in existing housing by targeting efforts not on individual children who are already exposed to lead but instead on housing that is likely to expose children to lead. This is a transition from an illness-based model, one predicated on identifying and treating clinically ill children, to a model of wellness promotion, one that seeks to prevent lead toxicity. Although physicians and other medical professionals continue to have a role to play, there is a much stronger role for environmental and housing experts and for community efforts to enforce housing codes (American Academy of Pediatrics, Committee on Environmental Health, 2005).

hierarchy similar in concept to primary and secondary prevention. From preferable to less preferable the hierarchy goes as follows:

- **Substitution**. Use safer chemicals, products, processes, or activities to eliminate the hazard from the workplace.
- **Engineering controls**. Use equipment that reduces or controls exposure in and around work areas.
- **Administrative controls**. Change the way that workers do their job to reduce or eliminate exposures to hazards.
- **Personal protective equipment** (PPE). Enforce the use of such equipment as respirators, hard hats, face and eye protection, hearing protection, gloves, and protective clothing and footwear that reduce or eliminate exposure to the hazard.

Pollution prevention is an approach to environmental health prevention akin to the concept of primary prevention. It extends approaches used in industrial hygiene to the general environment. The principles of pollution prevention as defined by the Pollution Prevention Act (1990) are as follows:

> "pollution should be prevented or reduced at the source whenever feasible;
> "pollution that cannot be prevented should be recycled in an environmentally safe manner whenever feasible;
> "pollution that cannot be prevented or recycled should be treated in an environmentally safe manner whenever feasible; and
> "disposal or other release into the environment should be employed only as a last resort and should be conducted in an environmentally safe manner."

Pollution prevention aims for increased efficiency in the use of raw materials, energy, water, or other resources, or protection of natural resources by conservation. Pollution prevention can be envisioned as a ladder of potential environmental health strategies, in order of most to least preferable:

- Source reduction
- Waste minimization
- Reuse of materials
- Recycling of materials
- Emission controls
- Proper waste disposal
- Cleanup of wastes and spills

Source reduction practices are varied and include equipment or technology modifications, process modifications, reformulation of materials, redesign of products, substitution of raw materials, and improvements in housekeeping, maintenance, training, or inventory control.

When all costs are taken into account, reduction of pollution at the source is generally less expensive than end-of-pipe efforts to control emissions or perform environmental cleanup. Pollution prevention strategies not only emphasize fundamental drivers (for example, population and technologies) and pressures that create the conditions that cause environmental health impacts, they also take a multimedia approach. It has long been recognized that efforts to address pollution one medium at a time can result in just moving pollutants from water to air to land to water. Multimedia approaches look at all impacts of decisions "from cradle to grave;" such an analysis, called a **life cycle analysis**, can result in the adoption of more effective preventive strategies. As shown in Figure 26.1, life cycle analysis is a systems approach that takes into consideration both inputs (raw materials and energy) and outputs (product, pollution, and waste). It attempts to encompass all related processes from the acquisition of raw materials and

FIGURE 26.1   Elements of a Life Cycle Analysis

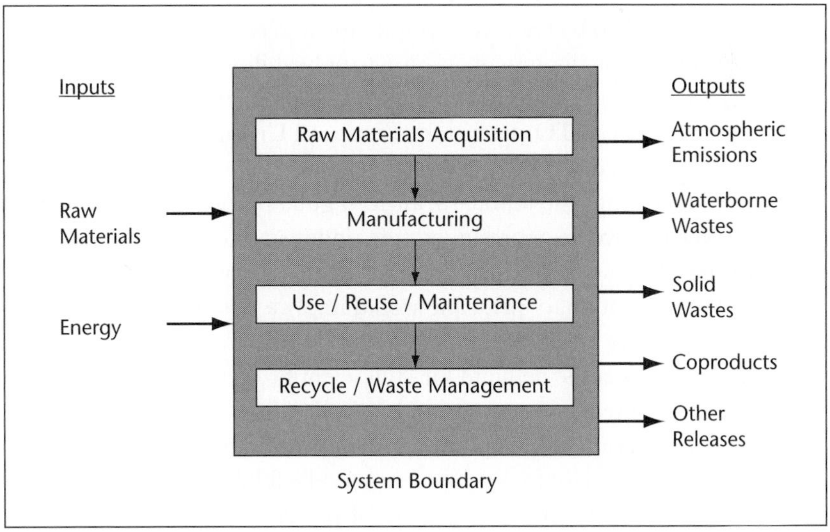

Source: Environmental Protection Agency, 1993.

the various steps in processing and manufacture to use and reuse and the ultimate fate of a product. Table 26.1 gives examples of elements that may need to be considered in a life cycle analysis.

PRINCIPLES OF PREVENTION

In 1992, more than 100 nations signed the United Nations Conference on Environment and Development (UNCED) treaty that formally adopted the goal of **sustainable development** and a number of principles of sustainable development, many of which have a direct bearing on prevention. Chief among these is principle 1, which states: "Human beings are at the center of concerns for sustainable development. They are entitled to a healthy and productive life in harmony with nature" (UNCED, 1992).

Another UNCED principle applicable to environmental public health is the **precautionary principle**. As governments agreed in 1992: "In order to protect the environment, the precautionary approach shall be widely applied by States according to their capabilities. Where there are threats of serious or irreversible damage, lack of full scientific certainty shall not be used as a reason for postponing cost-effective measures to prevent environmental degradation"(UNCED, 1992). For example, the pesticide dichlorodiphenyltrichloroethane (DDT) was banned in the United States long before its precise mechanisms of action had been described by scientists. Despite the agreement to this principle at UNCED, a great deal of disagreement on its applicability exists in other global contexts. For example, the United States and Canada filed a claim with the World Trade Organization (WTO) against the European Union's ban on hormones fed to farm animals (Carlarne, 2007). Another example is the tens of thousands of chemicals introduced into the market prior to regulation of chemicals. So-called existing chemicals have been presumed safe under statutory schemes that have required review of "new chemicals" but not chemicals previously on the market. Adoption of the precautionary principle would imply a duty to take "cost-effective" measures to reduce environmental degradation and prevent damage to health without having to meet the demand for "full scientific certainty" about the harm of toxic chemicals, greenhouse gases, and so forth.

A third principle that has a strong prevention focus is **intergenerational equity**: "The right to development must be fulfilled so as to equitably meet developmental and environmental needs of present and future generations" (UNCED, 1992).This principle emphasizes the responsibility of the present generation to take steps to prevent adverse circumstances for those that come after. For example,

TABLE 26.1 Commonly Used Impact Categories for Life Cycle Analysis

Impact Category	Scale	Examples of Data
Global warming	Global	Air releases of carbon dioxide (CO_2), nitrogen dioxide (NO_2), methane (CH_4), chlorofluorocarbons (CFCs), hydrochlorofluorocarbons (HCFCs), methyl bromide (CH_3Br)
Stratospheric ozone depletion	Global	Air releases of CFCs, HCFCs, halons, CH_3Br
Acidification	Regional, local	Air releases of sulfur oxides (SO_x), nitrogen oxides (NO_x), hydrochloric acid (HCl), hydrofluoric acid (HF), ammonia (NH_4)
Eutrophication	Local	Air releases of phosphate (PO_4), oxides of nitrogen (NOx), nitrates, ammonia (NH_4)
Photochemical smog	Local	Air releases of ozone, nonmethane hydrocarbon (NMHC), VOCs
Terrestrial toxicity	Local	Chemicals with toxicity to terrestrial species released to air, water and soil
Aquatic toxicity	Local	Chemicals with toxicity to aquatic species released to water
Human health	Global, regional, local	Chemicals with human toxicity released to air, water, and soil
Resource depletion	Global, regional, local	Quantity of minerals used Quantity of fossil fuels used Quantity of soils depleted Biological resources (fish, trees, and the like) depleted
Land use	Global, regional, local	Quantity disposed of in landfills or other land modifications Land area covered by impermeable surfaces Carbon sequestration potential of land use
Water use	Regional, local	Quantity of water used or consumed Alterations in water quality (for example, temperature, pH) Alterations in water dynamics (for example, subsidence, wetland depletion)

persistent organic pollutants (POPs), such as DDT, PCBs, methylmercury and dioxins, have contaminated agricultural and aquatic ecosystems, leaving a legacy of pollution for future generations. Emissions of greenhouse gases have set into motion processes that will alter the earth's climate for generations to come. From these and other examples we have learned that prevention needs to have a long time horizon. This principle contrasts with the perspective of monetary investment cycles, which have relatively short time frames and emphasize short-term gains over long-term earnings. Often false dichotomies are posed between environmental protection and jobs; there is little evidence of an association. However, there is a very real conflict between the approach taken by economists for rationally determining the rate of return for investments over time and the principle of intergenerational equity, which asks us to be willing to make sacrifices for the sake of the health and well-being of future generations as well as our own. A completely rational economic view argues that such actions need to be viewed as investments and judged against the expected economic return from other similar investments. In practice decision making needs to include both this kind of rational analysis and a consideration of principles such as our obligation to future generations, particularly for outcomes like global warming, for which there is no known remedy (other than prevention) and for which the consequences (and therefore the economic costs) are very difficult to predict but likely to be much larger than we recognize.

A fourth UNCED (1992) principle that is relevant in this context is *access to information and the decision-making process*: "At the national level, each individual shall have appropriate access to information concerning the environment that is held by public authorities, including information on hazardous materials and activities in their communities, and the opportunity to participate in decision-making processes. States shall facilitate and encourage public awareness and participation by making information widely available." Thus access to hazard information is an important element of prevention because not only environmental health experts but also many other actors—farmers, industries, utilities, developers, governmental agencies at all levels, and individual consumers—are involved in environmental decision making. It is also a key element of a democratic process to have shared information and input into decision-making processes. Finally, sharing information is often the preferred method of managing risks.

A fifth UNCED (1992) principle is **integrated decision making**: "In order to achieve sustainable development, environmental protection shall constitute an integral part of the development process and cannot be considered in isolation from it." This means that environmental considerations need to be incorporated into decision-making processes at all levels. In the United States, under the National Environmental Policy Act (NEPA), there is a responsibility for preparing **environmental impact reports** for all federally funded projects, and many states have such requirements as well. Such assessments seek to project possible negative impacts of proposed new projects so that such impacts can be avoided or mitigated. They have been successful in stopping projects that would have produced great environmental harm. A related tool, **health impact assessment**, focuses specifically on health consequences of decisions upstream from health (Kemm, Parry, and Palmer, 2004; Dannenberg and others, 2006). For example, a health impact assessment might assemble data comparing the health consequences of a highway expansion, a transit investment, and pedestrian infrastructure, to help a government reach the most health-promoting decision on the use of transportation funds.

Another important principle, adopted in many nations, is known as the **polluter pays principle**—the notion that those who cause and profit from pollution should pay the price for cleaning it up. In economic terms this is an effort to internalize the costs of externalities. More recently, this has evolved into the concept of economic instruments such as pollutant trading systems, which seek to shift the societal cost of pollution to the polluter in order to reduce the overall levels of pollution. Although these sound like secondary and tertiary prevention approaches, the ability to assign polluters the cost of emissions and cleanups serves as a powerful incentive for pollution prevention. (To put it another way, if polluting is "free" to the polluter and only society bears the price, then individuals and corporations have little incentive not to pollute.)

Even though the principles reviewed here have not been put in place consistently, they provide a strong policy framework for developing and implementing prevention strategies.

PUTTING PREVENTION INTO PRACTICE

In 1988, the U.S. Institute of Medicine published *The Future of Public Health*, a report that defined three major functions for **public health practice: assessment, policy development**, and **assurance** (Institute of Medicine, 1988).

Environmental public health assessment is discussed extensively in Chapter Four; this chapter focuses only on aspects of public health assessment having to do with prevention. The DPSEEA framework (described earlier) helps us to identify a number of potential targets for monitoring environmental conditions and associated health outcomes. As a tool for prevention, monitoring can provide data needed to

- Forecast the likely impacts of new technologies and population growth.
- Assess trends in drivers of environmental health (for example, human activities such as vehicle miles driven, construction of coal-fired power plants, automobile sales).
- Track trends in the state of the environment and human exposure levels.
- Track health trends.

Research is also an important component of the assessment process. All too often we do not have a strong enough understanding of the connection between environment and health to know what needs to be done to prevent some of the worst impacts of environmental exposures. Information about mechanisms of environmental health risks, including gene-environment interactions, will assist us in developing more informed and targeted strategies for disease prevention. Additionally, we have considerable uncertainty about the value of ecosystem services to human health and welfare. There have been serious disruptions in fundamental planetary processes—most famously in the carbon cycle, with a multitude of potential health effects (see Chapter Ten), but also in the nitrogen cycle, which has implications for agriculture and ecosystem productivity and pollution of sensitive water bodies. Species extinctions, overfishing, overfarming, and overirrigation have been documented in dramatic terms, but we do not fully understand their impacts on health.

Whether through monitoring and tracking efforts or through research, from the standpoint of prevention it is important to learn not only about the *proximate* causes of a problem but also the *root* causes. For example, scientists have identified in utero exposure to methylmercury as a risk factor for neurodevelopmental delays in children. This is definitely an issue involving intergeneration equity, and much of the policy effort has been directed toward protection of the fetus by advising women who are or may become pregnant to modify their fish consumption behaviors (because fish is an important pathway of exposure). However, completely different approaches could be taken. Going one step upstream, it would be possible for the government to set limits on the amount of mercury allowable in fish in order to protect the fetus from such exposures. Such an approach would not be politically popular, especially among industries that market these high-mercury fish. Going one step farther upstream one could try to identify all sources of mercury emissions, such as coal-fired power plants, and require the installation of pollution control equipment to remove the mercury from the air. Alternatively, it might be possible to address the root causes of the problem, such as mining and chemical manufacturing processes that generate mercury waste, use of mercury in compact fluorescent light bulbs, lack of any global commitments to cut mercury emissions (even though mercury circulates globally), and use of mercury-containing coal to generate energy. Examination of root causes might suggest a very different set of policy approaches than fish consumption advisories.

Environmental health policy has undergone major transformations over the years (see Chapter Thirty). There are numerous examples of environmental health policy failures over time, most reflecting an inability to predict, prepare for, and prevent adverse effects of new technologies. This includes the massive food safety and consumer products problems in the early 1900s (well documented by the author Upton Sinclair), the decision in the early part of the twentieth century to permit the use of lead in gasoline, the killer smog episodes in London caused by soot from coal burning in the mid-twentieth century, a very long-term problem with playing catch-up with the risks of industrial chemicals and pesticides (leading, for example, to epidemics of cancers from asbestos and vinyl chloride), and today, the continued construction of polluting industrial and energy plants that burn fossil fuels even while the evidence of global warming is incontrovertible. In addition, nanotechnology-based industries in the United States and elsewhere have expanded at a much more rapid pace than the development of a policy framework that would anticipate and mitigate the possible adverse consequences of this technology.

At the same time, there are many examples of successful prevention strategies. The National Environmental Protection Act and similar laws in the United States and internationally have required environmental impact studies that have been effective tools for pollution prevention. The Toxics Release Inventory in the United States is an example of a right-to-know approach to policy development that has promoted pollution prevention through informing industry and communities of toxic releases and driving pollution reduction and pollution prevention efforts; such efforts have been particularly effective in states such as Massachusetts that have toxic use reduction laws. In the United States, the Clean Air Act for new sources of pollution and the Food Quality Protection Act have been effective in preventing risks. An ethic of pollution prevention has caught hold in a number of sectors. The American Chemical Society, chemists, and many in the chemical industry have advanced the science of **green chemistry** and **green engineering** in order to develop new materials and processes that inherently are safe from cradle to grave. Builders and architects are increasingly embracing the green building movement, with voluntary certification programs stimulating customer demand for buildings that are more sustainable. Movements such as Health Care Without Harm have captured the imagination of the medical community, which is in turn evolving more environmentally benign ways to build and operate hospitals and other medical facilities. Many companies as well as governments at many levels have undertaken environmental purchasing policies. All of these voluntary approaches have been driven by the availability of information about the potential hazards associated with various alternatives.

A fundamental issue in environmental health policy development is the often great uncertainties in every aspect of it. Risk characterizations often include large ranges of potential risks, but there can be large uncertainties in risk management decisions as well. It is when decisions must be made in the face of uncertainty that principles such as precaution may be invoked. Technology-based approaches, such as the maximum available control technology (MACT) standards developed for hazardous air pollutants under the Clean Air Act, can be a useful strategy for preventing risks (of magnitude unknown) in the face of uncertainty by applying available technologies. The U.S. Environmental Protection Agency's hazardous air pollutant standards have been extolled for resulting in a 90 percent reduction of hazardous air emissions during the decade after passage of the 1990 Clean Air Act. Although such approaches do achieve prevention goals to an extent, failure to analyze and understand risk across the life cycle can have adverse consequences. For example, in the case of the hazardous air pollutant standards, control of ambient air emissions could come at the cost of greater exposures in the workplace, in discharges to water or waste, or even in a final product (Goldstein, 2004). Without an effort to reduce uncertainties about the risk of a substance, such exposures could go unnoticed, and uncontrolled, but the Clean Air Act does not drive the generation of such data. Conversely, excessive analysis can also have adverse and even paralyzing consequences; for example, the Environmental Protection Agency's dioxin assessment has been underway at this writing for more than twenty years, with no end in sight.

A second limitation in the ability to prevent environmental health risks is that all too often there are trade-offs among risks. An example of a **risk-risk trade-off** is the disinfection of drinking water with chlorine. Chlorine not only kills most pathogens in source waters but also leaves a residual level that protects against pathogens that may be introduced into the water distribution system later. Yet as described in Chapter Fifteen, chlorination can form disinfection by-products, some of which have chronic, low-level toxicity. It is almost axiomatic that as in the case of medicine, every environmental intervention that prevents one adverse effect is likely to have adverse side effects as well. A prevention strategy takes a careful look at all implications of alternative interventions.

Environmental public health assurance is covered in depth in Chapter Twenty-Seven, which addresses environmental health practice. Implementation of prevention strategies is complex because of the myriad parties who have a stake in environmental health issues or who must take action in order to implement policies. Few of those parties are environmental health experts. Additionally, in many cases policymakers in the executive, legislative, and judicial branches of government must be persuaded that the policy can be implemented. Thus it is critical that the public be engaged at every stage of the process and that there be broad agreement with the assessment of the problem as well as trust in the policymaking process. In other words, there needs to be a shared sense that there is a problem that needs to be addressed, a shared view of the magnitude of the problem and the uncertainties, and an assurance that a reasonable effort was made to develop fair, effective policies and to engage all involved parties. Vested interests may opt to oppose implementation of a new policy in any case, in which event it is particularly important to secure the agreement of other parties.

One particularly challenging aspect of implementing preventive policies is the difficulty of proving what would have happened in the absence of the policy. As has recently been observed in the case of climate change, some parties disbelieve the results of models and predictions of future scenarios, and they may be reluctant to invest in preventive strategies on that basis. Furthermore, for those who think primarily in economic terms, preventive interventions may appear to be bad investments. As already noted, because economists use a discount rate to calculate the future value of money that is invested in the present, economic analyses tend to downplay the value of measures that provide benefits in the remote future. Finally, the urgent may be the enemy of the important; more pressing and immediate issues may eclipse longer range concerns. Accordingly, it is crucial that preventive actions be accompanied by efforts to monitor the consequences of those actions, to link that information to policies that have been implemented, to modify actions based on this review, and to provide accurate and timely feedback to the public and policymakers about the success and failures of such actions.

SUMMARY

Prevention of illness, injury, premature death, and disability is a central mission of public health, and this is nowhere truer than in environmental public health. Prevention includes both the control of hazards—cleaning up a hazardous waste site or reducing air pollutants coming from a smokestack or tailpipe—but also health promotion through environmental strategies—providing parks, sidewalks, and bicycle paths. Prevention in environmental health extends upstream to such domains as energy, transportation, housing, and agriculture that eventually have an impact on human health and well-being. Primary prevention, such as the replacement of a hazardous chemical by a safe one, is a trademark environmental health approach, but secondary prevention (such as blood lead screening) and tertiary prevention (such as maintenance treatment of childhood asthma) are also relevant in environmental health. The prevention hierarchy ranges from definitive approaches such as completely removing a hazard, which are preferred, to administrative, behavioral, and end-of-pipeline approaches, which are less preferred. The precautionary principle proposes that cost-effective preventive measures should proceed even in the face of scientific uncertainty. In environmental public health practice, all the core functions of public health—in the categories of assessment, policy development, and assurance—are used to pursue prevention.

KEY TERMS

administrative controls

DPSEEA

  driving forces

  pressures

  state

  exposure

  effects

  actions

engineering controls

environmental health policy

environmental impact reports

green chemistry

green engineering

health impact assessment

health promotion

integrated decision making

intergenerational equity

life cycle analysis

personal protective equipment

polluter pays principle

pollution prevention

precautionary principle

prevention

primary prevention

secondary prevention

tertiary prevention

prevention hierarchy

public health practice

  assessment

  policy development

  assurance

risk-risk trade-offs

specific protection

substitution

sustainable development

DISCUSSION QUESTIONS

1. The old adage is that "an ounce of prevention is worth a pound of cure." Please identify an environmental health example and discuss whether this adage applies, giving your reasoning.

2. Sometimes, preventive goals seem to collide with each other. Examples include fish advisories, breast feeding advisories, and the use of DDT to control malaria. Please pick one of these, or another suitable example, and answer these questions. What are the trade-offs between the various possible preventive strategies for the issue you have chosen? How would you balance competing goals?

3. The precautionary principle has been the subject of considerable debate. Do some research on this principle, summarize supporting and opposing arguments, and draw conclusions.

4. Explain the prevention hierarchy as it applies both to occupational health and environmental health. Why are some strategies preferred to others?

5. Please discuss this statement: *Prevention is more effective upstream than downstream.*

REFERENCES

American Academy of Pediatrics, Committee on Environmental Health. "Lead Exposure in Children: Prevention, Detection, and Management." *Pediatrics*, 2005, *116*(4), 1036–1046.

Carlarne, C. "From the USA with Love: Sharing Home-Grown Hormones, GMOs, and Clones with a Reluctant Europe." *Environmental Law*, 2007, *37*(Spring), 301–336.

Dannenberg, A. L., and others. "Growing the Field of Health Impact Assessment in the United States: An Agenda for Research and Practice." *American Journal of Public Health*, 2006, *96*, 262–270.

Dubos, R. *Man Adapting*. New Haven, Conn.: Yale University Press, 1965.

Goldstein, B. D. "The Precautionary Principle, Toxicological Science, and European-U.S. Scientific Cooperation." *Drug Metabolism Reviews*, 2004, *36*(3–4), 487–495.

Institute of Medicine. *The Future of Public Health*. Washington, D.C.: National Academies Press, 1988.

Kemm, J., Parry, J., and Palmer, S. (eds.). *Health Impact Assessment: Concepts, Theory, Techniques, and Applications*. New York: Oxford University Press, 2004.

Leavell, H. R., and Clark, E. G. *Preventive Medicine for the Doctor in his Community*. New York: McGraw-Hill, 1958.

McMichael, A. J., Woodruff, R. E., and Hales, S. "Climate Change and Human Health: Present and Future Risks." *Lancet*, 2006, *367*(9513), 859–869.

Pollution Prevention Act. U.S. Code 42 (1990), §§ 13101–13102, et seq.

United Nations Conference on Environment and Development. *Rio Declaration on Environment and Development*. Rio de Janeiro: United Nations, 1992.

U.S. Environmental Protection Agency. *Life Cycle Assessment: Inventory: Guidelines and Principles*. Cincinnati, Ohio: U.S. Environmental Protection Agency, Office of Research and Development, 1993.

FOR FURTHER INFORMATION

Books, Reports, Articles, and Guidelines

Prevention in General

Centers for Disease Control and Prevention. *Guide to Community Preventive Services*. http://www.thecommunityguide.org/index.html. A unique and valuable Web-based resource that systematically evaluates programs and policies to improve health and prevent disease at the community level.

Wallace, R. (ed.). *Maxcy-Rosenau-Last Public Health and Preventive Medicine*. (15th ed.) New York: McGraw-Hill, 2007. A classic textbook in the medical specialty of preventive medicine.

Prevention in Environmental Health

Di Giulio, R. T., and Benson, W. H. (eds.). *Interconnections Between Human Health and Ecological Integrity.* Pensacola, Fla.: Society of Environmental Toxicology and Chemistry Foundation for Environmental Education, 2002.

O'Brien, M. *Making Better Environmental Decisions: An Alternative to Risk Assessment.* Cambridge, Mass.: MIT Press, 2000.

Pollution Prevention, Green Chemistry, and Engineering

One of the most promising aspects of prevention in environmental health is occurring in the chemical sector: the simultaneous growth of the concept of pollution prevention, the use of life cycle analysis and the emergence of green chemistry.

Allen, D. T., and Shonnard, D. R. *Green Engineering: Environmentally Conscious Design of Chemical Processes.* Upper Saddle River, N.J.: Prentice Hall, 2000.

Anastas, P. T., and Warner, J. C. *Green Chemistry: Theory and Practice.* New York: Oxford University Press, 2000.

Geiser, K. *Materials Matter: Toward a Sustainable Materials Policy (Urban and Industrial Environments).* Cambridge, Mass.: MIT Press, 2001.

Health Impact Assessment

Health impact assessment is emerging as an invaluable tool in applying preventive thinking upstream.

Dannenberg, A. L., and others. "Use of Health Impact Assessment in the U.S.: 27 Case Studies, 1999–2007." *American Journal of Preventive Medicine,* 2008, *34,* 241–256.

WHO Regional Office for Europe, European Centre for Health Policy. *Health Impact Assessment: Main Concepts and Suggested Approach.* Gothenburg Consensus Paper. http://www.euro.who.int/document/PAE/Gothenburgpaper.pdf, 1999.

World Health Organization. *Health Impact Assessment Guidelines.* http://www.who.int/hia/en, 2009.

Journal on Prevention in General

American Journal of Preventive Medicine. [Homepage.] http://www.journals.elsevierhealth.com/periodicals/amepre/home.

Agencies and Organizations

Prevention in General

American College of Preventive Medicine (ACPM). [Homepage.]. http://www.acpm.org.

Association for Prevention Teaching and Research (APTR). [Homepage.] http://www.aptrweb.org.

Partnership for Prevention. [Homepage.] http://www.prevent.org.

Prevention in Environmental Health

Centers for Disease Control and Prevention (CDC). "Environmental Health." http://www.cdc.gov/Environmental. A good starting point for further reading on prevention in environmental health.

Sustainability

International Institute for Sustainable Development (IISD). [Homepage.] http://www.iisd.ca. This useful source of information on sustainability publishes the *Earth Negotiations Bulletin* http://www.iisd.ca/enbvol/enb-background.htm.

UN Department of Economic and Social Affairs, Division for Sustainable Development. [Homepage.] http://www.un.org/esa/sustdev/documents/agenda21/index.htm. This organization's Web site provides information on Agenda 21 and the Commission on Sustainable Development.

Pollution Prevention, Green Chemistry, and Green Engineering

American Chemical Society. "ACS Green Chemistry Institute." http://www.acs.org/greenchemistry. A good starting point.

Beyond Benign Foundation. [Homepage.] http://www.beyondbenign.org. Another good starting point.

Health Care Without Harm. [Homepage.] http://www.noharm.org. This organization's Web site shows the application of green and pollution prevention concepts to the health care sector.

International Council of Chemical Associations (ICCA). "Responsible Care Project." http://www.responsiblecare.org/page.asp?p=6341&l=1. This and the next two Web sites are also good places to begin reading.

National Pollution Prevention Roundtable (NPPR). [Homepage.] http://www.p2.org.

UN Environment Programme (UNEP). "Cleaner Production Project." http://www.unep.fr/scp/cp/understanding/concept.htm.

U.S. Environmental Protection Agency (EPA), Office of Pollution Prevention and Toxics. "Pollution Prevention Information Clearinghouse." http://www.epa.gov/oppt/ppic.

U.S. Environmental Protection Agency (EPA), National Risk Management Research Laboratory. "Life-Cycle Assessment (LCA)." http://www.epa.gov/ord/NRMRL/lcaccess.

University of Massachusetts, Lowell. "Lowell Center for Sustainable Production." http://sustainable-production.org/publ.shtml.

CHAPTER TWENTY-SEVEN

ENVIRONMENTAL HEALTH PRACTICE

SARAH KOTCHIAN

ROBERT J. LAUMBACH

KEY CONCEPTS

- Environmental public health has deep historical roots in human efforts to assure clean food, water, and living conditions.

- Modern environmental public health includes a wide range of activities and responsibilities, such as food protection, water sanitation, air quality protection, safe and healthy housing, occupational health, injury prevention, and healthy community design.

- Many professions contribute to environmental public health, and many professional pathways can lead to successful careers.

- Environmental public health professionals collaborate with a wide range of other professionals in fields such as urban planning, engineering, law, emergency management, and law enforcement.

FROM earliest recorded times, human beings have recognized the need for guidelines, ordinances, and infrastructure to ensure the protection of the environment and human health. The practice of environmental health has grown and evolved as it has been informed over the years by the public health sciences of epidemiology and biostatistics and the emerging disciplines of toxicology and exposure and risk assessment. In addition, the public at large has demanded an increasing role in the design and delivery of community environmental health services. The practice of environmental health is carried out in a variety of settings, from local and state governments to federal and tribal governments and also in medical facilities and both the private and nonprofit sectors. This chapter begins with a historical overview of environmental public health services, from ancient times through modern recognition of the critical role of community participation. It then describes the organization and delivery of environmental health services, describes standards for service delivery, and outlines a process for community environmental health planning. The final portions of the chapter present case studies of environmental health practice in various settings and offer students information on career opportunities in environmental health.

A HISTORICAL OVERVIEW

The need for environmental health practices has been recognized since ancient times. The biblical book of *Leviticus* mentions food protection, housing quality, and quarantine. Engineers and public officials in ancient Rome planned for the water supply and waste disposal, and medieval England used quarantine to limit the spread of disease. Later, social reformers such as Edwin Chadwick in England advocated for improved housing conditions and clean drinking water in the 1842 Sanitary Report, and documented important environmental health protections in the 1871 Report of the Royal Sanitary Commission. Their counterparts in the United States published a similar report in Massachusetts, and campaigned effectively for the establishment of a Massachusetts state board of health in 1869. By the end of the nineteenth century, forty of the forty-five states in the United States at that time could claim health departments.

Sarah Kotchian declares receiving compensation from the National Environmental Health Association for work related to the national Environmental Public Health Performance Standards. NEHA receives a portion of its funding from the Centers for Disease Control and Prevention. Robert J. Laumbach declares no competing financial interests.

The Rise of Environmental Public Health

The late nineteenth century and the first six decades of the twentieth century saw the first of the modern eras of environmental health practice. C.E.A. Winslow, writing in 1923 in *The Evolution and Significance of the Public Health Campaign*, defined public health, which includes environmental health, this way: "Public health is not a concrete intellectual discipline, but a field of social activity. It includes applications of chemistry and bacteriology, of engineering and statistics, of physiology and pathology and epidemiology, and in some measure of sociology, and it builds upon these basic sciences a comprehensive program of community service" (Winslow, 1923). During the first fifty years of the twentieth century, states passed numerous public health laws regulating water and sewage treatment, protection of food, provision of safe housing and human and solid waste disposal, and reduction of insect- and rodent-borne diseases, resulting in a corresponding decrease in human morbidity and mortality and an increase in life expectancy.

During this same period, state legislatures expanded the resources available to state departments of health to assess the health status of citizens and environmental threats to health and to develop policies and programs to improve health and environmental quality. Health departments were normally headed by physicians, with nurses overseeing the immunization programs and sanitary engineers inspecting the construction and maintenance of safe water supplies, the purveyance of milk and meat, and the sanitary operation of food preparation and service facilities. Practitioners of environmental health services, known as *sanitarians*, were trained as generalists, with the capability to anticipate, prevent, and respond to a broad spectrum of environmental health threats with traditional functions in vector control, proper management and disposal of sewage, and food protection. Environmental health services and personal public health services (such as immunization programs) coexisted until the 1960s as partners in state health departments and in the increasing number of local health departments modeled after the state system.

New Legislation and New Accountability

The rapid industrialization that had begun during the late nineteenth century continued with the economic expansion that followed World War II. Additional widespread pollution of land, water and air, and the creation of new pollutants such as synthetic organic compounds helped to usher in the second modern era of environmental health protection. Scientists such as Rachel Carson and other environmental leaders brought public attention to the worsening condition of the environment and impacts on bird populations, natural habitats, and human health. As public outcry increased, the U.S. Congress responded over the next fifteen years by passing a great number of environmental laws, including the Safe Drinking Water Act, the Clean Air Act, the Occupational Safety and Health Act, the Consumer Product Safety Act, the Marine Mammal Protection Act, and the Toxic Substances Control Act (see also Chapter Thirty). These federal Acts were often complemented on the state level by similar state laws.

At the same time, the public demanded increased accountability by agencies responsible for environmental regulation. Public health professionals testified successfully before Congress for the establishment of the Environmental Protection Agency. On the state level, elected officials responded by creating separate environmental agencies, adding responsibility for enforcement of new environmental laws and regulations in air, water, and hazardous waste. In some cases, traditional environmental public health activities such as food protection and sanitary sewage disposal were also transferred to these new agencies. These agencies were variously known as Departments of Environment, Departments of Environmental Quality, Departments of Environmental Regulation, or Departments of Environmental Protection; most dropped the word *health* from their titles. These separate agencies benefited from increased visibility and enhanced funding and no longer faced the necessity of competing within a health department for environmental funds.

This combination of new legislation and increased public attention became a watershed period for the practice of environmental health, one that had both positive and negative consequences. Although the increased visibility and funding were important in supporting necessary environmental health programs, the separation from health agencies over the last forty years has resulted in the creation of separate data systems, uncoordinated planning, and the loss of a comprehensive picture of the community's health and environment. Whereas in the first half of the twentieth century, nurses and sanitarians were more closely connected to one another and to their small communities and familiar with the issues of the residents, population growth and the growth of agencies have interfered with this intimate local knowledge. In addition, many of these environmental health specialists, and indeed their agencies, became increasingly isolated from their public health counterparts in the state and local departments of health, losing valuable affiliations that would later take years to reestablish.

Along with the new, media-specific environmental laws came a new generation of environmental health specialists who devoted their careers to one specific area of the environment, such as solid waste, hazardous waste, air quality, or drinking water. Their training often did not include training in general public health concepts or in the use of public health tools such as epidemiology and effective public health campaigns. In addition, the specialized training and focus necessitated by complicated, single-media federal regulations on air and water made it more difficult for professionals in environmental health to have the time or the information to see the community's big picture. As a result, some of the programs developed by these professionals were not sensitive to community knowledge, culture, or concerns and were also not as effective as they might have been in addressing the overall connection between health and environment because they focused on one isolated component.

The Rise of Citizen Involvement

The 1970s and 1980s saw a convergence of a number of factors, including the ongoing negative impacts of rapid industrialization and urban growth, urban flight, and the disenfranchisement of citizens from environmental policymaking and enforcement decisions. In the wake of environmental disasters such as the widespread contamination at Love Canal in New York, Times Beach in Missouri, and Woburn in Massachusetts, average citizens demanded a stronger role in decision making and greater transparency and accountability of the governmental agencies that were supposed to be protecting their health and environment. Watchdog groups such as the Center for Health, Environment and Justice, headed by Lois Gibbs, and national environmental advocacy organizations such as the Natural Resources Defense Council gained membership and influence to ensure that agencies fulfilled their mandates and that citizen voices were heard and their input incorporated. Faith-based organizations, indigenous rights organizations, and other citizen groups combined their efforts and their strategies to create the **environmental justice** movement, insisting that social, economic, racial, and environmental concerns were interrelated and needed to be addressed with the central involvement of those who bore the greatest burden (see Chapter Eight). This became the third era of environmental health practice, in which agencies needed to learn how to address the environmental justice and equity concerns of their multicultural communities more effectively and in which they began to develop new techniques and to assign specific personnel for enhancing community participation and communicating risk. Federal laws were written or amended to require environmental impact statements, analysis of environmental justice, and public involvement in the development of policies, permits, and hazardous waste site remediation plans. In the academic community, researchers focused on effective community empowerment and strategies for effectively assessing and communicating risk in diverse communities, and they redirected research to include **community-based participatory research.** Agencies struggled with retraining their existing workforce to work in ways that were more culturally sensitive, and sought to hire employees drawn from the communities they served. In recent years citizen frustration over the inability of accountable agencies to document and address the link between environmental exposures and health outcomes has led to a number of initiatives intended to reconnect environmental and public health, a process aided greatly by the use of applied, computer-enhanced information in epidemiology, risk assessment, toxicology, and risk communication.

ORGANIZATION AND DELIVERY OF SERVICES

How is the practice of environmental health organized today? Not surprisingly, because of both universal and community-specific needs, environmental health services in the United States are provided at federal, tribal, state, and local levels and in the medical, academic, nonprofit, and private sectors. A set of federal laws governing various aspects of the environment are enforced by numerous federal agencies, including the U.S. Environmental Protection Agency (EPA), the U.S. Department of Agriculture (USDA), the U.S. Food and Drug Administration (FDA), and others. Many federal laws contain provisions that supersede state laws in order to provide equal environmental health protection to all citizens. Some of the federal Acts, such as the Clean Air Act, permit delegation of authority to states and, under certain circumstances of local home rule, to local jurisdictions. State governments have the authority to enact further environmental legislation, as long as it does not conflict with federal law. Many of these state laws provide additional protections or address areas not covered by federal law. Within states, municipalities and counties have the authority, usually given by their state legislature, to enact local laws to protect health and environment for their citizens.

Who decides what agencies should provide environmental health services, how they should be organized, and what services should be included? Historically, environmental health agencies are created through a combination of public health leadership, citizen advocacy, and political will. Their creation begins with the perception of a need to protect the public from environmental hazards and with the desire for a governmental unit charged with the provision of those services that will be responsive to elected officials and the public. The specific services provided are built around a core set of environmental health services, such as food protection, water sanitation, and air quality protection, with further services added as determined by public health data and public interest. Ideally, the community-specific tailoring of these agencies becomes a method of ensuring that the highest priority services for that community are provided. Yet this necessary and desirable local political process has also resulted in a patchwork of services that are not coordinated and that leave large gaps in the core public health functions of assessment, assurance, and policy development.

Because the authority for these services has developed over many decades and in multiple locations, the organization and delivery of environmental health services is now complex and is not easily understood by professionals themselves, much less the general public. In the early 1990s, the Health Resources and Services Administration (HRSA) of the U.S. Department of Health and Human Services commissioned two reports to catalogue the diversity of environmental health service organization and delivery. These reports analyzed the structure and function of state environmental health activities and found several pervasive problems. The first report (Burke, Shalauta, and Tran, 1995a) described the existing structure, authority, and funding for environmental health services at the state level. The researchers found that the federal environmental laws had driven the design and authority of state regulatory agencies but that there was no standardization in the organization for enforcement of these laws. Further, the report noted that many of the regulatory agencies had become oriented toward specific media and often lacked the necessary public health support, such as epidemiology, public health evaluation, or applied research, to allow a larger perspective on the environment and health.

The second report documented that regulatory enforcement generally took precedence over environmental health prevention, as reflected by approximately four times more funding. The report recommended reevaluation of this imbalance, a broader view of the relationship between health and the environment, better health training for environmental professionals, and "improved cooperation between the many health and environmental agencies in the complex 'Environmental Web' to assure that they do not lose sight of their fundamental mission—the protection of the public health" (Burke, Shalauta, and Tran, 1995b).

STANDARDS FOR SERVICE DELIVERY

Although many environmental health programs are indeed local, evolution across time and geographic location just described has resulted in a lack of consistency in the quality of programs and services provided to the public, and in an inability to measure effectiveness in order to continue to improve these services. In the last two decades of the twentieth century and the first part of the twenty-first, a number of reports have been prepared and initiatives undertaken to assess public health services and systems, to develop performance standards and indicators, and to design assessment tools with which agencies and the public can begin to assess and improve their public health system capacity.

In 1987, the Institute of Medicine (IOM) conducted a review of the U.S. public health system, and issued the *Future of Public Health*, a report that cited a number of problems within the system and made recommendations to strengthen it (IOM, 1988). This report outlined the three **core functions of public health**—assessment, policy development, and assurance (Exhibit 27.1).

EXHBIT 27.1
Core Functions of Public Health

Assessment

The committee recommends that every public health agency regularly and systematically collect, assemble, analyze, and make available information on the health of the community, including statistics on health status, community health needs, and epidemiologic and other studies of health problems.

Policy Development

The committee recommends that every public health agency exercise its responsibility to serve the public interest in the development of comprehensive public health policies by promoting use of the scientific knowledge base in decision making about public health and by leading in developing public health policy. Agencies must take a strategic approach, developed on the basis of a positive appreciation for the democratic political process.

Assurance

The committee recommends that public health agencies assure their constituents that services necessary to achieve agreed upon goals are provided, either by encouraging actions by other entities (private or public sector), by requiring such action through regulation, or by providing services directly.

The committee recommends that each public health agency involve key policymakers and the general public in determining a set of high-priority personal and communitywide health services that governments will guarantee to every member of the community. This guarantee should include subsidization or direct provision of high-priority personal health services for those unable to afford them.

Source: IOM, 1988, pp. 7–8.

Following the publication of that report, a group of federal agencies and organizations met to define the workforce competencies needed to carry out these three core functions, and further defined a set of ten **essential services of public health**, all of which are necessary to support the three core functions. Later, the wording of these ten essential services was modified slightly by the CDC's National Center for Environmental Health (NCEH) to create the **ten essential services of environmental health**, in order to be more relevant to the environmental health practice community. These services are shown in Table 27.1.

TABLE 27.1   The Essential Services

Ten Essential Services of Public Health	Ten Essential Services of Environmental Health
1. Monitor health status to identify and solve community health problems.	1. Monitor environmental and health status to identify and solve community environmental health problems.
2. Diagnose and investigate health problems and health hazards in the community.	2. Diagnose and investigate environmental health problems and health hazards in the community.
3. Inform, educate, and empower people about health issues.	3. Inform, educate, and empower people about environmental health issues.
4. Mobilize community partnerships and action to identify and solve health problems.	4. Mobilize community partnerships and actions to identify and solve environmental health problems.
5. Develop policies and plans that support individual and community health efforts.	5. Develop policies and plans that support individual and community environmental health efforts.
6. Enforce laws and regulations that protect health and ensure safety.	6. Enforce laws and regulations that protect environmental health and ensure safety.
7. Link people to needed personal health services and assure the provision of health care when otherwise unavailable.	7. Link people to needed environmental health services and assure the provision of health care when otherwise unavailable.
8. Assure a competent public and personal health care workforce.	8. Assure a competent public health and personal health care workforce.
9. Evaluate effectiveness, accessibility, and quality of personal and population-based health services.	9. Evaluate effectiveness, accessibility, and quality of personal and population-based environmental health services.
10. Research for new insights and innovative solutions to health problems.	10. Research for new insights and innovative solutions to environmental health problems.

Sources: CDC, 2008, n.d.

Each of these services represents an important component of the overall public health infrastructure. For instance, the first essential service requires the creation of an environmental health surveillance system, which is a priority in order to allow public health officials to detect environmental hazards and related illnesses, assess the need for additional services, develop necessary programs and regulations, and ensure that public health protection is provided. Using data from this system, public health professionals can advocate before policymaking bodies to obtain the necessary legal support and resources for programs to address community needs. In recent years the development of spatial data technology and its use in geographic information systems, has allowed public health officials to map the occurrence of hazards and illnesses in their communities and then to use these maps in dialogues with citizens and elected officials to create awareness and the political will to address these concerns (see Chapter Twenty-Eight). For example, in the Albuquerque Environmental Health Department in the 1990s, it was customary for the director to present each newly elected city councilor with an environmental health map of his or her district, with color-coded information on the location of restaurants inspected, mosquito complaints received, dog bites, noise complaints, and other public nuisances. The map was a visual reminder of the need for services as well as documentation of department services provided with taxpayer support.

To reinforce, support, and standardize public health systems, the CDC's Public Health Practice Program Office developed a set of performance standards tools that can be used to assess the capacity of state and local agencies and local boards of health to provide the ten essential services of public health. These free tools (available online from the **National Public Health Performance Standards Program** [NPHPSP] at http://www.cdc.gov/od/ocphp/nphpsp) describe the standard of performance, ask a series of questions, and provide indicators for each of the essential services, allowing public health professionals and their communities to assess their capacity to provide the ten essential services of public health and to identify service gaps that need to be filled. For example, there are questions about whether the local public health system maintains or contributes to population health registries for such data as environmental exposures and workplace injuries. A number of states and local communities have assessed their capacity using these performance standards tools. (Agencies can find many resources to assist in the implementation of the standards on the CDC Web site: http://www.cdc.gov/od/ocphp/nphpsp/General.htm.)

In cooperation with the National Public Health Performance Standards Program, the NCEH has developed a set of companion standards for environmental health based on the ten essential services of environmental health (available from http://www.cdc.gov/NCEH/ehs/EnvPHPS/default.htm). Through voluntary use of these standards at the federal, tribal, state, and local levels, the NCEH aims to enhance the capacity, consistency, and accountability of the nation's environmental health services. A number of local and state agencies have used these standards to improve their environmental health services.

As the challenges facing public health agencies have grown and available funding has become more constrained, there have been efforts over the last three decades of the twentieth century to define an effective public health agency and to set goals for the health of the nation. In order to support the development of consistent public health services and to raise public awareness of national public health goals, the U.S. Department of Health and Human Services, with broad input, created a set of model standards for public health services and established a set of national health indicators, published once each decade. The most recent health objectives for the nation, **Healthy People 2010**, include environmental quality among the top ten leading health indicators. Several specific objectives address environmental exposures. For example, one objective (8-1a) aims to reduce the proportion of persons exposed to excess ozone in the air, and another (27-10) aims to reduce the proportion of nonsmokers exposed to environmental tobacco smoke. Additional environmental objectives address outdoor air quality, water quality, toxics and waste, healthy homes and healthy communities, infrastructure and surveillance, and global environmental health. (Information on all of the Healthy People 2010 indicators, including specific, measurable environmental health indicators, can be found at http://www.healthypeople.gov.) Healthy People 2020 objectives are under development, and are scheduled to be released in 2010.

TOOLS FOR COMMUNITY PLANNING AND PRACTICE

With the increased emphasis on **community involvement**, agencies became interested in standard tools that could be used strategically, systematically, and meaningfully to involve their communities in policy and planning. The National Association of County and City Health Officials (NACCHO), in conjunction with other national public health organizations such as the American Public Health Association, the Association of Schools of Public Health, and the Association of State and Territorial Health Officials, took the lead in 1991 in publishing **APEX/ PH (Assessment Protocol for Excellence in Public Health)**, which guided public health agencies through a series of steps to assess their own strengths and needs and to work in partnership with their communities to respond to community health concerns and to design more effective health programs.

Environmental health agencies, while valuing the APEX tool, found that it did not fully address their need to identify specific community environmental health problems and to design environmental health programs in concert with the public that would build on community strengths and focus on community priorities. With funding from the NCEH, NACCHO supported a multiple-year effort by a committee of professionals in the field that resulted in ***PACE EH, Protocol for Assessing Community Excellence in Environmental Health:*** *A Guidebook for Local Health Officials* (NACCHO, 2004). This protocol takes local health departments and their communities through a thirteen-step process (see Table 27.2) of characterizing the community, assembling a community environmental health assessment team, generating a list of environmental issues for analysis, developing locally meaningful indicators for those issues, ranking the issues and setting priorities for action, and then evaluating progress and planning for the future. (PACE EH is available in English and Spanish, along with summaries of community success stories, on the NACCHO web site: http://www.naccho.org/publications/environmental/index.cfm.) NACCHO's MAPP process (Mobilizing for Action through Planning and Partnerships) is another tool for working with communities to improve health. The National Center for Environmental Health strongly supports the use of community environmental

TABLE 27.2   The PACE EH Process

Task 1	Determine community capacity
Task 2	Define and characterize the community
Task 3	Assemble a community-based environmental health assessment team
Task 4	Define the goals, objectives, and scope of the assessment
Task 5	Generate a list of community-specific environmental health issues
Task 6	Analyze the issues with a systems framework
Task 7	Develop locally appropriate indicators
Task 8	Select standards against which local status can be compared
Task 9	Create issue profiles
Task 10	Rank the issues
Task 11	Set priorities for action
Task 12	Develop an action plan
Task 13	Evaluate progress and plan for the future

Note: Detailed instructions for each of the thirteen tasks in the PACE EH process are outlined in *PACE EH, Protocol for Assessing Community Excellence in Environmental Health: A Guidebook for Local Health Officials* (NACCHO, 2004).

health assessments as a means to improve community health, and has provided a variety of resources and case studies (available on its Web site: http://www.cdc. gov/nceh/ehs/ceha/default.htm). A number of other agencies, such as the U.S. Environmental Protection Agency, have developed tools for community involvement, centering around the core value of community empowerment and voice in the design of environmental health services and healthier communities. The EPA's CARE program (Community Action for a Renewed Environment), is one such example (available at http://www.epa.gov/care).

NOTES FROM THE FIELD

What do environmental health professionals do? The next few pages offer visits with several practitioners from state and local health departments, clinical, corporate, and not-for-profit settings. They describe their career trajectories, their daily activities, and their places within the larger system of environmental public health.

Environmental Public Health in the Public Sector

Gerry Barron and Allegheny County: An Environmental Health Career in a Comprehensive Local Health Department
Large urban areas pose a broad set of challenges for the environmental health professional. Their dense populations and large geographic areas usually require that environmental health staff work out of several different locations, with a central coordinating office. An aging housing stock and crumbling public works infrastructure raise issues of lead exposures, rodent infestations, housing-related injuries, raw sewage, and potential drinking water contamination. Heavy workloads may result in fewer inspections of each site than might occur in smaller jurisdictions, and underscore the need to focus on education and on interventions that are most effective.

Urban environmental health services are often found within a larger department of health. Health department administrators must oversee a large number of separate issues in their department and are often unable to give much time and attention to environmental health when faced with other health crises. As a result, environmental health services have learned to operate fairly independently and must make a special effort to coordinate with other health services; this poses an ongoing challenge in creating a comprehensive collaborative approach to meeting community needs. Some departments have addressed this by co-locating staff from various programs in the same field offices to encourage communication and coordination of efforts. In this setting we look at the career of Gerry Barron, who worked in local environmental and public health for most of his life, and now teaches public health at the University of Pittsburgh's Graduate School of Public Health.

In 1970, with his undergraduate degree in biology in hand, Barron and his wife left Boston temporarily so that Gerry could pursue a master of public health degree at the University of Pittsburgh. Four and a half decades later, they are still in Pittsburgh, and Barron continues to innovate in the practice of local environmental health.

During his master's degree program, which had a concentration in environmental health, Barron came to know Al Brunwasser, the director of the Environmental Health Bureau in the Allegheny County Health Department. Al had an eye for students of promise, and he offered Barron a position as a **sanitarian** trainee. It was the 1970s, environmental issues were at the forefront, and Pittsburgh already had a long, proud history of civic involvement in collaborating to protect the environment. In the 1940s, with the city under a cloud of pollution from the steel and other manufacturing industries, David Lawrence, the mayor of Pittsburgh, and Richard King Mellon, a wealthy industrialist, called together the major industries, the health department, and other community leaders to develop solutions that would be healthy for both people and the economy; one of the results was the first smoke regulation in the country.

That community-wide awareness and support led to the growth of the comprehensive environmental health program into which Barron was hired, with traditional public health programs focused on food protection, housing sanitation, drinking water, wastewater, swimming pools, solid waste, plumbing oversight, and air pollution. Al was a good mentor, encouraging Barron to take on challenges, and Barron had the personality that allowed him to see these challenges as opportunities to learn. Over the next twenty years, he became chief of the food protection program, worked in housing and wastewater, and became deputy director for environmental health. When the opportunity arose to become the deputy director for medical services for the department, Barron took it, even though it represented a change in career orientation.

Over the years, with Barron's guidance and vision, the department reorganized to recognize the natural connections between the various public health programs. The food protection program is co-located with infectious diseases. Housing program personnel work alongside the lead, WIC, and dental programs, in recognition that these family and community health programs serve the same clientele. The department also administers federal programs in air quality and state programs in drinking water, wastewater, and solid waste, and has added injury control and school sanitation. The department regulates the licensure and training of plumbers in order to reduce the risk of cross-connections in the public drinking water supply. Barron insisted that department staff maintain dialogue with the regulated communities. The food protection, plumbing, air quality, and drinking water programs all have their own advisory committees, which include industry representation. The Allegheny County Health Department now has approximately 350 employees, and provides services to the 130 municipalities throughout the county, which has a population of 1.2 million. The department is now headed by Bruce Dixon, a full professor of medicine at the University of Pittsburgh who is employed by Allegheny County, another indication of a strong community partnership.

After twenty-five years with the health department, Barron became deputy director over all department operations, a position he held for another ten years. He continued to look forward to the challenges of environmental and public health. "Every day is different," he said of his supervisory position. "You're not sure what's going to happen that day." He ensured that the public health programs had a strong base in science. Entry-level field personnel are required to have an undergraduate major in science, and a master's degree in public health or public administration is required for upper-level administrative positions. He continued the tradition of mentoring staff and graduate students, looking for those willing to see challenges as opportunities and to move around to learn new skills. He enjoyed creative visioning; in his own words, "I like to spend time on what should be, and work to get there." He delegated the daily decision making in the programs and the management of personnel, purchasing, and contracting to the managers and supervisors, and spent much of his time in overseeing the implementation of strategic plans and in creating and maintaining an effective community network. Not only did this network allow him to gather the support for necessary programs, but also, Barron says, "you need to be able to respond quickly; you should have a system that will pick up and deal with community issues." His network served as a radar system that allowed him to listen and hear about issues and illnesses that provided information about new initiatives and interventions that were needed. The appointed board of health that oversees the Allegheny County Health Department provides an additional measure of citizen direction and involvement. As deputy director, Barron spearheaded a successful application for a community environmental health capacity-building grant from the CDC's National Center for Environmental Health. The funds from this grant allowed the department to hire Jo Ann Glad, a registered nurse with a master of public health degree, as a full-time epidemiologist who has begun to build the partnerships and the infrastructure to support a comprehensive community-wide health and environmental data system.

Barron continues to learn and develop his own skills. He retired from the Allegheny County Health Department after thirty-five years of service and now holds an associate professor position with the University of Pittsburgh's Graduate School of Public Health, where he serves as deputy director of the Center for Public Health Practice and director of the Pennsylvania Preparedness Leadership Institute. He is also a special assistant to the director of the Allegheny County Health Department in order to assist in the development of the department's strategic direction and to improve the collaboration between the graduate school and the department.

When asked what continues to bring him satisfaction after so many years, he replied, "It's all about social justice. Everyone has the same right to clean water, clean air, and access to health care. It's really about helping others who can't speak for themselves, who don't have as much say." There is a "nobility of service" in public health, he says, that is deeply satisfying. Gerry Barron is an example of the considerable number of outstanding leaders who have dedicated a lifetime of service to local environmental public health.

Ken Sharp, Iowa Department of Public Health: Assuring Improved Environment and Health Through Collaboration

States have unique challenges and opportunities when fulfilling their role of assuring the delivery of environmental health services to statewide populations, and are also organized in many different ways. The Iowa Department of Public Health, for instance, shares responsibility for various aspects of environmental health with sister departments of inspection and appeals and natural resources, much of this responsibility exercised through counties and local boards of health. Iowa is a home rule state, and Iowa Code requires counties to have county boards of health with five members, including a physician, appointed by each county's board of supervisors. Two cities with populations of over 25,000 have also established their own city boards of health, appointed by the city council. Therefore, Iowa, with 99 counties and two cities, has 101 local boards of health to address the needs of a state population of 2.9 million.

A person interested in working as an environmental health specialist has many options in Iowa. The Department of Inspections and Appeals regulates food safety, and has contracts with local environmental agencies to provide services that cover approximately 75 percent of the State of Iowa; department staff cover the remainder of the state. The Department of Natural Resources requires local boards of health to oversee construction of private wells and on-site septic systems and only has three staff members who directly support local boards of health in these programs. The Department of Public Health has direct responsibility to local boards of health and oversees indoor air quality, lead poisoning prevention, swimming pools, tattoo establishments, tanning facilities, and funeral homes. In addition, the Iowa Code places requirements on local boards of health to carry out on-site waste water and private well construction regulatory programs, and to address other issues such as vicious animals and dead animal disposal.

As director of the Division of Environmental Health in the Iowa Department of Public Health, Ken Sharp is responsible for oversight of the activities of the Bureau of Environmental Health Services, the Bureau of Lead Poisoning Prevention, the Bureau of Radiological Health, and the Office of Plumber and Mechanical Professional Licensure. In 2001, Sharp's office conducted an environmental health workforce survey, and estimated that 180 to 200 people are employed statewide in environmental health. Environmental health personnel at the county level may be located in a variety of offices; they may work in zoning, emergency management, weed control, engineering, or secondary roads as well as in health or environmental offices. There may be one person handling all of a county's environmental health issues, and that same person may work on other nonenvironmental issues as well. The survey found 50 percent of the workforce to have a four-year degree, and 25 percent of the workforce to have a degree in the sciences. Statewide, the workforce experiences an annual 10 to 15 percent turnover, which is costly in both economic and health terms. The Bureau of Environmental Health Services works directly with these county personnel to provide necessary training and support. The workforce training needs are great; many of the rural counties do not require a science degree, and the salaries are often low as well. Few resources are available at the county level for training. The bureau helps field staff to improve their skills, develop a local response to citizen requests on issues for which there is no established program, such as mold, nuisances, or landlord complaints, and improve the quality of services provided to citizens.

The Centers for Disease Control and Prevention has awarded several grants to the Iowa Department of Public Health to improve statewide capacity in environmental health services. Over the past seven years, the department has been able to give forty-two minigrants, totaling approximately $600,000, to counties to improve their environmental health services and to develop trainings, fact sheets, and other resources to help the often isolated field staff. With this assistance, these counties have been able to purchase equipment, develop plans and tools, and establish education and marketing programs that have given them greater capacity to carryout the core functions and essential services of environmental health. Through his leadership, Sharp's division obtained federal funds to focus on a three-year program to create healthier housing in Iowa, and it has been a state partner in the CDC's EHS-Net (Environmental Health Specialists Network) grant program, participating in studies to identify antecedents of foodborne illness outbreaks. The division's participation in the Emergency Management Assistance Compact (EMAC) and its active engagement in the national network of research, training, and planning in environmental health emergency response enabled it to recruit additional resources, such as a Florida EMAC team, to assist in the 2008 Iowa floods. In 2005, after Hurricane Katrina devastated the Gulf Coast, Iowa was the first state to respond to Louisiana with an environmental health emergency response team under EMAC.

Ken Sharp's own career reflects the variety of environmental health opportunities. After receiving a bachelor's degree in environmental science, he worked for almost two years on a flood recovery team in Iowa participating in a CDC nine-state well water quality survey and fieldwork, inspecting construction standards, and taking samples. He spent the next five years doing environmental case management in the lead poisoning prevention program, and was part of a team that established a training program for certification of lead inspectors and lead abatement contractors, before creating the Office of Technical Assistance. In April, 2007, he was appointed interim division director, and became division director in September of the same year. After fifteen challenging and interesting years in environmental health, Ken Sharp remains enthusiastic about his daily work. He says, "There have never been two days identical in the last fifteen years. I like the variety of the challenges, and the satisfaction of being able to help people." The profession itself is rewarding as well, Sharp says: "This profession seems to be unique in its willingness to help each other out. Other environmental health colleagues are willing to share their experiences, and to be called upon for technical assistance and guidance." It is because Iowa does not have stringent entry requirements, Sharp believes, that most of the field personnel have experienced the frustration of having to start from the ground up in their jurisdictions and are willing to acknowledge the challenges others face and to offer support. In one example, a public health nurse assumed responsibility for an environmental health program in one of Iowa's counties, and the bureau was able to support her in sorting out programs, procedures, and policies and setting guidelines on what qualifications to look for when hiring environmental health employees.

Sharp advises those interested in a career in environmental health to become familiar with the daily work involved and to develop an understanding of the kinds of skills necessary to do the job well. Sharp says, "There's a tremendous amount of public and professional interaction, and you have to be willing to talk to people." Sharp likes to hire employees who are diplomatic, honest, and open. He says:

> As we look more at the core competencies for environmental health and how they apply to the field, that set of competencies is as important as competencies in science and research. We need to be able to communicate the message. Faced with a scientist who is a poor communicator, I would rather take someone with

a desire and interest and strong interpersonal and problem-solving competencies and teach him or her the science. When we have done that, these people have done a fantastic job of creating a wonderful program. You can take all the science in the world, and if you can't communicate it, it is not going to do you a whole lot of good in real life practice.

Sharp's division has now incorporated questions related to these competencies in its interview process.

As is clear from the example of the State of Iowa, environmental health services are delivered at the state and local levels through a variety of settings. Environmental health personnel in most states can expect to be called upon for both their technical and interpersonal skills and to collaborate with citizens, other local and state agencies, private businesses, elected officials, and boards of health, as they seek to improve the public health and quality of life for the citizens they serve.

Stephanie Moraga-McHaley, Environmental Epidemiologist, Albuquerque, New Mexico Stephanie Moraga-McHaley knew what she was interested in, but she didn't know what it was called. During her coursework at the University of New Mexico, she had taken courses in geology and knew that she liked the science but that she didn't want to be a geologist. She was interested in the human aspects of science but didn't want to go into medicine. When she and her husband, Curtis, moved to Colorado with a small toddler, interrupting her undergraduate career, she began searching the various Web sites of Colorado universities and found the environmental health undergraduate program at Colorado State University in Fort Collins. The national and international media and popular press were full of stories of ebola, hantavirus, and other diseases, and here was the opportunity to study what she came to understand was the field of environmental health. She went back to school at age twenty-eight to take some additional preliminary courses, was accepted into the program, and completed both her undergraduate and graduate degrees there while raising two small children.

During her studies in environmental health, Moraga-McHaley took several courses in toxicology, organic chemistry, environmental health practice, epidemiology, and biostatistics. She also took a class in science communication, which trained her in how to communicate about science with the general public, a skill that has proven useful in her later work. As part of her program, she did an internship with the Colorado Department of Public Health and Environment, working on an EPA-funded childhood lead study and assembling a library of information on lead. She worked alongside community health workers and phlebotomists, conducting interviews with citizens on lead exposures and assisting with home environmental assessments. She visited homes that were in such poor condition that lead seemed to be the least of the resident's problems. She went on to complete her graduate work, concentrating in environmental epidemiology and writing her thesis on farm-related illness and injuries in children.

When she moved back to Albuquerque with her family, Moraga-McHaley was hired by the Albuquerque Environmental Health Department to conduct investigations of foodborne illness outbreaks and to perform other environmental health field activities such as inspection of food facilities, pools, and spas. Her fluency in Spanish was helpful in communicating desired improvements in some of the restaurants she visited. One of her outbreak investigations focused on hepatitis A in a day-care facility; another involved an outbreak of an environmentally transmitted skin condition at the local correctional facility. Following three years at the department, she and her family moved to Spain for a year, where her husband worked as an environmental engineer. Although she did not work during this time, she was able to observe occupational health issues, such as the musculoskeletal injuries related to the olive industry, and to add to her store of knowledge on the variety of ways in which environmental health is practiced. On moving back to New Mexico in 2003, she was hired as a project coordinator to help establish an occupational health registry for the State of New Mexico, a joint project of the University of New Mexico and the New Mexico Department of Health, funded by the National Institute for Occupational Safety and Health (NIOSH). She has worked in conjunction with the Council of State and Territorial Epidemiologists to develop a manual on how to create an occupational health surveillance system using occupational health indicators. To stay current in the field, she belongs to several listserves on issues such as pesticides and silicosis, attends workshops and seminars, and reads articles and information on the Internet.

She recommends the environmental health field to others interested in the intersection of sciences and health. "Environmental health is a good degree," she says, "because it has so many facets to it. There are so many possible career opportunities, from working with an oil company to a nonprofit or private environmental group to a public agency." Wherever they choose to work, she advises, environmental health professionals need to be able to see both sides to every story and to remain objective. She encourages interested students to find out as much as possible about the various opportunities to determine the work environment that is best suited to their personalities and interests. She also recommends that people consider learning more about international environmental health. When not engaged in occupational health, Moraga-McHaley loves to travel. Recently, she and her husband performed a health assessment of a village in Togo, Africa, as part of a water improvement project through the volunteer organization Engineers Without Borders. Moraga-McHaley says, "It's fascinating to see what's going on in other countries, how they address their environmental health issues, and what their epidemiologic focus is." She continues to find daily satisfaction in being able to study the science behind a health issue and to recommend interventions that will improve the situation. "There's nothing better," she says, "than bringing light to a public health problem and helping to find solutions." As an environmental epidemiologist, Moraga-McHaley obviously enjoys the challenges and rewards of an always changing field.

Environmental Health in Not-for-Profit Advocacy Organizations

Nsedu Obot Witherspoon, Executive Director, Children's Environmental Health Network (CEHN), Washington, D.C.   Nsedu Obot Witherspoon's first name in Ibibio (a language spoken in southeastern Nigeria) means "expected virtue." Known as Nse by most of her colleagues, she was born in the United States but spent her early toddler years in Nigeria, where reverence for the environment is a cultural and family virtue. Although her family later relocated to Buffalo, New York, her parents made sure that they maintained their connections to Nigeria, where Nse was encouraged to explore and value nature. Those passions for protecting the environment and her appreciation for enhancing people's connection to it have been strong themes throughout her professional and personal life.

Early in life Witherspoon believed she wanted to be a pediatrician, because of her deep concern for the health and well-being of children. She was a premed student and was awarded prestigious summer fellowships, with the National Heart, Lung, and Blood Institute, that involved minority students in clinical experiences. She attended a small college known for its sciences, but the only career options presented to her were medicine, research, or academia; public health was not mentioned. While taking her MCATs and applying to medical school, she stumbled across public health graduate schools on the Internet, applied, and was accepted to the George Washington University School of Public Health.

"It was one of the best decisions I ever made," Witherspoon says. During her graduate studies, she studied maternal and child health and was introduced through internships to nonprofit work. Her experiences through the graduate public health program helped her to make better career decisions on graduation. In 2000, she joined the Children's Environmental Health Network (CEHN), and has been there for the past eight years. As executive director she is responsible for the direction and oversight of this national nonprofit organization focused on protecting the fetus and child from environmental hazards affecting their health, and serves as a national spokesperson for child health advocacy. She travels around the country speaking about issues affecting this vulnerable population, and teaches stakeholders such as health care and child-care professionals, legislators, parents, public health advocates, and others how to incorporate environmental health into their practice. She gives testimony to policymakers and consults with her board members, staff, consultants, and advisory committees to equip them with the information to become effective advocates for children's environmental health policy.

Witherspoon values the support she receives from her board for activities that are important to her personally as well as professionally. Her board encourages her to be active in professional organizations such as the American Public Health Association (APHA), where she has served as the Section on Environment program planner, treasurer, and chair and also as chair of the student involvement committee for this section. She has also participated on many advisory committees for such agencies as the EPA and the National Institute of Environmental Health Sciences (NIEHS). She likes to travel and engage with the people on whose behalf she is working, and her position allows her to do that. She has organized many conferences, published papers on key issues, and has received a number of distinguished awards in recognition of her leadership.

Witherspoon's young children serve as daily reminders of how important it is to do environmental health work. She makes sure that her national leadership in environmental health does not interfere with her passion for spending time with her family. They continue to be active in the outdoors and in sports, and when possible her husband and children travel with her. Her nonprofit organization allows her the flexibility to be involved in school activities and to work from home one day a week so that she can spend more time with her daughter, who is a toddler. "They bring me such joy," she says. "Work can be demanding, so laughing and enjoying life with them helps me maintain balance and puts everything into perspective."

Witherspoon says that life is busy but that she is a very blessed person. She hopes to pass along her own strengths and gifts to others along the way. She has a number of recommendations for young people interested in environmental health:

1. Try always to identify potential mentors for yourself. You are not bothering them; they like to encourage up and coming professionals.
2. Try to expose yourself to interesting areas through fellowship, internships, and work in different settings. Try not to become pigeon-holed, but explore the many different environmental health settings that are available.
3. Be involved in at least one professional group that can be a point of resource for you and will help you refine your skills.
4. Think about your choices down the road a few years. Explore the emerging issues in environmental health, such as climate change, to discern whether there are career trends in which you might become involved. Think about the

areas in which there will be upcoming retirements to identify opportunities where your skills will be needed.

5. Seek positions that combine both personal and professional interests. Be sure that you are in a situation that will support your continued development as an individual. Witherspoon believes it is helpful to identify the skills you would like to develop; if, for instance, you are shy, she recommends seeking opportunities to do more public speaking.

Witherspoon believes that our current children and future generations are worth the effort. "I feel blessed every single day to be doing what I'm doing," she says. "I know that I am contributing in some little way by advocating for a population that is vulnerable and without its own voice."

Environmental Health in the Private Sector

Frank Ferko, Director of Distribution, Food Safety, and Quality Assurance, U.S. Foodservice   The private sector employs thousands of professionals in all aspects of environmental health, from food safety and quality to air quality, waste management, occupational health, water quality, and integrated vector management. Frank Ferko is one such professional who has spent his career working as a leader in the food safety industry, preventing foodborne illness, ensuring food quality, and partnering with professionals in other public health organizations to establish proactive food safety policies and practices across the country.

Ferko grew up in New Hampshire, close to nature, and developed a love for animals and for science that led him to major in microbiology at the University of Pennsylvania. During his senior year he took many business courses at the university's Wharton School of Business, which underscored for him the importance of being able to communicate the science in terms of the metrics that mattered to the listener, in this case, to company decision makers, from executives to managers. For the first twelve years after college, he worked in food safety and quality with food-processing companies, helping to implement the first USDA-approved Total Quality Control program in the Northeast, and assisting in the development of the time and temperature chart for cooking roast beef that is still used today. He earned his MBA degree from the University of New Hampshire while employed full time in his professional career.

He went on to work for another twenty years at leading food safety programs with national restaurant chains. When a local health department did not have the expertise or resources to properly investigate a foodborne illness outbreak, he became even more convinced of the importance of the food safety industry in providing leadership and influence to ensure food safety. "There are literally hundreds of thousands of people working in the food industry, tens of thousands in food processing and quality assurance, and many more working in food store chains across the country," Ferko says. "These food safety professionals in the industry directly impact food safety and public health, and are the natural allies of the professionals in public health agencies, with similar challenges of preventing illness, communicating the importance of prevention, and advocating for the necessary resources to protect health."

Over his career, Ferko worked for many different industry employers, and lived in multiple states, but was always involved in the food safety profession nationally. He invested time in numerous certifications and trainings, becoming a registered sanitarian, and earning certifications in HACCP (hazard analysis and critical control point) procedures, as a CFSP (certified food safety professional), and as a ServSafe Trainer, among others, that demonstrate recognition of his expertise in food safety. He has been committed to working on committees in partnership with local, state, and federal agencies to help them improve food safety and prevent illness; serving on the board of the national Conference for Food Protection; serving as a member of the Council to Improve Foodborne Outbreak Response (CIFOR) Industry Task Force, involved with the CDC's Epi-Ready program; and chairing the Conference for Food Protection's Committee on Food Borne Illness, the National Restaurant Association's QA Executive Group, and the National Council of Chain Restaurants' Food Safety Task Force, and many other committees. When he lived in Georgia, he was one of two industry representatives involved in helping the State of Georgia adopt a new food code based on the FDA model food code and using model forms developed by the Conference for Food Protection. He is now the director of distribution, food safety, and quality assurance for U.S. Foodservice, the second largest food service distributor in the United States, and oversees more than seventy distribution facilities.

Ferko advises students to look at the broad spectrum of career possibilities in environmental health, from industry to public health agencies, and to recognize the benefits of working in multiple organizations and locations. He would like students to know that by working in industry, they will have the ability to directly affect business operations that may prevent illness for thousands of people, and they will have the opportunity to become professionally involved in national organizations that develop effective policies and procedures to improve food safety. He feels strongly that mentoring is an important responsibility of professionals in environmental health. He himself was inspired by the leadership of industry food safety professionals Dee Clingman and Chet England, and encourages students to actively seek mentors throughout their careers and then to become mentors to those coming afterward.

Communication has continued to be a key theme for Ferko, who travels throughout the country speaking at conferences about improving food safety and quality. At the Conference for Food Protection in Boston, Ferko heard from a mother whose young son had died as a result of a foodborne illness. To a hushed crowd of 500 attendees, she told the painful story of how her young son died horribly after eating a common American hamburger. Ferko became even more determined to help food safety professionals put a human face on foodborne outbreaks in order to more effectively communicate the importance of adequate resources for prevention. "We need to personalize these experiences to give people an incentive to take action. People don't react to stories about bacteria; they respond to stories about people. When I teach about food safety, I sometimes ask people to take pictures of family members out of their wallets, and to ask themselves how they would feel if that family member became sick and died from something they ate. I remind them that what they do on a daily basis in food safety makes a difference that oftentimes they don't even know about." Because of his passion for people and his conviction about the importance of quality, Frank Ferko has devoted more than three decades of his life to making a great difference in food safety in both the private and public sectors throughout the United States.

Clinical Environmental Health

Although much of public health focuses on prevention, clinical care is also an essential part of the story. In primary care, clinicians diagnose illnesses, adminis-ter treatments, and help their patients with recovery and restoration of function. They also offer routine preventive services such as immunizations, screening, and education. In environmental and occupational health the clinical role is similar.

Diagnosing illnesses that relate to environmental exposures is an important clinical function, one that sometimes involves thorny questions: To what was the patient exposed? Did the exposure cause this case of illness? Treating environ-mentally related illnesses is often identical to treating the same illnesses when they occur from other causes, although some environmental ailments, such as lead poisoning, have specialized treatments. Finally, the clinician's public health role is broad and varied in environmental and occupational health, involving collaboration with many other professionals to achieve primary, secondary, and tertiary prevention.

What is the *environment* for a clinician? Historically, the care of patients with potentially hazardous exposures arose in the workplace environment. Occupational medicine traces its roots to an Italian clinician of the late Renaissance, Bernardino Ramazzini (1633–1714), who systematically observed the diseases of metalworkers, miners, painters, glassmakers, and others with work-related disorders. As the industrial revolution was beginning in England, Thomas Morson Legge (1633–1714), the first "medical inspector of factories," investigated poisoning by such substances as lead and arsenic among various occupational groups. Alice Hamilton (1869–1970), the first occupational medicine clinician in the United States and a crusader for safer workplaces, studied lead poisoning among bathtub enamellers, mercury poisoning among hatters, "vibration dead finger" in jackhammer operators, and anemia in workers exposed to benzene. Occupational nursing arose at about the same time. In 1888, a nurse named Betty Moulder cared for Pennsylvania coal miners and their families—and launched a profession. Occupational health nursing expanded as industry grew in the late nineteenth and early twentieth centuries, and *factory nurses* tended to workers injured and made ill on the job. It is easy to understand why these pioneering clinicians, beginning with Ramazzini, focused on the workplace. It was an environment with especially concentrated and long-term exposures. Workers, like the proverbial canaries in the coal mine, demonstrated some of the most severe environmental health problems.

More recently, clinical attention has broadened from the workplace to the general environment. Clinicians play roles in diagnosing and treating lead poisoning in substandard housing, asthma in polluted cities, and pesticide poisoning in farm children. In the environmental arena, clinicians also play an invaluable role in preventive efforts, ranging from advocacy for protective health standards to patient education.

The Clinician's Public Health Function   In addition to fulfilling traditional clinical roles of diagnosis and treatment, **occupational and environmental medicine** (OEM) clinicians play several important public health roles. First, they must always be alert for new conditions and particularly alert for new causes of recognized conditions. This requires a high index of suspicion, familiarity with the medical literature, and an orientation toward contributing new knowledge. Second, many clinicians conduct formal surveillance of different population groups, looking for indicators of exposure or disease. Surveillance is often targeted to populations known to have some potential for exposure to a hazardous agent or condition, and the surveillance aims to verify that the exposure is not causing a detectable increase in disease or injury. States or other entities may conduct surveillance for time-space clusters of disease (most often cancer); finding a cluster prompts evaluation that looks for an environmental or other cause. A related public health function is reporting. Many diseases with an environmental or occupational etiology, for example, metal poisonings and occupational lung diseases, are reportable to state or other authorities.

A key public health function is health education, and this is an important responsibility for OEM clinicians. Because the nuances of environmental disease causation are often not common knowledge, many environmental clinicians educate both their colleagues and their patients. Many serve in advisory roles for voluntary organizations such as the American Lung Association or on governmental boards and commissions that address environmental health issues. In these roles, clinicians make their expertise available to authorities responsible for public health decision making. Collaboration and coordination with state, local, and federal health officials are key functions of OEM clinicians in their roles as sentinels for and investigators of apparent disease outbreaks. Finally, clinicians collaborate with other professionals, such as industrial hygienists, to effect primary prevention—a core public health function.

Environmental Medicine Clinicians and Practice Venues   In some sense all clinicians are environmental clinicians because patients frequently relate information or ask questions about the relationship of their environment to their clinical state. However, only a minority of clinicians are actually trained in the disciplines of environmental medicine. Relatively few clinicians have a working knowledge of the disciplines that take a population approach to environmental health, such as toxicology, epidemiology, and environmental hygiene.

Nurses with special training in occupational and environmental medicine may become members of the American Association of Occupational Health Nurses (AAOHN), and gain certification for their added competencies. Many work in the occupational setting although federal, state, and local health authorities also employ many EOM nurses, along with nurses specializing in infectious disease and in general prevention.

Mental health professionals, especially neuropsychologists, sometimes specialize in problems related to toxic exposures. This specialization assists them in accurately determining whether observed effects are consistent with toxicity. Specialists in rehabilitation are often asked to participate in treatment of those recovering from toxic exposures, and they may need to deal not only with physical limitations but also with concerns related to potential future exposures to lower levels of a given agent.

In the United States and many other countries, following medical school and at least one year of general clinical training, a physician can continue training in a two-year residency in preventive medicine with a concentration in occupational medicine. Although this leads to an American Board of Preventive Medicine (ABPM) exam still formally called "occupational medicine," a majority of the residency programs in the United States have added the words and the focus of "environmental medicine" to this accredited residency training.

Many who choose to take the residencies leading to the ABPM exam have prior training or experience in a primary care specialty or in military medicine, which has a long record of emphasis on environmental and occupational exposures. Unfortunately, as stated earlier, most community practitioners, even those who are very sophisticated, are not well versed in occupational or environmental medicine. For various social and historical reasons, occupational medicine is better integrated with other medical specialties in many European and Asian countries than it is in the United States, although outside of workplace clinicians, a relative dearth of clinical expertise in environmental conditions is still the case around the world. Specialists in occupational and environmental medicine work in a variety of settings. A decreasing number are employees of large corporations, responsible for the health and safety of workers at either a clinical or an administrative level. Some are employed in clinics run by national, state or provincial, municipal, or labor organizations. Others work for private entities that contract their medical services to private businesses. Those employed in all these settings tend to practice in the occupational medicine sphere and may not even be available to address questions arising from the general environment.

Physicians who practice with a focus on environmental health tend to work either for government or in academic settings. Often they were originally trained in occupational medicine. In the United States the Centers for Disease Control and Prevention (along with the Agency for Toxic Substances and Disease Registry) has a relatively large number of clinicians who are trained in the scientific principles of public and environmental health, and most of the fifty states also have such capacity. International organizations, such as the World Health Organization, are also developing environmental health capabilities. Academic faculties are often engaged in research but also address issues of environmental disease in individuals or outbreaks. In the United States the Environmental Protection Agency is often the agency that takes the lead in characterizing an environmental problem, but it consults with clinicians from the CDC or nongovernmental entities in addressing clinical questions.

Robert Laumbach, Environmental Health Physician   As we have seen, environmental health professionals play diverse roles in governmental and nongovernmental agencies, private industry, and academia. Individual careers in environmental health often evolve through various stages, with new roles in different settings. The professional development of Robert Laumbach provides an example of such a series of metamorphoses.

Laumbach grew up in a suburban community in New Jersey, the son of two teachers, one an elementary school teacher and the other a special education teacher, who instilled in him a love of learning and an interest in serving the public good. Growing up in the 1960s and 1970s, he was exposed to the nascent environmental movement and developed an interest in environmental issues that ultimately led to his present career path. He recalls that as a teenager who mowed lawns in his neighborhood during summer vacations, he became concerned about air pollution from gasoline-powered lawn mowers and experimented with exhaust filters that he fashioned from various fabrics. He also designed a solar heating system for the swimming pool in his backyard. "But the path to my career in occupational and environmental medicine was not as obvious or direct as it appears in retrospect."

Having some talent for drawing and painting, he attended art school after graduating from high school. After studying fine art at the Cooper Union in New York City for two years, he decided he did not want to risk life as a "starving artist." He transferred to Rutgers University where he received a bachelor's degree in environmental science. Unsure of what he wanted to do after graduation, he followed a dean's advice to take a summer course at Rutgers that prepared sanitarians for the state licensing exam. He discovered that sanitarians worked on the "front lines" of public health and environmental health. At the local health departments where he subsequently worked, he enjoyed the variety and breadth of activities, which in these suburban and rural communities included inspections of food establishments, well water and surface water testing, inspection and testing for subsurface wastewater treatment (septic systems), investigations of foodborne illness outbreaks, infectious disease control, and a variety of other public health activities.

After several years working as a sanitarian, Laumbach was attracted to another area of environmental health, industrial hygiene (IH), which was growing rapidly in the mid-1980s. As the profession responsible for "anticipating, identifying, evaluating and controlling" workplace environmental hazards, this field offered opportunities to expand his technical knowledge and skill. He was fortunate to move to a starting position with a large pharmaceutical company in New York State, which provided on-the-job training. Here again, he enjoyed the diversity of activities, which included monitoring and evaluating airborne chemical hazards, noise, and radiation and implementing control measures, such as ventilation and personal protective equipment. A few years later he became an IH manager for a smaller specialty chemical company, where he worked in the corporate office. He traveled to locations across the United States, where he enjoyed assisting plant personnel in developing IH programs. Eventually, he became a certified industrial hygienist (CIH), a nationally recognized certification in the field of IH. While working as an industrial hygienist, with the support of his employers he attended classes in the MPH program at Columbia University, where he found that the academic public health courses complemented and synergized with his practical knowledge of IH.

After completing the MPH degree, Laumbach again looked for new ways to expand his knowledge and skills. As an industrial hygienist he had on occasion worked with physicians to design medical surveillance programs for employees. His interest in biology and medicine had been awakened by courses in toxicology in his MPH program. "I was very excited by the prospect of integrating clinical medicine with my background in population health and exposure science." So, at age thirty-one, he started medical school at Robert Wood Johnson Medical School (RWJMS) with the goal of ultimately contributing to the field of occupational and environmental medicine. Most of his medical school classmates had never heard of OEM, a relatively small medical specialty. The OEM residency program at RWJMS was next door to the medical school, and he was fortunate to have opportunities to attend clinical case conferences and other educational activities while attending medical school. After graduating from RWJMS, he decided to complete a three-year residency in family medicine before specializing in OEM. "For a physician interested in environmental health, family medicine is a natural fit. It is the field of medicine that is centered on the 'biopsychosocial' model of health, which recognizes the inseparability of the individual and the individual's family, work and environment." Completing an additional OEM residency required only one more *practicum year* of training because he had earlier acquired the requisite MPH degree.

After completing his residency, Laumbach joined the faculty in OEM at RWJMS and built an academic career that involves research, clinical practice, and teaching. He was fortunate to obtain a career development award from the NIH. With the support of strong mentors, this award has enabled him to conduct research with the goal of developing into an independent investigator. The research focuses on ways in which air pollution and psychological stress, which often occur together in urban areas, especially during activities such as commuting, may interact to affect respiratory and cardiovascular health. In order to conduct this type of interdisciplinary research, Laumbach is a member of a team that includes basic scientists in the fields of toxicology, exposure science, epidemiology, and psychology, as well as other OEM physicians. He works in the fertile, multidisciplinary environment of the Environmental and Occupational Health Sciences Institute, a joint institute of Rutgers University and RWJMS.

At this stage in his career, Laumbach is very gratified that environmental health has offered such varied and exciting opportunities to do important work in a scientific field that is constantly changing and developing. He looks forward to the challenges and opportunities that lie ahead for further personal and professional growth.

CAREERS IN ENVIRONMENTAL HEALTH

So you think you might enjoy a career in environmental health? You have many exciting options open to you! Environmental health services are delivered through a variety of federal, tribal, state, and local governmental agencies, within and outside of traditional departments, through nongovernmental organizations and through private businesses and academic institutions. The breadth of these services requires a diverse array of professionals in environmental health with undergraduate and graduate training in biology, chemistry, geology, engineering, public health education, public relations, nursing, epidemiology, statistics, public health administration and other disciplines. Technicians with associate degrees and community health workers are also valuable in delivering services and working with citizens to identify and resolve community environmental health concerns. Increasingly, as our understanding grows about the interconnections between the social, economic, and built environments and health and about the need to work collectively across disciplines to create healthy communities, the environmental health practice community is also coming to include those with backgrounds in architecture and planning, economic development, and community empowerment and capacity building.

Where do you find the training you need for a career in environmental health? You might begin by learning the location of accredited graduate and undergraduate environmental health programs near where you live. Accredited programs offer their students the advantage of a curriculum, faculty, and resources that meet nationally adopted standards. These programs are accredited by the National Environmental Health Science and Protection Accreditation Council (see the council's Web site, http://www.ehacoffice.org, for the accreditation criteria). Most of these programs require field practicums or internships with agencies as part of the student's preparation. The Bureau of Health Professions of the Health Resources & Services Administration of the U.S. Department of Health and Human Services has published a guide (White and Bock, 1996) that may be useful to both students and agencies in creating meaningful internship experiences.

You will want to be aware of the expectations of your future employers for the competencies they believe you should be bringing to their workforce. In 2001, the NCEH funded a workgroup to define the core competencies for local environmental health practitioners. In addition to expectations for technical competence, this group defined fourteen core competencies under three general skill headings: assessment, management, and communication (American Public Health Association and National Center for Environmental Health, CDC, 2001). Table 27.3 shows these fourteen competencies and their descriptions (more

TABLE 27.3   Core Competencies for Local Environmental Health

Assessment	
Information gathering	The capacity to identify sources and compile relevant and appropriate information when needed, and the knowledge of where to go to obtain the information.
Data analysis and interpretation	The capacity to analyze data, recognize meaningful test results, interpret results, and present the results in an appropriate way to different types of audiences.
Evaluation	The capacity to evaluate the effectiveness or performance of procedures, interventions, and programs.
Management	
Problem solving	The capacity to develop insight into and appropriate solutions to environmental health problems.
Economic and political issues	The capacity to understand and appropriately utilize information concerning the economic and political implications of decisions.
Organizational knowledge and behavior	The capacity to function effectively within the culture of the organization and to be an effective team player.
Project management	The capacity to plan, implement, and maintain fiscally responsible programs/projects using appropriate skills, and prioritize projects across the employee's entire workload.
Computer and information technology	The capacity to utilize information technology as needed to produce work products.
Reporting, documentation, and record-keeping	The capacity to produce reports to document actions, keep records, and inform appropriate parties.
Collaboration	The capacity to form partnerships and alliances with other individuals and organizations in order to enhance performance on the job.
Communication	
Educate	The capacity to use the environmental health practitioner's front-line role to effectively educate the public on environmental health issues and the public health rationale for recommendations.

Communicate	The capacity to effectively communicate risk and exchange information with colleagues, other practitioners, clients, policy-makers, interest groups, media, and the public through routine activities, public speaking, print and electronic media, and interpersonal relations.
Conflict resolution	The capacity to facilitate the resolution of conflicts within the agency, in the community, and with regulated parties.
Marketing	The capacity to articulate basic concepts of environmental health and public health and convey an understanding of their value and importance to clients and the public.

Source: American Public Health Association and National Center for Environmental Health, CDC, 2001.

detailed information can be found at http://www.cdc.gov/nceh/ehs/Corecomp/ Core_Competencies_EH_Practice.pdf).

When you graduate with a combination of these competencies and a degree in environmental health, or with a major in chemistry, biology, community health, health education, or another related discipline, there are a number of places you might seek to work. Local and state health departments and environmental health agencies, tribes, not-for-profit agencies, and industry are all looking for science-trained individuals to educate, advocate, monitor, assess, and assist with environmental health compliance. You might enter the field as a food protection specialist, inspecting all the various sources of food in a community, from bakeries and meat markets to grocery stores and food-processing plants. You might become an air or water quality technician or engineer, working with community pollution sources on engineering design, pollution prevention, plan review, air or water quality monitoring, calculation of emissions, and enforcement of regulations. If you are interested in the intersection of health, environment, economic development, and community planning, you might seek a position with an agency that focuses on land use and transportation planning, or you might offer those skills to an existing public health agency that is interested in expanding its efforts in community-based comprehensive health planning.

If you are interested in environmental health within the larger field of public health, you might consider a master's degree in public health or a medical degree. Graduate programs of public health accredited by the Council on Education for Public Health have a required core course in environmental health. The Council on Linkages Between Academia and Public Health Practice has adopted and regularly revises a list of skills and competencies expected of professionals in public health. With a graduate degree in public health, you might be employed as an epidemiologist in a mid- to large-sized agency, assessing exposures, estimating and communicating risk, investigating diseases caused by environmental factors, and working collaboratively with others across multiple agencies to develop policies and interventions to reduce exposures. Graduate public health training also prepares you for leadership of a program or agency and equips you with the skills to assess community needs, build constituencies, develop policies and plans, evaluate program effectiveness, and advocate for policy change. If you are a technology buff, you might enjoy working with data systems and geographic information and generating statistics and maps to assist community members and elected policymakers in improved decision making for health. One of the best ways to evaluate the many exciting work possibilities is to visit a variety of agencies and talk with the professionals about their daily job satisfaction and challenges.

Once you are working in the field of environmental health, you will want to plan for ongoing training and education to improve your skills and to enhance your own career development. Many of these training opportunities are available at low or no cost on line. Further detail on resources for career development, education, and training can be found on the Public Health Foundation's Web site (www.phf.org), and on its sponsored training Web site (www.train.org). One thing is certain: with the ever-changing environmental issues and emerging threats to community and environmental health, there will always be the opportunity to be challenged each day to provide the most effective environmental health services to keep your community healthy.

SUMMARY

Environmental public health has deep historical roots. Modern environmental public health includes a wide range of activities and functions, such as food protection, water sanitation, air quality protection, safe and healthy housing, occupational health, injury prevention, and healthy community design. Core functions include assessment, policy development, and assurance, and essential services range from data collection to communication to research (see Table 27.1). Many professionals perform these functions. Some have public health training and work in public health agencies, but others have a wide range of professional training (in civil engineering, transportation planning, environmental sciences, and many other fields) and work in a wide range of settings. Across these functions, certain shared characteristics are a constant: the need to base decisions on sound science, the need to collaborate across disciplines, the need to work closely with and be accountable to communities, and the need to assess needs systematically and to achieve measurable outcomes. In coming years, environmental public health will be an increasingly exciting field as it takes on expanded responsibilities, extending the traditional emphasis on sanitarian functions (clean water, sewage management, and waste management) to emerging issues such as disaster preparedness, community design, and climate change.

KEY TERMS

Assessment Protocol for Excellence in Public Health (APEX/HP)

Community-based participatory research

community involvement

core functions of public health

environmental and occupational medicine

environmental justice

essential services of environmental health

essential services of public health

Healthy People 2010

National Public Health Performance Standards

Protocol for Assessing Community Excellence in Environmental Health (PACE-EH)

sanitarian

DISCUSSION QUESTIONS

1. How would you tell someone else about the history of environmental health? How would you describe the link between environmental health and public health?

2. What were some of the factors that led to increased emphasis on the importance of community involvement in environmental health planning?

3. What are some of the common barriers to community environmental health planning?

4. What are some of the tools that are readily available to communities and agencies to conduct community environmental health planning?

5. Discuss the links among democracy, environment, economic development, and equity. What among remain to creating healthy people in healthy communities? Can you think of additional steps that need to be taken to address these barriers to achieve healthy environments for all?

6. What are some of the roles and practice settings for clinicians in environmental health?

REFERENCES

American Public Health Association and National Center for Environmental Health, Centers for Disease Control and Prevention. *Environmental Health Competency Project: Recommendations for Core Competencies for Local Environmental Health Practitioners*. Washington, D.C.: American Public Health Association, 2001.

Burke, T. A., Shalauta, N. M., and Tran, N. L. *The Environmental Web: Impact of Federal Statues on State Environmental Health & Protection, Services, Structure and Funding*. Rockville, Md.: U.S. Department of Health and Human Services, 1995a.

Burke, T. A., Shalauta, N. M., and Tran, N. L. *Who's in Charge? 50-State Profile of Environmental Health and Protection Services, Organization, Programs, Functions/Activities and State Budgets*. Rockville, Md.: U.S. Department of Health and Human Services, 1995b.

Centers for Disease Control and Prevention. "10 Essential Public Health Services." http://www.cdc. gov/od/ocphp/nphpsp/essentialphservices.htm, 2008.

Centers for Disease Control and Prevention. "10 Essential Environmental Public Health Services." http://www.cdc.gov/nceh/ehs/Home/HealthService.htm, n.d.

Institute of Medicine, *The Future of Public Health*. Washington, D.C.: National Academies Press, 1988.

National Association of City and County Health Officials. *PACE EH, Protocol for Assessing Community Excellence in Environmental Health: A Guidebook for Local Health Officials*. http://pace.naccho.org, 2004.

White, L. E., and Bock, S. *Designing Environmental Internships: A Guide for Successful Experiences*, HRSA Contract No. 240–930–0057. Rockville, Md.: U.S. Department of Health and Human Services, 1996.

Winslow, C.E.A. *The Evolution and Significance of the Modern Public Health Campaign*. New Haven, Conn.: Yale University Press, 1923.

FOR FURTHER INFORMATION

Books

In addition to the present volume, several other textbooks provide an introduction to environmental health.

Friis, R. *Essentials of Environmental Health*. Sudbury, Mass.: Jones & Bartlett, 2006.

Hilgenkamp, K. *Environmental Health: Ecological Perspectives*. Sudbury, Mass.: Jones & Bartlett, 2005.

Koren, H., and Bisesi, M. *Handbook of Environmental Health and Safety: Principles and Practice*. (2 vols., 4th ed.). Boca Raton, Fla.: Lewis, 2002.

Lippmann, M., Cohen, B. S., and Schlesinger, R. B. *Environmental Health Science: Recognition, Evaluation and Control of Chemical and Physical Health Hazards*. New York: Oxford University Press, 2003.

Moeller, D. W. *Environmental Health*. (3rd ed.) Cambridge, Mass.: Harvard University Press, 2004.

Moore, G. S. (ed.). *Living with the Earth: Concepts in Environmental Health Science*. (3rd ed.) Boca Raton, Fla.: CRC Press, 2007.

Morgan, M. T. *Environmental Health*. (3rd ed.) Pacific Grove, Calif.: Brooks Cole, 2002.

Nadakavukaren, A. *Our Global Environment: A Health Perspective.* (6th ed.) Long Grove, Ill.: Waveland Press, 2005.

Yassi, A., Kjellström, T., de Kok, T., and Guidotti, T. L. *Basic Environmental Health.* New York : Oxford University Press, 2001.

Agencies and Organizations

American Association of Occupational Health Nurses (AAOHN), http://www.aaohn.org. The professional association for occupational health nurses.

American College of Occupational and Environmental Medicine (ACOEM), http://www.acoem.org. A professional organization of more than 5,000 physicians and other health care professionals specializing in the field of occupational and environmental medicine.

American Public Health Association (APHA), http://www.apha.org. The largest U.S. organization of public health professionals, APHA has an active environmental health staff and membership section and related sections in such areas as occupational health.

Association of Occupational and Environmental Clinics (AOEC). http://www.aoec.org. A network of more than sixty clinics, many in academic medical centers, and more than 250 individuals committed to improving the practice of occupational and environmental medicine.

Association of State and Territorial Health Officials (ASTHO), http://www.astho.org. A national organization representing state and territorial public health agencies across the United States, ASTHO has an active environmental health program that supports states in a wide range of efforts.

National Association of County and City Health Officials (NACCHO), http://www.naccho.org. A national organization representing local public health agencies across the United States, NACCHO has an active environmental health program that supports county and city health departments in a wide range of efforts.

National Center for Environmental Health (NCEH), http://www.cdc.gov/nceh, and Agency for Toxic Substances and Disease Registry (ATSDR), http://www.atsdr.cdc.gov. Federal agencies that share environmental public health responsibility, with ATSDR focusing on hazardous chemical exposures and NCEH having a broader portfolio.

National Environmental Health Association (NEHA), http://www.neha.org. A national professional society for environmental health practitioners, NEHA emphasizes training and education, credentialing, advocacy; and organizational capacity building.

Educational Organizations

Association of Environmental Health Academic Programs (AEHAP), http://www.aehap.org. An association that promotes environmental health education at the undergraduate level and administratively supports the National Environmental Health Sciences and Protection Accreditation Council (EHAC).

Association of Schools of Public Health (ASPH), http://www.asph.org. An organization of public health schools and programs; these schools and programs offer graduate training in environmental health.

CHAPTER TWENTY-EIGHT

GEOGRAPHIC INFORMATION SYSTEMS

LANCE A. WALLER

KEY CONCEPTS

- Data relevant to environmental health are often place based and may be georeferenced, that is, associated with particular geographic locations.

- These data may include environmental exposures, health outcomes, and other information.

- Geographic information systems (GIS) allow mapping of these data, which in turn allows a range of useful analyses.

- A range of operations, such as layering, buffering, and spatial queries, are used in these analyses.

- GIS analyses are limited by data quality and availability and by other technical and methodological issues.

WHY GEOGRAPHY?

Georeferenced data, that is, data measurements associated with particular geographic locations, often play a critical role in environmental health. In fact, the phrase "global to local," used in the title of this book builds on a geographic concept, the notion of **spatial scale**. The spatial extent of a phenomenon—say, a chemical exposure—may in turn define the spatial extent of the health impacts and of potential remediation or other intervention efforts. Mapping spatially referenced exposure, populations at risk, and environmental factors (for example, stream flow, wind speed and direction, emissions locations, or monitoring sites) allows us to manage data geographically, identify the linkages among multiple indicators measured by different agencies over the same study area, and acquire valuable background information for interpreting the environmental context of public health data.

To begin to build ideas, consider the following key components of an environmental health response to an accidental release of a toxic agent: where is the exposure of interest, and where is the population at risk? The highest concern arises when areas of high exposure overlap areas of high population density. Although neither a quantitative exposure assessment nor an analytical epidemiological study, the simple act of overlaying a map of exposure with a map of population density provides a valuable exploratory tool for identifying areas of highest immediate concern.

The role of maps in public health extends at least to physician John Snow's famous maps of cholera mortality in London (Snow, [1853 and 1855] 1936). Most public health students have encountered the story of Snow, who mapped cholera deaths during the 1854 outbreak in London, noted an aggregation near a public water pump on Broad Street, and petitioned for the removal of the handle to the pump in the interest of public health. The story provides a powerful motivator for the potential of geographically linking data sets (in Snow's case, victims' homes and the locations of public pumps). Such a brief summary of the incident minimizes some of the nuances of the story and the role of maps plotted by Snow and others in the public health response, and Brody and others (2000), Koch (2005), and Johnson (2007) all provide insightful historical discussions regarding the variety of maps considered in the public health response to the 1854 epidemic.

Lance A. Waller reports receiving research funding from the National Institutes of Health (National Institute of Environmental Health Sciences, National Institute of Alcohol Abuse and Alcoholism), the U. S. Environmental Protection Agency, and the U. S. Centers for Disease Control and Prevention. The opinions expressed in this chapter reflect those of the author and do not necessarily reflect those of any funding agency.

The dramatic impact of the story of Snow's map often serves as a call for increased use of maps and mapping in environmental health, with the goal of identifying previously unknown connections between environmental exposures and public health problems. Indeed, if Snow could accomplish his study with little more than time, ink, and paper, many wonder what tools today's computers offer for such explorations.

A **geographic information system**, or GIS, is a computer software system (or more accurately, a set of linked software packages) that enables the collection, management, linkage, display, and analysis of georeferenced data. The first formal GISs arose out of the Canada Geographic Information System, devised in the 1960s to aid in the Canada Land Survey (Longley, Goodchild, Maguire, and Rhind, 2001, pp. 10–11). Since then, GISs have developed and evolved to address a wide spectrum of applications, grown to accommodate vast stores of georeferenced data, and advanced in both usability and versatility.

This chapter provides an introductory overview of the use of georeferenced data and geographic information systems within the field of environmental health. Important considerations include a general discussion of the role of maps in environmental health, the role of cartographic principles in an age of computer-generated maps, the basic features and operations of GISs, illustrations of the types of environmental health analyses enabled by GISs, and some limiting factors in such analyses.

COMPONENTS OF GEOREFERENCED DATA

Georeferenced data consist of **location**, **attributes**, and **support**. *Location* refers to the geographic location where a data measurement is taken. An *attribute* is a measurement taken at a given location. Note that several attributes may exist at a single location: for example, levels of particulate matter, oxides of nitrogen, and ozone may all be measured in one place. *Support* denotes the type of location associated with the attribute measurement. Geographic support is often classified in terms of *points* (a single location), *lines* (segments such as roads or rivers), and *areas* (typically political divisions such as states, counties, or census tracts, but also watersheds or ecologically-defined zones). Support provides a context for interpreting attribute values and a reference location for mapping. Data with point support are located as points on a map. Data with line support are associated with lines or curves on the map. Examples of the latter are traffic density on a particular road segment or contaminant levels in a stream.

To further illustrate these components it is helpful to think of a data set as consisting of a table of values (as in a spreadsheet) linked to a map of data locations.

Suppose each row in the data table corresponds to the set of attribute measurements associated with a single location. Each column corresponds to a particular type of attribute measurement across locations, for example, levels of particulate matter at each of a number of air sampling sites. The linkage between the table and map is such that selecting a location on the map results in selection of the associated row of attribute values in the table, and the selection of a row of the table corresponds to selection of the associated location on the map.

The multiple components of georeferenced data imply multiple components of data accuracy. In particular, quality assessments of georeferenced data must consider location accuracy and support accuracy as well as attribute accuracy. A precisely measured attribute value associated with the wrong location can be as misleading as a mismeasured attribute value.

BASIC GIS OPERATIONS

A variety of GIS packages are available, with a range of features, interfaces, and interoperability. However, all GISs contain certain core features allowing basic operations on spatial data, and we review three of these here, namely **layering**, **buffering**, and **spatial queries**.

As its name implies, *layering* refers to linking two or more separate databases by their underlying geography. For example, suppose we have a census database providing summary information on population demographics for census tracts in a given county. Suppose we obtain a second database providing the location and flow levels for a stream network in the same county. Finally, suppose we have a third database providing a point location for the residence of each case of a particular disease reported in the county for a given year and also concentration values for contaminant levels in tap-water samples from these homes. We have three different data sets but we can overlay the respective maps of locations by layering the data in a GIS. Conceptually, this corresponds to overlaying transparent maps of each set of locations so that we may view them together (see Figure 28.1). More important, we may now reference elements of one layer by their proximity to elements in another layer, for example, identify which streams are near homes with high tap-water concentration values.

Buffering involves selection of data items by their position relative to other locations. For example, suppose we wish to identify the census tracts falling within 1 km of a selected stream segment. We select the particular stream segment on our stream map, then define a *buffer* zone around it of the prescribed distance. Most GISs implement equidistant buffers around points, lines, and areas (see Figure 28.2 for examples), but some GISs allow the user to adjust for preferred directions corresponding to wind direction and the like.

FIGURE 28.1 Hypothetical Example of the Layering GIS Operation

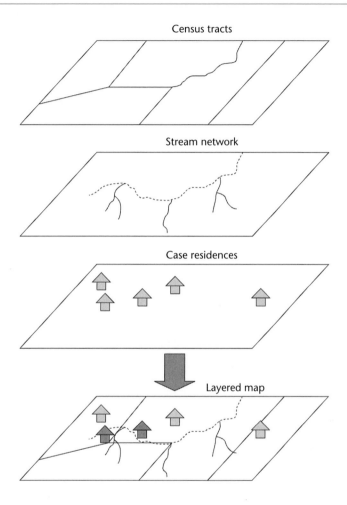

At its heart, any GIS either implements or accesses a relational database system allowing sorting, combining, and selecting data values. In addition to standard database queries such as, "Find all records with concentrations above 5 ppm," a GIS can also conduct *spatial queries*, such as, "Display all homes within 1 km of a selected stream segment." For example, suppose we wish to identify case residences within 1 km of the dashed stream segment in Figure 28.1. Layering our map of residences with our map of streams places the case residence data in geographic context with the stream data, and buffering identifies which case residences are within the prescribed distance (for example, the darker houses in Figure 28.1). One

FIGURE 28.2 Examples of Buffers Around Point (Top), Line (Middle), and Area (Bottom) Features

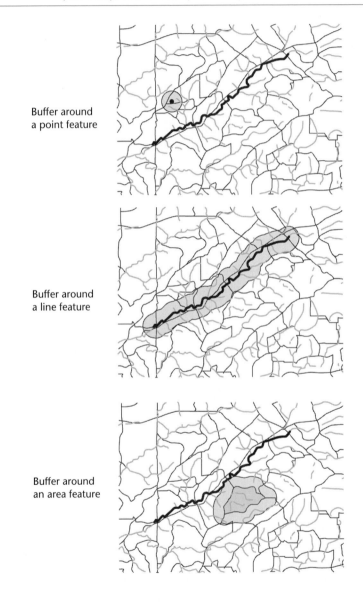

Buffer around a point feature

Buffer around a line feature

Buffer around an area feature

may also conduct combined queries incorporating both location and attribute data, such as, "Display all records with concentrations above 5 ppm [an attribute value] and within 1 km of the selected stream segment [a relative location value]."

Combining all three operations (layering, buffering, and spatial queries) allows complex queries such as, "Display all census tracts with disease rates above 5 cases per 100,000 person-years at risk, which are within 1 km of the selected stream segment and have concentration values above 5 ppm." This query requires layering to combine the stream, health, and population databases, buffering to identify census tracts within the prescribed distance of the stream, and a combined spatial and data query to identify the desired records.

WHY MAP EXPOSURE?

Having defined the basic structure of georeferenced data and basic GIS operations, we next consider the role of geography in environmental health science. Building on the earlier example of considering an appropriate public health response to an accidental toxic release, we find that spatial questions abound: Where was the release? Which way was the wind blowing? What streams are nearby? Where are exposures the highest? Who lives in that area? Who works in that area? What are the possible evacuation routes? Can the spill be contained? How can responders best reach the spill site? Expanding to other environmental health research questions we find similar sets of questions, for example: Where are pesticides applied? Which pesticides were applied where? How much? Who lives nearby? Who works nearby? Are environmental hazards sited in neighborhoods with high concentrations of minority residents? How many children live near a proposed landfill? An accurate map of exposure values would seem to answer, in whole or in part, many of these questions.

Several basic issues are involved in planning and creating exposure maps. To start, consider what information might be contained in a map of exposure. First, most exposure maps are maps of *ambient* exposures, the level of a contaminant existing at a given location. Note that the ambient exposure is only one component of the *personal* exposure sustained by a person at a given location. Other factors influencing a person's exposure include respiratory rate, the use of protective equipment, and behaviors such as smoking, among others, suggesting that two different people at the same location may receive very different personal exposures from the same ambient exposure (see Chapter Four).

Next, consider what data are required to map ambient exposures. In the case of airborne exposures, we might use point monitoring stations, which provide detailed ambient levels at those points. Construction of a map requires interpolation to all points within the study area based on the observed data. The accuracy of the monitoring data combined with the accuracy of the interpolation method will affect the accuracy of the overall exposure map. Many statistical techniques are used for spatial interpolation, and Webster and Oliver (2001) and Waller and Gotway (2004) provide details and additional references (also see the GIS discussion and sources in Chapter Eight).

In the absence of measured exposure values, it is common to use geographic *proximity* as a surrogate for relative exposure; that is, we generally assume that individuals residing or working closer to a source of contamination receive a higher exposure than individuals farther away. Even though proximity rarely (if ever) provides an accurate surrogate for exposure values, the relative ranking may be sufficiently accurate for some exploratory classifications, for example, into "high" and "low" exposure regions. Accurate exposure assessments strengthen the accuracy of any measured associations between exposure and health; however, the use of proximity may be acceptable for pilot studies, preliminary classifications, and other exploratory uses.

WHY MAP DISEASE?

Just as maps of exposure suggest answers to questions of interest in environmental health, maps of disease incidence and prevalence also provide insight into patterns and trends in the data. Questions of interest include these: Where is disease incidence or prevalence highest? Where is it lowest? How do observed local incidences or prevalences, or both, correspond to a map of exposure?

Maps of disease may be "dot maps," with point locations of each case, or **choropleth maps**, indicating counts or estimated rates from nonoverlapping regions such as states, counties, or census tracts. Choropleth maps are more common than point maps due to confidentiality restrictions—reporting aggregate counts of cases from census regions reveals less individual information than a map of case residence addresses does. Although not particularly cartographically progressive, choropleth maps summarize information and are easily created and (more important) interpreted by public health professionals (Pickle and others, 1994).

As with exposure, many factors complicate the construction of maps of health outcomes. First, most people move about during the day, making it difficult to assign individuals to fixed locations on a map. Especially important in environmental health is the difference between residential location (where one sleeps), and occupational location (where one works). The location of interest corresponds to the relevant exposures, but these are often unknown and under study. In addition, residential location may be more readily available from billing (or other mailing) records than occupational location. Another complication arises from increasing geographic resolution—choosing small regions often erodes the statistical precision of the local estimates within each region due to reduced local sample size. A variety of statistical methods exist for stabilizing local estimates from small sample sizes (Lawson and Williams, 2001; Waller and Gotway, 2004), but few are widely available in standard statistical software.

WHAT MAKES GOOD MAPS OF GOOD DATA?

The preceding sections suggest that mapping exposure and health data may provide answers to relevant questions. However, the discussion has also raised some worries regarding the accuracy of mapped values, such as for ambient versus personal exposures and for rate estimates from small areas. One of the greatest strengths of GIS is the ability to link disparate data sets collected over the same study area. For instance, we may wish to link exposure, health, and demographic data over the same region. These three data sets are likely to have been collected separately by different agencies, perhaps over different time periods, and for different reasons. As a result, the primary strength of GIS also entails an important weakness: the accuracy of any conclusions we draw from the map critically depends on the quality of the individual data components. Unlike a designed study in which a single research team is in charge of collecting, processing, analyzing, and interpreting the data, most GIS applications draw heavily from existing data sources for both location and attribute data such as census counts, stream locations, and the like, and as a result almost always involve multiple levels of data quality and accuracy.

In addition to quality data, creating a good map also requires careful thought and selection of cartographic symbols, colors, and other features. For instance, the standard order of hues in the spectrum (red, orange, yellow, green, blue, indigo, violet) may strike the novice mapmaker as a sensible way to display ordered categories in a map, but shifts from light to dark versions of the same hue (light red to dark red, for instance) are actually much easier for map readers to interpret as representing increasing values. As a test, try to decide quickly, without referencing the entire spectrum, if green is "bigger" than orange. Now, try to sort "light red" and "medium red" in terms of increasing value. (Monmonier, 1996, provides a readable introduction to important cartographic concepts and is essential reading for anyone planning to make wide use of GIS techniques or mapping in general.)

WHAT CAN WE DO WITH A GIS?

The previous discussion outlines data structures and operations in a GIS setting. Next, we briefly consider two examples of GIS applications addressing ongoing research programs in environmental health.

A Study of Physical Activity among Park Users

The first example is a comparison of physical activity levels between users and nonusers of parks in DeKalb County, Georgia. An important component of the study design is to sample park nonusers from neighborhoods that are demographically similar to and approximately the same distance from parks as the park users' neighborhoods in order to remove transportation time and demographics as potential confounding factors. The initial study design proposes sampling park users by interviewing individuals in the park, but it is not clear how to sample nonusers in a comparable manner.

We might use a two-stage approach. First, the sample of park users provides data regarding the geographic distribution of residences of park users, in effect defining a *catchment area* for the park. By mapping residence locations of sampled park users onto a street map layer in our GIS, then layering census block groups (subdivisions of census tracts), we assign each residence to its associated census block group. The U.S. Census provides summary demographic information for each block group, allowing us to identify additional block groups within the park's catchment area having demographics similar to the park users' and from which we can draw nonusers. More specifically, by buffering around park boundaries and applying a spatial query, we can identify the subset of the demographically matched block groups that are within the same geographic catchment area as the park users.

Note that this proposed study employs all three GIS operations and differs somewhat from the more typical conceptual use of GIS to identify proximity-based exposure surrogates to insert into a statistical model measuring links between the (surrogate) exposure and disease outcome. In addition, the use of GIS enhances implementation of a fairly standard epidemiological study design (a case-control study, as here where cases are the park users) by identifying potential controls (such as the park nonusers) via standard GIS operations.

An Analysis of Environmental Justice

Second, we consider the application of GIS operations as part of an assessment of an environmental justice claim. In June of 1998, Father Schmitter and Sister

Chiaverini of the St. Francis Prayer Center in Flint, Michigan, alleged environmental justice violations, under Title VI of the U.S. Civil Rights Act of 1964, relating to the proposed siting of a new steel recycling minimill proposed by the Select Steel Corporation of America. In August of 1998, the U.S. Environmental Protection Agency (EPA) agreed to investigate the claim. (A full collection of EPA documents relating to the case appear on the Web page of the EPA's Office of Civil Rights: http://www.epa.gov/civilrights/index.html.)

The proposed minimill was to produce up to 43 tons per hour of specialty metals and, according to the EPA's review, had the potential to emit 100 tons per year of criteria pollutants, including particulate matter, lead, carbon monoxide, and oxides of nitrogen. The complaint filed with the EPA alleged that "the vast majority of the people within 3 miles of the proposed site are minority Americans and will be burdened with a disparate impact of pollution in an already deeply polluted area." In reaction the *Detroit News* reported its own study, describing the "overwhelmingly white makeup of the surrounding neighborhood's demographics" and based on data for the neighborhood within a one-mile radius around the proposed site. The EPA reported demographic data based on one-, two-, three-, and four-mile radii, yielding 13.8 percent, 37.2 percent, 51.1 percent, and 55.2 percent minority, respectively.

How can a GIS help clarify the situation? Figure 28.3 displays a map of census block groups for the 1990 U.S. Census (the most recent census at the time of the EPA investigation), indicating the proposed minimill location and associated one-, two-, and three-mile buffers. We shade block groups according to the proportion of census responders who self-identified their race as "black" (the most common nonwhite racial classification for this county). The map immediately indicates the discrepancies between reports. The proposed location is northeast of the city of Flint, and a large proportion of the county's nonwhite population resides within the city. Within one mile, the population is predominantly white (as claimed in the newspaper reports) while the three-mile buffer begins to include the more densely populated block groups with higher proportions of nonwhite (predominantly black) residents. Although similar information is revealed in the EPA's report in the form of a table, a GIS quickly provides the same table accompanied by the map in Figure 28.3. As a result, the EPA has added tools to its Web sites linking EPA, Census, and U.S. Geological Survey (USGS) data and enabling users to create similar maps on line.

ARE THERE ANY LIMITATIONS?

Many introductions to the use of GISs in public health offer long lists of advantages and (often) little discussion of limitations or complications. The examples offered

FIGURE 28.3   Map of Genesee County, Michigan Block Groups (Census 1990), Shaded by the Percentage of Census Respondents Self-Identifying Race as "Black"

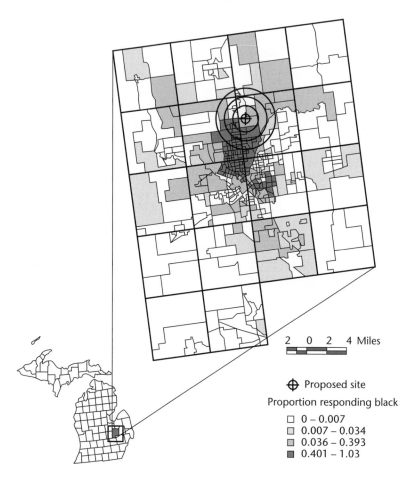

Note: The location of the proposed steel recycling minimill is also indicated, accompanied by one-, two-, and three-mile buffers.

here illustrate several compelling reasons to incorporate a GIS into the environmental health toolbox, and it is only fair to discuss the other side of the coin.

First and foremost, as mentioned above, the ability to combine multiple data sets collected by different agencies for different reasons is both a strength and a potential weakness of a GIS, because assessments of data quality often become murky when multiple data sets of differing quality are combined. In addition, we must consider data quality of *locations* as well as data quality of *attributes*.

Second, by their nature, most GIS studies are *observational* rather than *experimental*. That is, measures of associations are based on observed data, and epidemiological notions of the different types of bias, confounding, and effect modification should always define the suitable context for interpretation of results.

Third, spatial data often include spatial correlations between observations (nearby observations being more similar than those taken far apart). Such correlations violate many standard statistical assumptions and require specialized statistical techniques for analysis, many of which are not currently available in either GIS or standard statistical software packages (Cromley and McLafferty, 2002; Waller and Gotway, 2004).

Fourth, data availability (both location and attribute) varies widely. Some studies may require development of a *base map* of locations before any study data can be assigned locations on the map. The use of global positioning systems (GPSs) and aerial and satellite imaging aid in the development of such base maps, and relatively recent developments such as Google Earth provide growing access to base map imagery worldwide. That said, linking freely available images with GIS-based data can sometimes be a delicate task, and adding the standard GIS operations to Google Earth images is often not as straightforward as many users would like it to be.

Finally, basic GIS operations such as layering and buffering can be complicated when based on layers using different projections of the earth's surface to the map plane or on layers with different levels of resolution. For example, if we zoom in on the Mississippi River in a national map we may find a river defined by only a few line segments at the county level. As another example, consider that we may have population demographics for census block groups and hospital discharge data for hospital catchment areas whose borders do not coincide with block group boundaries. Combining data from such "misaligned" data often requires additional assumptions and calculations above and beyond standard GIS operations.

SUMMARY

In summary, geographic information systems provide a valuable set of tools for managing, merging, querying, and displaying geographically referenced data in environmental health. The basic operations outlined in this chapter may be combined in myriad ways, resulting in a broad set of tools for exploring, summarizing, and displaying such data.

However, as noted in the previous section, the use of GISs still requires appreciation of common limitations in both public health and geography. There is much to be gained by training public health professionals to "think spatially" and similarly much to be gained by training GIS professionals to "think epidemiologically." Innovative applications of GIS in environmental health most often occur as the result of collaboration between individuals familiar with GIS capabilities and individuals trained in public health research. A final consideration is that it is always helpful to frame research goals in terms of questions to be answered and analytical methods in terms of the questions they answer, then to carefully match capabilities.

KEY TERMS

attributes	georeferenced data	spatial scale
buffering	layering	support
choropleth maps	location	
geographic information system	spatial queries	

DISCUSSION QUESTIONS

1. The issue of *data quality* is always important in environmental health research, but do the structure and operations of a GIS raise other issues that might not arise in a controlled, laboratory setting?
2. How might the basic operations of a GIS help meet each of the following research needs?
   - Investigate the health impact of an accidental release of a toxic agent into a stream.
   - Design a targeted mosquito spraying program targeting control of the spread of West Nile virus.
   - Develop a sampling plan for controls in an environmental case-control study.
   - Evaluate and prioritize potential locations for new air monitoring stations.
   - Define commuting patterns from various development plans, and project the impact of lane blockages in various parts of the street network.

   In each case, discuss the data layers needed, the questions that various GIS operations might answer, and how close those questions are to the questions of primary interest in environmental health.

REFERENCES

Brody, H., and others. "Map-Making and Myth-Making in Broad Street: The London Cholera Epidemic, 1854." *Lancet*, 2000, *356*, 64–68.

Cromley, E. K., and McLafferty, S. L. *GIS and Public Health*. New York: Guilford Press, 2002.

Johnson, S. *The Ghost Map: The Story of London's Most Terrifying Epidemic—and How It Changed Science, Cities, and the Modern World*. New York: Riverhead Books, 2007.

Koch, T. *Cartographies of Disease: Maps, Mapping, and Medicine*. Redlands, Calif.: ESRI Press, 2005.

Lawson, A. B., and Williams, F. L. *An Introductory Guide to Disease Mapping*. Hoboken, N.J.: Wiley, 2001.

Longley, P. A., Goodchild, M. F., Maguire, D. J., and Rhind, D. W. *Geographic Information: Systems and Science*. Hoboken, N.J.: Wiley, 2001.

Monmonier, M. *How to Lie with Maps*. (2nd ed.) Chicago: University of Chicago Press, 1996.

Pickle, L. W., and others. "The Impact of Statistical Graphical Design on Interpretation of Disease Rate Maps." *Proceedings of the American Statistical Association's Section on Statistical Graphics*, 1994, pp. 111–116.

Snow, J. *Snow on Cholera*. New York: Oxford University Press, 1936. (Papers by Snow originally published 1853 and 1855.)

Waller, L. A., and Gotway, C. A. *Applied Spatial Statistics for Public Health Data*. Hoboken, N.J.: Wiley, 2004.

Webster, R., and Oliver, M. A. *Geostatistics for Environmental Scientists*. Hoboken, N.J.: Wiley, 2001.

FOR FURTHER INFORMATION

Albert, D. P., Gesler, W. M., and Levergood, B. (eds.). *Spatial Analysis, GIS, and Remote Sensing Applications in the Health Sciences*. Chelsea, Mich.: Ann Arbor Press, 2000.

Kahn, O., and Skinner, R. (eds.). *Geographic Information Systems and Health Applications*. Hershey, Pa.: Idea Group, 2002.

Kurland, K. S., and Gorr, W. L. *GIS Tutorial for Health*. (2nd ed.) Redlands, Calif.: ESRI Press, 2007. For those interested in hands-on examples, this tutorial workbook provides many examples and a time-limited version of ArcGIS by ESRI, one of the most common GIS packages in use.

Melnick, A. L., and Fleming, D. *Introduction to Geographic Information Systems for Public Health*. Sudbury, Mass.: Jones & Bartlett, 2002.

Mitchell, A. *The ESRI Guide to GIS Analysis*, Vol. 1: *Geographic Patterns and Relationships*. Redlands, Calif.: ESRI Press, 1999. This text and the next provide many examples of the types of spatial analysis enabled by GIS.

Mitchell, A. *The ESRI Guide to GIS Analysis*, Vol. 2: *Spatial Measurements and Statistics*. Redlands, Calif.: ESRI Press, 2005.

In addition, Longley and others (2001), cited in the References, provide many, many examples of the use of GISs in a broad array of disciplines, and Cromley and McLafferty (2002), also cited in the References, explore public health applications in more detail.

CHAPTER TWENTY-NINE

RISK ASSESSMENT

SCOTT BARTELL

KEY CONCEPTS

■ Risk assessment consists of hazard identification, dose-response assessment, exposure assessment, and risk characterization.

■ Animal experiments are often used along with statistical models to estimate the dose-response relationships for humans.

■ De minimis risk is a risk management concept commonly applied in the United States.

■ Risk assessment is a rapidly evolving, interdisciplinary endeavor that encompasses many philosophies and techniques.

R ISK assessment is the process of identifying and evaluating adverse events that could occur in defined scenarios. Scenarios may be broadly or narrowly defined and may include many possible events. One well-known risk assessor (Kaplan, 1997) describes risk assessment as an attempt to answer three questions for a particular scenario: What can happen? How likely is it to happen? and, What are the consequences if it does happen? Risk assessment is used in many fields, including public health, engineering, economics, computer science, medicine, and law.

In the environmental health setting, risk assessors focus on health impacts that might result from being exposed to a particular agent or from working in, living in, or visiting a particular environment. For example, risk assessors might analyze the health risks of drinking water with chemical and microbial contaminants, of eating fish contaminated with mercury or polychlorinated biphenyls (PCBs), of breathing particulate matter and other airborne contaminants, or of being exposed to natural and man-made sources of ionizing radiation. *Environmental health risk assessment* can be viewed as a quantitative framework for evaluating and combining evidence from toxicology, epidemiology, and other disciplines, with the goal of providing a basis for decision making.

PERSPECTIVE
Is Risk Assessment a Science?

Although it relies heavily on science-based information, risk assessment does not generate new empirical evidence on health effects in the way that toxicology and epidemiology do. Instead, risk assessment can be viewed as a synthesis of existing scientific information, often aimed at addressing specific regulatory or policy issues. This is why risk assessment has been referred to as a mixture of "science and judgment" (National Research Council [NRC], 1994).

Chloroform ingestion is used as an example throughout this chapter. Chloroform is a by-product of chlorinating drinking water (a disinfection by-product, or DBP, as explained in Chapter Fifteen), and appears at average concentrations

Scott Bartell reports receiving funding from the U.S. Environmental Protection Agency (grants), the National Institutes of Health (grants, travel expenses), the U.S. Centers for Disease Control and Prevention (travel expenses), the National Research Council (travel expenses), Emory University (salary, grants, subcontracts, and consulting fees), and Gradient Corporation (consulting fees).

of 1 to 90 µg/L in U.S. drinking-water systems (Toxicology Excellence for Risk Assessment, 1998). Although chlorination of drinking-water supplies is one of the most effective public health interventions ever conceived, due to its virtual elimination of cholera and other waterborne diseases, exposure to chloroform and other disinfection by-products may increase cancer rates in humans (U.S. Environmental Protection Agency [EPA], Integrated Risk Information System, 2001). What are the risks of consuming typical levels of chloroform in drinking water? This chapter illustrates approaches that risk assessors might use to answer that and other questions about environmental health risks.

THE ENVIRONMENTAL HEALTH RISK ASSESSMENT PROCESS

Although risk assessment did not blossom until probability theory was developed in the seventeenth century, gamblers and philosophers have grappled with the concept of risk since the time of ancient Greek civilization (Bernstein, 1996). The application of risk assessment to environmental health issues is much more recent, beginning largely in the 1970s, when new environmental laws in the United States created a need for science-based decisions on the questions raised by environmental pollution. It would be very costly, and probably impossible, to achieve a society entirely free of pollution, so risk assessment is used to help determine acceptable limits for concentrations of pollutants in air, water, soil, and biota and in emissions from vehicles and industry.

In 1983, the conceptual framework for environmental health risk assessment was formalized in a National Research Council (NRC) report, *Risk Assessment in the Federal Government*, commonly referred to as the **Red Book**. The Red Book divides risk assessment into four elements: hazard identification, dose-response assessment, exposure assessment, and risk characterization. Figure 29.1 shows how the four elements of risk assessment fit together.

Hazard Identification

Hazard identification is the process of identifying and selecting environmental agent(s) and health effect(s) for assessment. This process includes causal inference for particular health outcomes, based on the strength of the toxicological and epidemiological evidence for causation. Sometimes the scope of inquiry is limited to a single agent and single health effect from the outset, leading to a fairly straightforward hazard identification process. At other times, however, the scope of inquiry may be very broad, typically leading to the selection of key agents and their most important health effects for risk assessment purposes. In the 1970s, there was

FIGURE 29.1 Risk Assessment Framework

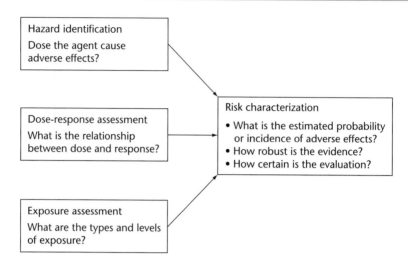

Hazard identification
Dose the agent cause adverse effects?

Dose-response assessment
What is the relationship between dose and response?

Exposure assessment
What are the types and levels of exposure?

Risk characterization
• What is the estimated probability or incidence of adverse effects?
• How robust is the evidence?
• How certain is the evaluation?

Source: Adapted from Omenn, 2003.

widespread concern about the potential contributions of environmental pollution to rising cancer rates, so early assessments focused primarily on cancer.

For example, there is clear evidence from controlled experiments that high levels of chloroform in drinking water can cause cancer in laboratory animals (EPA, 2001). In humans, a number of observational studies have associated chlorinated drinking-water consumption with a slight increase in bladder, rectal, and colon cancer; however, it is not clear how much, if any, of the cancer increase was caused by chloroform exposure, and studies that did not find an association between disinfection by-products and cancer may have been less likely to be published (EPA, 2001). Another example is chemical contaminants in fish. Although hundreds of contaminants, including pesticides, metals, dioxins, and PCBs, are typically present in low concentrations in fish and a wide variety of potential health effects are hypothesized from exposure to each of those contaminants, risk assessments for fish consumption tend to focus on the health outcomes of most concern or most clearly associated with the contaminants, such as neurodevelopmental deficits associated with methylmercury exposure (Rice, Schoeny, and Mahaffey, 2003).

Published reviews of the scientific literature can be helpful for identifying environmental hazards to health. The International Agency for Research on Cancer (IARC) has published over ninety monographs, each evaluating whether or not the **weight of evidence** suggests that human exposure to an agent or to a group of related agents causes cancer. IARC monographs classify agents according to five categories: carcinogenic to humans (Group 1), probably carcinogenic to humans (Group 2A), possibly carcinogenic to humans (Group 2B), not classifiable as to its carcinogenicity to humans (Group 3), and probably not carcinogenic to humans (Group 4) (IARC, 2004). The Agency for Toxic Substances and Disease Registry maintains and publicly distributes detailed toxicological profiles for over 250 hazardous substances commonly found at contaminated sites. Additional reviews are available from the U.S. Environmental Protection Agency's Integrated Risk Information System, from the National Academies, and from the National Institute for Occupational Safety and Health's Registry of Toxic Effects of Chemical Substances, and may also be found in scientific journals.

Dose-Response Assessment

Dose-response assessment attempts to describe the quantitative relationship between exposure and disease. In some cases direct evidence of the level of response at the dose of interest is available, and a mathematical dose-response model is unnecessary. However, that is rare; dose-response assessments frequently rely on mathematical models in order to estimate responses for exposures that fall between experimental dose groups, or for observational data for which doses are typically continuous with few or no repetitions. Mathematical models may also be used to adjust effect estimates for differences in species, gender, race, and other factors that may confound the observed dose-response relationship, or may be used to directly incorporate specific toxicological mechanisms that affect the shape of the dose-response curve.

One well-known dose-response model for cancer is the **linearized multistage model**. This model, like many other cancer dose-response models, assumes that every molecule of exposure adds more risk of cancer. In contrast, **threshold models** assume that nobody exposed at a level below a critical threshold dose will develop cancer as the result of exposure. At low risks the linearized multistage model predicts a nearly linear relationship between the dose (d) and the probability of response (π_d):

$$\pi_d \approx \pi_0 + \beta_1 d$$

where π_0 is the estimated probability of response without any exposure, and β_1 is the effect of the dose.

Table 29.1 shows the results of a toxicological study of kidney tumors in male rats exposed to chloroform. In this study rats were randomly assigned to

TABLE 29.1   Carcinogenic Effects of Chloroform on Male Rats

Dose	Number of Rats Tested	Number of Rats with Kidney Tumors	Proportion Affected
0	301	4	0.013
19	313	4	0.013
38	148	4	0.027
81	48	3	0.063
160	50	7	0.140

Source: Haas, 1994.

one of five groups, each of which was supplied with drinking water containing a different concentration of chloroform. The five concentrations were 0, 200, 400, 900, and 1,800 mg/L, corresponding to estimated doses of 0, 19, 38, 81, and 160 mg/kg/day (milligrams of chloroform per kilogram of body mass per day). Although other methods are sometimes used to extrapolate results from one species to another, many risk assessments assume equivalence on a mg/kg/day basis. A common statistical method called **maximum likelihood estimation** can be used to determine that $\beta_1 = 0.00011$ $(mg/kg/day)^{-1}$ provides the best fit to the rat data for the multistage model (Haas, 1994). In other words, the multistage model predicts that every mg/kg/day of chloroform exposure contributes an additional lifetime cancer risk of approximately 0.011 percent. Alternative dose-response models are described later in this chapter.

Exposure Assessment

Exposure assessment includes the estimation or measurement of the magnitude, duration, and timing of human exposures to the agent of concern (NRC, 1994). This requires explicit definition of the exposed population and the routes by which it might be exposed to the agent. Exposure assessment is often quite difficult to conduct, due to inherent difficulties in measuring complex, time-varying behavior such as the frequency and amounts of water consumed by an individual or the amounts and origins of soil and dust that she unintentionally ingests or inhales or that contacts her skin.

Although ideal exposure assessment would produce a full profile of each individual's exposures over time, in practice most exposure assessments are limited to estimating summary values, such as time-averaged exposure rates. In addition, many exposure assessments rely on default assumptions about media contact rates, such as water and soil ingestion rates, rather than attempting to estimate specific exposure factors for every individual or population of interest. (Exposure assessment is described in more detail in Chapter Four.)

Consider ingestion of chloroform in drinking water at a concentration of 90 µg/L, the upper end of the range described earlier in this chapter. Although skin absorption and inhalation during bathing and other water-related activities may contribute to overall chloroform exposure, first consider exposure through drinking-water ingestion alone. The U.S. Environmental Protection Agency (EPA) (1997) recommends a default assumption that adults drink two liters of water each day. This value is probably an overestimate for most people but is not unrealistic for those who drink lots of water and is commonly used in preliminary risk assessments. A 70 kg individual consuming two liters of drinking water containing 90 µg/L chloroform every day throughout his or her entire lifetime will have an average daily chloroform dose of $2 \times 90/70 = 2.6$ µg/kg/day, or 0.0026 mg/kg/day.

Risk Characterization

Risk characterization is the final step of risk assessment. It consists of combining the information from the other three steps in order to estimate the level of response for the identified health effects(s) at the specific level of exposure to the agent(s) of interest in the defined population. Mathematically, the approach consists of substituting the specific dose amount into the dose-response equation and computing the response level. The risk that is contributed by the exposure itself is often of more interest than the overall probability of response, so analysts often summarize the result in terms of the **relative risk** (π_d / π_0); the additional risk $(\pi_d - \pi_0)$, also known as the **attributable risk**; or the **excess risk** $[(\pi_d - \pi_0)/(1 - \pi_0)]$. Each of these risk measures adjusts the estimated probability of response in an exposed individual by the background probability of response (the response among the unexposed) in a different manner.

Combining the results of risk characterization, dose-response assessment, and exposure analysis in the chloroform example, one might conclude that chloroform in drinking water is a potential carcinogen in humans and estimate that the attributable risk of kidney cancer in a frequent consumer of drinking water containing 90 µg/L of chloroform might be about 0.0026 mg/kg/day $\times$ 0.00011 (mg/kg/day)$^{-1}$ = 3×10^{-8}, or about 3 in 100 million.

The Red Book (NRC, 1983) and subsequent reports (NRC, 1994) emphasize that uncertainties associated with risk estimation should be assessed and discussed as part of the risk characterization step. Qualitative uncertainties, such as those relating to the carcinogenicity of low exposures to chloroform, were mentioned in the hazard identification section of this chapter. Substantial uncertainty also exists regarding the true shape of the dose-response model, particularly its reliability at the extremely low dose used for the drinking-water example. Some toxicologists argue that chronic renal tubule injury is the likely mode of action for chloroform carcinogenicity and that a threshold model would be more appropriate for that mechanism, predicting no additional cancer risk at typical drinking-water exposure levels (EPA, 2001). The extrapolation from rats to humans on the basis of mg/kg/day of exposure introduces another major source of uncertainty. The exposure assessment example was stated for a hypothetical concentration and drinking-water ingestion rate, but the actual concentration and drinking-water ingestion rate might not be perfectly known for a specific population of interest.

PERSPECTIVE
Low-Dose Extrapolation: A Misnomer

A common feature of environmental health risk assessment is *extrapolation* from health outcomes at high exposures to predict health risks at lower exposure levels. In fact most toxicology and epidemiology studies include observations in individuals who are unexposed as well as in individuals who are exposed at higher doses. Risk estimation should actually be called low-dose *interpolation* when data for both lower and higher doses are used to fit the dose-response model.

Although qualitative uncertainty analysis is necessary and useful, the impacts and relative importance of the many sources of uncertainty are seldom obvious. In response, techniques for quantitatively characterizing the impacts of these uncertainties have proliferated during the past few decades. Quantitative uncertainty analysis techniques are summarized later in this chapter.

RISK MANAGEMENT

Risk managers are faced with the challenge of judging the significance of risks, comparing risks and costs for different risk management strategies, discussing these assessments with stakeholders, and finally, making appropriate decisions or recommendations. The Red Book (NRC, 1983) advises that risk assessment and risk management activities should be separated to ensure that the best science is used, although clearly risk assessment and risk management activities should be mutually informative.

Consider the chloroform example, which suggested an attributable kidney cancer risk of roughly 3 in 100 million. In comparison, the estimated lifetime risk of any type of cancer in the United States is about 38 percent in women and 46 percent in men (Ries, 2004). Although 3×10^{-8} is clearly a "drop in the bucket" compared to overall cancer rates, nobody would care to be among the few extra cases in that "drop." What should a risk manager do, faced with information like this? There are many different philosophies on risk management; several common approaches that rely on risk estimation are described here.

De Minimis Risk

Many risk managers and regulatory policies rely on the concept of **de minimis risk**, the idea that some risks are so small that they are acceptable or insignificant from a societal perspective. In practice the value of 1 in 1 million is often used as a threshold for excess cancer risks; activities that pose risks below this threshold are considered acceptable under this paradigm. However, activities or exposures that cause risks above the threshold are not necessarily unacceptable under this paradigm, which is sometimes used to screen out extremely small risks so that more attention can be paid to activities that pose larger risks. Using the cancer risk estimates in the chloroform example, a risk manager might conclude that the risks posed by chloroform are societally acceptable under the principle of de minimis risk.

Safety assessment relies on a similar principle. However, because procedures that do not directly assess the magnitude of risk are often employed in safety assessment, it might be more accurate to say that safety assessment relies on a philosophy of de minimis *exposure*.

Risk-Benefit Analysis

Some risks result from activities that are otherwise beneficial. For example, even though it may increase cancer risks, chlorination has the benefit of reducing the risk of waterborne diseases caused by a variety of microbes. Although an informal comparison between the magnitude of cholera risk from untreated water systems and the magnitude of cancer risk from disinfection by-products might produce figures sufficiently uneven to suggest that chlorination is preferable to no treatment of drinking water, sophisticated quantitative techniques, such as calculating quality-adjusted life years, are also available for comparing more risks and benefits for disparate health outcomes (Schwartz, Richardson, and Glasziou, 1993; Ponce and others, 2000). When conducting **risk-benefit analysis**, it is important to examine the risks and benefits in a balanced manner. For example, it would be

PERSPECTIVE
Risk Assessment Versus Safety Assessment

Although closely related, risk assessment and safety assessment differ in several important ways. **Safety assessment** (also referred to as **regulatory risk assessment** or **regulatory toxicology**) is commonly used by regulatory agencies to select reasonably safe exposure limits or concentration limits in food, water, air, or other parts of the environment. Although safety assessment often relies on hazard identification and dose-response modeling, its aim is to answer the question, What dose or concentration is safe? rather than to assess the likelihood of adverse health effects at a given dose or concentration. Historically, safety assessment for noncarcinogens has relied on the selection of a specifically tested dose that is not associated with statistically significant increases in adverse health effects. When this **no-observed-adverse-effect-level** (**NOAEL**) is derived from experiments in laboratory animals, it is typically divided by **uncertainty factors**, sometimes totaling as much as 1,000, in order to determine a reasonably safe reference dose. Typically, a factor of 10 is applied to account for potential differences in susceptibility across species (for example, rats versus humans), another factor of 10 is applied for potential individual differences in human susceptibility, and a third factor of 10 is applied when deriving a reference dose for children. In recent years many safety assessments have replaced the NOAEL with a model-based estimate of the dose at which the extra risk is 1 percent, 5 percent, or 10 percent, depending on the severity of the outcome. For carcinogens, recent EPA guidance suggests the use of linear interpolation from the lower bound on a benchmark dose to the origin in order to determine the lowest dose likely to be associated with a particular de minimis level of risk. In either case, identification of a safe dose relies on both dose-response modeling and a risk management decision regarding the acceptable level of risk for each health outcome.

more meaningful to compare cumulative risks from all disinfection by-products (not just the risks from chloroform) to the cumulative benefits of the variety of illnesses prevented by chlorination.

Cost-Benefit Analysis

Although the financial costs of risk abatement have always been of concern to affected businesses, they are increasingly considered by risk managers. In fact **cost-benefit analysis** is legally required in promulgating certain types of environmental health regulations (see Chapter Thirty). This approach is generally most useful—and most controversial—when abatement costs are compared to willingness-to-pay values (Tolley, Kenkel, and Fabian, 1994) or other estimates of the dollar value of those illnesses or deaths avoided by abating the risk.

Decision Analysis or Alternatives Analysis

It has been argued that the best decisions are made after considering all the relevant potential consequences of a variety of options, rather than focusing only on particular consequences of a single option (Clemen, 1997; O'Brien, 2000). For example, the financial costs, health risks, and health benefits of a variety of disinfection methods might be assessed and compared in order to make a thoroughly informed decision about what method to choose in a particular setting. This approach differs from the first three approaches discussed here in that the focus is on the comparison of options, rather than on a single activity or exposure. **Decision analysis** may contain elements of the other approaches, such as cost-benefit analysis, and may be done qualitatively or quantitatively.

The Precautionary Principle

The **precautionary principle** is the idea that serious risks should be avoided or mitigated when possible, even when those risks are unlikely or uncertain (see Chapter Twenty-Six). The precautionary principle may be most useful for situations in which little information is currently available to support risk estimation, situations such as global warming, bioterrorism, and the direct genetic modification of organisms. Although often advocated as an alternative to risk assessment, the precautionary principle is compatible with risk estimation and is perhaps better described as a risk management approach.

DOSE-RESPONSE MODELING

Dose-response models play an important role in environmental health risk assessment, as they determine interpolations between tested doses. Although the multistage linearized model is a commonly used dose-response model for carcinogenesis, there are many competing models. Ideally, model selection should be based on biological considerations and well-characterized mechanisms of toxicity. In practice this is more difficult than it might seem, and assessors often rely on the multistage model or other familiar approaches.

The multistage model postulates that a sequence of k critical subcellular events must occur for transformation from a normal cell to a tumor. Critical events might include mutation, changes in gene expression, or cell proliferation. Those events

$i = 1, 2,\ldots, k$ are modeled as independent Poisson processes with lifetime rates $(\alpha_i + \delta_i d)$, where α_i is the background rate of process i, δ_i is the rate change per unit dose for process i, and d is the dose. Under this model the probability of cancer (π_d) is equal to the probability that at least one event of each critical type occurs:

$$\pi_d = (1 - e^{-\alpha 1 - \delta 1 d})(1 - e^{-\alpha 2 - \delta 2 d}) \ldots (1 - e^{-\alpha k - \delta k d})$$

Rather than identifying specific critical events and estimating their rates, analysts typically rely on a linearized approximation to the model just displayed, one that uses a smaller number of parameters:

$$\pi_d \approx 1 - \exp(-\beta_0 - \beta_1 d - \beta_2 d^2 - \ldots - \beta_k d^k)$$

These parameters, $\beta, \beta_1, \ldots \beta_k$, are statistically estimable using dose-response data sets with at least $k + 1$ dose groups; this approach does not require external estimates of the specific event rates or even identification of the types of critical events (Guess and Crump, 1978). For data sets with few dose groups, β_1 typically dominates the function, and probabilities of cancer are nearly linear at low doses, resulting in the approximation shown earlier in this chapter. EPA risk assessments often refer to an upper bound estimate of β_1 called the **potency**, and use it in place of the best estimate of β_1 for estimating risk. Conservative regulatory assessments often rely on upper bound parameter estimates, intentionally overestimating health risks in order to be more protective of public health (EPA, 1990).

Although the multistage model is biologically motivated, the linearized version does not use quantitative information on specific toxic events. In contrast, **mechanistic dose-response models**, **biologically based dose-response models**, and **biologically motivated dose-response models** attempt to model the dose to disease process in more detail, in the hope of providing a better understanding of the true shape of the dose-response curve and a better basis for extrapolating results from laboratory animals to humans. Examples include **toxicodynamic dose-response models** that predict the influence of toxicants on critical events, such as stochastic cell proliferation models for carcinogenesis (Moolgavkar and Knudson, 1981) or neurodevelopment (Leroux, Leisenring, Moolgavkar, and Faustman, 1996); **toxicokinetic dose-response models** that model the transport, metabolism, and disposition of toxicants that enter the body (O'Flaherty, 1993); and models that include both toxicokinetic and toxicodynamic processes (Faustman, Lewandowski, Ponce, and Bartell, 1999). Although these models hold much promise, their development and use is often limited by poorly understood mechanisms of toxicity, the lack of supporting quantitative information to characterize parameters, and the computer programming effort needed for implementation.

All monotonic dose-response models can be expressed using a simple concept known as the **tolerance distribution** (Dobson, 1990). Assume that each individual has a specific tolerance for the toxicant. If exposed at or above that tolerance dose, the individual will develop the disease of interest. If exposed below that tolerance dose, she will not develop the disease. Although each individual's tolerance is unknown, the shape of the population distribution of tolerance values implies a specific dose-response curve, and vice versa. For example, assume that a population has a normal distribution of tolerance values for kidney cancer following chloroform exposure. The probability of kidney cancer for an individual randomly selected from that population is then the area under the tolerance distribution to the left of the dose, that is, the probability that the individual's tolerance is less than or equal to her dose (Figure 29.2). This model is known as the **probit model**, and it can be written as

$$\pi_d = \Phi[(d - \mu)/\sigma]$$

where π_d is the probability of disease, μ is the mean of the tolerance distribution, σ is the standard deviation of the tolerance distribution, and ρ is the cumulative standard normal distribution function; μ is also the ED_{50}, the expected dose at which 50 percent of the population develops the disease.

More generally, simple linear tolerance models can be written as

$$F^{-1}(\pi_d) = \beta_0 + \beta_1 d$$

FIGURE 29.2   Normal Tolerance Distribution (Probit Model)

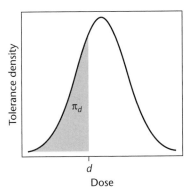

Note: The probability of response π_d is the area under the normal curve to the left of dose d.

where F^{-1} is an inverse cumulative distribution function for the tolerance distribution, and β_0 and β_1 are the distribution parameters. For the probit model, $\beta_0 = -\mu/\pi$ and $\beta_1 = 1/\sigma$.

These models are examples of binomial regression models. This class of models is popular among biostatisticians and epidemiologists, though they are not always aware of the tolerance distribution interpretation. The logistic tolerance distribution, with inverse cumulative distribution function $F^{-1}(\pi_d) = \log[\pi_d/(1-\pi_d)]$, is the basis for logistic regression.

Although *goodness-of-link* tests have been developed for choosing a tolerance distribution function that best fits the data (Collett, 1999), these tests are rarely helpful when there are few dose groups, as in the chloroform example. In such situations it is not uncommon for different dose-response models to fit the data equally well, as shown in Figure 29.3. Because these models predict roughly similar probabilities of cancer, the choice of model might not be very important for some applications. However, when interpolating to extremely low probabilities and using upper bounds on risk estimates, small differences in model predictions may become magnified (NRC, 1983). Although such differences in estimated risk may be small on an absolute scale, they can have large impacts on environmental policy and cleanup costs for contaminated sites.

Threshold dose-response models assume that there is no change in response at low exposures to an agent. In many toxicological experiments, the proportion of

FIGURE 29.3 Three Dose-Response Models (Logit, Probit, and Three-Parameter Multistage) Fit to the Chloroform Dose-Response Data in Rats

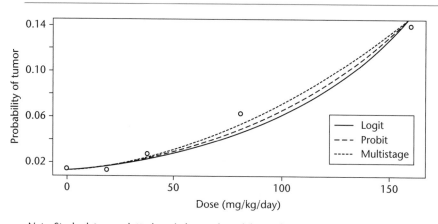

Note: Study data are plotted as circles, and models are shown as lines.

animals exhibiting a toxic response is similar for the unexposed group and one or more of the lowest exposure groups. For example, only about 1 percent of the rats given either 0 or 19 mg/kg/day of chloroform developed kidney tumors, compared to about 3 percent of the rats given 38 mg/kg/day. It is possible that there is a slight increase in the risk of kidney cancer throughout the 0 to 38 mg/kg/day range, as assumed by all three of the *nonthreshold* dose-response models shown in Figure 29.3. It is also possible that there is no additional risk of kidney cancer unless the chloroform dose exceeds a threshold somewhere between 19 and 38 mg/kg/day. Though the threshold model provides a theoretical basis for noncancer safety assessments based on the NOEL (no-observable-effect level), it is rarely used in mathematical dose-response modeling, as the threshold dose cannot be estimated with any useful degree of statistical precision.

A wide variety of dose-response models have been developed and continue to be developed for cancer and other end points. Recent innovations include fitting different mathematical models to different parts of the dose-response curve in an attempt to model low-dose mechanisms separately, and particularly to model hormesis (Hunt and Bowman, 2004) or carcinogens that act through cytotoxicity or other nonmutagenic mechanisms (EPA, 1996). **Hormesis** is a phenomenon in which a toxicant reduces the probability of an adverse response at low doses compared to the probability of the same response at a zero dose but increases the probability of an adverse response at higher doses, creating a dose-response curve that is not monotonic. Hormetic effects have long been debated in relation to alcohol and heart disease and in relation to radiation and cancer; some researchers have suggested that hormetic effects may exist for most or all toxicants (Calabrese, Baldwin, and Holland, 1999), but this hypothesis remains controversial.

Nonparametric regression (also called semiparametric regression) is an appealing but entirely different approach to dose-response modeling. Rather than relying on a mathematical function or functions to describe the shape of the dose-response curve, nonparametric regression relies heavily on the dose-response data set itself to determine the shape of the curve. One semiparametric regression approach uses a smoothing spline, a linked series of restricted cubic polynomial functions, to fit a dose-response curve to a data set. Figure 29.4 shows an example of a smoothing spline regression model for human lung cancer and silica exposure in a nested case-control analysis of 65,980 silica-exposed workers from ten cohorts (Steenland and others, 2001). A logistic regression model and a categorical analysis based on exposure quintiles for the same data are also plotted in the same figure. Note that the smoothing spline suggests some features that are hidden or less obvious in the other models, such as two slight dips in the dose-response curve.

FIGURE 29.4   Cubic Smoothing Spline, Logit Model, and Categorical Model Fit to Nested Case-Control Data on Silica Exposure and Lung Cancer

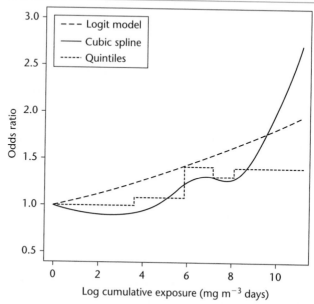

Note: The odds ratio is $\pi_d(1 - \pi_0)/[\pi_0(1 - \pi_d)]$, and is approximately equal to the relative risk when π_d and π_0 are small, as in this situation.

The primary advantage of nonparametric regression is its ability to show such features of data sets without imposing many a priori restrictions on the shape of the model. However, revealed "features" are sometimes just artifacts of study design or random error rather than reflections of the true dose-response curve. If confidence bounds for the dose-response curve rule out random error as a potential explanation for odd features, careful attention should be given to the data in those ranges, perhaps through suggesting new hypotheses about confounding or mechanisms of toxicity.

Nonparametric regression is rarely applied to data from controlled experiments in laboratory animals, as these studies typically rely on few dose groups, providing little information on the shape of the dose-response curve.

UNCERTAINTY ANALYSIS

Uncertainty analysis was highlighted as an important component of risk assessment in the Red Book, and has since been the subject of much interest from researchers and practitioners (Morgan, Henrion, and Small, 1990). At its simplest, uncertainty analysis consists of a qualitative description of the sources of uncertainty in a risk assessment and their potential impacts. However, uncertainty analysis is often quantitative, providing a range or distribution of reasonable risk estimates. Approaches to quantitative uncertainty analysis include probabilistic analysis and interval analysis.

Interval analysis (Alefeld and Herzberger, 1983; Ferson, 1996) is a relatively simple approach for describing uncertainty quantitatively. The idea of this approach is to estimate the risk twice, once using best-case parameter estimates and then again using worst-case parameter estimates. One advantage of this approach is its simplicity. It is relatively easy to conduct, does not require specialized software (although interval analysis software is available), is easy to explain, and provides potentially useful quantitative information about the uncertainty in the results of a given risk assessment. The primary disadvantage of this approach is that the interval provides no information about the relative plausibility of individual risk estimates within the interval. It is possible that every point in the interval is equally likely, but also possible that an estimate near the center of the interval is most likely and that estimates near the ends of the interval are less likely. Moreover, single points for the best-case and worst-case parameter estimates may be difficult to define when they are not bound by physical restrictions, such as proportions limited to the range of 0 to 100 percent.

Although they are seldom identified as such by risk analysts, statistical confidence intervals and prediction intervals are examples of another type of interval analysis. Such an interval, based on frequentist or Bayesian statistical methods, provides a range of estimates that is likely to include the true value. Procedures for finding these intervals are developed using mathematical statistics, resulting in intervals that seek to capture the true risk estimate with a fixed level of confidence (commonly 95 percent) (DeGroot, 1989). Frequentist methods dominated the statistical literature during the last century and serve as the basis for the most commonly used statistical software packages. However, frequentist statistical methods can be difficult to develop for complicated models, leading analysts to rely on approximations or to substitute simpler models. Moreover, traditional frequentist methods tend to divide model parameters into those that are known exactly and those that are completely unknown; there are few frequentist mechanisms for dealing with parameters that are partially understood or can only be guessed. Bayesian statistical methods, an alternative approach, readily handle parameter uncertainty, educated guesses, and complex models, and allow a formal probability-based interpretation of results (Greenland, 2001).

Probabilistic risk analysis describes risk using one or more probability distributions indicating the plausibility of an entire range of risk estimates. A number of philosophies and approaches are used to characterize these probability distributions, including formal statistical methods, but the most popular method among environmental health risk assessors is an informal approach called **Monte Carlo simulation**.

The Monte Carlo approach to probabilistic risk assessment requires additional steps after the initial quantitative risk assessment. First, probability distributions are selected to represent uncertainty, or variability, in the model parameters. Dependence among parameters may be specified using a variety of approaches, including multivariate distributions, conditional distributions, and rank correlations. Some analysts prefer to distinguish variability, which reflects known differences among individuals at risk, from uncertainty, which reflects lack of knowledge regarding the true values of model parameters. Next, plausible sets of parameter values are randomly and repeatedly selected according to the specified probability distributions and correlation structure. A risk estimate is calculated and recorded for each set of parameters. After risk estimates have been calculated for many (sometimes tens of thousands or hundreds of thousands) sets of parameters, the collection of risk estimates approximates the distribution of uncertainty regarding the risk. This Monte Carlo distribution shows the range and relative plausibility of various risk estimates after taking into account uncertainty in all the model parameters.

Although Monte Carlo simulation is a flexible method for conducting probabilistic risk assessment, it is sometimes not the most efficient approach. For some models, exact distributions can be determined explicitly. For example, the sum of a set of normal distributions is normally distributed, and the product of lognormal distributions is lognormally distributed. (Alternative methods for determining the exact or approximate distribution of functions of random variables are available in standard statistical references; see, for example, DeGroot, 1989; Evans, Hastings, and Peacock, 1993.)

Some argue that the relative plausibility of an entire range of risk estimates is impossible to determine reliably and that attempts to do so may mislead and confuse risk managers and stakeholders. Moreover, correlations between parameters are difficult to characterize and are often overlooked, introducing substantial errors in uncertainty propagation (Ferson, 1996).

AN ASSESSMENT OF RISK ASSESSMENT

Risk assessment has been widely criticized over the years. This may be inevitable for a process at the interface of science and policy, in which both evidence and judgment play important roles (NRC, 1994).

Some of the objections to risk assessment have been scientific. For example, critics have focused on the default assumptions (EPA, 1990, 2005) that are used when empirical data are not available, such as assumptions about the shape of the dose-response curve and implications for risk at low levels of exposure. The empirical data used have also come in for criticism. Skeptics question the accuracy of human health risk estimates derived from high-dose experiments in rodents. Epidemiological dose-response models can be equally controversial, as these studies are usually observational rather than experimental, raising doubts about causal interpretations. Moreover, in practice only a subset of possible illnesses is studied for any toxicant, implying that risk estimates for known diseases may underestimate the overall burden of health effects truly caused by a given exposure. Critics have also argued that the emphasis on single chemicals is inappropriate when the risk people experience reflects cumulative exposures to both chemicals and nonchemical conditions.

Other objections to risk assessment have turned on policy decisions, such as the selection of margins of safety. More broadly, critics of risk assessment have

PERSPECTIVE
Toxicology and Epidemiology in Environmental Health Risk Assessment

Although toxicology and epidemiology are both used to study the health effects of environmental pollution, each approach has several important limitations for supporting environmental regulations. Environmental epidemiology, for practical and ethical reasons, is usually observational rather than experimental, raising the potential for uncontrolled confounding. Moreover, pollutant exposures and health effects must have already occurred in large populations in order for epidemiologists to study their associations, yet environmental regulations often seek to prevent environmental health problems before they begin. Because careful epidemiological studies are often expensive, time consuming, and limited by ethical concerns, their widespread application to thousands of chemicals is impractical. Toxicological experiments are relatively quick and inexpensive to conduct in rodents, even for chronic health effects such as cancer. However, these experiments on rats, mice, or other laboratory animals may not always be relevant to humans. Viewed in isolation, neither observational human epidemiology nor experimental laboratory animal toxicology provides ideal information on environmental health. However, when observations in humans are confirmed by experimental evidence in laboratory animals, or vice versa, much stronger conclusions result.

argued that the practice seems to accept and even legitimate risk, when policy might be better directed to banning dangerous exposures or providing incentives for technological innovation (Commoner, 1990; Silbergeld, 1993; Montague, 2004).

Risk assessment is indeed at the interface of science and policy. In 2006, the Office of Management and Budget, a part of the Executive Office of the President that helps carry out presidential policy, proposed a major revision of risk assessment practices across the government. The proposal came in for intense criticism (as described in the Perspective on "explosive politics"). Some critics argued that the guidelines, if implemented, would contribute to "paralysis by analysis" and would hamstring agencies.

PERSPECTIVE
The Explosive Politics of Unified Risk Assessment

Risk assessment is widely used by various state and federal agencies, each applying its own standards. In early 2006, the U.S. Office of Management and Budget (OMB) proposed new guidelines for most federal risk assessments (OMB, 2006). Remarkably brief for such a far-reaching proposal, the twenty-six-page document included an unusually broad definition of risk assessment, and general standards requiring clear definition of the needs and scope of each risk assessment, a central or best estimate of risk, formal uncertainty analysis for influential risk assessments, objective evaluations based on weight of evidence, disclosure and impact analysis for critical assumptions, an executive summary, and cost-benefit analysis for regulations with large economic impacts. At the request of the OMB and seven other federal agencies and departments, the National Research Council convened an expert panel to review the proposed guidance. Although the NRC panel endorsed the goals of the OMB guidance and some of its good practice recommendations, it found the proposed guidelines scientifically unsound and "fundamentally flawed." The language was unusually strong; for example, the NRC panel wrote that "there is no scientific consensus to support the bulletin's universal prescriptions for how uncertainty should be evaluated. In the absence of clear guidance regarding the conduct of uncertainty analysis, there is a serious danger that agencies will produce ranges of meaningless and confusing risk estimates, which could result in risk assessments of reduced rather than enhanced quality and objectivity." Based this and similar observations, the panel recommended complete withdrawal of the OMB guidelines (NRC, Committee to Review the OMB Risk Assessment Bulletin, 2007).

In 2008, the National Research Council's Committee on Improving Risk Analysis Approaches Used by the U.S. EPA issued a landmark report, *Science and Decisions: Advancing Risk Assessment* (called the **Grey Book**, by analogy with the earlier Red Book). The report provided a comprehensive look at risk assessment since its inception in the 1980s, identified a series of problems, and recommended solutions (Table 29.2 and Figure 29.5). Although focused on the EPA, its findings were broadly applicable. Principal among the NRC findings was that risk assessment too often focuses on the narrowly technical task of quantifying risk and does not function optimally to guide decision making among various alternatives. The NRC also called for more attention to handling uncertainty and variability and to the use of default assumptions. These NRC recommendations are likely to guide risk assessment practice in coming years.

FIGURE 29.5 A Framework for Risk-Based Decision Making Designed to Maximize Risk Assessment Utility

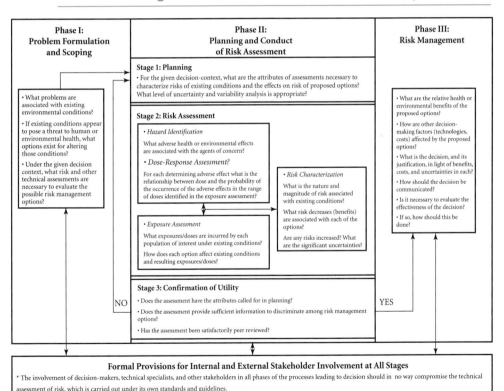

Source: NRC, Committee on Improving Risk Analysis Approaches Used by the U.S. EPA, 2008. Reprinted with permission from the National Academies Press, Copyright 2008, National Academy of Sciences.

TABLE 29.2   Problems with Risk Assessment
and Recommended Solutions

Problem	Recommended Solutions
Design of risk assessment: risk assessment often not conceived and planned to produce useful results that inform decision makers.	Increased attention to the design of risk assessment in its formative stages, including planning, scoping and problem formulation, and involving risk assessors, risk managers, and stakeholders.
Uncertainty and variability: these factors have not received enough attention and have been inconsistently handled in risk assessments.	Characterize and communicate uncertainty and variability in all key computational steps of risk assessment. Plan and manage uncertainty and variability analysis to reflect the needs for comparative evaluation of the risk management options.
Selection and use of defaults: default assumptions commonly used in the absence of data, but these are highly controversial. Some defaults are implicit.	Continue and expand use of the best, most current science to support and revise default assumptions. Replace implicit defaults with explicitly stated defaults. Develop clear, general standards for the level of evidence needed to justify the use of alternative assumptions in place of defaults, and describe specific criteria for the use of alternatives to each particular default assumption.
A unified approach to dose-response assessment: disparate approaches historically used for cancer and noncancer outcomes.	A unified dose-response assessment framework addressing background exposures and disease processes, possible vulnerable populations, and modes of action. Redefine *reference dose* (RfD) and *reference concentration* (RfC) as a risk-specific dose that provides information on the proportion of the population expected to be above or below a defined acceptable risk.
Cumulative risk assessment: risk assessment too often focuses on single agents when risk results from multiple exposures.	Promote cumulative risk assessment, including nonchemical stressors, using data from multiple fields.
Improving the utility of risk assessment: risk assessment too often focuses on quantifying a level of risk rather than guiding decision makers toward the best decision given various options.	Establish an expanded framework for risk-based decision making including initial problem formulation and scoping, up-front identification of risk management options, and use of risk assessment to discriminate among these options (see Figure 29.5).
Stakeholder involvement: stakeholders see risk assessment as lacking credibility and transparency.	Promote balanced participation of stakeholders, including affected communities and less advantaged stakeholders
Capacity building: need for retraining and expanding the risk assessment workforce.	Use training and capacity building to support risk-based decision making.

Source: Compiled from NRC, Committee on Improving Risk Analysis Approaches Used by the U.S. EPA, 2008.

SUMMARY

Risk assessment is a process that involves hazard identification, hazard characterization or dose-response assessment, exposure assessment, and risk characterization. Since it was formally defined in the 1983 Red Book, risk assessment has come to be a common practice. Data from human and animal studies are combined with assumptions and mathematical models to quantify the risk of various exposures and to guide decision making about those exposures. Risk assessment is inherently susceptible to criticism because it is, at heart, an attempt either to estimate an unmeasured past or present or to predict an unknown future, or to do both. There are many reasonable approaches that might be taken for any particular risk assessment, and people often disagree on the best approach. When risk assessment is used as the basis for environmental health regulations or other important decisions, even small changes in risk estimates can have large economic consequences. As long as risk assessment remains a central component of environmental health regulation, debate on its methods and predictions is sure to continue.

KEY TERMS

attributable risk

biologically-based dose-response models

biologically-motivated dose-response models

cost-benefit analysis

de minimis risk

decision analysis

dose-response assessment

excess risk

exposure assessment

Grey Book

hazard identification

hormesis

linearized multistage model

maximum likelihood estimation

mechanistic dose-response models

Monte Carlo simulation

no-observed-adverse-effect-level (NOAEL)

nonparametric regression

potency

precautionary principle

probit model

Red Book

relative risk

regulatory risk assessment

regulatory toxicology

risk-benefit analysis

risk characterization

safety assessment

threshold models

tolerance distribution

toxicodynamic dose-response models

toxicokinetic dose-response models

uncertainty factors

weight of evidence

DISCUSSION QUESTIONS

1. What role, if any, should risk assessment have in regulating pollution? Are small risks ever acceptable?
2. What are the advantages and disadvantages of the different risk management approaches described in this chapter?
3. Is it important for risk assessment and risk management to be separated, or is safety assessment a reasonable approach?

REFERENCES

Alefeld, G., and Herzberger, J. *Introduction to Interval Computations*. San Diego: Academic Press, 1983.

Bernstein, P. L. *Against the Gods: The Remarkable Story of Risk*. Hoboken, N.J.: Wiley, 1996.

Calabrese, E. J., Baldwin, L. A., and Holland, C. D. "Hormesis: A Highly Generalizable and Reproducible Phenomenon with Important Implications for Risk Assessment." *Risk Analysis*, 1999, *19*, 261–281.

Clemen, R. T. *Making Hard Decisions: An Introduction to Decision Analysis*. (2nd ed.) Pacific Grove, Calif.: Duxbury Press, 1997.

Collett, D. *Modelling Binary Data*. Boca Raton, Fla.: Chapman & Hall/CRC Press, 1999.

Commoner, B. "The Hazards of Risk Assessment." *Columbia Journal of Environmental Law*. 1990, *14*, 365–378.

DeGroot, M. H. *Probability and Statistics*. (2nd ed.) Upper Saddle River, N.J.: Addison-Wesley/Pearson Education, 1989.

Dobson, A. J. *An Introduction to Generalized Linear Models*. (2nd ed.) Boca Raton, Fla.: Chapman & Hall/CRC Press, 1990.

Evans, M., Hastings, N., and Peacock, B. *Statistical Distributions*. (2nd ed.) Hoboken, N.J.: Wiley, 1993.

Faustman, E. M., Lewandowski, T. A., Ponce, R. A., and Bartell, S. M. "Biologically Based Dose-Response Models for Developmental Toxicants: Lessons from Methylmercury." *Inhalation Toxicology*, 1999, *11*, 559–572.

Ferson, S. "What Monte Carlo Methods Cannot Do." *Human and Ecological Risk Assessment*, 1996, *2*, 990–1007.

Greenland, S. "Sensitivity Analysis, Monte Carlo Risk Analysis, and Bayesian Uncertainty Assessment." *Risk Analysis*, 2001, *21*(4), 579–583.

Guess, H. A., and Crump, K. S. "Best-Estimate Low-Dose Extrapolation of Carcinogenicity Data." *Environmental Health Perspectives*, 1978, *22*, 149–152.

Haas, C. N. "Dose-Response Analysis Using Spreadsheets." *Risk Analysis*, 1994, *14*(6), 1097–2000.

Hunt, D. L., and Bowman, D. "A Parametric Model for Detecting Hormetic Effects in Developmental Toxicity Studies." *Risk Analysis*, 2004, *24*(1), 65–72.

International Agency for Research on Cancer. *Complete List of Agents Evaluated and Their Classification*. http://monographs.iarc.fr/ENG/Classification/index.php, 2004.

Kaplan, S. "The Words of Risk Analysis." *Risk Analysis*, 1997, *17*(4), 407–417.

Leroux, B. G., Leisenring, W. M., Moolgavkar, S. H., and Faustman, E. M. "A Biologically-Based Dose-Response Model for Developmental Toxicology." *Risk Analysis*, 1996, *16*(4), 449–458.

Moolgavkar, S. H., and Knudson, A. G., Jr. "Mutation and Cancer: A Model for Human Carcinogenesis." *Journal of the National Cancer Institute*, 1981, *66*(6), 1037–1052.

Montague, P. "Reducing the Harms Associated with Risk Assessments." Environmental Impact Assessment Review, 2004, *24*, 733–748.

Morgan, M. G., Henrion, M., and Small, M. *Uncertainty: A Guide to Dealing with Uncertainty in Quantitative Risk and Policy Analysis.* New York: Cambridge University Press, 1990.

National Research Council. *Risk Assessment in the Federal Government: Managing the Process.* Washington, D.C.: National Academies Press, 1983.

National Research Council. *Science and Judgment in Risk Assessment.* Washington, D.C.: National Academies Press, 1994.

National Research Council, Committee on Improving Risk Analysis Approaches Used by the U.S. EPA. *Science and Decisions: Advancing Risk Assessment.* Washington, D.C.: National Academies Press, 2008.

National Research Council, Committee to Review the OMB Risk Assessment Bulletin. *Scientific Review of the Proposed Risk Assessment Bulletin from the Office of Management and Budget.* Washington, D.C.: National Academies Press, 2007.

O'Brien, M. *Making Better Environmental Decisions.* Cambridge, Mass.: MIT Press, 2000.

O'Flaherty, E. J. "Physiologically Based Models for Bone-Seeking Elements, 4: Kinetics of Lead Disposition in Humans." *Toxicology and Applied Pharmacology*, 1993, *118*, 16–29.

Omenn, G. S. "The Evolution of Risk Assessment and Risk Management." *Human and Ecological Risk Assessment*, 2003, *9*(5), 1155–1167.

Ponce, R. A., and others. "Use of Quality-Adjusted Life Year Weights with Dose-Response Models for Public Health Decisions: A Case Study of the Risks and Benefits of Fish Consumption." *Risk Analysis*, 2000, *20*(4), 529–542.

Rice, D. C., Schoeny, R., and Mahaffey, K. "Methods and Rationale for Derivation of a Reference Dose for Methylmercury by the US EPA." *Risk Analysis*, 2003, *23*(1), 107–115.

Ries, L.A.G., and others (eds.). *SEER Cancer Statistics Review, 1975–2001.* National Cancer Institute. http://seer.cancer.gov/csr/1975_2001, 2004.

Schwartz, S., Richardson, J., and Glasziou, P. P. "Quality-Adjusted Life Years: Origins, Measurements, Applications, Objectives." *Australian Journal of Public Health*, 1993, *17*(30), 272–278.

Silbergeld, E. K. "Risk Assessment: The Perspective and Experience of U.S. Environmentalists." *Environmental Health Perspectives*, 1993, *101*, 100–104.

Steenland, K., and others. "Pooled Exposure-Response Analyses and Risk Assessment for Lung Cancer in 10 Cohorts of Silica-Exposed Workers: An IARC Multicentre Study." *Cancer Causes & Control*, 2001, *12*, 773–784.

Tolley, G., Kenkel, D., and Fabian, R. (eds.). *Valuing Health for Policy.* Chicago: University of Chicago Press, 1994.

Toxicology Excellence for Risk Assessment. *Health Risk Assessment/Characterization of the Drinking Water Disinfection Byproduct Chloroform.* http://www.tera.org/news/Chloroform.PDF, 1998.

U.S. Environmental Protection Agency. *Risk Assessment Guidance for Superfund, Vol. 1: Human Health Evaluation Manual (Part A).* EPA/540/1–89/002. Washington, D.C.: U.S. Environmental Protection Agency, Office of Emergency and Remedial Response, 1990.

U.S. Environmental Protection Agency. "Proposed Guidelines for Carcinogen Risk Assessment." *Federal Register*, *61*, 17960–18011 (1996).

U.S. Environmental Protection Agency. *Exposure Factors Handbook, Vol. 1: General Factors*. Washington, D.C.: U.S. Environmental Protection Agency, 1997.

U.S. Environmental Protection Agency. *Guidelines for Carcinogen Risk Assessment*. EPA/630/P-03/001F. Washington, D.C.: U.S. Environmental Protection Agency, Risk Assessment Forum, 2005.

U.S. Environmental Protection Agency, Integrated Risk Information System. "Chloroform: CASRN 67663." http://www.epa.gov/iris/subst/0025.htm, 2001.

U.S. Office of Management and Budget. *Proposed Risk Assessment Bulletin*. Washington, D.C.: U.S. Office of Management and Budget, Office of Information and Regulatory Affairs, 2006.

FOR FURTHER INFORMATION

RiskWorld. [Homepage.] http://www.riskworld.com, 2005.

Society for Risk Analysis. [Homepage.] http://www.sra.org, 2005.

U.S. Environmental Protection Agency, Integrated Risk Information System. [Homepage.] http://www.epa.gov/iris, 2005.

CHAPTER THIRTY

ENVIRONMENTAL HEALTH POLICY

A. STANLEY MEIBURG

KEY CONCEPTS

- Many policies affect environmental health. Some explicitly target environmental health, but others that do not may still have profound health consequences.

- Federal environmental law grew rapidly in scope and complexity between 1970 and 1990, and it provides the foundation for many, though not all, environmental health policies.

- The institutions that administer laws at all levels of government have many tools to influence environmental health policy.

- Many actors shape environmental health policy. Understanding these actors and their motivations helps to explain particular policy choices.

WHO makes the rules that influence our common life? Many fields of study seek answers to this question, including sociology, psychology, anthropology, and political science.

These rules take many forms. Some are embodied in various types of law. **Statutory law** refers to rules enacted by a legislative body, **common law** grows out of court decisions that establish precedents, and **regulations** are rules issued by executive branch agencies and based on statutory law. In the United States the common law tradition goes back to colonial times. In the environmental arena, statutes and regulations specifically adopted by governments under our constitutional framework now hold a preeminent place in our society.

But statutory law, common law, and regulations are all influenced by cultural and institutional norms. These norms can change over time. For example, most people in the 1940s and 1950s took smoking for granted, including in public places. Now tobacco companies have settled billions of dollars worth of lawsuits against their products, many jurisdictions ban smoking in public buildings, and smoking is frowned upon socially in ways that would not have occurred to people fifty years ago.

WHAT IS ENVIRONMENTAL HEALTH POLICY?

We can think of policy as courses of action adopted, either formally or informally, to achieve social goals and determine community affairs. To be policy, these courses of action must affect human behavior. Ideas that do not affect behavior may be ideals or aspirations, but they are not policy. Policy enables certain activities and limits or forbids others. Policy is especially identified with the actions of government, and government is uniquely endowed with the authority to legitimately use coercion to accomplish policy objectives. Still, there are many other components of society that contribute to establishing social goals and carrying them out.

For the purpose of this chapter, environmental health policy refers to that subset of policies that affect the relationship between people's health and their environment. Because environment is everything around us, environmental health policy is a very broad subject! Here we will focus on the different types of policy, governmental institutions that develop policy, key actors and factors that influence policy, and environmental health policy trends.

Policy is not the same as practice. We usually think that practice follows policy, yet the relationship is more complex. Leaders may think they have established

A. Stanley Meiburg declares no competing financial interests.

policy, only to find that a lack of operational capability (or rebellion on the part of the operators) nullifies what they intended. Still, it is useful to start our analysis of environmental health policy by assuming that, at least for analytical purposes, decisions about *what* to do precede decisions about *how* to do it.

TYPES OF ENVIRONMENTAL HEALTH POLICY

Some environmental policies and laws directly target health outcomes. For example, the U.S. Environmental Protection Agency (EPA) establishes primary national ambient air quality standards under the Clean Air Act; the standards are those "requisite to protect the public health" (*U.S. Code*, 42, §S 7409(b)(1)). Areas with air quality worse than these standards must adopt measures to improve it. Other examples include standards for drinking water, garbage disposal, restaurant sanitation, and consumer products.

Although these policies seem clearly related to health, others may not appear at first glance to share such a connection. Consider zoning laws, for example. Zoning originated in the desire of communities to promote compatible uses of land and restrict the unfettered ability of property owners to do as they pleased with their property. Yet from its earliest days, one reason for zoning was to protect health by separating residential and industrial activities (Frumkin, Frank, and Jackson, 2004, p. 37). Now there is concern that by separating residential land uses from commercial uses like grocery stores and restaurants, specifying minimum lot sizes, or limiting multifamily housing, zoning can enable if not promote poor health by discouraging physical activity and creating dependency on automobile travel. Conversely, zoning requirements for sidewalks, green space, school siting, compact mixed use development, and interconnected street grids can promote health both by encouraging physical activity and by building social capital (Frumkin, Frank, and Jackson, 2004; Malizia, 2005).

Implicit environmental health policies may be at least as influential as explicit policies that directly target health outcomes. Just as the relationship between environment and health is a broad topic, so too is the range of policies that can influence the conditions around us and our health (Table 30.1).

Even well-intended policies may not work or may have unintended consequences. The widespread use of chemical pesticides and the draining of wetlands for agriculture and vector control in the years following World War II were seen at the time as major advances for public health, nutrition, and quality of life. Over time, however, these actions had detrimental consequences for the functioning of ecological systems and uncertain effects on public health and even safety (resulting in, for example, increased pesticide resistance in harmful insects and flooding

TABLE 30.1   Examples of Explicit and Implicit
Environmental Health Policies

Explicit Environmental Health Policies	Implicit Environmental Health Policies
Clean air standards	Residential and commercial zoning (for example, housing density, school locations, extension of water and sewer utilities, mixed use)
Water quality standards	
Drinking-water standards	
Solid waste collection and disposal	Building codes
Restaurant sanitation	Transportation planning and construction
Toxic chemical controls	Energy production
Pesticide regulation	Water quantity (for example, wells and reservoirs)
	Land conservation
	International trade and tariffs
	Agricultural commodity support pricing
	Land conservation and recreation

caused by wetland destruction and loss of absorptive capacity). On the one hand our inability to foresee all ends argues for prudence in adopting changes in policy. On the other hand an excess of prudence can also delay needed change. Balancing these imperatives is the most difficult judgment faced by those with policy responsibilities.

Policy Approaches to Environmental Health

There is no single policy approach to protecting environmental health. Policy interventions take many forms, but most fall into one of six categories. **Ambient standards** limit the concentration of environmentally harmful agents in air, water, or soil. **Emission standards**, or **effluent standards** limit the discharges from sources of pollution. **Technology standards** specify the use of a particular engineering design for a piece of equipment (specifying, for example, that landfills be lined with clay and plastic liners to prevent leakage). **Product standards** specify the permissible materials content of a given item. **Work practice standards** describe specific procedures that must be followed to limit releases of material (such as asbestos during demolition projects) or to reduce exposure (in occupational settings, for instance). **Exposure standards** are used when individual dosimeters (such as radiation badges) can measure with precision just how much contamination an individual is exposed to.

The choice of policy intervention type to use depends on circumstances, such as whether one can accurately measure levels of contamination in the environment or what the scale is of the desired outcome. For this reason, many efforts to protect environmental health use a combination of interventions. Recent years have also seen expanded use of market-based approaches, for example, allowing trading of emission rights (and varying emission standards) to meet an overall target for total loadings of sulfur emissions that contribute to acid rain. As new technologies such as biomonitoring develop, they will open new pathways for innovative tools and strategies to protect environmental health.

Science and Policy

Environmental health policy decisions are sometimes criticized as being driven by factors other than science. For example, in March 2008, the EPA lowered the National Ambient Air Quality Standard for ozone from 80 parts per billion (ppb) for eight-hour average exposures to 75 ppb. However, the EPA's Clean Air Act Scientific Advisory Committee had recommended that the standard be set at 70 ppb. The chair of the U.S. Senate Environment and Public Works Committee blasted EPA's decision, saying that the "administration would have us replace clean air standards driven by science with standards based on the interests of polluters." Another senator said that in contrast to EPA's decision, "standards must continue to be based solely on rigorous scientific study and our understanding of air pollution's impacts on our health and environment" (Boyle, 2008).

These criticisms assume that science can give unambiguous answers to questions such as what level of air pollution is "safe." The difficulty is that many factors enter into such determinations. For example the Clean Air Act states that the EPA administrator shall base air quality standards for a pollutant on "the latest scientific knowledge useful in indicating the kind and extent of all identifiable effects on public health or welfare which may be expected from the presence of such pollutant in the ambient air" (*U.S. Code*, 42, §S 7408 (a)(2)). Using this knowledge, the administrator is to set a standard, "allowing an adequate margin of safety" and "requisite to protect the public health" (*U.S. Code*, 42, §S 7409 (b)(1)). This leaves open such questions as these:

- What are "identifiable effects"? Do transient or reversible effects (such as a short-term cough) qualify?
- Individuals respond differently to the same level of air pollution, so whose health sets the standard for "public health"? Does this mean the most sensitive member of any subgroup of the population sets the standard? If not, how should this concept be understood?
- How can a "margin of safety" be properly defined?

Additional questions present themselves over how air quality is to be measured, how long an exposure to air pollution is too long, and what chemicals are the best indicators of what we think of as air pollution. Science has much to say about each of these questions; yet policy judgments are embedded in each of them. The most important aspects of the scientific method are a commitment to transparency in assumptions, rigor in methods, reliance on evidence, and willingness to subject judgments to scrutiny and criticism.

Few disagree that science, understood as knowledge obtained through the use of the scientific method, should inform environmental health policy. However, many considerations beyond scientific knowledge contribute to policy development. With issues such as equity, politics, economics, cultural and religious traditions to be considered, the list can be endless. Science by itself rarely determines environmental health policy.

THE INSTITUTIONAL FRAMEWORK

Although not unique among democratic societies, the federal structure established by the U.S. Constitution is complex. Even the term *federal government* can be confusing, but here it refers to the national government of the United States.

States are especially important in the American governmental structure. The tenth amendment to the Constitution reserves powers not delegated to the federal government to the states, or to the people. Of special note is that police powers are reserved to the states and, with these powers, the authority to govern many aspects of everyday behavior affecting environmental public health. State constitutions

EXHIBIT 30.1
Summary of Major Environmental Statutes

Clean Air Act (CAA) (Enacted 1963; Amended 1965, 1967, 1970, 1977, 1990)

The Clean Air Act (CAA) is the comprehensive federal law that regulates air emissions from stationary and mobile sources; the 1970 amendments dramatically increased the federal role in air pollution control. Among other things, this law authorizes the EPA to establish National Ambient Air Quality Standards (NAAQS) to protect public health can give state governments more powers than the U.S. Constitution gives to the federal government, for example, power over land use and water ownership and allocations.

Federal jurisdiction in environmental public health protection derives from Article I, section 8, of the U.S. Constitution, which gives Congress the authority to regulate commerce among the states. The U.S. Supreme Court has interpreted this "commerce clause" broadly, and it is the underpinning for the nation's environmental laws (Ashford and Caldart, 2008, pp. 245–247).

In the United States, the legislative, executive, and judicial branches of government all contribute to defining environmental health policy. Although there are many influences on environmental policy beyond the institutions of government, no understanding of policy can ignore the critical role that these institutions play. The following discussion draws on federal examples, but similar processes play out in the states.

Legislative Branch

The legislative branch influences environmental health policy largely through the passage of legislation and the actions of congressional committees.

Legislation   The years between 1970 and 1990 witnessed an outpouring of federal environmental law that dramatically increased the role of the federal government. In those years, Congress and its committees were heavily involved in the drafting and debating of environmental legislation (see the list in Exhibit 30.1; for more information about each law see EPA, 2009b). Following the 1990 Clean Air Act amendments the pace of new legislation slowed. However, Congress is capable of influencing policy in many ways other than passing laws.

and welfare, to regulate emissions of air pollutants from stationary and mobile sources of air pollution, to require permits for major sources of air pollution, to conduct research, and to support state and local air pollution control programs.

Clean Water Act (CWA) (Enacted 1948; Amended 1972, 1977, 1987)

The Clean Water Act (CWA) regulates discharges of pollutants into the waters of the United States; the 1972 amendments established a regulatory and financial assistance program far beyond previous law. Under the CWA, the EPA sets wastewater standards for industry and water quality standards for surface waters, requires permits for discharges to surface waters and (with the Army Corps of Engineers) discharges into wetlands, provides funding to state and local water pollution control agencies, and offers financial assistance for constructing wastewater treatment systems.

Comprehensive Environmental Response, Compensation, and Liability Act (CERCLA, or Superfund) (Enacted 1980; Amended 1986, 2002)

CERCLA provides a federal "superfund" to clean up uncontrolled or abandoned hazardous waste sites as well as spills and other releases of pollutants and contaminants into the environment. The EPA can seek out and enforce this law against parties responsible for any release, and it can clean up orphan sites when responsible parties cannot be found or fail to act. It can also recover costs from financially viable individuals and companies once a response action has been completed. This statute also created the Agency for Toxic Substances and Disease Registry in the U.S. Department of Health and Human Services.

Federal Insecticide, Fungicide, and Rodenticide Act (FIFRA) (Enacted 1947; Amended 1972, 1996)

FIFRA requires that all pesticides distributed or sold in the United States be registered (licensed) by the EPA. Before the EPA may register a pesticide under FIFRA, the applicant must show, among other things, that using the pesticide according to specifications "will not generally cause unreasonable adverse effects on the environment," defined as any unreasonable risk to humans or the environment, taking into account the economic, social, and environmental costs and benefits of the pesticide and any dietary risk from pesticide residues on any food inconsistent with the Federal Food, Drug, and Cosmetic Act.

National Environmental Policy Act (NEPA) (Enacted 1969)

NEPA establishes the broad national framework for protecting our environment. It requires agencies to evaluate the impact of any major federal action with significant potential environmental effects. Examples include federal activities involving airports, buildings, military complexes, highways, and parkland purchases. Federal agencies must prepare *environmental assessments* (EAs) or *environmental impact statements* (EISs), or sometimes both, to comply with NEPA requirements.

Oil Pollution Act (OPA) (Enacted 1990)

OPA created a trust fund, financed by a tax on oil, to clean up oil spills when the responsible party is incapable of doing so or unwilling to do so. It requires oil storage facilities and vessels to tell the federal government how they will respond to large discharges. The EPA and the Coast Guard share responsibility under OPA; EPA regulates aboveground storage facilities and the Coast Guard regulates oil tankers.

Resource Conservation and Recovery Act (RCRA) (Enacted 1976; Amended 1984)

RCRA gives the EPA the authority to control the generation, transportation, treatment, storage, and disposal of hazardous waste, and sets forth a framework for the management by state and local governments of nonhazardous solid wastes. This framework includes a manifest system for tracking off-site transport and disposal of hazardous waste and regulates on-site waste treatment and disposal. The 1984 amendments to RCRA promoted waste minimization and required the phasing out of land disposal (for example, in landfills or injection wells) of hazardous waste as well as corrective action for releases. The amendments also increased EPA's enforcement authority, tightened hazardous waste management standards, and established a comprehensive program to address environmental problems that could result from underground tanks used to store petroleum and other hazardous substances.

Safe Drinking Water Act (SDWA) (Enacted 1974; Amended 1996)

The SDWA protects the quality of drinking water in the United States by addressing all waters actually or potentially designed for drinking use, whether from aboveground or underground sources. The Act authorizes the EPA to establish minimum standards to protect tap water and requires all owners or operators of public water systems to comply with these primary (health-related) standards. The 1996 amendments require the EPA to consider a detailed risk and cost assessment and the best available peer-reviewed science when developing these standards. State governments, which can be approved to implement these rules for the EPA, also encourage attainment of secondary standards (nuisance related). The EPA also establishes minimum standards for state programs to protect underground sources of drinking water from endangerment by underground injection of fluids, and provides financial assistance to states in funding drinking-water supply systems.

Small Business Liability Relief and Brownfields Revitalization Act (Enacted 2002)

This statute codified and expanded the EPA's brownfields program by authorizing funding for assessment and cleanup of contaminated properties. It also exempted some owners and contributors from Superfund liability and authorized funding for state response programs.

Toxic Substances Control Act (TSCA) (Enacted 1976)

TSCA gives EPA the authority to track industrial chemicals produced in or imported into the United States. The EPA screens these chemicals and can require reporting or testing of those that may pose an environmental hazard or human health hazard. It can ban the manufacture and importation of chemicals that pose an unreasonable risk. The EPA also tracks new chemicals with either unknown or dangerous characteristics and can control these chemicals as necessary to protect human health and the environment. In general, regulatory programs under TSCA supplement control programs under other federal environmental statutes.

Congressional Committees   Both the U.S. House of Representatives and the U.S. Senate operate through committees with jurisdictions in many areas. In addition to their role in marking up and reporting legislation in their areas, these committees have many tools at their disposal, including requests for information, periodic oversight hearings, investigations, and reports.

Appropriations committees are a special case. Even though both houses of Congress officially frown on using appropriations legislation to modify authorizations (a prerogative jealously guarded by authorizing committees), there are few more effective ways to get the attention of an agency director than to challenge an agency's funding. Moreover, appropriations bills must be approved every year, and thus represent a routine and well-known opportunity to influence policy. This influence takes the form of *earmarks*, through which individual members add funds for issues that benefit their districts or support an issue of particular interest. Earmarks can work both ways; policies or decisions that irritate appropriations committee members can find themselves the subject of targeted cuts in funding.

Committee jurisdictions may change over time based on political developments, and many committees in both chambers have become involved in environmental health policy. For agencies charged with setting policy these overlapping jurisdictions can cause conflict or, at the least, be very time consuming. In 2008, the House of Representatives and the Senate each listed twenty separate committees

Other Statutes Relevant to Environmental Health

- Atomic Energy Act (AEA) (enacted 1946)
- Endangered Species Act (ESA) (enacted 1972)
- Energy Policy Act (EPA) (enacted 2005)
- Federal Food, Drug, and Cosmetic Act (FFDCA) (enacted 1938; many subsequent amendments)
- Marine Protection, Research, and Sanctuaries Act (MPRSA, also known as the Ocean Dumping Act) (enacted 1972, amended 1988)
- Nuclear Waste Policy Act (NWPA) (enacted 1982)
- Pollution Prevention Act (PPA) (enacted 1990)

Executive Orders

The EPA also operates under a large number of Executive Orders (information about them can be found at EPA, 2009b).

Source: Information drawn from EPA, 2009a.

and four joint committees (U.S. House of Representatives, 2009; U.S. Senate, 2009). To cite just one example, of these forty-four committees, seventeen claim jurisdiction over some aspect of the Environmental Protection Agency. Reformers and beleaguered agency heads have made periodic calls to streamline oversight and reduce the number of Congressional committees and overlapping jurisdictions, but neither political party has shown much interest.

Further complicating matters, most full committees establish specialized subcommittees. These subcommittees are especially important in the House of Representatives, as subcommittee chairmanships are a path to leadership for House members, and the larger size of the House leads members to build reputations as experts in specific public policy issues. The House of Representatives has a total of ninety-nine subcommittees, the Senate has sixty-eight, each with access to the tools described earlier. Twenty-nine of these subcommittees claim jurisdiction over EPA.

To enumerate each of the individual subcommittees and its role in environmental health policy would require a book in itself. Historically, the Senate committees with the most influence on environmental health have been Health, Education and Labor; Environment and Public Works; and of course, Appropriations. In the House of Representatives the Appropriations Committee has always been especially influential. Of the oversight or authorizing committees, the most influential has been the Energy and Commerce Committee and its Subcommittee on Health. However, the Science and Technology Committee and the Education and Labor Committee, among others, have also intervened in policy areas, such as the risks from exposure to formaldehyde in travel trailers used for temporary housing following Hurricane Katrina in 2005. On particular issues, almost any committee can find some link to environmental health.

Executive Branch

The executive branch consists of a bewildering array of agencies that influence environmental policy, making its methods of promulgating influence even more diverse than those of Congress. Table 30.2 lists some of these agencies, along with basic facts about each one's history, size, and mission.

Executive branch agencies, whether at the federal, state, or local level, play a tremendously important policy role because they ultimately determine what a policy really is by the way in which it is carried out. The best laws in the world are of little use if no one follows them. Therefore, whether the role of a specific unit of the Executive Branch is to develop the scientific basis for policy or to craft regulations of national, state, or local scope or to enforce particular rules, ultimately any policy will be only as good as the way it is carried out.

Reporting Relationships   Agencies differ widely in their placement within the executive branch. Some, such as the Centers for Disease Control and Prevention (CDC) or the Food and Drug Administration (FDA), are part of cabinet departments, those whose heads are members of the president's cabinet, in this case the Department of Health and Human Services. In contrast, the EPA is the largest independent federal regulatory agency. The EPA administrator is appointed by the president and confirmed by the Senate, and has had cabinet rank in the last several administrations. The EPA has thirteen presidentially appointed, Senate confirmed officials. The CDC, with a comparable budget, has none, although the CDC director serves at the pleasure of the Secretary of Health and Human Services.

Cultural and Professional Backgrounds   Agencies differ in the internal culture and in the professional backgrounds of their employees. For example, the CDC's leadership has historically been drawn from the medical profession. This agency grew out of institutions created to fight infectious diseases, such as malaria, that threatened American armed forces during World War II. Even though the CDC is now a far-reaching public health organization, it retains a strong focus on infectious diseases. However, CDC staff who focus on chronic or other noninfectious diseases or on the impacts of the built environment on health are likely to have somewhat different views of CDC's priorities.

TABLE 30.2 Selected U.S. Federal Agencies Involved in Environmental Health Policy

Agency (departments and independent agencies shown in bold)	Date Established	Annual Staff and Budget, Fiscal Year 2008 (subordinate agency budgets contained in department total)	Mission and Activities
Environmental Protection Agency (EPA)	1970	17,307 full-time equivalents (FTEs) $7.5 billion	Establishes and enforces national standards for clean air, drinking water, wastewater and stormwater; regulates pesticides and toxic chemicals; regulates disposal and cleanup of hazardous waste; assists state environmental agencies; funds water infrastructure; conducts environmental research; leads United States in international environmental agreements.
Department of Health and Human Services (DHHS)	1953: Department of Health, Education and Welfare 1980: DHHS	64,750 FTEs $715.8 billion; $636.9 billion are mandatory outlays, mostly Medicare and Medicaid	Conducts health and social science research, prevents disease, ensures food and drug safety, administers Medicare and Medicaid, develops health information technology; provides financial assistance and services for low-income families, and enhances medical preparedness.
Centers for Disease Control and Prevention (CDC) (includes National Center for Environmental Health)	1946	8,897 FTEs $9.2 billion	Assists state and local health agencies in developing and increasing their ability and capacity to address environmental health problems.
National Institute of Occupational Safety and Health	1970	1,188 FTEs $382 million	As a CDC unit, develops recommendations for occupational safety and health standards, conducts research on worker safety and health, conducts training and employee education, develops information on safe levels of exposure to harmful substances, conducts on-site investigations to determine the toxicity of materials used in workplaces, and funds research by other organizations.

(continued)

TABLE 30.2 (Continued)

Agency (departments and independent agencies shown in bold)	Date Established	Annual Staff and Budget, Fiscal Year 2008 (subordinate agency budgets contained in department total)	Mission and Activities
Agency for Toxic Substances and Disease Registry (ATSDR)	1980	330 FTEs $75 million	Conducts public health assessments and consultations around waste sites and releases of hazardous substances; maintains limited registries of exposed persons; maintains toxicological profiles of hazardous substances; develops and disseminates information, education and training about health impacts of hazardous substances.
Food and Drug Administration (FDA)	1927	10,070 FTEs $2.1 billion	Regulates the nation's blood supply; establishes product standards and develops testing methods for biological products; regulates safety and labeling of cosmetics, foods, and bottled water; approves drugs, regulates drug labeling, and sets drug manufacturing standards; regulates livestock feeds and pet foods; sets radiation safety performance standards.
National Institutes of Health (NIH)	1887: Laboratory of Hygiene 1930: NIH	17,138 FTEs $28.8 billion	Conducts and funds research related to human health.
National Institute of Environmental Health Sciences (NIEHS)	1967	658 FTEs $642.3 million	As an NIH institute, conducts and provides funding for environmental health research.
Department of Agriculture (USDA)	1889	104,682 FTEs $92.8 billion; $67 billion are mandatory payments, mostly food stamps and commodity payments	Provides leadership on food supply, agricultural, natural resource, and related issues.

Agency	Established	FTEs / Budget	Description
Food Safety and Inspection Service (FSIS)	1884: Bureau of Animal Industry 1977: Food Safety and Quality Service 1981: renamed FSIS	9,515 FTEs $937 million	Manages the National Advisory Committee on Meat and Poultry Inspection and the National Advisory Committee on Microbial Criteria for Foods; responsible for quality of the nation's commercial supply of meat, poultry, and egg products, including in-plant inspections.
Animal and Plant Health Inspection Service (APHIS)	1972	7,227 FTEs $1.1 billion	Responsible for ensuring the health and care of animals and plants; monitors plant and animal diseases, including inspection and potential quarantine of imports into the United States; regulates genetically engineered plants and animals; provides expertise to promote safe agricultural trade in plants and animals.
U.S. Forest Service (USFS)	1905	33,180 FTEs $5.8 billion	Manages public lands and national forests for conservation and multiple use; conducts forestry research; performs firefighting; provides financial and technical assistance to state and private organizations.
Department of Transportation (DOT)	1966	55,150 FTEs $63.4 billion, of which $41.2 billion is for highways and $7.8 billion is for transit	Responsible for all federal transportation programs, including highway, rail, air, and marine modes; organized primarily by type of transportation system, with the department serving to provide overall policy guidance and analysis.
Federal Highway Administration (FHWA)	1966	2,820 FTEs $42.2 billion, of which $41.2 billion is highway funding	Formulates policy regarding the national highway system; delivers federal-aid and federal lands highway programs; oversees state transportation planning and improvement programs, including safety and environmental impact analyses.
National Highway Traffic Safety Administration (NHTSA)	1970	635 FTEs $838 million	Conducts vehicle safety research; regulates automobiles; approves state highway safety measures; issues guidelines to states regarding drivers, automobiles, and highways; administers fleet mileage standards; uses financial leverage to encourage states to regulate motorcycle helmet use, drinking age, seat belt use.

(continued)

TABLE 30.2 (Continued)

Agency (departments and independent agencies shown in bold)	Date Established	Annual Staff and Budget, Fiscal Year 2008 (subordinate agency budgets contained in department total)	Mission and Activities
Department of Housing and Urban Development (HUD)	1965	9,428 FTEs $40.4 billion	Supports home ownership, community development, and access to affordable housing free from discrimination; provides grants, loans, subsidies, and other forms of assistance to leverage the private market.
Consumer Product Safety Commission	1972	420 FTEs $80.0 million	Protects the public from unreasonable risks of serious injury or death from consumer products, issues product recalls, develops voluntary standards with industry, issues and enforces mandatory standards or bans on consumer products, conducts research on potential product hazards, educates consumers.
Department of Homeland Security (DHS)	2002	195,579 FTEs $47.3 billion	Prevents terrorist attacks within the United States, reduces vulnerability of the United States to terrorism, minimizes the damage and assists in the recovery from disasters and terrorist attacks within the United States.
Federal Emergency Management Agency (FEMA)	1979	6,917 FTEs $8.0 billion	Reduces the loss of life and property and protects the nation from all hazards, including natural disasters, acts of terrorism, and other man-made disasters, by leading a national emergency management system of preparedness, protection, response, recovery, and mitigation; assists in recovery and rebuilding efforts, including temporary and long-term housing, crisis counseling, unemployment assistance, and legal aid.

Agency	Year	FTEs / Budget	Description
Department of Labor (DOL)	1913	16,142 FTEs $49.1 billion, of which $37.7 billion is in mandatory payments for unemployment insurance and pension benefit guarantees	Enforces fair labor practices; protects occupational health and safety; oversees worker's compensation and security of pension benefits; enforces worker protection and fairness laws, including family and medical leave, whistleblower protection, and right to organize.
Occupational Safety and Health Administration (OSHA)	1970	2,118 FTEs $486.0 million	Sets and enforces mandatory worker protection standards; conducts inspections, outreach, and training; promotes occupational safety through voluntary programs.
Chemical Safety and Hazard Investigation Board (CSB)	1990: authorized by CAA 1993: began operations	43 FTEs $9.3 million	A nonregulatory agency, CSB investigates chemical accidents and makes recommendations to facilities, regulatory agencies, industry groups, and labor unions.

Note: Many other agencies, most notably the Departments of Defense and Energy, affect environmental health. For example, these two departments spend significant funds cleaning up waste sites at military bases or facilities with legacy contamination from the nuclear weapons program.

In contrast, the EPA's political leaders have commonly (though not exclusively) been attorneys. EPA has few medical doctors on its staff but a large number of engineers, environmental scientists, and attorneys. Conflict arose early in the agency's history between engineers who advocated more incremental approaches to environmental protection and attorneys who saw in the new environmental statutes a mandate for "technology-forcing" regulation (Melnick, 1983). Other points of stress within the EPA include the division of the agency into separate units to address air, water, hazardous waste, and toxic chemical pollution, following the somewhat artificial distinctions set up in the enabling statutes (National Academy of Public Administration, 1995).

Legal Authority   Agencies also differ based on their underlying statutory authority. Some have very broad authority and can chart their own course, whereas others receive very specific legislative direction.

As with many agencies established in the 1930s and 1940s, organizations such as the CDC operate under broad authorities (in the CDC's case, the Public Health Service Act). Although these agencies are certainly subject to legislative direction, for example on specific diseases or disabilities, their authorities leave them with significant discretion in defining their mission. Such agencies tend to operate in an assistance mode, providing funding and expert support rather than exerting coercive authority (beyond the not insignificant leverage that comes from the power of the purse). Assistance can go directly to individuals, as in programs administered by the Natural Resources Conservation Service or other branches of the Department of Agriculture; it can go to state and local agencies, the primary customers historically of the CDC; or it can go to universities and academic research centers, historically the clients of the National Institutes of Health.

In the late 1960s, support diminished for broad agency discretion. Some state governments believed that the federal government was too intrusive in state matters under the Constitution. At the same time, public interest groups criticized the relationships that developed between agencies and their clients as being more oriented to their mutual benefit than to the public interest (McConnell, 1966; Lowi, 1969).

Agencies created in the wake of these critiques included the Occupational Safety and Health Administration, the Consumer Product Safety Commission, and the largest and most visible, the EPA. Congress gave these new agencies, and especially the EPA, regulatory and enforcement powers beyond those of traditional public health agencies. However, Congress also gave the new agencies detailed instructions and timetables to follow in implementing these authorities, using new tools of administrative law and of notice and comment rulemaking (Fiorino, 1995, pp. 34–35).

Environment and Health   Both federal and state organizational structures evolved along with the new federal statutes and agencies. When the EPA was formed in 1970, much of the agency came from the Department of Health, Education and Welfare. Prior to 1970, most states relied on their health departments to carry out pollution control efforts (Kotchian, 2005, p. 897). By 2009, only three state environmental agencies—those in Colorado, Kansas, and South Carolina—had *health* in their organizational name. Most states have created environmental agencies with structures either similar to the EPA's or expanded to include natural resource functions.

Judicial Branch

The expansion of federal environmental law also expanded the role of federal courts in setting environmental health policy, to the point where some have argued that the policy choices and even the management of agencies like EPA are essentially driven and determined by the courts (Melnick, 1983, p. 388). Although this view can be overstated (see Conglianese, 1997, pp. 1290–1301), two factors have extended the influence of the courts as actors in the environmental policy arena. First, new laws have contained expanded provisions for citizens to sue in federal court to address both noncompliance by other parties with the provisions of the various laws and failure by the government to meet various mandates contained in these laws. Second, the prescriptive and detailed nature of these laws has provided numerous opportunities for aggrieved parties to sue the federal government.

Federal district courts, courts of appeals, and ultimately the Supreme Court are the final arbiters of federal law. However, the federal courts are only one of the mechanisms available to actors seeking to use the court system to affect policy. States have their own systems of courts and their own laws governing environmental matters, and state courts can be venues for citizens seeking to affect policy. Several different types of court cases can set policy. The most common are tort cases, lawsuits over regulations, and civil or criminal enforcement cases.

Tort Cases   Lawsuits presenting private party claims for redress of injuries or damages resulting from environmental conditions, known as environmental *torts*, generally come under state law and fall within the jurisdiction of state courts. Tort lawsuits in the environmental health area can be difficult, especially in meeting the burden of proof required in such cases (for example, was a particular disease caused by a particular environmental exposure). Nevertheless, such lawsuits can be a powerful and appealing tool for persons who believe they have been injured from exposure to environmental contaminants, if these litigants can overcome barriers to entry such as standing and the cost of filing a case (Ashford and Caldart, 2008, pp. 228–233).

Litigation over Regulations Almost all regulations issued by federal environmental agencies are challenged in the courts. Challenges may be based on arguments that the regulations are inconsistent with the underlying statute or that the statute itself is unconstitutional. In either case the citizen suit provisions described previously and the procedural requirements of the Administrative Procedures Act, the Data Quality Act, and other laws give challengers many opportunities to sue and ready access to the court system. This adds to the burdens of agencies already facing prescriptive statutory deadlines that can overwhelm their capability and resources.

Some environmental statutes, notably the Clean Air Act, require that suits concerning national rules be brought in the D.C. Circuit Court of Appeals, to

---

EXHIBIT 30.2

Timeline: Review of the National Ambient Air Quality Standard (NAAQS) for Ozone

Clean Air Act, section 109(d)(1): "Not later than December 31, 1980, and at five-year intervals thereafter, the Administrator shall complete a thorough review of the criteria published under section 108 and the national ambient air quality standards promulgated under this section and shall make such revisions in such criteria and standards and promulgate such new standards as may be appropriate in accordance with section 108 and subsection (b) of this section. The Administrator may review and revise criteria or promulgate new standards earlier or more frequently than required under this paragraph."

July 1996	EPA publishes air quality criteria document for ozone and related photochemical oxidants.
December 1996	EPA proposes new 8-hour ozone NAAQS.
July 1997	EPA promulgates new 8-hour ozone NAAQS of .08 ppm.
May 1999	D.C. Circuit Court of Appeals, in split opinion, finds section 109(d) of the Clean Air Act gives an unconstitutional delegation of authority to EPA; says .08 standard cannot be enforced.

avoid "forum shopping." In both the federal and state governments, challenges to environmental rules or permits may have to proceed through an administrative process before being heard in court. In either instance, such litigation can last for many years. For example, the Clean Air Act requires the EPA to review the national ambient air quality standards (NAAQS) every five years. But litigation over the ozone NAAQS promulgated by EPA in 1997 lasted until January, 2003. By then, the EPA was already well behind its mandatory five-year review timetable. Environmental groups then sued the EPA in March 2003 to establish a *new* ozone NAAQS, even though the agency had barely implemented the 1997 revision (Exhibit 30.2).

January 2000	EPA petitions U.S. Supreme Court for review of D.C. Circuit decision.
February 2001	Supreme Court unanimously reverses D.C. Circuit; affirms standard; affirms administrator cannot consider cost; remands additional petition issues to D.C. Circuit.
March 2002	D.C. Circuit denies remaining petitions.
January 2003	EPA issues rulemaking establishing final .08 ozone standard.
March 2003	Environmental groups sue EPA to set a new ozone standard based on five-year review requirement in section 109(d).
June 2003	EPA proposes implementation rule for .08 ozone standard.
July 2003	EPA signs consent decree agreeing to timetable for revising the ozone standard.
April 2004	EPA promulgates final phase 1 ozone implementation rule.
March 2005	EPA issues final rule, the Clean Air Interstate Rule, to reduce interstate transport of air pollution.
November 2005	EPA promulgates final phase 2 ozone implementation rule.
March 2006	EPA releases final criteria document for new ozone standard.
December 2006	D.C. Circuit remands the ozone implementation rule to EPA.
July 2007	EPA proposes new ozone standard.
March 2008	EPA promulgates new ozone standard of .075 ppm.
July 2008	D.C. Circuit overturns Clean Air Interstate Rule.

Enforcement Cases   Other cases, brought by citizens or by government agencies and heard in U.S. District Courts around the nation, allege violations and seek to enforce rules or overturn permits in specific cases. Though such cases are less likely to have broad policy impact than litigation involving generally applicable rules, they can influence policy. Violations can be civil actions, but if willful violations of law can be established, federal prosecutors can bring criminal charges against corporations or individuals for environmental violations. (An example is presented in the Perspective concerning the city of Atlanta.)

PERSPECTIVE
City of Atlanta Sewer Consent Agreement

Municipal sewer systems around the United States are often taken for granted by both citizens and civic leaders. Yet the failure to build and maintain adequate wastewater collection and treatment facilities can create severe environmental problems and threaten health among people who come into contact with untreated or partially treated sewage.

Like many other large urban areas, the City of Atlanta has struggled with this issue. Atlanta has over 2,200 miles of sanitary sewers and four large wastewater treatment plants, serving over 1.5 million people. Some of this infrastructure is over 100 years old. Atlanta was the subject of one of the very first federal enforcement actions after the EPA was formed in 1970, but problems persisted, despite significant investments since the Clean Water Act passed in 1972. The oldest part of Atlanta's sewer system consists of combined sewers that carry both sewage and stormwater, and that can overflow during rainstorms. The rapid growth of Atlanta in the last part of the twentieth century has added additional stress to an aging system.

In 1995, an environmental organization, the Upper Chattahoochee Riverkeeper, filed a citizen suit in U.S. District Court against the City of Atlanta for violations of the Clean Water Act. Both the EPA and the Georgia Environmental Protection Division eventually joined this lawsuit. The lawsuit culminated in two federal consent agreements signed by the city and federal and state governments in 1998 and 1999. The consent agreements imposed a fine on the city, created requirements for removal of trash from urban streams and for the purchase of greenways, and established a schedule for the city to undertake a massive rehabilitation of the city's sewer system, build tighter controls on overflows from combined sewers, and add additional treatment capacity. This work will cost about $3 billion and is expected to be completed in 2012. In order to fund the work, the City of Atlanta substantially raised its water utility rates and instituted a special purpose local option sales tax. (For more information see Clean Water Atlanta, n.d.)

The Courts and Agency Discretion   Perhaps the biggest influence of courts on policy is whether they grant discretion to administrative agencies in interpreting ambiguous law. No matter how carefully Congress writes a law or an agency crafts regulations, it is impossible to eliminate all such ambiguities. The Clean Air Act vividly illustrates this point. One of the most frequently cited decisions in American administrative law, derived in a Clean Air Act case, is *Chevron* v. *NRDC* (467 U.S. 837 [1984]). In this case the U.S. Supreme Court held that if a statute was ambiguous, and if the agency's interpretation was reasonable, then the courts should defer to the agency's interpretation. But more recent court decisions have criticized the EPA for taking too much latitude in interpreting this Act. The D.C. Circuit Court of Appeals has refused to defer to the EPA in several major cases: for example, in *New Jersey* v. *EPA*, Case No. 05-1097 (D.C. Cir. Feb. 8, 2008), it overturned the EPA's mercury rule; in *North Carolina* v. *EPA*, Case No. 05-1244 (D.C. Cir. July 11, 2008), it overturned the Clean Air Interstate Rule; and in *New York* v. *EPA*, Case No. 03-1380 (D.C. Circuit, March 17, 2006), it vacated the EPA's regulation on excluding certain types of repair from scrutiny for tighter pollution controls and described the EPA's approach as "a Humpty-Dumpty world." Even the Supreme Court itself, in the landmark case of *Massachusetts* v. *EPA* (549 U.S. 497 [2007]), declined to defer to the agency over the question of whether greenhouse gases were "air pollutants" subject to regulation under the Clean Air Act.

Other Influences on Environmental Health Policy

As important as governments are in shaping environmental health policy, governments depend on outside parties for support. Legislators depend upon interest groups for contributions and for favorable publicity. Executive branch agencies seek allies who will advocate on behalf of their objectives, support their requests for funding, or at least not sue in response to an adverse decision. Even the courts, not usually thought of as subject to outside influence, do not operate in a vacuum. Peer pressure can have an effect. At a minimum, few district court judges want the reputation of having their opinions always overturned on appeal, not unlike scientists who would hope to avoid unfavorable peer reviews of their work.

Disasters can affect policy dramatically. As noted in the accompanying example, the accidental release in 1984 of a large quantity of the chemical methyl isocyanate from a Union Carbide facility in Bhopal, India, led directly to the creation of a national system for publicly reporting the release of hazardous substances. The burning Cuyahoga River in Cleveland, Ohio, became a symbol of the need for passage of the 1972 Clean Water Act, and the discovery of a large quantity of chemical waste at Love Canal in upstate New York promoted the passage of the Comprehensive Environmental Response, Compensation and Liability Act of 1980, usually known as Superfund (Landy, Roberts, and Thomas, 1990). Advocates for policy change can and do seize on such events to put public pressure on legislative and executive actors.

PERSPECTIVE
Bhopal

On December 3, 1984, a Union Carbide pesticide manufacturing plant in the center of Bhopal, India released a cloud of toxic gas into the surrounding neighborhood. Union Carbide identified the gas as forty metric tons of methyl isocyanate (MIC) (Bhopal Information Center, n.d.), though it may have included other chemicals as well (Eckerman, 2005).

The plant was situated in a densely populated, lower-income neighborhood. Casualty estimates range from 3,800 to 20,000 individuals killed, over 120,000 permanently injured, and as many as 520,000 exposed (Eckerman, 2005). Those living near the plant at the time of the release have been subject to significantly increased morbidity and mortality in subsequent years (Dhara and Dhara, 2002; Dhara, Dhara, Acquilla, and Cullinan, 2002). High-level MIC exposure may cause severe damage to the eyes, skin, and respiratory system and also death. At lower levels, the precise effects of MIC are not known, though it has been demonstrated to be an acute irritant (EPA, 2000). Long-term effects include persistent irritation and significant neurological and reproductive effects.

A water leak in the MIC storage tank caused the release. The resulting chemical reaction produced MIC gas, which could not be controlled by the plant's safety systems because they were poorly maintained, inadequate, or not in use (Dhara, Dhara, Acquilla, and Cullinan, 2002; Eckerman, 2005).

Following the incident, Union Carbide Corporation (UCC) sought to minimize its responsibility for the release (Dinham and Sarangi, 2002). In 1989, UCC settled with the Indian government for $470 million. (According to one analysis, by

ENVIRONMENTAL HEALTH POLICY ACTORS

Governments set the field of play and the rules for debate on environmental health policy choices, but energy comes from actors on the field. Given the broad scope of environmental health, it is hardly surprising that an enormous array of actors seeks to influence policy in this area.

Government Associations

Governmental agencies themselves are principal actors. For example, state and local governments have themselves formed associations for the purpose of advancing

Broughton (2005), had Bhopal victims received compensation comparable to that received by U.S. asbestos victims, UCC would have owed over $10 billion.) However, to date little funding has reached the victims themselves, and most health effects research in Bhopal has come from private organizations and initiatives (Acquilla and others, 2005). Survivors pursued legal action against UCC in the U.S. court system, resulting in a November 2001 ruling, in the U.S. Second Circuit Court of Appeals, affirming that the corporation is responsible for environmental damages (Dinham and Sarangi,. 2002). The plant site itself remains abandoned; on March 19, 2008, an Indian court issued orders for the government to initiate the cleanup of forty metric tons of chemical residues that had remained at the plant since 1984 ("40 Tonnes of Chemical Residues Removed from Bhopal Plant," 2008). As of 2009, criminal litigation continues in India against Dow Chemical, which bought UCC in September 2001 (Kripalani, 2008).

The Bhopal tragedy left an international legacy in public health and environmental policy. In the United States the Bhopal release and a subsequent chemical release from a Union Carbide facility in Kanawha, West Virginia, led Congress in 1986 to pass the Emergency Planning and Community Right-to-Know Act (EPCRA). This law, also known as Title III, required industrial facilities to report their releases of hazardous chemicals, plan for chemical emergencies, and inform local emergency planners and responders about chemicals these facilities used that might affect their communities. In Europe, the chemical release at Bhopal and earlier incidents at Flixborough, U.K., and Seveso, Italy, led the European Union to establish a Major Accident Hazards Bureau to analyze major industrial accidents and distribute information about lessons learned and risk prevention.

perceived common state interests in their interactions on environmental policy. Groups such as the Environmental Commissioners of the States and similar associations of state and local air, water, and waste officials not only gain influence through collective action but also give federal agencies a venue for exploring ideas and soliciting support for policy objectives.

Private Sector Associations

Private companies and organizations play a strong role in environmental health policy decisions, both individually and as members of trade associations to advance common interests. Business organizations such as the American

Chemistry Council, the American Petroleum Institute, the U.S. Chamber of Commerce, the American Motor Vehicle Manufacturers Association, the Edison Electric Institute, and the American Forest and Paper Association, to name just a few, engage vigorously with both Congress and executive branch agencies, up to and including lobbying and litigation involving regulations that they support or oppose. Although some businesses were initially slow to recognize the growth and enduring public support for environmental protection as it emerged in the 1960s and early 1970s, concern for environmental policy is now a mainstream (and a bottom-line) matter for virtually every business.

Nongovernmental Organizations

Nongovernmental organizations, or NGOs, also play an influential role. Even though few NGOs can match the resources available to large corporations, the citizen suit provisions of federal environmental law have been a powerful source of influence for many of them. More recently, NGOs have been aligning themselves in litigation with like-minded states; all of the recent Clean Air Act rule cases cited earlier, though styled as state-led cases, proceeded with substantial assistance from NGOs.

Active national environmental NGOs include the Natural Resources Defense Council, Sierra Club, Environmental Defense Fund, National Audubon Society, National Wildlife Federation, and League of Conservation Voters. As important as these national organizations are, however, countless groups have arisen and continue to arise in order to engage at the local level on issues important to their communities, such as a waste site or particular industrial facility. Community-based groups have been especially important in the environmental justice movement, and national environmental groups have recognized the need to reach out to such organizations (Sirianni and Friedlander, 2001; also see Chapter Eight).

Relationships among government, private firms and NGOs need not always be adversarial. Private companies can be sources of technical expertise as well as funding, and recent years have seen the emergence of partnerships between businesses and outside groups, as well as government, on environmental health matters of common concern. For example, the Environmental Defense Fund has entered into a partnership with Wal-Mart to "inform and influence Wal-Mart's sustainability goals and motivate change in the company, its supply chain and its customers to measurably reduce environmental impacts" (Environmental Defense Fund, 2009). Businesses and environmental groups have formed a coalition, the United States Climate Action Partnership, "to call on the federal government to quickly enact strong national legislation to require significant reductions of greenhouse gas emissions" (United States Climate Action Partnership, 2009). At the local level, groups such as the Civic Practices Network (CPN) seek "good neighbor agreements" with local industrial facilities as a means of promoting policy change. Although not all such relationships are smooth or sustainable in the long run, they provide another venue for groups whose interests might appear different to seek common ground (Civic Practices Network, n.d.).

Public Health Actors

Actors in environmental policy are being joined by others in the public health field. Although public health has been a key component of environmental protection, traditional public health agencies (as noted earlier) have felt somewhat left out by the explosive growth of environmental regulatory statutes and organizations. Organizations such as the American Public Health Association, Association of State and Territorial Health Officials, National Association of City and County Health Officials, and National Environmental Health Association have not engaged as actively in most environmental regulatory matters as the organizations already discussed here. At the same time, there is a growing desire, as one official put it, to see "well-developed environmental health and environmental protection functions reunified, especially at the local level" (Blake, 2008, p. 31). As convergence grows among such issues as community health, urban design and land use, energy consumption, rational transportation systems, and climate change, organizations that historically operated in different spheres may find themselves working together on related issues, living the ecological observation that everything is related to everything else.

INTERESTS, TOOLS, AND "GARBAGE CAN" POLICY

A famous public administration maxim is "Where you stand depends on where you sit" (Miles, 1978, p. 399). Although the maxim is about the behavior of government officials, it also applies more generally. In predicting the behavior of actors in environmental health policy areas, it is important to know where their interests lie.

That said, policy seldom results from the rational adjudication of interests by different actors. In virtually any policy arena, information can be unclear, ambiguous, or incomplete; short-term and long-term concerns collide with each other; time constraints and routine organizational processes may dictate actions that no one really wants; and actors may not fully understand where their interests lie. Not for nothing is public policy compared with making sausage! Far from policy processes forming a rational structure, students of these processes can describe them as "organized anarchy" or, more colorfully, as a "garbage can model" (Fiorino, 1995, pp. 15–16).

Tools of Policy Influence

Some of the tools that organizations use to participate in the policy process are

- Information
- Expertise
- Advocacy and lobbying
- Human capital
- Financial capital
- Networked alliances
- Public communication
- Legal authority
- Moral authority
- Formal processes

Different groups use different tools, depending on their own skill mix, strategic alignment, and base of support, and the same group may use different tools over time, depending on the needs of each situation. For instance, litigation can be effective, but it can also be costly. Moreover, it runs the risk of being a zero-sum game. A group like the Natural Resources Defense Council, historically a litigator, may rely on its expertise to participate actively in an agency's rulemaking, attempting to negotiate a satisfactory outcome and resorting to litigation only if talks break down. This was the case in a 2004 rulemaking to establish permissible levels of sulfur, a contaminant, in diesel fuel. The EPA conducted an extensive negotiation that led to a rule acceptable to the oil industry, the auto industry, NRDC, and state and local air pollution control agencies.

Other examples abound. Among NGOs, the League of Conservation Voters publishes a "Dirty Dozen" list of congressional representatives and senators that is based on environmental voting records in Congress. Greenpeace is noted for its use of oceangoing vessels to interfere with oceangoing whaling ships and for other nonviolent, high-profile efforts that attract media attention. Some groups will hold demonstrations; a few have adopted civil disobedience strategies, holding sit-ins on corporate lands. On some issues, such as global warming, national environmental groups may expand their strategies to include an emphasis on individual action as well as their traditional push for national legislation (Taylor, 2008).

For their part, private sector interests may conduct advertising campaigns aimed at the public or at politicians, contribute to political supporters, conduct extensive surveys and technical studies on matters of concern to them, set up support organizations of their own, and encourage their customers and employees to serve as advocates. This last tactic is now far easier. In days past, groups would demonstrate their displeasure with an official by organizing telephone and letter-writing campaigns. Now, groups can almost instantly react to developments through the Internet, bombarding officials (and sometimes disrupting organizations) with electronic communications. Like environmental groups, industries will litigate if they believe this to be in their interest, an interest that may include simply delaying high-cost investments to protect the time value of money.

The personal touch still matters, however. Both business groups and nongovernmental organizations work to identify and to acquaint themselves with elected and appointed policymakers and officials, gaining information about these individuals' needs and concerns.

The point is simply that there are many tools to influence policy. The choice of tools is always a decision, resources are always limited, and every participant in the policy process has to select which tools to use given their time, cost, and expected value in a particular situation. Sometimes groups choose well and sometimes poorly; sometimes rational factors govern such choices, and sometimes not. The nonlinear, constant, incremental application of all of these tools and techniques gives the garbage can model of policy development its power as an analogy. The wise response of policy officials to this swirl of circumstances is rightly described as a craft (Sparrow, 2000).

Policy Implementation and Feedback

Rational theories of organizations hold that once policy goals are established, all that is left is to decide how the goals are to be achieved, allocate resources to achieve them, apply the resources, and monitor the results. However, as Dan Fiorino has noted, "It takes very little experience in large organizations to realize that they do not work in this way" (Fiorino, 1995, p. 13).

Environmental health agencies can find themselves "bewildered by the number of conflicting priorities, statutory deadlines, court-imposed requirements, and public participation needs," as the National Academy of Public Administration described the EPA in 1995 (p. 40). To deal with this bewilderment, many agencies have worked to adopt systems to establish both more explicit priorities and better management and measurement systems to track performance and enable corrections to be made. In the federal government, this trend has been accelerated by the 1993 Government Performance and Results Act (GPRA) and the use of public scorecards such as the President's Management Agenda. In addition to the strategic plans and annual reports required by GPRA, the EPA,

PERSPECTIVE
PCB Contamination in Anniston, Alabama

The Solutia Inc. (formerly Monsanto) chemical plant sits on a seventy-acre lot near downtown Anniston, Alabama. Between 1929 and 1971, Monsanto produced polychlorinated biphenyls (PCBs) at the plant and dumped millions of tons of PCB-laden waste into local landfills and a drainage ditch that led to nearby Snow and Choccolocco Creeks.

PCBs were used as industrial coolants in transformers and capacitors as well as in flame retardants, sealants, paints, and adhesives. PCBs are highly toxic. As early as 1937, researchers reported liver damage from low-level PCB exposure, and by the 1940s these chemicals had been linked to cancer in animals. Other health effects include skin lesions, anemia, and immune and endocrine abnormalities. The EPA banned the manufacture of PCBs in 1979, and they have been phased out of most existing uses.

In 1970, Food and Drug Administration samplers found PCB-contaminated fish in Choccolocco Creek and observed that Snow Creek was entirely devoid of aquatic life. In 1993 a deformed bass was caught in Choccolocco Creek by a local resident. In response to litigation the facility purchased properties in the area surrounding the plant, and the Alabama Department of Environmental Management regulated the facility under the Resources Conservation and Recovery Act. However, in response to continued complaints by residents and environmental justice groups, in 1999 the U.S. Environmental Protection Agency began additional sampling for PCBs in Anniston. Soil sampling revealed high levels of PCBs in additional properties, and the EPA began

for example, has developed a quarterly management report to track progress against key management objectives (for a report example, see EPA, 2008). The Department of Health and Human Services, the CDC, and other agencies have adopted similar systems, sometimes referred to as *dashboards*.

These management systems can be somewhat unsatisfying in that they often rely on measures of organizational process, when the more satisfying measures would be of environmental and health outcomes. Both the EPA and CDC have embraced efforts to do the latter. The CDC publishes a national report on health statistics and is now on the fourth cycle of a biomonitoring report describing national average levels of hundreds of chemicals in body fluids. In May 2008, the EPA released its second *Report on the Environment*, a collection of national indicators of environmental quality.

This kind of tracking is important for policy. Air quality data on concentrations of ozone and fine particles made these two pollutants higher priority concerns to pursue a stronger course of action. In the meantime, members of the community brought additional private lawsuits against Monsanto, which by then had spun off the facility as part of a new company, Solutia Inc.

On March 25, 2002, EPA and Solutia agreed to a federal consent decree under which the agency would not list the Anniston site on the National Priority List (NPL) of Superfund sites if the company met a number of conditions, including that Solutia provide reimbursement for cleanup costs, begin a remedial investigation/feasibility study (RI/FS) within six months, and pay $3.2 million over twelve years to the community. Some citizen groups felt that the consent decree allowed Solutia to adhere to a less stringent cleanup requirement than a NPL listing would have mandated, and others felt that the agreement would give Solutia increased leverage in the ongoing private party litigation or that the payments to the community were insufficient. Litigants engaged in extensive outreach to national news media, receiving attention in the *New York Times* and the *Washington Post,* from national news organizations, and on the *60 Minutes* television show, and triggering a hearing by a Senate appropriations subcommittee of which Senator Richard Shelby of Alabama was a member.

The litigants succeeded in having a federal district judge delay accepting the consent decree between EPA and Solutia until after a further hearing. Eventually the judge facilitated a settlement in which the consent decree was entered, but only after a separate $600 million cash settlement was reached in the private party litigation between members of the community and Monsanto and Solutia.

By 2009, Solutia had completed cleanup on 500 residential properties and was conducting ongoing sampling. The Anniston plant continues to operate, producing polyphenyl compounds.

for the EPA and have allowed evaluation of whether current strategies are making progress in reducing air pollution. Debates on appropriate climate change policies are driven by information about changing atmospheric levels of greenhouse gases and shifts in global temperature. Surveillance to collect information about disease predictors and incidence is one of the critical tools of public health protection and can determine where and how to intervene to protect public health.

A full discussion of this topic is beyond the scope of this chapter. The point here is simply the importance of establishing feedback loops between policy decisions and their consequences. The best way to do this is to ask, at the beginning of policy formation, some simple questions:

- If this policy succeeded, how would we know?
- By when?
- Who would tell us?

If these questions can be answered, then it is likely that the policy in question has some hope of being an actual *policy*, something that affects behavior. If they cannot, that suggests that either more information would have to be collected to tell whether the policy was having the desired effect or that (more likely) policy objectives need clarification. When policy objectives are unclear, having more information about events in relation to the policy will not solve the problem; all it will do is to create, in the words of one observer, "dashboards as data dumps." In creating effective policy, too much information can be as damaging as not enough (Behn, 2008).

THE FUTURE: POLICY BY NETWORK

This chapter has made much of the formal processes and institutions that shape policy. It is perhaps fitting, therefore, to close by noting the importance of the informal networks that can frame if not always direct policy.

Networks have diverse origins (Goldsmith and Eggers, 2004). To give just a few examples: some are professional networks, of people with a common disciplinary background or specialty. Some result from common educational and training experiences or personal affinities. Others are oriented around issues, all the way from a neighborhood waste site to global climate change. Still others may result from common past experiences, for example, alumni of governmental agencies who, though now in private practice, retain connections to other past and present government officials. Among scientists, those with common research interests may form such networks. Conferences and workshops provide venues for the exchanging of information and reinforcing of personal ties among network members.

Such networks are growing in importance due to the immediacy of the Internet and electronic communications, which make it far easier to establish and maintain such networks and recruit new members. The importance of associations in American life dates from the founding of the republic, but it is now easier than ever to establish and maintain such groups (Friedman, 2007; Gladwell, 2002).

This does not mean that institutions are or will become irrelevant. Institutions provide structure and process for the operations of government. To the extent that we invoke government's coercive power to protect health (through quarantines, stop sale orders, vaccinations, mandatory evacuations, or enforcement against polluters, for example), institutions will be the means of exercising this power. Without the structure provided by institutions we have no assurance that this power will not be exercised arbitrarily or capriciously. At their best, institutions provide both accountability and transparency for policy choices: we should know who is responsible for making such choices, and why they did so. For all of their difficulties, institutions are the key to a free society.

Still, the growth of networks will challenge institutions, especially as networks decentralize control of communications and can respond more quickly than any institution. The full impact of this new "flat" world is unfolding before our eyes. Creative policy entrepreneurs can use these networks to achieve great good, disseminating vital information that might otherwise remain unknown and that citizens can use to empower their own policy choices. Private groups can get ahead of institutions, sharing information in ways that promote and enhance environmental health.

Experience to date with the Internet tells us, sadly, that the opposite possibility also exists. Networks can become the vehicle by which misinformation and poor science become widespread, at a minimum raising anxieties and pressure for policy choices that may not be in the long-term interest of environmental and public health. Promoting reflection, education, and understanding in an era of instant communications may be the greatest challenge facing future environmental health policy.

SUMMARY

Environmental health is shaped by a wide range of policies, including statutory law, common law, and regulations, at the federal, state, and local level. Some policies explicitly target environmental health, but others that do not—in transportation, agriculture, zoning, the environment itself, and other arenas—may still have profound health consequences. Federal environmental law grew rapidly in scope and complexity between 1970 and 1990 and provides the foundation for many, though not all, environmental health policies. The institutions that administer laws at all levels of government have many tools to influence environmental health policy; examples include ambient standards that limit the concentration of contaminants in air, water, or soil, emission standards that limit discharges from sources of pollution, and technology standards that specify a procedure or piece of equipment. Other tools, which may be used by government or private parties, range from information to litigation. An important issue is the extent to which such policies incorporate and reflect science; other factors invariably play a role as well. Many actors shape environmental health policy, including all three branches of the federal government, state and local governments, and civil society. Understanding these actors and their motivations helps to explain particular policy choices.

KEY TERMS

ambient standards	exposure standards	technology standards
common law	product standards	work practice standards
effluent standards	regulations	
emission standards	statutory law	

DISCUSSION QUESTIONS

1. How much scientific certainty would you need to support a change in a law or a regulation affecting environmental health? What criteria would you use in making such a judgment?

2. What policy changes today would likely produce the greatest environmental public health improvements? Why? Who would be the most important actors in bringing about such changes?

3. How important is it to set explicit regulatory limits for exposure to substances where there are no clear thresholds for health effects? What criteria would you use to set such limits?

4. When are national regulatory solutions appropriate for environmental health problems?

5. What role should scientists play in setting environmental health policy?

REFERENCES

"40 Tonnes of Chemical Residues Removed from Bhopal Plant." *Times of India.* http://timesofindia. indiatimes.com/Pollution/40_tonnes_of_chemical_residues_removed_from_Bhopal_plant/articleshow/3187249.cms, July 2, 2008.

Acquilla, S., and others. "Aftermath of the World's Worst Chemical Disaster: Bhopal, December 1984." *Journal of Loss Prevention in the Process Industries,* 2005, *18,* 268–273.

Ashford, N. A., and Caldart, C. C. *Environmental Law, Policy and Economics: Reclaiming the Environmental Agenda.* Cambridge, Mass.: MIT Press, 2008.

Behn, R. D. "Dashboards as Data Dumps." *Bob Behn's Public Management Report.* http://www.ksg.harvard.edu/TheBehnReport, July 2008.

Bhopal Information Center. "Incident Response and Settlement." http://www.bhopal.com/irs.htm, n.d.

Blake, R. "Remarriage of Environmental Health and Environmental Protection." *Journal of Environmental Health,* 2008, *70*(8), 30–31.

Boyle, K. "EPA's Clean Air Act Proposal Greeted with Jeers." *Energy and Environment Daily*. http://www.eenews.net/EEDaily/print/2008/03/13/1, Mar. 13, 2008.

Broughton, E. "The Bhopal Disaster and Its Aftermath: A Review." *Environmental Health: A Global Access Science Source*, 2005, *4*(1), 6.

Civic Practices Network. "Good Neighbor Agreements: A Tool for Environmental and Social Justice." http://www.cpn.org/topics/environment/goodneighbor.html, n.d.

Clean Water Atlanta. "The Goal of Clean Water Atlanta." http://www.cleanwateratlanta.org, n.d.

Conglianese, C. "Assessing Consensus: The Promise and Performance of Negotiated Rulemaking."*Duke Law Journal*. http://www.law.duke.edu/shell/cite.pl?46+Duke+L.+J.+1255, 1997.

Dhara, V. R., and Dhara, R. "The Union Carbide Disaster in Bhopal: A Review Of Health Effects." *Archives of Environmental Health*, 2002, *57*, 391–404.

Dhara, V. R., Dhara, R., Acquilla, S. D., and Cullinan, P. "Personal Exposure and Long-Term Health Effects in Survivors of the Union Carbide Disaster at Bhopal." *Environmental Health Perspectives*, 2002, *110*, 489–502.

Dinham, B., and Sarangi, S. "The Bhopal Gas Tragedy of 1984–? The Evasion of Corporate Responsibility." *Environment & Urbanization*, 2002, *14*(1), 89–99.

Eckerman, I. *The Bhopal Saga: Causes and Consequences of the World's Largest Industrial Disaster*. Hyderabad: Universities Press, 2005.

Environmental Defense Fund. "Corporate Partnerships." http://www.edf.org/page.cfm?tagID=1458, 2009.

Fiorino, D. J. *Making Environmental Policy*. Berkeley: University of California Press, 1995.

Friedman, T. *The World Is Flat 3.0*. New York: Picador, 2007.

Frumkin, H., Frank, L., and Jackson, R. *Urban Sprawl and Public Health*. Washington, D.C.: Island Press, 2004.

Gladwell, M. *The Tipping Point*. New York: Little, Brown, 2002.

Goldsmith, S., and Eggers, W. D. *Governing by Network: The New Shape of the Public Sector*. Washington, D.C.: Brookings Institution, 2004.

Kotchian, S. "The Practice of Environmental Health." In H. Frumkin (ed.), *Environmental Health: From Global to Local* (pp. 895–925). San Francisco: Jossey-Bass, 2005.

Kripalani, M. "Dow Chemical: Liable for Bhopal? The 1984 Disaster was Union Carbide's Fault, but Many Indians Want to Hold Dow Accountable." *BusinessWeek*, May 28, 2008.

Landy, M. K., Roberts, M. J., and Thomas, S. R. *The Environmental Protection Agency: Asking the Wrong Questions*. New York: Oxford University Press, 1990.

Lowi, T. J. *The End of Liberalism: Ideology, Policy, and the Crisis of Public Authority*. New York: Norton, 1969.

Malizia, E. "City and Regional Planning: A Primer for Public Health Officials." *American Journal of Health Promotion*, 2005, *19*(suppl.), 1–13.

McConnell, G. *Private Power and American Democracy*. New York: Vintage Books, 1966.

Melnick, R. S. *Regulation and the Courts: The Case of the Clean Air Act*. Washington, D.C.: Brookings Institution, 1983.

Miles, R. "The Origin and Meaning of Miles' Law." *Public Administration Review*, 1978, *38*(5), 399–403.

National Academy of Public Administration. *Setting Priorities, Getting Results: A New Direction for EPA*. Summary Report. Washington, D.C.: National Academy of Public Administration, Apr. 1995.

Sirianni, C., and Friedlander, L. *Civic Innovation in America*. Berkeley: University of California Press, 2001.

Sparrow, M. *The Regulatory Craft*. Washington, D.C.: Brookings Institution, 2000.

Taylor, K. D. "The Broadening Strategy of Environmental Organizations on the Issue of Global Warming." Paper presented at the 2008 Western Political Science Association Annual Conference, San Diego, Calif. http://www.allacademic.com/meta/p_mla_apa_research_citation/2/3/7/8/7/p237870_index.html, 2008.

United States Climate Action Partnership. [Homepage.] http://www.us-cap.org, 2009.

U.S. Environmental Protection Agency. Methyl Isocyanate Hazard Summary. 2000. http://www.epa.gov/ttn/uatw/hlthef/methylis.html#ref1

U.S. Environmental Protection Agency. *EPA Quarterly Management Report: January Through March 2008*. http://www.epa.gov/ocfo/qer/pdfs/fy08_q2_qmr.pdf, 2008.

U.S. Environmental Protection Agency. [Homepage.] www.epa.gov, 2009a.

U.S. Environmental Protection Agency. "Laws, Regulations, Guidance and Dockets." http://www.epa.gov/lawsregs/laws/index.html, 2009b.

U.S. House of Representatives. "Committee Offices." 111th Congress, 1st Session. http://www.house.gov/house/CommitteeWWW.shtml, 2009.

U.S. Senate. "Committees." http://www.senate.gov/pagelayout/committees/d_three_sections_with_teasers/committees_home.htm, 2009.

FOR FURTHER INFORMATION

Books

Johnson, B. *Environmental Policy and Public Health*. Boca Raton, Fla.: CRC Press, 2007. A detailed discussion of the various federal agencies involved in environmental and public health protection appears in chapter 3 of this book.

Rosenbaum, W. *Environmental Politics and Policy*. (7th ed.) Washington, D.C.: CQ Press, 2007. A widely used general introduction.

Vig, N., and Kraft, M. (eds.). *Environmental Policy: New Directions for the Twenty-First Century*. (6th ed.) Washington, D.C.: CQ Press, 2005. A comprehensive set of essays on the topic of environmental policy.

> In addition, two books listed in the References are especially useful. Though its description of EPA is a now a bit dated, Fiorino (1995) remains an excellent introduction to the federal laws and institutions that support environmental policy and the analytical frameworks available for policy analysis. Ashford and Caldart (2008) have compiled an extensive text on environmental and public health protection; chapter 4 on environmental torts is especially clear and accessible, even to nonlawyers.

Agency

U.S. Environmental Protection Agency. [Homepage.] http://www.epa.gov. The EPA's Web site contains extensive information on specific aspects of environmental policy and the history of EPA.

CHAPTER THIRTY-ONE

RISK COMMUNICATION

VINCENT T. COVELLO

KEY CONCEPTS

- Risk communication is the two-way exchange of information about environmental, health, and safety threats.

- Risk communication is a core public health function, designed to inform the public, achieve behavioral change and other effective public health protection, provide warnings of disasters and emergencies, and help in resolving conflicts.

- Risk communication may be applied in emergency situations or in the setting of long-term environmental exposures.

- Risk communication may be practiced by governmental agencies, nongovernmental organizations, and the private sector.

- Risk communication should be based on an understanding of the determinants of risk perception and the views and needs of the target audience(s).

OR public health professionals, including those in environmental public health, risk communication is a core practice. It corresponds to one of the ten essential public health services, "Inform, educate and empower people about health issues" (Centers for Disease Control and Prevention [CDC] . . ., 2008; also see Table 27.1 in Chapter Twenty-Seven). Risk communication is a special category of health communication. It consists of the two-way exchange of information about environmental, health, and safety threats, including threats such as hazardous waste, water contamination, air pollution, and radiation. The goals of risk communication are to enhance knowledge and understanding, build trust and credibility, encourage dialogue, and influence attitudes, decisions, and behaviors. These goals apply to all four major types of risk communication. Categorized by objective, these types are (1) information and education; (2) behavioral change and protective action; (3) disaster warning and emergency notification; and (4) joint problem solving and conflict resolution.

Effective risk communication is central to informed decision making. It establishes public confidence in the ability of individuals and organization to deal with an environmental, health, or safety risk. Numerous studies have highlighted the importance of risk communication in enabling individuals and organizations to make informed choices and participate in deciding how risks should be managed (see, for example, National Research Council, 1989, 1996; Covello, McCallum, and Pavlova, 1989; Covello, Peters, Wojtecki, and Hyde, 2001). Effective risk communication provides people with timely, accurate, clear, objective, consistent, and complete risk information. It is the starting point for creating an informed public that is

- Involved, interested, reasonable, thoughtful, solution oriented, cooperative, and collaborative
- Appropriately concerned about the risk
- More likely to engage in appropriate behaviors

Seven cardinal rules for effective risk communication are shown in Exhibit 31.1.

Vincent T. Covello declares no competing financial interests.

EXHIBIT 31.1
Seven Cardinal Rules of Risk Communication

1. Accept and involve the receiver of risk information as a legitimate partner. People have the right to participate in decisions that affect their lives.
2. Plan and tailor risk communication strategies. Different goals, audiences, and communication channels require different risk communication strategies.
3. Listen to your audience. People are usually more concerned about psychological factors, such as trust, credibility, control, voluntariness, dread, familiarity, uncertainty, ethics, responsiveness, fairness, caring, and compassion, than they are about the technical details of a risk. To identify real concerns, a risk communicator must be willing to listen carefully to and understand the audience.
4. Be honest, frank, and open. Trust and credibility are among the most valuable assets of a risk communicator.
5. Coordinate and collaborate with other credible sources. Communications about risks are enhanced when accompanied by referrals to credible, neutral sources of information. Few things hurt credibility more than conflicts and disagreements among information sources.
6. Plan for media influence. The media play a major role in transmitting risk information. It is critical to know what messages the media are delivering and how to deliver risk messages effectively through the media.
7. Speak clearly and with compassion. Technical language and jargon are major barriers to effective risk communication. Abstract and unfeeling language often offends people. Acknowledging emotions, such as fear, anger, and helplessness, is typically far more effective.

RISK COMMUNICATION MODELS

Effective risk communication is based on several models that describe how people form risk perceptions, process risk information, and make risk decisions. Together, these models provide the intellectual and theoretical foundation for effective risk communication.

The Risk Perception Model

One of the most important paradoxes identified in the **risk perception** litera-ture is that the risks that kill or harm people and the risks that alarm and upset people are often very different (see, for example, Sandman, 1989; Slovic, 2000). For example, there is virtually no correlation between the ranking of hazards according to statistics on expected annual mortality and the ranking of the same hazards by how upsetting they are to people. There are risks that make many people worried and upset but cause little harm. At the same time, there are risks that kill or harm many people but do not make people worried or upset.

This paradox is explained in part by the factors that affect how risks are perceived. Several of the most important risk perception factors are described in the following paragraphs. Because these risk perception factors often have high emotional content, they are often called *outrage factors* or *fear factors*.

Trust. Risks from activities associated with individuals, institutions, or organi-zations lacking in trust and credibility (such as organizations with poor health, safety, or environmental track records) are judged to be greater than risks from activities associated with entities that are trustworthy and credible (such as regula-tory agencies that achieve high levels of compliance among regulated groups).

Voluntariness. Risks from activities considered to be involuntary or imposed (for example, exposure to chemicals or radiation from a waste or industrial facility) are judged to be greater than risks from activities that are seen to be voluntary (for example, smoking, sunbathing, or mountain climbing).

Controllability. Risks from activities viewed as under the control of others (for example, releases of toxic agents by industrial facilities or bioterrorists) are judged to be greater than risks from activities that appear to be under the control of the individual (for example, driving an automobile or riding a bicycle).

Familiarity. Risks viewed as unfamiliar (for example, exposure to leaks of chemicals or radiation from waste disposal sites) are judged to be greater than risks viewed as familiar (for example, exposure to chemicals during household work).

Fairness. Risks from activities believed to be unfair or to involve unfair proc-esses (for example, inequitable siting of industrial facilities or landfills) are judged to be greater than risks from fair activities (for example, receiving vaccinations).

Benefits. Risks from activities that seem to have unclear, questionable, or dif-fused personal or economic benefits (for example, operating nuclear power plants or waste disposal facilities) are judged to be greater than risks from activities that have clear benefits (performing jobs, conducting actions with monetary benefits, or automobile driving).

Catastrophic potential. Risks viewed as having **catastrophic potential**, that is, the ability to cause a significant number of deaths and injuries closely grouped in time and space (for example, major industrial accidents), are judged to be greater than risks that cause scattered or random deaths and injuries (for example, automobile crashes).

Understanding. Poorly understood risks (for example, the health effects of long-term exposure to low doses of toxic chemicals or radiation) are judged to be greater than risks that are well understood or self-explanatory (for example, pedestrian accidents or slipping on ice).

Uncertainty. Risks that are relatively unknown or highly uncertain (for example, potential risks from biotechnology and genetic engineering) are judged to be greater than risks that appear to be relatively well known to science (for example, automobile crash risks that are known from actuarial data).

Delayed effects. Risks that may have delayed effects (for example, exposures that cause adverse health effects after long latency periods) are judged to be greater than risks having immediate effects (for example, exposures to poison).

Effects on children. Risks that appear to put children in harm's way (for example, contamination of milk with radiation or toxic chemicals or exposure of pregnant women to radiation or toxic chemicals) are judged to be greater than risks that do not (for example, workplace injury risks).

Effects on future generations. Risks that seem to pose a threat to future generations (for example, adverse genetic effects due to exposure to toxic chemicals or radiation) are judged to be greater than risks that do not (for example, musculoskeletal injuries from skiing accidents).

Victim identity. Risks from activities that produce identifiable victims (such as a worker exposed to high levels of toxic chemicals or radiation, a child who falls down a well, or a miner trapped in a mine) are judged to be greater than risks from activities that produce statistical victims (such as statistical profiles of automobile crash victims).

Dread. Risks from activities that evoke fear, terror, or anxiety (for example, exposures to cancer-causing agents, AIDS, or exotic diseases) are judged to be greater than risks from activities that do not arouse such feelings or emotions (for example, exposures to common colds and household accidents).

Media attention. Risks from activities that receive considerable media coverage (for example, accidents and leaks at nuclear power plants) are judged to be greater than risks from activities that receive little (for example, on-the-job injuries).

Accident history. Risks from activities with a history of major accidents or frequent minor accidents (for example, leaks at waste disposal facilities) are judged to be greater than risks from activities with little or no such history (for example, recombinant DNA experimentation).

Reversibility. Risks from activities considered to have potentially irreversible adverse effects (for example, exposures to a toxic substance that may cause birth defects) are judged to be greater than risks from activities considered to have reversible adverse effects (for example, engaging in sports that may result in muscle strains).

Personal stake. Risks from activities viewed by people as placing them (or their families) personally and directly at risk (for example, disposal of waste in a site near their homes) are judged to be greater than risks from activities that appear to pose no direct or personal threat (for example, disposal of waste in remote areas).

Ethical or moral nature. Risks from activities believed to be ethically objectionable or morally wrong (for example, foisting pollution on an economically distressed community) are judged to be greater than risks from ethically neutral activities (for example, taking medication that may have side effects).

Human versus natural origin. Risks generated by human action, failure or incompetence (for example, risks from industrial accidents caused by negligence, inadequate safeguards, or operator error) are judged to be greater than risks believed to be caused by nature or "acts of God" (for example, risks from earthquakes or cosmic rays).

These risk perception, or outrage, factors, together with actual risk numbers, determine a person's emotional response to risk information. For example, they affect levels of public fear, worry, concern, anxiety, and anger. Levels of fear, worry, concern, anxiety, and anger tend to be greatest and most intense when a risk is perceived to be involuntary, unfair, not beneficial, not under one's personal control, and managed by untrustworthy individuals or organizations. Research by Sandman (1989), Slovic (2000), Fischhoff (1995), and others reveals that people often assess risk more in terms of these perceived risk factors than in terms of actual potential for harm or hazard. For the public,

$$\text{Risk} = \text{Hazard} + \text{Outrage.}$$

This equation reflects the observation that an individual's perception or assessment of risk is based on a combination of hazard factors (for example, mortality and morbidity statistics) and outrage factors. When present, outrage often takes on strong emotional overtones. It predisposes an individual to react emotionally (for example, with fear or anger), which can in turn significantly amplify or deamplify levels of worry or concern.

The risk perception model is the key to understanding many risk controversies. For example, fairness is critical to understanding NIMBY (not in my backyard) controversies. An unfair risk is often perceived as more risky, and therefore less acceptable, than a fairly distributed risk. An activity providing minimal perceived benefits for the affected parties is perceived as more risky, and therefore less acceptable, than an activity providing large perceived benefits. An activity perceived as beyond the control of the affected parties—beyond voluntary choice, the sharing of power, or the acquisition of knowledge needed to make informed choices—is perceived as more risky, and therefore less acceptable, than an activity perceived as under the control of the affected parties.

The Mental Noise Model

The **mental noise** model focuses on how people process information under stress. Mental noise is caused by the stress and strong emotions associated with exposures to risks. When people are stressed and upset, their ability to process information can become severely impaired. In high-stress situations, people typically display a substantially reduced ability to process information. Exposure to risks associated with negative psychological attributes (for example, risks perceived to be involuntary, not under one's control, low in benefits, unfair, or dreaded) contributes greatly to mental noise.

People under stress typically

- Have difficulty hearing, understanding, and remembering information.
- Focus most on the first and last things they hear.
- Focus on the negative more than the positive.
- Process information at several levels below their educational level.
- Attend to no more than three messages at a time.
- Focus intensely on issues of trust, benefits, fairness, and control.
- Want to know that you care before they care what you know.

The Negative Dominance Model

The **negative dominance** model describes the processing of negative and positive information in high-concern and emotionally charged situations. In general, the relationship between negative and positive information is asymmetrical in high-stress situations, with negative information receiving significantly greater weight. The negative dominance model is consistent with a central theorem of modern psychology that people place greater value on losses (negative outcomes) than on gains (positive outcomes). One practical implication of the negative dominance model is it takes several positive or solution-oriented messages to counterbalance one negative message. On average, in high-concern or emotionally charged situations, it takes three or more positive messages to counterbalance a negative message. Another practical implication of negative dominance theory is that communications that contain negatives—words such as *no, not, never, nothing, none,* and other words with negative connotations—tend to receive closer attention,

FIGURE 31.1   Trust Factors in High-Stress Situations

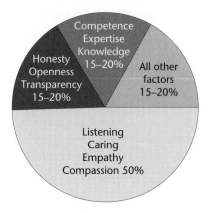

are remembered longer, and have greater impact than messages with positive words. As a result, the use of unnecessary negatives in high-concern or emotionally charged situations can have the unintended effect of drowning out positive or solution-oriented information. Risk communications are often most effective when they focus on positive, constructive actions; on what is being done, rather than on what is not being done.

The Trust Determination Model

A central theme in the risk communication literature is the importance of **trust** in effective risk communications. Trust is generally recognized as the single most important factor determining perceptions of risk. Only when trust has been established can other risk communication goals, such as consensus building and dialogue, be achieved.

Trust is typically built over long periods of time. Building trust is a long-term, cumulative process. Trust is easily lost. Once lost, it is difficult to regain.

Because of the importance of trust in effective risk communication, a significant part of the risk communication literature focuses on the determinants of trust. Research (see, for example, Peters, McCallum, and Covello, 1997) indicates that the most important trust determination factors are (1) listening, caring, empathy, and compassion; (2) competence, expertise, and knowledge; and (3) honesty, openness, and transparency (Figure 31.1). Other factors in trust determination are accountability, perseverance, dedication, commitment, responsiveness, objectivity, fairness, and consistency. Trust determinations are often made in fewer than thirty seconds and perhaps as few as nine seconds. Initial trust impressions are often lasting trust impressions.

Trust is created in part by a proven track record of caring, honesty, and competence. It can be substantially enhanced by endorsements from trustworthy sources. Trust in individuals varies greatly depending on their perceived attributes and their verbal and nonverbal communication skills. Trust in organizations also varies greatly. For example, surveys indicate that the most trustworthy individuals and organizations in many risk controversies are

- Informed citizen advisory panels
- Educators
- Firefighters
- Safety professionals
- Doctors
- Nurses
- Faith leaders

CHALLENGES TO EFFECTIVE RISK COMMUNICATION

These four models are the backdrop for two of the most important challenges to effective risk communication. The first consists of **media selectivity** and **media bias** in reporting about risk. The second consists of psychological, sociological, and cultural factors that create public misperceptions and misunderstandings about risks. Each challenge is discussed in this section.

Selectivity and Bias in Media Reporting

The media play a critical role in the delivery of risk information (see, for example, Hyer and Covello, 2007). However, journalists are often highly selective in their reporting about risks. For example, they often focus their attention on

- Controversy
- Conflict
- Events with high personal drama
- Failures
- Negligence
- Scandals and wrongdoing
- Risks or threats to children
- Stories about villains, victims, and heroes

Much of this selectivity stems from a host of professional and organizational factors. Several of the most important are described in the following paragraphs. Each factor contributes to distortions and inaccuracies in media reporting about risks.

Newsworthiness. Journalists typically look for **newsworthiness,** stories that will attract the largest number of readers, listeners, and viewers. Stories that attract the most attention typically have a high emotional content, involving people in unusual, dramatic, confrontational, conflicted, or negative situations (for example, emotionally charged town hall meetings). Attractive stories about risk typically involve dreaded events (for example, cancer among children), risks to future generations, involuntariness, unclear benefits, inequitable distribution of risks and benefits, potentially irreversible effects, and incompetent or untrustworthy risk managers. One result of this selectivity process is that many media stories about risk contain substantial omissions or present oversimplified, distorted, or inaccurate information. For example, media reports on cancer risks often fail to provide adequate statistics on general cancer rates for purposes of comparison.

Division of labor. In many cases the headline or the lead to a story about a risk is written by a person other than the journalist who covered the story. The headline or lead is often more sensational than the story. One reason for this is that a wide variety of tasks are carried out in the typical media organization, and these tasks are often performed by different individuals with different goals. An important goal for the headline writer is to attract readers, listeners, or viewers.

Generalist journalists. Most journalists are generalists rather than specialists, even in large media organizations. As a result, most journalists who cover risk stories lack expertise in sciences such as medicine, engineering, epidemiology, toxicology, ecology, and statistics where an understanding of risk is necessary. In addition, journalists are often shuffled among content areas (or *beats*). Shuffling often results in a journalist being assigned to cover a risk story for which he or she has little experience, background, or specialized knowledge. Lack of expertise and experience often leads to distortions and inaccuracies in media reporting about risks.

Resources. Most media organizations do not have the resources needed to conduct in-depth research on risk stories.

Objectivity and balance. Journalists typically attempt to achieve balance and objectivity by citing multiple sources with diverse viewpoints. However, the sources quoted are often highly variable in their expertise and objectivity.

Career advancement. Journalists typically advance their careers by moving from smaller media markets to larger media markets. As a result, media outlets often experience high staff turnover. Staff turnover, in turn, often results in stories written by journalists who are unfamiliar with the issues.

Watchdogs. Many journalists see themselves as watchdogs of industry and government and focus their attention on wrongdoing.

Source dependency. Journalists are highly dependent on individuals and organizations for a steady and reliable flow of newsworthy information. When a steady flow of information from authoritative sources is not forthcoming, journalists often turn to less authoritative sources. Additionally, journalists often look unfavorably on scientists or decision makers who use overly cautious or hedging language. In such cases, journalists may turn to sources willing to speak with certainty on the risk issue even though these sources are less reputable or less well informed.

Competition. Competition within and among media organizations (as well as among journalists) is often intense. Many news organizations compete zealously against one another for viewers, listeners, or readers. Much of this competition is centered on getting the story out first, and meeting this objective can lead to omissions and inaccuracies.

Deadlines. Journalists typically work under short deadlines. Short deadlines limit the ability of journalists to pursue accurate and credible information. Additionally, authoritative sources who do not respond to a journalist before his or her deadline are often looked on with disfavor and may be bypassed in the future.

Information compression. Because of the limited amount of time or space allocated for a story, journalists are limited in their ability to explore the complexities surrounding a risk issue.

Factors That Create Misperceptions and Misunderstandings

The second challenge to effective risk communication arises from the psychological, sociological, and cultural factors that create risk misperceptions and misunderstandings among the public. As a result of these factors, people may make biased judgments or use only a small amount of the available information to make risk decisions (see, for example, Kahneman, Slovic, and Tversky, 1982; Kahneman and Tversky, 1979).

One of the most important of these factors is **availability**. When an event has high availability (meaning that it is easily accessed or remembered), people tend to overestimate its frequency. That is, people tend to assign greater probability to events of which they are frequently reminded (for example, in the news media, scientific literature, or discussions among friends or colleagues) or to events that are easy to recall or imagine through concrete examples or dramatic images. For example, if the daily news coverage often includes accounts of violent crimes, then people may conclude that the risk of crime is high throughout the community, leading them to shun parks and public places and to drive rather than walk—choices that reduce opportunities for physical activity.

A second important factor is **conformity**. This is the tendency of people to behave in a particular way because everyone else is doing it or to believe something because everyone else believes it.

A third factor is overconfidence in one's ability to avoid harm. A majority of people, for example, consider themselves less likely than average to get cancer, get fired from their job, or get mugged. Overconfidence is most prevalent when high levels of perceived personal control lead to reduced feelings of susceptibility. Many people fail to use seat belts, for example, because of the unfounded belief that they are more skilled or safer than the average driver. In a similar vein, many teenagers often engage in high-risk behaviors such as drinking and driving, smoking, or unprotected sex because of perceptions, supported by peers, of invulnerability and overconfidence in their ability to avoid harm.

A fourth factor is **confirmatory bias**. People are exhibiting confirmatory bias when they (1) seek out and accept information that is consistent with their beliefs or biases, (2) ignore information that is not consistent with their beliefs or biases, or (3) interpret information to support or confirm their beliefs or biases.

Once a belief about a risk is formed, new evidence is generally made to fit, contrary information is filtered out, ambiguous data are interpreted as confirmation, and consistent information is seen as "proof."

A fifth factor is the public's aversion to **uncertainty**. This aversion often translates into a marked public preference and demand for statements of fact over statements of probability—that is, over the language of risk assessment. Despite statements by experts that precise information is seldom available, people

EXHIBIT 31.2

The 103 Questions Most Frequently Asked by Residents Affected by Environmental Cleanups and Hazardous Waste Sites

Health Risk Concerns

1. Am I at risk from the contamination?
2. What are the risks to my children?

often want absolute answers. For example, people often demand to know exactly what will happen, not what might happen.

A sixth factor is the reluctance of people to change strongly held beliefs. Strong beliefs about risks, once formed, change very slowly. They can be extraordinarily persistent in the face of contrary evidence.

STRATEGIES FOR EFFECTIVE RISK COMMUNICATION

Effective risk communication relies on several elements: having a **comprehensive risk and crisis communication plan** developed in advance, using message mapping, using and communicating high-quality information, and directly addressing the challenges just discussed that are presented by the media and by psychological, sociological, and cultural factors. These elements are described in the following sections.

Preparing a Comprehensive Risk and Crisis Communication Plan

Risk communicators, whether in governmental agencies, nongovernmental organizations, or the private sector, should plan for communication needs well in advance. This requires careful anticipation of what may need to be communicated and of available communication channels, both internally and externally. Exhibit 31.2 presents a list of questions most frequently asked by people directly affected by environmental cleanups and hazardous waste sites, drawn from public documents and media reports; such questions are useful in anticipating what information will be requested. Exhibit 31.3 presents twenty-five elements of a comprehensive risk and crisis communication plan.

3. What are the risks to my pets?
4. What are the impacts to the natural habitat (that is, fish and other species)?
5. Can my children and pets play in the soil?
6. What health effects can I expect to see if I've been exposed to site contaminants?
7. What are the short-term effects?
8. What are the long-term effects?
9. I have a recent health problem [for example, headaches or rashes] that I never had before; could the site contamination have caused this problem?
10. Have any health problems been reported so far?

11. How many people have become ill as a result of the site?
12. Are you going to test residents for exposure?
13. Can you set up a temporary, local health center or clinic where we can be tested?
14. I'm pregnant [or planning to become pregnant]. Will the contaminants affect my unborn child?
15. Is it safe to garden in my yard?
16. Is it safe to eat vegetables grown in my garden?
17. Is it safe to drink the water?
18. Will you provide us with bottled water?
19. Is it safe to bathe or shower in the water?
20. Is it safe to water our lawns with the potentially contaminated water?
21. Is it safe to mow our lawns if the soil underneath is potentially contaminated?
22. Is it safe to use the river for fishing and other recreational purposes?
23. Is it safe to eat the fish?
24. What's being done right now to protect my and my family's health?
25. Will capping the site protect my health?
26. How serious is the contamination?
27. What happens if my ventilation system shuts down?
28. Can I get sick from breathing the air?

Investigation and Data Concerns

1. Where did the contamination come from?
2. How bad is the problem?
3. How much contamination is there?
4. Is the contamination moving and, if so, in what direction?
5. Are there any other contaminants beside the ones we were told about?
6. How can you be sure there are no other contaminants?
7. Will you conduct testing [or sampling] to make sure the soil in my yard is free of contaminants?
8. How will you decide where to sample and where not to sample?
9. Who determines what levels of contamination are considered "safe"?
10. Why don't you clean up all of the contamination, instead of allowing some to remain?
11. How do you know whether my drinking water is contaminated?
12. How do you know whether my yard has contaminated soil?
13. How do you know that it's safe to breathe the air?
14. How do you know whether it's safe to go fishing?
15. Why hasn't my well been sampled?
16. Why have some people received bottled water and not others?

17. Can I see the results of the testing you've done on my property?
18. Can I see the results of testing you've done on other properties in the neighborhood?
19. Do I have to give you access to sample my property?
20. What if I refuse access to my property?
21. Do I need to be home and take time off work while you're sampling my property?
22. I'm moving into the area; can I see the results of sampling that's been done?
23. Who will be doing the sampling?
24. How can we be sure the sampling data are accurate?
25. How can we be sure that future sampling won't find things that you didn't find now?
26. Can you guarantee the accuracy of the sampling results?

Cleanup Concerns

1. How exactly are you going to clean up the site?
2. Why was this particular cleanup method chosen over other options?
3. How long will the cleanup take?
4. When are you going to start the cleanup?
5. Who is going to perform the cleanup?
6. What process was used [or will be used] to select contractors to perform the cleanup?
7. How will cleanup performance be monitored or evaluated?
8. How much will the cleanup cost?
9. Who will pay for the cleanup?
10. Will my tax dollars have to pay to address this problem that someone else caused?
11. Can taxpayers be reimbursed?
12. How will you know when everything is "clean"?
13. Why are you going to just "cap" everything and leave the contamination there?
14. Why not dig up the contamination?
15. Is dredging safe?
16. Won't dredging just "stir up" things and contaminate the water even more?
17. What if the cleanup doesn't work?
18. Can you guarantee that all of the contamination will be removed?
19. How will my quality of life be affected during the cleanup [with noise, traffic, odors, and so forth]?
20. After you finish the cleanup, then what [what happens next]?

21. After the cleanup, will you continue to test to make sure it's still working?
22. What happens if my water [or soil or other material] is still contaminated after the cleanup?

Communication Concerns

1. Why did it take you so long to tell us about the contamination?
2. How can I trust what you're telling me about the site?
3. How can I trust what you're telling me about my safety?
4. What happens if you find high concentrations of contaminants near my home—how will I know?
5. How will I be informed of what's going on?
6. Will you share the testing data with residents?
7. Will you let us know if something unexpected happens during the cleanup and things get worse?
8. Is there someone local residents can talk to if we have questions or concerns?
9. Where can I get more information about this site?
10. Where can I get more information about similar sites that have already been cleaned up?
11. If a cleanup plan is selected that residents disagree with, is there an appeal process?
12. How will you address public comments?
13. Will you address *all* of the public comments?
14. How do you decide which comments *not* to address?
15. If the majority of residents disagree with how the EPA [or other agency] is planning to clean up the site, will the EPA [or other agency] change its mind?
16. There's another site down the road; can you tell me what's going on there?
17. When you first discovered there *might* be a problem, why didn't you tell us then?

Message Mapping

An important aspect of effective communication is clarity on what is to be communicated. **Message mapping** is a useful tool for this purpose (see, for example, Covello, 2006). A risk communication message map consists of detailed and hierarchically organized information that can be used to respond to anticipated questions or concerns. It is a visual aid that provides, at a glance, the organization's messages on high-concern issues. The message map template enables spokespersons to meet the demands of the media as well as the public and other

Economic Concerns

1. If soil is excavated from my yard, will I receive financial assistance to replace plants and shrubbery?
2. My property value has decreased because of the site contamination problem. Will I be compensated for this?
3. I'm concerned that cost will be the driving force behind the agency's selected cleanup option; does community opinion really matter?
4. I was told residents might have to relocate during the site cleanup. Who will pay for my moving costs? What about other expenses I may be forced to incur [or costs of transporting my children to school because they won't be able to take the bus, or daily food costs because I won't have access to my stove and refrigerator, and so forth]?
5. The site has placed a "negative stigma" on our community that may affect potential investors, developers, or homeowners; what will be done about this?
6. Will this keep our community from developing?
7. Can we get jobs helping with the cleanup?
8. If we can't eat the fish anymore because of health risks, can you give us a food subsidy?
9. Do you have enough money to cover the cleanup costs?
10. What if you discover the cleanup is going to cost more than estimated; what happens then?

Source: J. Ross and V. Covello, 2007.

interested parties for timely, accurate, clear, concise, consistent, credible, and relevant information. A message map may be a port in a storm when questioning by journalists or others becomes intense or aggressive. Message maps also allow organizations to develop risk messages in advance. Once a message map is developed, its effectiveness can be tested through focus groups and other empirical studies.

Table 31.1 shows a general template for a message map. The top section of the message map identifies the stakeholder or audience for whom the messages

EXHIBIT 31.3

Elements of a Comprehensive Risk and Crisis
Communication Plan

1. Identify all anticipated scenarios for which risk, crisis, and emergency communication plans are needed, including worst cases and low-probability, high-
   consequence events.
2. Describe and designate staff roles and responsibilities for each of the different
   risk, crisis, or emergency scenarios.
3. Designate who in the organization is responsible and accountable for leading
   the crisis or emergency response.
4. Designate who is responsible and accountable for implementing various crisis
   and emergency actions.
5. Designate who needs to be consulted during the process.
6. Designate who needs to be informed about what is taking place.
7. Designate who will be the lead communication spokesperson and who will be
   the backup for each of the different scenarios.
8. Identify procedures for information verification, clearance, and approval.
9. Identify p rocedures for coordinating with important stakeholders and partners
   (for example, with other organizations, emergency responders, law enforcement, elected officials, state or provincial agencies, and federal government
   agencies).
10. Identify procedures to secure the required human, financial, logistical, and
    physical support and resources (such as staff, space, equipment, and food) for
    communication operations during a short, a medium, and a prolonged event
    (twenty-four hours a day, seven days a week if needed).
11. Identify agreements on releasing information and agreements on who releases
    what, when, and how policies and procedures for employee contacts with the
    media.
12. Include regularly checked and updated media contact lists (including after-
    hours news desks).
13. Include regularly checked and updated partner contact lists (day and night
    means of contact).
14. Identify schedule for exercises and drills for testing the communication plan,
    as part of larger preparedness and response training.
15. Identify subject-matter experts (for example, university professors) willing to
    collaborate during an emergency, and develop and test contact lists (day and
    night means of contact); know their perspectives in advance.
16. Identify target audiences.

17. Identify preferred communication channels (for example, telephone hotlines, radio announcements, news conferences, Web site updates, and faxes) for communicating with the public, key stakeholders, and partners.

18. Include message maps for core, informational, and challenge questions.

19. Include message maps with answers to frequently asked and anticipated questions from key stakeholders, including key internal and external audiences.

20. Include holding statements for each of the anticipated stages of the crisis.

21. Include fact sheets, question-and-answer sheets, talking points, maps, charts, graphics, and other supplementary communication materials.

22. Include a signed endorsement of the communication plan from the organization's director.

23. Include procedures for posting and updating information on the organization's Web site.

24. Include communication task checklists for the first two, four, eight, twelve, sixteen, twenty-four, forty-eight, and seventy-two hours.

25. Include procedures for evaluating, revising, and updating the risk and crisis communication plan on a regular basis.

TABLE 31.1 General Template for a Message Map

Stakeholder:		
Question or concern:		
Key Message 1	**Key Message 2**	**Key Message 3**
Supporting information 1-1	Supporting information 2-1	Supporting information 3-1
Supporting information 1-2	Supporting information 2-2	Supporting information 3-2
Supporting information 1-3	Supporting information 2-3	Supporting information 3-3

are intended as well as the specific question or concern being addressed. The next layer of the message map contains the three key messages that can function individually or collectively as a response to a stakeholder question or concern. These key messages are intended to address the information needs of a wide variety of audiences.

The three key messages can also serve individually or collectively as a media **sound bite**, a short, quotable message attributed to a spokesperson, played repeatedly by the media, and then also used by other sources of information. Speaking in sound bites helps to ensure that prepared key messages are carried in news stories. Reporters and editors almost always cut interview material into sound bites. The average length of a sound bite is twenty-seven words for print media and nine seconds for broadcast media.

The final section of the message map contains supporting information, arranged in blocks of three under each key message. This supporting information amplifies a key message by providing additional facts or details. Supporting information can also take the form of visuals, analogies, personal stories, or citations of credible information sources. An example of a message map, on the subject of smallpox, is shown in Table 31.2.

Message maps may also be produced in a bulleted list format. For example, Exhibit 31.4 displays a bulleted message map related to the use of chloramines as disinfectants for drinking water.

As a strategic tool, a message map provides multiple benefits. It is a handy reference for leaders and spokespersons who must respond swiftly to questions on topics where timeliness and accuracy are crucial. Multiple spokespersons can work from the same message map to ensure the rapid dissemination of consistent and core messages across a wide spectrum of communication outlets. Message maps provide a unifying framework for disseminating information on a wide range of public health issues. Message maps also minimize opportunities for "speaker's regret" after saying something inappropriate or not saying something that should have been said. Having a printed copy of the message map allows spokespersons being interviewed to check off the talking points they want to make in order of their importance. This helps to prevent omissions of key facts or misstatements that could provoke misunderstandings, controversy, or outrage.

One important lesson learned from message-mapping exercises is that the process of generating message maps can be as important as the end product. Message-mapping exercises involve teams of scientists, communication specialists, and individuals with policy expertise, and often reveal a diversity of viewpoints on a question, issue, or concern. Gaps in message maps are early warnings that messages are incomplete, providing scientists and issue-management teams with an opportunity to focus their efforts on filling the information gaps. Message-mapping

TABLE 31.2   Sample Message Map for Smallpox

Stakeholder: Public

Question or concern: How contagious is smallpox?

Key Message 1	Key Message 2	Key Message 3
Smallpox *spreads slowly* compared to many other diseases.	This allows *time to trace* those who have come into contact with the disease.	Those who have been traced *can be vaccinated*.
Supporting information 1-1	Supporting information 2-1	Supporting information 3-1
People are only infectious when the rash appears.	The incubation period for the disease is 10–14 days.	People who have never been vaccinated are the most important to vaccinate.
Supporting information 1-2	Supporting information 2-2	Supporting information 3-2
Smallpox spread typically requires hours of face-to-face contact.	Resources are available for tracing contacts.	Adults who were vaccinated as children may still have some immunity.
Supporting information 1-3	Supporting information 2-3	Supporting information 3-3
There are no carriers without symptoms.	Finding people who have been exposed and vaccinating them has proved successful in the past.	Adequate vaccine is on hand.

Note: Keywords for the map are shown in italics.

exercises also frequently identify changes needed in organizational strategies and policies.

The crucial final step in message map construction is systematic message testing using standardized procedures. Message testing should begin by asking subject-matter experts not directly involved in the original message-mapping process to validate the accuracy of the information given. Message testing should then be conducted with individuals or groups who have the characteristics to serve as surrogates for key internal and external target audiences. Finally, sharing and testing messages with partner organizations will promote message consistency and coordination. Once developed, message maps can be brought together to produce a media briefing book. They can also be used individually or collectively as aids during news conferences, media interviews, information forums and exchanges, and public meetings and their content can be used on Web sites, in telephone hotline scripts, and in fact sheets and brochures.

EXHIBIT 31.4
Sample Message Map for Chloramines

Stakeholder: Public
Question or Concern: What are chloramines?

Key Message 1: Chloramines are disinfectants used to treat drinking water

- Chloramines are most commonly formed when ammonia is added to chlorine to treat drinking water.
- The most typical purpose of chloramines is to protect water quality as it moves through pipes.
- Chloramines provide long-lasting protection as they do not break down quickly in water pipes.

Key Message 2: Chloramines of greatest regulatory interest are monochloramine, dichloramine, and trichloramine
- If chloramines are used to disinfect drinking water, monochloramine is the most common type.
- Dichloramine and trichloramine are produced when treating drinking water but at much lower levels than monochloramine.
- Trichloramines are typically associated with disinfected water used in swimming pools.

Key Message 3: The Environmental Protection Agency regulates the safe use of chloramines.*
- The EPA requires water utilities to meet strict health standards when using chloramines to treat water.
- EPA chloramine regulations are based on the average concentrations of chloramines found in a water system over time.
- The EPA regulates chemicals formed when chloramines react with natural organic matter in water.

---

*The drinking water standard for chloramines is four parts per million (ppm) measured as an annual average. More information on regulation of chloramines is available at http://www.epa.gov/safewater/disinfection/index.html.

Using and Communicating High-Quality Information

Risk data, especially numerical data, are only as good as the studies from which they are derived. The risk communicator should be clear about the source and quality of scientific and technical data being communicated. When discussing data with journalists or other stakeholders, risk communicators should address general questions, methods, and conclusions.

General questions to address include the following:

- Have the researchers found only a statistical correlation or have they found a difference that has actual implications?
- Have the findings been published yet in a peer-reviewed journal?
- Have the researchers published other research in this area?
- What are the institutional affiliations of the researchers?
- Are there any possible conflicts of interest?

Questions about research methods include the following:

- What research methods were used?
- Are the research methods conventional?
- Have the results been replicated by other researchers?
- What do other professionals in the field think about these methods?
- Is the sample size adequate to make a conclusion?
- If the research involves a diagnostic test, how often does the test produce a false negative or a false positive?

Questions about conclusions reached include the following:

- Have important caveats been made? For example, were there important variables that could not be, or were not, controlled?
- Are the findings preliminary or final?
- Are there other possible interpretations of the data?
- Do the findings differ markedly from those of previous studies?
- To what extent can the findings be generalized?

Fostering Comprehensive, Balanced Media Reporting

Ideally, journalists and risk communicators share many goals: informing and educating the public, getting the story out quickly, reaching major target audiences, rallying support, preventing undue fear and anxiety, providing accurate and needed information, and encouraging appropriate, protective behavior. Risk communicators can help journalists write better stories about risk by providing

- Accurate, truthful, evidence-based, and balanced information
- Early disclosure and regular updates of information
- Brief and concise information
- First-hand information
- Graphics and other visual information (for example, photographs, pictures, charts, timelines, diagrams, flowcharts, maps, drawings, videos, and animations)
- Simple statistics with explanations
- Human interest stories
- Access to experts and managers
- Information provided within media deadlines

A helpful starting point is to anticipate media questions. Journalists routinely ask six categories of questions: who, what, where, when, why, and how. Put more simply, in instances of environmental exposures, especially in emergency or crisis situations, journalists will want to know what happened, what caused it to happen, and what it means. Specific examples of questions asked by journalists are presented in Exhibit 31.5. Many of these correspond to general information needs among the public and other stakeholders, as shown in Exhibit 31.2.

As discussed earlier, risk communicators should anticipate selective or biased media reporting about risks. Here are seven strategies that can minimize these outcomes and help an organization achieve comprehensive, balanced reporting.

1. Accept the Media as a Legitimate Partner In an emergency or crisis, effective media communication enables the media to play a constructive role in protecting the public's health, enables public health officials to reach a wide range of stakeholders, and enables public health officials, in cooperation with the media, to build trust, calm a nervous public, provide needed information, encourage cooperative behaviors, and save lives. If you are in the role of risk communicator, you should demonstrate respect for the media by keeping them well informed of decisions and actions, establishing good working relationships with media contacts before an emergency arises, and including journalists in public emergency response planning exercises. Use a wide range of media communication channels to engage and involve people. When interacting with the media, be polite and courteous at all times, even if a reporter is not. Avoid embarrassing reporters,

EXHIBIT 31.5

Questions Commonly Asked by Journalists During an Emergency or Crisis

1. What is your name and title?
2. What are your job responsibilities?
3. What are your qualifications?
4. Can you tell us what happened?
5. When did it happen?
6. Where did it happen?
7. Who was harmed?
8. How many people were harmed [or injured, or killed]?
9. Are those who were harmed getting help?
10. How are those who were harmed getting help?
11. What can others do to help?
12. Is the situation under control?
13. Is there anything good that you can tell us?
14. Is there any immediate danger?
15. What is being done in response to what happened?
16. Who is in charge?
17. What can we expect next?
18. What are you advising people to do?
19. How long will it be before the situation returns to normal?
20. What help has been requested or offered from others?
21. What responses have you received?
22. Can you be specific about the types of harm that occurred?
23. What are the names of those who were harmed?
24. Can we talk to them?
25. How much damage occurred?
26. What other damage may have occurred?
27. How certain are you about damage?
28. How much damage do you expect?
29. What are you doing now?
30. Who else is involved in the response?
31. Why did this happen?
32. What was the cause?
33. Did you have any forewarning that this might happen?
34. Why wasn't this prevented from happening?
35. What else can go wrong?
36. If you are not sure of the cause, what is your best guess?

37. Who caused this to happen?
38. Who is to blame?
39. Could this have been avoided?
40. Do you think those involved handled the situation well enough?
41. When did your response to this begin?
42. When were you notified that something had happened?
43. Who is conducting the investigation?
44. What are you going to do after the investigation?
45. What have you found out so far?
46. Why wasn't more done to prevent this from happening?
47. What is your personal opinion?
48. What are you telling your own family?
49. Are all those involved in agreement?
50. Are people overreacting?
51. Which laws are applicable?
52. Has anyone broken the law?
53. What challenges are you facing?
54. Has anyone made mistakes?
55. What mistakes have been made?
56. Have you told us everything you know?
57. What are you not telling us?
58. What effects will this have on the people involved?
59. What precautionary measures were taken?
60. Do you accept responsibility for what happened?
61. Has this ever happened before?
62. Can this happen elsewhere?
63. What is the worst-case scenario?
64. What lessons were learned?
65. Were those lessons implemented?
66. What can be done to prevent this from happening again?
67. What would you like to say to those who have been harmed and to their families?
68. Is there any continuing danger?
69. Are people out of danger? Are people safe?
70. Will there be inconvenience to employees or to the public?
71. How much will all this cost?
72. Are you able and willing to pay the costs?
73. Who else will pay the costs?
74. When will we find out more?
75. What steps need to be taken to avoid a similar event?
76. Have these steps already been taken? If not, why not?
77. What does this all mean? Is there anything else you want to tell us?

and avoid being defensive or argumentative during interviews. To assist reporters, provide elements in interviews that make a story interesting, including examples. Offer to follow up on questions that cannot be addressed immediately. In general, such strategies help you to achieve win-win media outcomes, reflecting a constructive partnership.

2. Plan Thoroughly and Carefully for all Media Interactions   Part of the planning for media interactions involves reaching out to local journalists and editors in advance, providing educational opportunities for journalists to learn about the risk issue if appropriate. Another part of this planning is focused on the communication itself and includes proactively framing stories (rather than waiting until others have defined the story and then reacting); creating a written risk communication plan with clear, explicit goals (see Exhibit 31.3); identifying key messages based on message mapping; and anticipating questions (Exhibits 31.2 and 31.5). As a risk communicator, you should identify important stakeholders and subgroups within the audience as targets for your messages. Anticipate the cultural diversity, languages, and socioeconomic levels of the target populations, recognizing that all communication activities and materials should provide for a diverse public in a fair, representative, and inclusive manner. Prepare informational materials such as a briefing book and answers to frequently asked questions in advance. A limited number of key messages should also be prepared in advance, pretested before being used in interviews, and posted to the Web promptly.

Yet another part of the planning involves logistic considerations. Designate a lead spokesperson who has sufficient seniority, expertise, and experience to establish credibility with the media. He or she should be skilled in communicating risk and uncertainty. Other staff, including technical staff, should also be trained in media communication skills and should practice these skills regularly. One of these skills is never to say anything "off the record" that they would not want to see quoted and attributed to them, and another skill is to redirect an interview (or get it back on track) with such bridging phrases as "What is really important to know is . . ." In planning interviews, staff need to know to agree with the reporter on logistics and topic and to stick with that topic, but must also realize that the reporter may attempt to stray from the agreed topic.

Coordination should be established in advance when multiple agencies or organizations are involved. Establish a *joint information center* (JIC) in advance so it can function as the hub for media questions and inquiries during a disaster, emergency, or crisis. The JIC should have a room set up for daily media briefings. It should also have work room for public information officers from all partnering organizations.

Planning also involves allowing for flexibility as a situation unfolds and for follow-up afterward. Make needed changes in strategy and messages based on monitoring activities, evaluation efforts, and feedback. Carefully evaluate media communication efforts, learn from mistakes, and share with others what you have learned from working with the media.

3. Meet the Functional Needs of the Media   Inform on-site reporters of the location of electrical outlets, telephones, restrooms, hotels, restaurants, and other amenities. Be accessible to reporters and respect their deadlines. Accept that news reports will simplify and abbreviate your messages. Devise a schedule to brief the media regularly during an emergency and include frequent media events. Even if updates are not newsworthy by their standards, open and regular communication helps to build trust and fill information voids. Media availability sessions, where partners in the response effort are available for questioning in one place at one time, are very helpful to reporters. Provide accurate, appropriate, and useful information tailored to the needs of each medium, such as sound bites, background videotape, and other visual materials for television. Such materials can be provided both on a Web site and as part of media information packets and kits. While respecting the reporters' desire for information, strive for brevity.

If you do not know the answer to a question, focus on what you do know, tell reporters what actions you will take to get an answer, and follow up in a timely manner. If asked for information that is the responsibility of another individual or organization, refer reporters to that individual or organization. If a follow-up interview with a subject-matter expert would provide further clarity, offer this opportunity. Promise only what you can deliver, then follow through.

4. Be Candid and Open with Reporters   Be forthcoming, disclosing information about an emergency promptly and proactively. Be the first to share bad news about an issue or your organization but be sure to put it into context. Be accurate, supporting your messages with case studies and data. Avoid reassurance that is unwarranted by currently available information and also avoid exaggeration and speculation. Be careful when asked extreme or baseless what-if questions, especially when based on worst-case scenarios. Avoid speaking in absolutes, and be careful about comparing the risk of one event to the risk of another. Identify significant misinformation, being aware that repeating it may give it unwanted attention. Acknowledge uncertainty and data gaps, including those identified by other credible sources. If the answer to a question is unknown or uncertain, and if the reporter is not reporting in real time, express a willingness to get back to the reporter with a response by an agreed deadline. Recognize that saying "no comment" without explanation or qualification is often perceived as guilt or hiding something—consider saying instead, "I wish I could answer that. However . . . " Ask reporters to restate a question if you do not understand it. Be careful when providing numbers to reporters, as these can easily be misinterpreted or misunderstood; cite ranges of risk estimates when appropriate. If credible authorities disagree on the best course of action, be prepared to disclose the rationale for those disagreements, and why your agency has decided to take one particular course of action over another.

Recognize that most journalists maintain a "healthy skepticism" about sources and that trust you receive from the media must be earned; do not ask to be trusted. Tell the truth. Adhere to the highest ethical standards; recognize that people hold you professionally and ethically accountable. Make corrections quickly if errors are made or if the facts change.

5. Listen to the Target Audience Do not make assumptions about what viewers, listeners, and readers know, think, or want done about risks. Instead, if time and resources allow, prior to a media interview, review the available data and information on public perceptions, attitudes, opinions, beliefs, and likely responses regarding an event or risk. Such information may have been obtained through interviews, facilitated discussion groups, information exchanges, expert availability sessions, public hearings, advisory group meetings, hotline call-in logs, or surveys. As a situation unfolds, monitor and analyze information about the event appearing in media outlets, including the Internet. Use media channels that encourage listening, feedback, participation, and dialogue, and listen well. This information will help you as the risk communicator to identify with the **target audience**, and present information in a format that aids understanding and helps people to act accordingly.

During interviews and news conferences, acknowledge the validity of people's emotions and fears. Be empathetic. Recognize that competing agendas, symbolic meanings, and broad social, cultural, economic, and political considerations often complicate the task of effective media communication. For example, although public health officials may speak in terms of controlling "morbidity and mortality," more important issues for some audiences may be whether people are being treated fairly in terms of access to care and medical resources.

6. Coordinate, Collaborate, and Act in Partnership with Other Credible Sources Conflicting and uncoordinated messages from different agencies and organizations can confuse target audiences and create anxiety and cynicism. To avoid this problem, identify partner organizations in advance of potential emergencies, build bridges with them, develop procedures for information clearance and approval and for coordinating media spokesperson activities across multiple agencies and organizations (including procedures for reaching agreement on which organization should take the lead in responding to media enquiries and document the agreement reached), collaborate in developing messages, and encourage partner organizations to repeat, or "echo," messages in order to reinforce them. Establish links to the Web sites of partner organizations. Develop contact lists of authoritative sources of information, including external subject-matter experts able and willing to speak to the media on issues associated with potential emergencies, and cite these sources as part of your message.

These processes may not always be seamless; every organization has its own culture and this culture affects how and what it tries to communicate. If it is impossible to harmonize certain messages, be inclined to disclose the areas of disagreement and explain why your agency is choosing one course of action over another. Develop a contingency plan for times when partners cannot engage in consistent messaging; be prepared to make an extra effort to listen to their concerns, understand their point of view, negotiate differences, and apply pressure if required and appropriate.

7. Speak Clearly and with Compassion   Be aware that people want to know that you care before they care what you know. Express genuine empathy when responding to questions about loss; acknowledge the tragedy of illness, injury or death and avoid distant, abstract, and unfeeling language. Acknowledge and respond (in words, gestures, and actions) to the emotions people express, such as anxiety, fear, worry, anger, outrage, and helplessness. Similarly, acknowledge and respond to the distinctions people view as important in evaluating risks, such as perceived benefits, control, fairness, dread, effects on children, and whether the risk is natural or man-made. Be sensitive to local norms, such as those relating to speech and dress. Respect the unique information needs of special and diverse audiences. Always try to include in a media interview a discussion of actions being taken by the agency (to answer the "What are you doing?" question) and also a description of specific actions that can be taken by the public to protect themselves. The latter helps to empower people and restores a sense of control to them.

Use clear, nontechnical language. Use graphics or other pictorial material to clarify and strengthen messages. When medical or technical terms are used, explain them in clear language. Personalize risk data by using stories, narratives, examples, and anecdotes that make technical data easier to understand. Be careful to use risk comparisons only to help put risks in perspective and context and not to suggest that one risk is like another. Avoid comparisons that trivialize the problem, that attempt to minimize anxiety, or that appear to be trying to settle the question of whether a risk is acceptable.

Strategies for Overcoming Misperceptions and Misunderstandings

A broad range of strategies can be used to help avoid public misunderstandings about risk caused by psychological, sociological, and cultural factors. Several of the most important strategies derive from the risk perception model discussed earlier. For example, because risk perception (or outrage) factors such as fairness, familiarity, and voluntariness are as relevant as measures of hazard probability and magnitude in judging the acceptability of a risk, risk communicators should address these factors in their messages. Similarly, genuine efforts to share power, such as establishing and supporting community advisory committees or supporting third-party research, audits, inspections, and monitoring, can help organizations to achieve fairness, promote shared control, and build trust.

Risk communication is most successful when organizations are clear about their values and goals, open and transparent about their decisions, proactive in providing early warnings and bad news, prompt in acknowledging and acting on mistakes, open about uncertainty, and seen to be basing their decisions on science. It is important to take public values, concerns, and perceptions into account in decision making, and to convey to people that authorities share their values. Risk communicators should ensure that sufficient information is provided to allow individuals to make balanced, informed judgments; that excessive reassurance is avoided; that the legitimacy of fear and emotion is acknowledged; and that trusted voices are enlisted to support messages. It is essential that actions be consistent with words; judgments about trust often depend more on what is done than on what is said.

Leaders and risk communicators use a variety of specific tools for overcoming the psychological, sociological, and cultural factors that can create risk misperceptions and misunderstanding:

- Collecting and evaluating empirical information (for example, through surveys, focus groups, or interviews) about stakeholder judgments of each risk perception factor. To develop effective risk and crisis communication messages, it is necessary to develop a shared understanding of perceptions and expectations.
- Exchanging information with stakeholders on a regular basis about identified areas of concern.

- Developing only a limited number of key messages (ideally, three key messages or one key message with three parts) that address underlying concerns or specific questions.
- Developing messages that are clearly understandable by the target audience (typically at or below their average reading grade level) (CDC, National Center for Health Marketing, 2007).
- Adhering to the "primacy-recency," or "first-last," principle in developing information materials. This principle states that the most important messages should occupy the first and last position in lists. In high-stress and emotionally charged situations, listeners tend to focus most on (and remember) information that they hear first and last. Messages that are in the middle of a list are often not heard.
- Citing sources of information perceived as credible by the receiving audience. The greater the extent to which messages are supported and corroborated by credible third-party sources, the less likely it is that mental noise will interfere with the ability to comprehend messages.
- Providing information that indicates genuine empathy, listening, caring, and compassion, crucial factors in establishing trust in high-concern and emotionally charged situations. Again, when people are upset, they typically want to know that you care before they care what you know. The more individuals and organizations are perceived to be empathetic, caring, listening, and compassionate, the less likely it is that mental noise will interfere with comprehension.
- Using graphics, visual aids, analogies, and narratives (such as personal stories) to increase people's ability to hear, understand, and recall a message.
- Constructing messages that recognize the dominant role of negative thinking in high-concern and emotionally charged situations. As previously discussed, people tend to focus more on the negative than on the positive in emotionally charged situations, with resulting high levels of anxiety and exaggerated fears. Risk communication strategies related to this principle include
    - Avoiding unnecessary, indefensible, or unproductive uses of absolutes and of the words *no, not, never, nothing,* and *none.*
    - Balancing or countering a negative key message with positive, constructive, or solution-oriented key messages.
    - Providing three or more positive points to counter a single negative point or bad news. (Note that a trust-building message is a positive response and can count as one or more of the positives. Also recognize that the media control which messages will be cited, what visibility they will be

given, and how often they will be repeated. As a result many positive messages may fall by the wayside. This is especially likely to occur when the positives are hypothetical or predictive and the negatives are matters of fact.)

- Presenting the full message using the repetitive structure found in the "tell me, tell me more, tell me again" model (also called the triple T model):
  - Tell people the information in summary form (for example, use the three key messages).
  - Tell them more (give them the supporting information).
  - Tell them again what was told in summary form (repeat the three key messages). (The greater the extent to which messages are repeated and heard through various channels, the less likely it is that mental noise will interfere with people's ability to comprehend them.)
- Developing key messages and supporting information that address risk perception and outrage and fear factors such as trust, benefits, control, voluntariness, dread, fairness, reversibility, catastrophic potential, effects on children, morality, origin, and familiarity. Research indicates that the greater the extent to which these factors are addressed in messaging, the less likely it is that mental noise will interfere with understanding. (see, for example, National Research Council, 1989; Slovic, 2000; Covello and others, 2001).
- Providing people with understandable, concise, accurate, and reliable information at the outset so their first impressions are correct.
- Layering information according to individual needs. One recommendation for information materials is to provide multiple levels of information that can be targeted to various audiences. It is also important to recognize that information materials cannot replace the dialogue between stakeholders.
- Motivating people to understand risk information. When people are sufficiently motivated, they can learn even very complex material.
- Using message maps.
- Having an approved, comprehensive risk communication plan.

Risk comparisons are a common device used to help members of the public place risk in perspective. Although potentially useful, they carry their own risk, as described in the accompanying Perspective.

Because of institutional and other barriers, strong leadership is often required to implement risk communication strategies. An excellent example of such leadership occurred on September 11, 2001. An interviewer asked New York City mayor Rudolph Giuliani about the number of casualties sustained in the attack on the World Trade Center, before firm information was available. "The number

PERSPECTIVE
The Use and Abuse of Risk Comparisons

The goal of risk comparisons is to make a risk number more meaningful by comparing it to other numbers. Stand-alone probabilities are often difficult to conceptualize (just how small is "1 in 10 million" or a "probability of 0.00015"?). Although risk comparisons can provide a yardstick and are therefore useful for putting numbers in perspective, they can also create their own problems. For example, use of concentration comparisons can lead to disagreements. The statement "one part per million of a contaminant is equal to one drop in an Olympic-size swimming pool" is typically intended to help people understand how small an amount is. However, for some individuals, such comparisons appear to trivialize the problem and to prejudge their acceptability. Furthermore, concentration comparisons may be misleading because risk agents vary widely in potency—one drop of some biological agents in a community reservoir can kill many people whereas one drop of other biological agents will have no effect whatsoever.

Comparing the probabilities associated with different risks has many of the same problems. For example, a risk communicator may be tempted to make this type of assertion:

> The risk of situation A [for example, breathing polluted air] is lower than the risk of situation B [for example, injury or death caused by an automobile crash]. Since you [the target audience] find risk B acceptable, you are obliged to find risk A acceptable.

of casualties will be more than any of us can bear ultimately," he said. "And I don't think we want to speculate on the number of casualties. The effort now has to be to save as many people as possible." This response and Mayor Giuliani's statements in the ensuing days exemplified several key features of effective communication in an emergency situation:

- Take the first day of an emergency very seriously. Drop other obligations.
- Take ownership of the issue or problem.
- Be visible or readily available.
- Remain calm and in control, even in the face of public fear, anxiety, and uncertainty.
- Listen to, acknowledge, and respect the fears, anxieties, and uncertainties of the public and key stakeholders.

However, some audiences will respond to this assertion as follows:

> I do not have to accept the (small) added risk of breathing polluted air just because I accept the (perhaps larger, but voluntary and personally beneficial) risk of driving my car. In deciding about the acceptability of risks, I consider many factors, only one of them being the size of the risk; and I prefer to do my own evaluation.

Consequently, this risk comparison can severely damage trust and credibility.

The most difficult comparisons to communicate effectively are those that disregard the risk perception factors people consider important in evaluating risks. Probabilities are only one of many kinds of information upon which people base decisions about risk acceptability. Risk numbers cannot preempt those decisions. Explanations of risk numbers are unlikely to be successful when the explanation appears to be trying to settle the question of whether a risk is acceptable.

Many variables affect the success of using risk comparisons, including the context and also the trustworthiness of the source of the comparison. The most effective comparisons appear to be

- Comparisons of the same risk at two different times
- Comparisons with a regulatory standard
- Comparisons with different estimates of the same risk
- Comparisons of the risk of doing something versus not doing it
- Comparisons of alternative solutions to the same problem
- Comparisons with the same risk as experienced in other places

- Tell people what follow-up actions will be taken to get answers if a question cannot be answered immediately, or tell people where to get additional information.
- Offer authentic statements and actions that communicate compassion, conviction, and optimism.
- Acknowledge uncertainty.
- Avoid guessing. Check and double-check the accuracy of facts.
- Be honest, candid, transparent, ethical, frank, and open.
- Balance bad news with three or more positive, constructive, or solution-oriented messages.
- Avoid humor because it can be interpreted as uncaring or as trivializing the issue.
- Avoid saying anything that could be interpreted as an unqualified absolute (*never* or *always*). It takes only one exception to disprove an absolute.

Mayor Giuliani particularly understood the danger in making unfounded or premature reassuring statements. Such statements are often motivated by the desire of government officials to calm the public and avoid panic. Panic is a group phenomenon in which intense, contagious fear causes individuals to think only of themselves. Research indicates, however, that even though panic can erupt in emergencies and disasters, it is rare (see, for example, Clarke, 2002; Auf der Heide, 2004). Most people respond cooperatively and adaptively in emergencies and disasters. Among the factors that contribute to panic are

- Believing that chances of escape are small
- Seeing oneself at high risk of being seriously harmed or killed
- Being confronted by surprise and novelty
- Seeing available but limited resources for assistance
- Perceiving a "first come, first served" response system
- Perceiving a lack of effective risk management
- Perceiving a loss of credibility among authorities
- Lacking meaningful things to do (such as tasks that increase group interaction, increase connectedness, and rein in anxiety)

Another important risk communication skill demonstrated by Mayor Giuliani was the ability to communicate uncertainty. He recognized the challenge to effective risk communication caused by the complexity, incompleteness, and uncertainty of risk data. In addressing this challenge, Mayor Giuliani drew on the following risk communication principles for communicating uncertainty:

- Acknowledge, rather than hide, uncertainty.
- Explain that risks are often hard to assess and estimate.
- Explain how the risk estimates were obtained and by whom.
- Announce problems and share risk information promptly, with appropriate reservations about uncertainty.
- Tell people whether, in your estimation, what you currently have for information is
    - Certain
    - Nearly certain
    - Likely
    - Unlikely
    - Highly improbable
- Tell people when information is not currently known and may never be known.
- Tell people that what you believe now may turn out to be wrong later.
- Tell people about what is being done to reduce uncertainty.

Finally, Mayor Giuliani recognized the importance of risk communication planning, preparation, and practice. New York City had taken many such steps before this day, such as having prepared a risk and crisis communication plan.

SUMMARY

Without a great deal of forethought, prolonged training, and the development of systematic performances, drills, and tests for all participants, no organization can prepare itself adequately to meet the challenge of effective risk communication. When organizations prepare for risk communication, the efforts of all must be fitted into a coordinated system. Thinking ahead of time about risk communication decisions, activities, materials, and messages allows a timely and effective response. Each person or group who guides a part of the risk communication whole must have a clear concept of the working of all the other parts.

KEY TERMS

availability	familiarity	risk perception
catastrophic potential	media bias	sound bite
comprehensive risk and crisis communication plan	media selectivity	target audience
	mental noise	trust
confirmatory bias	message mapping	uncertainty
conformity	negative dominance	voluntariness
controllability	newsworthiness	
fairness	risk comparisons	

DISCUSSION QUESTIONS

1. What are decision makers to do when public risk perceptions are at odds with expert opinion?
2. Given the need to be extremely concise and clear when communicating in high-risk situations, how can one avoid oversimplification?

3. Given the importance of expressing empathy and caring when communicating in high-risk situations, what are decision makers to do if they feel no empathy?

4. Are there conditions that justify lying about or withholding risk information? What is the relationship between risk communication and ethics?

5. Is there an inherent conflict between the goals of risk communication and the goals of journalists? If so, can these conflicts be resolved?

REFERENCES

Auf der Heide, E. "Common Misconceptions About Disasters: Panic, the 'Disaster Syndrome,' and Looting." In M. O'Leary (ed.), *The First 72 Hours: A Community Approach to Disaster Preparedness* (pp. 340–380). Lincoln, Neb.: Universe, 2004.

Centers for Disease Control and Prevention, National Center for Health Marketing. *Plain English Thesaurus for Health Communication.* Document 07–151(NE)/092607. http://www.nphic.org/files/editor/file/thesaurus_1007.pdf, 2007.

Centers for Disease Control and Prevention, Office of the Chief of Public Health Practice, National Public Health Performance Standards Program. *10 Essential Public Health Services.* http://www.cdc.gov/od/ocphp/nphpsp/EssentialPHServices.htm, 2008.

Clarke, L. "Panic: Myth or Realty?" *Contexts*, Fall 2002, pp. 21–26.

Covello, V. T. "Risk Communication and Message Mapping: A New Tool for Communicating Effectively in Public Health Emergencies and Disasters." *Journal of Emergency Management*, 2006, *4*(3), 25–40.

Covello, V. T., McCallum, D. B., and Pavlova, M. T. (eds.). *Effective Risk Communication: The Role and Responsibility of Government and Nongovernment Organizations.* New York: Plenum, 1989.

Covello, V. T., Peters, R., Wojtecki, J., and Hyde, R. "Risk Communication, the West Nile Virus Epidemic, and Bio-Terrorism: Responding to the Communication Challenges Posed by the Intentional or Unintentional Release of a Pathogen in an Urban Setting." *Journal of Urban Health*, 2001, *78*(2), 382–391.

Fischhoff, B. "Risk Perception and Communication Unplugged: Twenty Years of Progress." *Risk Analysis*, 1995, *15*(2), 137–145.

Hyer, R. and Covello, V. T. *Effective Media Communication During Public Health Emergencies: A World Health Organization Handbook.* Geneva: World Health Organization, 2007.

Kahneman, D., Slovic, P., and Tversky, A. (eds.). *Judgment Under Uncertainty: Heuristics and Biases.* New York: Cambridge University Press, 1982.

Kahneman, D., and Tversky, A. "Prospect Theory: An Analysis of Decision Under Risk." *Econometrica*, 1979, *47*(2), 263–291.

National Research Council. *Improving Risk Communication.* Washington, D.C.: National Academies Press, 1989.

National Research Council. *Understanding Risk: Informing Decisions in a Democratic Society.* Washington, D.C.: National Academies Press, 1996.

Peters, R., McCallum, D., and Covello, V. T. "The Determinants of Trust and Credibility in Environmental Risk Communication: An Empirical Study." *Risk Analysis*, 1997, *17*(1), 43–54.

Ross, J., and Covello, T. "The 103 Most Frequently Asked Questions at Environmental Cleanups and Hazardous Waste Sites." Presented at the National Association of Remedial Project Managers (NARPM) Annual Training Conference, U.S. Environmental Protection Agency, Baltimore, Maryland, May 23, 2007.

Sandman, P. M. "Hazard Versus Outrage in the Public Perception of Risk." In V. T. Covello, D. B. McCallum, and M. T. Pavlova (eds.), *Effective Risk Communication: The Role and Responsibility of Government and Nongovernment Organizations* (pp. 45–49). New York: Plenum, 1989.

Slovic, P. (ed.). *The Perception of Risk.* London: Earthscan, 2000.

FOR FURTHER INFORMATION

Books, Articles, and Guides

Some key examples of the large literature on risk communication are listed here.

Agency for Toxic Substances and Disease Registry. *A Primer on Health Risk Communication.* http://www.atsdr.cdc.gov/risk/riskprimer/index.html, 1994.

Bennett, P., and Calman, K. (eds.). *Risk Communication and Public Health.* New York: Oxford University Press, 1999.

Bennett, P., Coles, D., and McDonald, A. "Risk Communication as a Decision Process." In P. Bennett and K. Calman (eds.). *Risk Communication and Public Health.* New York: Oxford University Press, 1999.

Chess C., Hance B. J., and Sandman P. M. *Planning Dialogue with Communities: A Risk Communication Workbook.* New Brunswick, N.J.: Rutgers University, Cook College, Environmental Media Communication Research Program, 1986.

Covello, V. T. "Best Practice in Public Health Risk and Crisis Communication." *Journal of Health Communication*, 2003, *8*(suppl. 1), 5–8.

Covello, V. T., and Allen, F. *Seven Cardinal Rules of Risk Communication.* Washington, D.C.: U.S. Environmental Protection Agency, 1992.

Covello, V. T., Clayton, K., and Minamyer, S. *Effective Risk and Crisis Communication During Water Security Emergencies: Summary Report of EPA Sponsored Message Mapping Workshops.* EPA Report No. EPA600/R-07/027. Cincinnati, Ohio: National Homeland Security Research Center, U.S. Environmental Protection Agency, 2007.

Covello, V. T., and Sandman, P. "Risk Communication: Evolution and Revolution." In A. Wolbarst (ed.), *Solutions to an Environment in Peril* (pp. 164–178). Baltimore, Md.: Johns Hopkins University Press, 2001.

Covello, V. T., Slovic, P., and von Winterfeldt, D. "Risk Communication: A Review of the Literature." *Risk Abstracts*, 1986 *3*(4), 171–182.

Cutlip, S. M., Center, A. H., and Broom, G. M. *Effective Public Relations.* (6th ed.) Upper Saddle River, N.J.: Prentice-Hall, 1985.

Douglas, M., and Wildavsky, A. *Risk and Culture: An Essay on the Selection of Technological and Environmental Dangers.* Berkeley: University of California Press, 1982.

Embrey, M., and Parkin, R. "Risk Communication." In M. Embrey and others (eds.), *Handbook of CCL Microbes in Drinking Water.* Denver, Colo.: American Water Works Association, 2002.

Hance, B. J., Chess, C., and Sandman, P. M. *Industry Risk Communication Manual.* Boca Raton, Fla.: CRC Press/Lewis, 1990.

Kasperson, R. E., and others. "The Social Amplification of Risk: A Conceptual Framework. *Risk Analysis,* 1987, *8*(1), 77–187.

Lundgren, R., and McKakin, A. *Risk Communication: A Handbook for Communicating Environmental, Safety, and Health Risks.* (3rd ed.) Columbus, Ohio: Batelle Press, 2004.

McKechnie, S., and Davies, S. "Consumers and Risk." In P. Bennett (ed.), *Risk Communication and Public Health.* New York: Oxford University Press, 1999.

Morgan, M. G., Fischhoff, B., Bostrom, A., and Atman, C. J. *Risk Communication: A Mental Models Approach.* New York: Cambridge University Press, 2001.

Stallen, P. J. M., and Tomas, A. "Public Concerns About Industrial Hazards." *Risk Analysis,* 1988, *8,* 235–245.

Substance Abuse and Mental Health Services Administration. *Communicating in a Crisis: Risk Communication Guidelines for Public Officials, 2002.* SMA02-3641. http://www.riskcommunication.samhsa.gov, 2002.

Weinstein, N. D. *Taking Care: Understanding and Encouraging Self-Protective Behavior.* New York: Cambridge University Press, 1987.

Articles for a Case Example

A recent public health emergency was the outbreak of severe acute respiratory syndrome (SARS) in Toronto in 2003. This episode provides a useful case study of risk communication. The following papers are exemplary.

Blendon, R. J., and others. "The Public's Response to Severe Acute Respiratory Syndrome in Toronto and the United States." *Clinical Infectious Diseases,* 2004, *38,* 925–931.

Brunk, D. "Top 10 Lessons Learned from Toronto SARS Outbreak: A Model for Preparedness." *Internal Medicine News,* 2003, *36*(21), 4.

Cava, M., and others. "Risk Perception and Compliance with Quarantine During the SARS Outbreak (Severe Acute Respiratory Syndrome)." *Journal of Nursing Scholarship,* 2005, *37*(4), 343–348.

Organizations and Individuals

Center for Risk Communication. [Homepage.] http://www.centerforriskcommunication.com. The Web site offers publications by center staff, suggested readings, and links to additional sources.

The Peter M. Sandman Risk Communication Web Site. [Homepage.] http://www.psandman.com. This Web site of an author, consultant, and former academic offers writings, videos, and other risk communication resources.

Academic Centers

Loyola University, New Orleans. Center for Environmental Communication. [Homepage.] http://www.loyno.edu/lucec.

University of Cincinnati. Center for Environmental Communication Studies. [Homepage.] http://www.uc.edu/cecs/cecs.html.

University of Maryland. Center for Risk Communication Research. [Homepage.] http://www.comm.riskcenter.umd.edu.

CHAPTER THIRTY-TWO

LEGAL REMEDIES

DOUGLAS A. HENDERSON

KEY CONCEPTS

- Legal remedies are the requirements and procedures to repair injury, collect and distribute compensation, and deter wrongs.

- Many injuries resulting from environmental exposures take years to manifest, complicating the legal remedies.

- Environmental exposures can involve personal injury or property damage.

- Common law theories for personal injury recovery address negligence, strict liability, nuisance, trespass, fraud, battery, slander, false imprisonment, and defamation.

- Damages in personal injury cases can include compensation for actual injury or disease, fear of disease (such as cancerphobia), increased risk of disease, or medical monitoring.

- Property damage claims can be addressed through common law claims such as trespass and nuisance or through statutory programs such as the Comprehensive Environmental Response, Compensation, and Liability Act.

- Three categories of statutes have been enacted to compensate people who have been harmed in specific circumstances: no-fault programs, such as workers' compensation; partial-fault programs, such as the Federal Employers' Liability Act; and compensation funds.

IN 1998, while filling your car with gasoline, you notice a warning on the
pump that gasoline vapors have been "shown to cause cancer in laboratory
animals." Three years later you are diagnosed with fatal lung cancer. Can you
sue the gas station for your medical expenses, pain, suffering, and likely death?
Or is it medically—and legally—unreasonable to think that you developed cancer
by simply filling your car with gasoline? And what if you don't have cancer? Can
you still sue just for inhaling vapors? Can you sue for cancerphobia, the fear of
getting cancer? Now suppose the truck delivering gasoline to the station crashes
near your home, spilling 5,000 gallons of gasoline on your front lawn. Can you
force the trucking company to clean up the spill? Or is that the responsibility of
the U.S. Environmental Protection Agency (EPA)? And to what extent can you
recover the decrease in the value of your property caused by the spill?

All of these questions address the legal remedies available to exposed individuals and property owners. **Remedies** are the requirements and procedures
to repair injury, collect and distribute **compensation**, and deter wrongs. As a
subject of inquiry, legal remedies appear disordered and confusing. They reflect a
patchwork of laws: cases decided during the industrial revolution, confusing statutes enacted by Congress and state legislatures, both slanted and sincere judicial
interpretations, and bewildering regulations promulgated by multiple regulatory
agencies. From another perspective, remedies are what happen when prevention—
the main focus of environmental and public health—fails and an exposure occurs
that results in some damage to human health and the environment.

Unfortunately, for even the simplest of environmental exposures, it is difficult
to know which laws apply, how they apply, when they apply, and where they apply.
A sixty-five-year-old retired coal miner suffering from pneumoconiosis (black lung
disease) is presumptively entitled to compensation and his family to death benefits,
if warranted, under the Black Lung Benefits Act. But a sixty-five-year-old retired
ship worker suffering from mesothelioma has no such remedy available under
any law, even though his mesothelioma indisputably resulted from his employment. Unlike the coal miner the ship worker must hire a lawyer, file a lawsuit, and

Douglas A. Henderson is an attorney whose practice includes environmental law, toxic tort litigation, and property rights litigation. He reports having represented both plaintiffs and defendants in chemical exposure and groundwater contamination cases, contract disputes involving
environmental issues, condemnation cases involving endangered species, and similar cases.
These cases often involve issues covered in this chapter. In several cases Henderson represented
associations and interest groups as amicus or interested parties, including the Georgia Chamber
of Commerce, the Washington Legal Foundation, and the Georgia Industry Association. None
of his clients financed or contributed in any way to this chapter.

spend years fighting for information about his asbestos exposure—just to have the chance to present his case to a jury, assuming of course the defendant has not filed for bankruptcy.

The same confusion arises in property exposure cases. A leak of perchloroethylene (PERC) from an underground storage tank is regulated under the Resource Conservation and Recovery Act (RCRA), the federal hazardous waste law, but a spill of polychlorinated biphenyls (PCBs) from an aboveground electrical transformer is regulated by the Toxic Substances Control Act (TSCA). To recover cleanup costs for the PERC spill, a property owner might file a cost recovery lawsuit, not under RCRA but under another law, the Comprehensive Environmental Response, Compensation, and Liability Act (CERCLA). As enacted by Congress, RCRA cannot be used to recover cleanup costs; it permits an individual only to seek an injunction in a federal court to force compliance with the applicable regulatory requirements. And adding to the legal confusion, CERCLA does not provide the actual cleanup standard for the PCB spill, because that is set by the TSCA, which controls the cleanup of certain substances, namely, PCBs and asbestos.

The legal system in the United States, as in many nations, offers two general approaches to remedies. First, a citizen can demand that another citizen or firm compensate him for his losses. This is known as the *tort system*, and claimants generally have to go to great lengths to prove their tort claims have merit. Second, if a group of victims is considered deserving, society can set up mechanisms to compensate them more or less automatically, relieving them of some of the burdens of proving their case, and delivering more rapid relief.

Both of these general approaches to remedies are discussed in this chapter. The focus here is not prevention but exposure—what remedies, if any, does the legal system offer to those exposed or about to be exposed? These remedies, it turns out, differ considerably for personal injury and property damage, both of which are addressed, in separate sections. Following this the chapter turns to the reasons why the tort system, with the concept of fault as its foundation and with transactional costs eating up much of the compensation, continues to survive over various no-fault alternatives that distribute compensation largely without blame and for far lower costs. Not covered in this chapter are two related issues—the legal rights and remedies available to federal, state, and local governments to remedy harms, and the laws and regulations designed to prevent environmental exposures. Rather, the goal here is to consider why Congress and the states provide guaranteed compensation to certain individuals with certain environmental diseases but leave other individuals with diseases that are just as deadly to battle their way through an expensive and arbitrary legal process.

REMEDIES FOR POTENTIALLY DANGEROUS EXPOSURES

Environmental exposures prompt thousands of lawsuits every year in the United States. At issue in these lawsuits is a range of both toxic and nontoxic chemicals, substances, and conditions. They involve natural substances such as asbestos, lead, arsenic, chromium, manganese, and silica; they involve synthetic substances such as paint thinners, pesticides, dry-cleaning solvents, and nail polish remover. The lawsuits also involve exposures to drugs such as Rezulin, Propulsid, Prozac, and Baycol and to "defective" medical devices such as breast implants, hair transplants, and tooth fillings. The exposures in these lawsuits derive from everyday occurrences—from talking on a cell phone, inhaling urban air, and smelling carpet emissions to eradicating cockroaches, drinking water, eating hamburgers, and wearing latex gloves.

But exposure lawsuits are not just about chemicals. In Eastern Pennsylvania, one hepatitis-infected carton of lettuce at one Chi-Chi's restaurant killed several individuals, sickened thousands, generated concern in restaurants throughout the world—and prompted more than 800 lawsuits. Mold, ubiquitous throughout the world, is today the subject of thousands of lawsuits in the United States. A more recent development is lawsuits against fast-food restaurants owing to their alleged contribution to obesity.

Challenges of Exposure Lawsuits

Exposure lawsuits differ from traditional personal injury and property damage lawsuits in several ways. Instead of, for example, acute, immediate physical injuries resulting from an automobile accident, the harm in the typical exposure lawsuit is a disease, sickness, condition, or in some instances, a fear resulting from the exposure. Still other differences raise fundamental legal issues (Cranor, 1993). For example, environmental exposures are often invisible to the naked eye, and concentrations as low as one part per million (a measurement equivalent to one inch in sixteen miles) may cause some physical irritation or injury.

Another distinguishing factor in exposure lawsuits is timing. Injuries resulting from environmental exposures typically take years or decades to manifest. For instance, it may take ten to twenty years for exposure to asbestos to result in asbestosis and thirty to fifty years for it to result in mesothelioma. Complicating matters further, some individuals exposed to asbestos never experience a related injury or disease. In addition, the diseases caused by environmental exposures are frequently indistinguishable from naturally occurring illnesses, a unique challenge for a legal system based on the plaintiff's proving his or her case. Compounding all this is a serious lack of basic knowledge about the thousands of chemicals and compounds to which people may be exposed. Although hundreds of thousands of substances are used in commerce, very little is known about the majority of these substances, contrary to what many people would assume. For many substances, even fundamental questions about carcinogenicity remain unanswered. All these unique circumstances challenge a legal system founded on examining direct, immediate, and easily detectable impacts.

Factors Affecting Remedies

For every potential lawsuit, a range of factors determine whether, when, where, and how it can it can be filed. For environmental exposures, several additional issues are important, including

- Whether the exposure or injury involves personal injury or property damage—this is the key screening variable in remedy law
- For personal injury or property damage, the specific substances or media involved (for example, dioxin, soil, and so forth)
- For personal injury or property damage, the type of relief being sought (for example, monetary damages, an injunction to stop certain behavior, and so forth)
- For personal injury or property damage, the means through which injury or exposure occurred (for example, a vaccine, air release, and so forth)
- For personal injury, the type of damage that occurred (for example, black lung disease, birth-related brain injury, AIDS, and so forth)
- For personal injury, whether the exposure or injury occurred while the person was at work and, if so, the position of that person (for example, employee, coal miner, and so forth)

Largely as a result of these differences, learning which remedies are available for a particular type of case is complicated (Kole and Nye, 1999).

TORT REMEDIES FOR PERSONAL INJURY

Several types of remedies may be available to an environmentally exposed or injured individual attempting to recover expenses, seek compensation, and punish wrongdoers. No single remedy works for all exposures; a wide variety of factors influence which remedies are legally permitted. By far the most frequently used remedies for **personal injury** recovery are tort remedies—and negligence in particular. Any exposed or injured individual, however, needs to consider whether one or more of the no-fault compensation programs covers his or her damage.

Common Law Theories of Recovery

A **tort** is simply a civil wrong, distinguished from wrongs resulting from criminal behavior and wrongs resulting from a breach of contract. A tort is legal shorthand for a number of theories of **common law** recovery. Negligence is the best known of these; among the others are nuisance, trespass, fraud, battery, slander, false imprisonment, and defamation. The tort system is based largely on the concept of fault. The driving principal in tort law is that the person or entity causing the injury should pay to remedy the harm.

Traditional Tort Theories to Remedy Personal Harms   The most common theory of recovery in environmental exposure cases is **negligence**. To establish a claim for negligence, a plaintiff must prove several key elements by a preponderance of the evidence. Namely, a **plaintiff** must prove the **defendant** had a duty to conform to a standard of care to protect others, the defendant breached that duty, the plaintiff sustained actual damages, and the breach of the duty by the defendant actually caused the plaintiff's injuries. Stated differently, negligent behavior is behavior that falls below what a reasonably prudent person would do confronting the same facts and circumstances.

Perhaps the most common negligence lawsuit is one for medical malpractice. While intending to remove a bunion from a left toe, a surgeon cuts off the right toe—and the patient is a professional athlete. In this case all the elements of negligence are met. The surgeon owed a duty of care to remove the correct bunion, and the loss of a toe damages the professional athlete. As for other elements of liability, it is clear that the surgeon's breach of the duty to remove the correct bunion caused the damage. With these findings a jury would likely find the surgeon liable for negligence.

Injured parties also rely on other tort theories. In virtually all states, when a manufacturer puts a product into the stream of commerce (that is, sells a product), the legal system typically holds the manufacturer of a product that is defective or unreasonably dangerous to a standard of **strict liability**. When a product injures somebody owing to a design or manufacturing defect, the injured party may have a claim against the manufacturer under the law of **product liability**, as this area of the law is known. When a hot water heater explodes, spraying scalding water across a porch, the injured owner may be able to sue the manufacturer for defective design or manufacturing. And subject to several limited defenses, the manufacturer may be strictly liable for the defect; in other words, the manufacturer may have no defenses to liability. Contrary to what many might think, a manufacturer may be liable for a product's defective design even if the manufacturer is not negligent. The goal of product liability law is to force manufacturers to internalize the costs of any damage caused by their products. The focus is not on the reasonableness of the manufacturer but on the adequacy of the product.

Under product liability law an injured party may claim the manufacturer failed to warn or inadequately warned about the dangers of its products, even if those products were designed and manufactured properly. A claim of **failure to warn** is a common cause of action for injuries sustained from prescription drugs, over-the-counter drugs, and chemical exposures. Failure-to-warn cases are, however, legally complex, with often unpredictable results. For example, even though it unquestionably complied with Food and Drug Administration labeling requirements for a particular drug, a drug manufacturer may still be liable for failure to warn if a jury concludes the labeling was insufficient. If a defendant can establish that its actions were in compliance with law, that demonstration will not usually constitute a complete defense to liability but rather represents only strong evidence that the defendant's actions were reasonable.

In many exposure cases, however, the law of product liability provides no remedy because the exposure may result from a substance, chemical, or other exposure not considered a product. In mold exposure cases, for example, the mold is not a product placed into commerce, although product liability claims may be brought against the manufacturer of the equipment, flooring, or furniture where mold is growing. Wet plasterboard, a defective heating and ventilation system, or a leaking window may have visible mold, but mold in itself is likely not a product. In addition, in a successful product liability case, an injured party must identify the type of product causing the harm and know the manufacturer of the product. For lead or asbestos exposure, it is often impossible to know which company produced the lead or asbestos, even assuming the lead and asbestos would be considered a product subject to product liability law.

Old and New Damages   Under any theory of liability—product liability, negligence, or fraud—if there are no **damages**, a plaintiff has no case. In a personal injury action the damages sought by plaintiffs are often relatively straightforward. Plaintiffs may seek to recover medical costs and lost wages (both past and future); they may seek recompense for pain and suffering, wrongful death (if applicable), and attorney fees; and they may seek **punitive damages**. Assuming liability has been established, the calculation of damages for personal injury—although sometimes challenging for certain individuals—is usually not the most difficult issue in an exposure case involving personal injury. In addition to monetary relief, an exposed or injured person may seek **equitable relief**, which usually means an order from the court that the defendant must take some action or refrain from taking some action. The sought-after relief may be a temporary restraining order, a temporary injunction, or a permanent injunction. Finally, in the context of environmental health, several innovative kinds of damages have been the subject of lawsuits, especially when the medical outcome of an exposure has not (yet) appeared. In the aftermath of a hazardous environmental exposure, lawsuits have sought damages for such things as a fear of future disease, such as a fear of developing cancer (known as **cancerphobia**); an increased risk of future disease; and costs of ongoing or future medical monitoring.

Cancerphobia   Along with traditional damages, some plaintiffs seek recovery for cancerphobia in environmental health cases. Here the damages sought by a plaintiff are not for getting cancer and not for being at an increased risk for cancer from an exposure. Rather, a cancerphobia claim is about the fear of contracting cancer, and the money damages are intended to compensate for that fear. For these plaintiffs, in other words, the emotional distress resulting from an environmental exposure is as real as the actual disease, assuming it were to materialize.

For centuries the common law has permitted plaintiffs to recover for the emotional distress resulting from a physical injury. For instance, the emotional distress of seeing a toe severed by a defective lawn mower is traditionally permitted to be recovered in a tort suit. In other instances, known as bystander cases, individuals may recover for emotional distress if they were not personally injured but were near family members or close friends when those individuals were injured. It is under this line of cases that a parent may be able to recover for emotional distress after seeing a child killed or significantly injured.

Courts are reluctant about, but not adamantly opposed to, awarding damages for *fear-of* claims, whether the fear in question is fear of cancer, fear of AIDS, or fear of becoming a lawyer. A few courts have held that "mere" exposure is sufficient to establish a claim for cancerphobia. But most courts reject this approach, noting that in today's modern civilization, exposure to potentially hazardous substances is a fact of life and that permitting plaintiffs to win damages for mere exposure would cripple the economy and debilitate an already troubled judicial system. For this reason many courts require plaintiffs to show at least a physical impact to recover for cancerphobia or other emotional distress lawsuits, and among these courts, most require a plaintiff to prove a resulting physical injury of some sort, such as a rash, headache, or related injury. The physical impact requirement is simply a device to make sure only meritorious claims for emotional distress are compensated. Individuals believing they have been exposed to a hazardous substance and filing a lawsuit to recover for fear of exposure but lacking any evidence of exposure are not likely to prevail in most jurisdictions in the United States. Still other courts, perhaps a majority, require a plaintiff to show more than impact to claim damage in fear-of cases. In these jurisdictions a plaintiff not only must prove a physical injury, such as a rash or headache, resulting from the emotional distress but also must prove that his or her reaction was reasonable under the circumstances. For instance, a court is unlikely to conclude that simply by pumping gas a plaintiff could suffer the requisite physical injury and the requisite reasonable emotional distress to establish the elements of a claim for cancerphobia.

For most courts considering a fear-of claim, simple exposure to a hazardous or toxic substance, product, or condition does not constitute damage under the law. Has an individual been damaged when there are absolutely no signs or symptoms after exposure to a toxic substance? For most courts, the answer is no. In most AIDS needlestick cases, unless the plaintiff can show evidence of HIV infection, it is unlikely the plaintiff can recover for a fear of AIDS cause of action. In the asbestos context, if a plaintiff can show only pleural thickening and not asbestosis, a claim for fear of disease likely, though not always, will fail legally.

Increased Risk of Disease   Along with cancerphobia claims, exposed individuals sometimes file increased risk of disease claims. Here the damage is the probability that through one or more exposures caused by the defendant, the plaintiff faces an increased risk of contracting a disease. In these cases plaintiffs present no symptoms or physical indications of the disease, only the knowledge of being at an increased probability of getting the disease. Legally, this is a claim for risk of future injury, not present exposure. As a general rule courts are reluctant to accept increased risk of disease cases. Most courts believe that if increased risk claims were permitted, those who do not develop the illness would be overcompensated and those who do would be undercompensated, at least over the long run (Kanner, 2000).

The few courts that accept these claims invoke a number of legal tests to screen out unmeritorious claims. A few require plaintiffs to prove to a *reasonable medical certainty* that they will develop the disease, although offering no definition of this concept. Other courts, perhaps a majority, require plaintiffs to prove they will "more probably than not" contract the disease, a threshold established through expert testimony that the disease is more than 50 percent likely to occur. In most cases, largely because of the enormous technical challenges involved, experts are unwilling or unable to opine that an individual's risk of contracting a disease has increased by a set percentage.

Medical Monitoring   Rather than fighting over fear of cancer or increased risk, many exposed but unaffected plaintiffs seek to recover the costs of medical surveillance, also known as **medical monitoring** costs. The award of medical monitoring costs to asymptomatic plaintiffs is a difficult issue philosophically, medically, and legally. The results in court cases range across the board, from a simple no to elaborate multipart tests for calculating medical monitoring costs. At this point in the development of the case law, the majority rule appears to be that medical monitoring claims for the asymptomatic claimant are likely not legally recognized, even if those individuals are undeniably exposed to highly toxic or hazardous substances. For most courts it makes more sense legally and economically for a plaintiff to wait until symptoms of the disease manifest before any recovery is permitted through the legal system. If a plaintiff has undertaken medical monitoring prior to actually exhibiting symptoms, that individual should be able to recover the costs for that surveillance at the time the symptoms appear.

In interpreting an asbestos case, for example, the U.S. Supreme Court rejected a claim for medical monitoring. After reviewing the available case law and considering the policy implications of awarding damages to asymptomatic plaintiffs, the Court declined to award medical monitoring costs. The Court held that without symptoms, a plaintiff has no claim for medical monitoring. According to the Court, the fundamental reason for not permitting medical monitoring costs was that health care funds would then be used to monitor currently healthy individuals when those funds would be better reserved for assisting the truly injured. For other courts the benefits of medical monitoring for individuals exposed to environmental exposures have warranted recovery, even if the individuals have no symptoms of the disease or injury. However, before a recovery for medical surveillance is permitted, a number of requirements must be met, and these requirements vary from court to court. Generally, however, these courts have required a plaintiff to establish the following to recover on a medical monitoring claim:

- Exposure was greater than normal background levels of an established hazardous substance.
- Exposure was caused by defendant's negligence.
- Exposure has resulted in a "significantly increased risk of contracting the disease."
- Monitoring procedures exist that make early detection possible.
- Monitoring is different from what would ordinarily be carried out during routine medical care.
- Early detection has an established clinical value.

With each of these conditions established, courts will sometimes award lump sum payments for medical surveillance. Usually, though, courts award only periodic payments or funds to cover limited medical monitoring.

Challenges of the Common Law Tort System

As suggested by the range of innovative damages sought by plaintiffs today, exposure cases raise significant problems for the traditional tort system.

Causation   Without question the most difficult issue in exposure law is **causation**—that is, did the exposure (or repeated exposures or a combination of exposures) actually cause the injury? Exposure cases are won and lost on the issue of causation, because a defendant will be held liable only for those harms actually and legally caused by the defendant. Causation is generally not an issue when an individual breaks a leg during an automobile accident. But for the accident, the leg would not have been broken. Environmental exposure cases are, however, different. Causation is difficult to prove for numerous reasons (Kanner, 2002):

- The toxic properties of many hazardous substances are not known.
- Information on the plaintiff's frequency, duration, and amount of past exposures to most substances is not available.
- Not all individuals react the same way to similar exposures to disease-producing agents or chemicals.
- Multiple exposures in a variety of settings have contributed to or caused the injury.

For these and other reasons, juries in exposure cases are often at a loss when trying to assess the weight and importance of scientific evidence.

In environmental exposure cases, courts typically break causation into two components: (1) general causation, and (2) specific causation. **General causation** is the requirement that the specific substance, exposure, or process is capable of producing the general type of injury. Does benzene exposure cause cancer generally? If so, the court will proceed to the second element, specific causation. **Specific causation** is the requirement that under the specific facts of the case in dispute, the actual exposure more likely than not caused the disease. Did low-level exposure to benzene while filling up a car with unleaded gasoline cause cancer in that individual—who also smoked a pack of cigarettes a day and who worked in a dry-cleaning store where perchloroethylene, a suspected carcinogen, was used regularly?

The 200 or so reported legal decisions addressing causality in environmental exposure cases defy easy description. Just as scientists disagree over the fundamental meaning of causation, courts struggle with the type and sufficiency of evidence necessary to prove or capable of proving causation, and often the battleground—as in science—is epidemiological research studies. A few courts are reluctant to delve into the meaning of epidemiology, toxicology, and the scientific method. These courts, believing these issues to be a fundamental fact question, permit parties to explain the science to a jury and let the decision fall where it may. For many courts, epidemiological studies that do not address the substance at issue in the case or the disease or injury at issue in the case will be considered uninformative. Epidemiological findings that are not statistically significant may likewise be rejected. If the reported cases are any measure, the judicial system's reliance on epidemiology has not made causation decisions any easier.

Yet a majority of courts, especially federal courts, operating under stricter rules of civil procedure regarding the testimony of experts (see the Perspective

PERSPECTIVE
Who Is an Expert in Exposure Cases?

Under the evidentiary laws of almost every state, if a matter is beyond the ken of the ordinary citizen, then an expert is required to clarify the issues and offer opinions regarding those issues. Before or after trial the distinction between an expert witness and a fact witness is critical in exposure cases, as in all other cases. A **fact witness** testifies to personal knowledge, and a fact witness is not usually permitted to present opinions, which essentially amount to speculation. In contrast, an **expert witness** offers opinions, which may or may not be based on facts admitted into evidence. An expert is someone who through experience, expertise, or education has gained a unique perspective on an area of technical subject matter.

In exposure lawsuits, experts are necessary to offer opinions on whether the exposure caused the damage and, if so, to what extent. Establishing causation in toxic exposure cases is the number one area where expert testimony is critical. Expert testimony is also critical in establishing damage—whether the contamination interferes with the use of the property or whether filling up a car with gasoline could lead to cancer.

For many years courts took a relaxed view of the definition of expert. Then, in 1993, the Supreme Court, in **Daubert v. Merrill Dow**, held that a plaintiff must prove that the opinion of its expert witness is (1) relevant and (2) reliable. And perhaps more important, the Court held that the trial court was required to act as a gatekeeper to screen out expert testimony that did not meet this standard. The

Court also provided a nonexclusive list of factors a trial court should consider in this gatekeeping function:

- Whether the theory or technique used by the expert can be, and has been, tested
- Whether the theory or technique has been subjected to peer review and publication
- What the known or potential error rate of the theory or technique used is
- The degree to which the theory or technique or conclusion is accepted in the relevant scientific community

Daubert has become the standard in federal courts, but not all states have accepted *Daubert*. Several have specifically rejected *Daubert*, finding that judges are not required to scrutinize experts closely, leaving those matters for the jury. These courts have continued to rely on a general acceptance standard, meaning that if a plaintiff can show its theory meets a general acceptance standard it can be admitted.

The Supreme Court's decision in *Daubert*, subsequently explained in two additional cases, *Joiner* and *Kumho Tire*, now forms the most important standard for expert testimony in federal courts. Lawsuits in federal court regularly include numerous motions trying to strike experts or limit their testimony. To be reliable, all testimony must be by an expert with appropriate qualifications, experience, and knowledge, and the particular method used by the expert must be acceptable scientifically. If a plaintiff cannot convince a court that its expert testimony is both relevant and reliable, then that testimony will not be admitted for use in the proceeding. If the defense is successful in striking the testimony of the plaintiff's expert witness, the case may be over, because the plaintiff may not be able to offer another expert to testify on this issue.

titled "Who Is an Expert in Exposure Cases?"), take their role as gatekeepers more seriously. For these courts, *relative risk*—a standard measure in epidemiology—constitutes fair game for the legal system. Among the reported decisions interpreting relative risk in environmental exposure cases, the bottom line is not clear. Some courts require plaintiffs to show a relative risk greater than 2.0 (that is, a doubling of the risk), whereas still other courts require a showing of a relative risk greater than 4.0. Still other courts, perhaps the most sophisticated of the pack, look to relative risk only as a measure of causality that should be considered in the context of other factors, especially those developed by A. B. Hill (see Chapter Three).

In lawsuits over environmental exposures, proving causation is challenging for yet another reason: the existence of multiple defendants. In the typical exposure case numerous defendants may have produced the substance or equipment at issue. At trial the plaintiff is required to prove that one or more of the defendants caused the injury. But this is often a difficult burden, especially given the historical conditions at work. For example, fifty different companies may have produced the lead-based paint used in apartment buildings, making it impossible to tell which company produced the paint at issue in a particular lawsuit. To prove his or her case, however, a plaintiff must make a case for liability against a manufacturer of lead-based paint.

A final reason causation is so difficult to establish in exposure cases is just as basic. In proving an exposure caused a disease, injury, or condition, a plaintiff is required to offer expert testimony that none of the plaintiff's own prior exposures, eating habits, drug habits, exercise habits, family history, or risk-taking behaviors caused the very disease attributed to the defendant's actions or omissions. Canceling out competing explanations for the injury, an element of the plaintiff's case, is often technically and legally challenging. It will be tough for a plaintiff to prove that his or her cancer resulted from the benzene vapors escaping from the service station pump when the plaintiff also works at a dry-cleaning shop that uses PERC and when he or she smokes a pack of cigarettes a day.

Latency   The second major legal challenge presented by environmental exposures is latency. In an automobile accident, the exposure (the crash) and the damage (the broken leg or dented fender) occur nearly simultaneously. But in an exposure case it may take years or decades for the exposure to result in a symptom, disease, or disorder. It may take thirty years for exposure to asbestos to result in pleural thickening, which may—or may not—be a result of asbestos exposure and may—or may not—result in asbestosis that likely resulted from asbestos exposure.

The delay between initial exposure and discernable injury creates a fundamental problem for the legal system. The legal system is premised on the notion that if a party has a legally recognizable claim, that party should bring the claim when he or she discovers or should have discovered the injury or learns about the claim—or the party should forever waive that right after a set period of time. As a matter of public policy a defendant should not have to worry about any past exposures it may have caused after a reasonable period of time has run.

Statutes of limitations are the legal barriers created to bar stale claims. A **statute of limitations** is nothing more than a time frame within which a legal claim must be brought, and these statutes vary widely from state to state. In some states the statute of limitations for personal injury claims allows only a year from the date the individual "discovered" or "should reasonably have discovered" the injury, but other states allow as long as three years for the very same exposure. The period allowed by a statute of limitations for a property damage case may be as short as four years from the time the injury occurred to the property, irrespective of when the damage was discovered. Every year in every state, plaintiffs lose their cases because they failed to file their claims before the statute of limitations period expired. Once that period is over a plaintiff is forever barred from bringing the claim. Given the implications, lengthy legal battles frequently occur over the time when an injury was discovered or reasonably should have been discovered.

The potential delay between toxic exposures and injuries or damage creates two perverse results. First, exposed individuals may be prevented from recovering medical expenses related to an environmental exposure because they waited too long to file a claim, even though they may have been symptom free and may never have been told by a physician that they had a disease. Second, knowing the harsh effects of statutes of limitations, exposed individuals often race to file lawsuits so they do not miss the limitation period, even when it is clear to all involved they do not have any real symptoms or injury. The end result is that precautionary filers clog the courts while the truly injured wait for their day in court. Nowhere is there a better example of this than in asbestos lawsuits (see the accompanying Perspective).

PERSPECTIVE
The Elephantine Mass of Asbestos Litigation

Asbestos exposure has been called the worst occupational health disaster in U.S. history, and asbestos litigation in turn represents a legal crisis of unprecedented proportions. As of 2002, 600,000 individuals had filed personal injury lawsuits involving asbestos (Carroll and others, 2002; American Academy of Actuaries . . . , 2003). Between 1999 and 2001, the number of claims for asbestos exposure tripled, and between 2000 and 2002, roughly 50,000 to 70,000 new claims were filed (American Academy of Actuaries . . . , 2003; Congressional Budget Office, 2003).

The costs of this process are staggering. One estimate puts the total spent by defendants and insurers at $70 billion. Of that $70 billion, $21 billion went to defendants' lawyers and $20 billion went to plaintiffs' lawyers (White, 2004). As a point of reference, the total amount paid to lawyers in the tobacco settlement was only $13 billion, paid out over twenty-five years.

The asbestos cases are different from other mass tort cases involving environmental exposures for a number of reasons (White, 2004). First, the sheer number of plaintiffs distinguishes asbestos litigation. According to one estimate, 1 to 3 million people will eventually file asbestos lawsuits. In comparison, the breast implant litigation involved only 440,000 plaintiffs (White, 2004).

Second, the number of defendants is unparalleled. Upward of 8,000 companies in the United States are now defendants in asbestos exposure lawsuits. No other mass tort has had more than twenty or so major defendants. This list of defendants has grown along with the number of cases. Three hundred companies were targeted by plaintiffs in the 1980s; more than 8,400 companies have been named as defendants in asbestos cases today. At least one company in nearly every U.S. industrial sector is now involved in asbestos litigation (American Academy of Actuaries . . . , 2003).

Third, the ease of forum shopping, of seeking a favorable venue, is making the crisis worse. For example, although Mississippi has only 1 percent of the U.S. population, approximately 20 percent of the pending cases have been filed in Mississippi, because Mississippi courts are believed to be more pro-plaintiff (American Academy of Actuaries . . . , 2003). Apparently, this forum shopping does pay off. Asbestos verdicts in Mississippi, West Virginia, and Texas were on average $3 million higher than awards in other jurisdictions (White, 2004). Elected judges, variable procedural rules, sympathetic juries, and an active plaintiffs' bar likely explain these regional differences.

Fourth, unimpaired plaintiffs have had significant success in asbestos lawsuits to date. In fact most asbestos plaintiffs today are unimpaired, showing no signs of serious asbestos impact, a perverse result of the impact of statutes of limitations on filings (White, 2004). Indeed, the number of mesothelioma cases, which virtually everyone recognizes as caused by asbestos, represent only a tiny fraction of all asbestos cases (Carroll and others, 2002). To date, about 65 percent of the compensation in asbestos lawsuits has gone to nonmalignant claimants (Carroll and others, 2002).

Fifth, unlike what has happened in other mass torts, the procedural options for resolving difficult exposure cases have failed to work. For example, the bankruptcy of asbestos manufacturers has slowed but not stemmed the filing of asbestos lawsuits. After asbestos manufacturers were bankrupt, plaintiffs targeted other companies handling asbestos. Likewise, class action settlements, a procedural device that has been successful in certain other settings, have not worked to resolve the asbestos crisis. Even though the Supreme Court has called for a national solution to the problem, on at least two occasions when the Court has reviewed massive settlement class actions for asbestos claims, it has rejected the settlements on legal grounds, noting that future asbestos claimants would be compromised by the settlement.

For more than thirty years there have been repeated calls to resolve the asbestos litigation crisis, but to date, none of the proposals has been successful, According to Michael Green (U.S. Congress, Senate . . . ,1999), professor of law at Wake Forest University, "Everyone knows that the system is broken, judges know it, commentators know it, asbestos victims know it, their families know it, the experts who testify over and over and over again know it, and the lawyers who are litigating these cases know it."

The 1980s saw several proposals by asbestos defendants, insurers, and Congress to resolve the crisis (American Academy of Actuaries . . . , 2003). The best known have been the proposal to form the Center for Claims Resolution (CCR), an entity created by twenty-one asbestos producers in 1988 to resolve asbestos claims, and the Georgine settlement of 1993, a class action settlement intended to resolve the vast majority of claims. The Georgine settlement, and the similar Fibreboard settlement, were overturned by the U.S. Supreme Court, and the CCR stopped settling new asbestos claims in 2001.

Legislative attempts to control asbestos litigation have been largely unsuccessful to date (O'Malley, 2008). In 2003, the Fairness in Asbestos Injury Resolution Act (FAIR Act) of 2003 was introduced by Senator Orrin Hatch. The FAIR Act proposed an elaborate administrative compensation framework to make payments to individuals suffering from—or alleged to be suffering from—diseases associated with asbestos exposure. With no final agreement on the details of the FAIR Act of 2003, Congress adjourned without voting on the Act. The Act fared no better in 2004 or 2005.

Since 2005, the lack of legislative focus on asbestos is largely explained by an unexpected phenomenon—the decline of asbestos lawsuits, especially the decline in filings by individuals with no specific asbestos-related diseases (Hanlon, 2007). Apparently, state-by-state efforts for "tort reform"—an effort to enact caps on damages, slow the filings of tort lawsuits, and enact other measures—have been slowing the asbestos filings, which has reduced the pressure on Congress to develop a federal fix for the asbestos crisis. Today, individuals claiming injuries from asbestos exposure must still look to the courts. But strange as it may seem given the history of asbestos litigation and legislation, the use of asbestos is still legal in the United States, a fact that boggles the minds of many observers of the asbestos litigation crisis.

Procedural Innovations

A few courts have developed procedural solutions to address these issues. With respect to the harsh implications resulting from short limitation periods for personal injury, some courts in some asbestos cases have held that exposure is not damage for purposes of the statute of limitations. For these courts a plaintiff can file a claim only when he or she shows concrete symptoms of a disease. To ensure that asbestos-exposed but symptom-free plaintiffs are not barred from filing their claims by a statute of limitation, other courts have created pleural registries, which permit plaintiffs to sign up as potential plaintiffs, after which the case is administratively frozen. These registries permit symptom-free plaintiffs to preserve their cases without currently clogging the judicial system with their claims.

Another procedural technique used by judges in tort cases is **bifurcation**—separating some issues from others, especially contentious ones, and considering them sequentially. In tort cases the general rule has been for courts to bifurcate issues of causality from issues of damages. Procedurally, this means a plaintiff first has to prove that an exposure caused an injury, before offering evidence and making arguments about damages. If a plaintiff proves exposure, then another trial is held to determine damages. In asbestos cases some judges have employed reverse bifurcation, which requires a plaintiff to prove damages first, followed by a trial on liability. The goal in reverse bifurcation is to ensure that damage has occurred before considering the issue of responsibility.

Another procedure, used for many types of cases, not only exposure cases, is to file a class action in order to pursue a large number of claims at once. The key legal issue in a **class action lawsuit** is whether common issues of law and fact predominate. In environmental exposure cases, putative members of a class may differ considerably from each other. For example, among people exposed to groundwater contamination, there are salient differences between smokers and nonsmokers and between those who use pesticides in their backyards and those who do not.

STATUTORY REMEDIES FOR PERSONAL INJURY

For certain exposures and health outcomes, Congress and state legislatures have enacted specific statutes to compensate people who have been harmed. These statutory remedies fall into three general types: **no-fault programs**, such as workers' compensation; partial-fault programs, such as the federal Employers' Liability Act; and compensation funds. These three approaches vary in their eligibility requirements, claims processing, and exclusivity (that is, whether or not claimants can also file tort suits).

No-Fault Programs: Workers' Compensation

Largely because of the limitations of the traditional tort system, the U.S. Congress and state legislatures have enacted several no-fault programs. These programs, which differ widely in scope and structure, address only a few personal injuries, diseases, and exposures.

The best known of the administrative no-fault systems for personal injury is the **workers' compensation** system. Workers' compensation guarantees medical and income benefits to those who are injured on the job, regardless of who is at fault. All states have workers' compensation systems, although they differ in many respects from state to state.

Workers' compensation is an **exclusive remedy**. In exchange for the no-fault provision of this remedy—for being relieved of the burden of proving fault in cases of workplace injury or illness—workers are barred from suing their employers in tort. Following a workplace injury or illness, an employee cannot sue the employer for negligence, cannot receive compensation for pain and suffering, and cannot receive punitive damages. However, at least in theory, workers receive their compensation, including medical costs and lost wage replacement, promptly and without the need for extensive legal maneuvers. This was the trade-off crafted by state legislatures in the early twentieth century when workers' compensation systems originated.

To be covered under most workers' compensation statutes, an injury must "arise out of and be in the course of employment." Both the injury and the "in course of employment" elements are at issue in these cases. As a general rule an injury may be the result of a single traumatic event, the result of an aggravation of an existing condition, or the result of a cumulative traumatic activity. Injuries arising from inherently personal risk factors—attributes such as epilepsy, drug addictions, or physical deformities—are not covered under the definition of injuries. Death occurring during the course of employment is covered under the workers' compensation program. For injuries covered by the workers' compensation system, the employer must pay all work-related costs, including doctor bills, therapy costs, and travel expenses, and death benefits may be available in certain instances. If an employer does not provide the workers' compensation coverage sought by an employee, the employee may seek a hearing before an administrative law judge.

Workers' compensation programs may also cover occupational diseases. Under most state workers' compensation programs, an employee can recover for an occupational disease provided certain basic conditions are met:

- The work or employment condition directly caused the disease.
- The disease "naturally resulted" from the work experience.

- The disease is one that does not ordinarily result from an employee's exposure to conditions outside the work setting.
- The disease is not a normal disease of life endured by the general public.

If a worker contracts a disease meeting these conditions, the medical expenses and disability resulting from that disease are covered under the workers' compensation program.

Still other issues arise in determining coverage under workers' compensation programs. By definition, only employees are covered by these programs. An independent contractor, for example, someone hired for a specific job, is not an employee and is not covered. In many states additional categories of workers, such as domestic servants and farm laborers, are not covered by workers' compensation programs.

Workers' compensation systems, like all legal frameworks, contain certain exceptions. Although the workers' compensation system bars employees from suing their employers, employees are free to sue third parties. Accordingly, if an employee severs his hand while using an electric saw at work, he can sue the saw manufacturer (say, in a product liability claim). And under certain circumstances—injury arising from an intentional act by the employer or while in the hire of an employer who has not been participating in the workers' compensation insurance program—the employee is permitted to sue the employer in the tort system.

Some workers' compensation systems cover only a few types of employees. For example, civilian federal employees are covered by the Federal Employees' Compensation Act (FECA), and longshore and harbor workers are covered by the Longshore and Harbor Workers' Compensation Act (LHWCA). Another workers' compensation law that covers a specific category of worker is the Federal Mine Safety and Health Act, and a specific title of this Act, Black Lung Benefits,, addresses a certain type of injury. Under this title, coal miners, railroad workers hauling coal, and others involved with coal mining who demonstrate that they have pneumoconiosis (black lung disease) are compensated by the Federal Black Lung Program, which provides monthly payments to them and their surviving dependents. To establish eligibility, a coal miner must show, by chest X-ray or a "physician's reasoned medical opinion," that he or she has black lung and is totally disabled. The Black Lung Program is administered by the U.S. Department of Labor.

Partial-Fault Programs: FELA and the Jones Act

The remedy for certain other injured workers is not a no-fault workers' compensation program but other similar programs. For example, injured interstate railroad workers are required to seek recovery under the Federal Employers' Liability Act

(FELA). Like a workers' compensation program, FELA was enacted to reduce the inefficiencies of the tort system. But unlike a workers' compensation program, FELA is not a true no-fault program. FELA is best thought of as a partial-fault workers' compensation program or a relaxation of certain tort requirements. Although an injured employee must prove that the railroad was negligent, FELA contains several mechanisms to make proof of negligence easier than it is under a classic tort system. If an injured employee can show that the railroad violated certain federal laws, for instance, FELA becomes a strict fault system. The Jones Act, a section of the Merchant Marine Act of 1920, is a FELA-like program for merchant marines.

Compensation Funds

Other statutes attempt to take certain exposures, certain substances, and certain injuries out of the tort system completely or at least to significantly limit the tort liability associated with these exposures. These statutory remedies may be in addition to those provided by the tort system, but often they take the place of tort remedies. Of these administrative compensation programs, the most important for environmental health are the

- Smallpox Emergency Personnel Protection Act of 2003
- September 11th Victim Compensation Fund of 2001
- Radiation Exposure Compensation Act of 1990 (as amended, 2000)
- Florida Birth-Related Neurological Injury Compensation Act of 1988
- Virginia Birth-Related Neurological Injury Compensation Act of 1987
- California AIDS Vaccine Victims Compensation Fund of 1986
- National Childhood Vaccine Injury Act of 1986
- Agent Orange Veterans Payment Program of 1984
- National Influenza [Swine Flu] Immunization Program of 1976
- Price-Anderson Act of 1957, an amendment to the Atomic Energy Act of 1954

These compensation frameworks vary in their breadth and structure, and few generalizations are possible (Mullenix and Stewart, 2002–2003). In all these programs, when claimants meet the program requirements, they receive compensation for their injury or exposure, without needing to prove that a defendant caused the injury.

Some of these programs have exclusivity provisions like those of workers' compensation plans. For example, the National Influenza Immunization Program limited people contracting swine flu from a vaccine to recovery from the fund. But in other programs a claimant may be able to file a tort suit despite being covered by an administrative fund. The National Childhood Vaccine Injury Act bars civil suits that allege inadequate product warnings from the manufacturer of the vaccine. Under this Act a claimant who wants to bring other tort claims must adjudicate these claims under the National Childhood Vaccine Injury Act and then waive an award before filing a civil action to recover damages under the tort system. Under the Smallpox Emergency Personnel Protection Act a claimant may sue in tort only after exhausting that Act's program.

Other programs implement their own brand of exclusivity. Under the Agent Orange program, for example, disputes over recovery must be submitted to binding arbitration. The California AIDS fund permits plaintiffs to file tort suits along with seeking compensation from the fund, but provides that the fund is subrogated to any recovery, meaning the fund may recover if the claimant is successful in the tort suit. Under the Price-Anderson Act, claimants are required to waive all defenses in the event of a substantial nuclear accident.

Although purportedly no-fault, each of these programs differs widely in its approach to causality. For example, under the National Childhood Vaccine Injury Act a claimant does not have to prove causation. If the claimant received one of the vaccines covered by the Act and has one of diseases identified on the vaccine table, the court will award damages. Instead of causality the legal issue becomes whether an injury is included on the vaccine table. If it is not on the table, the Act may still cover the injury but to a lesser extent and then only if the claimant presents expert testimony that the injury resulted from the vaccine exposure. Under the LHWCA a worker can receive compensation without proving negligence because there is a presumption of causation if a worker can show both exposure to an injurious substance and a disease and if the exposure could have caused the disease. Under the Radiation Exposure Compensation Act (RECA) Amendments of 2000, the standards of eligibility differ by an individual's status. Uranium miners, millers, and ore transporters may receive $100,000 if they can establish certain basic criteria. Under RECA, any individuals who "participated" in any atmospheric testing of nuclear weapons can receive $75,000 payment for certain diseases. In addition, RECA provides that downwinders, those individuals physically present in one of the areas downwind from the Nevada Test Site during atmospheric testing, can receive $50,000. There are no periodic payments under RECA. If eligible, the person receives a one-time payment.

These programs exhibit still other differences, including the ways in which funds are distributed. For some the U.S. District Courts administer funds, whereas for the Agent Orange program the administrator is Aetna Technical Services, Inc., a private company. For the September 11th Victim Compensation Fund a special master determines eligibility and awards compensation. Under the National Childhood Vaccine Injury Act a special master for the U.S. Court of Federal Claims issues awards, which are appealable to that court.

Statutes Providing Limited Private Remedies

Individuals exposed to certain substances or hazardous situations may be able to seek certain other relief short of compensation. The two best-known examples of legislation that enables such relief are the federal Occupational Safety and Health Act and a California law known as Proposition 65.

Occupational Safety and Health Act   Even though the Occupational Safety and Health Act (OSH Act) was intended to provide the Occupational Safety and Health Administration (OSHA) with significant statutory authority to protect workers, the OSH Act also provides employees with certain, although limited, direct remedies to address occupational exposure. When construction workers are exposed to certain lead concentrations, for example, the employer may be required to provide certain medical monitoring tests. And under the lead standard, if employees notify their employer that they have developed symptoms associated with a lead-related disease or that they desire medical advice concerning the effects of past or current lead exposure on pregnancy, those employees can seek medical monitoring that must be funded by the employer. Beyond requiring the employer to provide certain monitoring, OSHA does not guarantee workers any relief for damages. However, following a request for medical monitoring, an employee may also file a workers' compensation claim related to the lead exposure.

Proposition 65   California's Safe Drinking Water and Toxic Enforcement Act of 1986, also known as Proposition 65, prohibits the discharge of listed chemicals to potential drinking-water sources and prohibits exposing persons to listed chemicals without prior warning of the risks created by those substances. The Office of the California Attorney General and certain city attorney offices enforce the Act. In addition, Proposition 65 permits private citizens to file enforcement actions, provided appropriate notice is given to the offending party. Proposition 65's citizen suit provision is similar to the citizen suit provisions of other environmental statutes discussed later in this chapter. If a citizen believes that consumers—including the citizen who wishes to file the complaint—are being exposed to certain substances without proper warning of the risks of those substances, that citizen is permitted to file a complaint intended to cause the proper warnings to be displayed.

Sovereign Immunity

The exclusive remedy provisions of workers' compensation programs are not the only barrier to lawsuits against certain defendants, especially government defendants. Exposure claims against federal or state governments may also be barred by the concept of **sovereign immunity**. Under the Constitution of the United States and the constitutions of most states, the government can be sued only when that action is specifically permitted and in no situations can punitive damages be recovered from a government entity. Under the Federal Tort Claims Act, the federal government has waived its sovereign immunity for negligent acts of agents of the United States, and states have enacted comparable state Tort Claims Acts. Before a claimant files suit in court, these Acts typically require that claimant to present an administrative claim to the appropriate agency identifying the negligent act and damages sought. If the agency does not admit or deny the claim within six months, the claimant can then file a negligence claim.

These Tort Claims Acts permit negligence suits only in a few narrow situations. If a government employee's alleged negligent activities resulted from the "exercise or performance or the failure to exercise or perform a discretionary function or duty," those claims are not permitted by the Tort Claims Act. For example, a claim relating to the negligent design of a federal wastewater treatment system that permitted the cross-contamination of stormwater and sewage would probably be barred by the Federal Tort Claims Act. Suits based on misrepresentation are also specifically not permitted by most Tort Claims Acts. Claims against government employees who maintain that lead ingestion does not harm adults would also probably be barred. So when considering who can be sued, it is always critical to know whether the defendant has sovereign immunity.

REMEDIES FOR PROPERTY DAMAGE

The remedies for **property damage** resulting from environmental exposures differ fundamentally from the remedies for personal injury, as one might expect. But still there are parallels, particularly the concern over whether the tort system can handle the difficult issues created by environmental exposures. For example, just as several no-fault programs were enacted to correct the tort system's failure to remedy certain personal injuries, numerous environmental laws were enacted in the 1970s and 1980s to correct the tort system's failure to protect the environment.

Tort Remedies for Property Damage

In considering the available remedies for property damage, the first question is to determine what relief is being sought. If the goal is to recover the costs of cleaning up contamination, one set of laws applies. If the goal is to recover the diminution in property value caused by contamination, another set of laws applies. And if the goal is to force compliance with already existing laws and regulations, still another set of laws applies.

Traditional Tort Claims   Traditional tort law provides several theories of recovery to remedy property damage. An owner of property next to a leaking underground storage tank may file a claim for nuisance, trespass, negligence, strict liability, fraudulent or negligent concealment, or similar tort claims. The standard elements of negligence in a personal injury setting (for example, duty, breach, cause, and damages) also apply when the negligence involves property damage, and all the limitations of the tort system (including those concerning proof of causation, expert testimony, and statutes of limitations) likewise apply. Under a negligence theory, a gasoline station owes a duty of care to adjacent property owners to prevent leaks from underground storage tanks, and some courts would regard that duty as having been breached when the tanks leak.

The adjacent property owner may also be able to bring a **nuisance** claim, one of the most common claims brought to remedy property contamination. Nuisance comes in two types, public nuisance and private nuisance. A cause of action for **private nuisance** is a claim that the leaking underground storage tank on the adjacent property "substantially and unreasonably" interferes with the adjacent property owner's use of his property. The issue is whether the activity actually constitutes a substantial and unreasonable interference. In the case of a leaking underground storage tank, does the presence of contaminated groundwater actually constitute a substantial and unreasonable interference with the land if the property is served by a public drinking-water system and there are no streams or other water receptors on the property? A claim for **public nuisance** differs in the rights that are harmed. A public nuisance is an injury to some public good, not to private property, and the party bringing a public nuisance claim must do so on behalf of the public. Traditionally, governments brought public nuisance claims to stop the open dumping of waste materials on public lands or to prohibit some land uses. In recent years, however, public nuisance has become a favorite choice for states and municipalities trying to influence public health and environmental health policy. In the war against tobacco, for example, the attorneys general of several states filed public nuisance claims against the tobacco companies, arguing that these companies were creating a public nuisance. Several states and cities have filed public nuisance claims to stop the sale of handguns, to force the cleanup of lead-based paint, and most recently, to force electric utilities to stop burning coal and thus to reduce global climate change (see the accompanying Perspective). Often simply the filing of these public nuisance claims prompts discussions, which may in turn lead to settlement. Instead of trying to enact statutes or promulgate regulations, these states and municipalities prefer to fight these significant public health issues in the courts. The strategy of filing a lawsuit to address thorny public health issues—where no statute or regulation seems to work—has been called "regulation by litigation." It is a subject with its own set of issues and concerns.

PERSPECTIVE
Climate Change and the Law

Historically, the creation and management of carbon dioxide and other *greenhouse gases* (GHGs) slipped through the cracks in existing environmental law and regulation in the United States. But that has changed. Although the legal details concerning climate change are still being shaped in Congress and the courts, one thing has become clear: carbon dioxide and other GHGs will likely become the most widely regulated chemical compounds in the United States.

Ironically, the most recent and perhaps most effective push to regulate carbon dioxide and other greenhouse gases has come from the U.S. Supreme Court. In its 2007 *Massachusetts* v. *EPA* decision, the Court ruled (1) that GHG emissions were "pollutants" under Title II of the Clean Air Act (CAA), which addresses automobile emissions, and (2) that the U.S. Environmental Protection Agency must regulate GHG emissions from new motor vehicles if the EPA administrator finds that such emissions cause or contribute to air pollution that may endanger public health or welfare (called an *endangerment finding*). With its decision, the Supreme Court put climate change on the legal map.

Under *Mass.* v. *EPA*, the U.S. Environmental Protection Agency's options were either to make the endangerment finding and regulate GHGs or to find that science did not justify the conclusion that GHGs endanger public health and welfare. In 2008, toward the end of the Bush administration, the EPA released an "advance notice of proposed rulemaking" on the regulation of climate change. In that proposal, the EPA concluded that the CAA, as currently drafted, was not appropriate to regulate climate change. And because the issue was of such great complexity, controversy, and legislative debate, the EPA sought to collect the views and opinions of other governmental agencies. From a practical perspective, the EPA concluded it was for Congress to decide how the United States should respond to global warming.

In 2009, with a new administration and new leadership, the EPA moved climate change to the forefront of environmental issues. In April 2009, in response to the *Mass.* v. *EPA* decision, the agency concluded that carbon dioxide and five other GHGs were contributing to climate change, finding specifically that these substances "endangered human health and the environment." Having made the endangerment finding, the agency now could turn toward developing a wide-ranging regulatory framework to slow climate change.

As of 2010, the actual details of the EPA's approach to regulating climate change are still not well known. Initially, the agency issued regulations aimed at reducing GHG emissions from automobiles. When finalized, however, the EPA's proposed regulations will affect more than the automobile industry. Electricity generators using fossil fuels, chemical companies, and other large industrial facilities will likely be affected, as will hundreds of thousands of smaller GHG emitters, such as landfills, farms, hospitals, and office buildings.

Even before these recent agency developments, Congress was moving to regulate climate change. In early 2009, comprehensive energy and climate legislation, known as the Waxman-Markey bill, passed the U.S. House of Representatives. If passed by the Senate and enacted into law, this legislation would ratchet down GHG emissions significantly. For instance, it would mandate an 83 percent reduction in GHG emissions by 2050, a measure that would leave virtually no sector of the economy untouched. It would also address increased promotion of renewable energy technologies, the adoption of new energy-saving standards, and several other related measures.

Except for *Mass.* v. *EPA*, which unquestionably prompted the EPA to focus on climate change, litigation approaches to climate change regulation have been largely unsuccessful. Several years before the *Mass.* v. *EPA* decision, eight states and New York City had filed a public nuisance lawsuit against several electric utilities, claiming their carbon dioxide emissions would cause flooding and other damages. In rejecting the suit, the U.S. federal court for the Southern District of New York found that any solution to climate change was not for the judiciary but for Congress. Several residents in Louisiana filed a similar suit against chemical and other industries, claiming industrial emissions caused global warming, which caused hurricanes, which caused the flooding that destroyed their properties. In this case, the U.S. federal court for the Southern District of Mississippi likewise held that it was a political question for the legislatures to decide. As a general rule, few courts have been willing to decide climate change issues, finding the subject warrants a legislative remedy.

While the EPA and Congress consider alternative approaches for regulating carbon dioxide, several state governments already regulate climate change. States in the Northeast created the Regional Greenhouse Gas Initiative in order to establish a regional *cap-and-trade* program for carbon dioxide. Western states created the Western Climate Initiative and states in the Midwest created the Midwestern Greenhouse Reduction Accord to develop similar cap-and-trade systems. California enacted the California Global Warming Solutions Act of 2006, which implemented carbon caps that will take effect in 2012. Still other states have passed other measures to reduce global warming, from requiring carbon dioxide emission limitations on power plants, to implementing renewable energy portfolio standards, to providing climate friendly fuel incentives. At the state level several coal-fired power plants have been shelved completely because their air quality permits failed to include emission limitations for carbon dioxide.

Judging by the regulatory and legislative proposals put forth so far, climate change may rewrite environmental law in the United States as no other issue, chemical, or condition has before. Ultimately at issue in addressing climate change will be the regulation of energy use, international trade, and personal habits. No matter the legal approach taken, whether a carbon tax, a cap-and-trade allocation of GHGs, or a more standard regulatory approach, the regulation of climate change will require a fundamental reordering of how individuals, governments, and private companies conduct their lives and run their businesses.

A number of other common law torts may be available to address property damage claims. A trespass claim may be available to the adjacent property owner, assuming the gasoline from the underground tank has in fact migrated onto his or her property. A **trespass** is an intentional, reckless, or negligent entry onto land owned by another. A trespass can occur when a party permits a "thing or third person" to enter the land of another. If during the construction of a shopping center the developer fails to install soil and erosion control and thus permits silt to run onto the adjacent property, the developer may be liable for trespass. The unpermitted entry of chemicals onto property is also a trespass. For a successful nuisance claim, however, contamination need not physically affect the property. Simply being next door to a contaminated site may be enough for a successful nuisance claim.

Under a strict liability claim a defendant may be liable for activities that are considered **abnormally dangerous** or ultrahazardous—a situation where no amount of care would prevent the harm. In these cases the focus is on the activity, not the injury. The prototypical abnormally dangerous activity is blasting. If a prudent person takes every known precaution prior to blasting dynamite, it is still possible that windows in the area will be cracked and dishes destroyed. Legally, because no amount of precaution can prevent the harm, the blasting becomes an abnormally dangerous activity, and the defendant has no defenses to liability.

Just what other activities are abnormally dangerous remains unclear. In a few cases a spill of hazardous substances has been held to be an abnormally dangerous activity, but in the majority of cases it has not. Just because a landfill leaks toxic waste, it does not necessarily follow that the landfill is an abnormally dangerous activity imposing strict liability. The defining activity for a landfill is not such leaking, which clearly is a significant environmental harm, but the depositing of waste. For most courts the determining factor is whether a regulatory agency would issue a permit or license to conduct the activity. Accordingly, a leaking underground storage tank is generally not an abnormally dangerous activity for most courts, because an underground storage tank is permitted by federal and state regulations. And for many courts, if a state agency will issue a permit for the activity, it cannot be abnormally dangerous, by definition.

Property Damage Valuation   A key issue in contaminated property cases is **valuation**. Under the common law the measure of damage for contaminated property depends on whether the injury is defined as permanent or abatable. If the property damage is considered permanent, the measure of damage will be the diminution in value of the property, calculated from the fair market values before and after the injury. But if the contamination is considered abatable, the measure of damages is the cost of repair. This legal difference can be significant. If a leaking underground storage tank is considered an abatable nuisance, then an affected property owner may be able to recover only the costs of repair. And if someone is already correcting the problems with the underground storage tank, there may be no damages for the cost of repair, even if the contamination remains in place. In this instance the arcane nature of tort law, which is keyed to the permanent versus abatable distinction, would also prevent the property owner from recovering the decrease in value to his or her property caused by the abatable contamination from the underground storage tank.

The difference between a permanent and an abatable nuisance raises still other issues in the context of contaminated property. A state statute of limitations for claiming permanent property damage may offer periods as short as two years or as long as six years. As a general rule these periods run from the time the property is first damaged, not from the time the property owner discovers the damage, which is the standard rule in personal injury cases. Under this rule, when a leak or other exposure first occurs it triggers the running of the period in which a claim of permanent property damage may be filed, assuming the leak is considered permanent.

But in the case of most contamination, the time of the first leak, release, or spill can be difficult or impossible to establish. When an underground storage tank is leaking, the first injury may be many years past, preventing an adjacent property owner from filing suit to seek damages. For many courts, however, this result is unacceptably harsh, and they have developed a fiction that the damage from the contamination is still continuing, assuming some of the contamination remains, even though the leak may have occurred several years in the past. Courts therefore often characterize contamination as a continuing nuisance so that the statute of limitations for permanent property damage will not bar meritorious claims.

Stigma Damages   Another issue raised in property damage cases is whether a plaintiff can recover stigma damages. **Stigma damages** come in several varieties. A property owner may claim that simply by being located near some undesirable activity, such as a landfill or industrial facility, his or her property has been stigmatized. Or the owner of a property contaminated by a leaking underground gasoline storage tank may claim that his or her property is stigmatized even though the leaking tanks and contamination have been removed and the regulatory agency has issued a letter stating "no further action" is required. The more difficult case is where property has been cleaned up but some residual contamination below the regulatory standard remains. Does this constitute stigma? For many courts it is an open legal question whether the presence of contamination below the regulatory standard constitutes property damage.

In the context of environmental exposures the case law on stigma damages is anything but clear on whether contamination—even after it has been cleaned up—creates long-term valuation issues. A majority of courts seem to hold that if even one molecule of a substance affects a property, the owner can seek stigma damages and that the jury should determine whether and how much that stigma affects the value of the property. A few courts have permitted stigma claims where there is no physical impact, focusing on whether it is reasonable to believe the property is affected, but this is likely a minority position. For most courts, however, the simple act of being located next to a hazardous waste landfill or a leaking underground storage tank cannot constitute a stigma claim when nothing from the landfill or the tank has affected the property. Otherwise, simply living next to a morgue or a strip club might imply stigma damages, a result with negative public policy implications. This proximity may, however, be a nuisance if the elements of a nuisance are met.

Statutory Remedies for Property Damage

The perceived failure of the tort system—including the failure of claims of nuisance and trespass—to protect human health and the environment was a main reason why Congress enacted a wide range of environmental laws in the 1960s, 1970s, and 1980s. These laws empowered certain regulatory agencies—in particular, the U.S. Environmental Protection Agency—to take action to protect human health and the environment. Under these environmental laws, federal and state environmental agencies were given the responsibility and resources to protect the environment. (These laws and agency functions are discussed in Chapter Thirty.)

Citizen Suits   In certain situations environmental statutes permit private citizens to become, in effect, private attorneys general and to enforce the environmental requirements as if they were the regulatory authorities. Under these **citizen suit** provisions, private parties can enforce environmental regulations, traditionally the province of regulatory agencies. Although they differ from statute to statute, in general the citizen suit provisions limit a private party's action to those situations where the agency in charge has taken no action or has taken inadequate action. In the case of the leaking underground storage tank contaminating groundwater, for example, it may be possible to file a citizen suit under the Resource Conservation and Recovery Act (RCRA) to seek an injunction to force the remediation of contaminated groundwater when the groundwater concentrations are above the maximum contaminant level. Under RCRA's citizen suit provision, an adjacent property owner may be able to force the operator of the underground storage tank to install new monitoring devices or take other remedial action. Under these citizen suit provisions, attorney fees and expert witness expenses may be awarded to the prevailing party, an attractive feature to many plaintiffs.

Cost Recovery Actions   Other environmental statutes permit private parties to seek compensation for cleanup costs. Take the case of a shopping center contaminated by a tenant's improper waste disposal from a dry-cleaning facility. If required to clean up dry-cleaning solvent contamination in soil or groundwater, the landlord may be able to file a cost recovery claim against the tenant under CERCLA or a state Superfund regulation to recover the costs necessary to investigate or clean up the groundwater. Under CERCLA a private party can recover the costs incurred in investigating and remediating contaminated sites.

In fact the most common environmental lawsuit throughout the 1980s and 1990s was the **cost recovery action**, brought by the government and by private parties. As thousands of contaminated sites were identified in the 1980s and 1990s, the U.S. Environmental Protection Agency took action to force potentially responsible parties (PRPs) to clean up these sites. If these PRPs would not assist in the cleanup, the EPA would clean up the site itself and then file a cost recovery action. PRPs that settled with the EPA would then file a cost recovery action against the nonsettling parties to recover their share of the cleanup. To win a cost recovery claim, the claimant must meet a number of procedural and substantive requirements, including the requirement of public notice prior to cleanup.

COMPLEXITY OF ENVIRONMENTAL LAWS

Whether the subject is contaminated sites, wetlands, or air quality, the applicable environmental statutes are complex. Few environmental laws are intuitive. Almost all the standard environmental laws contain intricate liability frameworks, complex technical definitions, and numerous exclusions, all often implemented by an agency through formal and informal guidance. To illustrate, a spill of PCBs on a concrete floor would be governed by the Toxic Substances Control Act, but a spill of PERC on unpaved soil might be governed by CERCLA, depending on the quantity of PERC released. A release of either PERC or PCBs from an underground storage tank would be regulated by the Resource Conservation and Recovery Act, but a release of PERC from an aboveground storage tank would not be regulated by that Act. At the same time, an airborne release of PERC or PCBs would be regulated by CERCLA or the Clean Air Act, or both, depending on the quantity of PERC and PCBs and on the molecular weight of the PCBs released. Unfortunately, the only way to know these differences is to know the fine technical distinctions in the law.

For private parties seeking to clean up a contaminated site, the hypertechnical hurdles contained in most environmental laws create very real legal challenges. Because petroleum products are excluded from CERCLA's definition of hazardous substances, CERCLA cannot be used to recover cleanup costs when the cleanup involves only petroleum contamination. Legally, this means the owner of property contaminated by a leaking underground gasoline storage tank on an adjacent property cannot use CERCLA to recover associated cleanup costs. However, if lead, which is included in CERCLA's hazardous substance definition, were also contained in the groundwater plume from the underground storage tank, it might be possible to use CERCLA to recover costs associated with the contamination. But CERCLA has additional limitations. It cannot be used to recover for diminution in property value resulting from contamination or to recover medical monitoring expenses. To recover the petroleum contamination cleanup costs, a property owner would be required to file a tort claim, such as negligence, nuisance, or trespass. To effect a complete recovery for many property damages, accordingly, an injured party must file both common law and statutory claims.

IMPLICATIONS AND DISCUSSION

The first and chief complaint about the tort system is its ineffectiveness. According to the Congressional Budget Office (2003), available data show that people who file claims under the tort system receive an average of forty-six cents from each direct dollar spent (with the other fifty-four cents going to attorney's fees and insurance expenses). Others estimate that 54 percent of total tort costs are expenses rather than transfers: 19 percent to claimant's attorney fees, 14 percent to defense costs, and 21 percent to defense administrative costs. Of the 46 percent of the funds that is actually compensation for injured parties, 22 percent is for awards for economic loss and 24 percent is for awards for pain and suffering (Tillinghast-Towers Perrin, 2004).

Second, along with this perceived inequity, the tort system also appears to overcompensate less-injured claimants and undercompensate more-injured claimants. In the context of automobile accidents, it has been estimated that for losses less than $500, people receive almost four and a half times their loss in the tort system, but people with over $25,000 in expenses receive only about a third of their costs (Hager, 1998). That litigation costs in the tort system add up quickly is not surprising. A board-certified toxicologist typically charges $250 to $500 per hour, and it is not unusual for a toxicologist to spend several weeks reviewing medical records, researching the scientific and medical literature, and otherwise preparing for a deposition or a trial. If the toxicologist spends two weeks on a case, the cost of this one expert may exceed $18,000. With the typical exposure case having ten to fifteen experts on each side, the costs skyrocket.

A third criticism leveled against the tort system is its arbitrariness. An individual claiming asbestos exposure in a Mississippi court is, other things being equal, far more likely to recover damages than is an individual claiming asbestos exposure in a New Jersey court. A fourth criticism concerns the tort system's lack of speed. It is not unusual for lawsuits to take years to reach final resolution. It may be seven to fifteen years from the time the case is filed before an asbestos exposure claimant has his day in court. Yet another criticism is the nature of the participants. Under the tort system, judges and juries decide the key issues, legal and technical, although they may have absolutely no expertise or experience with the subject matter at hand. Particularly in the context of punitive damage, awards by juries often do not reflect the true state of the scientific literature.

Largely as a result of these perceived shortcomings, a number of changes to the current tort system have been proposed. Several state legislatures have taken measures to reduce the filing of claims by shortening statutes of limitations, capping legal fees, and setting limits for punitive damage and noneconomic loss awards (Furrow and others, 2000). Strategies taken by other state legislatures to control the tort system include increasing the plaintiff's **burden of proof**, forcing more pretrial review of cases, and requiring mandatory alternative dispute resolution.

What Is the Status of No-Fault Programs?

Theoretically a strong medicine for the tort system, no-fault programs have turned out to be no panacea, and the actual strengths and weaknesses of these programs remain largely undocumented. Ironically, in one empirical evaluation of no-fault automobile accident programs, the number of collisions actually increased following the enactment of a no-fault liability program (Cummins, Phillips, and Weiss, 2001). Apparently, without the threat of tort liability, drivers actually acted more carelessly. This may explain why no-fault programs exist in only twenty-six states plus the District of Columbia and Puerto Rico, and it may also explain why several other states have recently repealed no-fault automobile insurance programs (Hager, 1998).

The lack of strong evidence one way or the other on the efficiency and effectiveness of no-fault programs reflects the small universe of substances, injuries, and damages covered by these programs. The best available data show that the transaction costs for no-fault systems are proportionately much smaller than in the tort system. According to the National Academy of Social Insurance, only twenty-three cents out of every dollar of workers' compensation claims goes to administrative costs. Under the National Childhood Vaccine Injury Act, administrative costs are estimated to be 15 percent of the total compensation award

(Congressional Budget Office, 2003). In an assessment of the Virginia Birth-Related Neurological Injury Compensation Act of 1987, only 10.3 percent of total spending went to dispute resolution (Bovbjerg, Sloan, and Rankin, 1997).

Despite the main selling point of more dollars going to compensation, the existence of a no-fault program may not equate to less litigation. The best example of this may be the National Childhood Vaccine Injury Act, the most frequently cited example of a model no-fault program. As of 1999, there were more than 1,000 published decisions, including one by the U.S. Supreme Court and 38 from U.S. Courts of Appeals (Ridgway, 1999). At issue in these disputes are challenges to an applicant's compliance with the filing requirements, disagreement over the cause of the injury, doubts over the credibility of witnesses, and disputes over the amount of compensation (Mariner, 1992). Similarly, a leading assessment of the Florida Birth-Related Neurological Injury Compensation Act concludes its success as a no-fault program is only "modest" (Studdert, Fritz, and Brennan, 2000). Implementation of this no-fault program failed to steer cases away from the tort system; litigation over negligence in birth-related neurological injuries occurred almost as frequently in the years after the plan as before it.

Why Does the Tort System Survive?

Why are some injuries or exposures covered by a no-fault administrative compensation fund while others are not? Clearly, no single event motivates Congress or state legislatures to move certain injuries out of the tort system (Culhane, 2003). One cynical explanation is that plaintiffs' lawyers exert undue influence on policy. No doubt special interests influence how Congress and state legislatures enact public policy, but in the case of no-fault programs, it is doubtful that one group holds the legislative reins tightly enough to perpetuate the tort system.

A more likely basic explanation for the continued survival of the tort system is legislative inertia. The tort system is the default system in the United States, for better or worse, and unless or until a legal crisis comes along that forces elected officials on both sides of the aisle to believe that change is required, that system will not change. In the case of asbestos litigation—a situation that everyone agrees is a crisis—the lack of any legislative change to the tort system and the lack of a no-fault system are probably explained by several realities, including the absence of congressional agreement on the elements of a no-fault system for asbestos claims and the continued success of plaintiffs' lawyers in filing lawsuits under the current system. For many environmental exposures, advocates of no-fault systems or administrative compensation funds have been unable to organize enough votes to revise the system.

However, reluctance to alter the tort system may also simply reflect the superior theory underlying tort law—deterrence and corrective justice. In the tort system a plaintiff files suit to compensate a loss, and if the plaintiff wins, the culpable party pays for the injury, not the plaintiff and not the federal government. And if society knows the culpable party paid for the injury, that result will deter others from committing the same type of injury, at least theoretically.

In contrast, the theory driving no-fault systems is equality in distribution of compensation. The costs of remedying a wrong are paid out of a common fund funded by taxes or other mechanisms. The main attribute is efficient compensation allocation, not blame, not deterrence, and not corrective justice. A second attribute is a framework in which professionals, whether special masters, bureaucrats, or claims processors, make the key decisions. A no-fault or administrative compensation system focuses on addressing the victim's injuries. It does not address whether all the losses—economic and noneconomic—are being recovered.

In deciding to keep the tort system, Congress and the state legislatures may simply be embracing the tort system's fundamental focus on deterrence and corrective justice. Even with its ineffectiveness in getting compensation to the truly injured, the tort system may be preferred over a no-fault framework on the purely philosophical grounds that no administrative system should replace the tort system when culpable parties are available to pay for the wrongdoing causing the harm. Because no-fault offers little deterrence, it is unlikely to replace the tort system.

Similarly, it may be that the tort system survives because it guarantees that an individual will have his or her day in court. Few legal protections in the United States are as sacred as a citizen's day in court, and it may be that any displacement of the tort system by no-fault programs impermissibly undermines that protection. Other things being equal, Congress probably views juries as more fundamental to democracy than regulatory decision makers. Again, it may be that Congress continues to keep the tort system because it keeps the jury system at the forefront of legal decision making. It may be that Congress and the state legislatures realize that but for plaintiffs' lawyers operating in the tort system, tobacco reform would have been unlikely. Given a choice between the tort system with judges and juries making decisions and a bureaucracy charged with operating an administrative compensation framework, Congress apparently gives the nod to juries.

What Prompts No-Fault Frameworks and Administrative Compensation Funds?

The main reason some injuries are taken out of the tort system is apparently a legislative concern about the survival of a class of defendants if a no-fault or compensation system is not implemented. In the case of the National Childhood Vaccine Injury Act, for example, Congress was concerned that a safe and effective supply of vaccines could not be established if vaccine producers were defending lawsuits. In some cases, Congress enacts a social insurance program, such as the Price-Anderson Act, or an administrative compensation fund, but the motivation is the same.

Concern for the financial health of a certain category of defendants prompted the creation of the September 11th Victim Compensation Fund. A few days after the September 11, 2001, tragedy, Congress enacted the Air Transportation Safety and Stabilization Act, which provided substantial financial incentives to the airline industry and limited the personal injury liability associated with the terrorist hijackings and crashes. In return for limiting the airline industry's liability, Democrats in Congress pushed for a no-fault compensation fund, which became the September 11th Victim Compensation Fund. According to one observer, the fund was part of the bailout of the airline industry following the disaster (Diller, 2003). The fund provides that victims of the September 11 attack can receive an allocated compensation provided they agree not to file claims against the airline industry.

By enacting any administrative compensation program, legislatures are also sending a message. By protecting those with personal losses resulting from the September 11 attack, for example, Congress was also reassuring Americans that if they were to fall victim to a terrorist attack, their families would be well cared for (Diller, 2003). The same can be said about the smallpox vaccine program for emergency workers. Congress wanted to ensure that if any of these workers died from the vaccine, their families would at least not be destroyed financially.

Historically, Congress has also enacted no-fault or administrative compensation programs to encourage certain behaviors. In the case of the smallpox vaccinations, Congress wanted to assure that anyone receiving the smallpox vaccination would not be required to pursue claims through the normal tort system. In the case of black lung and certain other diseases, Congress enacted administrative compensation funds because of concern for workers so clearly affected by one exposure. But it is still difficult to understand why dock workers exposed to asbestos have no administrative compensation system while miners exposed to coal dust do.

No matter how many perspectives are considered, there are still no logical explanations for addressing some matters outside the tort system and leaving others matter within the tort system. For example, emergency workers exposed to asbestos more than seventy-two hours after the September 11, 2001, World Trade Center collapse were not provided compensation as a matter of law, but those exposed to asbestos-containing dust a few hours after the collapse were. Victims of the Oklahoma City bombings received no compensation from the U.S. government; their families were required to file suit to try to collect damages. Yet the average award from the September 11th Victim Compensation Fund is $1.6 million per estate.

SUMMARY

Environmental public health aims to prevent hazardous exposures and to control the risks of those exposures that do occur. And when these exposures occur, appropriate remedies serve important purposes. As a matter of social justice, remedies help to compensate people who have been harmed. And as a matter of public health, remedies can represent incentives that prevent additional exposures.

Remedies may result from private actions in the tort law system or from social mechanisms such as compensation funds. Neither approach is perfect. Tort law has been criticized for being inefficient, costly, and arbitrary, although tort actions have provided compensation to many harmed by environmental exposures and may be credited with helping to reduce exposures to such hazards as asbestos and secondhand cigarette smoke. Administrative compensation schemes may also appear inconsistent and arbitrary. Individuals with nearly identical diseases and exposed to nearly identical substances often have vastly different legal remedies available. An individual with a work-related disease is eligible for workers' compensation, and an individual with the identical disease resulting from environmental exposures may end up with no recovery options. Nevertheless, systems such as the Black Lung Program have provided compensation to thousands of disease victims in a manner that is generally equitable, transparent, and economically efficient. Each of these approaches to remedies needs to be improved. Despite the best preventive efforts, hazardous exposures are likely to continue to occur, and fair and efficient remedies remain necessary.

KEY TERMS

abnormally dangerous

bifurcation

burden of proof

cancerphobia

causation

citizen suits

class-action lawsuit

common law

compensation

cost recovery actions

damages

Daubert v. *Merrill Dow*

defendant

equitable relief

exclusive remedy

expert witness

fact witness

failure to warn

general causation

medical monitoring

negligence

no-fault programs

nuisance

personal injury

plaintiff

private nuisance

product liability

property damage

public nuisance

punitive damages

remedies	stigma damages	valuation
sovereign immunity	strict liability	workers' compensation
specific causation	tort	
statute of limitations	trespass	

DISCUSSION QUESTIONS

1. Should judges or juries decide issues of causation in exposure cases, or is that decision best left to professionals?
2. Who has improved environmental health more: plaintiffs' lawyers, regulators, or elected representatives?
3. Why does the tort system survive, given that a no-fault liability framework has demonstrably lower costs?
4. Is there really a litigation crisis in mass tort exposure cases—involving, say, breast implants, asbestos, or tobacco—or is the problem simply that too many hazardous exposures are permitted to occur?

REFERENCES

American Academy of Actuaries, Committee on Property/Casualty Insurance, National Conference of Insurance Legislators. *Hearing on "Proposed Resolution Regarding the Need for Effective Asbestos Reform": Statement of Jennifer L. Biggs, FCAS, MAAA, Chairperson, Mass Torts Subcommittee, American Academy of Actuaries, July 10, 2003.* Washington, D.C.: American Academy of Actuaries, 2003.

Bovbjerg, R. R., Sloan, F. A., and Rankin, P. J. "Administrative Performance of 'No-Fault' Compensation for Medical Injury." *Law & Contemporary Problems,* 1997, *60,* 71–115.

Carroll, S. J., and others. *Asbestos Litigation Costs and Compensation: An Interim Report.* Santa Monica, Calif.: Rand, 2002.

Congressional Budget Office. *The Economics of U.S. Tort Liability: A Primer.* Washington, D.C.: Congressional Budget Office, 2003.

Cranor, C. F. *Regulating Toxic Substances: A Philosophy of Science and the Law.* New York: Oxford University Press, 1993.

Culhane, J. G. "Tort, Compensation, and Two Kinds of Justice." *Rutgers Law Review,* 2003, *55,* 1027–1107.

Cummins, J. D., Phillips, R. D., and Weiss, M. A. "The Incentive Effects of No-Fault Automobile Insurance." *Journal of Law & Economics,* 2001, *44,* 427–461.

Diller, M. "Tort and Social Welfare Principles in the Victim Compensation Fund." *DePaul Law Review,* 2003, *53,* 719–768.

Furrow, B. R., and others. *Health Law.* (2nd ed.) St. Paul, Minn.: West, 2000.

Hager, M. M. "No-Fault Drives Again: A Contemporary Primer." *University of Miami Law Review,* 1998, *52,* 793–830.

Hanlon, P. M. "Federal Asbestos Legislation: Wrestling with the Medical Issues." *Brooklyn Journal of Law and Policy,* 2007, pp. 1171–1208.

Kanner, A. "Theories of Recovery in Toxic Tort Litigation." *Trial Lawyer,* 2000, *23,* 130–158.

Kanner, A. *Environmental and Toxic Tort Trials.* Dayton, Ohio: LexisNexis, 2002.

Kole, J. S., and Nye, S. *Environmental Litigation.* (2nd ed.) Chicago: American Bar Association, 1999.

Mariner, W. K. "The National Vaccine Injury Compensation Program." *Health Affairs,* 1992, *11*(1), 255–265.

Mullenix, L. S., and Stewart, K. B. "The September 11th Victim Compensation Fund: Fund Approaches to Resolving Mass Tort Litigation." *Connecticut Insurance Law Journal,* 2002–2003, *9,* 121–152.

O'Malley, C. J. "Breaking Asbestos Litigation's Chokehold on the American Judiciary." *University of Illinois Law Review,* 2008, pp. 1101–1124.

Ridgway, D. "No-Fault Vaccine Insurance: Lessons from the National Vaccine Injury Compensation Program." *Journal of Health Politics, Policy and Law,* 1999, *24,* 59–90.

Studdert, D. M., Fritz, L. A., and Brennan, T. A. "The Jury Is Still In: Florida's Birth-Related Neurological Injury Compensation Plan After a Decade." *Journal of Health Politics, Policy and Law,* 2000, *25,* 499–526.

Tillinghast-Towers Perrin. *U.S. Tort Costs: 2003 Update: Trends and Findings on the Costs of the U.S. Tort System.* New York: Tillinghast-Towers Perrin, 2004.

U.S. Congress. Senate. Subcommittee on Administrative Oversight and the Courts of the Senate Committees on the Judiciary. "Prepared Statement of Michael Green." In *Finding Solutions to the Asbestos Litigation Problem: The Fairness in Asbestos Compensation Act of 1999: Hearing Before the Subcommittee on Administrative Oversight and the Courts of the Committee on the Judiciary, United States Senate.* 106th Congress, 1st Session. http://frwebgate.access.gpo.gov/cgi-bin/getdoc.cgi?dbname5106_senate_hearings&docid5f:70244.pdf, Oct. 5, 1999.

White, M. J. *Asbestos and the Future of Mass Torts.* NBER Working Paper 10308. http://papers.nber.org/papers/w10308.pdf, Feb. 2004.

FOR FURTHER INFORMATION

Books and Film

Eggen, J. M. *Toxic Torts in a Nutshell.* (3rd ed.). St. Paul, Minn.: West, 2005. A succinct overview of environmental torts.

Erin Brockovich. Universal Pictures, 2000. A film about a lawsuit arising from an environmental tort.

Farber, D. A., and Chen, J. *Disasters and the Law: Katrina and Beyond.* New York: Aspen, 2006. An in-depth discussion of mechanisms for compensation and risk spreading in the context of major natural disasters.

Harr, J. *A Civil Action*. New York: Random House, 1995. A popular account of a lawsuit arising from
     an environmental tort.
Prosser, W. L., and others. *Prosser and Keeton on the Law of Torts*. (5th ed.) St. Paul, Minn.: West, 1984.
     The classic legal treatise on torts.
Stern, G. M. *The Buffalo Creek Disaster: How the Survivors of One of the Worst Disasters in Coal-Mining History
     Brought Suit Against the Coal Company—and Won*. New York: Random House, 1976. Another
     popular account of a specific lawsuit.

Codes and Public Laws

Selected Environmental Law Statutes. (Educational ed..) St. Paul, Minn.: West. An annual compilation of the
     major federal environmental statutes and a useful resource for in-depth research into particu-
     lar laws (although all these statutes are available from other sources as well).
U.S. Code (USC), http://www.gpoaccess.gov/uscode/index.html. The entire *United States Code*, which
     collates all current provisions of federal environmental statutes by topic, is available online
     from the U.S. Government Printing Office.
Code of Federal Regulations (CFR), http://www.gpoaccess.gov/cfr/index.html. The *CFR*, containing the
     rules established by the agencies in the executive branch of the federal government, is also
     available online from the Government Printing Office.

Agencies and Organizations

American Association for Justice, http://www.justice.org. An association of plaintiffs' counsel; there
     is no corresponding national association for defense lawyers, but many states have such
     associations.
American Bar Association (ABA), http://www.abanet.org. A voluntary organization for lawyers of
     all types. The Section of Environment, Energy, and Resources; Section of Litigation; and
     Section of Tort Trial and Insurance Practice have numerous committees and task forces,
     many of which address issues surrounding environmental exposures.
Findlaw, http://www.findlaw.com. A good source of general information about a variety of legal areas,
     as well as a portal to state legal materials such as statutes and administrative codes.
Occupational Safety and Health Administration (OSHA), http://www.osha.gov. OSHA's Web site pro-
     vides information about statutory programs for compensation for those harmed by environ-
     mental exposures in the workplace.
U.S. Environmental Protection Agency (EPA), http://www.epa.gov. The EPA's Web site offers informa-
     tion about statutory programs that provide compensation to injured parties.

INDEX

Page references followed by *fig* indicate an illustrated figure; followed by *t* indicate a table; followed by *e* indicate an exhibit.